W0257300

HANDBUCH DER MEDIZINISCHEN RADIOLOGIE

ENCYCLOPEDIA OF MEDICAL RADIOLOGY

HERAUSGEGEBEN VON · EDITED BY

L. DIETHELM
MAINZ

O. OLSSON
LUND

F. STRNAD
FRANKFURT/M.

H. VIETEN
DÜSSELDORF

A. ZUPPINGER
BERN

BAND/VOLUME XIX
TEIL/PART 3

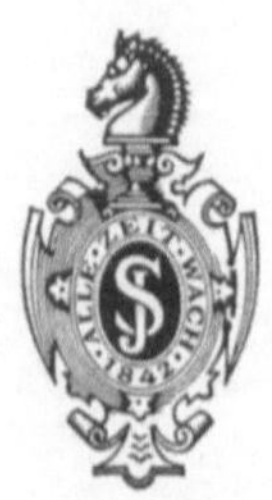

SPRINGER-VERLAG BERLIN · HEIDELBERG · NEW YORK 1971

SPEZIELLE STRAHLENTHERAPIE MALIGNER TUMOREN
Teil 3

RADIATION THERAPY OF MALIGNANT TUMOURS
Part 3

VON · BY

H. J. G. BLOOM · W. DIETZ · S. DISCHE · F. EDSMYR · H.-J. FRISCHBIER
R. FRISCHKORN · F. GAUWERKY · H.-L. KOTTMEIER · D. M. WALLACE
B. WINDEYER

REDIGIERT VON · EDITED BY

A. ZUPPINGER
BERN

MIT 179 ABBILDUNGEN
WITH 179 FIGURES

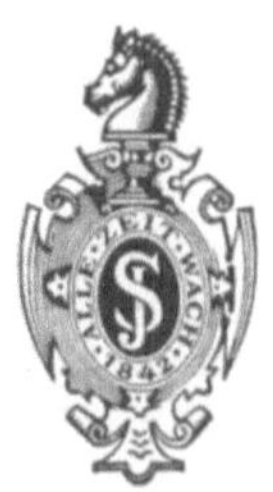

SPRINGER-VERLAG BERLIN · HEIDELBERG · NEW YORK 1971

ISBN-13: 978-3-642-80567-7   e-ISBN-13: 978-3-642-80566-0
DOI: 10.1007/978-3-642-80566-0

Vorwort

Stahl und Strahl sind, trotz aller Fortschritte auf dem Gebiet der Biologie und der pharmakologischen und hormonalen Beeinflussung bösartiger Geschwülste, immer noch die Hauptwaffen im Bemühen, maligne Erkrankungen zu beherrschen. Die wesentlichen Verbesserungen der Heilungsquoten beruhen auf dem systematischen Ausbau beider Methoden, die sowohl biologische Erkenntnisse als auch selbstverständlich medikamentöse Möglichkeiten sinngemäß zu berücksichtigen haben. Der edle Wettstreit zwischen Chirurgie und Strahlenbehandlung hat viel dazu beigetragen, die Leistungsfähigkeit beider Vorgehen klarzustellen und zu steigern und führte schließlich zu einer grundlegenden Änderung der Strategie. Beide Verfahren, die grundsätzlich lokale Beeinflussungen darstellen, stehen überall, wo fortschrittlich gedacht wird, nicht mehr in Konkurrenz zu einander, sondern werden sinnvoll koordiniert. Diese Entwicklungstendenz kann kaum eindrücklicher dargestellt werden als bei der Behandlung maligner Erkrankungen des weiblichen Genitaltrakts.

Bei den Erkrankungen der männlichen Geschlechtsorgane ist der Weg ein ähnlicher, wenn auch etwas weniger augenfällig. Bei den Geschwülsten der Nieren und abführenden Harnwege ist das therapeutische Vorgehen in voller Entwicklung. Noch sind längst nicht alle Möglichkeiten der Kombination und Assoziation erschöpft.

Man hört oft kritische Äußerungen über den Wert von Handbuchdarstellungen, zumal durch die gelegentlich nicht zu vermeidenden Verzögerungen der Drucklegung die Darstellungen bei der sehr raschen Entwicklung manchmal nicht mehr ganz dem neuesten Stand entsprechen. Der Ausbau beider Methoden und die Verbesserung von für gut befundenen Behandlungen erfolgt meistens schrittweise, wobei es von großem Vorteil ist, wenn auf früheren Erfahrungen aufgebaut werden kann. Hierin sehen wir eine der bedeutendsten Aufgaben der enzyklopädischen Darstellung, die als solche niemals erschöpfend sein kann. In diesem Sinn hoffen wir, daß auch dieser Band als Basis allen denjenigen dienen möge, die sich auf dem Gebiet der Tumorbehandlung nicht nur strahlentherapeutisch sondern auch chirurgisch betätigen und sich für die verschiedenen Methoden, Möglichkeiten und weiteren Entwicklungen interessieren.

Bern, Januar 1971 A. Zuppinger

Preface

Despite all the advances in biology and in understanding the action of drugs and hormones on malignant tumours, the chief weapons in the fight against cancer are still the surgeon's knife and irradiation. The very real improvements in the rate of cure are due to the fact that these two methods have been systematically extended with a proper appreciation of both the new biological knowledge and, of course, the potentialities of drugs. The noble contest between surgery and radiology has done much to clarify and amplify the capabilities of both and has finally brought about a basic change in strategy. The two procedures, both, in principle, local treatments, are no longer seen by progressive thinkers as competing with one another, but are coordinated in a rational manner. There can hardly be a better illustration of this trend than the treatment of malignant diseases of the female genital tract.

A similar, if less striking, revolution has occurred with diseases of the male sex organs. As regards tumours of the kidneys and urinary tract, the therapeutic procedure is in full development. The many possibilities of combination and association are still far from being exhausted.

Critical remarks are frequently heard about the value of encyclopedic presentations, in particular that, because delays in publication are inevitable, they tend to be out-of-date in fast developing fields. However, advances in surgery and radiology and improvements in established forms of treatment usually come about gradually and here it is very useful to be able to build upon earlier experience. We regard this as one of the most important functions of the encyclopedic presentation which, as such, can never be exhaustive. It is in this sense that we hope this volume, too, will provide a base for all engaged in treating cancer, whether by surgery or by radiotherapy, who take an interest in the range of methods, possibilities and prospective developments.

Bern, January 1971   A. ZUPPINGER

Inhaltsverzeichnis — Contents

Mitarbeiter von Band XIX/3 — Contributors to Volume XIX/3

Dr. H. J. G. Bloom, The Royal Marsden Hospital, Radiotherapy Department, Fulham Road, London S.W. 3 (England)

Professor Dr. Werner Dietz, 7800 Freiburg, Kaiser-Joseph-Str. 178

Dr. Stanley Dische, Regional Radiotherapy Centre, Mount Vernon Hospital, Northwood, Middlesex (England)

Dr. F. Edsmyr, Radiumhemmet, Karolinska sjukhuset, 10401 Stockholm 60 (Schweden)

Professor Dr. H.-J. Frischbier, Strahlenabteilung der Universitäts-Frauenklinik und Poliklinik, 2000 Hamburg 20, Martinistr. 52

Professor Dr. Rolf Frischkorn, Strahlenabteilung der Universitäts-Frauenklinik, 3400 Göttingen, Humboldtallee 3

Professor Dr. F. Gauwerky, Chefarzt am Institut für Strahlentherapie und Nuklearmedizin im Allgemeinen Krankenhaus St. Georg, 2000 Hamburg 1, Lohmühlenstr. 5

Dr. H.-L. Kottmeier, Radiumhemmet, Karolinska sjukhuset, 10401 Stockholm 60 (Schweden)

David Wallace, The Royal Marsden Hospital, Radiotherapy Department, Fulham Road, London S.W. 3 (England)

Professor Sir Brian Windeyer, Meyerstein Institute of Radiotherapy, The Middlesex Hospital, London W. 1 (England)

A. Tumoren des weiblichen Genitale

I. Carcinoma of the vulva

By

F. Edsmyr and H.-L. Kottmeier

With 3 Figures

1. Introduction

Cancer vulva is among the more rare of the neoplastic diseases, constituting less than 1% of all cancers and 3–5% of all gynecological cancers. In 1962 the Swedish Cancer Registry reports 107 new cases of carcinoma of the vulva. It amounts to 0.93% of all female cancers and 2.0% of all new malignant tumours of the genital tract.

The literature contains reports of numerous series demonstrating the incidence of vulva cancer in relation to all malignant tumours of the genital tract. HUBER (1951) gives a figure of 2.7%, LANGFELT-ANDERSEN (1959) of 3.8% and INSTRE (1959) of 7.7%. During the years 1922 through 1952 inclusive 708 new cases of malignant neoplasms of the vulva were admitted to the Radiumhemmet. Out of these, 44 were malignant melanoblastomas, five sarcomas and two adenocarcinomas. Of the remaining 657 vulva carcinomas 560 cases proved to have histopathologically verified squamous cell carcinomas. These cases will be presented in this paper.

2. Anatomy

The vulva region embraces the mons veneris, the labia minora and majora, the clitoris, the large vestibular glands and the area of the posterior commissure. The external urethral orifice also is situated in the same region (WAY, 1948 and HAFFERL, 1957).

The study of the lymphatics in the vulva is of fundamental importance to the treatment of vulvar carcinoma.

The vulva has an extraordinarily ample lymphatic system; the channels forming a fine network. The fine network gives occasion to ample anastomosing, in part between the two sides of the vulva by way of the commissures and in part by the ample lymphatic network in the mons pubis. It is not rare to see trunks of one side reaching the nodes of the opposite side. Consequently contralateral metastases are seen. WAY (1951) has divided the lymph nodes draining the vulva into six groups:

1. Superficial inguinal nodes.
2. Superficial femoral nodes grouped around the saphenous vein.
3. Deep inguinal nodes.
4. Deep femoral nodes along the femoral vessels, the most important of these being the node of Cloquet or Rosenmueller, which lies at the upper end of the femoral canal.
5. External iliac nodes, the most important of which lying inframedial to the external iliac vein.
6. Presymphyseal nodes usual around the root of the clitoris.

Opinions differ whether deep lymph nodes could be involved directly without passing through the superficial inguinal group. PARRY-JONES (1963) has demonstrated a lymphatic trunk coming from the midline following the pudendal artery directly to the hypogastric nodes.

3. Different data

a) Age

Cancer of the vulva is predominantly a disease of advanced age and, in those series that have been reported, is comparatively rare before the age of forty. The mean age usually exceeds sixty (TAUSSIG, 1940; ELLIS, 1949; BERVEN, 1949; GREEN, 1958; and LUNDVALL, 1961).

In our series of 560 patients 7 (1.7%) were under 30 years, 30 (5.4%) under 40, 65% over 60 and 32% over 70 years. The youngest was 23 and the oldest 92 years. The mean age was 63.7 years.

b) Marital status

In 337 of the present cases the number of childbirths were annotated in the records. It is remarkable that five-year survival was lower in patients who had had three childbirths or more.

Table 1

Number of childbirths	0	I	II	III	IV–VI	VI–IX	X
No of patients	94	57	46	34	63	27	16
Five-year survival number	46	26	24	15	19	7	10
Five-year survival in per cent	48.9	45.6	52.2	44.1	30.2	25.9	(62.5)
		48.5				36.4	

The table gives the number of childbirths in 337 patients and their relation to 5-year survival.

c) Predisposing factors

Predisposing factors are important in the discussion of any malignant tumour. Several factors have been annotated as to carcinoma of the vulva.

α) Atrophy of the vulvar tissue

Atrophy of the vulvar tissue secondary to ovarian failure is of importance in the etiology of malignant tumours in this area. Pruritus is a common symptom in women more than 50 years of age. It is accompanied by atrophy of the vulvar tissue. Many patients with carcinoma in the vulva have suffered for a long time from pruritus. In literature figures of 20–50% are given for cases of vulvar carcinoma with symptoms of pruritus.

β) Diabetes mellitus

Pruritus is occasionally the first symptom of diabetes. Numerous authors consider this disease to be a factor predisposing to carcinoma of the vulva (BIRTH and COLLINS, 1960). SMITH and POLLACK (1947) report a figure of 4.4%, PALMER (1949) of 1.2%, GREEN (1958) of 8.8% and LANGFELT-ANDERSEN (1958) of 2.4%. In the Radiumhemmet series of 560 patients the incidence of diabetes was 2.9%. However, whether the diabetic state is of any etiological significance to the development of leukoplakia is questionable.

γ) Leukoplakia

Leukoplakia heads the list as a local precursor. Leukoplakia begins as a chronic inflammatory and hyperplastic process. The first manifestation appears on the labial folds around the vaginal outlet. Although leukoplakia may appear simultaneously with kraurosis it is important to distinguish these two lesions. As a rule leukoplakia appears as a slightly elevated, discrete white patch on the surface of the mucosa. It may occur many years before cancer develops. Reports vary as to the actual incidence from 12–70 % association. Authorities as BERVEN (1949), TAUSSIG (1940), WAY (1960), STENNING (1959) design leukoplakia as precancerous. It was seen in 33 % of the Radiumhemmet 560 patients and in 58 % in the series of 238 patients reported by GREEN *et al.* (1958).

δ) *Syphilis and other venereal diseases*

Leukoplakia has a strong epidemiologic relation to venereal disease, particularly syphilis and lymphogranuloma venereum or granuloma inguinale. However, the connection between leukoplakia respectively vulvar cancer and veneral infections have not been generally established. Only five patients in the Radiumhemmet series had a history of venereal disease. A small group of patients with vulvar lesions may have positive serologic test for syphilis. We consider it important to check the Wassermann reaction in all patients prior to therapy.

ε) *Kraurosis vulvae*

Kraurosis vulvae is a distinct condition, occupying mostly the vestibulae and not the labia majora which are the usual seat of leukoplakia. Kraurosis is a condition of atrophy, and frequently the subepithelial vessels are dilated which yields to a brown-reddish colour of the surface. It is rarely the precursor of carcinoma.

ζ) *Condylomata accuminata*

In literature there have been reported a number of cases with condylomata that have developed into frank invasive cancer. The Radiumhemmet series includes five such cases.

η) *Papillomata*

The vulvar region is sometimes the site of papillomata which may in due course become malignant (MÜLLER, 1946; HUBER, 1951). We have seen 14 patients (12.5 %) with papillomas which after a period of one to 30 years had developed into carcinoma.

ϑ) *Pernicious anemia, Plummer-Vinson syndrom, and Grave secondary anemia*

It is likely that patients suffering from severe anemia may have a reduced resistance of the mucous membrane of the vulvar region. The Radiumhemmet series includes 19 patients with severe blood-dyscrasia. Six patients had a typical history of Plummer-Vinson syndrom.

d) Multiple malignancies and heredity

SHIELD WARREN (1940) analyzed multiple tumour cases in a series of 1149 cases of skin cancer. 77 patients showed evidence of carcinoma in other organs of the body (6.7 %). TAUSSIG (1940) reports 6.4 % and GREEN (1958) 13.5 % multiple carcinomas in their series of vulva cancer. In our series multiple malignancies were seen in 37 (6.6 %) of the 560 patients. Sixty-one of the patients had a family history of malignancy (10.9 %). GREEN gives a corresponding figure of 21 %, LUNDVALL of 20 %.

4. Symptomatology

The symptomatology may include pruritus, ulceration—usually as a result of intensive scratching—the development of a nodule or "pimple" in the vulvar region; pain when seated, formication in the vulvar area, eczema, symptoms associated with micturation and frequently caused by contact of the urine with ulcerated areas; haemorrhages and discharges from the vulva and vagina (HUBER, 1951; GREEN, 1958; LANGFELT-ANDERSEN, 1959). In this series the major symptom was nodule and ulcerations. Worthy of note is the fact that so few of the patients reported pruritus as a symptom that had led them to consult a physician.

1*

Table 2 gives a summary of symptoms, which led the patient to consult a physician.

In the total series of patients 4.5% had felt enlarged inguinal nodes but had not sought medical advice on that score. The duration of symptoms varied considerably.

Table 2

Symptoms	Percentage of patients
Nodule	44.1%
Ulcerations	23.9%
Pruritus	8.2%
Smarting pain	5.2%
Dysuria	4.8%
Vaginal discharge	4.3%
Hemorrhages	2.5%
Vulvar pain	2.1%

Tumour size. Many of the carcinomas in this series had already attained a considerable size at the time of admission to the Radiumhemmet. 45.4% of the tumours were more than 4 cm in diameter (Table 3).

Table 3

Tumour diameter on admission	< 2 cm	2–4 cm	4–6 cm	> 6 cm
Number of patients	57	198	86	126
%	12.2	42.4	18.4	27.0

Table 3 gives the size of the tumour at first examination.

a) Extension of primary tumour

Vulvar carcinomas are characterized in general by lesions ranging from superficial ulcerations or papillary fungoid growths to large ulcerous craters with secondary infection and frequent involvement of a large portion of the vulva and adjacent tissues. The great majority of these carcinomas arise in the labia majora and minora, but sometimes it originates in the clitoris (Taussig, 1940; Berven, 1949; Huber, 1951; Green, 1958). Tumours originating from the clitoris are considered more malignant than others.

In this series it was a high incidence of cancerous infection of the clitoris region. However, in many cases the extension of the growth to the clitoris occurred at a late stage. Many times it is difficult to tell from which anatomic area the carcinoma has originated (Table 4).

Table 4

Site	Percentage of cases
Labia	84.1%
Clitoris	40.9%
Post. com.	16.6%
Vagina	15.9%
Urethra	11.4%
Rectovag. sept.	7.1%
Ant. com.	6.3%
Anal sphincter	6.3%
Rectal mucosa	4 cases
Invas. of the bladder	1 case

Table 4 gives the anatomic location of the primary lesion.

b) Diagnosis

As a rule, the diagnosis by inspection or palpation is easy. In a case of a small early lesion the diagnosis may be difficult especially if it is associated with leukoplakia. Biopsy confirmation should be made routinely.

Clinical palpation of inguinal nodes is a poor method of determining whether or not they contain cancer. Not every enlarged node is enlarged because of neoplasm. WAY has shown that 43 % of impalpable nodes do actually contain cancer. *Needle biopsy* has proven to be of considerably value in deciding the nature of a lymphnode.

α) Lymphography

Pelvic lymphography permits direct radiographic visualization of the lymph-nodes of the para-iliac and the caudal para-aortic areas. Opinions differ concerning the practical value of roentgenologic evidence of lymph node metastasis and many authors consider lymphography as an unreliable method. FUCHS (1965) thinks that metastases from a vulvar cancer can be diagnosed by lymphography first when the regional nodes are deeply involved by the growth.

β) Histology

The majority of malignant tumours of the vulva consist of squamous cell carcinomas with various degree of keratinization and differentiation (Fig. 1). ELLIS (1949) gives a figure of 95 %, CORSCADEN (1956) of 80 %, and LANGFELT-ANDERSEN (1959) of 92 % in

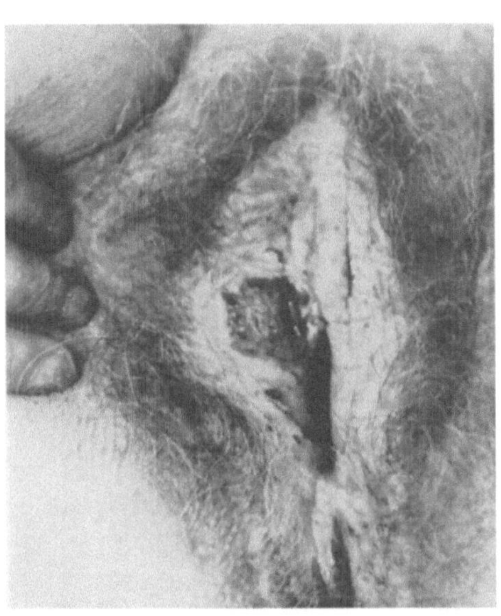

Fig. 1. Epidermoid carcinoma of the vulva

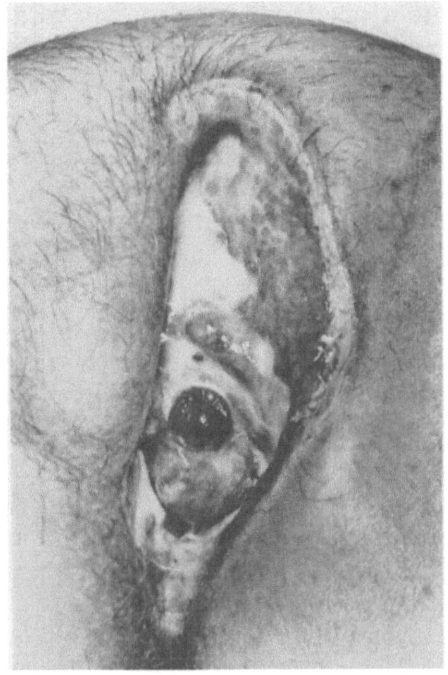

Fig. 2. Melanoblastoma of the vulva

their series of cases. All tumours in this series of 560 patients were squamous cell carcinomas with various degree of keratinization and differentiation. All the neoplasms were examined at the Institute of Radiopathology why evaluation and classification were uniform.

c) Differential diagnosis

α) Condyloma

Condyloma is a common lesion which is seen especially in young women. The growth is soft, occasionally pedunculated and usually associated with an infectious disease.

β) Veneral lymphogranuloma

Veneral lymphogranuloma may occasionally resemble a cancer. As a rule it is soft and attended by rectal ulcers. Frei's laboratory test permits the differential diagnosis. It is essential to bear in mind, however, that a veneral disease may co-exist with a carcinoma of the vulva.

γ) Bartholonitis

Benign tumours as hemangiomas, lipomas and fibromas. They are of slow growth and not ulcerated.

Hidroadenoma is frequently confused with cancer. It takes origin from the sweat glands in the vulvar skin. The hidroadenoma is usually small, papillary, and reddish gray in appearance. It tends to be sharply circumscribed. It is rarely ulcerated.

Bowens disease, also called erythroplasia Quegrat. This lesion is similar to carcinoma in situ of the cervix and vagina and may be considered as the earliest form of epidermoid carcinoma in the vulvar region. Bowens disease may present as red slightly raised placques with a finally granular surface or as superficial ulcerations. It is designated as TIS in the UICC classification (page 7).

Pagets disease arises most likely from the apocrine glands. Typical large clear Paget's cells are seen in the basal portions of the epidermis. The clinical features vary considerably, but as a rule the disease appears with white or reddened patches.

δ) Basal cell carcinoma

Basal cell carcinoma represents 2–5 % of all vulvar tumours and assumes two different forms—one superficial and one that usually produces a crateriform ulcer. At Radium-hemmet we have observed basal cell carcinoma in less than 1 % of vulva tumour cases. Hultberg (1960) pointed out that basal cell carcinoma in the vulva may be more malignant than its counterparts in other areas of skin.

ε) Malignant melanoblastoma

Malignant melanoblastoma is relatively common in the vulvar region. Its usually blue-black appearance will render the diagnosis easy. Further regard will be paid to this very malignant tumour on page 14.

ζ) Other gynecologic cancer

Malignant tumours of the uterus or ovary may extend or metastasize to the vulva. A careful gynecological examination, may be a curettage, should be carried out in every case of carcinoma of the vulva.

d) Classification

Comparison of reported therapeutic results and evaluation of different methods of therapy is possible only if all cases examined with a view to therapy at the institution are reported and if they are classified and staged in accordance with rules internationally accepted. Many authors have employed clinical stage-classifications and/or histopathological classifications (Simon, 1932; Taussig, 1940; Berven, 1949; Cosbie, 1951; Gylling, 1958; Stenning, 1959; Way, 1960; Lundvall, 1961), but none of the methods proposed has facilitated an adequate comparison of different series.

The Committee on Clinical Stage Classification of the UICC has considered it important to reach an agreement as to description of the anatomical extent of growth until a clinical staging is applied. The Committee has developed the TNM system, and has in 1967 proposed a TNM classification for carcinoma of the vulva. This classification follows the rules that previously have been established for carcinoma of the breast, gynecological cancers etc. The clinical TNM classification for carcinoma of the vulva reads as follows:

Carcinoma of the vulva

T   *Primary tumour*

TIS   Preinvasive carcinoma. Carcinoma in situ
T0   No evidence of primary tumour
T1   Single tumour not more than 2 cm in its largest dimension
T2   Single tumour more than 2 cm, but not more than 5 cm in its largest dimension
T3   Single tumour more than 5 cm in its largest dimension *or* tumour of any size with extension to vagina not more than 2 cm in length *or* to anal canal without involvement of mucosa, *or* with extension to urethra
T3m   Multiple tumours covering an area of not more than 10 cm in diameter
T4   Single tumour of any size with extension to vagina more than 2 cm in length
       or to anal canal with involvement of the mucosa
       or to recto-vaginal septum
       or to other neighbouring structures
T4m   Multiple tumours covering an area more than 10 cm in diameter

N   *Regional nodes*

N0   No palpable nodes
N1   Movable homolateral nodes
     N1a   Nodes not considered to contain growth
     N1b   Nodes considered to contain growth
N2   Movable contralateral or bilateral nodes
     N2a   Nodes not considered to contain growth
     N2b   Nodes considered to contain growth
N3   Fixed nodes

M   *Distant metastases*

M0   No distant metastases
M1   Distant metastases present

      Clinical staging

With regard to the TNM classification a clinical staging is rendered possible. It is necessary that four stages be used in accordance with the staging of ovarian, uterine, and vaginal carcinoma. The following staging is proposed:

Stage I:	T1, N0, M0	Stage IV:	T1, N3, M0
Stage II:	T1, N1, M0		T2, N3, M0
	T2, N0, M0		T3, N3, M0
	T2, N1, M0		T4, N0, M0
Stage III:	T1, N2, M0		T4, N1, M0
	T2, N2, M0		T4, N2, M0
	T3, N0, M0		T4, N3, M0
	T3, N1, M0	All cases with M1	
	T3, N2, M0		

5. Methods of treatment

Two essentially different procedures are to be dealt with in the treatment of vulvar cancer, i.e. surgery and radiotherapy or a combination of surgery and radiation. Chemotherapy in the form of perfusion or infusion of derivates of nitrogen mustard or methotrexate has been tried in cases too advanced to be treated by surgery (MASTERSON and NELSON, 1965) but is valuable only from a palliative point of view.

a) Surgery

α) Local removal

Local removal of the growth or *simple vulvectomy* is indicated only in patients considered as very poor operative risk. Such a surgical procedure is inadequate. Local excision should never be carried out. The carcinoma is often multiple and tumours frequently involve both labia. Such growths are designed as kisstumours.

β) Electrocoagulation

Electrocoagulation was introduced by MATTHAELI (1921) and perfected by BERVEN (1922) and has been widely used in many countries.

γ) Radical surgery

Adequate radical surgery must be defined as a wide resection of the vulva and its surrounding tissue combined with bilateral dissection of superficial and deep inguinal nodes. Experience has shown that if possible, the operation should be performed in one stage. Various surgical techniques have been developed (RUPPRECHT, 1893; GOSSET, 1909; BASSET, 1912; TAUSSIG, 1929; BARANOFSKY, 1948; WAY, 1948; MACAFEE, 1962; BOUTSELIS, ULLERY and TETERIS, 1963; McKELVEY, 1965; TWOMBLY, 1966). A curved incision is made beginning medial to each anterior superior iliac spine. The dissection is continued inferiorly separating all tissue from the fascia and underlying muscle. As much excess skin as possible is removed. This extended vulvectomy is the standard surgical procedure. McKELVEY has stressed that two teams, one on each side, work simultaneously to shorten the required time. The most unsatisfactory aspect, however, of the wide excision is the often long time it takes for the raw surface left by the vulvectomy to heal. Plastic surgeons have developed skin grafting methods, which have been of benefit in the healing process (McGREGOR, 1966).

From studies performed by many authors especially in recent years, it is evident that dissection of superficial and deep inguinal and femoral nodes should be routinely carried out in all patients in whom vulvectomy is considered as an adequate therapy if good results are to be achieved (BORIA and GRAHAM, 1960; GOSLING, 1961). WAY and GREEN among others have shown that metastases to the inguinal lymph nodes are frequently seen in the clinical absence of lymphnode metastases.

It is, however, a highly controversial point whether the pelvic lymphnodes above Poupart's ligament should be dissected routinely. WAY has shown that lesions arising in the midline, especially in the area of the clitoris, could metastasize directly to hypogastric and iliac nodes. GREEN on the other hand points out that, in his series, although the deep pelvic nodes were frequently involved there were no instances of deep pelvic node spread in the absence of superficial inguinal or femoral node involvement. In earlier years WAY recommended dissection of deep pelvis nodes as a routine procedure. This extensive operation was followed by a high risk of primary mortality. The operative mortality ran up to 12 % for this extended operation. As a consequence of this experience WAY, in 1952, altered his technique and carried out a deep lymph-node dissection only if smear taken from inguinal nodes during operation demonstrated malignant cells.

Nevertheless, some surgeons recommend still extended dissection of deep pelvic lymph nodes as a routine procedure, but there is a tendency to individualize the surgical approach in carcinoma of the vulva.

The operability rate varies. WAY (1960) gives a figure of 83 %, McKELVEY (1965) of 93.5 %.

δ) Exenteration

BRUNSCHWIG (1956) has discussed the value of exenteration in cases of vulva carcinoma. He performed such an operation in 27 instances. The operation may be justified in selected cases of advanced slowly growing tumour.

b) Radiotherapy

Authorities do agree that radiation therapy whether by local or irradiation by roentgen therapy is of little benefit in the curative treatment of vulvar cancer especially as it is difficult to apply cancericidal doses to this area. The normal tissue in the vulva has a reduced tolerance to radiation. In general, radiation therapy is indicated in cases not suitable for surgery either because of the general condition of the patient or the extent of the disease. In cases of involvement of the urethra radiotherapy may be indicated as a preoperative procedure. Inplantation of lowintensity radium needles or treatment with radium moulage has been tried (BERVEN, 1949; TOD, 1940; BAUD, 1949; COSBIE, 1952; CUCCIA, 1966) but in general the results are unsatisfactory. In recent years German gynaecologists especially, have employed electron beam irradiation in cases of both circumscript and advanced vulvar carcinoma (KEPP, 1951; OBERHEUSER, 1965).

In 1949 SCHUBERT, KEPP, PAUL and SCHMERMUND reported preliminary experience with electron-therapy of vulvar cancer from a 6-MeV Betatron. The Hamburg-clinic has developed this method further and in 1965 OBERHEUSER gave a survey of the present experience. The local growth is treated through one large portal, which irrespective of the size of the growth always covers the vulva. A dose of 4 500–5 300 rad is applied from a 15 MeV Betatron. The daily dose amounts to 300 rad. In addition electron-therapy is given to the inguinal regions with a similar technique and dose. At the Radiumhemmet electron-therapy has been tried in selected patients of young age. The primary reaction is unpleasant for the patient, and late prolonged ulceration or necrosis may arise in the irradiated mucosa.

At the Radiumhemmet external cobalt-60 irradiation has been given in advanced cases of inoperable vulvar carcinoma with metastases. The therapy should be carefully planned. A dose of 6 000–6 500 rad has been delivered in 5–7 weeks. The results have been remarkably satisfactory.

c) Radiotherapy and surgical treatment

Several authors have proposed a combined treatment of radiation and surgery in vulvar carcinomas. ANTOINE and MAIER (1942) for instance, performed a primary electro-coagulation of the local disease, but implanted radium needles in the growth around the urethra. Teleradium or conventional X-ray therapy was delivered to the inguinal nodes in addition to the surgical procedure by several specialists. As a rule the series of cases presented are small. At the Radiumhemmet the treatment of choice has been, for years, an electrocoagulation of the local growth followed by irradiation to the area of inguinal lymphnodes.

In this paper it will be impossible to discuss in detail therapeutic aspects. The authors will concentrate the description to their own method.

d) Radiumhemmet method

In 1922 BERVEN introduced bipolar electrocoagulation to the treatment of primary vulvar carcinoma. The coagulation has been carried out with appartus from the Wapper Electrical Co., New York, in recent years during spinal anaesthesia. It is important to perform repeated irrigation of infected tumours, proper anticeptics prior to the operation. In general, round electrodes with uniform diameters of 0.5–1 cm are used. The infected and, frequently, disintegrated tumour is coagulated first. The coagulation starts in the anterior portion and terminates in the posterior part of the vulvar region. It is important to coagulate all vulvar tissue. Via an incision in the coagulated tissue it can be ascertained whether the coagulation is sufficiently deep. It is important to start the coagulation far out in the periphery in order to initially coagulate and block the patent lymphatics. To obviate overheating and charring of the operative field, reducing the deep effects, the entire field is irrigated with cold water. A piece of ice is introduced into the rectum for cooling the mucosa. Berven (1941) and Edsmyr (1962) have described the technique; for further details the reader is referred to their publications.

α) Postoperative complications

Sixteen of 535 patients operated upon (3.0 %) died within one month after the operation. The mean age of these patient was 73.1 years; 9.4 years greater than for the total series. Twelve of the deaths occurred prior to 1940 and only four after that year. This result demonstrates the value of the measures taken in recent years, i.e. more stringent pre-operative medical treatment and more advanced anestesiology.

Postoperative moderate haemorrhage occurred in eight cases from the coagulation area.

β) Recurrences in the vulvar region

In the years 1922 to 1952, 535 patients with vulvar carcinoma were subjected to primary electrocoagulation. In 83 of these patients (15.9 %) fresh tumours later developed either as local recurrences or as new growths elsewhere in the vulva. Nineteen of the tumours were not histo-pathologically verified, but were considered clinically as obvious recurrences. In 1941, Berven gave a figure of 11.3 % local recurrences.

γ) Time of onset of recurrences

Fifty per cent of the recurrences occurred within two years after electrocoagulation and more than 70 % within five years. It is likely that many of the recurrences diagnosed two years or more after electrocoagulation actually were new tumours as they appeared in other parts of the vulva than did the primary tumour.

δ) Site of tumour

The majority of "recurrences" were localized to the labia, the clitoris, the posterior commissure or/and the area of the urethra. It is worthy to note that no recurrences were observed in those cases where the primary tumour had extended to the sphincter ani (36 cases).

ε) Subjective symptoms

The present series was studied with special regard to whether or not electrocoagulation had been followed by subjective distress—various type of prolaps, manifestation of vesical and anal incontinence and sexual discomfort. Green (1958) had reported prolaps in 12 % and stress incontinence in 7 % of patients in whom radical vulvectomy had been performed.

ζ) Prolapses

Prolaps of the urethra was recorded in seven patients, cystocele in eight, prolaps of the vagina in six, prolaps of the uterus in seven, and proctocele in seven patients. In brief, prolapses were observed in 5.6 % of 535 patients who had undergone primary electrocoagulation. The prolapses observed in this series affected elderly patients, whose tissues had already lost much of their tonus and elasticity.

η) Stenosis of the lower vagina

The patients in this series were subjected to a special follow-up investigation in order to establish what symptoms referable to the genito-urinary tract had occurred as a sequel of the electrocoagulation. Adequate information was obtained from 76 of the 101 patients interviewed and examined. Fourteen of the 76 patients (18.4%) reported that intercourse was impossible at least partly due to stenosis of the vestibulum. Five of these patients suffered from dysuria. As a rule information as to sexual disturbances occurring after vulvectomy is not given in literature.

Rectovaginal fistule occurred in three cases in which the carcinoma had extended to the posterior wall and commissure as well as to the sphincter ani. The three patients are living free from evidence of the disease.

Urethro- and vesico-vaginal fistule occurred in two patients in whom conventional X-ray therapy had been given towards the carcinoma prior to the electrocoagulation.

Damage to the symphysis with osteitis occurred in two patients. Swelling of the legs is frequently seen as a sequel of radical vulvectomy. We have not observed any such complications in cases in which electrocoagulation had been carried out.

It is of interest to observe that, although half the sphincter muscle had been coagulated, the functional effect of the sphincter remained satisfactorily in the vast majority of patients.

ϑ) Treatment of regional lymph nodes

Following primary electrocoagulation of the vulvar tumour and an interval of two to three weeks, during which the coagulated tissues usually sloughed off, prophylactic teleradium-radiation was given to inguinal and femoral nodes in the cases reported in this series. Two fields were radiated on each side. The size of each field amounted to 6 cm and the distance between the center of each field to 6–7 cm. A dose of 2 700–3 600 rad was delivered to each field over a period of 10–20 days (BERVEN, 1931, 1932; SIEVERT, 1933, 1937; BENNER, 1947; EDSMYR and WALSTAM, 1959). In cases of palpable clinically suspicious metastases 2 700–3 600 rad were delivered to each field in 8–10 days preoperatively. In general dissection of inguinal and femoral nodes was performed following the radiation.

Since 1954 the radiation technique has been modified. In 1959 EDSMYR and WALSTAM introduced the overlapping field technique with a short-distance ^{60}Co unit, which proved to be of great value both from a clinical and a physical point of view. Each treatment area comprises ten fields in a row with the field centers at intervals of one cm. The size of the deca-curie field is 6×6 cm. A dose of 800 rad is delivered to each of the ten fields.

ι) Diagnosis by cytological puncture of inguinal lymph nodes

The diagnostic methods formerly available for detecting metastases in the inguinal regions were palpation and, in certain cases, biopsy. In recent years cytological puncture of lymph nodes has been added to our diagnostic aids. This method was introduced by FRANZÉN in 1953. The puncture is made with thin needles of special design (LAGER-HOLM, 1960).

At the Radiumhemmet many thousands punctures have been performed. Implantation metastases occurred in only one case of melanoblastoma pulmones. The cytologic puncture of inguinal nodes has proved to be of great value, and we do feel that it should be used as a routine procedure. Negative cytologic findings cannot be considered conclusive. The puncture should be repeated in clinically suspicious cases.

e) Results

α) Surgery

Most authorities agree that the standard procedure is radical vulvectomy with bilateral inguinal and femoral lymphadenectomy. WAY (1957) analysed the 5-year survival rates in cases treated by local vulvectomy, vulvectomy and unilateral node dissection or vulvectomy and bilateral superficial node dissection. A 5-year cure rate of 23.6% was reached in 123 cases treated by any of these techniques. All node involved cases died before five years had elapsed. The credit of having worked out modern surgical techniques is due to Way's research. In 1954 he was able to publish the results of his technique in 79 unselected and consecutive patients followed for at least 5 years. Sixty-five patients were operated upon. Forty-eight patients were alive and well at 5 years, i.e. an absolute five year survival rate of 61%. The five-year cure rate was 86% in 44 cases with negative nodes and 48% in 21 cases with positive nodes. Eight patients died following the operation.

Way (1960) has analysed in detail the presence of lymph node involvement in 143 consecutive operations. The incidence of node involvement was 42%. Table 5 demonstrates that there were twice as many cases with involvement of the superficial nodes as there were with involvement of the superficial and deep nodes together. Metastases to the deep nodes alone were seen in only 3%. As a consequence of this low incidence of deep node involvement Way has modified his surgical technique as previously mentioned.

Table 5. *Lymph node involvement at operation in carcinoma of the vulva*

Total operations	143
Nodes involved	60 (42%)
Nodes not involved	83
Superficial nodes only involved	37 (26%)
Superficial and deep nodes involved	18 (13%)
Deep nodes only involved	5 (3%)

Several series of therapeutic results have been published in recent years, but, in general, it is difficult to draw substantial conclusions from statistics presented. Way (1966) reports that out of 69 patients operated on prior to 1950, 42 survived for 5 years (61%), 32, for 10 years (46%) and 23, for 15 years (33%) McKelvey (1965) has achieved a 5-year cure rate of 54% in 124 consecutive cases of vulvar cancer. Two patients were not treated. McKelvey's series is of special interest, as he divides the cases into four stages with regard to the anatomical extent of the disease.

Stage 1. Tumour of 10 sq cm or less not involving the urethra, vagina or anus; 64 patients, 5-year cure rate 70.3%.

Stage 2. Tumour of more than 10 sq. cm, not involving the urethra, vagina or anus: 35 patients, 5-year cure rate 48.5%.

Stage 3. Tumour of any size which also involves the urethra, vagina or anus: 22 patients, 5-year cure rate 22.7%.

Stage 4. Tumour of any size with clinically demonstrable intra-abdominal or distant metastases = 3 patients.

A 5-year cure rate of 68.2% was obtained in cases with negative lymphnodes while the corresponding rate was 26.4% in cases with positive nodes.

Ten patients died from intercurrent disease within 5 years following surgery.

β) Radiotherapy

Stoeckel collected 126 cases irradiated at different institutions. A five-year cure rate of 11.9% was achieved. Local application of radium, infiltration of platinum needles or irradiation by orthovoltage roentgen therapy have been tried in selected cases. Berven gives a 5-year survival rate of 13%, Baud of 14 and Tod of 25%. Oberheuser has from literature collected a series of 1384 cases which had received different kind of radiation. 401 patients survived for 5 years or more (28.9%). In recent years electron-beam therapy has been tried by German authors, in particular. In 1965 Schubert and Höhne reported a 44% 5-year cure rate in 27 patients. Oberheuser has in 1965 collected a series of 116 patients, who have received exclusively electrontherapy from a 12–16 MeV Betatron.

In 92 cases the carcinoma was rather advanced (79 %). A 5-year cure rate of 47 % was achieved in 54 patients, treated at least 5 years ago. The results are remarkably satisfactory why the Radiumhemmet very recently has started to use electron-therapy more extensively.

In 1959 to 1966 at the Radiumhemmet external cobalt-60 irradiation has been used in 19 cases of external vulva carcinoma with lymph-node metastases in the inguinal regions, histologically proven by needle biopsy. A dose of 6000–6500 rad has been delivered in 5–7 weeks. The primary results have been satisfactory and 3 patients have survived for 5 years.

γ) Electrocoagulation—Radiumhemmet method

657 cases of malignant neoplasms of the vulva were examined with a view to therapy at the Radiumhemmet in the years 1922 to 1952 incl. 560 patients of vulvar carcinoma were treated. These cases will be studied with regard to the stage-classification in 1967 proposed by the UICC and the International Federation of Gynecology and Obstetrics.

Table 6

Classification	Number of cases	Living at		Intercurrent death within		Cure rate	
		5 years	10 years	5 years	10 years	5 years	10 years
T 1 N 0	49	33	27	2	7	67%	55%
T 1 N 1	16	12	9	1	4	76%	56%
T 1 N 2	40	31	21	4	11	70%	53%
T 1 N 3	5	—	—	—	—	—	—
T 2 N 0	68	31	19	9	16	46%	28%
T 2 N 1	31	18	10	5	8	58%	32%
T 2 N 2	81	40	31	10	19	49%	38%
T 2 N 3	26	2	2	1	1	8%	8%
T 3 N 0	24	13	10	4	4	54%	42%
T 3 N 1	31	11	8	3	4	36%	26%
T 3 N 2	79	32	24	11	15	41%	30%
T 3 N 3	33	4	4	—	—	12%	12%
T 4 N 0	2	1	1	—	—		
T 4 N 1	15	1	—	—	—		
T 4 N 2	25	3	—	2	4		
T 4 N 3	35	1	1	—	—		

Table 6 gives the 560 cases of carcinoma of the vulva divided into the T and N groups as described on page 7 in this paper. The classification is based entirely on the clinical findings prior to therapy. The table reports the 5- and 10-year cure rate in per cent.

Table 6 presents 560 cases of carcinoma of the vulva treated at Radiumhemmet in 1922 to 1952 incl. TNM classification. 5- and 10-year cure rate.

In Table 7 the 560 cases classified in accordance with the TNM method have been allotted to stages (page 7). The relative 5-year apparent recovery rate amounts to 41.6 %, the 10-year, to 29.7 %. The corresponding recovery rates are for Stage I 67 and 55 %, for Stage II 53 and 33 %, for Stage III 50 and 37 %, and for Stage IV 8 and 6 %. Carcinoma of the vulva is a disease of elderly women. Consequently it is not remarkable that 52 patients have died from intercurrent disease within 5 years after initial therapy (9 %). Ninety-three patients have died from intercurrent disease within 10 years. considering the facts just mentioned the correlated survival rate for 5 years amounts to 45 % and for 10 years to 36 %.

Ninety-seven patients were not accepted for treatment because of very poor general condition or presence of distant metastases. The absolute 5-year survival rate amounts to 35.5 %, and the corresponding 10-year rate to 25.4 %.

It is of interest to review cases of metastases to inguinal and femoral nodes and correlate the findings to the TNM stage-classification. Only cases of lymph-node metastases proved by histologic examination or clinical progress are included in Tables 8 and 9. The presence of metastases increases with the size of the primary tumour. The majority of cases allotted to Stage IV have positive lymph nodes.

Table 7

Stage	Number of cases	Living at		Dead from intercurrent disease within		Cure rate	
		5 years	10 years	5 years	10 years	5 years	10 years
I	49	33	27	2	7	67%	55%
II	115	61	38	15	28	53%	33%
III	255	127	94	32	53	50%	37%
IV	141	12	8	3	5	8%	6%
Total number treated	560	233	167	52	93 16.6%	41.6%	29.7%
Absolute cure rate	657	233	167			35.5%	25.4%

Table 8. *Presence of lymph-node metastases in relation to TNM classification*

Type of lesion	Number of cases	Percentage of proved metastases to inguinal or femoral lymph-nodes
T 1 N 1	16	6%
T 2 N 1	31	35%
T 3 N 1	31	58%
T 4 N 1	15	86%
T 1 N 2	40	15%
T 2 N 2	81	41%
T 3 N 2	79	51%
T 4 N 2	25	68%
T 1 N 3	5	100%
T 2 N 3	26	91%
T 3 N 3	33	94%
T 4 N 3	35	97%

Table 9. *Presence of lymph-node metastases in relation to clinical staging*

Stage	Percentage of proved metastases to inguinal and femoral lymph-nodes
I	0%
II	10%
III	38%
IV	89%

6. Sarcoma vulvae

Sarcoma vulvae is a rare disease, but nevertheless it is of importance to give some statements about this growth. At the Radiumhemmet, 62 patients with sarcoma vulvae were seen in the years 1922 to 1963. This amounts to about 5% of vulvar neoplasms.

Malignant melanoblastoma is the most common of vulvar neoplasms besides cancer. In 56 of the 62 cases the growth was of this type.

Many authors have pointed out that 40–80 % of patients with melanoblastoma had previously observed a naevus, which degenerated into a malignant growth. Only in 7 of our 56 cases the records give information that the patient had observed a naevus in earlier years. The melanoblastoma was localized to the area of the clitoris in 14 cases, to the anterior commissure in 3 cases and to the labia in 38 cases. No information is given as to the anatomical region in one case.

Verified metastases to the inguinal lymph nodes occurred in 15 cases (27 %).

Surgery is the treatment of choice in cases of malignant melanoblastoma.

Most authorities recommend radical vulvectomy (p. 8), but in general the results are unsatisfactory. At the Radiumhemmet the treatment has been individualized with regard to the local extension of the growth, the presence of metastases and the condition of the patient. Primary electrocoagulation was carried out in 34 cases. In 14 of these 34 patients also an excision was performed of superficial and deep inguinal and femoral nodes. Examination of the nodes revealed malignant growth in 11 of the 14 cases.

Local excision of the tumour was carried out in 15 cases, vulvectomy, in 5.

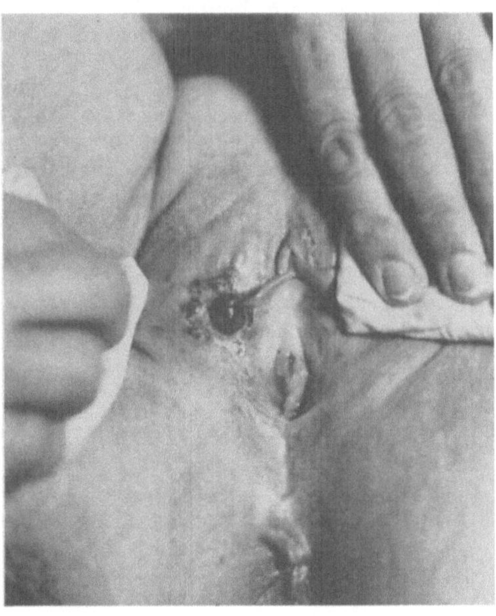

Fig. 3. Melanoblastoma of the vulva

Twelve of the 56 patients with malignant melanoblastoma are living at 5 years or more, i.e. 5-year survival rate of about 21 %. Four of these 12 patients later succumbed from the disease. None of the patients with positive metastases to inguinal nodes survived 5-years. The average survival time for these 15 patients was one year and one month.

References

ANTOINE, T., MAIER, E.: Die Elektrokoagulation des Vulvacarcinoms. Arch. Gynäk. **172**, 487 (1942).

— — Behandlung des Vulvacarcinoms mit Diathermie. Arch. Gynäk. **173**, 109 (1942).

BARANOFSKY, D.: Technique of inguinal node dissection. Surgery **24**, 555 (1948).

BASSET, A.: L'épithélioma primitif du clitoris. Thèse de Paris, 1912.

BAUD, J.: Le traitement des épithéliomas de la vulva. Bull. Cancer **36**, 104 (1949).

BERVEN, E.: The treatment of cancer of the vulva. Brit. J. Radiol. **22**, 498 (1949).

BORIA, M. N., GRAHAM, J. B.: Squamous carcinoma of the vulva. N. Y. J. Med. **60**, 398 (1960).

BOUTSELIS, J. G., ULLERY, J. C., TETERIS, N. J.: Epidermoid carcinoma of the vulva. Obstet. and Gynec. **22**, 713 (1963).

BRUNSCHWIG, A., DANIEL, W.: Total and anterior pelvic exenteration. Surg. Gynec. Obstet. **99**, 324 (1954).

— — Pelvic exenteration for advanced carcinoma of vulva. Amer. J. Obstet. Gynec. **72**, 489 (1956).

BYRON, R. L., JR., MISHELL, D. R., JR., YONEMOTO, R. H.: The surgical treatment of invasive carcinoma of the vulva. Surg. Gynec. Obstet. **121**, 1243 (1965).

COLLINS, C. G., COLLINS, J. H., NELSON, E. W., SMITH, R. C., McCALLUM, E. A.: Malignant tumors involving the vulva. Amer. J. Obstet. Gynec. **62**, 1198 (1951).

COLLINS, J. H., BARCLAY, D. L., COLLINS, C. G.: Vulvectomy. Amer. J. Obstet. Gynec. **84**, 1135 (1962).

CORSCADEN, J. A.: Gynecologic cancer, third ed., Cancer of the vulva, p. 101. Baltimore: William & Wilkins Co. 1962.

COSBIE, W. G.: The treatment of cancer of the vulva. Amer. J. Obstet. Gynec. **63**, 251 (1952).

CUCCIA, C. A.: Radiation therapy in the treatment of carcinoma of the vulva. New concept. gynec. oncology by LEWIS, WENTZ and JAFFE, p. 405. Philadelphia: Davis Comp. 1966.

EDSMYR, F.: Carcinoma of the vulva. Acta radiol. (Stockh.), Suppl. **217**, 132 (1962).

— ÅSÉN, P.: Inguinal irradiation and lymph-node excision in carcinoma of the vulva. Acta chir. scand. **120**, 447 (1961).

— WALSTAM, R.: Method for irradiation of parasternal lymph-node metastases. Acta radiol. (Stockh.) **51**, 308 (1959).

FUCHS, W. A.: Lymphographie und Tumordiagnostik, S. 54. Berlin-Heidelberg-New York: Springer 1965.

Göbel, A., Hamann, A.: Zur Klinik und Therapie der Karzinome am äußeren Genitale. Zbl. Gynäk. **61**, 1394 (1937).

Green, T. H.: Carcinoma of the vulva. Meigs and Sturgis, Progress in gynec., vol. III, p. 507. New York: Grune & Stratton 1957.

— Ulfelder, H., Meigs, J. V.: Epidermoid carcinoma of the vulva. Amer. J. Obstet. Gynec. **75**, 834, 848 (1958).

Gylling, T.: Primary cancer of the vulva. An. Chir. Gynaec. Fenn., Suppl. **81**, 17 (1958).

Hodari, A. A., Hodgkinson, C. P.: Lymphography as a Diagnostic aid in female genital malignancy. Obstet. and Gynec. **29**, 34 (1967).

Hultberg, S.: Personal communication, 1962.

International Union Against Cancer. The T.N.M. system general rules. Geneva 2.

Johnsson, J. E.: Malignant neoplasms of the vulva. Acta radiol. (Stockh.) **56**, 385 (1961).

Kepp, R. K., Paul, W., Schermund, H. J., Schubert, G.: Neue Methoden in der Behandlung des Vulvakarzinom. Geburtsh. u. Frauenheilk. **11**, 298 (1951).

Langfelt-Andersen, B.: Cancer of the vulva. Acta radiol. (Stockh.) **51**, 369 (1959).

Lundvall, F.: Cancer of the vulva. A clinical review. Acta radiol. (Stockh.), Suppl. **208**, 326 (1961).

Macafee, C. H. G.: Some aspects of vulvar cancer. J. Obstet. Gynaec. Brit. Cwlth **49**, 177 (1962).

McGregor, I. A.: Skin grafting after radical vulvectomy. J. Obstet. Gynaec. Brit. Cwlth **73**, 599 (1966).

McKelvey, J. L.: The treatment of carcinoma of the vulva. Amer. J. Obstet. Gynec. **54**, 626 (1947).

— Adcock, L. L.: Cancer of the vulva. Obstet. and Gynec. **26**, 455 (1965).

Minet, P., Chevalier, Ph., Closon, J., Garson, J.: Preliminary report about electrontherapy of the tumours of the vulva, p. 376. Symp. High Energy Electrons. Berlin-Göttingen-Heidelberg: Springer 1965.

Oberheuser, F.: Klinische Gesichtspunkte bei der Elektronentherapie des Vulvacarcinoms, S. 372. Symp. High Energy Electrons. Berlin-Göttingen-Heidelberg: Springer 1965.

Palmer, I. P., Sadugor, M. G., Reinhard, M. C.: Carcinoma of the vulva. Surg. Gynec. Obstet. **88**, 435 (1949).

Parry-Jones, E.: Lymphatics of vulva. J. Obstet. Gynaec. Brit. Cwlth **67**, 919 (1960).

Paterson, E., Tod, M.: The treatment of malignant disease by radium and X-ray. London: Edward Arnold Co. 1948.

Renner, K.: Behandlungsergebnisse an der Strahlenklinik Janker unter besonderer Berücksichtigung der Ergebnisse mit energiereichen Strahlen. Sonderbd. Strahlentherapie **61**, 138 (1965).

Scherman, A. S.: Cancer of the female reproductive organs, p. 243. St. Louis: C. V. Mosby Comp. 1963.

Schubert, G., Höhne, G.: Spätergebnisse nach Supervolt-Therapie gynäkologischer Karzinome. Sonderbd. Strahlentherapie **61**, 143 (1965).

Smith, F., Pollack, R.: Carcinoma of the vulva. Surg. Gynec. Obstet. **84**, 98 (1947).

Stenning, M., Elliott, P.: Primary carcinoma of the vulva with special reference to "leucoplakia". J. Obstet. Gynaec. Brit. Cwlth **66**, 897 (1959).

Stoeckel, W.: Zur Therapie des Vulvakarzinoms. Zbl. Gynäk. **54**, 47 (1930).

Taussig, F. J.: Primary cancer of the vulva, vagina and female urethra. Five years results. Surg. Gynec. Obstet. **60**, 477 (1935).

— Late results in the treatment of leucoplakic vulvitis and cancer of the vulva. Amer. J. Obstet. Gynec. **31**, 746 (1936).

— Cancer of the vulva. Analysis of 155 cases. Amer. J. Obstet. Gynec. **40**, 764 (1940).

Tod, M.: Radium implantation treatment of carcinoma vulvae. Brit. J. Radiol. **22**, 508 (1949).

Twombley, G. H.: Surgical treatment of vulvar cancer. New conc. gynec. oncology by Lewis, Wentz and Jaffe, p. 395. Philadelphia: Davis Comp. 1966.

Way, S.: The anatomy of the lymphatic drainage of the vulva and its influence on the radical operation for carcinoma. Ann. Roy. Coll. Surg. Engl. **3**, 187 (1948).

— Results of a planned attack on carcinoma of the vulva. Brit. J. Med. **2**, 780 (1954).

— Carcinoma of the vulva. Meigs and Sturgis, Progress in gynec., vol. III, p. 489. New York: Grune and Stratton 1957.

— Carcinoma of the vulva. Amer. J. Obstet. Gynec. **79**, 692 (1960).

— Carcinoma of the vulva: the problem of recurrence. New conc. gynec. oncology by Lewis, Wentz and Jaffe, p. 417. Philadelphia: Davis Comp. 1966.

— Personal communication 1967.

Woodruff, J. D., Hildebrandt, E. E.: Carcinoma in Situ of the vulva. Obstet. and Gynec. **12**, 414 (1958).

— The significance of premalignant lesions of the vulva. New conc. gynec. oncology by Lewis, Wentz and Jaffe, p. 375. Philadelphia: Davis Comp. 1966.

II. Tumoren der Vagina

Von

F. Gauwerky

Mit 9 Abbildungen

1. Klinik

a) Häufigkeit

Die bösartigen Neubildungen der Scheide sind so selten, daß Berichte über 100 oder mehr Fälle aus einer einzigen Klinik nicht gerade häufig sind. Die meisten Veröffentlichungen stellen also in der Regel entweder kasuistische Beobachtungen oder Erfahrungsberichte über eine kleinere Anzahl von Patientinnen dar. Gewöhnlich wird mit einer Häufigkeit zwischen 1—3 % aller bösartigen Genitaltumoren der Frau gerechnet.

EMMERT, St. Louis, stellte unter 1546 bösartigen Tumoren des weiblichen Genitale 37 Vaginalcarcinome zusammen, das sind 1,9 %. Bei anderen Autoren liegen ganz ähnliche Häufigkeiten vor:

PALMER u. BIBACK	112 bei 8312 Genitalcarcinomen	= 1,3 %
NÜRNBERGER	226 bei 9430 Genitalcarcinomen	= 2,4 %
W. R. LANG	77 bei 5399 Genitalcarcinomen	= 1,4 %
MARTIUS	42 bei 1400 Genitalcarcinomen	= 3,0 %
MILLAR	40 bei 1600 Genitalcarcinomen	= 2,5 %
MÖBIUS	194 bei 6076 Genitalcarcinomen	= 3,2 %

Neuerdings hat RUTLEDGE auf Grund des großen Krankenguts des Anderson Hospital, Houston, Texas, und auf Grund seines Literaturstudiums relative Häufigkeiten, wie folgt, konstatiert:

Auf 1 Vaginalcarcinom kommen in der Regel 3 Vulvacarcinome, 12 Korpuscarcinome des Uterus und 60 Collumcarcinome. Unter solchen Umständen ist es nicht überraschend, daß ins einzelne gehende klinische Erfahrungen am Vaginalcarcinom nur von wenigen Autoren gesammelt werden können. Das ist um so bedauerlicher, als die Heilbarkeit des Scheidencarcinoms auch in sonst sehr fachkundigen ärztlichen Kreisen nicht genügend bewußt geworden ist. Daß die Kurabilität der Vaginalcarcinome ebenso wie die anderer bösartiger Tumoren von der Erfahrung der behandelnden Ärzte in hohem Maße abhängig ist, bedarf keiner besonderen Betonung.

Altersverteilung der primären Vaginalcarcinome

1. Jahrzehnt	1 =	0,15%
2. Jahrzehnt	5 =	0,70%
3. Jahrzehnt	43 =	6,45%
4. Jahrzehnt	103 =	16,00%
5. Jahrzehnt	127 =	19,10%
6. Jahrzehnt	175 =	26,40%
7. Jahrzehnt	137 =	20,70%
8. Jahrzehnt	58 =	8,70%
9. Jahrzehnt	12 =	1,80%
Zusammen	661 =	100,00%

b) Lebensalter

Bösartige Scheidentumoren, in erster Linie Plattenepithelcarcinome, kommen in allen Lebensaltern vor und sind sogar gelegentlich im Kleinkindesalter beobachtet worden (beispielsweise HUBER). Übersichten über die Altersverteilung sind u. a. gegeben worden von E. SCHLUND, W. R. LANG u. Mitarb., J. H. KAISER, H. HUBER, PALMER und BIBACK. Die Beobachtungen dieser Autoren unterscheiden sich nicht wesentlich, so daß die von ihnen berichteten Fälle durchaus in der nebenstehenden Tabelle summiert werden konnten.

c) Klinische Symptomatik

Die Patientinnen kommen zum Arzt mit Fluor und Blutungen, gelegentlich Kohabitationsblutungen, ferner Schmerzen, in selteneren Fällen mit Stuhl- und Urinbeschwerden. In den 75 Fällen von Palmer u. Biback kamen 65 mit Blutungen, 20 mit Schmerzen, 9 mit Ausfluß, 4 mit Miktionsbeschwerden, 3 hatten den Tumor selbst unmittelbar bemerkt; 10 Fälle ohne subjektive Symptome sind besonders erwähnenswert, weil sie auf den Wert der vorbeugenden Krebsuntersuchung eindringlich hinweisen.

Bei den 76 Fällen von Lang u. Mitarb. waren die ersten Symptome folgende: 36mal Blutungen, 17mal Blutung und Ausfluß, 12mal Ausfluß, 11 Fälle mit sonstigen Beschwerden.

Die klinische Symptomatik unterscheidet sich somit nicht wesentlich von derjenigen des Collumcarcinoms des Uterus. Bemerkenswert ist hier nur der Umstand, daß die Patientinnen sich unter Umständen noch recht lange Zeit in einem Zustand des subjektiven Wohlbefindens fühlen können und hierdurch unter Umständen der erste Gang zum Arzt verzögert wird. In den Fällen von W. R. Lang waren nur 22% innerhalb eines Monates zum Arzt gegangen und in 53% der Fälle war die Anamnese bis zur Diagnose länger als ein Vierteljahr. Verantwortlich für die Verzögerung vom ersten Symptom bis zum Stellen der Diagnose ist natürlich nicht nur der Patient, sondern auch leider nicht allzu selten der Arzt; in Langs Fällen rechnet er bei ca. 30% der Verzögerungen der notwendigen Behandlung dem ersten Arzt die Verantwortung zu. Daß mehrmonatige Versuche zur Blutstillung mit medikamentöser Therapie ohne gynäkologische Untersuchung eine Katastrophe für die Patientin darstellen, kann nicht oft und eindringlich genug gesagt werden.

d) Abgrenzung und Klassifikation

Nach dem Annual Report on the Results of Treatment in Carcinoma of the Uterus, 13. Band 1963, ist schon wegen der verschiedenen Ausbreitungstypen die größte Sorgfalt auf die Abtrennung des primären Vaginalcarcinoms von den Tumoren des Gebärmutterhalses, der Vulva und Urethra und selbstverständlich auch von den sekundären Tumorabsiedlungen an der Scheidenschleimhaut zu verwenden. Danach sind Tumorfälle dann als Vaginalcarcinom einzuordnen, wenn:

1. der Sitz der Geschwulst in der Vagina liegt,
2. die klinische Untersuchung zeigt, daß der Gebärmutterhals intakt ist,
3. kein Grund für die Annahme besteht, daß das Carcinom ein anderes als eine primäre Geschwulst in der Scheide ist.

In jenen Fällen, in denen das Carcinom den Gebärmutterhals einbezieht, muß der Fall als ein Collumcarcinom betrachtet werden. In diesem Grundsatz liegt die einzige echte Schwierigkeit. Man gibt ja z.B. andererseits zu, daß es ratsam (ja notwendig) sein kann, solche Fälle als Vaginalcarcinom zu klassifizieren, in denen die Peripherie einer mehr oder minder konzentrisch sich ausbreitenden Tumormasse in der Scheidenschleimhaut die Außenseite der Portio erreicht. Die Diskussion über die Grenzfälle geht aber noch weiter:

Als *Carcinoma vaginae et cervicis* ist ein Tumor zu bezeichnen, wenn nicht entschieden werden kann, ob es sich um einen Primärtumor der Vagina oder des Collum handelt, z.B. auch dann, wenn bei Behandlungsbeginn die Portio nicht untersucht werden kann.

Als *Carcinoma vaginae et vulvae* ist ein Tumor zu bezeichnen, wenn es unmöglich ist, zwischen einem primären Vaginalcarcinom und einem Vulvacarcinom zu unterscheiden.

Als ein *Urethralcarcinom* ist ein Tumor zu bezeichnen, wenn der Sitz der Geschwulst in der Harnröhre oder in den Geweben unmittelbar neben der Harnröhrenmündung liegt und wenn kein Grund für die Annahme besteht, daß es sich um eine metastatische Geschwulst handelt.

Über diese allgemeinen Grundsätze hinaus, die für die Einordnung von bösartigen Tumoren der Scheidenschleimhaut und deren unmittelbare Nachbarschaft beachtet werden sollen, hat die Internationale Gesellschaft für Gynäkologie und Geburtshilfe erstmals im 13. Annual Report versuchsweise eine eigene Stadieneinteilung der Scheidentumoren angenommen. In welchem Umfang diese Einteilung von den zusammenarbeitenden Kliniken in der Zukunft verwendet werden kann, ist noch nicht völlig zu übersehen. Die bereits angedeuteten Schwierigkeiten, z.B. auch im Hinblick auf eine etwaige Anwendung des TNM-Systems, zwingen offensichtlich zu einer zurückhaltenden Beurteilung. Eine Reihe von erfahrenen Autoren benutzen daher auch heute noch eigene Klassifikationen.

Die Klassifikation von ST. SIMON von 1930 unterscheidet:

Gruppe I: Infiltrate der Scheidenschleimhaut oder Knoten bis zu einem Durchmesser von 2,5 cm.

Gruppe II: Tumoren größer als 2,5 cm Durchmesser, aber nicht mehr als $^1/_3$ des Scheidenumfanges erfassend. Das paravaginale Gewebe ist nicht mehr frei, aber noch ohne deutliche Infiltration; auch kleine ulceröse Tumoren gehören zu dieser Gruppe.

Gruppe III: Tumoren, die fast zirkulär den Scheidenumfang umfassen, mehr als die halbe Scheidenlänge ergriffen haben. Infiltration des paravaginalen oder parametranen Gewebes, eventuell bis zur Beckenwand; inguinaler Lymphknotenbefall.

Gruppe IV: Befall der ganzen Scheidenlänge oder des ganzen Scheidenumfanges; Übergreifen auf Blase oder Mastdarm; knotige Infiltrationen des Parakolpiums bis zur Beckenwand; ein- oder beidseitig ausgesprochene Drüsenmetastasen, auch bei kleinem Primärtumor.

In französischen und angelsächsischen Schriften ist die Stadieneinteilung von COURTIAL weit verbreitet:

Stadium I: Auf die Vagina beschränkte Tumoren bis zu einem Durchmesser von 3 cm; kein Durchbruch in die Muscularis mucosae.

Stadium II: Einbruch in Nachbargewebe durch die Muscularis hindurch. Tumoren, die größer als 3 cm Durchmesser sind, aber keine Fixation an der Beckenwand.

Stadium III: Fixation an der Beckenwand durch parakolpische oder parametrane Tumorinfiltration, Einbruch in Blase oder Rectum oder Urethra.

Bemerkung. BIVENS berichtet bei seinen 46 Fällen über 100% 5-Jahresheilungen beim Stadium I, 30% beim Stadium II und 0% beim Stadium III nach COURTIAL.

Die Stadieneinteilung nach MILLAR ist derjenigen von COURTIAL ähnlich, grenzt aber vom Stadium III noch die Fälle mit Einbruch in Blase, Mastdarm und außerhalb des kleinen Beckens als Stadium IV ab.

MURPHY hat 1957 und 1959 seine Klassifikation anhand von 135 eigenen Fällen erprobt:

Stadium I: 79 Fälle, Begrenzung des Tumors auf die Vagina und das unmittelbar anschließende paravaginale Gewebe.

Stadium II: 45 Fälle. a) Manifeste paravaginale Ausbreitung; b) Einbruch in Urethra, Blase, Rectum oder Vulva; c) Beteiligung regionärer Lymphknoten außerhalb des kleinen Beckens.

Stadium III: 11 Fälle. Auswärtig vorbehandelte Patientinnen.

Die Stadieneinteilung der Münchener Universitäts-Frauenklinik, vor allem von RIES und BREITNER vertreten, zeichnet sich durch besondere Klarheit und durch die konsequent eingehaltene Analogie zur international anerkannten Stadieneinteilung des Collumcarcinoms aus. Sie ist nach eindeutig definierten anatomischen Kriterien geordnet, und zwar so, daß prognostisch zusammengehörige Gruppen in das gleiche Stadium fallen.

Stadium I: Das Carcinom ist auf die Vagina beschränkt.

Stadium II: Das Carcinom geht über die Scheide hinaus (Septum recto- bzw. vesico-vaginale, parakolpisches Gewebe, Teile des Parametriums, Portio), dringt aber nicht bis zur Beckenwand vor.

Stadium III: Das Carcinom erreicht die Beckenwand, überschreitet aber den Scheideneingang nicht.

Stadium IV: Das Carcinom infiltriert die Blase oder das Rectum oder greift über die Grenze des kleinen Beckens und des Scheideneingangs hinaus. Fernmetastasen.

Ein Stadium 0 wird, obwohl es zweifellos Einzelfälle von präinvasiven Carcinomen der Vagina gibt, nicht geführt. Ries legt besonderen Wert darauf, Klassifikations-irrtümer zu vermeiden und sich in der Bezeichnung als Vaginalcarcinom streng an die vom Annual Report on the Results of Treatment in Carcinoma of the Uterus (s. oben) festgelegten Regeln zu halten.

Die nunmehr empfohlene internationale Klassifikation unterscheidet folgendes:

Stadium 0: Präinvasives Vaginalcarcinom, intraepitheliales Carcinom, Carcinoma in situ.

Invasives Vaginalcarcinom:

Stadium I: Das Carcinom ist auf die Scheidenwand begrenzt.

Stadium II: Das Carcinom hat das subvaginale Gewebe ergriffen, ist aber nicht bis zur Beckenwand ausgebreitet.

Stadium III: Das Carcinom hat die Beckenwand erreicht.

Stadium IV: Das Carcinom hat sich über das kleine Becken hinaus ausgebreitet oder die Schleimhaut von Blase oder Mastdarm ergriffen. Ein bullöses Ödem gestattet nicht die Einordnung eines Falles zum Stadium IV.

Der 13. Annual Report enthält Beiträge von 58 Kliniken mit 1199 Vaginalcarcinomen für die Jahre 1953—1957 noch ohne Stadieneinteilung. 387 Patienten dieses Berichtes waren nach 5 Jahren am Leben, einer Überlebensziffer von 33,5% entsprechend. In welchem Umfang die beschriebene Stadieneinteilung sich endgültig bewähren kann, muß zunächst, wie gesagt, noch offenbleiben. Wenngleich eine Stadieneinteilung sich defini-torisch ausschließlich an den Kriterien der anatomischen Ausbreitung orientieren muß, so ist doch zu fragen, ob die Beschreibungen nicht gerade für das Vaginalcarcinom prognostisch außerordentlich unterschiedliche Fälle in einem Stadium zusammenfassen. Das gilt insbesondere für die Stadien I und II, in welchen sehr kleine, bis sehr ausgedehnte Ausbreitungen über die Scheidenschleimhaut jeweils enthalten sind. Die Erfahrungen am eigenen Krankengut legen die Vermutung nahe, daß der spezielle anatomische Sitz innerhalb des befallenen Organs für die Prognose von ausschlaggebender Bedeutung sein kann. Es ist daher einer detaillierten Beschreibung des eigenen Krankenguts mit einer listenmäßigen Kasuistik von 82 Fällen der Vorzug gegeben worden. Ein solches Verfahren erschien vor allem auch darum zweckmäßig, weil eine nachträgliche Klassifikation bekanntermaßen grundsätzliche Nachteile aufweist.

e) Makroskopischer Tumorbefund

Das primäre Scheidencarcinom kann, wie auch Tumoren anderen Sitzes, die histo-logisch überwiegend Plattenepithelcarcinome sind, in drei verschiedenen makroskopischen Formen auftreten, nämlich

1. als *exophytisch-papillärer Tumor*, unter Umständen mit sekundär zentraler Er-weichung und Vertiefung, so daß es zur zentralen Nekrose bei fortwucherndem exo-phytischem Randwall kommt.

Diese exophytischen Scheidencarcinome sind oft stark zerklüftet, blumenkohlartig in das Scheidenlumen vorspringend, pilzartig auf der Oberfläche sitzend. Meist treten sie in der Einzahl auf; primäre Mehrfachgeschwülste der Scheide kommen gelegentlich vor;

2. als *flächenhafte Infiltration* der Scheidenschleimhaut, meist wenig infiltrierend, geröteter samtartiger, häufig auch landkartenartig angeordneter Schleimhautüberzug. Diese Form ist nicht häufig und geht gewöhnlich von einer leukoplakischen Präcancerose aus. Der als samtartiger Belag der Schleimhaut sich ausbildende Tumor ist häufig der Ausläufer eines Tumorzentrums mit tieferer Tumorinfiltration. Bei dieser Tumorform muß also besonders sorgfältig nach einem Primärtumor außerhalb des typischen Sitzes der Scheidencarcinome gesucht werden, insbesondere auch nach kleinen Carcinomen der Portio, der Vulva und Urethra, die, falls vorhanden, in diesen Fällen als Primärtumor zu gelten haben.

Zunächst ist die Scheidenschleimhaut bei dieser Tumorform normalerweise elastisch und wird erst bei fortgeschritteneren Fällen steif infiltriert;

3. als unregelmäßig *kraterförmiges Geschwür*, wobei der Schleimhautsubstanzdefekt gelegentlich kleiner als der eigentliche Geschwürsgrund ist, so daß die Ränder überlappen. Bei dieser Tumorform ist die Wachstumsrichtung in die Peripherie von vornherein anzunehmen, d.h. also in das Septum recto- und vesicovaginale, das Parakolpium und Parametrium, den Blasenboden und in den Urethralwulst.

Die beschriebenen makroskopischen Formen gehen häufig ineinander über, so daß dieses Einteilungsprinzip sowohl zur klinischen Beschreibung notwendig, zur prognostischen Beurteilung wie zur therapeutischen Entscheidung nützlich ist, andererseits aber zur Klassifikation im engeren Sinne schlecht dienen kann. Einer der wenigen Autoren, die unter dem Gesichtspunkt der makroskopischen Tumorform eingeteilt haben, sind BUSSE und SOERGEL, die unter ihren 29 Fällen 18mal ulcerierte Kraterbildungen, 8mal exophytisches Tumorwachstum und 3mal knotige Tumorbildungen beschrieben haben.

Auffallend häufig ist die Scheidenhinterwand, und zwar das obere Drittel der *Tumorsitz*. Auf diesen Umstand hat bereits O. KÜSTNER 1876 hingewiesen. Auch neuere Mitteilungen bestätigen ihn.

EMMERT fand z.B. 14mal das hintere Scheidengewölbe, 5mal die Scheidenvorderwand, 13mal eine der Seitenwände befallen und 6mal eine ringförmige Tumorausbreitung.

ROHDE (zitiert nach EMMERT) beobachtete 71mal Hinterwandbefall, 23mal Vorderwand-, 13mal Seitenwandtumoren und 16mal ringförmige Ausbreitung. Ähnliche Beobachtungen machte BIVENS.

NÜRNBERGER hat 1930 die Zusammenstellungen von HECHT und SCHLUND zusammengefaßt, welche von insgesamt 261 primären Scheidencarcinomen an der Hinterwand 146, an der Vorderwand 48, an der rechten Wand 10, an der linken Wand 9, an der vorderen und hinteren Wand 1, an beiden Seitenwänden 1, im Scheidengewölbe 6, an der rechten und hinteren Wand 2, an der rechten und vorderen Wand 1, an der linken und hinteren Wand 3 und ringförmig 34 Fälle beobachtet haben.

Eine ebenso ins einzelne gehende Lokalisationsgliederung der Vaginalcarcinome haben in jüngerer Zeit PALMER und BIBACK gegeben. Die Beobachtungen sind immer wieder die gleichen, so daß auf die Wiedergabe hier verzichtet werden kann.

Die Lokalisation, die Ausdehnung und Ausbreitung von 82 Vaginalcarcinomen, die im Allgemeinen Krankenhaus St. Georg, Hamburg, von 1935—1959 beobachtet worden sind, geht aus der kasuistischen Tabelle 1 hervor.

Die Lokalisationsverteilung der Tabelle 1 ist offensichtlich typisch. Abweichende Verhältnisse hat eigentlich nur RUTLEDGE beschrieben, der in seinem Krankengut von 70 Fällen ein bevorzugtes Befallensein der Vorderwand (22) gegenüber Hinterwand (15), Seitenwand rechts (12), links (8) gefunden hat.

Tabelle 1. *Kasuistische Übersicht über Ausbreitung, Behandlungsmethodik und Behandlungsergebnis von 82 Vaginalcarcinomen im A.K. St. Georg 1935—1959*

Nr.	Jahr	Lokalbefund	Alter Jahre	Vorgeschichte	Radium vaginal und uterin	Röntgen	Kompli-kationen	Metastasen	Überlebenszeit
1	1935		59	5 Monate	Ø	Ø	—	—	1 Jahr
2	1935		40	2 Monate	vaginal und uterin	Ø	—	—	7 Jahre
3	1935		70	3 Jahre	Ø	+ 2 Serien	—	—	2 Jahre
4	1936		47	5 Monate	Ø	+ 1 Serie	—	Leber	4 Monate

5	1936	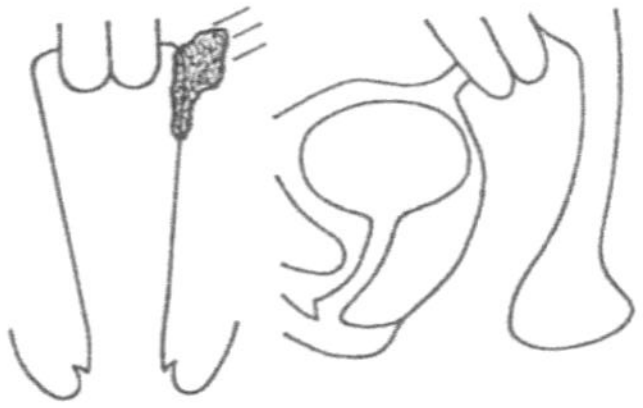	60	2 Wochen	+ vaginal	+ 1 Serie	—	—	nach 7 Jahren symptomfrei
6	1936	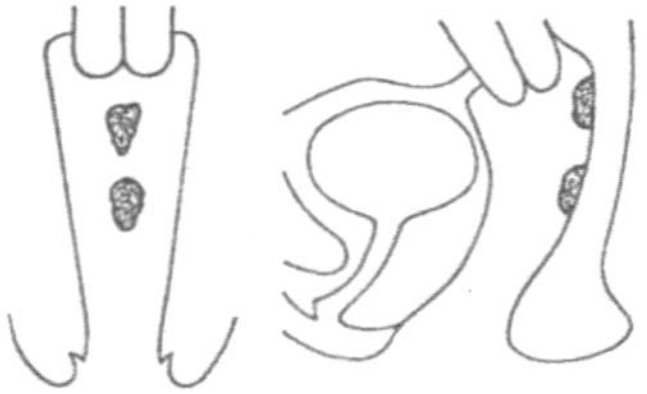	29	4 Monate	+ vaginal	1 Serie	—	—	nach 17 Jahren symptomfrei
7	1936	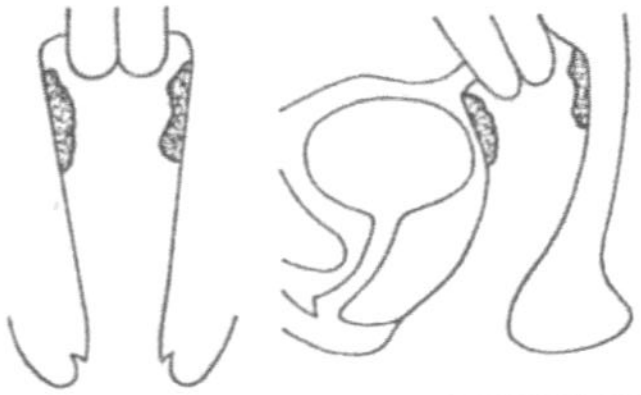	59	unbekannt	vaginal und uterin	1 Serie	—	—	nach 15 Jahren symptomfrei
8	1936	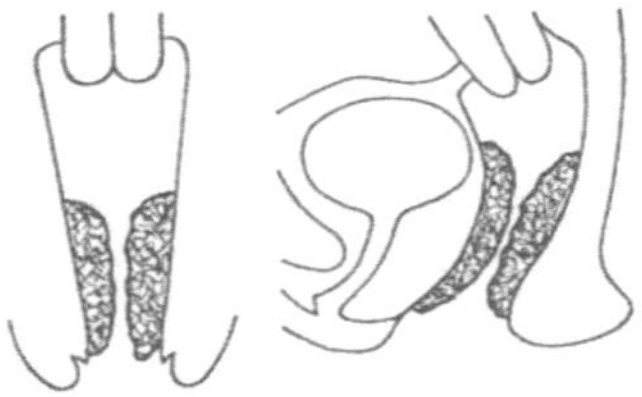	69	1 Jahr	Ø	1 Serie	—	—	im 1. Jahr †
9	1936	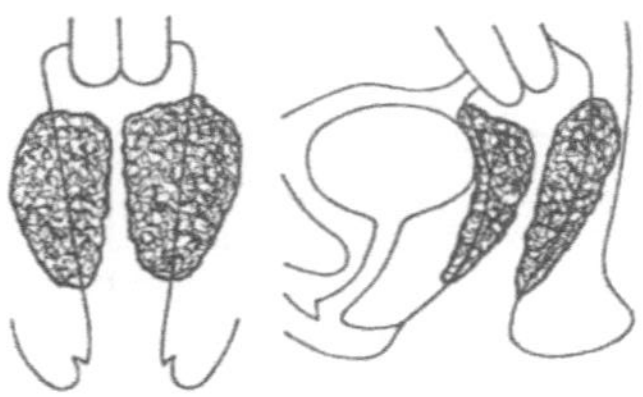	54	2 Wochen	vaginal und uterin	1 Serie	Vesico-vaginal-fistel	—	nach 2 Jahren †

Tabelle 1 (Fortsetzung)

Nr.	Jahr	Lokalbefund	Alter Jahre	Vorgeschichte	Radium vaginal und uterin	Röntgen	Kompli-kationen	Metastasen	Überlebenszeit	
10	1937	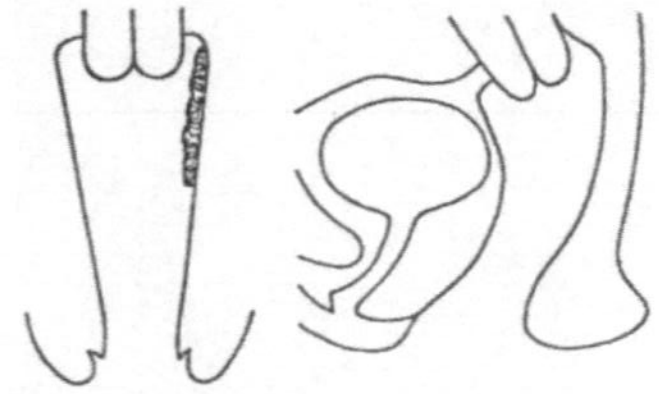	69	3 Wochen Pessar 10 Jahre getragen	vaginal und uterin	1 Serie	—	—	nach 1 Jahr †	Einbruch in Blase, Rectum, Para-metrien
11	1937	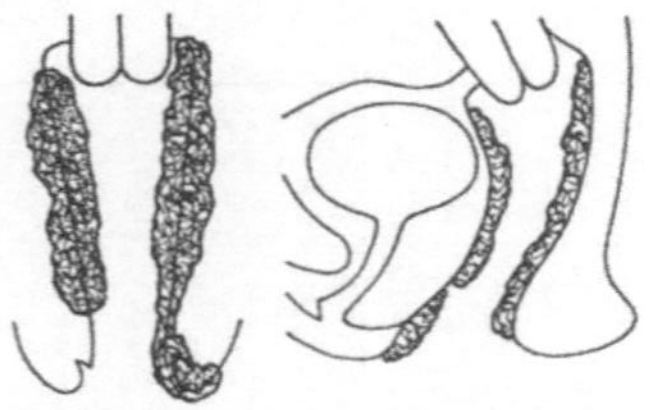	43	3 Monate	—	—	Recto-vaginal fistel	—	im 1. Jahr †	
12	1937	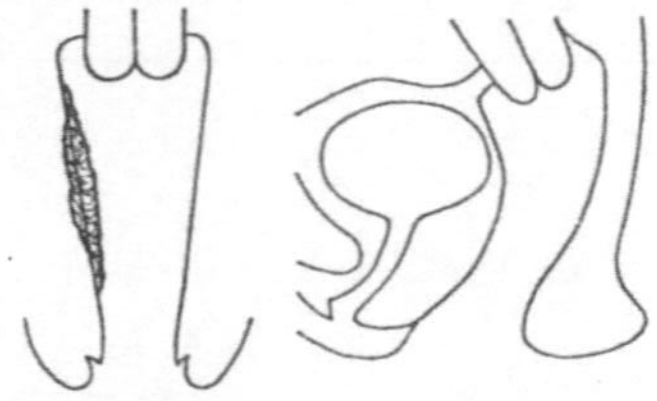	71	6 Monate	vaginal und uterin	1 Serie	—	rechte Leistenbeuge	im 1. Jahr †	
13	1937	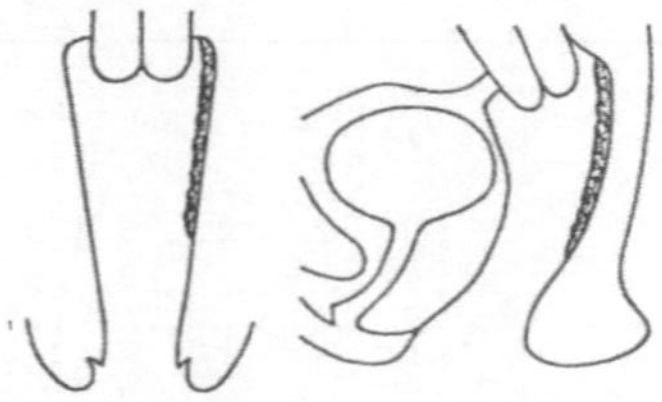	50	3 Wochen	vaginal und uterin	—	—	Lenden-wirbelsäule und Hüftgelenk	im 6. Jahr †	

14	1938	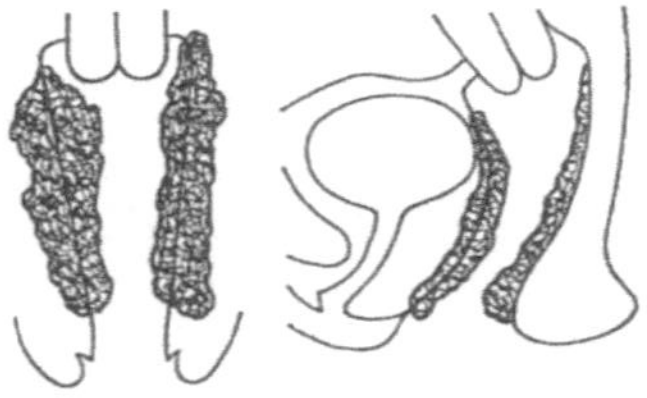 72	mehrere Jahre	vaginal	1 Serie	—	—	im 3. Jahr †
15	1940	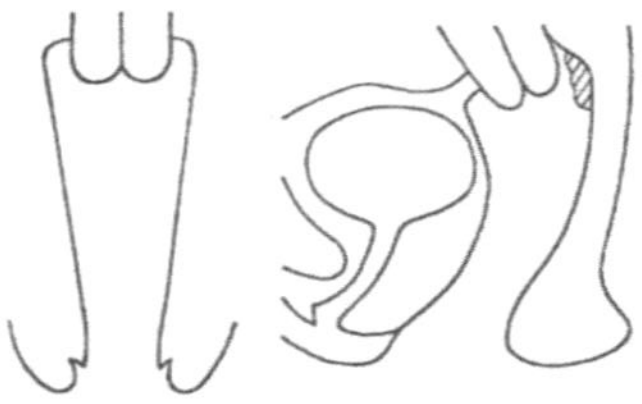 53	2 Monate 1½ Jahre Pessar getragen!	vaginal	1 Serie	—	—	nach 9 Jahren symptomfrei
16	1940	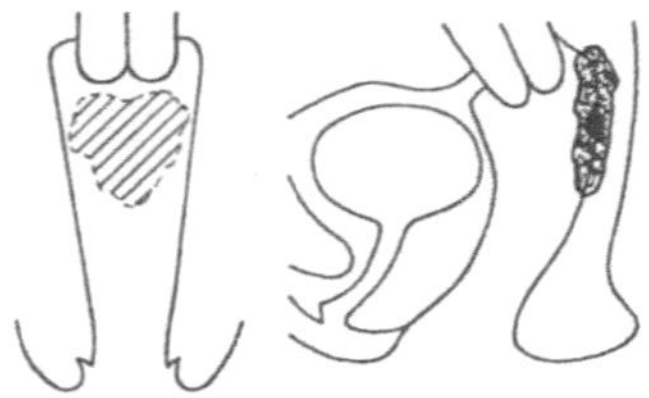 55	8 Wochen	vaginal und uterin	1 Serie	—	—	nach 6 Jahren symptomfrei
17	1940	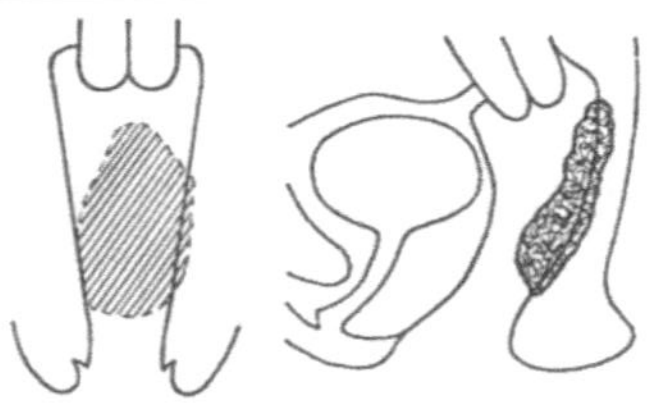 44	2 Monate	—	unvollständig	—	—	im 1. Jahr † desolater Ausgangszustand
18	1940	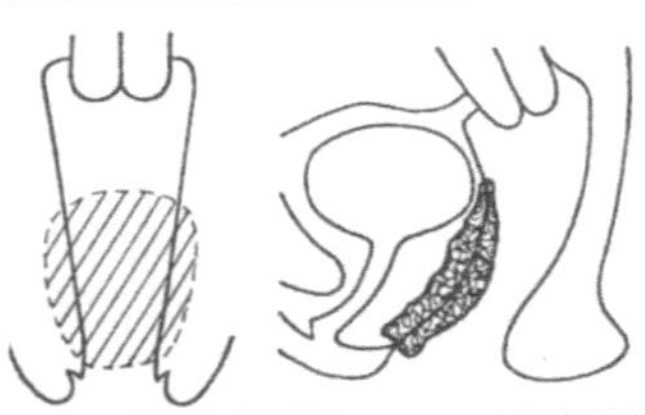 61	6 Monate vor 20 Jahren Röntgen Menolyse	vaginal	1 Serie	—	—	im 1. Jahr †

Tabelle 1 (Fortsetzung)

Nr.	Jahr	Lokalbefund	Alter Jahre	Vorgeschichte	Radium vaginal und uterin	Röntgen	Kompli- kationen	Metastasen	Überlebenszeit
19	1940	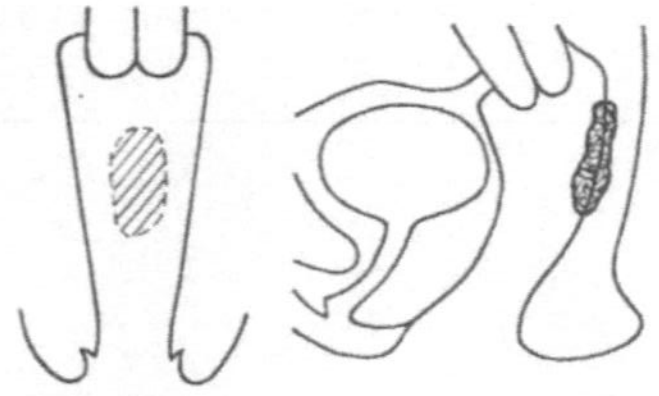	65	1 Jahr	vaginal	1 Serie	—	—	nach 4 Jahren noch symptomfrei
20	1940	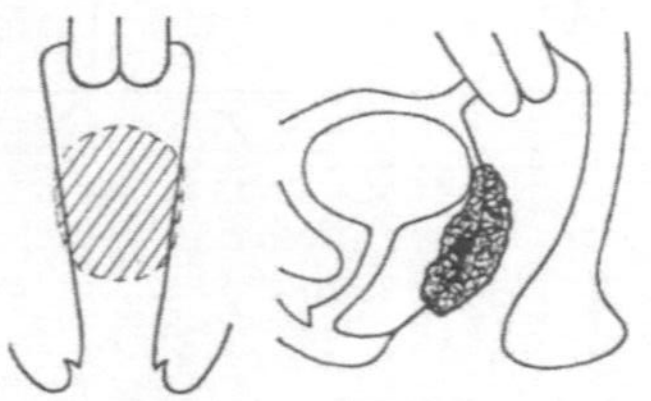	39	1 Jahr	—	1 Serie percutan 1 Serie vaginal	—	—	nach 15 Jahren symptomfrei
21	1941	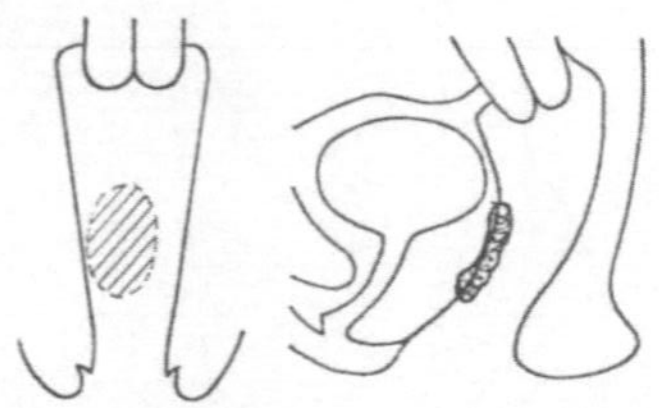	60	?	vaginal (Spickung)	—	—	—	nach 12 Jahren symptomfrei
22	1941	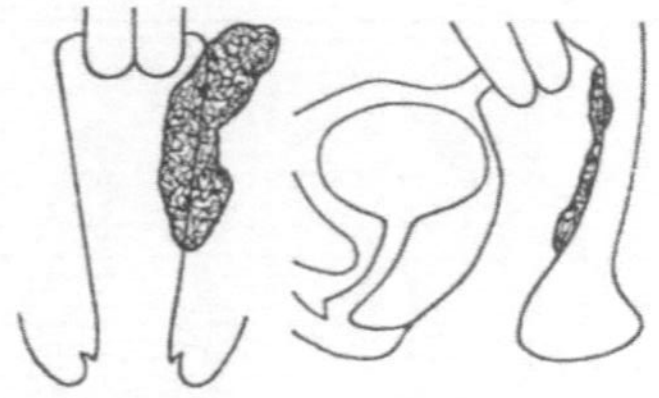	50	6 Monate	—	2 Serien	Recto- vaginal- fistel	—	nach 1 Jahr †

23	1941	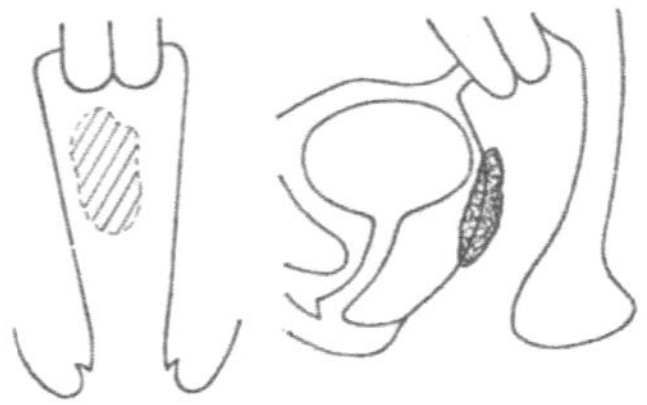	62	1 Woche	vaginale Spickung	1 Serie	Vesico-vaginal-fistel	—	nach 1 Jahr †
24	1941	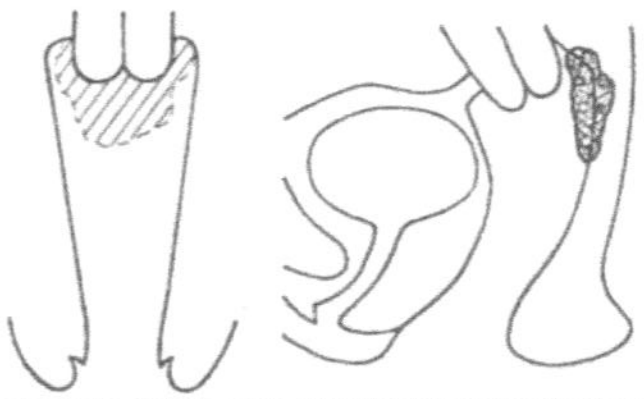	36	5 min	vaginal	1 Serie	—	—	nach 10 Jahren symptomfrei
25	1942	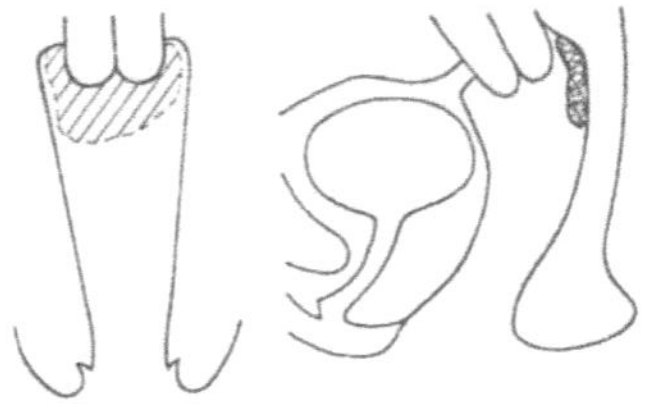	40	2 Jahre	—	—	—	—	1 Std postop. †
26	1942	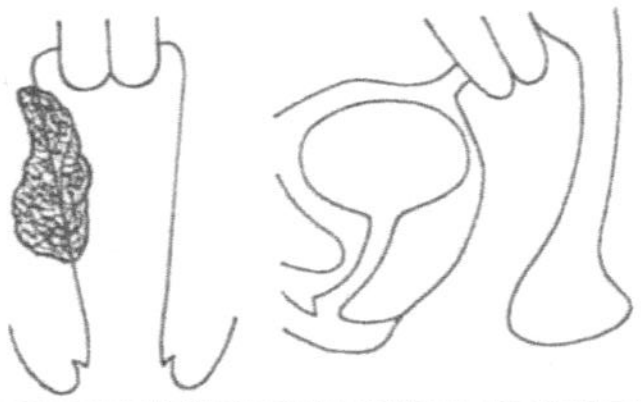	67	2 Jahre	vaginal	1 Serie	—	—	nach 1 Jahr verschollen
27	1942	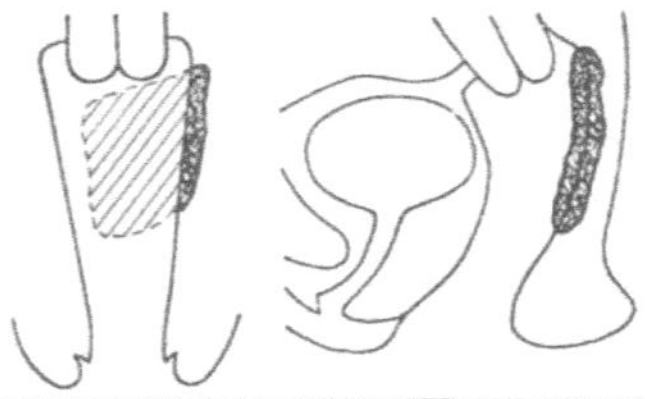	64	2 Wochen	vaginal	1 Serie	—	—	im 2. Jahr †

Tabelle 1 (Fortsetzung)

Nr.	Jahr	Lokalbefund	Alter Jahre	Vorgeschichte	Radium vaginal und uterin	Röntgen	Kompli- kationen	Metastasen	Überlebenszeit
28	1943		64	Röntgen- Menolyse vor 22 Jahren Uterus- exstirpation vor 5 Jahren	vaginal	2 Serien	—	—	nach 2 Jahren †
29	1940		37	3 Wochen	vaginal und uterin	1 Serie	nach 17 Jahren Myo-Sa der Bauchhaut op.	—	nach 20 Jahren symptomfrei
30	1944		39	6 Monate	vaginal und uterin	1 Serie	—	—	im 1. Jahr †
31	1945		77	3 Monate	vaginale Spickung	1 Serie	—	—	verschollen

32	1946	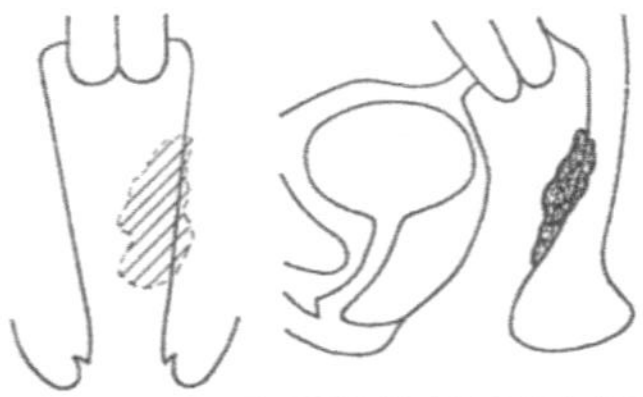 86	3 Monate	vaginal	1 Serie	—	—	nach 2 Jahren interkkurrent †
33	1946	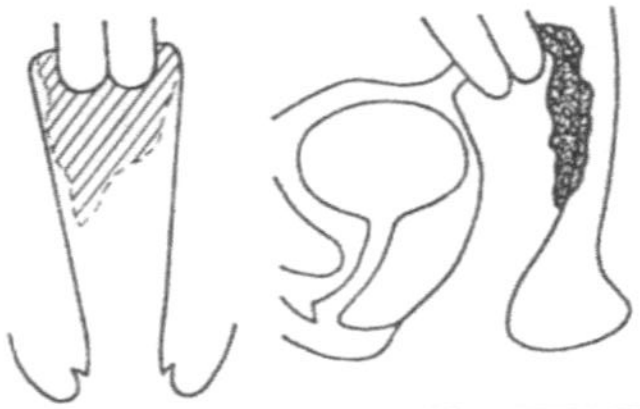 43	6 Monate	vaginal	1 Serie percutan 1 Serie vaginal	Recto-vaginal-fistel	—	nach 1 Jahr †
34	1946	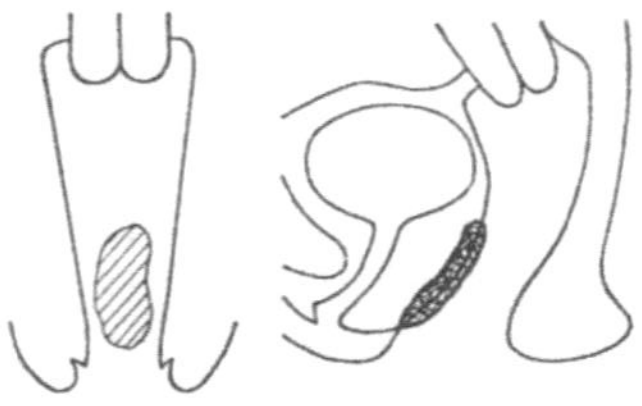 68	2 Monate	vaginale Spickung	1 Serie	—	Leistenbeugen, op. entfernt	nach 1 Jahr verschollen
35	1947	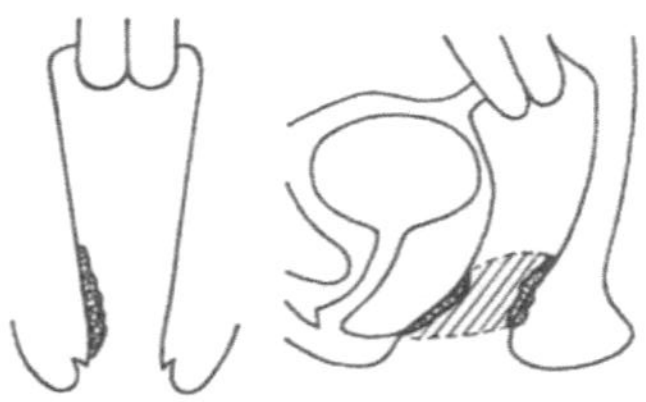 47	4 Monate	vaginal	1 Serie	—	—	im 1. Jahr †
36	1948	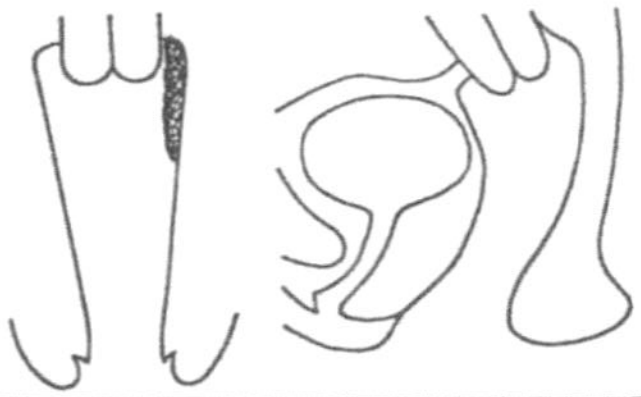 59	?	vaginal und uterin	—	—	—	nach 6 Jahren symptomfrei

Tabelle 1 (Fortsetzung)

Nr.	Jahr	Lokalbefund	Alter Jahre	Vorgeschichte	Radium vaginal und uterin	Röntgen	Kompli- kationen	Metastasen	Überlebenszeit	
37	1948	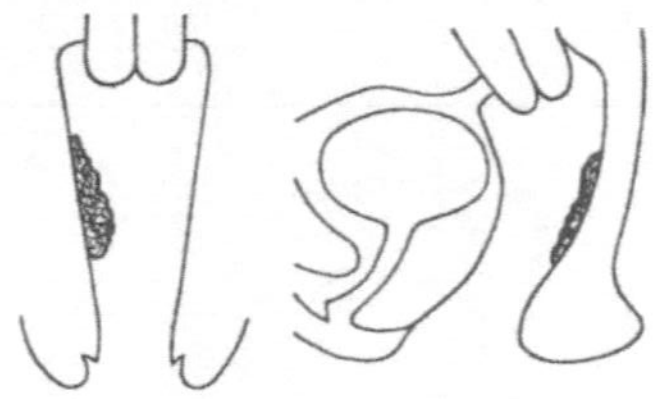	57	2 Monate	—	1 Serie percutan 1 Serie vaginal	Rectovaginal- fistel	—	nach 11 Jahren symptomfrei	Fistel spontan geheilt!
38	1948	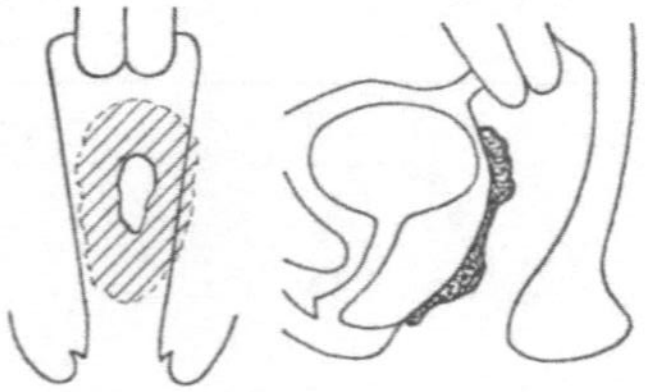	49	5 Monate	vaginal	1 Serie	—	—	im 1. Jahr †	
39	1948	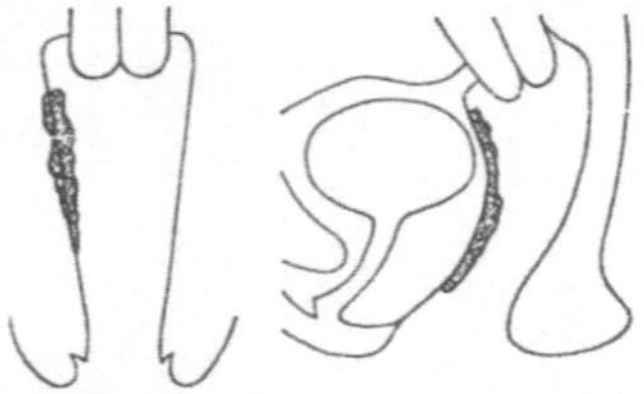	56	2 Monate	vaginal und Spickung	2 Serien	—	—	nach 1 Jahr †	
40	1947	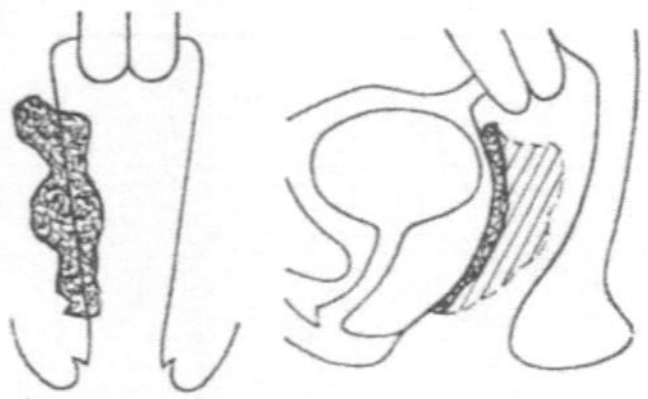	50	2 Jahre	vaginal	1 Serie	—	—	im 1. Jahr †	

41	1948		57	3 Monate	vaginal Spickung	1 Serie	—	—	im 1. Jahr †
42	1948		53	1 Jahr	vaginal	1 Serie	—	—	nach 11 Jahren symptomfrei †
43	1949		59	?	vaginal Spickung	1 Serie	—	—	nach 1 Jahr ausgewandert
44	1949		51	4 Wochen	—	1 Serie percutan 1 Serie intravaginal	—	—	nach 7 Jahren symptomfrei
45	1949		70	4 Wochen	vaginal	1 Serie	—	—	

Tabelle 1 (Fortsetzung)

Nr.	Jahr	Lokalbefund	Alter Jahre	Vorgeschichte	Radium vaginal und uterin	Röntgen	Kompli- kationen	Metastasen	Überlebenszeit
46	1950	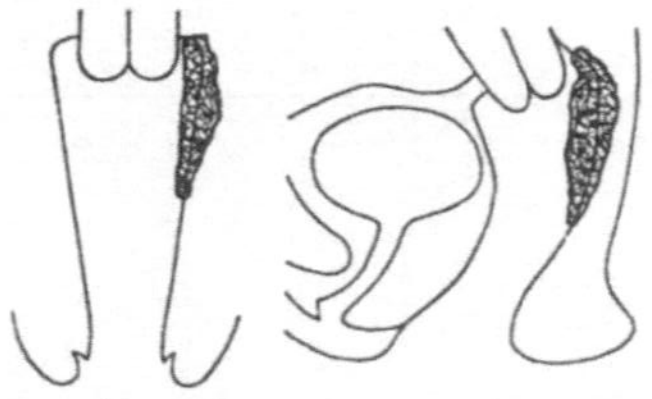	63	4 Monate	vaginal	1 Serie	—	—	im 1. Jahr †
47	1950	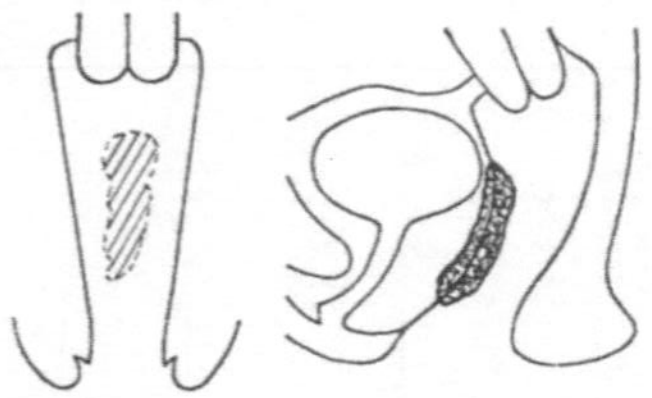	66	6 Monate	vaginal und Spickung	1 Serie	—	—	nach 3 Monaten †
48	1951	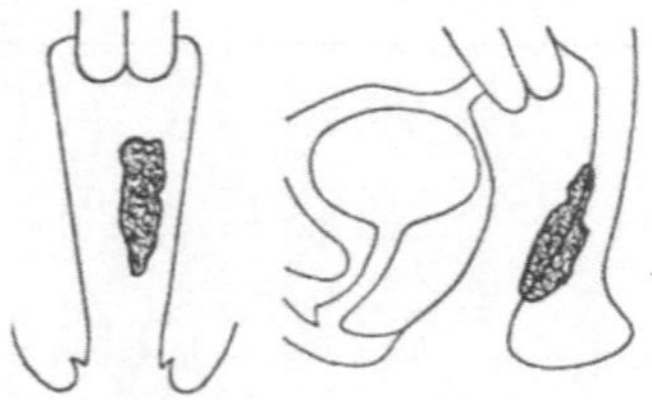	74	3 Monate	vaginal und Spickung	1 Serie	Thrombose	—	nach 1 Jahr †
49	1951	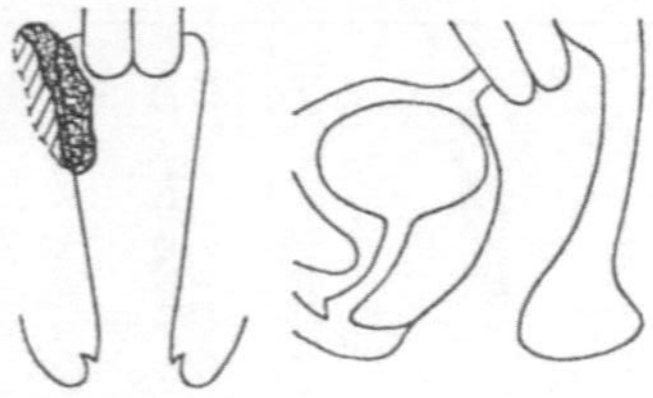	65	1 Woche	vaginal und uterin	1 Serie	—	—	nach 8 Jahren symptomfrei

50	1951	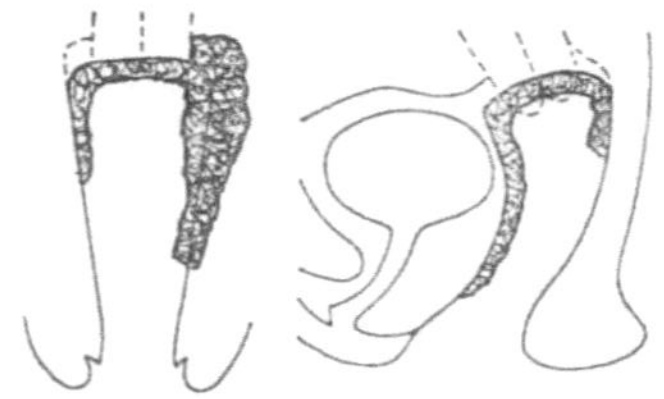	56	4 Wochen Total- exstirpation vor 12 Jahren	vaginal	2 Serien	—	—	im 1. Jahr †
51	1952	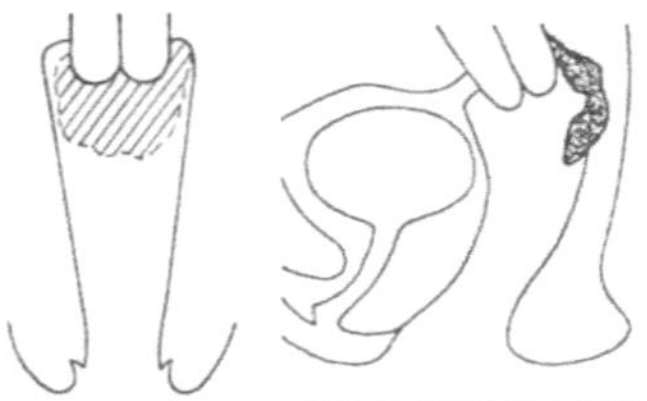	40	2 Monate	vaginal und uterin	1 Serie	—	—	nach 6 Jahren symptomfrei
52	1953	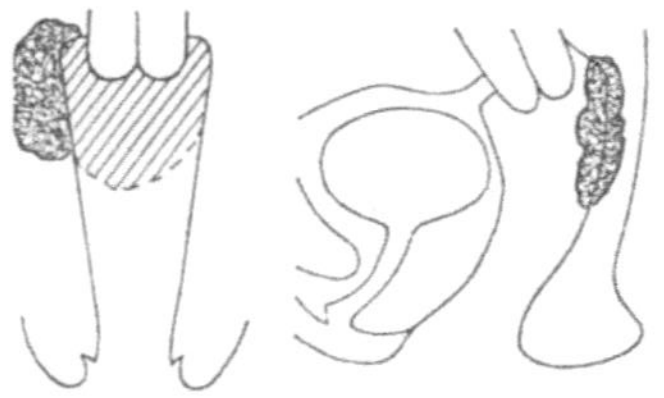	46	6 Monate	vaginal und uterin	1 Serie	Recto- vaginal- fistel	—	im 3. Jahr †
53	1953	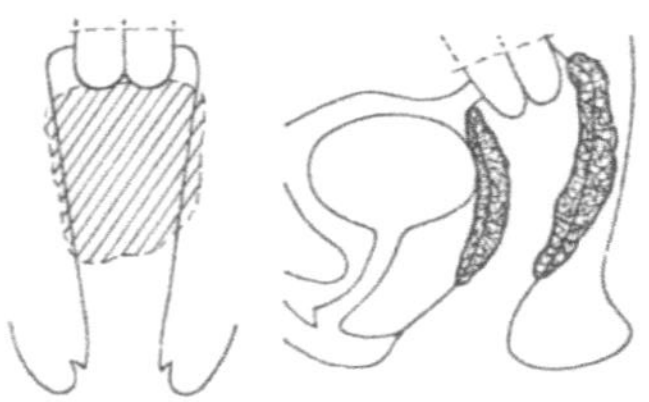	42	3 Monate	vaginal	1 Serie	Recto- vaginal- fistel	—	im 2. Jahr †
54	1953	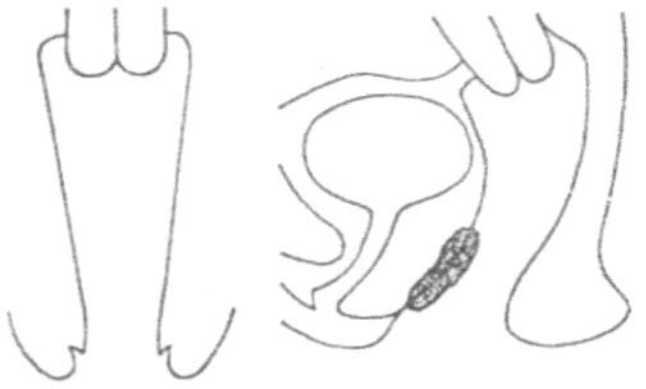	64	1 Monat	vaginal und uterin	2 Serien	—	Leisten- beugen	im 6. Jahr †

Tabelle 1 (Fortsetzung)

Nr.	Jahr	Lokalbefund	Alter Jahre	Vorgeschichte	Radium vaginal und uterin	Röntgen	Kompli-kationen	Metastasen	Überlebenszeit
55	1954		35	1 Jahr	vaginal und uterin	1 Serie	—	—	im 1. Jahr †
56	1954		55	2 Wochen	keine Therapie		—	Inguinal, iliacal, axillär, mediastinal	im 1. Jahr †
57	1954		75	1 Jahr	vaginal und uterin	1 Serie	—	—	nach 5 Jahren symptomfrei!
58	1954		57	4 Monate	vaginal und uterin	1 Serie	—	—	im 1. Jahr †

59	1954	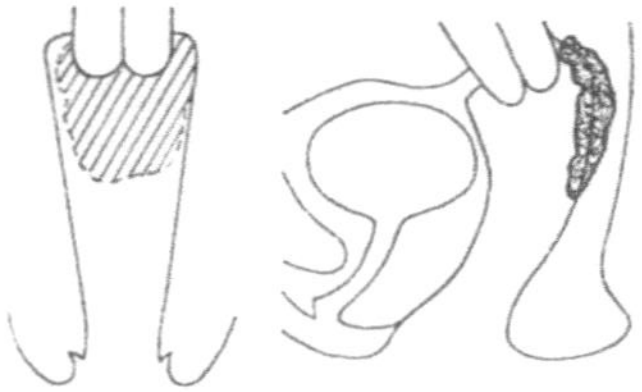	58	3 Wochen	vaginal und uterin	1 Serie	—	—	im 3. Jahr †
60	1954	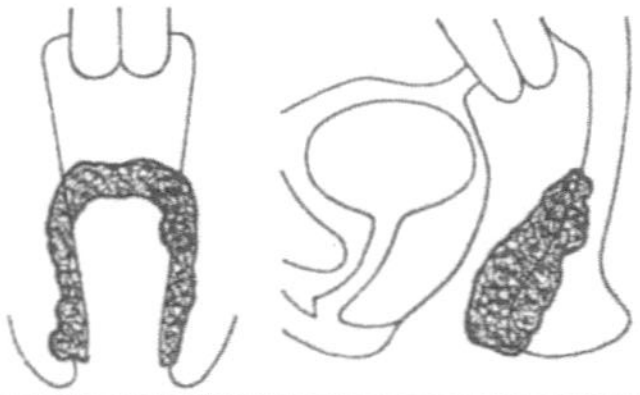	46	3 Monate	vaginal und Spickung und ^{198}Au	1 Serie	—	—	im 2. Jahren †
61	1955	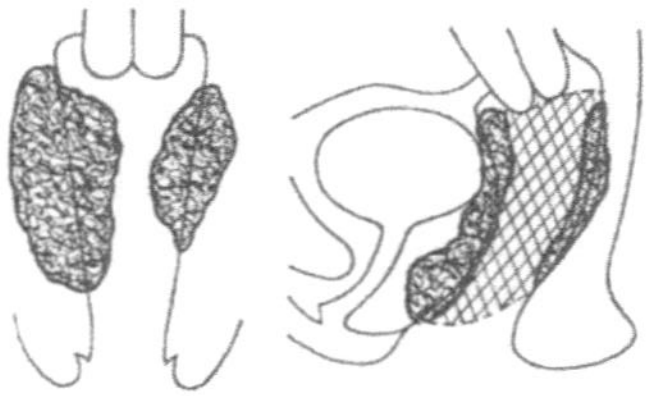	47	2 Jahre	vaginal	1 Serie	—	—	im 1. Jahr †
62	1955	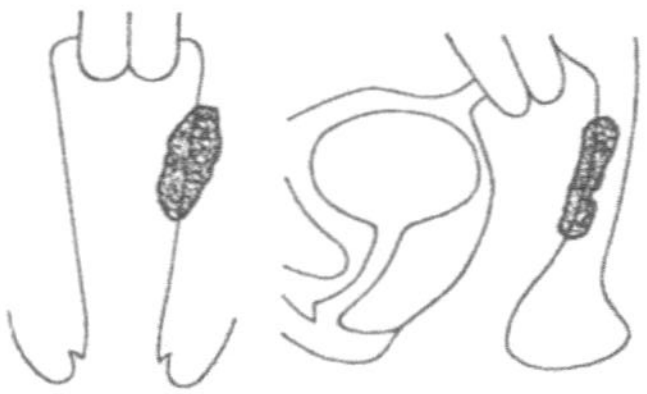	51	1 Jahr	vaginal und uterin	—	—	—	nach 7 Jahren symptomfrei
63	1955	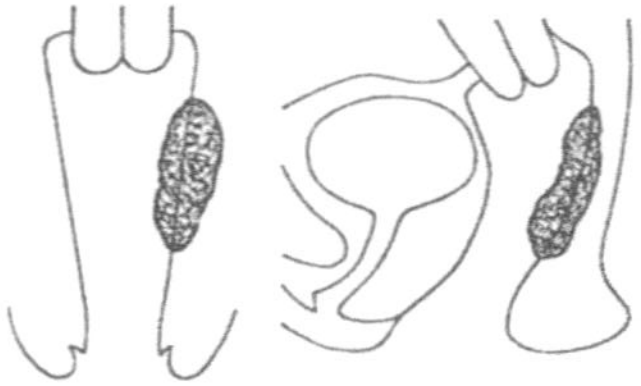	35	5 Monate	vaginale Spickung, ^{137}Cs Spickung uterin	2 Serien	—	—	im 4. Jahr †

Tabelle 1 (Fortsetzung)

Nr.	Jahr	Lokalbefund	Alter Jahre	Vorgeschichte	Radium vaginal und uterin	Röntgen	Kompli-kationen	Metastasen	Überlebenszeit
64	1955	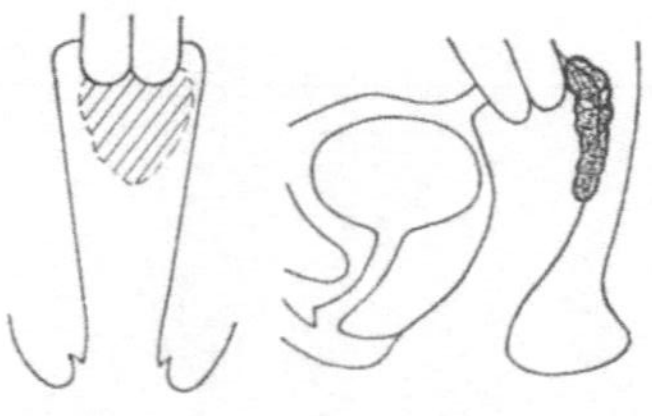	32	2 Wochen	vaginal und uterin	1 Serie	—	—	nach 7 Jahren symptomfrei
65	1956	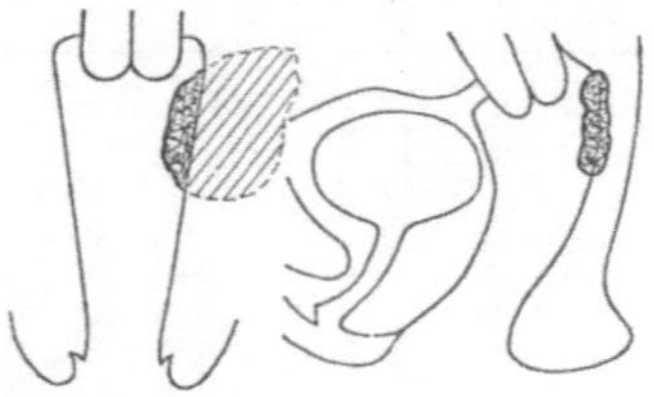	74	6 Wochen	vaginal Cs und uterin	1 Serie	—	—	nach 6 Jahren symptomfrei
66	1957	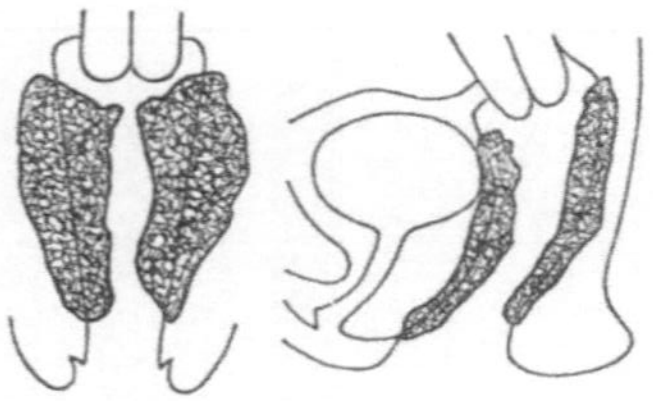	55	?	vaginal und uterin	1 Serie	—	—	im 1. Jahr †
67	1957	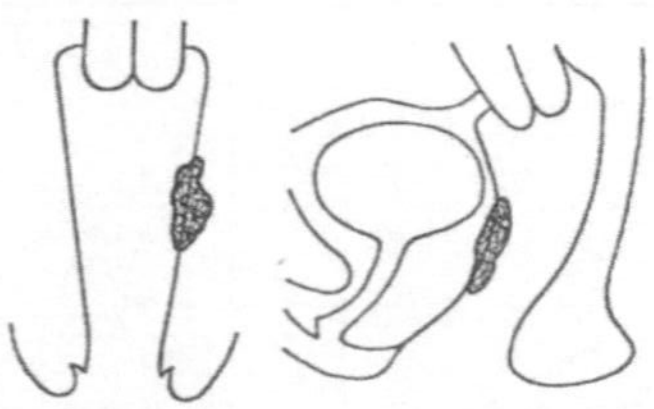	70	3 Monate	vaginal Cs und uterin Spickung	—	—	Lungen metastasen	im 3. Jahr †

68	1957	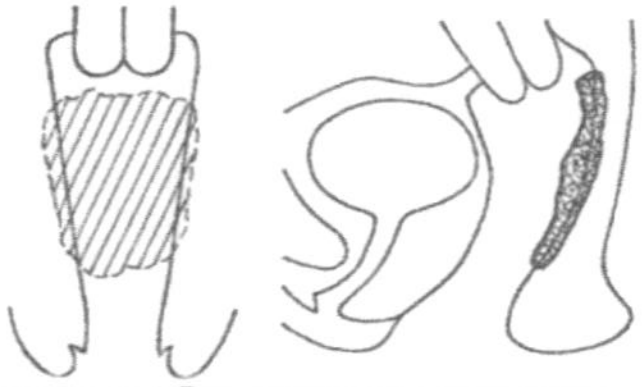	37	3 Wochen	vaginal Cs und uterin	1 Serie	—	—	nach 5 Jahren symptomfrei
69	1957	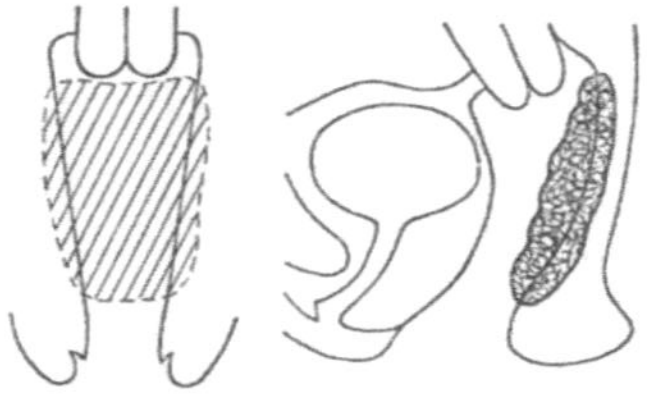	51	2 Monate	vaginal Cs und uterin	1 Serie	Recto-vaginal-fistel Rektumstenose Anuspraeter	—	nach 6 Jahren symptomfrei
70	1957	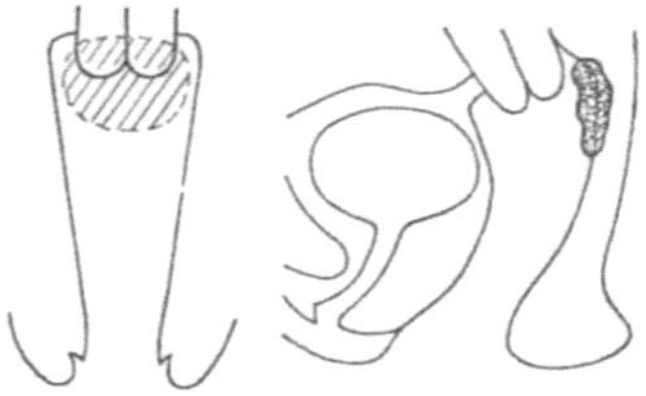	30	4 Wochen	vaginal Cs und Ra und uterin	1 Serie	—	—	im 2. Jahr †
71	1957	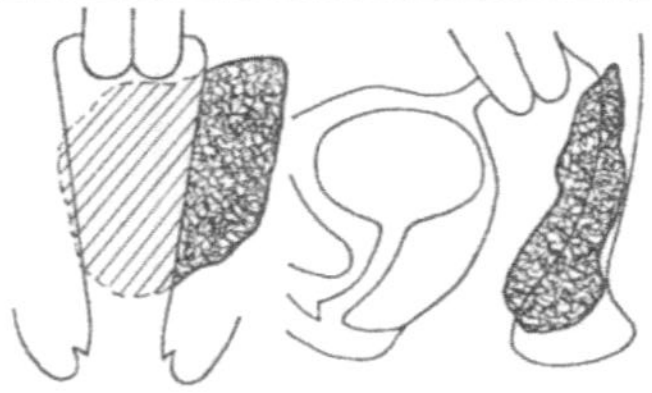	51	2 Wochen	vaginal Cs und uterin	1 Serie	—	—	im 1. Jahr †
72	1958	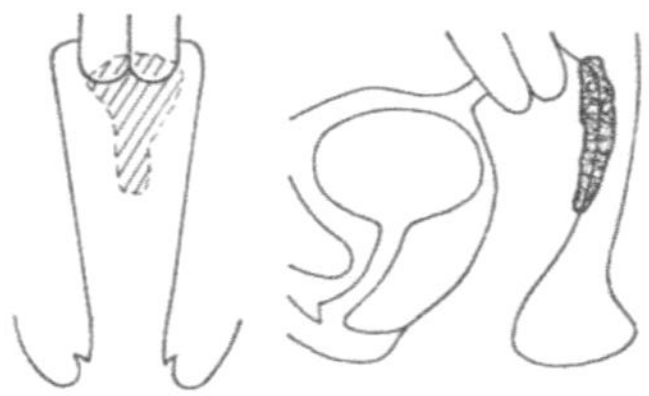	60	3 Wochen	op. vaginal Ra	1 Serie	—	—	nach 6 Jahren symptomfrei

Tabelle 1 (Fortsetzung)

Nr.	Jahr	Lokalbefund	Alter Jahre	Vorgeschichte	Radium vaginal und uterin	Röntgen	Kompli- kationen	Metastasen	Überlebenszeit
73	1958	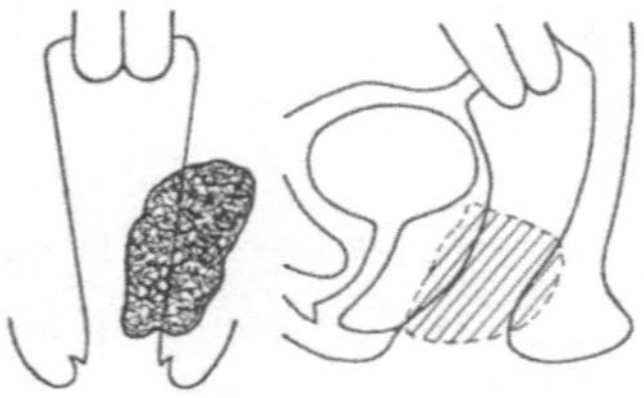	73	?	vaginal Cs Spickung	1 Serie	—	—	nach 5 Jahren symptomfrei
74	1958	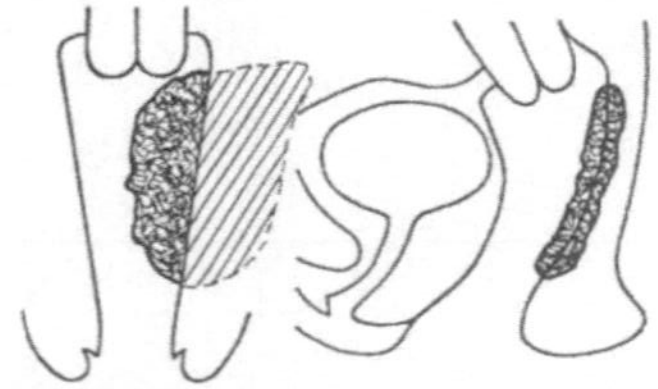	60	?	—	palliativ 1 Serie	—	—	im 1. Jahr †
75	1958	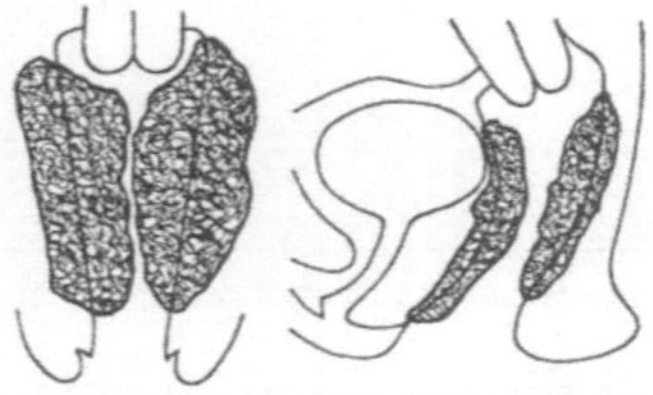	60	1 Monat	vaginal Cs	1 Serie	—	—	im 2. Jahr †
76	1958	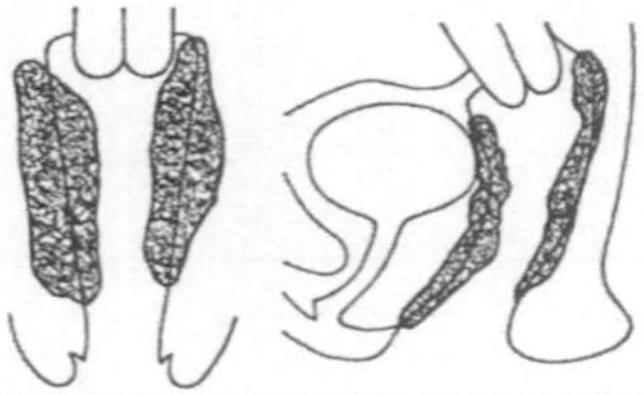	69	6 Wochen	vaginal Cs	1 Serie	—	Leisten- beugen- metastasen	im 1. Jahr †
77	1959	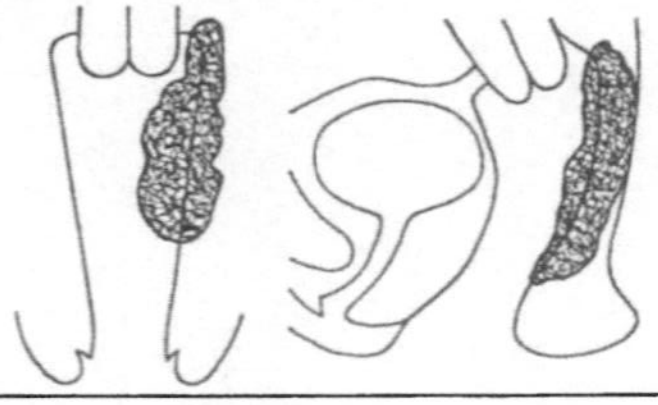	52	3 Wochen	vaginal Cs	1 Serie	Anuspraeter wegen riesiger intrapelviner Tumor- ausbreitung	—	im 2. Jahr †

78	1959	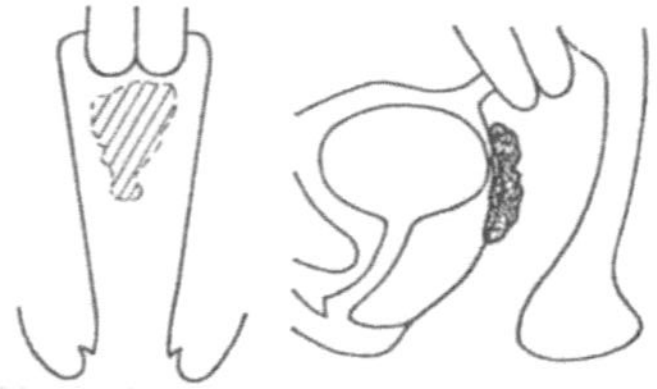	39	1 Jahr	vaginal und uterin	1 Serie	—	—	nach 6 Jahren symptomfrei
79	1959	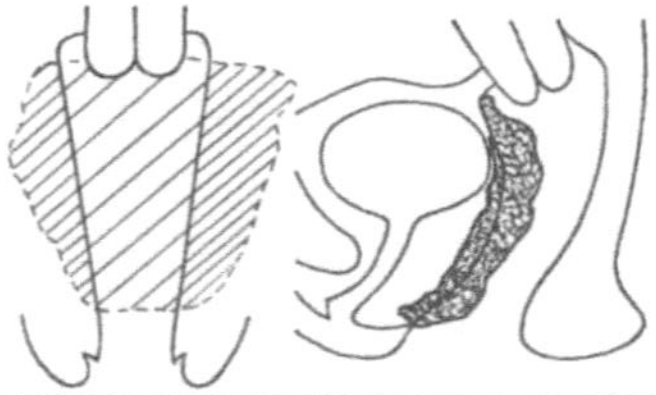	59	4 Monate	vaginal Cs und Ra	1 Serie	—	—	im 1. Jahr †
80	1959	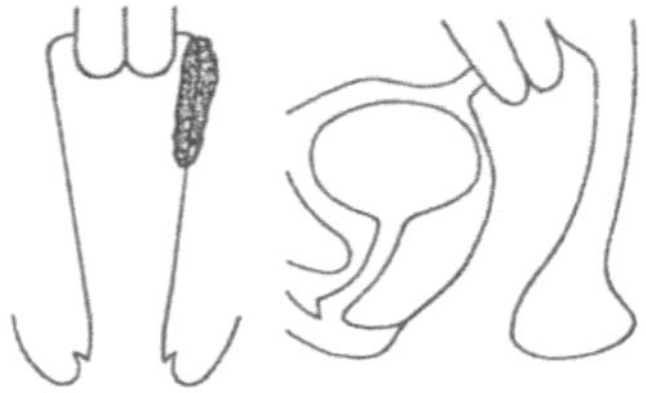	67	6 Monate	vaginal Cs und uterin Ra	1 Serie	—	—	im 1. Jahr †
81	1959	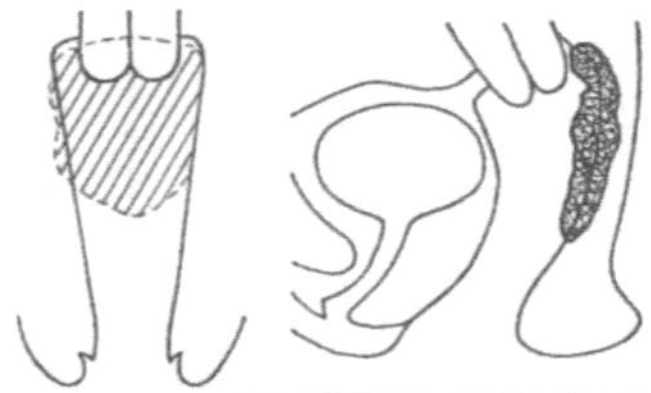	54	6 Monate	vaginal Cs und uterin Ra	1 Serie	—	—	im 1. Jahr †
82	1959	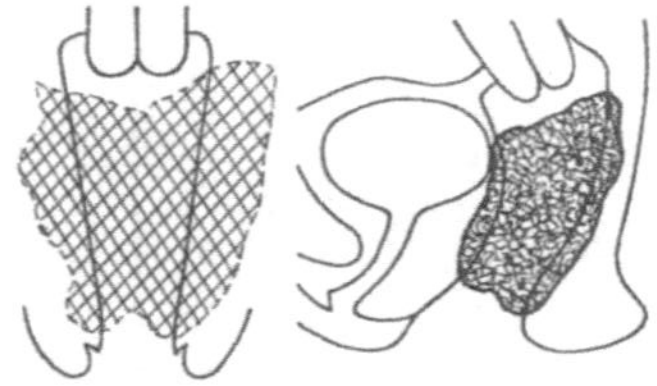	74	4 Jahre	—	1 Serie palliativ	—	—	im 1. Jahr †

f) Mikroskopische Beschaffenheit der Scheidentumoren

Wie bereits erwähnt, sind die Scheidentumoren mit wenigen Ausnahmen vom Typ des Plattenepithelcarcinoms mit oder ohne Verhornung. Tumoren anderen mikroskopisch-anatomischen Typs stellen Seltenheiten dar, sind jedoch nicht völlig ausgeschlossen, so daß bei der Aufnahmeuntersuchung einschlägiger Patientinnen an diese Möglichkeiten, die prognostisch unter Umständen von ausschlaggebender Bedeutung sind, gedacht werden muß.

Abgesehen vom Plattenepithelcarcinom kommen Adenocarcinome vor, welche hervorgehen können aus Resten des Müllerschen, des Wolffschen und des Gartnerschen Ganges, ferner vom sog. Vestibulumepithel, von drüsigen Ausstülpungen der Rectumschleimhaut und schließlich von Schleimdrüsen der Vagina; alles dies natürlich unter der Voraussetzung, daß es sich nicht um die Metastase eines endocervicalen Collumcarcinoms, eines Korpuscarcinoms des Uterus oder eines Ovarialcarcinoms handelt.

Gelegentlich kommen auch Tumoren nicht epithelialer Herkunft an der Vagina vor, z.B. Sarkome; letztere auch beim Kleinkind, wobei alle histologischen Typen vom Rundzellsarkom bis zum Hämangioendotheliom beschrieben worden sind. Hypernephrommetastasen, Chorionepitheliome sind zu erwähnen. Vereinzelte Scheidenmelanome sind beobachtet worden, meist bei älteren Frauen auf der Grundlage einer Melanosis mucosae entwickelt, mit praktisch stets infauster Prognose. Im eigenen Krankengut der letzten 15 Jahre sind 4 Scheidenmelanome beobachtet worden. Bei Rutledge fanden sich neben 70 Plattenepithelcarcinomen 5 Adenocarcinome, 4 Sarkome verschiedener Typen, 2 Melanome, 1 mesodermales Sarkom, außerdem 31 Fälle mit intraepithelialen Carcinomen, die nach der internationalen Regel als Stadium 0 bezeichnet werden müssen.

Zuletzt sind zu erwähnen kasuistische Mitteilungen über benigne oder semimaligne Mischgeschwülste, Teratome, Dermoidcysten. Appelberg hat kürzlich sogar ein Plasmocytom der Scheidenschleimhaut veröffentlicht, das sich als auffallend radiosensibel erwies. Über die Melanome sind gelegentlich günstigere Erfahrungen berichtet worden, die im Gegensatz zu den eigenen Beobachtungen stehen. Allen und Spitz sahen unter 25 Melanomen des weiblichen Genitale, also nicht nur an der Vaginalschleimhaut, 5 Fünfjahresheilungen nach operativen Behandlungen.

Eine typische Häufigkeitsverteilung der verschiedenen histologischen Typen der Vaginaltumoren bietet auch das Krankengut von W. R. Lang, der unter 76 Fällen 68 Plattenepithelcarcinome, 4 Adenocarcinome, 1 undifferenzierten bösartigen Tumor, 1 Sarkom, 1 Melanom, 1 Hämangioendotheliom beobachtete.

In diesem Zusammenhang sind einige seltenere Einzelbeobachtungen von Interesse, z.B. der Umstand, daß Freund u. Mitarb. in der gesamten, ihnen 1959 zugänglichen Weltliteratur nur 28 Fälle von Scheidenmelanomen fanden. Das ist mit Sicherheit nicht repräsentativ für die tatsächliche Häufigkeit. Wir können wahrscheinlich mit 2—4% Melanomen unter allen Scheidenmalignomen rechnen.

Bemerkenswert ist auch ein Bericht von Ariel über eine erfolgreiche radiologische Behandlung des primären Scheidenmelanoms. Er hat 1956 bei seiner Patientin 3mal eine intratumorale Radiophosphorinjektion als ^{32}P-Chromphosphatsuspension ausgeführt, daran anschließend eine Radonspickung des submukösen Gewebes und schließlich eine Tamponade des Scheidengrundes mit ^{32}P getränktem Löschpapier. Die nachträglich vom Autor errechnete Totalstrahlendosis an der Scheidenwand soll etwa 400 000 Rö.-Äquivalente betragen haben. Die Patientin war im Mai 1961 noch rezidivfrei. Der Fall ist sicherlich nicht charakteristisch für die durchweg schicksalhaft ungünstigen Verläufe der Scheidenmelanome.

Fricke u. Mitarb. betonen die Radiosensibilität des Hämangioendothelioms. Abgesehen von ihren beiden gut beeinflußbaren Hämangioendotheliomen haben sie 2mal 1 Leiomyosarkom, 1mal 1 Sarcoma botryoides, 1mal 1 Melanoepitheliom und 1mal ein Spindelzellmelanom behandelt. Alle diese Sarkome und Melanome waren radioresistent und sind ungünstig verlaufen.

g) Ätiologie

Über die Ätiologie des Vaginalcarcinoms ist ebenso wenig Sicheres auszusagen wie über die Carcinome im allgemeinen. Daß lokale Reizmomente, der Druck eines jahrelang getragenen Pessars oder auch eine chronische Kolpitis, Scheuern der Kleidung bei Prolapszuständen, eine mitverursachende Rolle spielen können (NEUGEBAUER, HUBER u.v.a.), wird nicht bestritten. Auch die Beobachtung, daß ein Plattenepithelcarcinom sich aus einer Leukoplakie entwickelt, kann an der Scheidenschleimhaut wie bei anderem Tumorsitz gemacht werden.

Eine ausgeprägte Seltenheit ist offensichtlich das Entstehen eines Vaginalcarcinoms in einem irreponiblen Totalprolaps des Uterus, wie 1955 von D. B. BROWN berichtet. Die Patientin konnte durch Cervixamputation geheilt werden. Im London Hospital war innerhalb von 45 Jahren nur ein einziger vergleichbarer Fall aufgetreten.

Völlig unbekannt sind die Ursachen für den Befall des oberen Drittels der hinteren Vaginalwand. Man müßte schon an die starke mechanische Beanspruchung dieses Gebietes in den letzten Wochen der Schwangerschaft und intra partum denken: Die gleiche Überlegung also anstellen, die zur Erklärung der relativ hohen Häufigkeit der Collumcarcinome bei Mehrgebärenden herangezogen worden ist.

h) Ausbreitung des Scheidencarcinoms

Die Tatsache, daß das Scheidenrohr, besonders im Vergleich mit dem Uterus, ein verhältnismäßig dünnwandiges Hohlorgan darstellt, führt dazu, daß hier auftretende infiltrierende Carcinome die Scheidenwand frühzeitig durchbrechen können und in der Lage sind, sich per continuitatem oder auf dem Lymphwege auszubreiten. Man kann daher in Übereinstimmung mit zahlreichen klinischen und pathologisch-anatomischen Beobachtungen prinzipielle Ausbreitungsrichtungen feststellen:

1. Kontinuierliche Ausbreitung in das *Parakolpium* und *Parametrium*, ferner in das Septum rectovaginale und *Rectum*, in das Septum vesicovaginale und die *Harnblase*.

2. Ausbreitung auf dem Lymphwege in die inneren *Lymphknoten der Leistenbeugen*. Dieser Ausbreitungsweg steht insbesondere den Carcinomen des *unteren Vaginaldrittels* und hier wiederum der Seitenwand offen. Es ist dies der gleiche Weg, den Carcinome der Vulva, der Clitoris und Urethra auf dem Lymphwege nehmen (Abb. 1).

3. Ausbreitung auf dem Lymphwege in die *Obturatorius-„drüse"*, ferner die Lymphknotengruppen entlang der Vena und *Arteria ilica interna*, der *Ilica communis* und schließlich in die *präsacralen Lymphknoten*. Diese letzteren drei Ausbreitungswege werden gewöhnlich von Tumoren des *mittleren und oberen Scheidendrittels* beschritten, sie sind weitgehend die gleichen wie der Metastasierungsweg des Collumcarcinoms.

Für den behandelnden Arzt ist das Wissen um die in Abb. 1 dargestellten Ausbreitungsmöglichkeiten der weiblichen Genitalcarcinome von entscheidender Bedeutung, ergibt sich doch daraus die therapeutische Methodik und häufig sogar die prognostische Beurteilung für den Einzelfall. Für das Vaginalcarcinom ist daher, ähnlich wie für das Collumcarcinom des Uterus, von verschiedenen Autoren, insbesondere von GERTEIS, REIFFENSTUHL, FRISCHBIER u.a. der klinische Wert der Röntgenlymphographie betont worden. Freilich fehlt es nicht an kritischen Stimmen, die darauf hinweisen, daß die lymphographische Darstellung mit der heute üblichen Technik nicht notwendigerweise jedes erkrankte Lymphom im Raum des kleinen Beckens mit Sicherheit nachzuweisen vermag. Die Erfahrungen am Vaginalcarcinom sind begrenzt. FRISCHBIER fand unter 4 Vaginalcarcinomen, daß in 3 Fällen die klinische und die lymphographische Untersuchung das gleiche Ergebnis und in einem Falle die klinische Untersuchung einen größeren Befall als die Lymphographie nachweisen konnte. Eine endgültige Beurteilung über die Leistungsfähigkeit der Lymphographie auf diesem Gebiet ist verfrüht. Der Autor ist zu einer zurückhaltenden Skepsis geneigt, zumal in der Regel aus den klinischen und lymphographischen Befunden therapeutische Konsequenzen nicht möglich sind, wenn man bereits von Beginn an sich zu einer radikalen oder palliativen Behandlung hat entscheiden müssen.

Unabhängig von den Ausbreitungswegen eines primären Scheidencarcinoms muß bei jedem beobachteten Tumorbefall in der Scheidenschleimhaut an die Möglichkeit gedacht werden, daß diese Manifestation nicht die einzige zu sein braucht, sondern die Metastase eines außerhalb der Vagina gelegenen Primärtumors des weiblichen Genitaltrakts oder anderer Organe sein könnte. Aber auch mit der Möglichkeit einer primären multizentrischen Tumorentstehung des weiblichen Genitalcarcinoms ist im Prinzip in, wenn auch seltenen Fällen zu rechnen.

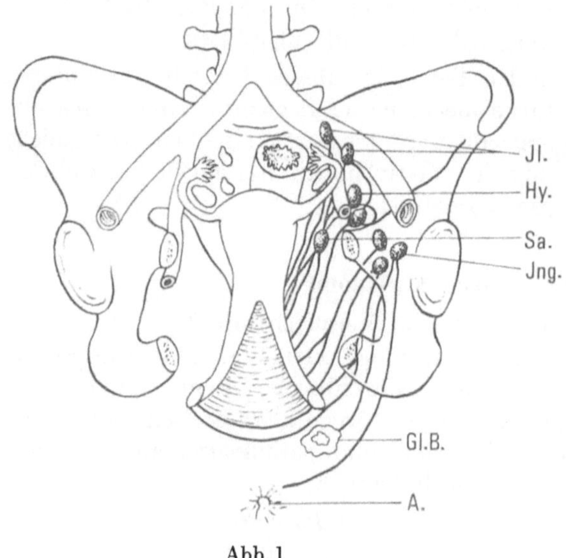

Abb. 1

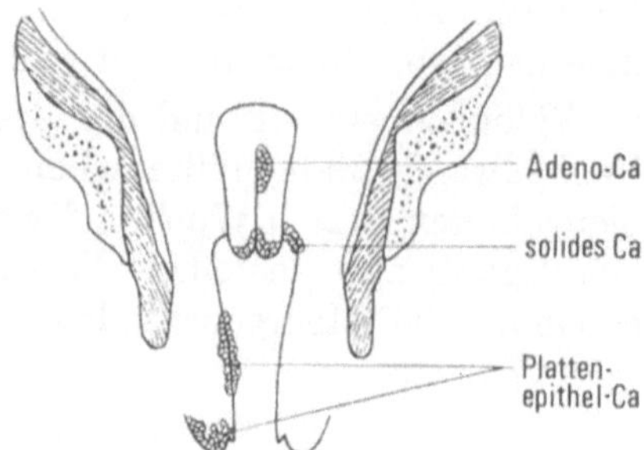

Abb. 2. Multizentrisches Carcinom im weiblichen Genitaltrakt

Abb. 1. Lymphausbreitungsgebiet der Vaginalcarcinome

Ein typisches Beispiel hierfür wird in Abb. 2 wiedergegeben: Ein multizentrisches Carcinom an 4 voneinander getrennten anatomischen Primärsitzen mit 3 verschiedenen histologischen Beschaffenheiten, nämlich

1. ein Adenocarcinom der Fundusschleimhaut des Corpus uteri,

2. ein unreifes, solides Carcinom des Collum, offenbar vom äußeren Muttermund ausgehend, mit Übergriff auf das linke Scheidengewölbe,

3. ein verhornendes Plattenepithelcarcinom an der rechten Seitenwand im mittleren Scheidendrittel,

4. ein ebenfalls verhornendes Plattenepithelcarcinom in der Falte zwischen Labium und Labium majus rechts.

Auch dieser Fall ist im übrigen ein Hinweis auf die Berechtigung der Auffassungen von SMITHERS über die prinzipielle Genese der Tumorkrankheit, in der er nicht etwa allein den cytologischen Aspekt auf Grund einer prinzipiellen Umwandlung der cellulären Eigenschaften, sondern vor allem den Gesichtspunkt der zur Tumorentstehung notwendigen Desorganisation des Organismus (lokal, regional oder allgemein) in den Vordergrund gestellt hat.

2. Die bisherigen Formen der Therapie des Vaginalcarcinoms

a) Operative Behandlung

Vor Beginn der strahlentherapeutischen Ära und vor der Entwicklung angemessener Strahlenbehandlungsmethoden stand ausschließlich das operative Behandlungsverfahren zur Verfügung. Zahlreiche Operationsmethoden wurden geschaffen, so von C. SCHRÖDER (1878), OLSHAUSEN (1889) und DÜHRSSEN (1895). Leider waren diese Operationen, im einzelnen beispielsweise bei NÜRNBERGER beschrieben, meist nicht erfolgreich, so daß SCHLUND (1913) feststellen mußte, daß von den bis dahin operierten Scheidencarcinomen innerhalb eines Monats bis zu 3 Jahren die übergroße Mehrzahl rezidiviert hatte. FRANZ fand 1925 nur eine von seinen 7 operierten Patientinnen rezidivfrei. Ähnlich ging es nahezu allen Autoren. So hat z.B. GIESECKE (1922) festgestellt, daß von 11 in den Jahren 1910—1916 operierten Vaginalcarcinomen der Kieler Universitäts-Frauenklinik nur eine Patientin die 5-Jahresgrenze erreichte.

Seit etwa der Jahrhundertwende kommt als chirurgische Methode lediglich in Frage

1. die abdominale Radikaloperation nach WERTHEIM mit entsprechender Erweiterung auf das Scheidenrohr und das parakolpische Gewebe;

2. die vaginale Radikaloperation nach SCHAUTA, STOECKEL und AMREICH.

Dabei wird es ebenfalls als selbstverständlich angesehen, daß der größere oder sogar der größte Teil des Scheidenrohres mitentfernt wird.

Auch hierdurch sind die Heilungsergebnisse nach dem bisherigen Wissen nicht wesentlich besser geworden, so daß auch hochangesehene, überwiegend operativ tätige Gynäkologen beim Vaginalcarcinom der primären Strahlentherapie den Vorzug zu geben bereit sind. Für diese Einstellung besonders charakteristisch sind bereits die frühen Ausführungen von O. KÜSTNER (1927):

„Denn, selbst wenn man dem Rektum und der Blase gegenüber mit äußerster Rücksichtslosigkeit, mit äußerstem Radikalismus vorgeht, so ist wieder ein gleicher Radikalismus dem paravaginalen Gewebe gegenüber nicht möglich wie gegenüber dem Parametrium bei der Exstirpation des karzinomatösen Uterus. Hier können wir tatsächlich beträchtliche Gewebsmassen mitnehmen und uns so voraussichtlich im Gesunden halten. Das verbietet sich aber bei dem viel kürzeren, von der Scheide aus breit in das Becken ausstrahlenden Parakolpium. Waren wir im Rektum, den retrorektalen Drüsen und der Blase gegenüber noch so radikal und wurde der Eingriff vertragen, hier im paravaginalen Gewebe lauert doch noch das Rezidiv. Das ist in Rechnung zu ziehen. Das muß unserem künftigen therapeutischen Verhalten Richtung geben und uns die Frage vorlegen, ob wir überhaupt noch die Scheidenkarzinome operieren oder sie nicht lieber prinzipiell der Strahlentherapie anheimgeben wollen.“

Diese Stellungnahme KÜSTNERS ist eindeutig und wegen ihrer grundsätzlichen, durch die Anatomie gegebenen Gesichtspunkte auch heute gültig geblieben. Er wird aber noch eindringlicher und begründet seinen Standpunkt mit beispielhaften Ausführungen:

„Wenn, um nur ein Beispiel heranzuziehen, eine Kranke, welche ein Karzinom des Vaginalgewölbes aufwies, welches zwar nicht umfänglich, so doch eine Induration darstellte, die in beachtenswerter Weise das paravaginale Gewebe ergriffen hatte und bei welcher von anderer Seite die Operation als nicht mehr erfolgversprechend abgelehnt war, auch von uns nicht operiert, sondern bestrahlt wurde, nach 5 Jahren einen Befund darbot, der, mit den früheren verglichen, nicht nur eine beträchtliche Umfangsreduktion bis zu einem kleinen narbenartigen Gebilde erkennen ließ, sondern vielleicht sogar radikale Heilung bedeutete, wenn diese Kranke zudem bei Zunahme des Körpergewichts sich äußersten Wohlbefindens erfreute, so steht diesem Erfolg die hohe Wahrscheinlichkeit gegenüber, daß sie, operiert, dem Rezidiv längst erlegen wäre.“

Durch diese sehr charakteristische Einstellung des bedeutenden Operateurs ist die eingeschränkte Bedeutung der operativen Behandlung des Scheidencarcinoms gekennzeichnet, wenngleich von anderer Seite in ausgewählten Fällen Operationen ausgeführt worden sind. Es fehlt verständlicherweise an Erfahrungen, die systematisch an einem größeren operierten Krankengut gewonnen worden sein könnten, und es ist wohl richtig, daß man sich im allgemeinen mit der Operation des Scheidencarcinoms zurückhielt. Die kleinräumige vaginale Exstirpation kleinerer Scheidencarcinome wird allseits als praktisch stets unzureichender Eingriff abgelehnt.

An dieser grundsätzlichen Einstellung hat sich auch durch die neuzeitlichen Fortschritte der operativen Technik mit der Herabsetzung der Risiken durch Antibioticaschutz, Operationsvorbereitung und moderne Technik der Anaesthesie nicht das geringste geändert.

b) Die Strahlenbehandlung des Vaginalcarcinoms

Die ersten Mitteilungen über mehr oder weniger erfolgreiche Strahlenbehandlungen des Vaginalcarcinoms, hier im allgemeinen als eine lokalisierte Radiumapplikation ausgeführt, stammen von Bumm, Weibel, Singer und wenigen anderen Autoren. Bumm hatte 1919 5 von 22 Fällen 3—6 Jahre geheilt, davon 2 von ihm als inoperabel bezeichnete Patientinnen.

Weibel behandelte 1926 ein inoperables, isoliertes, handtellergroßes Carcinom der hinteren Vaginalwand mit etwa 3 000 mg-Elementstunden Radium. Das Carcinom bildete sich unter Zurücklassen einer großen Scheiden-Mastdarmfistel vollkommen zurück. Die Fistel konnte 4 Jahre später operativ geschlossen werden. Singer berichtete 1927 über eine Radiumspätschädigung (Fistelbildung) im Falle eines vor 13 Jahren behandelten Scheidenkrebses. Eine ausführliche Beschreibung der damaligen Radiumbehandlungstechnik stammt von B. Bienenfeld, die 1926 34 Fälle der Literatur sammelte, die als durch Strahlenbehandlung geheilt bezeichnet wurden. Sie schildert dann einen Einzelfall, bei dem ein einziges Dominiciröhrchen, enthaltend 50 mg Radiumelement, unmittelbar auf dem Carcinom durch Tamponade fixiert wurde, so daß etwa 2 000 mg-Elementstunden wirksam wurden. Anscheinend ist es zu einer Heilung dieses Falles nicht gekommen. Überhaupt ist die Leistungsfähigkeit der Strahlenbehandlung jener Tage heute schwer zu beurteilen, weil nur in wenigen Fällen eine ausreichende Beobachtungszeit vorlag und es sich immer nur um Einzelfälle gehandelt hat.

Aber auch aus jenen Darstellungen geht bereits hervor, daß für das Scheidencarcinom längst nicht gleich gute Heilbarkeit wie für das Collumcarcinom des Uterus angenommen werden konnte. Eine bessere Leistungsfähigkeit der Strahlenbehandlung ist erst nach den Jahrzehnten einer systematischen Fortentwicklung der curietherapeutischen Methoden und unter Einbeziehung einer modernen Dosimetrie mit physikalischer Grundlage zustande gekommen. Die moderneren Methoden sollen daher in kurzen Zügen geschildert werden, wobei auch von deren historischer Entwicklung ausgegangen wird.

3. Moderne Methoden der Strahlenbehandlung

a) Röntgen-Therapie

Seitz und Wintz haben auch für das Vaginalcarcinom die Erlanger „Konzentrationsmethode" angewendet, wobei in kürzester Zeit, möglichst an einem Tag, alle Einfallsfelder bestrahlt wurden mit je 90—100% der HED (Hauteinheitsdosis nach Wintz). Sie haben unterschieden zwischen den Carcinomen des unteren und des oberen Scheidenabschnitts. Für den unteren Scheidenabschnitt, bei dessen Befall wie beim Vulvacarcinom bestrahlt wurde, ist ein Vulvafeld, zwei Inguinalfelder, ein dorsales Feld auf den Tumor gerichtet, gegeben worden. Bei Tumoren des oberen Scheidenabschnittes, bei denen entsprechend dem Collumcarcinom bestrahlt wurde, wählten die Autoren ein Vulvadammfeld, zwei suprasymphysäre, ein Steißbeinfeld und zwei parasacrale Felder, sämtliche Felder zum Tumorzentrum gerichtet. Wintz betrachtete diese von ihm und seinen Mitarbeitern inaugurierte Methode der Röntgentiefenbestrahlung als die Hauptmethode und auch die von ihm nicht vollkommen verschmähte Radiumapplikation (2 000 mg-Elementstunden) in Kontakt mit dem Scheidentumor als eine zusätzliche Behandlung. Es ist bemerkenswert, daß unter dieser Behandlung an der Erlanger Universitäts-Frauenklinik in den Jahren bis 1929 unter 52 so behandelten Patientinnen 10 5-Jahresheilungen zu verzeichnen waren, entsprechend einer absoluten Heilung von 19,6%. Das ist ein Ergebnis, das den Erfolgen der damaligen chirurgischen Behandlung überlegen war.

In den meisten Strahlenkliniken ist jedoch die Röntgenbestrahlung von außen, die bei WINTZ und seinen Schülern unter völligem Verzicht auf die Vorteile, die eine höhere Fraktionierung bietet, in 1—2 Tagen appliziert wurde und damit eine viel zu hohe Belastung für die Patientinnen bedeutete, nicht als Hauptbehandlungsverfahren akzeptiert worden.

Im Mittelpunkt des Interesses stand von allem Anfang an die lokalisierte Radiumanwendung, gefördert vor allem durch die eindrucksvollen Erfahrungen, die man an der Universitäts-Frauenklinik München, unter DÖDERLEIN, am Radiumhemmet in Stockholm, unter FORSSELL und HEYMAN, an der Fondation Curie, Paris, unter LACASSAGNE und REGAUD gesammelt hatte. Dieses Interesse konnte aber nicht den Verzicht auf zusätzliche *Röntgentiefentherapie* bedeuten, da auch bei maximaler Ausnutzung des gesamten verfügbaren intrakavitären Raumes im weiblichen Genitaltrakt an den potentiell tumortragenden Lymphknotengebieten des kleinen Beckens, an der Beckenwand, höchstens 2000—3000 rad erzielt werden konnten, also eine Dosis, die nicht in der Lage war, etwaige Lymphknotenmetastasen im Obturatoriusgebiet oder entlang der ilicalen Gefäße ausreichend zu bestrahlen, geschweige denn, die inguinalen Lymphknotengebiete, welche für tiefsitzende Vaginalcarcinome von Bedeutung werden. Neben der intrakavitären Radiotherapie, auf deren Methodik noch eingegangen werden soll, mußte also, wie beim Collumcarcinom des Uterus, eine fraktionierte Tiefenbestrahlung der seitlichen Abschnitte des kleinen Beckens unter Einschluß der Inguinalgegend ausgeführt werden, und zwar in der Regel von 2 Unterbauch- und 2 Sacralfeldern aus.

Über die zweckmäßige Anordnung und Größe dieser Einfallsfelder ist viel geschrieben worden, so z.B. in den zusammenfassenden Darstellungen von OESER und KEPP sowie in jüngster Zeit von WEISHAAR u. Mitarb. Sicher muß erkannt werden, daß die Aufgabe einer solchen Zusatzbehandlung bzw. -bestrahlung der seitlichen Abschnitte des kleinen Beckens als Ergänzung der Radiumbestrahlung der axial oder paraaxial gelegenen Tumoren nicht die Aufgabe haben kann, weit seitlich vom knöchernen Beckenring gelegene Gewebeabschnitte mitzuerfassen. Da der Querdurchmesser des kleinen Beckens praktisch konstant ca. 12 cm beträgt und außerdem ein in der Mittellinie gelegener Bereich mit Rücksicht auf die dort durch die Radiumapplikation erzeugte hohe Strahlendosis geschont werden muß, empfiehlt es sich, die Feldbreite der ventro-dorsalen Einfallsstrahlenkegel auf 6, höchstens 8 cm zu begrenzen. Die Feldlänge ist abhängig von dem Ausmaß, in dem die entlang der Arteria ilica interna und im Bereich der Ilica communis gelegenen potentiell tumortragenden Lymphknoten nach cranial miterfaßt werden sollen. Es ist gewiß unmöglich, jeden potentiell tumortragenden Lymphknotenbezirk bis hinauf zur Bifurkation der Aorta und darüber hinaus durch percutane Röntgentherapie mit einer ausreichend hochdosierten Strahlendosis ebenso wie den Primärtumor, den man kennen und in seiner Größe einigermaßen realistisch abschätzen kann, zu erfassen. Das Eingehen von Kompromissen unter behandlungstaktischen Gesichtspunkten ist also notwendig, wobei auf Miterfassung weniger häufig auftretender Metastasierungssitze und entfernterer Lymphknotenabschnitte bewußt verzichtet wird.

Zurück zur Technik der percutanen Röntgentherapie: De facto entsteht somit eine *Stufenbestrahlung*, welche auf 3 räumliche anatomische Bereiche gerichtet ist, nämlich

1. den sicher vom Tumor befallenen Bereichen der Vagina mit höchster Strahlendosis durch die Curietherapie belegt, beispielsweise 8000—10000 rad, eventuell an einzelnen „heißen" Punkten mehr;

2. den potentiell tumortragenden Bereich, Parakolpium, typische Lymphknotenausbreitungsgebiete, von Curietherapie unzureichend bis ca. 2500 rad bestrahlt, mit einer Zusatzdosis durch percutane Therapie auf 4500—6000 rad aufgefüllt;

3. den direkt durch percutane Therapie mitbestrahlten Bereich außerhalb des sicher oder potentiell tumortragenden Gebiets, ein Gebiet also, in dem die Strahlenexposition an sich nicht notwendig, aber unvermeidlich stattfindet, in dem auch unerwünschte Nebenmaxima der räumlichen Dosisverteilung auftreten können.

Unter solchen Überlegungen und unter Berücksichtigung des Wissens um typische Tumorausbreitungsformen erscheint es ratsam, das Lymphausbreitungsgebiet höchstens bis hinauf zur Bifurkation der Arteria ilica communis mitzuerfassen, also den Bereich, der auch bei der Behandlung des Collumcarcinoms im Rahmen der kombinierten Strahlentherapie mit hoher Strahlendosis belegt wird, den gleichen Bereich, der bei einer erweiterten Wertheimschen Operation in toto entfernt werden kann unter Verzicht auf Überradikalität, deren therapeutischer Nutzen problematisch sein würde.

Die Feldlänge der abdomino-sacralen Einfallsfelder braucht daher keinesfalls größer als 15 cm zu sein. Sie kann dann kleiner sein, beispielsweise 12 cm betragen, wenn Tumorsitz und Ausdehnung auch in der Längsrichtung des Patienten besonders gut bekannt sind. Im Allgemeinen Krankenhaus St. Georg wird also, sofern diese *Vierfeldertechnik* noch benutzt wird, die Feldgröße 8×15 cm bevorzugt.

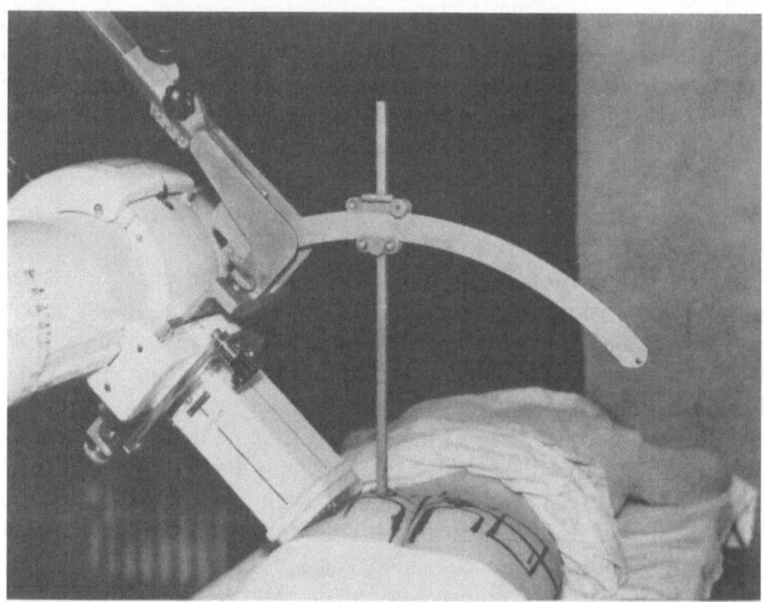

Abb. 3. 8-Felder-Bestrahlungstechnik. Einstellung von dorsal mit dem Bogenlotzeiger und Orthovoltröntgentherapiegerät

Untersuchungen von Röntgenaufnahmen, mit der Therapieröhre angefertigt, ferner Überlegungen, die z.B. Winternitz, G. Fletcher u.v.a. vorwiegend für das Collumcarcinom, aber auch für das Vaginalcarcinom gültig, angestellt haben, zeigen jedoch, daß es bei dieser *Vierfelderbestrahlungstechnik* kaum möglich ist, eine wesentliche Mitbestrahlung des medialen Abschnittes des Schenkelhalses zu vermeiden, wenn man eine genügend hohe Herddosis in den seitlichen Abschnitten des kleinen Beckens, beispielsweise in Punkt B nach Margaret Tod, erzielen will. Da von der intrakavitären Radiumanordnung aus hier nicht mit einer größeren Gesamtdosis als etwa 2000 rad gerechnet werden kann, ist eine Zusatzdosis im Parakolpium und auch in den Punkten B und H (geometrischer Punkt, 4 cm oberhalb Punkt B, anatomisch etwa entsprechend der Birfurkation der Arteria ilica interna, Gauwerky) von wenigstens 3000 rad anzustreben. Wenn dieses Ziel mit Hilfe der vielerorts üblichen Vierfelderbestrahlungstechnik erreicht werden soll, dann muß allerdings auch bei normalem Sagittaldurchmesser nicht korpulenter Patientinnen (Durchschnitt in Hamburg 22 cm) ein sehr kräftiges Hauterythem und unter Umständen eine exsudative Reaktion in Kauf genommen werden. Bei korpulenten Patientinnen mit Sagittaldurchmessern von 25 cm und mehr ist das erwähnte Ziel mit dieser Technik kaum erreichbar.

Man bevorzugte daher im Allgemeinen Krankenhaus St. Georg, bevor ultraharte Strahlenenergien, Telekobaltgerät und Betatron verfügbar waren, ebenso wie von WINTERNITZ (1948) und GILBERT FLETCHER (1950) angegeben, die Anwendung einer *8-Feldertechnik:*

2 Abdominalfelder 8×15 cm. Medialer Feldrand 2 cm lateral der Mittellinie. Unterer Feldrand 1 cm unterhalb der Symphyse, 10° nach caudal gekippter Zentralstrahl.

2 Sacralfelder 6×10 cm. Medialer Feldrand 2 cm lateral der Mittellinie. Unterer Feldrand 2 cm oberhalb der Verbindungslinie zwischen den Trochanteren, Zentralstrahl 30° nach caudal gekippt.

2 Glutealfelder. Senkrecht unterhalb der beiden Sacralfelder angeordnet, Feldgröße 6×10 cm, medialer Feldrand 2 cm von der Mittellinie entfernt, oberer Feldrand 2 cm unterhalb der Trochanterlinie, Zentralstrahl 35—40° nach cranial gekippt.

2 laterale Sacralfelder. Feldgröße 6×12 cm, Zentralstrahl auf die Trochanterlinie gesetzt, medialer Feldrand 2 cm lateral der oben angegebenen dorsalen Felder, Zentralstrahl 45° nach medial gekippt.

Alle Zentralstrahlen werden auf Punkt B gerichtet. Das Bestrahlen mit dieser Technik kann verhältnismäßig gut reproduzierbar eingestellt werden, wenn die 4 erstgenannten dorsalen Felder mit Hilfe einer Schablone auf der Haut der Patientin aufgezeichnet und die genaue Winkeleinstellung der beiden lateralen Sacralfelder unter Hinzuziehung eines individuellen Körperquerschnitts der Patientin mit Hilfe eines Bogenlotgeräts (pin and arc) vorgenommen wird (Abb. 3).

Diese auch beim Collumcarcinom angewandte Methodik der Röntgenzusatzbestrahlung des kleinen Beckens gilt für Scheidencarcinome der oberen Vaginalhälfte und der Hinterwand, deren Lymphausbreitungsrichtung praktisch die gleiche wie beim Collumcarcinom ist. Für die Carcinome des unteren Vaginalabschnittes, deren Lymphausbreitung wie beim Vulvacarcinom und beim Urethralcarcinom zunächst in die Leistenbeugen erfolgt, ist eine Röntgenzusatzbestrahlung der Inguinalregion vorzuziehen.

b) Radiumbestrahlung

Das Scheidenrohr und die hier gelegenen Tumoren bieten sich für eine lokalisierte Anwendung radioaktiver Substanzen, in erster Linie des Radiums selbst und in früheren Jahren, als noch nicht überall Radiumpräparate in ausreichender Zahl zur Verfügung standen, auch des Mesothoriums, geradezu an. Während in den ersten Jahren der Strahlenära sog. *Dominiciröhrchen,* d.h. verhältnismäßig stark beladene Messingfilter von ca. 5 mm Durchmesser, die bis zu 50 mg Radium enthielten, unmittelbar auf den Tumor gelegt und dort fest tamponiert wurden, haben sich anstelle dieser ersten Beispiele einer intrakavitären Radiumtherapie, deren Dosierung rein empirisch bemessen wurde und im allgemeinen 2000—3000 mg-Elementstunden betrug, fortschrittlichere Methoden entwickelt, wobei meist von schwächeren Einzelpräparaten ausgegangen wurde und unter Ausnutzung des Zeitfaktors eine protrahierte und gleichzeitig auf 2—5 Sitzungen über 3—5 Wochen verteilte fraktionierte Behandlung stattfindet.

Man unterscheidet:

α) Die vaginale Kontakttherapie

Sie wird nur bei zirkulären, stark stenosierenden Prozessen noch als einzelnes Dominiciröhrchen gegeben (siehe z.B. MARTIUS). Nahezu überall, beispielsweise auch im Radiumhemmet Stockholm, im Radiuminstitut in Kopenhagen unter JENS NIELSEN und auch im eigenen Krankenhaus St. Georg, werden ,,schmale" rechteckige *Radiumplatten* (Kantenverhältnis 1:2 bis 1:5) unmittelbar auf die Tumorfläche aufgelegt, wobei zur Erzielung einer günstigeren, d.h. etwas höheren relativen Dosis in 10—15 mm Gewebetiefe die Abstände der Radiumtuben zur Schleimhautoberfläche ca. 5 mm betragen, im Unterschied zum historischen, unmittelbar aufgelegten einzelnen Dominiciröhrchen.

Dennoch hat auch dieses Verfahren der kurzen Distanzen den Vorteil des sehr steilen Dosisabfalls der Kleinvolumenbestrahlung und bietet gleichzeitig die Möglichkeit, den durch Tamponade distanzierten gegenüberliegenden Teil der Scheidenschleimhaut, ebenso aber die unmittelbar angrenzenden Organe, wie Rectum und Blase, weitgehend zu schonen. Voraussetzung für die Verwendung dieser Methode ist ein verhältnismäßig oberflächlicher Tumorbefall ohne tiefere Infiltration. Die Rectum- und Blasendosis ist abhängig von der recto-vaginalen bzw. vesico-vaginalen Distanz, die individuell verschieden zwischen wenigen Millimetern und Zentimetern liegt und außerdem abhängig von der lokalen Tumorausbreitung ist.

Eine ordnungsmäßige Radiumanwendung dieses Typs erfordert außerdem sorgfältige vollständige Bedeckung des erkrankten Gebietes, unter Einbeziehung eines genügend großen Sicherheitsrands gesunder Scheidenschleimhaut, in der Regel wenigstens 10 bis 15 mm nach allen Seiten. Jahrzehnte hindurch betrug nach der üblichen empirischen Anwendung die „Dosis" 2-, meist 3mal 2 000 mg-Elementstunden innerhalb 3 bis 4 Wochen. Das bedeutet nach heutigem Wissen je Applikation eine Oberflächendosis im Kontakt zum Applikator von 3 500—4 000 rad pro Sitzung, also eine Gesamtdosis von 7 000—12 000 rad.

β) Vaginal-Zylinder

Vaginal-Zylinder mit axialer Anordnung der strahlenden Substanz, entweder in vorgeformten zylindrischen Strahlungsträgern aus Kunststoff oder als zylindrische Moulage aus Stentsmasse, vermeiden die erwähnte Unsicherheit der angedeuteten einfachen Kontakttherapietechnik.

Vaginal-Zylinder zur Radiumanwendung bei axialer Anordnung sind schon in frühester Zeit konstruiert worden, z.B. von Voltz beschrieben, von Ries und anderen Repräsentanten der Münchner Schule benutzt. Entsprechende Applikatoren, wie auch diejenigen von Weigand und Neeff, sind im Laufe der Jahre oft konstruiert und beschrieben worden. Ein besonders gutes Beispiel hierfür sind die Perspex-Applikatoren von Blomfield. Auch in jüngerer Zeit, beispielsweise von Swyngedouw u. Mitarb., Lederman und Mayneord, sind Verfahren zur Herstellung individueller Radiumapplikatoren (Moulagen) beschrieben. Besonders interessant erscheint die Lösung von Focht u. Mitarb., die ein durchsichtiges Kunststoffrohr einführen, um anschließend, nach Orientierung über den genauen Sitz des Scheidencarcinoms hinter der durchsichtigen Wand des Rohres, den eigentlichen Radiumträger in zylindrischer Anordnung einzuführen, und dabei ist es möglich, je nach Wunsch entweder die axiale oder die periphere Anordnung von Radiumröhrchen zu bevorzugen, je nachdem, ob man bei relativ oberflächlichem Tumor einen steilen Dosisabfall nach der Tiefe zu wünscht oder ob man durch Einhalten eines Abstandes einen weniger steilen Abfall erreichen will (Abb. 4). Auch die an der Universitäts-Frauenklinik München jetzt gebräuchlichen Neeff-Rohre gestatten eine entweder zentrale oder periphere Radiumanordnung. Eine sowohl zentrale als auch periphere Anordnung erreicht E. Maier durch Verwenden eines intravaginal applizierten Gummiklotzes, ein Verfahren, das dem in den 50er Jahren durch Becker und Scheer vorgeschlagenen Plastobalt bzw. Makrobalt infolge der bei multiplen eintretenden „Nullpunktunterdrückung" ähnlich ist.

Das Verfahren axialer Strahlenquellen ist im allgemeinen bei tiefer in das Paravaginalgewebe infiltrierenden Tumoren zu bevorzugen, zumal man auch hierbei individuell dosieren und die räumliche Dosisverteilung modifizieren kann.

γ) Intrauterine Radiumbehandlung

Die Radiumbehandlung des Scheidencarcinoms wäre in der überwiegenden Mehrzahl der Fälle unvollständig ohne eine mit der intravaginalen Applikation kombinierten *intrauterinen Radiumeinlage*.

Dieses Zusatzverfahren ist unbedingt zu fordern für die im oberen Vaginalabschnitt gelegenen Tumoren, welche, wie betont, den gleichen Lymphausbreitungsweg wie die Collumcarcinome aufweisen. Wenn man in Kombination mit der erwähnten vaginalen Radiumeinlage durch zusätzliche Intrauterinbehandlung den gesamten verfügbaren intrakavitären Raum des weiblichen Genitale zur Radiumbehandlung ausnutzt, entstehen

Summationsisodosen, welche weiter nach lateral ausladen und auch im Hypogastrica-
gebiet (Punkt H. GAUWERKY) eine nicht vernachlässigbare Gammastrahlendosis (1 800 bis
2 000 rad) wirksam werden lassen. Hierdurch wird somit in letzter Konsequenz die Geo-

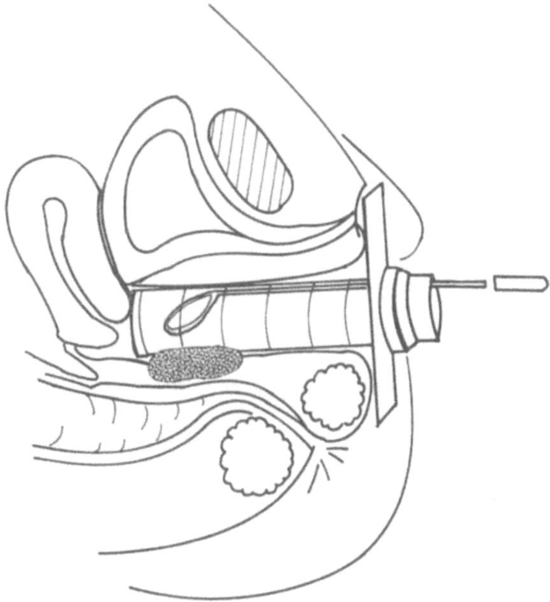

Abb. 4. Vaginaler Radiumapplikator nach FOCHT u. Mitarb. Einstelltechnik unter Spiegelbeleuchtung des
Tumors

metrie des „mandrin par source axial" nach SWYNGEDOUW ausgenutzt. Nur dann, wenn
es sich um einen sehr kleinen, eng umschriebenen Tumor handelt, von dem wegen seiner
geringen Ausdehnung nicht erwartet wird, daß er sich collumcarcinomähnlich ausbreiten
könnte, oder wenn der Tumor im unteren Scheidendrittel sitzt, kann es verantwortet
werden, auf die intrauterine Radiumbehandlung zu verzichten. Abb. 5a zeigt relative
Tiefendosen verschiedener vaginaler Curieanordnungen, Abb. 5b Summationsisodosen
einer vaginalen und intrauterinen Kombination.

δ) Radiumspickung

Diese Methode, bereits durch die Pariser Schule der Radiotherapie unter REGAUD
in die Strahlenbehandlung eingeführt, eignet sich ganz besonders für kleinere Vaginalcarcinome des mittleren und unteren Scheidendrittels, welche nicht allzu tief in das
paravaginale Gewebe hinein infiltrieren und vor allem hinsichtlich Größe und Ausdehnung völlig übersichtlich sind. Auch dieses Verfahren, das zunächst unmethodisch,
d. h. mit empirischer Anordnung der Radiumnadeln und empirischer Dosierung angewendet
wurde, hat durch die verdienstvollen Arbeiten von R. PATERSON und PARKER (1934,
1938) sowie MINDER (1944) und E. QUIMBY (1944) eine systematische Ordnung erfahren
und vor allem ein Dosierungssystem in physikalischen Einheiten erhalten. Das in graphischen Tafeln und Tabellen wiedergegebene Dosierungssystem gibt für definierte geo-
metrische Radiumanordnungen und Abmessungen, auch für Spickungen in einer oder
zwei Ebenen und schließlich für Volumenspickungen die für 1 000 R Minimaldosis im
gespickten Bereich erforderlichen mg-Elementstunden Radium an.

Man kann somit leicht die Liegedauer für eine gewünschte physikalische Minimaldosis
im Bereich eines Scheidencarcinoms ermitteln, wenn man die Regeln für die von PATERSON
und PARKER beschriebene Radiumimplantationstechnik beachtet. Im allgemeinen werden
hier Spickungen nur in einer Ebene in Betracht kommen, wobei die Spicknadelanordnung

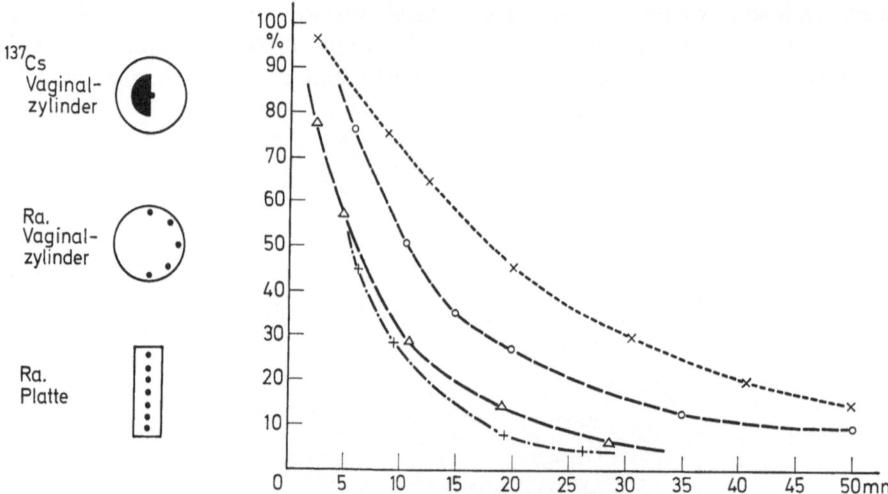

Abb. 5a. Tiefendosen bei verschiedenen Formen vaginaler Curietherapie. Die Abbildung zeigt deutlich die Erhöhung der relativen Tiefendosis bei Ausnutzung des gesamten verfügbaren Genitaltrakts als Träger einer axial angeordneten intrakavitären Curietherapie, aber auch die dadurch bedingte Erhöhung der Gesamtvolumendosis. ×······× Axial vaginal+intrauterin; ○————○ axial vaginal ^{137}Cs; △———△ Ra 5 mm Abstand (Platte 12 cm²); +—·—·—·+ Ra 3 mm Abstand (Platte 5 cm²)

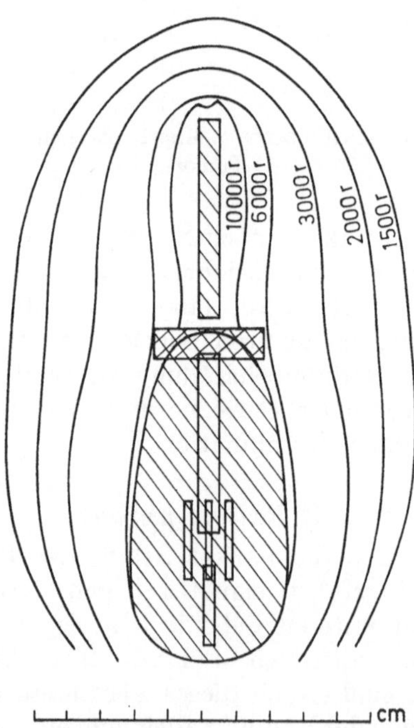

Abb. 5b. Kombination intrauteriner und vaginaler Radiumeinlagen mit zugehörigen Isodosen bei fraktionierter Anwendung

parallel zueinander und zur Scheidenachse gelegen sein wird. Eine quer zur Scheidenrichtung zum Abschluß einer bespickten Ebene vorgesehene Radiumnadel wird wegen der räumlichen Enge häufig nicht gut genug zu plazieren sein. Darum ist es bei der Spickung des Scheidencarcinoms besonders wichtig, daß die freien Enden der Spicknadel in der Längsrichtung das makroskopisch erkennbare Tumorgebiet deutlich überschreiten, um unter allen Umständen eine unterdosierte offene Endzone zu vermeiden. Eine Spikkung in 2 Ebenen (two plane implant) nach Paterson und Parker, wie sie z.B. auch von Murphy für ausgedehntere, auch für ringförmige Scheidencarcinome in Betracht gezogen wird, ist im deutschen Sprachgebiet im allgemeinen nicht üblich gewesen, weil man sich für diese Indikationen meist dazu entschieden hat, unter Ausnutzung der Zeitfaktorvorteile fraktioniert zu behandeln, d.h. schichtweise oder schrittweise abzutragen, was mit einer der intrakavitären Radiummethoden unter gleichzeitiger Beobachtung des Fortschritts der Heilung leicht möglich ist. Die bei Spickmethoden angewandten durchschnittlichen Strahlendosen liegen in der Größenordnung von 8000—9000 rad in 6 bis 10 Tagen. Auch die Höhe dieser Dosen, die für eine sichere Anwendung der Spickmethode und eine vollständige Tumorvernichtung notwendig sind, betont die Notwendigkeit, die Spickmethode auf kleinere und bei Inspektion übersichtliche Geschwülste zu begrenzen, um katastrophale Schädigungen an Nachbargeweben und Organen zu vermeiden. Jedenfalls müssen Scheidenkrebse von mehr als 3 cm Durchmesser als nicht mehr spickbar gelten. Sie sollten einer Kombination intrakavitärer Curietherapie mit percutanen Bestrahlungsmethoden zugeführt werden.

Abweichungen von diesen Grundsätzen sind unter der Voraussetzung besonderer Umstände gelegentlich statthaft. MURPHY aus dem Roswell Park Memorial Institute, Buffalo, berichtete beispielsweise über einen einschlägigen Fall, bei dem etwa $1/_2$ Jahr vor der Krankenhausaufnahme durch den behandelnden Arzt eine kleine Tumormasse hoch oben im Septum recto-vaginale gefunden worden war. Die Patientin erschien mit einer vergrößerten Tumormasse, die sich histologisch als Plattenepithelcarcinom erwies, und war gleichzeitig im 3. Monat gravide. Die Behandlung bestand in einer Radongoldseeds-Implantation in einer Fläche von etwa 8 cm². Die Gesamtdosis betrug bei $8 \times 1,3$ mCi nach den Dosistafeln von QUIMBY ca. 20000 R in 0,5 cm oberhalb des Zentrums der umspickten Fläche. Der Tumor bildete sich vollkommen zurück, $4^1/_2$ Monate später wurde ein normales Kind auf normalem Wege zur Welt gebracht. Auch 14 Jahre später war kein Tumorrezidiv feststellbar.

c) Intravaginale Röntgenbestrahlung

In dem bekannten Lehrbuch der „Strahlenbehandlung des Krebses mit Radium- und Röntgenstrahlen" betonen R. PATERSON und M. TOD am Ende des Abschnitts über die Behandlung des Scheidenkrebses:

"X-ray treatment is never indicated for cancer of the vagina. Local radium application is superior for the primary growth and the method of spread is too uncertain to justify the irradiation of large volumes."

Als diese Worte 1948 gedruckt wurden, lag die Einführung des Hohlanodenrohres durch SCHÄFER und WITTE in die Strahlentherapie gynäkologischer Carcinome bereits 16 Jahre zurück. Das Verfahren der intravaginalen Röntgenbestrahlung mit Hilfe des Körperhöhlenrohres hatte in den Händen erfahrener Strahlentherapeuten der Göttinger Universitäts-Frauenklinik unter MARTIUS mit seinen Mitarbeitern, ERICHSEN, KEPP u.a., seine Bewährungsprobe längst bestanden. Vor allem R. K. KEPP hat sich mit besonderem Nachdruck für die Verwendung des Körperhöhlenrohres gerade auch beim Scheidencarcinom eingesetzt und betont, welche großen Vorteile darin liegen können, mit einem ähnlich steilen Dosisabfall wie bei der Radiumkontaktbestrahlung gezielt zu bestrahlen und gleichzeitig eine hohe Fraktionierung anzuwenden. Ähnlich wie bei der Göttinger Methode zur Bestrahlung des Collumcarcinoms des Uterus haben MARTIUS und seine Schüler auf die Tumorgrenzfläche zum normalen Umgebungsgewebe, d.h. hier aber in 2—5 cm Tiefe von der Vaginalschleimhaut gerechnet, 12×200 R beim Scheidencarcinom häufig auch unter Einsatz des sog. „Abflachtubus" gegeben, eine Dosis, die, je nach der Tiefenlage, die für die Grenze zwischen Tumor und Normalgewebe angenommen wurde, das 5—10fache an dem höchstbelasteten Gebiet der Scheidenschleimhaut bedeuten kann. Die Göttinger Schule beschreibt die Abheilung der Vaginalcarcinome über einen grünlichweißlich belegten „Strahlenschorf"; sie betont außerdem die besonders hohe Strahlenresistenz der Vaginalschleimhaut unter den Bedingungen der fraktionierten Kleinraumbestrahlung, d.h. mit der intravaginalen Nahbestrahlung. Sie gibt die Toleranzgrenze für die Scheidenschleimhaut mit 30000—40000 R in 4—6 Wochen an, wobei eine exsudative Reaktion, eine vorübergehende nekrotisierende Ulceration, die unter entsprechender Pflege abheilt, in Kauf genommen wird. Es leuchtet ein, daß dieses Verfahren, der Radiumspickung vergleichbar, sich für örtlich begrenzte Scheidentumoren besonders

4*

gut eignet. Für größere Scheidencarcinome, vor allem aber auch für zirkulär wachsende Tumoren, wurde auch von dieser Schule, deren Technik in Deutschland in den 40er und 50er Jahren von vielen mit Vorliebe angewandt wurde, die intravaginale Radiumeinlage bevorzugt.

Im übrigen plädiert Kepp 1941 für die alleinige intravaginale und damit kombinierte percutane Röntgentherapie unter Verzicht auf Radium, wenn es sich nicht um zirkulär wachsende Tumoren handelt. Gute erste Erfahrungen mit der alleinigen Schäfer-Witte-Behandlung berichtet u.a. Weibel, der 3 von 5 inoperablen Scheidencarcinomen 1 Jahr nach Behandlungsbeginn ohne Rezidiv sah; ferner Herold aus Prag 1956, der 1935—1944 mit kombinierter Radium-Röntgenbehandlung 11 von 38 Fällen heilen konnte: 28,9% 5-Jahresheilungen. 1940—1944, d.h. nach Einführung des Körperhöhlenrohres, betrug die Heilungsziffer 41% (7 von 17 so behandelte Patientinnen). Herold glaubte somit, auf die Überlegenheit des Körperhöhlenrohres schließen zu können.

Kepp hat immer wieder betont, daß das Verfahren des Körperhöhlenrohres nicht verwechselt werden dürfte mit einem intravaginalen Konus, angeschlossen an eine Tiefen-therapieröhre, wie von amerikanischen Autoren, z.B. Twombly und Chamberlain, zur Behandlung des Collumcarcinoms beschrieben. Der grundlegende Unterschied ist durch den beim Hohlanodenrohr vorhandenen kurzen Focus-Schleimhautabstand von höchstens 5 cm gegeben, der den gewünschten steilen Dosisabfall gewährleistet.

Mit dem Aufkommen differenzierterer lokalisierter Curietherapie, der Lösung der hierbei auftretenden dosimetrischen Probleme und mit zunehmender Verfügbarkeit der sehr wirksamen Megavolttherapie ist das Interesse an der Verwendung des Körperhöhlenrohres wieder in den Hintergrund getreten.

d) Behandlung mit künstlich radioaktiven Stoffen

Auch das Scheidencarcinom ist, wie mit Radium und anderen natürlich radioaktiven Substanzen, mit künstlichen Gammastrahlern behandelt worden. Die Gesichtspunkte, die zu einer Bevorzugung der künstlichen Radioisotope gegenüber dem klassischen Radium führen könnten, liegen

a) in der guten Verfügbarkeit,

b) in der Wählbarkeit von Strahlenenergie und

c) in der Wählbarkeit der physikalischen Halbwertzeit, so daß bei kurzlebigen Präparaten permanente Implantationen und Inkorporationen möglich werden.

Sofern es sich also bei der Wahl künstlich radioaktiver Stoffe zur Behandlung des Scheidencarcinoms nicht nur um einen einfachen Ersatz des nicht leicht verfügbaren Radiums handelte, so sind einige physikalische und technische Gesichtspunkte ausschlaggebend für die Wahl gewesen. Dabei wurde an folgendes gedacht:

α) Plastobalt bzw. Makrobalt (nach Becker und Scheer)

Bei Makrobalt handelt es sich um mit Radiokobaltpulver durchmischte Plexiglaskügelchen, die in eine knetbare plastische Masse eingebettet sind und daher in jede der Anatomie angepaßte, für die Therapie notwendige äußere Form leicht gebracht werden können. Makrobalt ist daher, in Cellophansäckchen eingepackt, auch für die Behandlung des Scheidencarcinoms verwendet worden.

Die Deformierung von Makrobalt in die gewünschte Form ist offenbar bequemer und geht wesentlich rascher vonstatten als die Anfertigung von Radiummoulagen aus Stentsmasse, die hier allenfalls als Konkurrenzmethode mit natürlichen Strahlern in Betracht kommen.

Es ist im Zusammenhang mit dem Makrobalt zu erwähnen, daß praktisch die gesamte Masse homogen strahlt, ohne daß eine wesentliche Autoabsorption im Strahler selbst stattfände. Die Methode stellt also, ähnlich wie der Vaginalradiumapplikator von E. Maier, ein System dar, mit dessen Hilfe der gelegentlich allzu steile Dosisabfall bei einer Kontakttherapie abgemildert wird. Als einen Nachteil der Anwendung von Makrobalt beim Scheidencarcinom muß man gewiß die Tatsache ansehen, daß die knetbare Masse allseitig und homogen strahlt. Die Dosisleistung des Strahlers wird nur an jenen Teilen der Oberfläche niedriger, wo die strahlende Substanz dünner ist, d.h. also, daß Makrobalt sich im wesentlichen dort bewähren kann, wo die ganze Scheidenlänge in ein starres Carcinomrohr umgewandelt ist. Bei einseitig gelegenen Scheidencarcinomen wäre es nicht möglich, die gegenüberliegende Scheidenwand in wünschenswerter Weise zu schonen, es sei denn, daß man den Strahler als Ersatz für eine Radiumpräparation plattenförmig deformiert nach der gewünschten räumlichen Strahlungsverteilung, gegebenenfalls auch asymmetrisch verdickt oder verdünnt und wie eine Radiumplatte im Kontakt anwendet, d.h. die gegenüberliegenden Abschnitte der Scheidenwand durch Tamponade distanziert. Hiermit wäre aber der ursprüngliche Verwendungszweck des Makrobalt bereits variiert. Größere Erfahrungen über die Anwendung von Makrobalt beim Scheidencarcinom sind bisher nicht bekanntgeworden, wohl wegen der großen Seltenheit der Scheidencarcinome und der in den großen Behandlungszentren selbstverständlichen Verfügbarkeit ausreichender Radiummengen.

Als Nachteil ist die Tatsache anzusehen, daß es sich bei diesen radioaktiven Präparaten nicht um ein nach der Begriffsbestimmung der 1. Strahlenschutzverordnung umschlossenes Präparat handelt; daß Spuren radioaktiven Antriebs nicht auszuschließen sind, das ist wohl der wesentliche Grund, weshalb der Hersteller seit einigen Jahren dieses sehr interessante Produkt nicht mehr anbietet. Es repräsentiert in der Tat eine der interessantesten Ideen der modernen Radionuklidära der medizinischen Radiologie.

β) Spickung mit Radionukliden

Da Radoncapillaren, welche als kurzlebige Strahler zur *permanenten Implantation* beim Scheidencarcinom dienen konnten, wegen der Abschaffung der notwendigen Abpumpanlagen nicht mehr in genügendem Umfange zu erhalten sind, lag es nahe, einen kurzlebigen Gammastrahler, nämlich *metallisches* ^{198}Au für den gleichen Zweck zu benutzen, entsprechend den Vorschlägen von W. G. Myers und B. H. Colmery. Diese bereits 1951 eingeführte Methode ist in den nachfolgenden Jahren besonders von H. Henschke u. Mitarb. und anschließend von vielen anderen vervollkommnet und zuletzt für das Scheidencarcinom von Kapp-Schwoerer und Busch gegenüber anderen Methoden der lokalisierten Curietherapie bevorzugt worden. Die physikalische Halbwertszeit von 2,7 Tagen, der hohe Neutroneneinfangquerschnitt von ^{197}Au und damit die leichte Herstellbarkeit von ^{198}Au, dessen monochromatische Gammastrahlung von 411 keV, die leichte Abschirmbarkeit der Betastrahlung des Radiogolds durch einen metallischen Überzug aus Platin-Iridium und nicht zuletzt die günstigen metallurgischen Eigenschaften des leicht zu bearbeitenden Edelmetalles stellen sehr günstige Eigenschaften dar. Es kommt hinzu, daß durch mehrere Autoren, in Deutschland durch W. Hellriegel, in England durch den Hoed und Sinclair, geeignete Instrumente für die Radiogoldimplantation geschaffen wurden („Implantationspistole"). In Deutschland haben sich besonders Becker und Scheer sowie Schumacher und Frost für die Radiogoldspickmethoden eingesetzt.

Günstige klinische Erfahrungen hatten, wie gesagt, Kapp-Schwoerer u. Mitarb. beim Scheidencarcinom. Dabei wird eine Gewebeminimaldosis, die nach den Verfahren von Minder, von Frost und schließlich von Kapp-Schwoerer und Busch berechnet werden kann, in der Höhe von 6000—8000 rad einzeitig bei entsprechend den physikalischen Konstanten der Radionuklide fallender Dosisleistung in praktisch 3—4 Halbwertzeiten angestrebt. In Einzelfällen, besonders bei kleineren Tumoren, sind wohl auch 10000 rad eine noch tragbare Gewebebelastung. Als ein besonderer Vorteil der Radiogoldspickung des Scheidencarcinoms hat Kapp-Schwoerer die Möglichkeit hervorgehoben, unmittelbar benachbarte empfindliche Organe, trotz der sehr hohen Strahlenexposition des Tumors, verhältnismäßig niedrigen Dosen auszusetzen. Das von ihm demonstrierte Beispiel eines nahezu die gesamte Scheidenlänge an der Vorderwand einnehmenden Carcinoms könnte so behandelt werden, daß im Tumor die Strahlendosis zwischen ca. 6 000 und 10 000 R betrug, während der Blasenboden weniger als 5 000 R, die Mastdarmvorderwand mit nur 3 000—4 000 R belastet wurden. Der Autor hat hier aber offenbar eine intrauterine Curietherapie nicht ausgeführt. Eine Zusatzbehandlung der vom Primärtumor entfernter gelegenen Gewebeteile des kleinen Beckens hat er offensichtlich mit Hilfe eines Telekobaltgeräts angestrebt, in die von ihm vorgelegten Darstellungen der Dosisverteilung aber nicht einbezogen.

Außer ^{198}Au sind von Henschke (USA) und Pierquin (Frankreich) modernere Methoden der interstitiellen Curietherapie mit ^{192}Ir-Drähten, von F. Ellis (England) mit ^{182}Ta auch für das Vaginalcarcinom ausgearbeitet worden. Die systematisierte Weiterentwicklung der von Henschke inaugurierten Afterloading-Technik hat am Institut Gustave Roussy, Villejuif, durch B. Pierquin stattgefunden, dessen Methoden die besonderen metallurgischen und radiophysikalischen Vorteile des ^{192}Ir ausnutzt (Halbwertzeit 74d, maximale β-Energie 0,67 MeV, mittlere γ-Energie 0,3 MeV, Dosisleistungskonstante 5 R/h in 1 cm/mCi).

Bei aller Eleganz aller Spickmethoden, die ganz gewiß ihren endgültigen Platz in der modernen Radiotherapie behalten werden, sind auch einige prinzipielle Nachteile nicht zu übersehen, nämlich die dabei unvermeidliche, sehr stark inhomogene räumliche Dosisverteilung. Günstige Erfahrungen bei der percutanen Siebbestrahlung völlig inkurabler Tumoren können hier nicht als Vergleichsmodell dienen. Dosislücken kleineren Ausmaßes bei nicht erreichbarer Idealgeometrie der Verteilung der Strahler müssen bei kurablen Tumoren sich unter Umständen als Katastrophe auswirken. Darüber täuschen auch nicht computerproduzierte Isodosenbilder hinweg, in denen die erwähnten Dosislücken zeichnerisch elegant überdeckt oder infolge der nicht genügend engmaschigen Darstellung verwischt sind.

γ) Intrakavitäre Caesium-Therapie

Die unmittelbare Nachbarschaft strahlenempfindlicher Organe, wie Blase und Mastdarm, aber auch die Notwendigkeit, etwa vorhandene Tumorausläufer im paravaginalen Bindegewebe mit ausreichender Strahlendosis zu erfassen, haben zu dem Wunsche geführt, der Tumorform angepaßte und reproduzierbare räumliche Dosisverteilungen zu verwirklichen (ohne gleichzeitig durch eine Implantations- oder Injektionsmethode das Tumorgebiet selbst zu traumatisieren). Für diesen Zweck eignete sich ein Strahler besonders gut, der ähnlich wie Radium in Vaginalzylindern aus leichtatomigem Material, beispielsweise aus Plexiglas oder besser noch aus einem kochbaren Kunststoff, axial angeordnet werden kann. Die Strahlenqualität sollte gleichzeitig so weich sein, daß sie durch Schwermetallschichten nicht allzu großer Dicke, d.h. akzeptablen Gewichtes, auf wenigstens ein Drittel der Ausgangsdosisleistung geschwächt werden kann. Auf diese Weise wird die räumliche Dosisverteilung um einen solchen Zylinder durch Lage und Stärke der radioaktiven Röhrchen, ferner durch Einschalten oder Fortlassen einer Gammastrahlen absorbierenden Schicht modellierbar. Wichtig war für die Wahl des Strahlers die Bedingung auch einer nicht zu kurzen physikalischen Halbwertzeit, um ein allzu häufiges Erneuern des radioaktiven Materials zu vermeiden. Unter den leicht erhältlichen Gammastrahlern mittlerer Quantenenergie kommt den genannten Wünschen am ehesten das ^{137}Cs nahe, das als ein Spaltprodukt des Urans mit einer Häufigkeit von etwa 6 % anfällt und dessen physikalische Halbwertzeit mit etwa 30 Jahren angegeben wird. ^{137}Cs ist zwar ein reiner Betastrahler, aber sein kurzlebiges Übergangsprodukt ^{137}Barium, mit dem das ^{137}Cs im Gleichgewicht steht, sendet eine mittelharte monochromatische Gammastrahlung von 0,662 MeV aus.

Die Halbwertschichtdicke in Wolfram für ^{137}Cs-Gammastrahlungspräparate beträgt 3,9 mm. ^{137}Cs-Sulfat ist in 15 mm langen Monel-Normalröhrchen mit 0,3 mm Wandstärke und einer Beladung von 50 mCi ^{137}Cs pro Röhrchen erhältlich.

Die für die Strahlenbehandlung vaginaler Tumorausbreitungen konstruierten Kunststoff-Vaginalzylinder nach GAUWERKY gestatten eine axiale Belegung bis zu 6 Caesium-Normalröhrchen. Durch entsprechend geformte Abschirmkörper aus Wolfram-Metall von 6 mm effektiver Dicke kann die Strahlung entweder in einem Winkel von 180° oder 270° bis auf ein Drittel geschwächt werden, so daß es möglich ist, eine Reihe von stets gleichen Isodosen zu verwirklichen (Abb. 6a). Zwei verschiedene Stärken von Vaginalzylindern mit

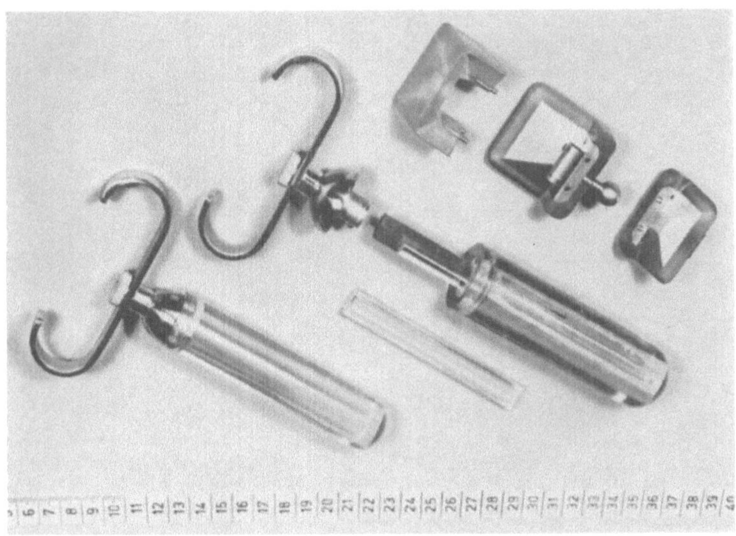

Abb. 6a. Caesiumvaginalzylinder aus kochbarem Kunststoff

Tabelle 2. *Dosierungstabelle zur Behandlung mit* ^{137}Cs*-Vaginalzylinder. Die in der Tabelle wiedergegebene Dosisleistung gilt nur für einen definierten Zeitpunkt. Entsprechend dem physikalischen Zerfall muß der Tabellenwert und damit die Dauer für eine gewünschte Dosis am Punkte des Interesses einmal jährlich korrigiert werden. (Dosisleistung der Vaginalzylinder in R/h; Kontaktmessungen über Mitte der Aktivität)*

⌀	mCi ^{137}Cs	D_{max}	D_{min}	D_{wo}
2,5 cm	300 (6)	175	135	50
	150 (3)	150	120	42
	100 (2)	115	92	30
3,0 cm	300 (6)	135	110	40
	150 (3)	115	92	35
	100 (2)	90	72	25

Durchmessern von 2,5 bzw. 3 cm ermöglichen volle Ausnutzung des zur Verfügung stehenden Vaginalraums. Musterbeispiele sind bildlich wiedergegeben (Abb. 6b). Man muß sich darüber im klaren sein, daß solche Dosisverteilungsfiguren bei Verwendung der harten Gammastrahlung des ^{60}Co oder des Radiums nur bei Verwendung von Schwermetall-abschirmkörpern unzumutbaren Gewichtes zustande kämen. Die dargestellten Möglichkeiten der Variation können noch vermehrt werden durch Änderung der Verteilung der radioaktiven Substanz, ferner durch Kombination mit anderen Strahlern, beispielsweise mit Radiumkontakttherapie oder Intrauterinbehandlung. Das Dosierungssystem kann sich aus der Dosisleistung an der „heißesten" Stelle an der Oberfläche des Caesium-Vaginal-zylinders ergeben. Dabei erfordert die um 1,5 mm paraaxial gelegene Bohrung der Caesium-Zylinder, welche die Tube mit der Radioaktivität aufnimmt, eine Mitteilung über die Oberfläche, woraus sich eine einfache tabellarisch ablesbare Korrektur ergibt (Tabelle 2).

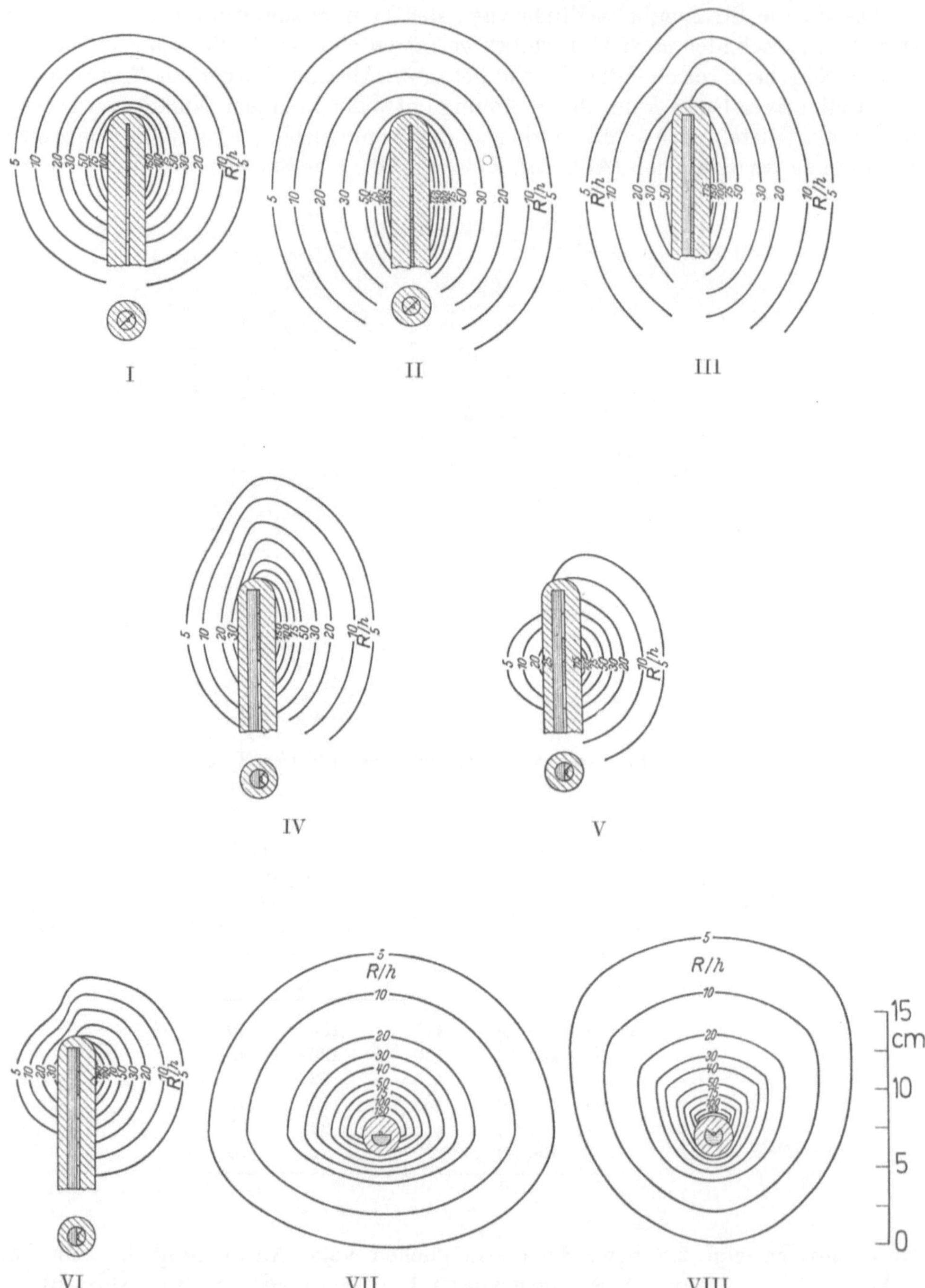

Abb. 6b. Einige Isodosen um den Caesiumvaginalzylinder mit voller oder teilweiser Belegung mit und ohne einseitige Wolframabschirmung. I: Längsschnitt durch den Vaginalzylinder. Isodosen in R/h bei 150 mCi ^{137}Caesium. Keine Abschirmung. II: Längsschnitt durch den Vaginalzylinder. Isodosen in R/h bei 300 mCi ^{137}Caesium. Keine Abschirmung. III: Längsschnitt durch den Vaginalzylinder. Isodosen in R/h bei 300 mCi ^{137}Caesium. Halbseitenabschirmung mit 6 mm Wolfram. IV: Längsschnitt durch den Vaginalzylinder. Isodosen in R/h bei 150 mCi ^{137}Caesium. 180° oder 27° Abschirmung mit 6 mm Wolfram. V: Längsschnitt durch den Vaginalzylinder. Isodosen in R/h bei 100 mCi ^{137}Caesium. 180° oder 270° Abschirmung mit 6 mm Wolfram. VI: Längsschnitt durch den Vaginalzylinder. Isodosen in R/h bei 100 mCi ^{137}Caesium. 180° oder 270° Abschirmung mit 6 mm Wolfram. VII: Querschnitt durch den Vaginalzylinder. Isodosen in R/h bei 300 mCi ^{137}Caesium. 270° Abschirmung mit 6 mm Wolfram. VIII: Querschnitt durch den Vaginalzylinder. Isodosen in R/h bei 300 mCi ^{137}Caesium. 180° Abschirmung mit 6 mm Wolfram

Als ein besonderer Vorteil der Anwendung von Caesium-Vaginalzylindern mag zusammenfassend hervorgehoben werden:

1. die eindeutig reproduzierte räumliche Dosisverteilung, auch bei mehreren zeitlich getrennten Applikationen, ohne unübersichtliche Dosisinhomogenitäten;

2. die Einfachheit und Sicherheit der Handhabung, welche die unangenehme und unhygienische Scheidentamponade überflüssig macht;

3. die Sicherheit, mit der das tumortragende und das potentiell tumortragende Gebiet erfaßt wird;

4. die Schonsamkeit des Verfahrens für das nicht mit Höchstdosen belastete Gewebe.

e) Ultraharte Tiefentherapie beim Scheidencarcinom

Die hohen relativen Tiefendosen, die Möglichkeit, infolge eines physikalischen Aufbaueffektes die Oberhaut und bei ultraharten Photonen eines Vielfachbeschleunigers auch das Unterhautgebiet zu schonen, die bessere Verträglichkeit im Hinblick auf die allgemeinen Reaktionen und schließlich die Vermeidung höherer Strahlenabsorption im Knochen lassen es beim Carcinom im weiblichen Genitaltrakt und somit auch beim Scheidencarcinom geraten erscheinen, ultraharte Strahlenqualitäten, d.h. Photonen mit einer Quantenenergie von 1 MeV und mehr, wo irgend verfügbar, zu bevorzugen. Dabei wird man aber nur bei sehr ausgedehnten Tumoren auf die Möglichkeit, eine hohe lokale Dosis durch Curietherapie zu applizieren, verzichten wollen. Ausschließliche percutane Bestrahlung des Scheidencarcinoms ist also ein Ausnahmefall, eine Behandlungsmaßnahme mit meist begrenztem, palliativem Ziel. Dieser Gesichtspunkt gilt — von wenigen Ausnahmen abgesehen — um so mehr, als bei alleiniger Bestrahlung von außen auf ausgedehnte Tumoren eine vollständige Erfassung des erkrankten Gebietes nur durch eine gleichmäßige Durchstrahlung großer Abschnitte des kleinen Beckens erzielt werden kann. Die an sich wünschenswerte Taktik mit dem Ziel, den Tumor selbst mit sehr hoher Strahlendosis in der Größenordnung von 8 000—10 000 R, seine Ausläufer und das potentiell tumortragende Gebiet aber mit einer kleineren Dosis, d.h. mit etwa 4 000—6 000 R zu bestrahlen („Stufenbestrahlung"), ist hier nicht mehr erreichbar. Aus solchen Überlegungen ergibt sich, daß die Bestrahlung von außen mit ultraharten Photonen für die Mehrzahl der Fälle von Vaginalcarcinomen eine Zusatzbehandlung zur lokalen Curietherapie darstellt.

Unter den heutigen technischen Voraussetzungen wird die percutane Zusatzbestrahlung am besten ausgeführt mit Beschleunigungsmaschinen vom Typ des Linearaccellerators oder durch einen Kreisbeschleuniger (Betatron). Eine Alternative stellt der Einsatz einer Telekobaltbestrahlungsanlage dar. Sehr häufig sind beim gynäkologischen Carcinom das ganze kleine Becken erfassende ventro-dorsale Gegenfelder verwendet worden, mit deren Hilfe, bei Kreisbeschleunigern gelegentlich auch unter Zuhilfenahme von seitlichen Gegenfeldern ergänzt, eine homogene Durchstrahlung des Raumes des kleinen Beckens erzielt wird. Dabei ist es aber, ebenso wie bei der Telekobalttherapie, mit ventro-dorsalen Gegenfeldern unmöglich, eine erhebliche Mitbestrahlung sicher nicht tumortragender Gewebe zu vermeiden (s. Abb. 7). Das gilt besonders dann, wenn es sich um ^{60}Co-Photonen handelt, bei deren Anwendung in Gegenfeldern ein vom Patientendurchmesser abhängiger, mehr oder minder großer zentraler „Durchhang" (Abb. 8) zustande kommt. Diese Nachteile lassen sich durch den Einsatz von Rotationsbestrahlungsmethoden individueller Technik, beispielsweise durch Zweizentrenrotation mit verschiedenem Abstand der Rotationsachsen oder aber durch die von HEINZEL vorgeschlagene Vierzentrenrotation herabsetzen bzw. ausschließen, gewiß auch durch die Methode der biaxialen Pendelung nach den Vorschlägen von FRISCHBIER. Die Vierzentrenrotation bewährt sich in unserem Hause bei allen gynäkologischen Carcinomen (gegenseitiger Abstand der Rotationsachsen von

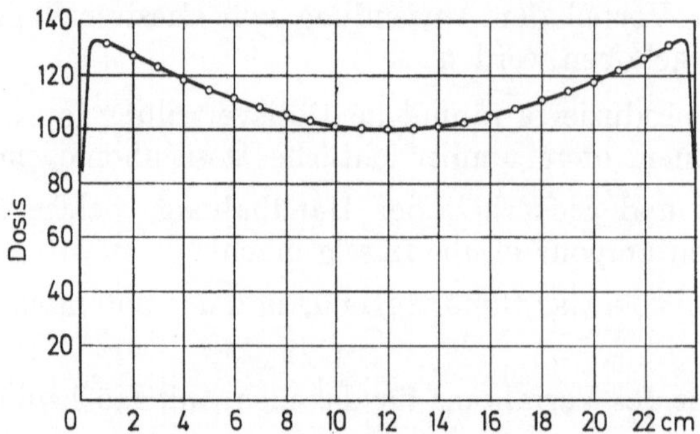

Abb. 7. Dosisverteilung im Wasserphantom mit 24 cm Durchmesser bei parallel opponierenden Feldern, ^{60}Co und Feldgröße 10×10. Bemerkenswert ist der Dosisdurchhang in Phantommitte

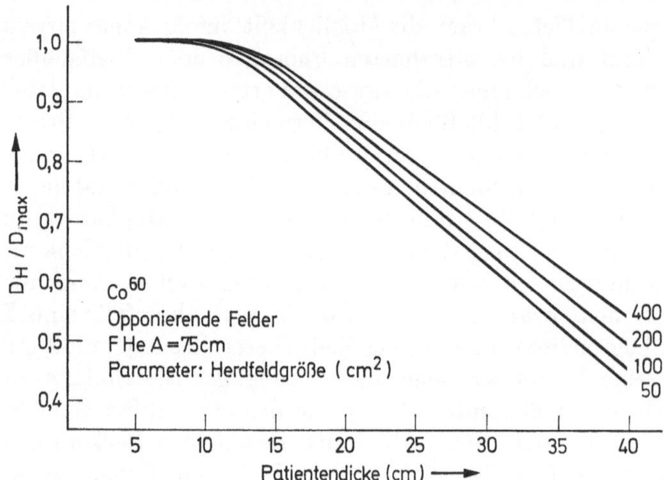

Abb. 8. Relative Dosis in der Achse eines Phantoms oder im Patientenkörper bei opponierender Einstrahlung mit dem Telekobaltgerät in Abhängigkeit vom Patientendurchmesser und der Herdfeldgröße in Quadratzentimetern. Man erkennt, daß der in Patientenmitte vorliegende Dosisdurchhang oberhalb von 12 cm Durchmesser kritische Größen annehmen kann und bei gegebener Zentraldosis unerwünscht hohe Maxima im Unterhautgebiet auftreten können (Gefahr der Unterhautfibrose)

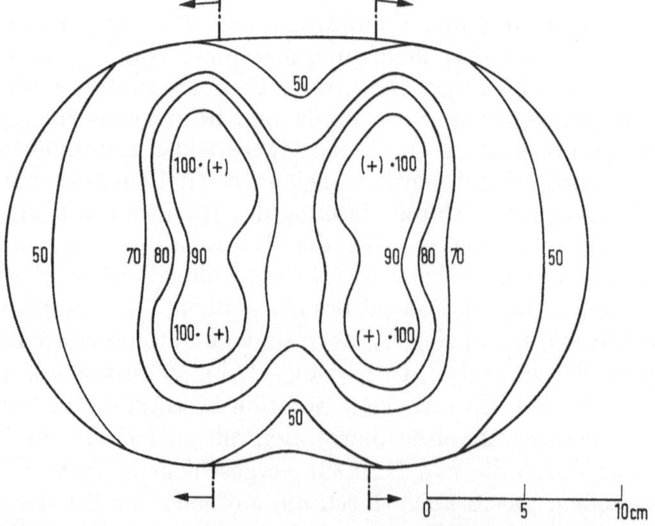

Abb. 9 a. Isodosendiagramm bei Vierzentrenrotation mit Telekobaltteilrotation um 4 Zentren um je 180°, Feldbreite 5 cm. Die in einer Ebene liegenden Rotationszentren sind 8 cm voneinander entfernt. (Nach Heinzel)

4 cm), bei denen eine zentrale Radium- oder Caesium-Applikation in Kombination durchgeführt wird. Die Vorteile des Verfahrens werden aus der Isodosenabbildung deutlich. Individuelle Variationen sind zulässig und gegebenenfalls empfehlenswert (Abb. 9a und b).

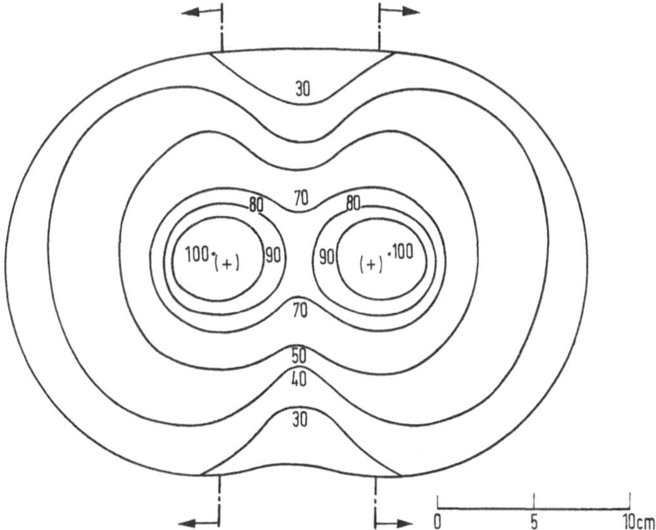

Abb. 9b. Isodosendiagramm bei Telekobaltzweizentrenrotation nach HEINZEL. Diese Anordnung wird bei schlanken Patientinnen gegenüber der Vierzentrenrotation bevorzugt

f) Bestrahlungsmethoden von Scheidencarcinomen im Allgemeinen Krankenhaus St. Georg

Im Mittelpunkt der Behandlung steht eine *lokalisierte Curietherapie*. Bei sehr *kleinen Tumoren* bis zu einem Durchmesser von 3 cm bei Sitz im unteren Scheidendrittel kann sie als Radiumspickung oder als Radioiridiumspickung ausgeführt werden, wobei die lokale „Minimal"-Dosis nicht mehr als 8000—9000 R betragen darf.

Bei *mittelgroßen* und ausgedehnteren *Tumoren* mit Sitz im mittleren und erstrecht bei Sitz im oberen Scheidendrittel, ferner bei Tumoren, die die Scheidenlänge zu $^2/_3$ oder mehr ergriffen haben, *Caesium-Vaginalzylinder* mit Belegung der ganzen Länge oder eines Teiles der verfügbaren Achse mit oder ohne Schwermetallabschirmung nach der nicht vom Tumor befallenen Scheidenwand mit einer Dosis von 3mal 1500 R an der maximal belasteten Schleimhautstelle im Verlaufe von 4 Wochen, kombiniert mit *Radium-Intrauterinbehandlung* (33 mg ^{226}Ra für 120 h) und mit percutaner *Tiefenbestrahlung* des kleinen Beckens nach der Methode der Vierzentrenrotation mit der Telekobaltanlage bis zu einer zusätzlichen Herddosis im Parametrium und Parakolpium von etwa 3000 R im Verlaufe von 3 Wochen, bei sehr schlanken Patientinnen ausnahmsweise nach der oben beschriebenen 8-Feldertechnik mit Orthovolt-Röntgentiefentherapie (200—300 kV Röhrenspannung). Individuelle Abweichungen von den symmetrischen Verfahren sind entsprechend dem Tumorsitz möglich.

Tumoren des hinteren Scheidengewölbes werden wie Collumcarcinome bestrahlt. Im Tumor werden auf diese Weise Herddosen von 6000—7000 rad in 4 Wochen erreicht, während im potentiell tumortragenden Gewebe außerhalb des Primärtumors, d.h. in den regionalen Lymphknotengebieten, niedrigere Gewebedosen zustande kommen. Dieses von der klassischen Forderung nach homogener Dosis im gesamten Zielgebiet abweichende Verfahren ist bei der großräumigen Abmessung des regionalen Lymphknotengebietes im kleinen Becken unvermeidlich und gelegentlich als Stufenbestrahlung (GAUWERKY) bezeichnet worden. Die Stufenbestrahlung erlaubt außerdem die dringend erforderliche Schonung von Blase und Mastdarm in ausreichendem Umfang.

Pendelkonvergenzbestrahlung, beispielsweise mit dem TU 1 als Zusatzbestrahlung zur lokalen Curietherapie, wird z.Z. nicht angewendet, weil die mit dieser Technik möglichen Zielvolumina im allgemeinen zu klein sind.

Es ist im A. K. St. Georg, Hamburg, selbstverständlich, daß jede Tiefenbestrahlung, insbesondere auch die Telekobalttherapie, nach Anfertigung eines individuellen Körperquerschnitts mit dem Zeichengerät geplant und berechnet wird.

4. Klinische Verläufe, Komplikationen

a) Normale Verläufe im günstigen Fall

Fall 1. 53jährige Hausfrau, bei der seit einem Vierteljahr nach körperlichen Anstrengungen über hexenschußartige Rückenschmerzen geklagt wird.

Bei gynäkologischer Untersuchung wird ein Scheidentumor festgestellt, der zur Klinikeinweisung führt. An der Scheidenhinterwand ein zungenförmiger, sulziger, länglicher, ulcerierter Tumor mit aufgeworfenen Rändern, der etwa die obere Hälfte der Scheide einnimmt und gleich unterhalb der Portio im Vaginalgewölbe beginnt. Die Portio selbst ist gerötet, blutet bei Berührung, ist jedoch von Tumormassen frei. Histologisch: nicht verhornendes Plattenepithelcarcinom.

Behandlung: Lange, schmale Radiumplatte (69,3 mg Ra.El.) 24 h direkt auf den Tumor der hinteren Scheidenwand tamponiert, gleichzeitig kleine Platte (2×6,6 mg Ra.El.) 26 h vor die Portio aufrecht tamponiert. Reaktion mit erheblichen Durchfällen etwa eine Woche nach Behandlungsbeginn und für eine Woche anhaltend. 4 Wochen später Wiederholung der individuell geplanten Radiumapplikation auf die Vaginalhinterwand sowie vor die Portio aufrecht. Dosismessungen im Rectum mit dem Bomke-Momentan-Dosimeter ergaben eine Gesamtdosis von etwa 8000 R, so daß an der Tumoroberfläche etwa 10000 R vermutet werden müssen. Ferner wurde eine Röntgentiefenbestrahlung der Leistenbeugen mit 10×300 R ausgeführt, da hier beiderseits, rechts mehr als links, kleine derbe Lymphome zu tasten waren. Bei Behandlungsabschluß bestand eine kräftige exsudative Strahlenreaktion der Mucosa mit weißlichen Fibrinbelägen, während die Tumormassen sich in die Vagina abgestoßen hatten. Die Patientin ist 9 Jahre nach Behandlungsbeginn beobachtet worden und während dieser Zeit rezidivfrei geblieben.

Kommentar. Erfolgreiche klassische Radiumbehandlung eines ausgedehnten Carcinoms der Scheidenhinterwand ohne Komplikationen.

Fall 2. 29jährige Patientin mit 2 gut erbsgroßen Knoten an der hinteren Scheidenwand im unteren Drittel. Die Probeexcision ergab ein nicht verhornendes Plattenepithelcarcinom.

Behandlung: Radiumspickung mit 3 Nadeln zu je 4,5 mg Radiumelement für 120 h, entsprechend einer lokalen Durchschnittsdosis von nahezu 20000 R auf kleinstem Raum. Abheilen der kleinen Tumoren über eine örtliche exsudative Reaktion (ohne Ulcusbildung!). 3 Monate später ist von den vorher beschriebenen Knoten nichts mehr zu sehen oder zu fühlen. Nachuntersuchungen: Prophylaktische Bestrahlung der Leistenbeugen unter Tiefentherapiebedingungen von 8×300 R. Nachbeobachtung: 17 Jahre rezidivfrei geblieben.

Kommentar. Erfolgreiche Radiumspickung eines kleinen Scheidencarcinoms des unteren Drittels der vaginalen Hinterwand.

Fall 3. 42jährige Frau mit teilweise exophytischem, teils exulceriertem Tumor im oberen Drittel der hinteren Vaginalwand und geringer Infiltration des Septum recto-vaginale, ferner einem feinen samtartigen Tumorüberzug auf der hinteren Muttermundslippe. Parametrien und Parakolpien palpatorisch frei.

Histologie: Verhornendes Plattenepithelcarcinom. Behandlung: 2mal ^{137}Cs-Vaginalzylinder mit Wolfram-Abschirmung nach ventral, freier Strahlung nach dorsal = zusammen 5000 R; 1mal mittlere Stockholmer Platte (9×6,6 mg Ra.El.) 25 h vor die Portio tamponiert, Intrauterinstift mit 33 mg Ra.El. für 120 h. Röntgenbestrahlung der Parametrien mit Herddosen von etwa 2000 R pro Parametrium.

Abheilen des Tumors über kräftige exsudative Strahlenreaktion, in diesem Falle ohne wesentliche Proktitis. Endzustand: Narbige Obliteration der oberen Scheidenhälfte. Beobachtung bis zu 6 Jahren; kein Rezidiv.

Kommentar. Erfolgreiche Radiocaesiumbehandlung eines ausgedehnten Scheidencarcinoms des oberen Drittels ohne Komplikationen.

b) Mit Komplikationen verbundene Verläufe

Fall 4. 70jährige Frau. Im oberen Vaginaldrittel, nach dorsal und links gelegen, ein längliches, blutendes Tumorulcus von 3—4 cm Längsausdehnung. Portio frei. Tumor vom Rectum her tastbar bei derber Infiltration des linken Parametriums bis an die Beckenwand.

Histologie: Plattenepithelcarcinom.

Behandlung: Caesium-Vaginalzylinder mit 200 mCi ^{137}Cs, Wolfram-Abschirmung nach rechts, freie Strahlung nach links; maximale Oberflächendosis 3000 R; gleichzeitig Radium-Intrauterinstift 33 mg Ra.El. für 120 h, der im Tumor zusätzlich 1500 R zur Wirkung gebracht haben dürfte. 3 Wochen später erhebliche Mastdarmbeschwerden mit Blut- und Schleimabgang sowie Tenesmen. Gleichzeitig hatte sich das Tumorulcus in der Scheide wesentlich zurückgebildet, die Infiltration des linken Parametriums war aber noch vorhanden, so daß das linke Parametrium mit Pendelkonvergenzbestrahlungen auf ein 3,5×7 cm großes Herdfeld zusätzlich behandelt wurde bis zu 3000 R HD. Weitere 4 Wochen später hat die Mastdarmblutung zunächst aufgehört, aber auch in den folgenden Jahren immer wieder gelegentliche Blutabgänge, ohne daß am Rectum ein objektiver Befund noch nachweisbar wäre. 5 Jahre später kein Rezidiv.

Beurteilung. Ausgeprägte empfindliche Mastdarmreaktion bei noch unvollständiger lokaler Curietherapie eines primären Vaginalcarcinoms. Trotz der Unvollständigkeit der Therapie vollständige Tumorrückbildung bei besonders empfindlicher Gewebereaktion.

Fall 5. 60jährige Patientin mit einem etwa 2 cm langen Carcinomulcus an der linken Scheidenseitenwand ohne nachbarschaftliche Gewebeinfiltration.

Histologie: Solides Carcinom.

Behandlung: Röntgentiefentherapie nach Vierfeldertechnik. Intrauterinstift 33 mg Ra.El. für 120 h, ^{137}Caesium-Vaginalzylinder in ganzer Länge, zirkulär strahlend = 2000 R. Einen Monat später sehr erhebliche Strahlenreaktion der Scheidenschleimhaut mit exsudativem Charakter, gleichzeitig erhebliche Blasentenesmen auf Grund hämorrhagischer Cystitis. Verzicht auf weitere Curietherapie. Scheidenpflege mit Hydrocortison-Suspensionen, Blasenpflege nach urologischen Grundsätzen. Abheilen der Reaktion über 3 Monate. Scheide ist jetzt verengt und hat unelastische Wände, für den Finger aber noch gut durchgängig. 2 Jahre später am Scheideneingang links ein kleines Rezidivulcus, das mit 3 kleinen Radiumnadeln gespickt wird und ebenfalls über eine exsudative Lokalreaktion, diesmal aber im Verlaufe von 3 Wochen, abheilt. Bis heute, 6 Jahre nach Beginn der ersten Behandlung, rezidivfrei geblieben.

Beurteilung. Außergewöhnlich kräftige Schleimhautreaktion nach Radio-Cäsiumbestrahlung der gesamten Scheidenlänge mit 2000 R in einer Sitzung, gleichzeitig hämorrhagische Radiocystitis, in etwa 3 Monaten abgeheilt.

Bei heutiger Behandlungstechnik wäre eine Abschirmung der Radium-Caesiumbestrahlung nach rechts und eine Beschränkung der Beladung des Caesium-Vaginalzylinders auf das mittlere Drittel erfolgt.

Fall. 6. 52jährige Patientin mit einem nahezu über die gesamte Scheidenhinterwand ausgedehnten Plattenepithelcarcinom, das plattenförmig teils exophytisch ausgebildet, teils in das Septum recto-vaginale infiltriert hatte. Ferner fand sich an der hinteren Muttermundslippe ein erosionsartiger Epitheldefekt und eine straffere Konsistenz des rechten Parakolpiums.

Histologie: Stark verhornendes Plattenepithelcarcinom.

Behandlung: Intrauterinstift 33 mg Ra.El. für 120 h; 2mal ^{137}Caesium-Vaginalzylinder im Abstand von 3 Wochen mit 6×50 mCi ^{137}Cs nach ventral mit Wolfram-Abschirmung, nach dorsal 2mal 3000 R.

Ungewöhnlich kräftige lokale Strahlenreaktion des gesamten Scheidenrohres mit eitrigen Absonderungen, Blasen- und Mastdarmtenesmen bei entsprechenden erheblichen Schmerzen. Nach 2 Monaten kein Anhalt für Tumor, Vaginalverklebungen müssen gelöst werden. Vaginalbehandlung mit reizlosen Salben und Sitzbädern noch für ein halbes Jahr erforderlich, dann aber endlich Abklingen der erheblichen Reaktion.

Jetzt 5 Jahre nach dieser Behandlung noch rezidivfrei.

Beurteilung. Ungewöhnlich kräftige Strahlenreaktion der gesamten Scheidenschleimhaut, der Mastdarmschleimhaut und der Blasenschleimhaut bei zu hoher Einzeldosis nach Radio-Caesiumbehandlung.

Die vorstehenden Beispiele, die schließlich noch durch Beobachtungen über die Bildung ausgedehnter Recto-Vaginal-Fisteln nach erfolgreicher Bestrahlung eines ausgedehnten Tumors im Septum recto-vaginale vermehrt werden könnten, zeigen deutlich, daß hohe Einzeldosen in der Größe von 2000 und 3000 R von der Scheidenwand im mittleren Drittel häufig längst nicht so gut toleriert werden wie im oberen Drittel und im Bereich der Vaginalgewölbe. Die von KEPP u.a. angenommene Strahlentoleranz der Vagina in Größe von 30000—40000 R ist mit Sicherheit nur unter den Bedingungen der hochfraktionierten Kleinraumbestrahlung und nur im oberen Vaginalabschnitt, d.h. in den Scheidengewölben und an der Portio selbst gültig. Im mittleren und unteren Scheidendrittel dagegen bestehen andere Voraussetzungen für die Strahlenbelastbarkeit. Wir verabfolgen daher jetzt in diesem Bezirk mit Hilfe der Caesium-Vaginalzylinder Einzeldosen von 1500 R in 14tägigen Abständen 3- bis höchstens 4mal und haben seither ähnliche Erscheinungen, wie beschrieben, nicht mehr erleben müssen. Es wird trotzdem ausreichender Tumorschwund erreicht.

Die Beobachtung, daß lokale Curietherapie mit 3 Einzeldosen von je 1500R ausreichen, um einen sicheren Tumorschwund des Vaginalcarcinoms zu erreichen, haben uns anfangs sehr überrascht, weil von der Radiumkontaktbehandlung der Collum- und Vaginalcarcinome her bekannt war, daß Oberflächenwirkungsdosen am Tumor zwischen 3mal 2500 R bis 3mal 4000 R innerhalb von 4 Wochen durchaus üblich und notwendig sind. Es ist offensichtlich die mit zunehmendem Abstand der strahlenden Achse von der zu bestrahlenden Oberfläche und bei zirkulärer Einstrahlung von uterinem und vaginalem Strahler aus erheblich anwachsende Volumendosis bei mäßig anwachsender relativer Tiefendosis, welche diese auffallenden Wirkungen hervorruft: Siehe auch Abb. 4. Die klinische Beobachtung ausreichenden Tumorschwunds, bei der kleineren Oberflächendosis durch Caesium-Vaginalzylinder eine ausreichende Rückbildung zu erzielen und die Notwendigkeit, das Risiko einer Schädigung an Blase, Mastdarm und Scheidenwand klein zu halten, hat dazu gezwungen, über die Empirie hinaus in den Bezugssystemen der Strahlenphysik und Strahlenbiologie dieses Neue zu lernen.

5. Behandlungsergebnisse der Literatur

Die in der bisherigen Fachliteratur veröffentlichten Behandlungsergebnisse des primären Vaginalcarcinoms, mit wenigen Ausnahmen (beispielsweise die Fälle von Giesecke) Ergebnisse der alleinigen Strahlenbehandlung, sind zu einem großen Teil in der folgenden Tabelle 3 zusammengestellt. Aus dieser Sammelstatistik über 2278 Fälle geht vor allem hervor, daß aus einer kleinen Zahl von Beobachtungen, gewiß auch aus Beobachtungsziffern von weniger als 100 Fällen, eine Schlußfolgerung über die Güte der stattgefundenen Behandlung nicht gezogen werden kann. Gewiß sind die meisten in der Tabelle enthaltenen Unterschiede der Ergebnisse nicht signifikant. Auch ein so glänzendes Ergebnis wie die von Courtial erzielten 45,4 % 5-Jahresheilungen kann nicht als ein Nachweis für die Unterlegenheit anderer in dieser Zeit veröffentlichter Behandlungsverfahren anerkannt werden.

Außerdem ist der Tabelle 3 aber eine allgemeine Tendenz zu einer verhältnismäßig geringen Besserung der Heilungsergebnisse in jüngerer Zeit zu entnehmen. Wenn man das dargestellte Krankengut zahlenmäßig etwa halbiert und beim Jahreswechsel 1950/51 eine Grenze setzt, bekommt man für die ältere Gruppe von 1218 Fällen eine Sammelheilungsziffer von 17,6 % und für die jüngere Gruppe von 1951/1961 eine Sammelheilungsziffer von 22,1 %.

Die durchschnittlichen Heilungsziffern betragen im ganzen gesehen immer noch etwa 20 %, werden gelegentlich von Therapeuten, vom Glück begünstigt, überschritten und können nur verbessert werden bei sehr sorgfältiger Beschäftigung mit den anatomischen Eigenheiten des Scheidencarcinoms und einem individuellen Eingehen auf die Besonderheiten des einzelnen Falles.

6. Eigenes Krankengut von 1935—1959

Das Krankengut des Allgemeinen Krankenhauses St. Georg, Hamburg, an primären Scheidencarcinomen aus den Jahren 1935—1959 ist in der kasuistischen Tabelle 1 enthalten. Sie enthält, abgesehen von dem Lebensalter der Patientinnen und dem Jahre des Behandlungsbeginns, eine Skizze über die anatomische Tumorausbreitung, auf das Vorhandensein von Metastasen bei Behandlungsbeginn, die Formen der Therapie und das endgültige Behandlungsergebnis. Es handelt sich um insgesamt 82 Fälle.

Die *Altersverteilung* des eigenen Krankengutes unterscheidet sich, wie Tabelle 4 zeigt, nicht von den Beobachtungen anderer Autoren. Die Mehrzahl der Kranken stehen im 6. und 7. Lebensjahrzehnt. Die „besten" Heilungsziffern sind in den beiden jüngsten tabellarisch dargestellten Gruppen erreicht worden. Natürlich wird es nicht ratsam sein, aus solch einer Beobachtung ein Rechtsgefälle der Heilungsziffern in Abhängigkeit vom Lebensalter zu folgern.

Eine Übersicht über die *Lokalisation* und Größe des Primärbefundes bei Behandlungsbeginn, ferner über die Tumorausbreitung außerhalb des primären Sitzes wird in Tabelle 5 gegeben. Auch diese Beobachtungen bestätigen bereits oben wiedergegebene Erfahrungen anderer Kliniker. Rutledge (1967) allerdings hat hiervon abweichende Verhältnisse bezüglich der Verteilung auf Vorder- (22), Hinter- (15) und Seitenwand berichtet.

Tabelle 3. *Primäres Vaginalcarcinom. Behandlungsergebnisse. Sammelstatistik*

	Autor	Jahr der Veröffentlichung	geheilt beobachtet	5-Jahres-Heilungsziffer
1.	E. Bumm	1919	5/22	21,7%
2.	F. Gál	1920	5/29	17,2%
3.	A. Giesecke	1920	1/11	—
4.	Bailey and Bagg	1921	0/18	—
5.	Broders	1922	2/18	11,1%
6.	Moench u. Stacy	1922	3/37	8,1%
7.	J. Heyman	1926	2/16 ⎫	16,7%
8.	J. Heyman	1930	3/14 ⎭	
9.	F. Voltz	1930	4/89	4,5%
10.	P. Feldweg	1930	2/32	6,2%
11.	J. v. Büben	1931	2/29	6,9%
12.	E. Philipp	1932	13/83	15,7%
13.	Healy	1933	21/99	21,2%
14.	Nelson	1933	0/26	—
15.	Masson	1934	18/80	22,5%
16.	H. Wintz u. F. Wittenbeck	1934	10/51	19,6%
17.	H. Burckhardt	1935	10/31	32,2%
18.	Taussig	1935	2/27	7,4%
19.	E. Berven u. J. Heyman	1936	6/58	10,4%
20.	D. den Hoed	1936	7/21	33,3%
21.	F. V. Emmert	1938	4/33	12,0%
22.	J. Courtial	1938	10/22	45,5%
23.	E. Maier	1941	10/38	26,3%
24.	R. K. Kepp	1941	5/25	20,0%
25.	Johnston	1942	0/3	—
26.	M. Lederman u. W. V. Mayneord	1942	1/7	—
27.	R. G. Livingstone	1947	8/76	10,5%
28.	S. Way	1948	5/25	20,0%
29.	R. Paterson, zit. nach Blomfield	1950	7/51	14,0%
30.	H. Huber	1950	18/104	17,3%
31.	R. E. Fricke et al.	1950	10/32	31,2%
32.	F. Buschke u. S. Cantril	1951	5/10	—
33.	R. Paterson	1951	7/51	14,0%
34.	O. T. Messelt	1952	17/78	22,7%
35.	Singh	1952	0/21	—
36.	J. H. Kaiser	1952	9/38	22,7%
37.	M. D. Bivens	1953	11/40	27,5%
38.	J. P. Palmer u. S. M. Biback	1953	24/75	32,0%
39.	O. Millar	1954	15/52	28,8%
40.	F. R. Smith	1955	14/109	12,8%
41.	W. Möbius	1956	29/119	24,4%
42.	J. Herold	1956	18/55	32,7%
43.	J. Swyngedouw et al.	1956	8/16	—
44.	W. T. Murphy	1957	24/103	23,3%
45.	J. A. Merrill u. W. T. Bender	1958	7/25	28,0%
46.	O. Busse u. W. Soergel	1959	4/29	13,8%
47.	J. Ries u. J. Breitner	1959	30/130	23,1%
48.	St. L. Marcus	1960	4/20	20,0%
49.	W. R. Lang	1960	11/76	14,0%
50.	G. H. Arronet et al.	1960	11/25	44,0%
51.	M. D. Schtscherbina et al.	1960	5/15	33,3%
52.	R. Scheele	1961	8/24	33,3%
53.	F. N. Rutledge	1967	25/70	35,0%
54.	H. C. Frick, H. W. Jacox, H. C. Taylor	1968	11/34	32,4%
	1919/50		214/1218 =	17,6%
	1951/61		266/1181 =	22,5%
		zusammen	480/2399 =	20,0%

Aus diesen Darstellungen ergibt sich aber auch die Güte des Krankengutes, bei dem aus prinzipiellen Erwägungen auf eine nachträgliche Klassifikation in Stadien verzichtet worden ist. Mehr als die Hälfte der Tumoren hatte eine Längenausdehnung über die Hälfte des Scheidenrohres und mehr. Über 35 % der Patientinnen wiesen bei Behandlungsbeginn eine Tumorausbreitung über den Primärsitz hinaus in das paravaginale Gewebe, in die Leistenbeugen oder sogar Fernmetastasen auf. Auch die Erfahrung, daß Vaginalcarcinome

Tabelle 4. *Vaginalcarcinom A. K. St. Georg, Hamburg, 1935—1959. Relative Heilung in Abhängigkeit vom Lebensalter*

20—29	30—39	40—49	50—59	60—69	70—79	80—89
1/1	6/10	2/13	8/26	6/20	4/11	0/1

der Hinterwand und der Seitenwände leichter als die Tumoren der Vorderwand und selbstverständlich leichter als die mehr oder weniger zirkulär ausgebreiteten Carcinome heilbar sind, bestätigt sich am vorliegenden Krankengut des Allgemeinen Krankenhauses St. Georg; während die Carcinome der Hinterwand und der Seitenwände zu mehr als 51 % einer Heilung zugeführt werden konnten, betrug die Heilungsziffer bei der Restgruppe nur 12,8 % (Tabelle 6), für das Gesamtkrankengut 33 %.

Tabelle 5. Vaginalcarcinom *A. K. St. Georg, Hamburg, 1935—1959. Häufigkeiten spezieller Lokalisation und Ausdehnung*

Primärbefund (Lokalisation):

Hinterwand	Seitenwand	Vorderwand	Semizirkulär	Zirkulär	Gesamt
34	9	13	13	13	82

Oberes Drittel	Mittleres Drittel	Unteres Drittel	Gesamt
36	35	11	82

Ausdehnung des Primärtumors:

Bis zu $^1/_3$ Länge der Vagina	Bis zu $^2/_3$ Länge der Vagina	Bis ganze Länge der Vagina	Gesamt
41	30	11	82

Ausbreitung des Primärtumors:

Im paravaginalen Gewebe	Metastasen in der Leistenbeuge	Fernmetastasen
22	8	2

Die günstige Erfahrung über die Scheidencarcinome der Hinterwand und des oberen Scheidendrittels entspricht also sehr guten Behandlungsergebnissen beim Collumcarcinom, während die weiter ausgebreiteten Scheidencarcinome und diejenigen des mittleren und unteren Scheidendrittels die Prognose der Gesamtgruppe belasten.

An einer Gruppe von 60 vor Jahren zusammengestellten Vaginalcarcinomen der Jahrgänge 1935—1954 ist der Wert der einzelnen Behandlungsmethoden geprüft worden und wird in Tabelle 7 wiedergegeben. Es war eindrucksvoll, daß die einer vaginalen *und* intrauterinen Radiumbehandlung zugeführten Carcinome eine wesentlich höhere Heilungsziffer als die Fälle ohne intrauterine Behandlung aufwiesen. Ohne allzu weitreichende Schlußfolgerungen aus dieser Beobachtung ziehen zu wollen, hat dies unsere Auffassung über die Notwendigkeit der intrauterinen Radiumbehandlung bestätigt.

Nach Hinzufügen eines nachträglich gefundenen geheilten Falles ergibt sich für die 61 Fälle der Jahre 1935—1954 eine absolute 5-Jahresheilung von 17 Fällen = 28%. Für die gesamte Gruppe von 83 Fällen der Jahre 1935—1959 ergeben sich bei 28 Fällen 5-Jahresheilungen eine Gesamtheilungsziffer von 33,7%.

Tabelle 6. *Vaginalcarcinom A. K. St. Georg, Hamburg, 1935—1959. Heilungsziffern in Abhängigkeit vom speziellen Tumorsitz*

5-Jahres-Heilungsziffern in Abhängigkeit vom speziellen Tumorsitz		Relative Heilung
Hinterwand	16/34	51,0%
Seitenwand	6/9	
Vorderwand	2/13	
Semizirkulär	1/13	12,8%
Zirkulär	2/13	
Zusammen	27/82 =	33,0%

Tabelle 7. *60 Vaginalcarcinome 1935—1954. Spezielle Behandlungsmethode und 5-Jahresheilung*

Radium, vaginal und uterin	7/16	43,8%
Radium, vaginal	6/22	27,3%
Radium, Spickmethode	1/10	
Körperhöhlenrohr	2/3	
Röntgentiefentherapie	0/5	
Konservativ	0/3	
Operativ	0/1	
Gesamt	16/60	

7. Die heutige Problematik bei der Strahlentherapie des Scheidenkrebses

Es ist dargestellt worden, daß die sorgfältig durchgeführte Strahlenbehandlung für das primäre Vaginalcarcinom die Methode der Wahl darstellt und daß operative Eingriffe nur ganz selten als Primärbehandlung in Betracht kommen. Die allgemeinen Grundsätze einer kurativen Strahlentherapie gelten somit auch für das Vaginalcarcinom. Ebenso wie die Krebschirurgie ist die Strahlentherapie bestrebt, das vom Primärtumor eingenommene Gebiet und, wo irgend möglich, auch das potentiell tumortragende Nachbargebiet voll mit einer Tumorvernichtungsdosis zu erfassen. Für die Krebse in der Nähe des hinteren Scheidengewölbes, die sich nach dem Typ des Collumcarcinoms auszubreiten vermögen, wäre dies das gleiche anatomische Gebiet, welches bei der erweiterten Wertheimschen Operation entfernt wird.

Daß diesem Streben nach Radikalität der Strahlenbehandlung nach oben Grenzen gesetzt sind, wurde angedeutet. Dem Streben nach Radikalität steht auch konkurrierend gegenüber die Notwendigkeit, strahlenempfindliche Nachbarorgane, wie Harnblase, Harnleiter und Mastdarm, so gut wie möglich zu schonen; dies um so mehr, als die genannten Organe lebenswichtige Funktionen auszuüben haben.

Auch dem Streben des Strahlentherapeuten, eine standardisierte Behandlungsmethode zu entwickeln, sind — wie dargelegt — infolge der Variabilität der anatomischen Tumorausbreitung Grenzen gesetzt. Anstelle der Standardisierung, welche sich infolge der konstanten

Anatomie des kleinen Beckens wiederum vorzugsweise für die im oberen Scheidendrittel gelegenen Tumoren anbietet, tritt daher außerordentlich häufig die Notwendigkeit einer individuellen Anpassung des strahlentherapeutischen Vorgehens an die tatsächliche Größe und den Sitz des Tumors.

Der Strahlentherapeut hat bei der Planung einer kurativen Behandlung zu unterscheiden und zu definieren

1. das vom *Tumor* befallene *Volumen;*

2. das *Zielvolumen.* Das ist jenes Gewebevolumen, welches das tatsächlich vom Tumor befallene Gebiet, einschließlich eines ausreichend breiten Sicherheitsrandes, enthält und in welchem die verordnete Dosis in der verordneten Zeit wirksam werden soll;

3. das *bestrahlte Volumen;* das ist Tumorvolumen + Zielvolumen + unvermeidlich mitbestrahlte Gewebevolumina, wobei die außerhalb des Zielvolumens gelegenen Gebiete eine möglichst kleine Dosis erhalten sollen, insbesondere dann, wenn in ihr kritische Organe und deren Toleranzgrenzen zu berücksichtigen sind;

4. das *indirekt bestrahlte Volumen,* welches praktisch den ganzen Patientenkörper umfaßt.

Die Besonderheiten der anatomischen Lage der Scheide zwischen Blase und Mastdarm, ihrer Einbettung in mehr oder weniger lockeres Bindegewebe des Parakolpiums sind für eine rücksichtslos radikale Strahlenbehandlung, besonders bei intravaginaler Applikation eines radioaktiven Strahlungsträgers oder des Hohlanodenrohres nicht zu unterschätzende Hindernisse. Die unterschiedliche Radiotoleranz verschiedener Abschnitte der Vaginalschleimhaut kann auf Grund von zahlreichen klinischen Erfahrungen und Beobachtungen festgestellt werden. Während in der Göttinger Schule und auch an anderer Stelle, z.B. auch an einzelnen Fällen des eigenen Krankengutes für kleine bestrahlte Volumina mit einer Toleranzgrenze bis zu etwa 30000—35000 R in 6 Wochen gerechnet worden ist, muß man die Toleranzgrenze für den mittleren und unteren Abschnitt weit geringer einschätzen, sie dürfte auch bei fraktionierter Bestrahlung und Verteilung auf 4—5 Wochen nicht höher als etwa 6000—8000 R liegen. Man ist geradezu versucht, von einem *cranio-caudalen Gefälle der Strahlentoleranz der Scheidenschleimhaut* zu sprechen.

Bei solcher Feststellung muß man sich aber gewiß dessen bewußt bleiben, daß die obigen Zahlenangaben nur sehr näherungsweise gelten können. Abgesehen von der Fraktionierung, d.h. dem Zeitfaktor, sind sie auch abhängig von der bestrahlten Feldgröße und damit vom bestrahlten Gewebevolumen. Im Falle der Curietherapie wächst bekanntlich die Integraldosis mit dem Quadrat des Abstandes, wenn gleiche Oberflächendosen der Schleimhaut zugrunde gelegt werden. Solche Umstände, aber auch die zusätzlich durchgeführte Strahlenbehandlung von außen, sind beim Festlegen der Behandlungspläne des Scheidenkrebses sorgsam zu berücksichtigen.

Verbesserungsmöglichkeiten für die im großen und ganzen recht verschiedenen Dauerergebnisse der Strahlenbehandlung des Scheidencarcinoms kann der Strahlentherapeut nur dort erhoffen, wo eine ausreichende, auch für dieses Organgebiet spezielle Erfahrung dadurch gewonnen werden kann, daß immer wieder einschlägige Krankheitsfälle auftreten. Daraus ergibt sich für Ärzte, Fachärzte und kleinere Krankenanstalten, in denen primäre Vaginalcarcinome entdeckt werden, der Hinweis, daß diese kranken Frauen nicht Behandlungsversuchen mit unzureichenden Mitteln zugeführt werden dürfen, daß deren Behandlung vielmehr in die Hände der größeren radiotherapeutischen Schwerpunktinstitute gehört.

Die tabellarische Zusammenstellung des eigenen Krankengutes verdankt der Verfasser Herrn Dr. Wilfried Wannovius, jetzt Rendsburg, dem auch an dieser Stelle für seine Mitarbeit sehr herzlich gedankt werden soll.

Literatur

ALLEN, A. C., SPITZ, S.: Malignant melanoma. A clinico-pathological analysis of the criteria for diagnosis and prognosis. Cancer (Philad.) 6, 1 (1953).

APPELBERG, G.: Plasmocytoma of the vagina: Case report. Acta radiol. (Stockh.) 39, 83 (1953).

AMREICH, A. J.: Das Karzinom der Frau. Wien. klin. Wschr. 55, 801 (1942).

Annual Report on the Results of Treatment in Carcinoma of the Uterus. XII. Vol. 1960.

ARIEL, J. M.: Five-year cure of a primary malignant melanoma of the vagina by local radioactive isotope therapy. Amer. J. Obstet. Gynec. 82, 405 (1961).

ARRONET, G. H., LATOUR, J. P., TREMBLAY, P. C.: Primary carcinoma of the vagina. Amer. J. Obstet. Gynec. 79, 455 (1960).

BASU, SATGEN, MAZUMDAR, JIBAN, ROY, DILIP (Calcutta): Treatment of primary cancer of vagina with radium. Brit. J. Radiol. 28, 111 (1955).

BECKER, J., SCHEER, K. E.: Radiokobalt als plastisches Präparat zur Strahlenbehandlung. Strahlentherapie 85, 581 (1951).

BIENENFELD, B.: Primäres Scheidenkarzinom. Gebh.-Gynäkol. Ges. zu Wien, 22. 6. 26. Ref. Zbl. Gynäk. 1926, 2974.

BIVENS, M. D.: Primary carcinoma of the vagina. Amer. Obstet. Gynec. 65, 390 (1953).

BLOMFIELD, G. W.: Diseases of the vagina, urethra and vulva. In: Rock Carling, Windeyer and Smithers, British practice in radiotherapy. London: Butterworth & Co. 1955.

BROWN, D. B.: Procidentia with primary carcinoma of the vagina. Proc. roy. Soc. Med. 48, 1091 (1955).

BÜBEN, J. v.: Die Radiumtherapie des Scheidenkrebses. Strahlentherapie 36, 503 (1930).

— Radium in the treatment of cancer of the vagina. Surg. Gynec. Obstet. 52, 884 (1931).

BUMM, E.: Sechs Jahre Radium. Zbl. Gynäk. 1919, 1.

BURCKHARDT, H.: Die Ergebnisse der Behandlung der weiblichen Genitalkarzinome an der Staatl. Frauenklinik Dresden 1925—1929. Strahlentherapie 54, 377 (1935).

BUSCHKE, F., CANTRIL, S. T.: Radiation therapy of carcinoma of vagina. Radiology 56, 193 (1951).

BUSSE, O., SOERGEL, W.: Bericht über 800 maligne Erkrankungen des weiblichen Genitale der Jahre 1947—1952. Geburth. u. Frauenheilk. 19, 201 (1959).

CORSCADEN, J. A.: Gynecologic cancer, 3rd ed. Baltimore: Williams & Wilkins Co. 1962.

COURTIAL, JEAN: La radiothérapie des épithéliomas primitifs du vagin. Arch. Électr. méd. 46, 193 (1938).

DANIEL, W. W., KOSS, L. G., BRUNSCHWIG, A.: Sarcoma botryoides of the vagina. Cancer (Philad.) 12, 74 (1959).

DIEHL, W. K.: Sarcoma of the vagina. Amer. J. Obstet. Gynec. 52, 302 (1946).

DOBBIE, B. M. W.: Vaginal recurrences in carcinoma of body of uterus and their prevention by radium therapy. J. Obstet. Gynaec. Brit. Emp. 60, 702 (1953).

DOUGAL, D.: Primary carcinoma of the vagina treated by hysterovaginectomy. J. Obstet. Gynaec. Brit. Emp. 30, 38 (1923).

DOUGLAS, G. W.: Observations on the pathology of primary carcinoma of the vagina and its relation to therapy. Surg. Gynec. Obstet. 98, 456 (1954).

ELLIS, F., OLIVER, R.: A new technique for treating papillomatosis of the bladder with colloidal gold and some unusual applications of tantalum wire. Radioisotope Conference 1954, p. 22—29. London: Butterworth 1954.

EMMERT, F. V.: Primary cancer of the vagina. Amer. J. Obstet. 36, 1058 (1938).

FELDWEG, P.: Die Behandlungserfolge der Genitalkarzinome. Zbl. Gynäk. 1930, 779.

FLETCHER, G. H.: The planning of external irradiation in pelvic cancer. Amer. J. Roentgenol. 64, 95 (1950).

FOCHT, E. F., MARINELLI, L. D., TWOMBLY, G. H.: A cylindrical radium applicator for the treatment of surface vaginal lesions. Amer. J. Roentgenol. 56, 751 (1946).

FREUND, D. R., KEGEL, E. E., DUGGER, J. H.: Primary malignant melanoma of the vagina. Amer. J. Obstet. Gynaec. 78, 290 (1959).

FRICK, H. C., JACOX, H. W., TAYLOR, H. C., JR.: Primary carcinoma of the vagina. Amer. J Obstet. Gynec. 101, 695—705 (1968).

FRICKE, R. E., BOWING, H. H., DECKER, D. G.: Radium therapy of primary carcinoma and other malignant lesions of the vagina. Amer. J. Roentgenol. 64, 86 (1950).

— HERIK, M. VAN, SOULE, E. H.: Treatment of rare lesions of the uterus and vagina. Radiology 63, 353 (1954).

FRISCHBIER, H. J.: Experience with lymphography in diagnosis of recurrent female genital carcinoma. In: A. RÜTTIMANN, Progress in lymphology, p. 221. Stuttgart: Thieme 1967.

GÁL, F.: Durch Strahlenbehandlung erzielte Dauerresultate beim Karzinom der weiblichen Geschlechtsorgane. Strahlentherapie 27, 27 (1920).

GAUWERKY, F.: Gezielte Tiefentherapie mit feststehenden Feldern. Fortschr. Röntgenstr. 83, 802 (1955).

— Caesium[137] zur gerichteten intrakavitären Curietherapie gynäkologischer Karzinome. Sonderbd. Strahlentherapie 36, 211 (1956).

— Standardisierung und individuelle Anpassung bei der Strahlenbehandlung der Gebärmutter- und Scheidenkarzinome. Strahlentherapie 103, 16 (1957).

— Erfahrungen mit der Verwendung von Caesium[137] bei der intrakavitären Curietherapie gynäkologischer Karzinome. Strahlentherapie 105, 107 (1958).

— Special applications of caesium[137] in radiotherapy of short distance. Sec. Un. Nat. Int. Conf. on the Peaceful Uses of Atomic Energy a/Conf. 15 P 974, 17. June 1958.

— HEINZEL, F., LEETZ, H. K.: Die Abteilung für ultraharte Strahlung im Therapeutischen Strahleninstitut des Allgemeinen Krankenhauses St. Georg, Hamburg. Fortschr. Röntgenstr. 95, 291 (1961).

Gerteis, W.: Diskussionsbemerkung in A. Rüttimann, Progress in lymphology, p. 224—225. Stuttgart: Thieme 1967.

Giesecke, A.: Die Dauerresultate nach operativer und Strahlenbehandlung des Uterus- und Scheidenkarzinoms. Arch. Gynäk. 115, 435 (1922).

Hecht, A.: Der primäre Scheidenkrebs. Inaug.-Diss. München 1891. Zbl. Gynäk. 15, 779 (1891).

Heinzel, F.: Über die Notwendigkeit der Rotationsbestrahlung in der Telekobalttherapie. Strahlentherapie 116, 180 (1961).

Hellriegel, W.: Methode der Radiogold-Implantationstherapie. Strahlentherapie 102, 511 (1957).

Henschke, U. K., James, A. G., Myers, W. G.: Radiogold seeds for cancer therapy. Nucleonics 11, 46 (1953).

— — — Radiogold seeds in clinical therapy. Radiology 63, 390 (1954).

Herold, J.: Contact X-ray treatment of vaginal carcinoma. Čs. Gynek. 21, (35), 256 (1956). Ref. Ber. ges. Gynäk. Geburtsh. 60, 46 (1956).

Heyman, J.: Über die Behandlung der inoperablen Carcinome der weiblichen Beckenorgane. Strahlentherapie 23, 15 (1926).

— Die Strahlenbehandlung als vollständiger oder teilweiser Ersatz der Operation bei der Behandlung von Karzinomen des Uterus. Strahlentherapie 37, 254 (1930).

Hoed, D. den: Results obtained in treatment of malignant tumors of vagina, vulva and urethra. Acta radiol. (Stockh.) 17, 569 (1936).

Holthusen, H., Gauwerky, F.: Ergebnisse der Strahlentherapie gynäkologischer Karzinome im Krankenhaus St. Georg. In: Aktuelle Probleme der Pathologie und Therapie, S. 153—167. Stuttgart: Thieme 1949.

Huber, H.: Das primäre Carcinom der Vagina. Geburtsh. u. Frauenheilk. 10, 879 (1950).

James, A. G., Henschke, U. K., Myers, W. G.: The clinical use of radioactive gold (Au 198) seeds. Cancer (Philad.) 6, 1034 (1953).

Kaiser, J. H.: Primary carcinoma of the vagina. Cancer (Philad.) 5, 1146 (1952).

Kapp-Schwoerer, H., Busch, M.: Über die Anwendung von Radiogoldseeds (Au 198) bei der gynäkologischen Strahlentherapie mit Untersuchungen der Isodosenverläufe und Belastung kritischer Organe. Strahlentherapie 120, 481 (1963).

Kepp, R. K.: Über die Anwendung der intravaginalen Röntgenbestrahlung bei der Therapie des Vaginalkarzinoms. Geburtsh. u. Frauenheilk. 3, 228 (1941).

— Gynäkologische Strahlentherapie. Stuttgart: Thieme 1952.

— Methoden und Ergebnisse der Behandlung der Uteruskrebse in der Göttinger UniversitätsFrauenklinik. Strahlentherapie 86, 353 (1952).

Klvaua, M.: Erweiterung zur Methodik der Radiumbehandlung des Scheidenkarzinoms mit zylindrischem Applikator. Čs. Onkol. 3, 116 (1956). Ref. Ber. Geburtsh. Gynäk. 61, 333 (1957).

Küstner, O.: Die bösartigen Geschwülste der Vagina: In Zweifel-Payr, Klinik der bösartigen Geschwülste, Bd. 3, S. 356. Leipzig: Hirsch 1927.

Lang, W. R., Menduke, H., Golub, L. J.: The delay period in carcinoma of the vagina. Amer. J. Obstet. Gynec. 80, 341 (1960).

Lederman, M., Mayneord, W. V.: Radium treatment of cancer of the vagina. Brit. J. Radiol. 15, 307 (1942).

Livingstone, R. G.: Primary carcinoma of the vagina. Springfield, Ill.: Ch. G. Thomas 1950.

McFarland, J.: Dysontogenetic and mexed tumors of the urogenital region. Surg. Gynec. Obstet. 61, 42 (1935).

Maier, E.: Die Radiumtherapie der malignen Tumoren des weiblichen Genitales. Strahlentherapie 69, 141 (1941).

Marck, A., Wirthwein, C., Melamed, A.: Hemangioendothelioma of the vagina. Amer. J. Obstet. Gynec. 66, 436 (1953).

Marcus, St. L.: Primary carcinoma of vagina. Obstet. and Gynec. 15, 673 (1960).

Martius, H.: Die Strahlenbehandlung der inoperablen Portio-Carcinome. Dtsch. med. Wschr. 1922I, 977.

— Lehrbuch der Gynäkologie, 2. Aufl., S. 139. Stuttgart: Thieme 1949.

— Kepp, R. K.: Die Behandlung der bösartigen Genitaltumoren an der Universitäts-Frauenklinik Göttingen. Strahlentherapie 71, 627 (1941).

Martzloff, K. H., Manlove, Ch. H.: Vaginal and ovarian metastases from hyponephroma. Surg. Gynec. Obstet. 88, 145 (1949).

Merill, J. A., Bender, W. T.: Primary carcinoma of the vagina. Obstet. and Gynec. 11, 3—11 (1958).

Messelt, O. T.: Primary carcinoma of vagina. Surg. Gynec. Obstet. 95, 51 (1952).

Milatz, W.: Die Anfertigung einer Radiummoulage zur Bestrahlung eines Vaginalkarzinoms. Zbl. Gynäk. 82, 873 (1960).

Millar, Owen: Primary carcinoma of vagina. J. Canad. Ass. Radiol. 5, 23 (1954).

Minder, W.: Dosimetrie der Strahlungen radioaktiver Stoffe. Wien: Springer 1961.

Möbius, W.: Über das primäre Scheidenkarzinom und seine Behandlung. Z. Geburtsh. Gynäk. 145, 253 (1956).

— Die Röntgenintensivbestrahlung in der Gynäkologie. Strahlentherapie 93, 73 (1954).

Moluch, L. M.: Primary epithelioma of the vagina. Amer. J. Obstet. Gynec. 22, 837 (1931).

Murphy, G. H., Du Shane, J. W.: Mesodermal mixed tumor of the vagina; report of case. Amer. J. Obstet. Gynec. 55, 527 (1948).

Murphy, W. T.: Primary vaginal cancer: irradiation, management and end results. Radiology 68, 157 (1957).

— Radiation therapy. Philadelphia-London: W. B. Saunders Company 1959.

Myers, W. G., Colmery, B. H.: Radioactive Au[198] in gold seeds for cancer therapy. Cancer Res. 12, 285 (1952).

— — McLellon, W. M.: Radioactive gold[198] for gamma radiation therapy. Amer. J. Roentgenol. 70, 258 (1953).

Neugebauer, F. L.: Zur Warnung beim Gebrauch von Scheidenpessarien. Arch. Gynäk. 43, 373 (1893).

NÜRNBERGER, L.: Die Erkrankungen der Scheide. In: W. STÖCKEL, Handbuch der Gynäkologie, Bd. V, 2. Hälfte, S. 603—657: Das Karzinom der Scheide. München: J. F. Bergmann 1930.

OESER, H.: Strahlenbehandlung der Geschwülste. Technik, Ergebnisse und Probleme. München u. Berlin: Urban Schwarzenberg 1954.

PALMER, J. P., BIBACK, S. M.: Primary cancer of vagina. Amer. J. Obstet. Gynec. 67, 377 (1954).

PATERSON, R., PARKER, H. M.: Dosage system for gamma ray therapy. Brit. J. Radiol. 7, 592 (1934).

— — Dosage system for interstitial radium therapy. Brit. J. Radiol. 11, 252 (1938).

— TOD, MARGARET: In the treatment of malignant disease by radium and X-rays. London: Edward Arnold 1948.

— — RUSSELL, M.: The results of radium and X-ray therapy in malignant disease. Third Statistical Report from the Manchester Radium Institute, p. 146. Edinburgh: Livingstone 1950.

PHILIPP, E.: Statistik der Karzinome des Collum uteri und der Vagina aus den Jahren 1923—1925. Zbl. Gynäk. 1932, 212.

PIERQUIN, B.: Précis de Curiethérapie, p. 269—272. Paris: Masson & Cie. 1964.

POMERANCE, W.: Vesicorectostomy for primary vaginal carcinoma. Obstet. and Gynec. 11, 12 (1958).

QUIMBY, E. H.: Dosage table for linear radium sources. Radiology 43, 572 (1944).

REIFFENSTUHL, G.: Diskussionsbemerkungen in A. RÜTTIMANN, Progress in lymphology, p. 197—223. Stuttgart: Thieme 1967.

REITER, E.: Ergebnisse der Strahlenbehandlung beim primären Vaginalkarzinom. Diss. München 1937.

RIES, J., BREITNER, J.: Strahlenbehandlung in der Gynäkologie. Sonderbd. Strahlentherapie 40, 127 (1959).

ROCHA PITTA, H. DA: Carcinoma primitivo da vagina e Gestacao. An. bras. Ginec. 45, 247 (1958).

ROUVIÈRE, H.: Anatomy of the human lymphatic system. Ann. Arbor, Mich.: Edwards Bros. Inc. 1958.

RUTLEDGE, F. N.: Cancer of vagina. Amer. J. Obstet. Gynec. 97, 635 (1967).

— FLETCHER, G. A.: Transperitoneal lymphaden-estomy following supervoltage irradiation for squamous carcinoma of the cervix. Amer. J. Obstet. 76, 321 (1958).

SANDLER, B.: An investigation into the dosage delivered by certain techniques in the radiation therapy of carcinoma cervix. Brit. J. Radiol. 11, 623 (1938).

— Preliminary note on planning of combined radio-therapy of carcinoma of cervix uteri. Brit. J. Radiol. 16, 331 (1943).

SAMUELS, B., BRADBURN, D. M., JOHNSON, C. G.: Primary carcinoma in site of the vagina. Amer. J. Obstet. Gynec. 82, 393 (1961).

SCHÄFER, W., WITTE, E.: Über eine neue Körperhöhlenröntgenröhre zur Bestrahlung von Uterustumoren. Strahlentherapie 44, 283 (1932).

SCHEELE, R.: Die Behandlungsergebnisse bösartiger Geschwülste der Jahre 1944—1955. Geburtsh. u. Frauenheilk. 21, 845 (1961).

SCHLUND, E.: Über das primäre Carcinom der Vagina. Diss. Freiburg 1913.

SCHMERMUND, H. J., OBERHEUSER, F., KUTTIG, A.: Geschwülste der weiblichen Genitalorgane. In: J. BECKER u. O. SCHUBERT, Die Supervolttherapie, S. 445ff. Stuttgart: Thieme 1961.

SCHRAM, M.: Leiomyosarcoma of the vagina: Report of a case and review of the literature. Obstet. and Gynec. 12, 195 (1958).

SCOKEL, P. W., COLLIER, F. C., JONES, W. N., McMANNS, J. F. A., HUTCHINS, K.: Relation of carcinoma in site of the vagina to the early diagnosis of vaginnal cancer. Amer. J. Obstet. Gynec. 82, 397 (1961).

SHCHERBINA, M. D., STUKOVA, L. M., STRUTSOVSKAYA, S. V., REPINA, V. A.: Treatment of primary carcinoma of the vagina with Co 60 and its remote results. Med. Radiol. (Mosk.) 5, 67—70 (1960).

SIDDALL, R.: Vaginal carcinoma in a girl of 14 years, treated by radiation. Amer. J. Obstet. Gynec. 57, 396 (1949).

SIMON, ST.: Die Bestrahlungsergebnisse beim Carcinoma vulvae. Strahlentherapie 43, 273 (1932).

— Die Curie-Röntgentherapie bösartiger Frauenleiden. Leipzig: Thieme 1933.

SINGER, H.: Späte Radiumschädigung im Falle eines vor Jahren behandelten Scheidenkrebses. Klin. Wschr. 1927 I, 857.

SINGH, B. P.: Primary carcinoma of the vagina. Cancer (Philad.) 4, 1073 (1951).

SMITH, FRANK R.: Primary carcinoma of vagina. Amer. J. Obstet. Gynec. 69, 525 (1955).

STARK, F.: Ergebnisse der Strahlenbehandlung des Vaginalkarzinoms. Diss. Hamburg 1949.

STRACHAU, G. I.: Primary adenocarcinoma of vagina (2 cases). J. Obstet. Gynaec. Brit. Emp. 39, 566 (1932).

STUDDIFORD, W. E.: Vaginal lesions of adenomatous origin. Amer. J. Obstet. Gynec. 73, 641 (1957).

SWYNGEDOUW, J., ROHART, J., DELATTRE, R.: La radiothérapie du cancer primitif du vagin (Roentgen- et curie thérapie). J. de Radiol. 37, 893 (1956).

TAUSSIG, F. J.: Primary cancer of the vulva, vagina, and female urethra. Five year results. Surg. Gynec. Obstet. 60, 477 (1935).

TOD, M. C., MEREDITH, W. J.: Dosage system for use in treatment of cancer of uterine cervix. Brit. J. Radiol. 11, 809 (1938).

TRUSKETT, I. D., CONSTABLE, W. C.: Clean cell adeno-carcinoma of the cervix and vaginal vault of mesonephric origin. Cancer (Philad.) 21, 249—254 (1968).

TWOMBLY, G. H., CAMBERLAIN, J. A.: Intravaginal roentgen therapy in cancer of cervix uteri. Radiology 52, 14 (1949).

VOLTZ, F.: Die Strahlenbehandlung der weiblichen Genitalkarzinome: Methoden und Ergebnisse. Sonderbd. Strahlentherapie 13, 113 (1930).

WAY, S.: Primary carcinoma of the vagina. J. Obstet. Gynec. Brit. Emp. 55, 739 (1948).

— Vaginal metastases of carcinoma of the body of the uterus. J. Obstet. Gynaec. Brit. Emp. 58, 558 (1951).

Weibel, W.: Das Karzinom der Scheide, in: Die Krebskrankheit, S. 331. Wien: Springer 1925.

— Ergebnisse der Kontaktbestrahlung nach Schäfer-Witte bei Karzinom der Frauenorgane. Strahlentherapie 58, 609 (1937).

Weigand, H.: Zur Technik der Radiumapplikation in der Gynäkologie. Strahlentherapie 27, 54 (1920).

Weishaar, J., Keller, R.: Experimentelle Untersuchungen zur Frage der Feldgröße und prozentualen Dosisverteilung bei der zusätzlichen perkutanen Röntgen- und Kobaltbestrahlung des Kollum-Karzinom (Messungen am Phantom). 2. Mitt. Strahlentherapie 119, 525 (1962).

Wichmann, H., Heinzel, F.: Leitfaden der Bewegungsbestrahlung. Teil I: Physikalische und methodische Grundlagen. Berlin-Göttingen-Heidelberg: Springer 1959.

Williams, J. J.: Primary carcinoma of vagina. New Engl. J. Med. 212, 156 (1935).

Winternitz, J. G.: Carcinoma of cervix; discussion on value and techniques of supplementary x-ray therapy. Brit. J. Radiol. 21, 27 (1948).

Wintz, H., Wittenbeck, F.: Klinik der gynäkologischen Röntgentherapie. Handbuch Veit-Stoeckel, Bd. IV, 2. Hälfte, Teil 2, S. 542—565. Behandlung der bösartigen Geschwülste, 3. völlig umgearbeitete und erweiterte Auflage. München: Bergmann 1935.

III. Die Strahlenbehandlung des Korpuscarcinoms

Von

R. Frischkorn

Mit 27 Abbildungen

1. Biologie des Korpuscarcinoms

Das Carcinoma corporis uteri, das Korpuscarcinom, im angelsächsischen Schrifttum zumeist als Endometriumcarcinom bezeichnet, geht von der Schleimhaut des Corpus uteri aus. Es zeigt gegenüber dem häufigeren Cervixcarcinom pathogenetische, histologische, anatomische und klinische Eigenheiten, die eine gesonderte Darstellung bedingen.

Zunächst einmal ist es gegenüber dem Cervixcarcinom seltener; es wird aber in den letzten Jahren eine relative und absolute Zunahme festgestellt. So betrug das Verhältnis Korpus- zu Cervixcarcinom nach HUBER (1949) noch 1:7,4, im Material der Universitäts-Frauenklinik Göttingen nach KIRCHHOFF 1950 1:5,7, 1959 aber 1:2,8. BUSSE und SOERGEL gaben 1959 dagegen noch ein Verhältnis von 1:5 an und v. MIKULICZ-RADECKI und GANSAU 1962 1:3,6. HUNT fand dagegen bereits 1956 ein Verhältnis von 1:1,7 und J. H. MÜLLER im Material der Universitäts-Frauenklinik Zürich sogar schon für die Jahre 1921—1923 ein Verhältnis von 1:3.

Die Unterschiedlichkeit dieser Zahlen ist sicherlich zum Teil durch strukturelle Besonderheiten der einzelnen Klinik bedingt. KOTTMEIER (1969) weist darauf hin, daß das Verhältnis altersabhängig ist und bei Frauen vor der Menopause 1:6 beträgt, in den siebziger Jahren dagegen 3:1. Es ist also denkbar, daß eine Klinik mit vorwiegend operativer Richtung eine andere Verhältniszahl finden wird, als eine solche mit vorwiegender oder ausschließlicher radiologischer Therapie, da das operative Krankengut vielfach jünger ist als das radiologische (PETERSEN).

Immerhin ist auch an der absoluten Zunahme nicht zu zweifeln. Da das Korpuscarcinom eine Erkrankung des höheren Lebensalters ist und die Lebenserwartung gestiegen ist, erleben mehr Frauen das Carcinom. Der Häufigkeitsgipfel ist nach den meisten Autoren heute um das 60. Lebensjahr anzunehmen. Er zeigte in den letzten Jahren eine Verschiebung zum höheren Alter. Allerdings finden sich auch hier noch niedrigere Altersangaben, die aber ebenfalls durch die Zusammensetzung des Materials abhängig von den Besonderheiten der einzelnen Klinik erklärbar sein können. v. MIKULICZ-RADECKI und GANSAU fanden für die Jahre 1925—1948 ein Durchschnittsalter von 56,5 Jahren, POCKRANDT an der gleichen Klinik 1955 eine Verschiebung zum 60. Lebensjahr. Hier ist oftmals entscheidend, welche Zeiträume dabei abgegrenzt werden. So gibt JAVERT für die Zeit von 1919—1960 55,7 Jahre als Durchschnittsalter an, BICKENBACH, LOCHMÜLLER und FLACH dagegen für die Jahre 1948—1958 60 Jahre und RANDALL und GODDARD 1956 59,2 Jahre.

Vor dem 5. Lebensjahrzehnt ist das Korpuscarcinom selten. Man kann damit rechnen, daß etwa 2 % oder wenig mehr unter 40 Jahren sind (RIMBACH; HUBER (1949); AMREICH). Einzelne Fälle werden aber auch schon im 3. Lebensjahrzehnt angegeben (AMREICH, CHIARI, HUBER, 1949), und schließlich fand DIECKHOFF 1963 ein Zusammentreffen von Korpuscarcinom und Gravidität in 8 Fällen in der Literatur.

Als Grund für die Zunahme des Korpuscarcinoms werden neben der ansteigenden Lebenserwartung noch andere ursächliche Möglichkeiten diskutiert, die die Frage der Entstehungsursache des Korpuscarcinoms unmittelbar berühren. So finden sich im

Schrifttum zahlreiche Untersuchungen über das Zusammentreffen des Korpuscarcinoms mit hormonalen Störungen, insbesondere einer vermehrten Oestrogenbildung. Auch die Frage, ob bei Korpuscarcinom-Patientinnen gleichzeitig oder anamnestisch häufiger eine glanduläre Hyperplasie des Endometriums gefunden wird, wird diskutiert. Immerhin deutet manches darauf hin, daß unter Oestrogeneinfluß ein Korpuscarcinom früher in Erscheinung tritt und schneller wächst. Gusberg (1954) empfiehlt aus diesem Grunde, Patientinnen mit einer glandulären Hyperplasie sorgfältig weiter zu überwachen. Andere Untersuchungen zeigen, daß bei Korpuscarcinom-Patientinnen auch in der Menopause noch in zahlreicheren Fällen eine Oestrogenaktivität gefunden wird als in Vergleichs-kollektiven. Dementsprechend sind die Gonadotropine eher vermindert. Auch eine Be-ziehung zu den Gestationsvorgängen erscheint manchen Autoren möglich, da die Kinder-zahl bei den Korpuscarcinom-Trägerinnen unter dem Durchschnitt liegen soll. Die mit-geteilten Ergebnisse sind aber uneinheitlich, ebenso wie ein Zusammenhang zwischen früherer Strahlentherapie wegen gutartiger Erkrankungen des Uterus und dem späteren Auftreten eines Korpuscarcinoms nicht bewiesen werden konnte (Abou-Daoud; Arneson, 1964; Behrens; Charles; Charles, Bell, Loraine u. Harkness; Cianfrani; O'Con-nor; Fuchs; Goecke u. Stüper; Goetschel; Greenblatt, Stoddard u. King; Gusberg, 1954; Hofmann u. Künzler; Huber, 1949 u. 1959; Husslein; Javert u. Renning; Kaiser; Kepp, 1961; Kistner; Kottmeier, 1959; Lynch, Krush, Larsen u. Magnuson; E. G. Mayer, 1960 u. 1961; Østergaard; Paroli; Ries, 1954; Rimbach; Roux u. Marchal; Rubin, Ryplanski u. Dutton; H. H. Schmid; Sherman; Sommers; Te Linde, Jones u. Galvin).

Die nicht bestrittene Zunahme des Korpuscarcinoms muß aber, sowohl absolut ge-sehen als auch hinsichtlich ihrer Relation zum Cervixcarcinom, Veranlassung sein, dieser Krankheit mehr Beachtung zu schenken. Dies um so mehr, als die weit verbreitete An-sicht, das Korpuscarcinom habe eine bessere Prognose als das Cervixcarcinom, wegen der Verbesserung der Heilungsergebnisse des Gebärmutterhalskrebses, zumindest für vergleichbare Ausbreitungsstadien, nicht mehr aufrecht erhalten werden kann.

Die Korpuscarcinome gehen — unabhängig von der histologischen Struktur — vom Endometrium aus. Sie sollen bevorzugt im Bereich der Tubenwinkel, des Fundus und isthmusnahe entstehen. Histologisch handelt es sich in der überwiegenden Mehrzahl um Adenocarcinome ($\sim$ 90%). Es werden aber auch solide Carcinome, Plattenepithel-carcinome und Adenocancroide, im angelsächsischen Schrifttum als Adenoakanthome bezeichnet, beobachtet. So fanden Busse und Soergel in ihrem Material neben 98 Adeno-carcinomen 6 solide und 4 Plattenepithelcarcinome. Die Häufigkeit der Adenocancroide wechselt von Autor zu Autor außerordentlich stark. Es ist sicherlich die Annahme be-rechtigt, daß diese Frequenzunterschiede nicht immer durch eine andersartige Zusammen-setzung des Krankengutes, als vielmehr durch Variationen in der Deutung bzw. der Untersuchungstechnik bedingt sind (Charles; Chiari; Strauss u. Hiersche). Es kommt hinzu, daß die histologische Beurteilung, insbesondere bei den unreiferen Formen, große Schwierigkeiten machen und in manchen Fällen mit letzter Exaktheit sogar unmöglich sein kann. Immerhin wird der histologischen Differenzierung von einer Reihe von Autoren besondere Bedeutung hinsichtlich der Prognose und der Strahlensensibilität beigemessen. Es wird daher auch in diesem Zusammenhang noch näher darauf einzugehen sein (s. Tabelle 5 und 6).

Das Adenocarcinom des Corpus uteri kann — vielleicht abhängig von seiner histo-logischen Dignität — längere Zeit auf das Endometrium beschränkt bleiben, bevor es schließlich in das Myometrium infiltriert. Es besteht daher auch gelegentlich die Möglich-keit, daß es allein durch eine Abrasio vollständig entfernt und z.B. im Operations-präparat kein Carcinom mehr gefunden wird (Chiari; Amreich; Martius). Auch eine Ausheilung durch alleinige Abrasio ist beschrieben (Hofmann u. Baldus). Unter Um-ständen erst nach längerer, im Einzelfall naturgemäß nicht sicher anzugebender Zeit kommt es zur Infiltration der Uterusmuskulatur, schließlich bis zur Serosa. Mit dem

Grad dieser Infiltration nimmt die Wahrscheinlichkeit einer Ausbreitung auf dem Lymphwege ebenfalls zu (AMREICH). Hier ist offenbar eine Revision der Ansicht angebracht, daß die primären Abflußstationen des Endometriumcarcinoms vorwiegend die aortalen Lymphknoten seien (CHIARI; HENRIKSEN; DU MESNIL DE ROCHEMONT). Obwohl hierüber schon lange eindrucksvolle Befunde vorliegen, ist die Tatsache, daß auch beim Korpuscarcinom Metastasen in den parametranen und iliacalen Lymphknoten häufiger sind als in den aortalen nicht recht zur Kenntnis genommen worden. Dies betont vor allem JAVERT. Er fand bei zumeist partieller Lymphonodektomie in 28% Metastasen in den pelvinen Lymphknoten, dagegen nur in 4% in den aortalen. GRÜNBERGER fand nur in 7,5% (80 Pat.) iliacale Lymphknotenmetastasen. Aber auch KÄSER weist auf die Häufigkeit von iliacalen Lymphknotenmetastasen beim Korpuscarcinom hin. HOLZAEPFEL und EZELL fanden bei Sektionen ein Verhältnis zwischen iliacalen und paraaortalen Lymphknotenmetastasen von 5:3. WALTHER hatte Lymphknotenmetastasen beim Collum- und Korpuscarcinom in gleicher Häufigkeit gefunden. Auch KEPP und HOFMANN weisen auf die größere Häufigkeit der pelvinen Ausbreitung des Korpuscarcinoms hin, was, wie JAVERT ausdrücklich betont, schon vor der Jahrhundertwende bekannt war. Nach AMREICH besteht in etwa 10% der Fälle eine lymphogene Verschleppung in die Parametrien, die diffus und daher nicht tastbar ist. Erst bei Befall der Cervix bilden sich auch tastbare Infiltrate. Die Ausbreitung im kleinen Becken ist aber nicht an die Voraussetzung geknüpft, daß das Carcinom auf die Cervix übergegriffen hat. Die Ursache ist vielmehr in der Anatomie der Lymphwege (REIFFENSTUHL; GERTEIS), sowie in der Möglichkeit einer Umkehrung des Lymphstromes zu sehen (BUTTENBERG; RUBIN; GERLE, QUICK u. GREENLAW; RUTLEDGE, TAN u. FLETCHER, 1958).

Schließlich hat die Lymphographie hier weiteren Aufschluß gebracht. Zwar sind die mitgeteilten Untersuchungszahlen speziell beim Korpuscarcinom noch nicht sehr groß, aber es liegen doch auch schon Hinweise über den häufigen Befall der pelvinen Lymphknoten vor, die größenordnungsmäßig den Befunden von JAVERT nahekommen (FUCHS, DAVIDSON u. FISCHER; FRISCHBIER). Die Lymphographie hat zugleich klargestellt (FUCHS; GERTEIS), daß auch bei frühen Stadien bereits häufig Metastasen in den regionären Lymphknoten gefunden werden, so nach GERTEIS (1966) beim Stadium I in 20%. GERTEIS folgert daraus, daß die bisherige Ansicht über die relative Gutartigkeit des Korpuscarcinoms infolge einer, wie früher angenommen, erst spät erfolgenden Metastasierung revidiert werden müsse. Damit bedarf dann auch die Angabe in der Stadieneinteilung der UICC: „Die regionären Lymphknoten (des Korpuscarcinoms) sind die intraabdominalen subdiaphragmatischen Knoten" der Revision.

Daß auch eine hämatogene Metastasierung schon relativ früh erfolgen kann, machen die Untersuchungen JAVERTS wahrscheinlich, der in 57% einen Venenbefall im Operationspräparat fand.

Demgegenüber treten die anderen Ausbreitungswege zahlenmäßig zurück. Hier ist zunächst das direkte Einwachsen des Carcinoms in benachbarte Organabschnitte zu nennen, so in die Tuben, wobei offenbar eine Tubenendometriose, die in den Altersklassen der Korpuscarcinom-Patientinnen häufig gefunden wird, eine Rolle spielen kann (HUBER, 1949; PHILIPP u. HUBER; TREITE). Von besonderer Bedeutung ist das Übergreifen auf die Cervix, mit dem nach LOUROS in 15,6% der Fälle zu rechnen ist. Diese Fälle sind nach übereinstimmender Meinung zahlreicher Autoren prognostisch anders einzustufen als das auf das Korpus beschränkte Carcinom. So fand z.B. KOTTMEIER (1969) bei 8 Patientinnen mit einem Carcinoma corporis et endocervicis in 4 Fällen Lymphknotenmetastasen im Becken, sonst jedoch bei den operierten Korpuscarcinom-Patientinnen nur im Verhältnis 1:50. GRÜNBERGER berichtet über 10 Fälle (von 80), bei denen das Carcinom in den Cervicalkanal vordrang. Lymphknotenmetastasen hatten von diesen nur 2.

Die nächsten Metastasenlokalisationen betreffen die Ovarien und die Vagina. JAVERT fand Adnexmetastasen in 10—12%, SCHIEFERSTEIN dagegen nur in 2%. Der letztere fand in Übereinstimmung mit JAVERT Scheidenmetastasen in 8%. Die Angaben in der

Literatur über die Häufigkeit von Scheidenmetastasen schwanken nach J. H. Müller (1941) zwischen 8 und 18%. Kottmeier (1959) rechnet mit 12% und Soergel fand 45,5% der überhaupt beobachteten Metastasen in der Vagina. Scheidenrezidive treten nach Price, Hahn und Rominger in 72% im Scheidengewölbe und in 12% im unteren Scheidendrittel auf.

Schließlich berichten Dede, Plentl und Moore über 124 Rezidivpatientinnen mit insgesamt 233 festgestellten Rezidiv- bzw. Metastasenlokalisationen (Tabelle 1).

Die Lokalisation der Metastasen im Material der Universitäts-Frauenklinik Göttingen (1942—1961) ist in Tabelle 2 dargestellt.

Tabelle 1. *Tumorlokalisationen bei 124 Rezidivpatientinnen. (Nach* Dede, Plentl *und* Moore*)*

Uterus	18	Kleines Becken	35
Scheidengewölbe	24	Rectosigmoid	17
Obere Vagina	20	Abdomen	31
Untere Vagina	6	Skelet	11
Rechtes Parametrium	21	Lunge	19
Linkes Parametrium	26	Kopf und Hals	5

Tabelle 2. *Die Häufigkeit der verschiedenen Metastasenlokalisationen (Universitäts-Frauenklinik Göttingen, 1942—1961). (Nach* Bernds*)*

Vagina	31	Ileum	1
Ovar	15	Coecum	1
Nodi lymph. ing.	9	Colon	1
Tuben	1	Vulva	2
Beckenwand	8	Lunge	5
Excavatio recto- vesicalis	8	Gehirn	2
Peritoneum	2	Leber	1
Omentum	6	Nodi, lymph. cerv. prof.	2
Harnröhre	2	Wirbelsäule	2
Blase	3	Femur	2
Rectum	3	Schambein	1
Mamma	1	Bauchwand	1

Die 110 Fälle der Tabelle 2 beziehen sich auf ein Krankengut von 615 Patientinnen und betreffen sowohl Primärbehandlungen als auch Rezidive. Da diese 615 Patientinnen nur zu einem Teil bei Auftreten von Metastasen wieder in die Klinik zurückkamen, kann unterstellt werden, daß die wirkliche Metastasenzahl bei lückenloser Erfassung wesentlich höher gewesen wäre. Immerhin ist dies für die Beurteilung des Verteilungsmusters von geringerer Bedeutung. Die auffällige Häufigkeit der Scheidenmetastasen und hier besonders der Lokalisationen im oberen Scheidenabschnitt ist immer wieder Gegenstand der Diskussion gewesen. Hier lassen sich verschiedene Gründe anführen und Zusammenhänge aufdecken, die im wesentlichen mit der Operation zusammenhängen. Es wird daher in dem Kapitel über die Rezidive und ihre Behandlung noch mehr darauf eingegangen, ebenso wie dort noch einmal Stellung genommen wird zu der Frage, wann beim Korpuscarcinom vom Rezidiv oder sogar vom Lokalrezidiv und wann von Metastasen gesprochen werden sollte.

Schwierigkeiten bestehen bei gleichzeitigem Befall der Ovarien in der Abgrenzung zum Ovarialcarcinom, weil histologisch nicht immer zu entscheiden ist, ob es sich um ein in das Korpus metastasierendes Ovarialcarcinom handelt oder ob der Ausbreitungsweg umgekehrt anzunehmen ist. Bergsjö (1962) entschied sich bei der Untersuchung von

430 Korpus- und 454 Ovarialcarcinomen, von denen insgesamt 115 Fälle Carcinom in beiden Organen hatten, dafür, daß in $^3/_4$ der Fälle die Ovarien der Ausgangspunkt und 3 echte Doppeltumoren waren.

Von den metastatischen Tumoren sind nach HUBER die Fälle primärer Tumormultiplizität abzutrennen, bei denen es infolge gleicher Ansprechbarkeit verschiedener Organe auf einen gemeinsamen geschwulstbildenden Reiz zur gleichzeitigen Tumorentstehung in mehreren Organen kommt. Da die Prognose solcher Befunde günstiger ist als die metastatischer Tumoren, kommt dieser Ansicht auch eine praktische Bedeutung für die Therapie zu (BAILAR; BERGSJÖ; GIBEL, BERNDT u. SCHWARZ; HUBER, 1949 und 1951; KIRCHHOFF, 1962).

2. Die Stadieneinteilung

Während sich die Stadieneinteilung des Cervixcarcinoms allgemein durchgesetzt hat, ist dies beim Korpuscarcinom bisher nicht in gleicher Weise der Fall. Es wurden viele Einteilungsvorschläge gemacht, zum Teil wieder verworfen oder immer wieder abgeändert. Die Schwierigkeit der Einteilung ist durch die Unmöglichkeit, den Ausbreitungsgrad durch die gynäkologische Untersuchung und den bei einer Abrasio erhobenen Befund wirklich zu erkennen, bedingt, da das Carcinom vom Uterus aus zumeist ohne eine tastbare Infiltration des Beckenbindegewebes in die verschiedenen Lymphknotengruppen metastasiert.

Diese befallenen Lymphknoten könnten vor Therapiebeginn mit großer Sicherheit durch die Lymphographie entdeckt werden (FRISCHBIER; FUCHS; SIEBER). Es liegt daher der Gedanke nahe, die Lymphographie für die Stadieneinteilung mit heranzuziehen. Weitere Aussagen kann die Cavographie in dieser Richtung machen und schließlich in manchen Fällen auch die Ausscheidungsurographie mit guter Darstellung des Ureterverlaufs, also am besten in Form des Infusionsurogramms.

Es kann aber nicht ernst genug davor gewarnt werden, Untersuchungen, die nicht überall im gleichen Umfang angewandt werden und werden können, für die Stadieneinteilung zu verwenden. Die Kollektive würden dann noch weniger vergleichbar und Rückschlüsse auf die Wirksamkeit des zugrunde liegenden Behandlungsverfahrens noch weiter erschwert werden. Es wäre zum jetzigen Zeitpunkt unrealistisch zu erwarten, diese Diagnostikverfahren ständen an allen Kliniken zur Verfügung, wie eine Umfrage bei den Frauenkliniken der Bundesrepublik ergab.

Schon die Änderung der Stadieneinteilung für das Korpuscarcinom im Annual Report ab 1962 ist verwirrend genug, und es muß unbedingt bei Berichten verlangt werden, daß angegeben wird, welche Stadieneinteilung Verwendung findet. Bezüglich der Zulässigkeit der verschiedenen diagnostischen Methoden für die Stadieneinteilung sollte unbedingt Einhelligkeit bestehen. So gibt die UICC in ihren entsprechenden Empfehlungen zur TNM-Klassifikation (1968) für das Collum- und das Korpuscarcinom ganz klar folgende Richtlinien für die Beurteilung der Ausdehnung des Prozesses:

a) Methoden, die für die Stadieneinteilung angewandt werden *müssen:* Inspektion, Palpation und einfache Röntgenuntersuchungen, wie z.B. Lungen- und Skeletaufnahmen.

b) Methoden, die zusätzlich angewandt werden *können:* Abrasio, Konisation oder Cervixamputation.

c) Methoden, deren Anwendung zwar empfohlen wird, die aber bis jetzt *nicht* für die Stadieneinteilung *berücksichtigt werden dürfen:* Kolposkopie, Urographie, Pelveographie, Lymphographie, Phlebographie, Arteriographie.

Im Widerspruch dazu soll für die am Annual Report mitarbeitenden Kliniken Vorschrift sein, daß bei einem Collumcarcinom mit Hydronephrose oder stummer Niere, unabhängig vom sonstigen Tastbefund, eine Zuordnung zum Stadium III erfolgt (Handbook for the guidance of collaborators when reporting cases of carcinoma of the cervix, Stockholm 1968).

Der Übersichtlichkeit halber sollen die TNM-Klassifikation (Tabelle 3) und die Stadieneinteilung (Tabelle 4) hier dargestellt werden. Es ist aber nach dem Gesagten eindeutig, daß jede Stadieneinteilung unbefriedigend bleiben muß und daher immer wieder variiert werden wird. Daher erscheint es uns, zumindest für den Gebrauch in unserer Klinik, günstiger, auch alle Feststellungen, die über die Ausdehnung des Tumors gemacht wurden, mit zu erfassen und zu dokumentieren. Das ermöglicht dann zu jedem späteren Zeitpunkt eine Zuordnung der Fälle auch zu einer anderen Stadieneinteilung. Das ist bei

Tabelle 3. *TNM-Klassifikation des Korpuscarcinoms (UICC 1966)*

T	Primärtumor	N	Regionäre Lymphknoten	M	Fernmetastasen	G	Histopathologische Einteilung
T1S	prae-invasives Carcinom, sog. Carcinoma in situ	NX	Beckenlymphknoten nicht zu beurteilen	M0	kein Anhalt für Fernmetastasen	G1	Tumor stark differenziert
T1	auf das Corpus uteri beschränktes Carcinom	NX −	(histologische Untersuchung exstirpierter Lymphknoten negativ)	M1	Fernmetastasen gesichert (Metastasen in den inguinalen Lymphknoten gelten als Fernmetastasen)	G2	Tumor mit mäßig ausgeprägter Differenzierung
T1a	das Cavum uteri ist nicht vergrößert					G3	anaplastischer Tumor
T1b	das Cavum uteri ist vergrößert	NX +	(histologische Untersuchung exstirpierter Lymphknoten positiv)				
T2	das Carcinom greift auf die Cervix über						
T3	Carcinomausbreitung außerhalb des Uterus einschließlich Vaginalmetastasen. Tumor beschränkt auf das kleine Becken	N0	keine Veränderungen der *regionären* Lymphknoten bei der Lymphographie				
T4	Carcinomausbreitung außerhalb des kleinen Beckens *oder* Befall der Blasenschleimhaut *oder* der Rectumschleimhaut. Der Nachweis eines bullösen Ödems reicht allein nicht für die Zuordnung des Tumors zum Stadium T4 aus!	N1	spezifische Veränderungen der *regionären* Lymphknoten bei der Lymphographie festgestellt				

Tabelle 4. *Stadieneinteilung des Korpuscarcinoms. (Nach dem „Annual Report on the results of treatment in carcinoma of the uterus and vagina", 1967)*

0	Histologische Befunde verdächtig auf Malignität, aber eine Bestätigung liegt nicht vor
I	Das Carcinom ist auf das Korpus beschränkt
II	Das Carcinom hat Korpus und Cervix befallen
III	Das Carcinom hat sich über den Uterus ausgebreitet, aber nicht über das kleine Becken hinaus
IV	Das Carcinom hat sich über das kleine Becken hinaus ausgebreitet oder hat die Schleimhaut von Blase und Rectum befallen

elektronischer Datenverarbeitung dann leicht durch Variierung des entsprechenden Programms möglich. Wir haben daher maschinenlesbare Belege entworfen, deren Druckvorlagen in Abb. 1 und 2 dargestellt sind. Durch eine einfache Strichmarkierung der Befunde kann die Stadienzuordnung von der Maschine vorgenommen oder bei zusätzlicher Angabe des Stadiums oder der TNM-Klassifikation auf dem Bogen von der Maschine eine Plausibilitätskontrolle durchgeführt werden.

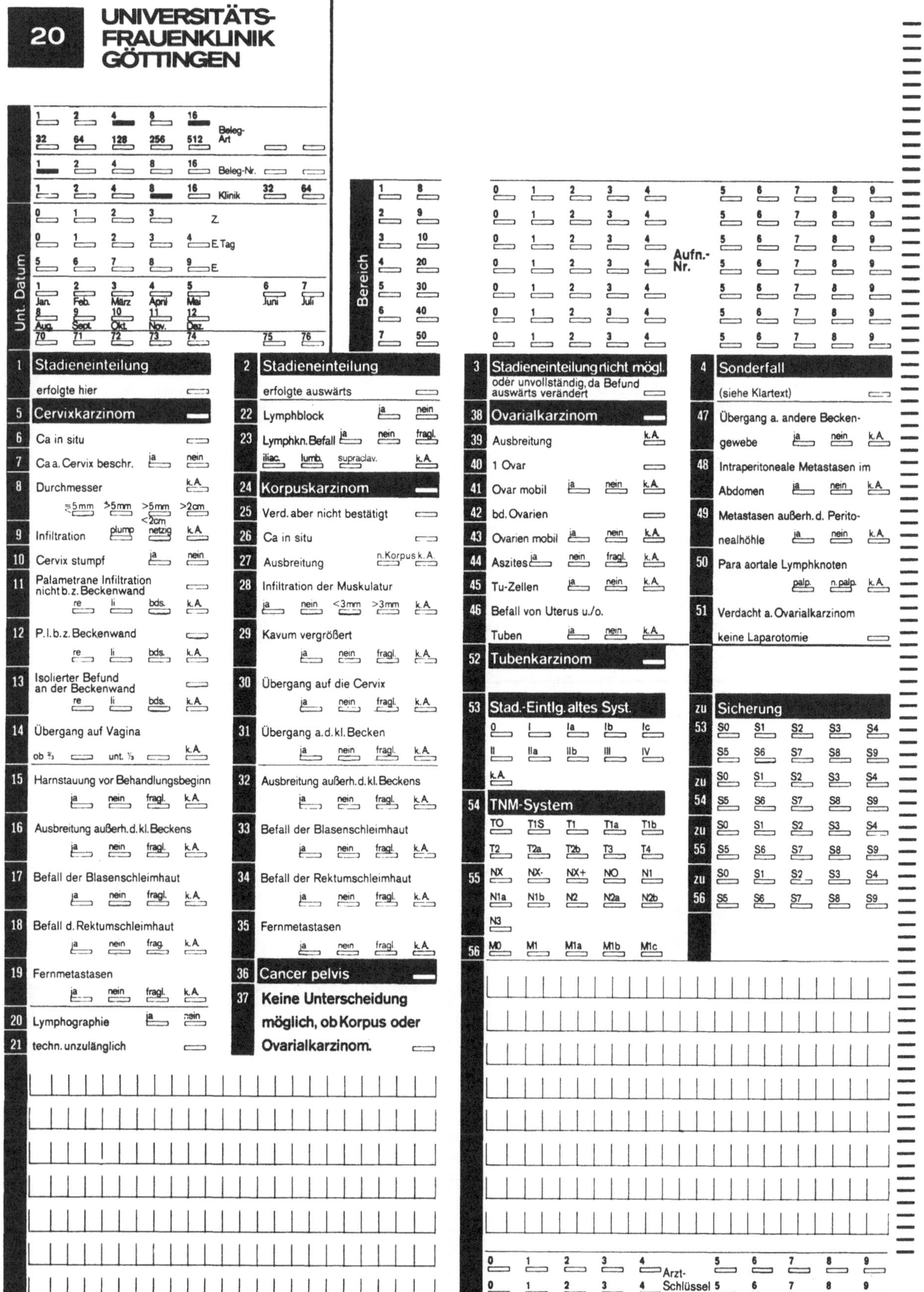

Abb. 1. Markierungsbeleg I: Stadieneinteilung für Cervixcarcinom, Korpuscarcinom, Ovarialcarcinom und Tubencarcinom für optischen Belegleser

21 UNIVERSITÄTS-FRAUENKLINIK GÖTTINGEN

1 2 4 8 16 · 32 64 128 256 512 — Beleg-Art
1 2 4 8 16 — Beleg-Nr.
1 2 4 8 16 32 64 — Klinik
0 1 2 3 — Z
0 1 2 3 4 — E.Tag
5 6 7 8 9 — E.
Unter.-Datum — 1 Jan. 2 Feb. 3 März 4 April 5 Mai 6 Juni 7 Juli / 8 9 10 11 12 Aug. Sept. Okt. Nov. Dez. — Monat / 70 71 72 73 74 75 76 — Jahr

Bereich — 1 8 / 2 9 / 3 10 / 4 20 / 5 30 / 6 40 / 7 50

Aufn.-Nr. — 0 1 2 3 4 5 6 7 8 9 (repeated rows)

1 Stadieneinteilung
erfolgte hier

5 Vaginalkarzinom
6 Ca in situ
7 Ausbreitung k.A.
8 Prim.-Tumor n. sichtbar
9 Ca a. Scheidenwand beschränkt — Tumor Ø <2cm >2cm
10 Befall paravaginalen Gewebes — ja nein frag. k.A.
11 Ausbreitung bis zur Becken-wand rechts — ja nein k.A.
12 links — ja nein k.A.
13 Ausbreitung außerh. des klein. Beck. — ja nein frag. k.A.
14 Befall der Blasenschleimhaut — ja nein frag. k.A.
15 Befall der Rektumschleimhaut — ja nein frag. k.A.
16 Fernmetastasen — ja nein frag. k.A.

33 Lymphographie ja nein
34 technisch unzulänglich
35 Lymphblock — ja nein
36 Lymphknoten Befall — ja nein frag. / iliac. lumb. supraclav. k.A.

2 Stadieneinteilung
erfolgte auswärts

17 Vulvakarzinom
18 Ca in situ
19 Ausbreitung k.A.
20 Prim.-Tumor n. sichtbar
21 Vulva-Tumor Ø — ≤2cm >2cm <5cm 75cm
22 Multiple Tumoren Ø — >10cm <10cm k.A.
23 Ausdehnung a. Vagina — ≤2cm >2cm k.A.
24 Befall der Urethra — ja nein frag.
25 Befall des Anus — ja nein frag. k.A.
26 Befall der Rektumschleimhaut — ja nein frag. k.A.
27 Befall d. Septum rektrovaginale — ja nein frag. k.A.
28 Befall anderer benachbarter Bezirke — ja nein frag. k.A.
29 Lymphknoten — palp. n.palp. bewg. fix. k.A.
30 Seite — glei. and. bd
31 Lymphknoten — Tu.-verd. u.-verd.
32 Fernmetastasen — ja nein frag. k.A.

3 Stadieneinteilung
nicht möglich o. unvollständig da Bfd. auswärts veränd.

37 Urethralkarzinom
38 Ca in situ
39 Tumor — bewg. fix. k.A.
40 Ausbreitung k.A.
41 Hälfte d. Urethra — unt. ob.
42 Befall der Blase — ja nein frag. k.A.
43 Befall der Vulva — ja nein frag. k.A.

48 Mammakarzinom re. li. bds.
49 Ausbreitung k.A.
50 Prim.-Tumor n. sichtbar
51 Durchmesser — ≤2cm >2cm <5cm -5cm <10cm >10cm k.A.
52 Hautbeteiligung — gesp. m.Gr. fix. A.-Ph. ja nein k.A.
53 Mam. eingez. — ja nein k.A.
54 Paget in Umgebung der Mamille — ja nein k.A.
55 M. pect. fix. — ja nein k.A.
56 Fixierung an der Brustwand — ja nein k.A.

64 Stad.-Eintlg. altes Syst.
0 I Ia Ib Ic / II IIa IIb III IV / k.A.

65 TNM-System
T0 T1S T1 T1a T1b / T2 T2a T2b T3 T4
66 NX NX- NX+ N0 N1 / N1a N1b N2 N2a N2b / N3
67 M0 M1 M1a M1b M1c
0 1 2 3 4 5 6 7 8 9

4 Stadieneinteilung
Siehe Klartext

44 Befall anderer Gewebsbezirke — ja nein frag. k.A.
45 Leistenlymphknoten k.A. — palp. n.palp. bewg. fix.
46 Seite — re. li. bds. k.A. / tumorverd. unverd.
47 Fernmetastasen — ja nein frag. k.A.
57 Lymphknoten gl. Seite Axilla — palp. n.palp. bewg. fix. k.A.
58 Lymphknoten verd. a. Beteilig. k.A. — ja nein verback. fix.
59 Lymphkn. gleiche Seite supra — o. infracavicular palpabel — ja nein bewg. fix. k.A.
60 Armödem — ja nein k.A.
61 Hautbeteiligung außerh. der Brust — ja nein frag. k.A.
62 Befall der anderen Seite — Mamma ja nein frag. k.A. / Lymphk. ja nein frag. k.A.
63 Fernmetastasen — ja nein frag. k.A.

Sicherung
zu — S0 S1 S2 S3 S4 / **64** S5 S6 S7 S8 S9
zu — S0 S1 S2 S3 S4 / **65** S5 S6 S7 S8 S9
zu — S0 S1 S2 S3 S4 / **66** S5 S6 S7 S8 S9
zu — S0 S1 S2 S3 S4 / **67** S5 S6 S7 S8 S9

0 1 2 3 4 5 6 7 8 9 — Arzt-Schl.

Abb. 2. Markierungsbeleg II: Stadieneinteilung für Vaginalcarcinom, Vulvacarcinom, Urethralcarcinom und Mammacarcinom für optischen Belegleser

Ein weiteres Problem stellt die Schwierigkeit der Zuordnung der oben schon beschriebenen Fälle dar, in denen die Endocervix und/oder die Ovarien befallen sind. Hier sind nach dem Annual Report (bzw. der UICC) folgende Richtlinien zu berücksichtigen:

1. Ein Carcinom soll als Cervixcarcinom eingruppiert werden, wenn der Sitz des Primärtumors die Cervix ist.

2. Ein Carcinom soll als Korpuscarcinom eingruppiert werden, wenn der Sitz des Primärtumors im Corpus uteri ist (damit sollte auch die früher vorgeschriebene Aussonderung der Fälle von Carcinoma uteri et ovarii bis auf wenige Ausnahmen hinfällig sein).

3. Kann bei einem Carcinom des Korpus und der Cervix nicht entschieden werden, ob der Ausgangspunkt die Cervix oder das Korpus ist, soll ein Adenocarcinom als Korpus- und ein Plattenepithelcarcinom als Cervixcarcinom eingruppiert werden.

4. Ein Carcinom im Corpus uteri, das sich nach früherer Adnexexstirpation wegen eines Ovarialcarcinoms entwickelt hat, soll nur dann als Korpuscarcinom eingestuft werden, wenn ein rezidivfreier Zeitraum von mindestens 5 Jahren dazwischenliegt.

Ebenso wie von der UICC (Tabelle 3) wurden von zahlreichen Autoren weitergehende Unterscheidungen nach histologischen Kriterien versucht und angegeben, um den Malignitätsgrad eines Tumors, sowohl für die Prognose als auch für die Auswahl der Therapie, heranzuziehen. Diese Versuche, die zum Teil schon sehr lange zurückliegen (MAHLE, 1923; BRODERS, 1925), haben für die Praxis nur wenig Bedeutung erlangt, obwohl sich daraus gewisse Schlüsse ziehen lassen. So hat, ähnlich wie HEALY und CUTLER (1930), z.B. J. H. MÜLLER (1941) eine Einteilung nach histologischen Kriterien in vier Gruppen, je nach dem Differenzierungs- bzw. Ausreifungsgrad, angegeben:

1. Adenocarcinoma Grad I (adenoma malignum),
2. Adenocarcinoma Grad II,
3. Carcinoma glandulare partim solidum Grad III,
4. Carcinoma solidum (cylindrocellulare) Grad IV.

PÜSCHEL und MÖBIUS schlagen 1967 in Anlehnung an v. ALBERTINI und DALLENBACH-HELLWEG und BRÄHLER folgende Einteilung vor:

1. Hochdifferenziertes Adenocarcinom,
2. Carcinoma adenomatoides,
3. schleimbildendes Adenocarcinom,
4. Adenocancroid,
5. mucoepidermoides Carcinom,
6. solides Carcinom.

Eine Übersicht bringt die Tabelle 5 von P. HOFMANN, auf der zugleich in Spalte 2 die an unserer Klinik übliche Einteilung aufgeführt ist.

Trotz verschiedener Nomenklaturen, Begriffsbestimmungen und auch Beurteilung einzelner histologischer Kriterien im Schrifttum besteht eine gewisse Übereinstimmung darüber, daß die reiferen, ausdifferenzierten Tumoren ein langsameres Wachstum und eine bessere Prognose zeigen als die anaplastischen Formen. So fand LINDGREN in 525 Fällen bei ausdifferenzierten Formen ein Verhältnis zwischen oberflächlicher und tieferer Infiltration der Uterusmuskulatur von 3:1, bei anaplastischen Tumoren aber von 1,5:1. LINDSAY fand, daß bei den unreifen Formen (Grad IV) mit der Strahlentherapie bessere Ergebnisse als mit der Operation erzielt wurden. Ähnliche Äußerungen, auch aus neuerer Zeit, liegen neben den obengenannten von einer ganzen Reihe weiterer Autoren vor, so von ARNESON (1964), von GUSBERG und YANNOPOULOS, von HEALY und CUTLER, KAMNIKER, KOTTMEIER (1959) und von RENNING und JAVERT. STRICKLAND (1965) sah dagegen keine Korrelation zwischen dem histologischen Bild und der Prognose. Tabelle 6 zeigt hierzu eine übersichtliche Zusammenstellung von HOFMANN und SIMMENROTH.

Tabelle 5. *Vorschläge verschiedener Autoren zur histologischen Klassi-*

	BRODERS (1925)	GÖTTINGEN (1968)	W. PÜSCHEL, G. MÖBIUS (1967)	J. A. RANDALL, et al. (1951)	P. FELDWEG (1935), SCHRÖDER-CORDUA (1922)	J. A. CORSCADEN (1962)	v. FRANQUÉ (1930), H. D. KLEINE (1930)	E. KAUFMANN (1911)	SCHOTTLÄNDER, KERMAUNER (1912)
Entdifferenzierung	Grad 1 bis 25% solid	Gruppe I hochdifferenziertes Adeno-Ca.	hoch-differenziertes Adeno-Ca.	Gruppe I malignes Adenom	reifes Ca.	Grad 1 malignes Adenom	reifes Adeno-Ca. (malignes Adenom)	malignes Adenom	malignes Adenom
		Gruppe II solide Anteile ≦ 25%	kernisomorph Carcinoma adenomatoides	Gruppe II teilweise solides papilläres Wachstum beträchtliche Verzweigung	mittelreifes Ca.	Grad 2 Carcinoma adenomatoides	mittelreifes Adeno-Ca.	Adeno-Ca. und das papilläre Adeno-Ca.	Adeno-Ca. mit Zellschichtung und Bildung solider Nester, jedoch Wahrung des ursprünglichen Drüsentypes
	Grad 2 25—50% solid	Gruppe III solide Anteile zwischen 25 und 75%							
	Grad 3 50—75% solid		kern-poly-morph	Gruppe III mehr solides Wachstum, aber glanduläre Struktur ist noch deutlich	unreifes Ca.				
	Grad 4 über 75% solid	Gruppe IV solide Anteile > 75%	Carcinoma solidum	Gruppe IV Carcinoma solidum	strukturloses Ca.	Grad 3 völlig undifferenziertes Ca.	völlig unreifes Ca.	solides Adeno-Ca.	Carcinoma glandulare, „bei denen durch primäre Ausfüllung des Drüsenlumens der drüsige Charakter schnell verlorengeht"
Sonderformen		Adenocancroid mucoepidermoides Ca. schleimbildendes Ca.	Adenocancroid mucoepidermoides Ca. schleimbildendes Ca.	Plattenepithelmetaplasie				Adeno-Ca. mit Plattenepithelmetaplasie	

Schließlich sei noch erwähnt, daß vereinzelt die histologische Differenzierung bei der Festsetzung des Bestrahlungsplanes und besonders der Dosis berücksichtigt wird (FLETCHER). Darüber hinaus wurden Untersuchungen angegeben, um die Dignität des Carcinoms in der Gewebekultur zu beurteilen und daraus prognostische Schlüsse zu ziehen (RUBIN). Die Versuche, die Strahlensensibilität von Korpuscarcinomen in gleicher Weise zu testen wie bei Collumcarcinomen (Radiation response), führten zu keinem Ergebnis (FEINER und GARIN). Immerhin ist nach dem Vorstehenden ARNESON (1964) beizupflichten, daß beim Korpuscarcinom eine größere Übereinstimmung zwischen der histologischen Beurteilung und dem Verlauf, sowohl bei der Operation als auch bei der Strahlentherapie, festzustellen ist als bei anderen Tumorlokalisationen. Auch JAVERT und RENNING fanden bei 610 Patientinnen der Jahre 1909—1960 die Überlebensrate abhängig vom histologischen Differenzierungsgrad. Sie betrug bei Adenoma malignum 81,9%, bei Adenocarcinom 53,9% und bei Adenoakanthom 35,9%. PRICE, HAHN und ROMINGER fanden die größte Rezidivhäufung bei den unreifen Formen und RUBIN, GERLE, QUICK und GREENLAW geben an, daß die Adenoakanthome auffällig häufig in die Scheide metastasieren.

Es ist also sicherlich berechtigt, die histologische Differenzierung des einzelnen Falles in die therapeutischen und prognostischen Überlegungen mit einzubeziehen. Eine all-

fizierung des Korpuscarcinoms. (Nach P. HOFMANN und H. SIMMENROTH)

LINDSAY (1927), LAHM (1927), KEHRER (1920)	E. DAVIS (1964)	A. V. ALBERTINI (1955)	J. EWING (1940)	SCHEFFEY et al. (1943)	G. DÖDERLEIN, A. DÖDERLEIN, F. VOLZ (1926)	PALUGYAY (1925), FRANKEL u. KRAUL (1925)	L. ADLER (1916)	CARMICHAEL (1967), G. DALLENBACH-HELLWEG (1962)
malignes Adenom	malignes Adenom	malignes Adenom	papilläres malignes Adenom malignes Adenom	gut differenziertes Ca.	gut gereiftes Adeno-Ca.	hohe Reife	höhere Reife	gut differenziertes Adeno-Ca.
sekundär solides Adeno-Ca.	Adeno-Ca.	Carcinoma adenomatoides	Gruppe 3 Adeno-Ca. alveolär oder solide	mittleres Ca.	mittelgereiftes Adeno-Ca.	mittlere Reife	mittleer Reife	anaplastisches (unreifes) Adeno-Ca.
			Gruppe 4 diffuses Ca.	undifferenziertes Ca.	unreifes Ca.	niedere Reife	niedere Reife	
Adenocancroid Plattenepithel-Ca. (LAHM)	Adenoakanthom maligne Polypen des Endometriums		Adenoakanthom					Adenoakanthom, Carcinosarkom

gemeinere Bedeutung für das praktische Vorgehen, wie GUSBERG und YANNOPOULOS es vorschlagen, haben diese Dinge allerdings bisher nicht erlangt. Die histologische Differenzierung etwa bei der Stadieneinteilung zusätzlich zugrunde zu legen, ist abzulehnen, da hierbei keine Einheitlichkeit gewährleistet wäre (HOFMANN; BLAIKLEY, KOTTMEIER, MARTIUS und MEIGS). Für die Stadieneinteilung des Korpuscarcinoms sollte nach Ansicht mancher Autoren auch die Uterusgröße Berücksichtigung finden (DELCLOS, FLETCHER, GUTIERREZ u. RUTLEDGE; FLETCHER; GUSBERG u. YANNOPOULOS, UICC). GUSBERG und YANNOPOULOS sowie HEALY und BROWN fanden die Prognose um so schlechter, je größer der Uterus war und PRICE, HAHN und ROMINGER sahen eine dreimal höhere Rezidivhäufigkeit bei primär vergrößertem Uterus. Zur Beurteilung solcher Angaben müßte allerdings auch das gewählte Behandlungsverfahren berücksichtigt werden, insbesondere, ob bei einer eventuellen intrauterinen Radiumtherapie die Dosisverteilung der Uterusgröße angemessen war.

Für die Uterusgröße gilt das gleiche, was oben für die histologische Differenzierung gesagt wurde. Sie sollte bei der Prognose berücksichtigt und protokolliert werden, was ohnehin schon immer praktiziert wurde, dagegen nicht als Kriterium bei der Stadieneinteilung Verwendung finden. Daß sie für die Auswahl des Behandlungsverfahrens eine Rolle spielt, ist einleuchtend.

Tabelle 6. *5-Jahres-Heilung des Korpuscarcinoms innerhalb der einzelnen histologischen*

W. Püschel u. G. Möbius (1967)				J. A. Randall, D. F. Mirik u. E. E. Wieben (1951)				E. L. Renning u. C. T. Javert (1964) (Ewing-System)			K. W. Barber, H. B. Hunt et al. (1962) (Broders-System)		
	Fälle	5-Jahres-Heilung	in %		Fälle	5-Jahres-Heilung	in %		Fälle	5-Jahres-Heilung in %		Fälle	5-Jahres-Heilung in %
hochdifferenz. Adeno-Ca.	29	25	86	Adenoma malignum	26	23	88,4	Adenoma malignum	76	81,9	Grad 1	179	91
Carcinoma adenomatoides kernisomorph	72	57	79	teilweise solides Wachstum aber glandul. Struktu-ren zu erkennen — Drüsenschläuche dos à dos dicht gepackt und verzweigt	117	70	59,8	Adeno-Ca. papillär	386	53,9	Grad 2	63	81
kernpolymorph	31	18	58		132	68	51,5	Adeno-Ca. alveolär	38	54,8	Grad 3	27	52
Ca. solidum	3	2	—	solides Ca.	38	10	26,3	Acanthom	96	35,9	Grad 4	8	62

3. Die Symptome

Über die Symptomatologie des Korpuscarcinoms ist an dieser Stelle nur wenig zu sagen. Hier steht die vaginale Blutung als wichtigstes Zeichen an erster Stelle. Nach Amreich sind unregelmäßige Blutungen nach der Menopause in 42—60% Zeichen eines Korpuscarcinoms. Nach Kottmeier (1959) haben wenigstens 6 von 10 Patientinnen, die nach zweijähriger oder längerer Amenorrhoe wegen Spontanblutungen den Arzt aufsuchen, ein Genitalmalignom. Den Blutungen kann mehr oder weniger lange ein hartnäckiger Ausfluß vorausgehen, nach Amreich in 21—28% als erstes Zeichen. Neben den Blutungen können Cervixpolypen, eine tastbare Uterusvergrößerung, eine Pyometra und in Zusammenhang damit wehenartige Schmerzen einen Hinweis geben. Uteruspolypen sind im Klimakterium nach Amreich u.a. in etwa 30% mit einem Carcinom vergesellschaftet.

Auffällig ist, daß man bei den Korpuscarcinom-Patientinnen überdurchschnittlich häufig weitere Störungen oder Krankheiten findet, die auf eine Beteiligung des Endokriniums hindeuten und die auch zu Spekulationen hinsichtlich der Ursache der Korpuscarcinome geführt haben (s. a. Abschnitt „Biologie des Korpuscarcinoms", S. 72). So finden sich nach v. Mikulicz-Radecki in 26,8% gleichzeitig Myome. Bekannt ist auch der große Anteil an übergewichtigen Patientinnen. Kottmeier (1959) sah 7% mit einem Gewicht über 100 kg, 36% über 80 kg. Soergel fand sogar 76% über 85 kg. Die Häufigkeit eines Diabetes wird von den gleichen Autoren mit 7% (Kottmeier) bzw. 13% angegeben. Überdurchschnittlich häufig soll auch die Zahl der Hypertonikerinnen sein. Im gleichen Sinne und mit Zahlen ähnlicher Größenordnung äußerten sich Charles, Bell, Loraine und Harkness; Dibbelt, Müller und Ehlers; Garnet; Goetschel; Grimm; Weber. Grimm geht so weit, zu formulieren, daß das Zusammentreffen von

Gruppen nach verschiedenen Autoren. (Nach P. Hofmann und H. Simmenroth)

G. Franz (1965) (Broders-System)				A. E. Mahle (1923) (Broders-System)			T. N. Roman, R. P. Beck u. J. P. A. Latour (1967) (Broders-System)				T. N. Roman, R. P. Beck u. J. P. A. Latour (1967) (Einteil. Royal Victoria Hosp.)				Göttingen (1968)			
	Fälle	5-Jahres-Heilung	in %		Fälle	5-Jahres-Heilung in %		Fälle	5-Jahres-Heilung	in %		Fälle	5 Jahres-Heilung	in %		Fälle	5-Jahres-Heilung	in %
Grad 1	68	68	100	Grad 1	10	100	Grad 1	38	33	86,8	hoch	47	41	87,2	Gruppe I	29	21	72,4
Grad 2	64	52	81	Grad 2	114	71,6	Grad 2	56	46	82,4	mittel	116	83	78,3	Gruppe II	96	55	57,3
Grad 3	52	17	33	Grad 3	54	38,0	Grad 3	89	65	73,3					Gruppe III	52	24	46,2
Grad 4	19	3	16	Grad 4	8	0,0	Grad 4	83	38	45,8	niedrig	113	58	51,5	Gruppe IV	11	3	27,3

Blutungen in der Menopause mit Endokrinopathien den besonderen Verdacht auf Vorliegen eines Korpuscarcinoms erwecken müßte. Frühsymptome oder auch spezifische Symptome des Korpuscarcinoms gibt es nicht. In jedem verdächtigen Falle muß den Symptomen nachgegangen und eine histologische Verifizierung vorgenommen werden.

4. Die Diagnose

Die Diagnose des Korpuscarcinoms wird ausschließlich durch die histologische Untersuchung des durch Abrasio gewonnenen Gewebes gestellt. Da es wichtig ist, zu wissen, ob das Carcinom auf das Corpus uteri beschränkt ist oder aber ob es sich um ein Carcinom des Korpus und der Endocervix handelt, sollte stets eine fraktionierte Abrasio vorgenommen werden. Dabei soll zunächst nur der Cervicalkanal dilatiert und abradiert werden. Danach erfolgt die Dilatation des inneren Muttermundes und die Abrasio des Cavum uteri. Bei getrennter Untersuchung des gewonnenen Materials ist so eine Entscheidung über den Befall der Cervix möglich. Die noch weitergehende Fraktionierung der Abrasio, wie sie von Heyman vorgeschlagen wurde, hat sich nicht durchgesetzt und ist auch kaum von Bedeutung. Die Situation wird außerdem dadurch erschwert, daß bei den meisten Patientinnen schon vor der Aufnahme in die Klinik eine Abrasio vorgenommen wurde. Eine Therapie des Korpuscarcinoms — sei sie chirurgisch, radiologisch oder kombiniert — darf erst dann durchgeführt werden, wenn die histologische Diagnose vorliegt.

Auf keinen Fall kann diese histologische Verifizierung des Geschwulstleidens durch eine andere Untersuchungsmethode ersetzt werden. Die Cytologie, als Fährtensuchmethode beim Cervixcarcinom unentbehrlich, hat beim Korpuscarcinom bisher nicht befriedigen können (v. Mikulicz-Radecki). Auch die offenbar höhere Treffsicherheit besonderer Techniken der Materialentnahme, so durch Absaugen (Soost) oder durch Verwendung eines bürstenartigen Instrumentes (Boschann; MacLean; Wenig), ändert nichts daran, daß in jedem verdächtigen Falle eine Abrasio unerläßlich ist.

Die Hysterographie kommt ebenfalls als primäre diagnostische Maßnahme nicht in Betracht. Sie ist jedoch in hervorragender Weise geeignet, für die Therapie und die Prognose weitere wertvolle Informationen für den Einzelfall zu geben, wie die Abb. 3—6 zeigen. Die Lokalisation und die Ausdehnung der Geschwulst, die Konfiguration und die räumliche Lage des Uteruscavums und nicht zuletzt eventuelle Mißbildungen, z.B. ein

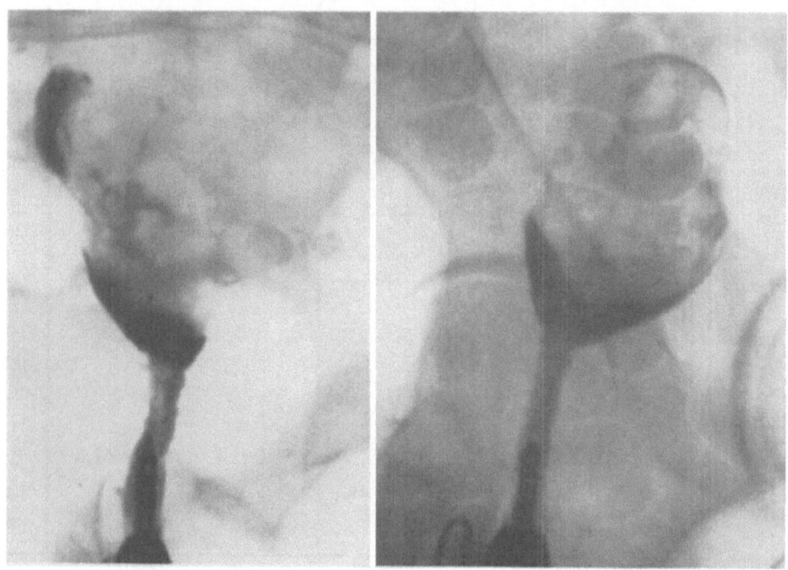

Abb. 3. Hysterogramm eines ausgedehnten Korpuscarcinoms (links sagittal, rechts seitlich)

Uterus bicornis, lassen sich, insbesondere im Hinblick auf die Packmethode, beurteilen, nach Reinermann auch beschränkte Rückschlüsse auf den Reifegrad des Tumors ziehen. Der praktische Wert der Hysterographie für die Therapie des Korpuscarcinoms wird von zahlreichen Autoren betont (Castaño-Almendral u. Frischkorn; Dalsace u. Garcia-Caldéron; Graziani u. Caturani; Hilfrich, Castaño-Almendral, Flaskamp u. Hofmann; Kepp; du Mesnil de Rochemont, Ringleb, Scherer u. Schmitt; J. H. Müller, 1941; Norman; Obolensky u. Zürcher; Petersen; Zsolnai u. Nyirö). Ein Teil der Autoren betont auch den Wert der Hysterographie für die Verlaufskontrolle. Dagegen möchte Kottmeier (1959) sie wegen der Gefahr der Infektion und der Tumorzellverschleppung nur in bestimmten Fällen angewendet wissen.

In diesem Zusammenhang ist noch die Hysteroskopie zu nennen (Silander; Lyon; Schmidt-Matthiesen). Es handelt sich dabei um die Betrachtung des Uteruscavums durch ein cystoskopähnliches Instrument, dessen Objektiv und Beleuchtungsquelle sich innerhalb eines dehnbaren, mit Wasser zu füllenden Gummibläschens mit durchsichtiger Wand befinden. Nach Einführen des Instrumentes in das Uteruscavum wird das Bläschen mit Wasser gefüllt und distanziert dabei die Uteruswand. Hiermit lassen sich Tumoren direkt betrachten und ihre Lokalisation und Ausdehnung erkennen. Auch für andere Zwecke — gedacht sei an die Erkennung einer Uterusperforation — ist diese Methode brauchbar.

Erneut erwähnt werden müssen aber auch die Angiographien. Die Arterio- und die Phlebographien haben beim Korpuscarcinom vorwiegend in der Rezidivdiagnostik und bei der Untersuchung spezieller Folgezustände nach der Behandlung eine Bedeutung

(BREIT; FERNSTRÖM; FRISCHKORN, 1965, 1966; KOTTMEIER, 1959). Dabei ist aber die Einschränkung zu machen, daß die Cavographie es durchaus gestatten kann, prä- und paracavale Lymphknotenmetastasen nachzuweisen (FUCHS). Die wesentlichste Bedeutung kommt hier aber der Lymphographie zu, sowohl für die Auswahl der Therapie als auch für die Prognose. Gerade beim Korpuscarcinom, bei dem sich eine weitergehende

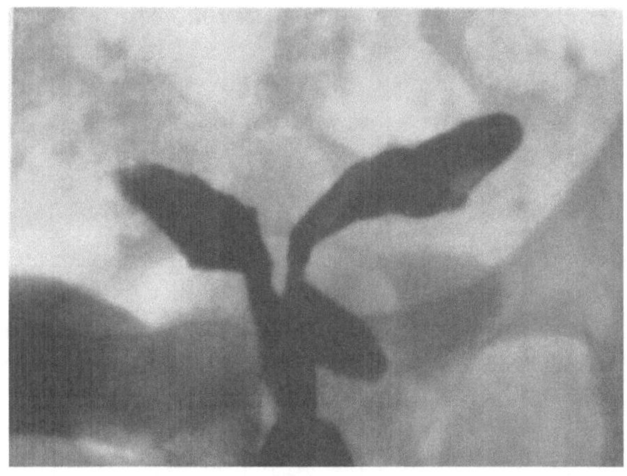

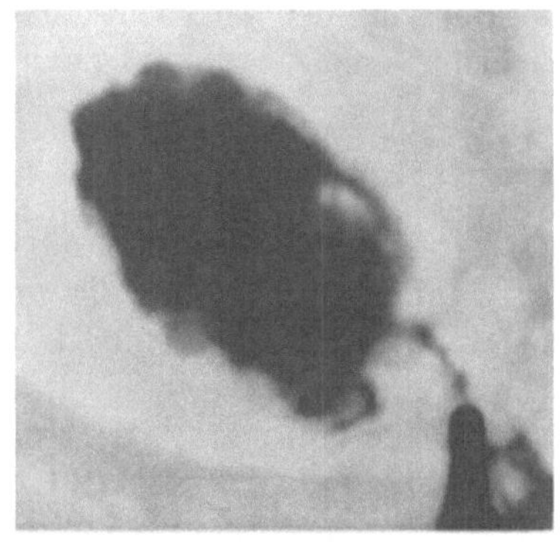

Abb. 4   Abb. 5

Abb. 4. Hysterogramm: Uterus bicornis unicollis. Endometriumcarcinom histologisch in beiden Uterushörnern bestätigt. Röntgenbefund nur im rechten Horn verdächtig. Gartnergangcyste links an der Cervix

Abb. 5. Hysterogramm: Endometriumcarcinom, mehr flächenhaft wachsend, weites Uteruscavum

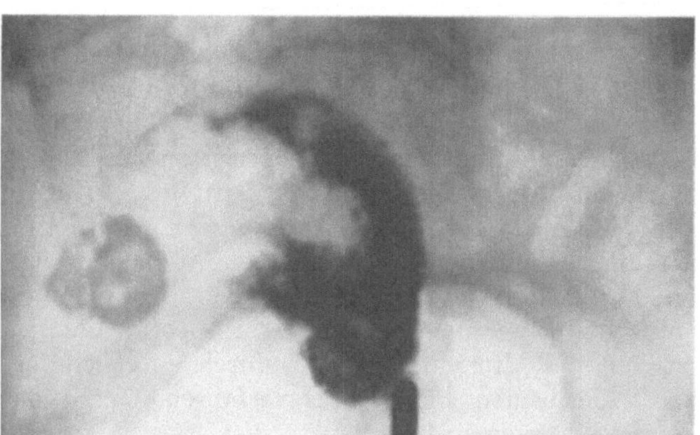

Abb. 6. Hysterogramm: Korpuscarcinom, vorwiegend rechtsseitig entwickelt. Befall des rechten Tubenwinkels (Kalkschatten rechts neben dem Uterus)

Ausbreitung nur sehr selten an einem parametranen Infiltrat erkennen läßt, im Gegensatz zum Collumcarcinom, stellt die Lymphographie nahezu die einzige Möglichkeit dar, mit großer Zuverlässigkeit einen Befall der regionären Lymphknoten zu erkennen. Die Lymphographie ist daher an zahlreichen Kliniken inzwischen eine obligatorische Untersuchung vor Therapiebeginn. Schließlich ist noch bei der Besprechung der Diagnostik zu erwähnen, daß auch in einem Ausscheidungsurogramm Hinweise für eine Lymphknotenmetastasierung im Retroperitonealraum gefunden werden können. Hier handelt es sich im wesentlichen um Verdrängung des Ureters oder auch der Niere, die schließlich zu einer Achsendrehung führen kann, und um Stauungszeichen. Die Darstellung carcinomatöser Lymphknoten ermöglicht sowohl deren systematische Entfernung mit anschließender röntgenologischer Kontrolle des Operationserfolges wie die gezielte Bestrahlung (AVERETTE, HUDSON, VIAMONTE, PARKS u. FERGUSON; FUCHS u. ZUPPINGER; GERTEIS; REIFFENSTUHL; RÜTTIMANN).

Es sei auf die entsprechenden Ausführungen in diesem Handbuch verwiesen.

Mit den geschilderten diagnostischen Verfahren läßt sich in typischen Fällen ein komplexes Bild des vorliegenden Geschwulstwachstums gewinnen, das nicht nur zur Indikationsstellung erforderlich ist, sondern darüber hinaus auch wertvolle Hinweise für Einzelheiten der Therapie liefert. In den Fällen aber, in denen aus dem Abradat histologisch nur der Verdacht auf Malignität zu entnehmen ist, sollte unter genauer Beobachtung abgewartet und nach 4—6 Wochen erneut curettiert werden.

5. Therapie

Trotz der Fortschritte, die die Strahlentherapie auch bei der Behandlung der Korpuscarcinome gemacht hat, ist die am weitesten verbreitete Ansicht die, daß das Korpuscarcinom nach Möglichkeit operiert werden sollte (BOCK, LATOUR u. BOURNE; BUSSE u. SOERGEL; GUSBERG u. YANNOPOULOS; HOFMANN; JAVERT u. RENNING; KEPP u. HOFMANN; KIRCHHOFF, 1962; KRAATZ; DU MESNIL DE ROCHEMONT, RINGLEB, SCHERER u. SCHMITT; von MIKULICZ-RADECKI u. GANSAU; J. H. MÜLLER, 1941; PRICE, HAHN u. ROMINGER; SCHEELE; SOERGEL). Allerdings betont KIRCHHOFF aufgrund der Arbeit von WIMHÖFER, ZEITZ und RUNGE, daß die Strahlentherapie neben der Operation als gleichwertig anzusehen sei und nur bestimmte Befunde, wie Myome, vergrößerte Uteri mit weitgehend carcinomatös durchsetzter Wand und Adnextumoren, günstiger für ein operatives Vorgehen sind. Wie schon GUSBERG feststellt, ist aus dem Schrifttum keinerlei Einmütigkeit hinsichtlich des besten Verfahrens zu erkennen. Erschwerend kommt hinzu, daß die Statistiken nach Material und Ansatz so uneinheitlich sind, daß ein Vergleich der Behandlungserfolge zwischen Operation und Bestrahlung kaum möglich ist. Immerhin weisen neben WIMHÖFER, ZEITZ und RUNGE auch GROSSE-HOLZ, SCHULZE und VOGELGESANG darauf hin, daß bei Berücksichtigung des Alters beide Methoden offenbar Gleiches zu leisten imstande sind. Daß dieser Faktor ganz beträchtlich sein kann, zeigt z.B. PETERSEN, der das Durchschnittsalter der Operierten mit 52,6, das der Bestrahlten aber mit 64 Jahren angab. Ein weiterer Faktor wird von v. MIKULICZ-RADECKI und GANSAU erwähnt. Sie weisen darauf hin, daß gut operable Patientinnen mit günstigem Befund oftmals die großen Kliniken gar nicht erreichen, weil sie in umliegenden kleineren Häusern operiert und nur die lokal und allgemein schlecht operablen weitergeleitet werden. Schließlich zeigt auch die Untersuchung von BICKENBACH, LOCHMÜLLER und FLACH, daß bei Berücksichtigung des Altersunterschiedes durch Vergleich der Kollektive mit der „Normalsterblichkeit" die beiden Behandlungsverfahren, Operation und Bestrahlung, offenbar zu gleich guten Ergebnissen führen.

In den letzten Jahren wird aber mehr und mehr die Kombination beider Methoden in Form der *Vor*bestrahlung mit Operation nach unterschiedlich angegebenem zeitlichen Zwischenraum befürwortet. Hierauf wird weiter unten noch eingegangen.

In diesen Diskussionen wird auch immer wieder geltend gemacht, daß das Adenocarcinom weniger strahlensensibel sei als das Plattenepithelcarcinom. Das veranlaßt beim Collumcarcinom vielfach zu einer höheren Dosierung, wenn es sich histologisch um ein Adenocarcinom handelt (FRISCHBIER in diesem Band, Kap. IV, S. 144). Es ist sicher so, daß bei der Beurteilung der Behandlungsergebnisse das Patientenalter und die Ausbreitungsstadien nicht immer genügend berücksichtigt werden. Daß verschiedene Differenzierungsgrade eventuell eine entsprechend unterschiedliche Prognose haben (Tabelle 6), ist bekannt. Ein Anlaß, das Korpuscarcinom als nicht ausreichend strahlensensibel anzusehen, besteht aber, wie die Erfolge zeigen, auf keinen Fall. Ob bei wirklich vergleichbaren Bedingungen zur Erzielung desselben Effektes beim Adenocarcinom eine höhere Dosis erforderlich ist als beim Plattenepithelcarcinom, ist zumindest nicht erwiesen.

Wie unterschiedlich die Auffassungen hinsichtlich der Therapie sind, geht vielleicht am besten aus dem „Annual Report" hervor, wo im 14. Band die Häufigkeit der Uterusexstirpation — mit oder ohne Vorbestrahlung — von Klinik zu Klinik zwischen 0 und 100% schwankt (Tabelle 18). Wenn somit auch keine klare Entscheidung im Sinne eines Entweder/Oder zwischen Operation und Bestrahlung möglich ist, vielmehr beide Methoden, wie auch Kirchhoff betont, sich gegenseitig ergänzen, so sind doch auch in einem radiologischen Handbuch die Gesichtspunkte zu besprechen, die für oder gegen eine operative Behandlung einer Korpuscarcinom-Patientin sprechen können.

Wie schon bei den Symptomen aufgeführt, ist das Korpuscarcinom oftmals mit mannigfachen anderen Störungen verbunden, die zusätzlich zu dem meist relativ hohen Alter der Patientinnen die Allgemeinoperabilität ganz wesentlich einschränken. Da, wie erwähnt, der Anteil der operierten Patientinnen im Krankengut der einzelnen Kliniken außerordentlich unterschiedlich ist, scheint die Beurteilung der Operabilität gerade beim Korpuscarcinom aber doch nach sehr verschiedenen Kriterien vorgenommen zu werden. Bei der Auswahl der Methode helfen auch die Zahlenangaben über die primäre Mortalität nicht weiter, da sie sich sehr angenähert haben. Nach Amreich bewegen sie sich bei der operativen Behandlung zwischen 0 und etwa 6%.

Unabhängig von der persönlichen Auffassung des Therapeuten gibt es aber ganz zweifellos Gesichtspunkte, die für die Operation sprechen müssen und bei deren Vorliegen die Unterlassung der Operation für die Patientin von Nachteil sein muß. Der diesbezügliche Standpunkt von Kirchhoff ist schon weiter oben gegeben worden. Huber betont, zum Teil in Übereinstimmung mit Kirchhoff, daß bei ausgedehnter Zerstörung der Uteruswand, Einbruch in den interstitiellen Tubenabschnitt, Beteiligung von Tube, Peritoneum, Ovar und Kombination mit gutartigen Tumorbildungen der Operation der Vorzug gegeben werden sollte. Das gleiche sollte unseres Erachtens auch für Uterusmißbildungen gelten. Nach Bickenbach besteht aber keine Notwendigkeit, die Operation zu forcieren. Auf die Kombination beider Methoden wird unten im Kapitel über die Vor- und Nachbestrahlung noch einzugehen sein. Die Operationsmethode ist die Exstirpation des Uterus auf abdominalem oder vaginalem Wege, bei Übergang des Carcinoms auf die Endocervix die erweiterte abdominelle Totalexstirpation des Uterus und der Anhänge nach Wertheim oder auf vaginalem Wege nach Schauta. Im allgemeinen wird wegen der Übersichtlichkeit und der Möglichkeit der Lymphknotenexstirpation heute der abdominale Weg bevorzugt, zumal dabei der Uterus nicht so stark traumatisiert wird (Gefahr der Tumorzellaussaat). Die gegenüber den Collumcarcinom-Patientinnen im allgemeinen wesentlich schlechtere Allgemeinoperabilität wird aber in zahlreichen Fällen veranlassen, den schonenderen vaginalen Weg zu wählen.

Die Ovarien müssen in jedem Fall mit entfernt werden, da in ihnen nach Price, Hahn und Rominger u.a. in 5—18% der Fälle Metastasen gefunden werden. Auch makroskopisch unverdächtige Ovarien dürfen nicht belassen werden, da nach Virieux bei 100 Sektionen 56,8% der Ovarialmetastasen nur mikroskopisch erkannt werden konnten.

a) Die primäre Strahlentherapie des Korpuscarcinoms

Das primäre Ausbreitungsgebiet des Carcinoms, das Cavum uteri, stellt ursprünglich einen dreizipfligen, in sagittaler Richtung abgeplatteten Hohlraum dar, an den sich nach caudal der mehr röhrenförmige Cervicalkanal anschließt. Dieser Raum wird durch das Geschwulstwachstum im allgemeinen eine Größenzunahme, besonders aber auch eine Formveränderung, erfahren, über die quantitativ und qualitativ, abgesehen von einer Sondierung und instrumentellen Austastung des Uterus, nur eine Hysterographie etwas aussagen kann (Abb. 3—6). Ein derartiges mehr oder weniger kompliziertes Raumgebilde homogen zu bestrahlen, wäre an sich nur mit einer Tiefentherapie möglich. Da diese wegen der gesamten räumlichen Dosisverteilung und der geringen in der Uteruswand erzielbaren Dosis bisher als alleinige Therapie nicht in Frage kommt, besteht die Notwendigkeit, mit Hilfe einer intrauterin eingelegten Strahlenquelle entsprechender Form der idealen Dosisverteilung möglichst nahe zu kommen. Daß dies mit einem einfachen Röhrenfilter nicht möglich ist, geht aus der schematischen Abb. 7 hervor, zumal wenn selbst bei annähernd regelmäßig geformtem Cavum das Filter eventuell nicht symmetrisch liegt. Der besonders filternahe, außerordentlich steile Dosisabfall führt zwangsläufig im Bereich der Tubenwinkel, also gerade in Bezirken, in denen das Carcinom in einem höheren Prozentsatz lokalisiert ist, zu sehr viel niedrigeren Strahlendosen als in anderen Bezirken der Uteruswand. Trotz dieser Probleme hat das Radium seine dominierende Stellung in der Strahlentherapie der Korpuscarcinome behalten, weil in Form der von Heymann 1936 eingeführten Packmethode die Möglichkeit besteht, sich jeder Uteruskonfiguration mit der Strahlenquelle anzupassen. Es hat bis in die neueste Zeit nicht an Versuchen gefehlt, besondere Filter zu entwickeln, die den räumlichen Anforderungen

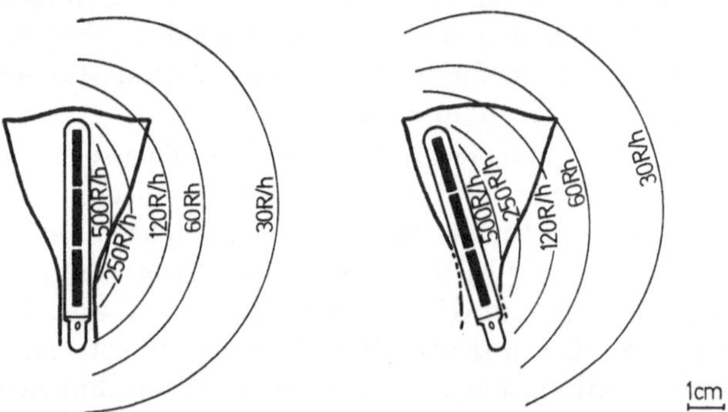

Abb. 7. Bestrahlung des Corpus uteri mit einem Röhrenfilter (3×30 mCi Ra). Schematische Darstellung der ungenügenden Ausleuchtung der Tubenwinkel, insbesondere bei asymmetrischer Lage des Filters

gerecht werden sollten. Erinnert sei an die Triangel- und Bukettform von Dietel und den Versuch von Henschke, durch Vermehrung der Aktivität in der Spitze des Röhrenfilters die Konfiguration der Isodosen entsprechend der Cavumform zu beeinflussen. In letzter Zeit haben noch Granone und Juliani einen entsprechenden Hysterostaten angegeben und Schmitz (1952) einen sog. Y-Applikator. Es ist aber J. H. Müller beizupflichten, wenn er sagt, daß bei deformiertem Uterus alle diese Filter weniger brauchbar sind.

Wenn sich diese Erkenntnisse auch nur zögernd durchgesetzt haben und zum Teil auch heute noch Korpuscarcinome bei vergrößertem Uterus mit Röhrenfiltern bestrahlt werden, so kann doch zum jetzigen Zeitpunkt gesagt werden, daß die Radium- und eventuell Isotopentherapie in Form der Packmethode das Verfahren der Wahl ist (Arneson, 1964; Bickenbach, Gärtner u. Zoeppritz; Busse u. Soergel; Costolow, Nolan, Budenz u. Du Sault; Fletcher; Frischkorn, 1964; Gross und Veillon; Gusberg u. Yannopoulos; Hess u. Rosendahl; Hofmann; Kepp; Kirchhoff; Kottmeier; Martin u. Martin; J. H. Müller).

Wenn nachfolgend die einzelnen strahlentherapeutischen Methoden besprochen werden, dann muß man sich darüber im klaren sein, daß gerade beim Korpuscarcinom eine strenge Unterscheidung zwischen alleiniger Strahlentherapie und operativer Behandlung mit Vor- und/oder Nachbestrahlung gar nicht möglich ist. Eine primär operierte Korpuscarcinom-Patientin wird immer sorgfältig darauf zu prüfen sein, in welchem Umfang zusätzliche strahlentherapeutische Maßnahmen erforderlich sind, die ja, besonders bei fortgeschrittenen Fällen, auch noch als kurative und nicht als prophylaktische Maßnahmen aufzufassen sind. Ebenso wird eine primär bestrahlte Patientin in vielen Fällen nach kürzerem oder längerem Zwischenraum der Operation zuzuführen sein.

α) Die Radium-Packmethode

Die von HEYMAN 1936 eingeführte Packmethode unter Verwendung von Radium basiert auf der Auffüllung des Uteruscavums und eventuell auch des Cervicalkanals mit einer Reihe kleinerer eiförmiger oder auch zylindrischer Filter, die im allgemeinen jeweils ein Radiumröhrchen enthalten. Abhängig von Größe und Gestalt dieser Filter ist es mehr oder weniger vollkommen möglich, eine räumliche Angleichung der Aktivität an die Form des Uteruscavums zu erzielen. Die Unterschiede zwischen den an den einzelnen Kliniken angewandten Methoden bestehen, abgesehen von der Dosierung, vor allem in der Form und den äußeren Abmessungen der verwendeten Filter (Tabelle 7, Abb. 8). J. H. MÜLLER verwendet z. B. Filter mit einer Länge von 33 mm, während die kürzesten von RIES nur 8,5 mm lang sind. Die Dicke schwankt von 5,0—13,8 mm. Je umfangreicher

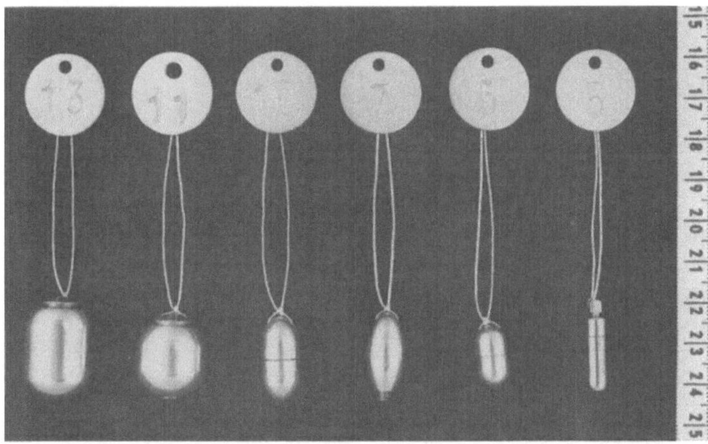

Abb. 8. Verschiedene Formen von Radiumfiltern für die Packmethode. Ganz rechts die zumeist gebräuchliche Zylinderform (Buchler & Co., Braunschweig)

das einzelne Filter, um so weniger läßt sich die Verteilung der Aktivität dem Ideal annähern. Größere Filterdurchmesser benötigen zudem eine weitergehende Dilatation des Cervicalkanals, was bei der Rigidität der Cervix älterer Frauen ein wesentlicher Nachteil sein und das Risiko des Eingriffs erhöhen kann. Kleinere Filter können dagegen eine größere Perforationsgefahr bedingen. Diese Filter werden entweder untereinander verbunden und als Kette in den Uterus eingeführt, was die Komplikationsmöglichkeiten beim Ziehen des Radiums vermindert (RIES), oder sie werden mittels Draht oder Faden einzeln mit Nummernschildern versehen, die es ermöglichen, sie bei Beendigung der Bestrahlung in umgekehrter Reihenfolge wieder zu ziehen (Göttingen, Houston, Stockholm). Dabei dürfte das Einführen einzelner Filter hinsichtlich des Strahlenschutzes günstiger sein, da jeweils nur ein Filter außerhalb des Schutzbehälters zu sein braucht. Weitere Einzelheiten sind aus der Tabelle 7 zu ersehen.

Die unterschiedlichen Methoden der einzelnen Kliniken und Institute (Tabelle 8) sind dabei zum Teil nicht durch Zweckmäßigkeitsgründe bedingt, sondern einfach aus ihrer historischen Entwicklung zu verstehen. Es kommen allerdings auch abweichende oder sogar gegensätzliche Gesichtspunkte zum Tragen. So z. B., wenn im Radiumhemmet in Stockholm auf eine möglichst starke Filterung Wert gelegt, an der I. Universitäts-Frauenklinik München dagegen eine möglichst geringe vorgezogen wird, die es gestattet, auch weichere Anteile des γ-Spektrums noch zur Wirkung kommen zu lassen. Hier wird schließlich sogar die zusätzliche Anwendung von β-Strahlern erwogen, um das Endometrium mit einer noch höheren Dosis zu belegen (RIES und BREITNER). Die Form der von RIES verwendeten Filter ist dazu dem Isodosenverlauf angepaßt.

Tabelle 7. *Übersicht über die an einigen Kliniken für*

Klinik	Strahlen-quelle und Aktivität des einzelnen Filters	Filterform	Applikation als Kette oder einzeln
Radiumhemmet, Stockholm	Radium 10 mCi 8 mCi	Zylinder	einzeln
I. Universitäts-Frauenklinik, München	Radium a) 2—6 mCi b) 10—20 mCi	Eiform	Kette
	^{60}Co-Perlen	Kugel	Kette
Universitäts-Frauenklinik, Zürich	Radium	Zylinder	einzeln
Los Angeles Tumor-Institut	Radium 10 mCi	Zylinder	einzeln
Universitäts-Strahlenklinik, Marburg	Radium 10 mCi ^{60}Co-Perlen	Zylinder	Kette
Universitäts-Frauenklinik, Göttingen	Radium 10 mCi	Zylinder	einzeln
M.D. Anderson Hospital and Tumor Institute, Houston	Radium 5, 10 und 15 mCi	Zylinder	einzeln

Der differenzierteste Behandlungsplan für das Korpuscarcinom ist zweifellos von Fletcher angegeben worden, dessen Tabellen daher hier vollständig wiedergegeben werden sollen (Tabelle 9—14). Hierbei wird ausdrücklich das Adenocarcinom der Cervix einbezogen, da vielfach hinsichtlich der Stadieneinteilung und der Abgrenzung und damit auch der Therapie Unklarheiten bestehen. Im übrigen sei aber bezüglich des Adenocarcinoms der Cervix uteri auf das Kapitel von Frischbier, S. 137 verwiesen.

Die Packmethode scheint auf den ersten Blick alle Komplikationsmöglichkeiten, die sich aus der Form des Uteruscavums und seiner tumorbedingten räumlichen Veränderung für die Dosisverteilung ergeben können, zu beseitigen. Hier sind jedoch Einschränkungen zu machen. Einmal kann der Uterus so klein sein, daß bei Anwendung der Packmethode nur eine sehr geringe Aktivität appliziert werden könnte, wobei außerdem je nach Abmessung der Filter wieder größere Inhomogenitäten der Dosisverteilung in Kauf genommen werden müßten. In derartigen Fällen wird allgemein die Applikation eines Röhrenfilters vorgezogen. Außerdem besteht auch bei der Packmethode notwendigerweise an den Stellen des Bestrahlungsraumes ein kritischer Dosisbereich im Sinne eines Defizits, an denen er eine zipflige Ausziehung aufweist. Dies ist im Bereich der Tubenwinkel und des Os internum der Fall. Durch Einlegen von Radium auch in den Cervicalkanal läßt sich eine zu geringe Bestrahlungsdosis im unteren Pol des Uteruscavums vermeiden, in den Tubenwinkeln dagegen nicht in erwünschtem Maße. Hinzu kommt die Schwierigkeit, daß niemals mit absoluter Sicherheit gewährleistet ist, daß die im allgemeinen zu Beginn der Applikation in die Tubenwinkel eingelegten Filter hier auch tatsächlich verbleiben. Die Abbildung läßt dies klar erkennen und unterstreicht die Notwendigkeit, auf die Tubenwinkel besonders zu achten. Hier kann aber auch die Röntgenkontrollaufnahme (Abb. 9—11) die Beurteilung erleichtern.

Die für besonders große Uteri mit erhöhter Perforationsgefahr von Kottmeier (1959) angegebene Methode, zunächst ein Röhrenfilter in das Korpus einzulegen und durch ständigen Lagewechsel der Patientin („Rollkur") zu erreichen, daß das Filter mit den

die Packmethode verwendeten Filter und Aktivitäten

Äußere Abmessungen	Wandstärke	Material	Gesamt-filterung Platin	Anmerkungen
mm	mm		mm	
5,1 — 6,3 × 18 7,8 —13,8 × 27,0 — 32,0	—	—	1,25 —1,3	nach Möglichkeit Verwendung der kleinsten Filter (max. 20)
5,0 × 8,5 10,0 × 19,0 ∅ 6,0	—	Aluminium Kobalt mit Gold- mantel	0,63	
8,0 × 33,0	1,2	Silber vergoldet	1,0	
Länge 23,0	—	—	1,37	
5,0 × 19,0	—	—	1,0	
5,5 × 22,0	1,5	Messing	0,87	
4 verschiedene Stärken	—	—	1,0	

verschiedensten Wandteilen des Uterus Kontakt bekommt, hat keine Bedeutung erlangt. Die so angestrebte gleichmäßige Bestrahlung des Uterus läßt sich heute besser durch eine Supervolttherapie erreichen. Die Methode von KOTTMEIER hatte bei einer Dosierung von 3000 mgeh eine Verkleinerung des Corpus uteri zum Ziele, so daß dann 2—3 Wochen später die übliche Packmethode erfolgen konnte. Auch bei primärer Anwendung der Packmethode ergibt sich im Laufe der Behandlung eine Verkleinerung des Cavum uteri wie die Abb. 9—11 zeigen, die alle von der gleichen Patientin stammen. Interessant ist beim Betrachten der Bilder auch die offenbar von der Tamponade abhängige unterschiedliche Lage des Uterus auf Abb. 10 im Vergleich zu den beiden anderen Abbildungen.

Die Radiumdosierung bei der Bestrahlung des Korpuscarcinoms wird heute noch fast ausschließlich nach Milligrammelementstunden (mgeh) vorgenommen. Da bei der Packmethode die unterschiedlichsten Aktivitäten ganz verschiedenartige räumliche Anordnungen erfahren, im Einzelfall die Aktivität im Uterus also jeweils eine Strahlenquelle unbekannter Dosisleistung darstellt, die dazu noch an geometrisch gleichwertigen Raumpunkten stark variieren kann, ist es praktisch nicht möglich, mit Strahlendosen an bestimmten Bezugspunkten, wie bei der Behandlung des Collumcarcinoms (TOD u. MEREDITH; FRISCHKORN, 1964; GAUWERKY, 1957), zu arbeiten. Abgesehen von direkten Meßverfahren ist daher nur eine „Dosierung in Größenordnungen" möglich, wie sie auch zumeist praktiziert wird. So wird bei der Stockholmer Methode angestrebt, mit zwei Einlagen insgesamt etwa 3000 R in 1,5 cm Tiefe, gerechnet von der Uterusinnenfläche, einzustrahlen (KOTTMEIER, 1959), eine Distanz, die etwa der Wandstärke des Uterus entspricht. Diese — vergleichsweise außerordentlich niedrige — Dosis entspricht dabei einer mgeh-Zahl von 3000 bis maximal 4080. Die mgeh-Rechnung wird aber von KOTTMEIER abgelehnt. Für die verschiedenartigen dort verwendeten Filter und ihre jeweiligen Anzahlen wird die Bestrahlungszeit Tabellen entnommen. Die Belastung von Blase und Darm wird durch direkte Messung kontrolliert.

Tabelle 8. *Beispiele für die Bestrahlungsmethoden einiger Kliniken*

Klinik	Primäre Strahlentherapie				Postoperative Nachbestrahlung	Obligatorische histologische Nachkontrolle
	Radium			zusätzliche Percutanbestrahlung		
	intrauterin (^{60}Co-Perlen)	cervical	vaginal			
Radiumhemmet, Stockholm	Packmethode, zweimal fraktioniert 3000 R/1,5 cm (etwa 3000 bis maximal 4080 mgeh). Je nach verwendeter Aktivität wird die Bestrahlungsdauer Dosistabellen entnommen	ja, mit gleicher Methode	ja, bei einer intrauterinen Einlage wie bei der postoperativen Nachbestrahlung. Bei Carcinom der Endocervix eine weitere Einlage vor die Portio. Bei Scheidenmetastasen eine zusätzliche Einlage auf diesen Bezirk	nur bei fortgeschrittenen Fällen und bei Carcinom der Endocervix	obligatorisch: zylindrischer Applikator mit 100—150 mCi Radium. Dosis 2500—3000 R/1 cm Gewebstiefe. Zusätzliche Percutanbestrahlung bei tieferer Infiltration des Carcinoms empfohlen	ja
I. UniversitätsFrauenklinik, München	Radium-Packmethode, 3mal fraktioniert im Abstand von 2—3 Wochen. 6000 mgeh werden angestrebt, aber auf keinen Fall werden 6—7000 R Blasen- oder Rectumbelastung überschritten. Bei kleinen Uteri auch Kobaltperlen: 3×1300 R/3 cm Tiefe, etwa 3×8 Std Bestrahlungsdauer	ja, mit gleicher Methode	zusätzliche Einlage einer Portioplatte mit 30—50 mCi Radium bei einer der drei intrauterinen Einlagen	nur bei den weniger adipösen Patientinnen: 8—10 mal 200—300 ROD (190 kV, 16 mA, HWS 1,0 Cu, 10×15 cm, 50 cm FHA) 4 Felder. Fortgeschrittene Fälle konventionelle Pendelbestrahlung bis 4000 RHD an der Beckenwand	obligatorisch: Rundfilter in das Scheidengewölbe, 30—50 mg Radium für 20—25 Std. 14 Tage später Bestrahlung der gesamten Vagina mit Röhrenfilter in Hartgummi-Distanzrohr	—
UniversitätsFrauenklinik, Zürich	Packmethode mit wenigen großen Filtern (zumeist 4), 4000—5500 mgeh, je nach Uterusgröße	Röhrenfilter zusätzlich, 8 mm ⌀ 5,1—9 cm lang	Federbügelkolpostat, 2×40 mCi Radium für 25 Std 5—7 Tage nach der zweiten intrauterinen Applikation	1 ventrales und 1 dorsales Feld 18×18 cm 80 cm FHA, 2 Seitenfelder 8×16 cm, 50 cm FHA. Ab 1000 ROD wird 5 cm breiter Mittelstreifen ausgespart. 6 Tage steigende Dosen. Ventral und dorsal 2400 ROD, Seitenfelder 2000 ROD. Konventionelle Tiefentherapie, Thoraeusfilter	obligatorisch: Radium, Pariser Kolpostat, 2000—2500 mgeh. Percutanbestrahlung wie bei primärer Strahlentherapie	—

Los Angeles Tumor Institut	Packmethode, Radium, mindestens zweimal fraktioniert, je 24—48 Std, meist 30 Std 6000—8000 mgeh, vaginales Radium eingeschlossen	Röhrenfilter mit 20 mCi Radium	Gummi- oder Kunststoffapplikatoren, 25 mCi Radium beiderseits im Scheidengewölbe	nur, wenn keine Uterusexstirpation vorgesehen ist: 4 Felder 10 × 15 cm, 1800—2100 RED pro Feld (500 kV, 4 mA, 1 mm Pb-Äquivalent-Filter, HWS 6 mm Cu)	—	wenn möglich und angezeigt Uterusexstirpation nach 4—6 Wochen
Universitäts-Strahlenklinik, Marburg	Radium-Packmethode, zweimal fraktioniert. Dominiciröhrchen je 10 mCi, 7000 bis 8000 R/1 cm (im allgemeinen 10 Filter) (gelegentlich ^{60}Co-Perlen)	bei einer Einlage ein Röhrenfilter, das äußeren Muttermund überragt	—	grundsätzlich ja, nur bei sehr adipösen Patientinnen mit sehr günstigem Befund wird verzichtet. „Marburger Methode" Felderanordnung radiär um die durch die Portio gehende Querachse des Beckens, aber Ziellinie beim Corpuscarcinom 2—3 cm nach cranial verlegt. Herddosis 2500 R. (Telekobalt)	Percutanbestrahlung 3000 RHD, Technik wie nebenstehend	ja
Universitäts-Frauenklinik, Göttingen	Radium-Packmethode, dreimal fraktioniert. Gesamtbestrahlungsdauer maximal 60 Std (werden zumeist unterschritten). 6000 R in Blase oder/und Rectum werden insgesamt nicht überschritten	ja, mit gleicher Methode. Bei Carcinoma endocervicis Röhrenfilter	nein (außer bei Befall der Vagina)	ja, wenn keine Gegenindikation (hohes Alter, Adipositas, schlechter Allgemeinzustand) Telekobalt, 4 Felder 6 × 14 cm, 50 cm FHA, täglich 2 Felder mit je 300 ROD (max.), 2500 RHD pro Parametrium	obligatorisch: Radium in den Scheidenstumpf, Kunststoff-Filter, 50 mCi, 2000 R/1 cm. Percutanbestrahlung bei Infiltration der Uterusmuskulatur, 4 Felder, 8 × 14 cm, 50 cm FHA, Telekobalt, täglich 2 Felder, je 300 ROD (max.), 3000—4000 RHD. Palliativ operierte Patientinnen: Homogenbestrahlung des kleinen Beckens bis maximal 6000 RHD (4 konvergente Felder 10 × 14 cm)	ja
M. D. Anderson Hospital and Tumor Institute, Houston	s. Tabellen 9—14					

Tabelle 9. *Adeno-Carcinom des Uterus. Behandlungsrichtlinien des M.D. Anderson Hospital and Tumor Institute. (Nach* Fletcher, *Textbook of Radiotherapy)*

Klinische Situation	Korpus	Korpus und Collum	Cervix-Carcinom
Kleiner Tumor	*Operation* Zusätzlich präoperativ Radium intrauterin und vaginal	*Operation* Zusätzlich präoperativ Radium intrauterin und vaginal (wie beim Platten-epithel-Carcinom der Cervix) *Bestrahlung der Para-metrien*	*Strahlentherapie* Behandlung wie beim Plattenepithel-Carcinom
Großer zentraler Tumor	*Operation* Zusätzliche Percutan-bestrahlung und Radium intrauterin und vaginal	*Operation* Zusätzlich präoperativ Percutanbestrahlung und Radium intrauterin und vaginal (wie beim Platten-epithel-Carcinom der Cervix)	*Strahlentherapie* Behandlung wie beim Plattenepithel-Carcinom. Zusätzlich Totalexstir-pation nach der Bestrah·lung
Fortgeschrittener Tumor oder allgemein inoperabel	*Strahlentherapie* Percutanbestrahlung; Radium wenn möglich	*Strahlentherapie* Percutanbestrahlung; Radium, wenn möglich	*Strahlentherapie* Percutanbestrahlung; Radium, wenn möglich

Tabelle 10. *Adeno-Carcinom der Cervix. Behandlungsrichtlinien des M. D. Anderson Hospital and Tumor Institute. (Nach* Fletcher, *Textbook of Radiotherapy)*

Klinische Situation	Behandlung
Stadium I und II Kleine Tumoren	*Behandlung wie Plattenepithel-Carcinom* Tandem und Kolpostat 2 × 72 Std, 2 Wochen Abstand ? Bestrahlung der Parametrien
Stadium I und II Große zentrale Tumoren	4000 rad auf das ganze Becken; Tandem und Kolpostat 72 Std; Uterusexstirpation 4—6 Wochen nach Bestrahlung; Allgemein inoperabel: 4000 rad auf das ganze Becken; Tandem und Kolopostat 2 × 48 Std, 3 Wochen Abstand
Stadium II und III Beteiligung der Parametrien oder Fixierung	*Behandlung wie Plattenepithel-Carcinom* Percutanbestrahlung; 4000 rad auf das ganze Becken; Tandem und Kolpostat 2 × 48 Std, 2 oder 3 Wochen Abstand oder 6000 rad auf das ganze Becken Tandem und Kolpostat 72 Std

Von Czech wurde 1951 eine einfache Methode einer Dosierung angegeben, die bei unterschiedlichen Uterusgrößen und Filterzahlen gewissermaßen der jeweiligen Eigen-absorption und Distanzierung von der Uteruswand Rechnung tragen sollte. Er schlug vor, daß sich die Anzahl der eingelegten Filter mit je 10 mCi Radium und die Liegezeit in Stunden zu 30 ergänzen sollte. Das heißt also:

    8 Filter sollten 22 Std liegen = 1 760 mgeh,
   10 Filter sollten 20 Std liegen = 2 000 mgeh,
   15 Filter sollten 15 Std liegen = 2 250 mgeh.

Bei höheren Filterzahlen sollte dann die Zeit von 15 Std aber nicht mehr überschritten werden.

Tabelle 11. *Adeno-Carcinom des Endometriums, lokal und allgemein operabel. Behandlungsrichtlinien des M.D. Anderson Hospital and Tumor Institute. (Nach* FLETCHER, *Textbook of Radiotherapy)*

Klinische Situation	Behandlung des Uterus	Behandlung der Vagina
Kleiner Uterus gut ausdifferenzierter Tumor	Nur Totalexstirpation	Mitnahme einer Scheidenmanschette
Uterus *wenig vergrößert* gut ausdifferentzierter Tumor	Radium 1 × 72 Std Tandem oder 3000—3500 mgeh Packmethode Totalexstirpation	Kolpostat 7000 rad Oberflächendosis in 1 Applikation
Mäßig vergrößerter Uterus gut ausdifferenzierter Tumor	Radium 2 × 2000 mgeh, 2—3 Wochen Abstand oder 4000 rad auf das ganze Becken und Radium entweder 1 × Packmethode 2500 mgeh oder Tandem 72 Std mit 15—10 mg Radiumröhrchen Totalexstirpation	Kolpostat 2 × 4000 rad Oberflächendosis, 3 Wochen Abstand 4000 rad Oberflächendosis 1 Applikation
Großer Uterus oder anaplastischer Tumor	4000 rad auf das ganze Becken und Radium entweder 1 × Packmethode 2500 mgeh oder Tandem 72 Std mit 15—10 mg Radiumröhrchen Totalexstirpation	Kolpostat 4000 rad Oberflächendosis 1 Applikation

Tabelle 12. *Adeno-Carcinom des Endometriums, lokal operal, aber allgemein inoperabel oder lokal inoperabel. Behandlungsrichtlinien des M.D. Anderson Hospital and Tumor Institute. (Nach* FLETCHER, *Textbook of Radiotherapy)*

Klinische Situation	Behandlung des Uterus	Behandlung der Vagina
Kleiner Uterus gut ausdifferenzierter Tumor	Tandem (20—15—10 mg), 2 × 72 Std (6000 mgeh)	*Kolpostat* 2 × 4000 rad Oberflächendosis
Uterus *wenig vergrößert* gut ausdifferenzierter Tumor	*Packmethode* 2 × 3000 mgeh oder 3 × 2500 mgeh	*Kolpostat* 2 × 4000 rad Oberflächendosis
Mäßig vergrößerter Uterus oder anaplastischer Tumor	*Percutanbestrahlung* 4000 rad auf das ganze Becken; Packmethode oder Tandem 3500—4000 mgeh	*Kolpostat* 4000 rad Oberflächendosis
Großer Uterus	*Percutanbestrahlung* 4000—6000 rad auf das ganze Becken. ? Eventuell zusätzlich 1 oder 2 Radiumeinlagen, abhängig von der Reaktion des Tumors	*Kolpostat* 4000 rad Oberflächensdosis, falls Percutanbestrahlung mit 5000 rad beendet wird
Lokal inoperabel	*Percutanbestrahlung* 4000 rad/4000—6000 rad/6 Wochen. Eventuell zusätzlich 1 × Radium; Packmethode, wenn der Tumor auf die äußere Bestrahlung befriedigend anspricht	Oberflächendosis 2500—4000 rad abhängig von der Percutanbestrahlung

J. H. MÜLLER variierte die Bestrahlungszeit nur wenig nach Uterusgröße und verabfolgte im allgemeinen 5000—6500 mgeh. DU MESNIL DE ROCHEMONT strebt 7000—8000 R in 1 cm Gewebstiefe auf zwei Einlagen verteilt an. FREED und PENDERGRASS halten 7000—15000 R an der Uterusaußenfläche für erforderlich. Zahlreiche weitere Autoren

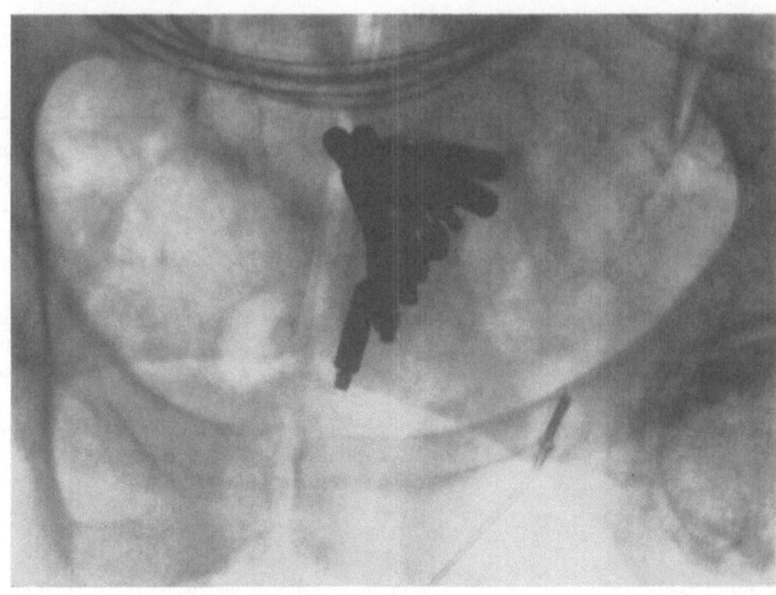

a

Abb. 9a u. b. Stereoaufnahmepaar der ersten Radiumeinlage. Zugehöriges Hysterogramm Abb. 12

Tabelle 13. *Adeno-Carcinom des Korpus und der Cervix. Behandlungsrichtlinien des M. D. Anderson Hospital and Tumor Institute. (Nach* Fletcher, *Textbook of Radiotherapy)*

Klinische Situation	Behandlung
Uteruscavum *klein oder normal groß*	Tandem und Kolpostat 72 Std und 48 Std (wie bei Plattenepithel-Carcinom der Cervix) 2 Wochen Abstand ? Bestrahlung der Parametrien Uterusexstirpation nach 4—6 Wochen Abstand
Uteruscavum vergrößert Keine Ausbreitung über den Uterus hinaus	4000 rad auf das ganze Becken; Tandem und Kolpostat 72 Std (wie bei Plattenepithel-Carcinom der Cervix) Uterusexstirpation nach 4—6 Wochen; Allgemein Inoperabel: 4000 rad auf das ganze Becken; Tandem und Kolpostat 2 × 48 Std, 3 Wochen
Ausbreitung über den Uterus hinaus und allgemein inoperabel	4000—6000 rad auf das ganze Becken Packmethode oder Tandem und Kolpostat; 3500—4000 mgeh auf den Uterus, 4000 rad Oberflächendosis auf die Vagina

geben in ihren Mitteilungen die Dosierung in Milligrammelementstunden an (Costolow, Nolan, Budenz u. Du Sault; Fletcher; Grimm; Hofmann; Kirchhoff; Kraatz; Laborde u. Montagnon; v. Mikulicz-Radecki u. Gansau; Montgomery, Lang, Farell u. Hahn; Ries). Costolow u. Mitarb. definierten aber außerdem einen Punkt „C" 5 cm oberhalb des äußeren Muttermundes und 2,5 cm lateral der Mittellinie, der der Peripherie eines normalen Corpus uteri entsprechen soll. Sie fanden eine Beziehung zwischen der in diesem Punkt nach größenordnungsmäßiger Schätzung applizierten Dosis und dem Behandlungserfolg.

Eine übersichtliche Darstellung der von Fletcher u. Mitarb. angewandten Dosen ist in den Tabellen 11—14 dargestellt.

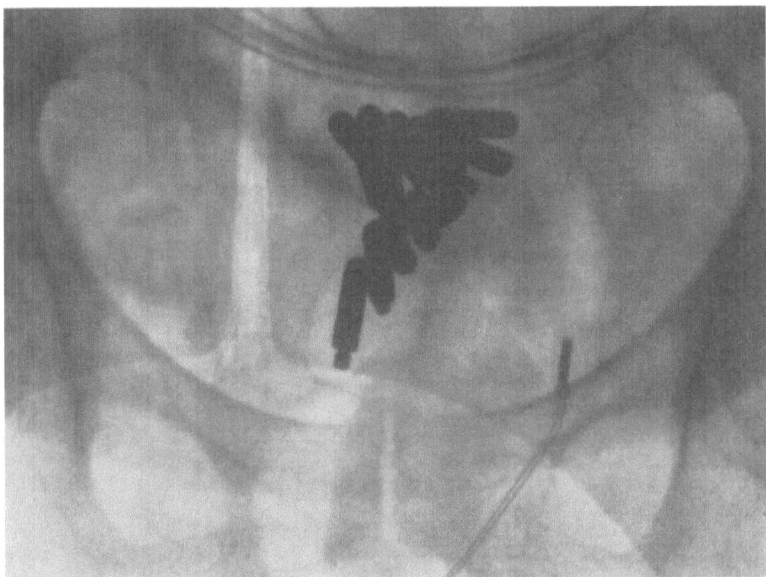

Abb. 9b

Eine wesentliche Grundlage der Dosierung ist heute jedoch nicht mehr nur die Berechnung der Dosisleistung der eingelegten Aktivität oder ihre Abschätzung nach Phantommessungen, sondern die direkte Kontrolle der Strahlenbelastung in Blase und Darm (FRISCHKORN; RIES). Ist der Uterus nur wenig deformiert, dann ist das Uteruscavum ein in sagittaler Richtung abgeplatteter Hohlraum. Wird diese Konfiguration des Cavums bei der Tamponade mit Radiumfiltern annähernd beibehalten, dann müssen

Tabelle 14. *Adeno-Carcinom des Endometriums, postoperative Bestrahlung. Behandlungsrichtlinien des M.D.Anderson Hospital and Tumor Institute. (Nach* FLETCHER, *Textbook of Radiotherapy)*

Klinische Situation	Bestrahlung des ganzen Beckens	Vagina
Normal großer Uterus mit gut ausdifferenziertem Oberflächentumor	—	—
Normal großer Uterus mit gut ausdifferenziertem Tumor, begrenzte Infiltration des Myometriums	—	*Kolpostat* 7000 rad Oberflächendosis 1 Applikation
Vergrößerter Uterus, tiefe Infiltration in das Myometrium; Anaplatischer Tumor, Restbefund	5000 rad/5 Wochen bis 7000 rad/7 Wochen (Verkleinerung der Felder nach 5000 rad)	*Kolpostat* 4000 rad Oberflächendosis (Voraussetzung, daß die Percutanbestrahlung mit 5000 rad beendet wird)

die Isodosen ventral und dorsal stärker ausbiegen und damit weiter entfernt von der Mitte des Cavums verlaufen als an den Seitenkanten, denn die Eigenabsorption und die durchschnittliche Distanzierung wird nach ventral und dorsal entsprechend kleiner sein. Da sich dem Uterus ventral und dorsal in Form von Blase und Rectum sehr wandschwache Hohlräume anlagern, kann hier die Strahlung direkt gemessen werden. Sie wird größenordnungsmäßig im allgemeinen über derjenigen liegen, die an der Seitenkante des Uterus oder etwa in der Gegend der Adnexabgänge anzunehmen ist. Es ist daher naheliegend, die Applikationsdauer überhaupt nach diesen Meßergebnissen festzulegen, zumal die Meßsonde wegen der geringen Wandstärke von Blase und Darm der Uterusoberfläche ja sehr stark angenähert werden kann. So verabfolgten RIES, FRISCHKORN u.a. maximal etwa 6 000 R auf Blase und/oder Rectum bei dreimaliger Fraktionierung. Dabei wird die maximale Bestrahlungsdauer beispielsweise auf 20 Std begrenzt, im allgemeinen

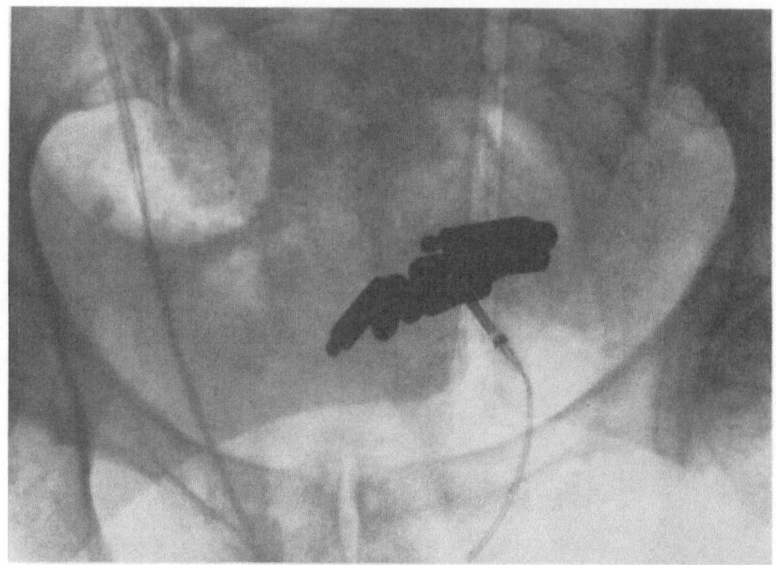

Abb. 10. Röntgenaufnahme der zweiten Radiumeinlage (gleiche Patientin wie Abb. 9)

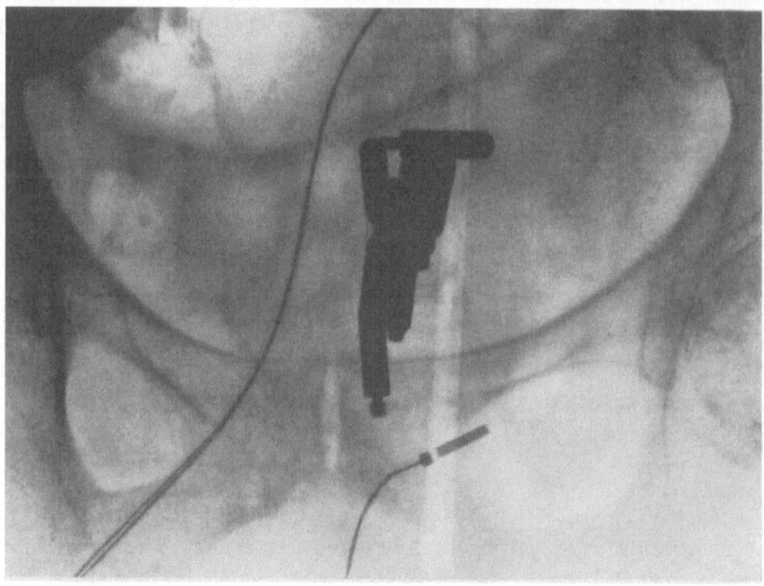

Abb. 11. Röntgenaufnahme der dritten Radiumeinlage (gleiche Patientin wie Abb. 9)

aber etwas unterschritten (Frischkorn). Ries (1950) weist außerdem auf die Bedeutung der Protrahierung für die Höhe der Toleranzdosis hin. Die Messung erfolgte früher in Deutschland zumeist mit dem Dosimeter nach Bomke und Eberle, heute aber vorwiegend mit dem sehr einfach und schnell zu handhabenden „Gammameter" der Siemens AG. Während das Prinzip der ersteren auf der Messung der Luftionisation beruht, enthält das letztere ein Cadmiumsulfidkristall als Meßelement. Es kann sowohl bei Radium als auch bei ^{60}Co Verwendung finden, da eine entsprechende Wellenlängenunabhängigkeit besteht (Bomke u. Eberle; Joelsson u. Bäckström; Reuss, Plesch, Mayer u. v. Muschwitz; Reuss u. Brunner; Ries; Zeitz u. Zitzmann). Es sind darüber hinaus auch neue Ionisationskammern der verschiedensten Fabrikate, neuerdings auch andere Meßelemente verwendet worden, wie z.B. Lithiumfluorid (Thermoluminescenzdosimetrie) und silberaktiviertes Phosphatglas (Radiophotoluminescenzdosimetrie). Es sei in diesem Zusammenhang auf das Kapitel „Festkörperdosimetrie" im Band XVI, Teil 1, dieses Handbuchs verwiesen. Die letztgenannten Dosimeter eignen sich aber im Rahmen der Radiumtherapie weniger für eine sofortige Feststellung der Strahlenbelastung der Organe als vielmehr für eine Integrierung der Strahlendosen an verschiedenen Punkten während der ganzen Dauer der Einlage, z.B. auch in den Ureteren.

Für die praktischen Erfordernisse der klinischen Radiumdosierung dürfte ein Gerät wie das „Gammameter" infolge seiner leichten Handhabung und unmittelbaren Anzeige am geeignetsten sein, nicht zuletzt auch wegen seiner geringen Störanfälligkeit. Daß der Momentanmeßwert nicht repräsentativ für die gesamte Dauer der Radiumbestrahlung ist, wurde mehrfach durch entsprechende Kontrollmessungen erwiesen. Hierfür wird als Ursache das Zusammensintern der Tamponade, wechselnder Füllungszustand der Organe des kleinen Beckens und die Änderung der Körperlage verantwortlich gemacht. Am grundsätzlichen Wert der Messung ändert sich aber dadurch nichts, wenn man als ihr Ziel lediglich die Vermeidung unerwünschter Dosisspitzen ansieht. Wenn STRICKLAND und GREGORY keine Korrelation zwischen gemessener Dosis und aufgetretenen Rectumschäden sahen, so widerspricht das der allgemeinen praktischen Erfahrung, daß nach Einführung der routinemäßigen Kontrollmessung Strahlenreaktionen des Rectums — ebenso wie die Blasenschäden — als alleinige Folge der Radiumbehandlung selten geworden sind.

Die Dosismessung kann nicht davon befreien, einen Gesamtbestrahlungsplan aufzustellen, der auch die räumliche Lage des Radiums zu berücksichtigen hat. Hierzu kann die Messung in Blase und Darm allerdings kaum beitragen, da die gefundenen Werte bei gleicher Aktivität große Unterschiede zeigen (Tabelle 15). Immerhin ist es mit Hilfe der Stereoaufnahme (Abb. 9) leicht möglich, die Lage des Uteruscavums zu ermitteln und

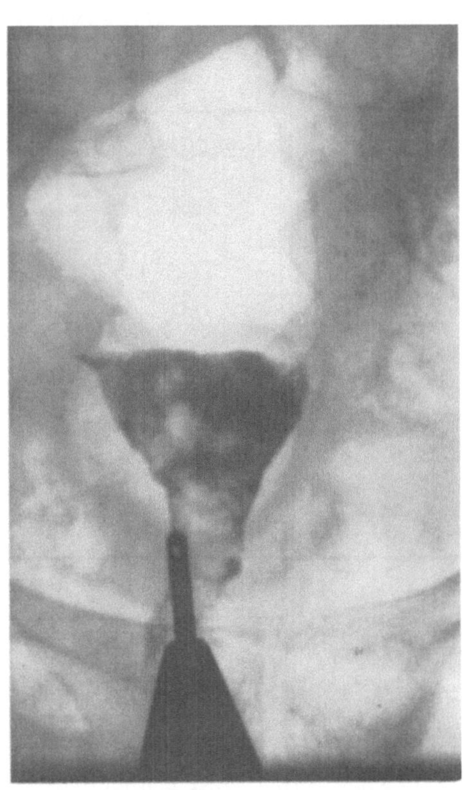

Abb. 12. Hysterogramm zu den Radiumeinlagen Abb. 9—11

in Form einer einfachen Formel auszudrücken. Abb. 13 zeigt unsere Methode für Röhrenfilter. Bei der Packmethode werden statt dessen das höchste und das tiefste Filter angemessen. Das Lageprotokoll, für die in den Abb. 9—11 gezeigten Einlagen, wird in der Tabelle 16 wiedergegeben. Dies sind dann zugleich die Grundlagen für das angeschlossene elektronische Rechenprogramm zur Ermittlung und Darstellung der räumlichen Dosisverteilung.

Der Radiumpackmethode prinzipiell vergleichbar ist die Einlage von ^{60}Co-Perlen in den Uterus. BECKER und SCHEER haben 1952 ihre Verwendung für die Behandlung des Korpuscarcinoms vorgeschlagen. Mit Hilfe dieser von einem Goldmantel umhüllten Perlen mit einem Durchmesser von 6 mm läßt sich eine noch gleichmäßigere Verteilung der Aktivität erreichen. Falls eine protrahiertere Bestrahlung erwünscht ist, kann durch Zwischenschaltung von inaktiven Perlen die Gesamtaktivität bei immer noch gleichmäßiger Verteilung verringert werden. BICKENBACH, GÄRTNER und ZOEPPRITZ führten 1955 Vergleichsmessungen an einem exstirpierten Uterus durch, den sie einmal mit einem Radiumröhrenfilter mit 120 mCi, dann mit 26 ^{60}Co-Perlen zu je 5 mCi beschickten. Die gemessenen Dosiswerte verhielten sich (^{60}Co:Ra) wie 4:1 bis 2:1. Die Vergleichbarkeit ist dabei allerdings auf die gewählten Bedingungen beschränkt. Bickenbach, Gärtner und Zoeppritz folgerten, daß bei Verwendung von Radiokobaltperlen die Bestrahlungsdauer gegenüber dem Radium etwa halbiert werden könnte. Bemerkenswert ist dabei aber die hohe Strahlenintensität in der Blase, die bereits nach 8 Std zum Erreichen der Toleranzgrenze von etwa 2000 R führte.

Nachdem gewisse technische Probleme der ^{60}Co-Perlenherstellung gelöst waren (Becker, Scheer u. Schick; v. Braunbehrens, Bunde u. Wittenzellner; Frost), haben auch andere Kliniken und Institute die Therapie des Korpuscarcinoms hiermit aufgenommen (Bocci, Tetti, Barbanti u. Davitti; Hendricks, Callendine u. Morton; Hess u. Rosendahl; Kuhn; du Mesnil de Rochemont; Picha u. Weghaupt; Ries

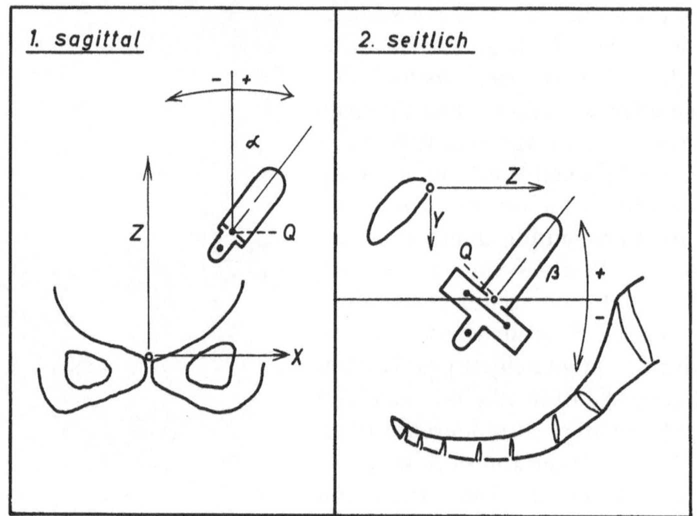

Abb. 13. Röntgenstereophotogrammetrie der Radiumfilterlage. Darstellung der gemessenen Größen zu Abb. 9—11 und Tabelle 16

u.a.). Auch dabei wird schließlich, ebenso wie bei der Radiumpackmethode, nach dem Meßergebnis in Blase und Darm dosiert (Bocci, Tetti, Barbanti u. Davitti; Kuhn). Der Nachteil der Kobaltperlen ist in dem Aktivitätsverlust von monatlich 1% zu sehen. Dieser läßt sich zwar rechnerisch leicht berücksichtigen, er bedingt aber die Notwendigkeit, in relativ kurzen Abständen die Aktivitäten zu erneuern, wobei jeweils nicht unbeträchtliche Kosten entstehen. Der Vorteil der Kobaltperlen ist insbesondere für die Bestrahlung kleiner Uteri nicht zu bezweifeln. Auch die Tatsache, daß damit größere relative Tiefendosen, hier also z.B. höhere Dosen an der Beckenwand, zu erzielen sind, wird von manchen Autoren betont. Ein prinzipieller Vorteil gegenüber der Radiumpackmethode mit nicht zu voluminösen Filtern dürfte aber kaum bestehen.

Erwähnenswert ist noch der Versuch J. H. Müllers, flüssige Aktivitäten mittels eines Ballons in das Uteruscavum zu bringen. Er verwendete dazu ^{60}Co (J. H. Müller, 1949 und 1951). Obwohl eine solche Methode, insbesondere bei großen Uteri mit tiefer Wandinfiltration, die Perforationsgefahr vermindern würde, mußte sie wegen der außerordentlich hohen Kontaminationsgefahr mit einem langlebigen Strahler wieder aufgegeben werden. Wallace, Walton und Sinclair beschrieben 1948 ebenfalls einen solchen Versuch unter Verwendung von ^{24}Na.

Auch die vielfach zitierte ^{60}Co-Spirale nach Jones, die in ihrer räumlichen Anordnung dem Triangel von Dietel ähnelt und der entsprechenden Modifikation von Strickland, sei lediglich erwähnt. Gegenüber der Packmethode wird sie allgemein als weniger geeignet

Tabelle 15. *Schwankungsbereiche der Meßwerte in Blase und Darm bei der Radium-Packmethode. (94 Patienten mit unterschiedlichen Aktivitäten) (Siemens-Gammameter)*

Anzahl der Korpus-filter	Radium mg	Liege-zeit h	mgeh	Patienten-zahl	Blase			Rectum		
					min. R	max. R	Mittel R	min. R	max. R	Mittel R
7	70	23	1610	1			460			184
8	80	22	1760	2	460	880	670	2200	2480	2340
9	90	21	1890	5	820	2940	1064	630	2730	1642
10	100	20	2000	9	700	2920	1827	520	2960	1544
11	110	19	2090	7	1440	4280	2417	610	3320	1422
12	120	18	2160	15	600	4200	2057	288	3670	1477
13	130	17	2210	6	1420	4200	2852	782	3400	2010
14	140	16	2240	9	576	2650	1794	273	1700	1068
15	150	15	2250	28	540	3375	1893	270	2100	986
16	160	15	2400	1			1364			432
17	170	15	2550	5	2290	4125	3142	347	3380	1251
18	180	15	2700	5	735	1980	1317	780	2230	1283
26	260	15	3900	1			4125			2850

Tabelle 16. *Auswertung der Stereophotogramme (Abb. 9-11). Angabe der Größen siehe Abb. 13. Es wird die Lage des Punktes „Q" am Filter, der im allgemeinen der Lage des äußeren Muttermundes entspricht, in dem in Abb. 13 dargestellten Koordinatensystem angegeben, also sein Abstand in 3 Richtungen vom oberen Symphysenrand sowie 2 Neigungswinkel gegen die Z-Achse*

	Radiumeinlage Nr.		
	I	II	III
Datum	14. 8. 69	27. 8. 69	10. 9. 69
Bezeichnung des Filters	12 Korpusfilter	10 Korpusfilter	9 Korpusfilter
X Abweichung nach rechts —; nach links +	− 0,1 cm	+ 1,5 cm	0,0 cm
Y Entfernung von der Symphyse nach dorsal	9,6 cm	9,2 cm	10,1 cm
Z Entfernung vom oberen Symphysenrand nach cranial +; nach caudal −	+ 0,4 cm	+ 1,7 cm	− 1,1 cm
∢α Neigung zur Seite nach rechts —; nach links +	+ 11°	+ 57°	+ 13°
∢β Neigung nach ventral +; nach dorsal −	+ 41°	+ 64°	+ 40°

angesehen. SCHULTE, HINMAN und LOW-BEER verwandten eine in einem Wasserballon zentral befestigte Strahlenquelle, die so gleichmäßig von der Wand distanziert war. Schließlich sei noch die von BECKER angegebene „Makrosuspension" von kleinsten Kunststoffperlen, die ^{60}Co enthielten, berichtet. Alle diese zumeist für die Behandlung des Blasencarcinoms entwickelten Verfahren und auch andere in der gynäkologischen Strahlentherapie angewandte Isotope (^{24}Na, ^{32}P, ^{137}Cs, ^{90}Y, ^{182}Ta, ^{192}Ir, ^{198}Au, ^{131}J) haben für das Korpuscarcinom bisher keine größere Bedeutung erlangt (BECKER u. SCHEER; GAUWERKY, 1957; IKLÉ; KAPP-SCHWOERER; PICARD, GONGORA, SZIGETI; PIERQUIN; SCHEER; WALKER; WALTER, JONES u. FISHER).

β) Komplikationen bei der Anwendung der Packmethode

Gegen die Packmethode wird immer wieder angeführt, daß sie mit einer erhöhten Perforationsgefahr des Uterus verbunden sei. Sicherlich besteht für jeden, der Erfahrung mit dieser Methode hat, kein Zweifel, daß sich eine solche Uterusperforation in einer Anzahl von Fällen ereignet. Die Erfahrung lehrt aber, daß ein solches Ereignis zumeist ohne Komplikationen bleibt und daß eine Perforation im allgemeinen keinen operativen Eingriff erforderlich macht (Kirchhoff, 1962; Kottmeier, 1959; Picha u. Weghaupt, 1961). Das gilt natürlich nur dann, wenn anzunehmen ist, daß es nicht zu einer größeren Zerreißung der Uteruswand gekommen ist und kein Anhalt für eine innere Blutung besteht. Kottmeier gibt die Häufigkeit der Uterusperforation bei der Packmethode mit

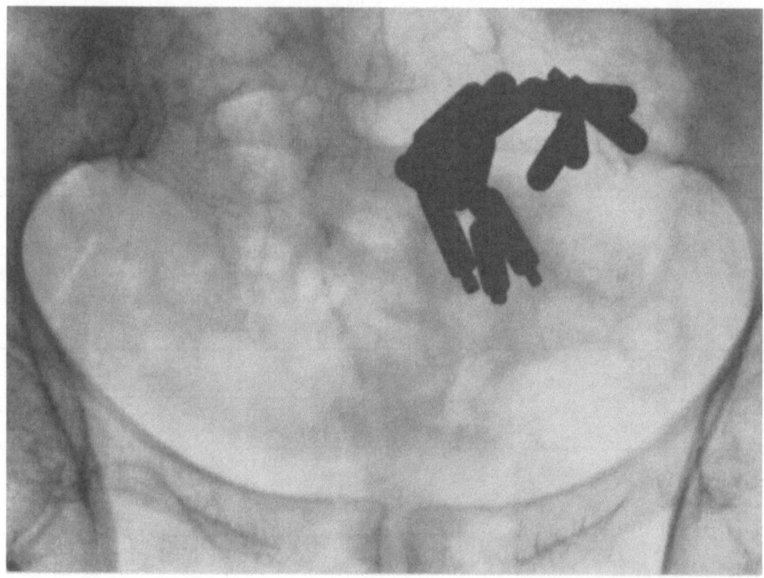

Abb. 14. Uterusperforation bei der Radiumeinlage. Die oberen seitlichen Filter liegen in der freien Bauchhöhle (sofortige vaginale Totalexstirpation des Uterus, glatter Verlauf)

4,4% an. Kottmeier und Kirchhoff haben keine Bedenken, nach einer reaktionslosen Perforation nach 10 Tagen bis wenigen Wochen die intrauterine Radiumapplikation doch durchzuführen. Dabei kann die Zwischenzeit durch die percutane Bestrahlung überbrückt werden. Die Vermeidung solcher Zwischenfälle wird aber durch eine möglichst weitgehende Abklärung der Carcinomausdehnung, wie sie weiter oben in dem Abschnitt über die Diagnostik dargestellt ist, erleichtert. Kritisch kann es dann werden, wenn eine solche Perforation nicht entdeckt wird und die Filter auch nicht wieder entfernt werden. Das ungewollte Einbringen von Korpusfiltern in die freie Bauchhöhle wird aber im allgemeinen aus einer Röntgenkontrollaufnahme, wie sie J. H. Müller schon 1941 für erforderlich hielt, erkennbar sein (Abb. 14). Auch Kottmeier und du Mesnil de Rochemont sprechen sich für die Anfertigung solcher Kontrollaufnahmen aus.

Wir selbst haben unseren Radiumoperationstisch mit einer Zwillingsröhre versehen und fertigen mit konstanter Strahlengeometrie Stereobildpaare an, die, wie oben dargestellt, anschließend ausgemessen werden (Abb. 15). Der Vergleich dieser Aufnahmen mit einem etwa vorher angefertigten Hysterogramm (Abb. 12) kann in dieser Richtung noch weitere Aufschlüsse geben. Die zunehmende Einrichtung der Radiumabteilungen mit Röntgenlokalisationseinrichtungen wird diesen Möglichkeiten weitere Verbreitung verschaffen. Darüber hinaus kann auch die automatische Fernkontrolle von Puls, Temperatur und Blutdruck die Gefahren einer eventuellen Perforation weiter verringern.

Die Frage des Strahlenschutzes ist in diesem Zusammenhang immer wieder aufgeworfen worden. Die „afterloading technique" ist bei der Packmethode bisher nicht praktikabel. Außerdem stehen wir auf dem Standpunkt, daß bis jetzt die technischen Möglichkeiten des Strahlenschutzes nicht ausgenutzt sind. Es würde in diesem Zusammenhang zu weit führen, auf den Strahlenschutz bei der Radiumtherapie näher einzugehen. Immerhin ist aber gerade bei der Packmethode der Strahlenschutz besonders wichtig, da das Manipulieren der Aktivität hierbei längere Zeit erfordert als bei der Einlage eines anderen Radiumfilters. Die bei uns neu entwickelten Schutzeinrichtungen seien in Abb. 16 teilweise dargestellt. Das Bild zeigt, daß der Radiumoperateur auf einem Strahlenschutzstuhl (mit elektrischem Antrieb) mit Bleiglasfenster als Augenschutz (5 cm Pb-Äquivalent) und seitlichem Gonadenschutz sehr gut abgeschirmt ist. Die Abbildung läßt gleichzeitig die Röntgeneinrichtung erkennen. Für die erforderlichen Röntgenstereoaufnahmen wird die Patientin gestreckt gelagert. Das Aufnahmepaar wird mittels einer Spezialkassettenhalterung unter Anwendung der Belichtungsautomatik ohne wesentlichen zusätzlichen Zeitaufwand angefertigt. Schließlich erleichtert der in unserer Klinik zusammen mit der Firma H. Wälischmiller entwickelte Operationstisch mit teilbarer Tischplatte das strahlengeschützte Umlagern der Patientin ins Bett (Abb. 15 und 16). Mit dieser und weiteren technischen Neuentwicklungen kann bei uns konsequent dafür gesorgt werden, daß jede mittels technischer Einrichtungen vermeidbare Belastung auch tatsächlich ausgeschaltet wird.

γ) Die zusätzliche Bestrahlung der Cervix und der Vagina

Es war schon erwähnt worden, daß LOUROS in 15,6 % seiner Fälle einen Mitbefall der Cervix fand. KOTTMEIER berichtet im 14. Band des „Annual Report", daß im Radiumhemmet in den Jahren 1951—1960 neben 1 278 Fällen von Korpuscarcinom 382 Fälle von Carcinoma corporis et endocervicis behandelt wurden. Wenn hiervon auch nach der jetzt geltenden Einteilung möglicherweise einige dem Collumcarcinom zuzurechnen sind, so geht doch auch daraus hervor, daß bis zu 20 % aller Patientinnen, bei denen ein Carcinom des Korpus gefunden wird, gleichzeitig eine Mitbeteiligung der Cervix aufweisen. Es wird daher von zahlreichen Autoren immer wieder die Forderung erhoben, den Cervicalkanal ebenfalls mit Radium zu bestrahlen. Daß dies bei Anwendung der Packmethode allein möglicherweise nicht ausreicht, lassen die Isodosen (Abb. 17) erkennen. Die kleinen Korpusfilter haben immerhin schon einen Durchmesser von 5 mm oder mehr. Es werden sich also kaum mehrere nebeneinander in den Cervicalkanal legen lassen. Gegenüber einer cervicalen Radiumeinlage mit einem Röhrenfilter, bei dem in jeder Etage z. B. drei 10-mCi-Röhrchen nebeneinander liegen können, bei einem Gesamtdurchmesser von 8 mm, beträgt die in den Cervicalkanal eingelegte Aktivität mit der Packmethode unter Umständen nur ein Drittel der sonst üblichen. Da die Bestrahlungsdauer durch die korporal eingelegte Aktivität und die von ihr ausgehende Blasen- und

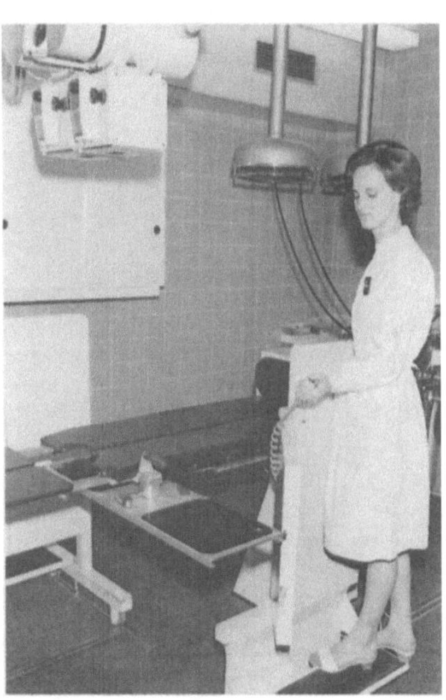

Abb. 15. Radiumapplikationstisch mit angesteckten Beinauflagen (nach Entfernung der gynäkologischen Beinhalter). Zwillingsröhre, drehbare Kassettenhalterung für zwei Kassetten 24 × 30 cm in Aufnahmestellung. Die Assistentin löst den ersten Schuß aus. Die Drehung der Kassettenhalterung und die Auslösung des zweiten Schusses erfolgen automatisch. Belichtungsautomatik. Strahlenschutz durch motorisch fahrbare Bleiwand (Siemens AG, Erlangen; Firma H. Wälischmiller, Markdorf/Baden und Eigenentwicklung der Strahlenabteilung der Universitäts-Frauenklinik Göttingen)

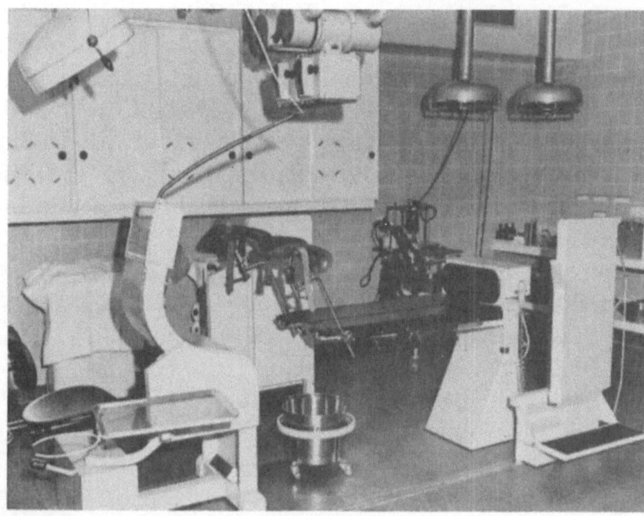

Abb. 16. Strahlenschutzeinrichtungen am Radiumapplikationstisch. Operationstisch mit teilbarer Tischplatte, Strahlenschutzschilde (5 cm), der vordere motorisch angetrieben. Strahlenschutzstuhl (Vor- und Rückwärtsfahrt durch Fußkippschalter) mit angelenktem Instrumententisch, Bleiglasfenster mit 5 cm Pb-Äquivalent (Firma H. Wälischmiller, Markdorf/Baden; Eigenentwicklung der Strahlenabteilung der Universitäts-Frauenklinik Göttingen)

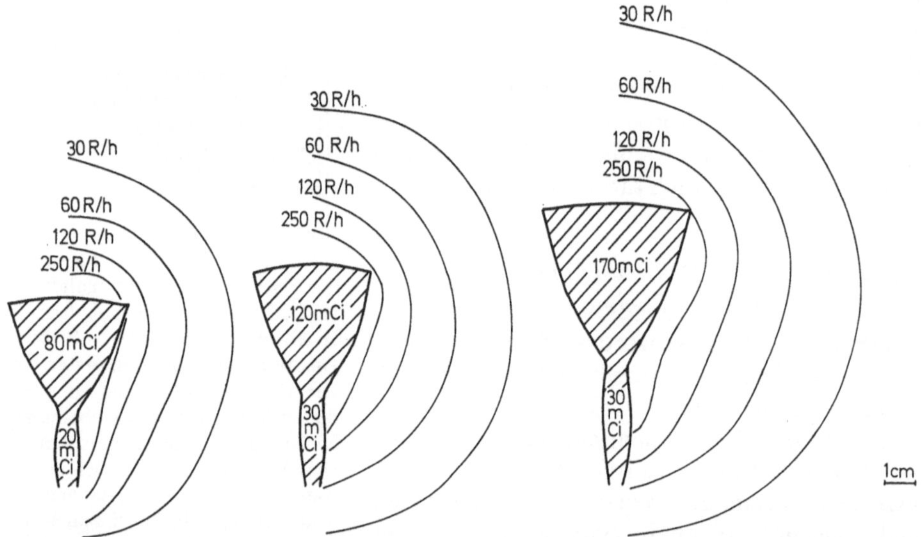

Abb. 17. Der Isodosenverlauf bei der Radiumpackmethode zeigt, daß die Gefahr einer Unterdosierung vor allem im Bereich der Tubenwinkel und des unteren Cervicalkanals besteht. Phantommessung mit drei verschiedenen Aktivitäten bei unterschiedlichen Uterusgrößen (10, 15 und 20 Korpusfilter zu je 10 mCi Ra)

Darmbelastung bestimmt wird, ist eine entsprechende Verlängerung der Bestrahlungszeit nicht möglich. Es besteht daher die Notwendigkeit, in den Cervicalkanal zusätzlich ein Röhrenfilter der erforderlichen Länge einzulegen. Diese Notwendigkeit wird allgemein betont, zum Teil wird allerdings nur in den Fällen so verfahren, in denen die fraktionierte Abrasio einen Übergang auf den Cervicalkanal nachgewiesen hat.

Etwas anders liegen die Verhältnisse hinsichtlich der Vagina. Da in 8—10% mit dem Auftreten von Scheidenmetastasen gerechnet werden muß, wird vielfach von vornherein zusammen mit der intrauterinen Radiumtherapie auch eine Einlage in die Vagina vorgenommen. Hier ist das Vorgehen allerdings noch weniger einheitlich. Während z.B. an der Universitäts-Frauenklinik Göttingen eine vaginale Radiumeinlage nur bei besonderer Indikation erfolgt, also bei festgestellter Metastasierung, legt KOTTMEIER (1957 und 1959) grundsätzlich vaginal Radium. Er verwendet dabei je nach den räumlichen Verhältnissen zylindrische Applikatoren verschiedener Größe, die mit 100—150 mCi Radium beschickt sind. Die applizierte Dosis beträgt 1800 R in 1 cm Tiefe von der Scheidenhaut. Diese vaginale Einlage wird mit einer der intrauterinen Einlagen verbunden. Falls das Carcinom auf die Cervix übergeht, wird eine weitere Einlage vor die Portio vorgenommen wie bei der Radiumbehandlung des Collumcarcinoms, also mit einer Stockholmer Platte.

RIES legt ebenfalls bei einer der drei intrauterinen Einlagen einmal Radium vor die Portio mit einem der für die Bestrahlung des Collumcarcinoms verwendeten Rundfilter, das mit 30—50 mg Radiumelement bestückt ist.

J. H. MÜLLER verwendete einen modifizierten Federbügel-Kolpostaten der Pariser Methode. Dabei können in jeden der beiden aus Kunststoff gefertigten Applikatoren 40 mCi Radium eingebracht werden. Die vaginale Applikation wird 5—7 Tage nach Abschluß der zweiten intrauterinen Bestrahlung durchgeführt. Bei einer Liegezeit von 25 Std werden so zusätzlich noch einmal 2000 mgeh verabfolgt.

Auch FLETCHER u. Mitarb. legen grundsätzlich beim Korpuscarcinom — wenn überhaupt bestrahlt wird — (Tabelle 11 und 12) Radium in die Vagina mittels Kolpostat. Dabei werden zweimal 4000 rad Oberflächendosis im Abstand von 3 Wochen verabfolgt oder aber, wenn außerdem eine Percutanbestrahlung des Beckens erfolgt, einmal 4000 rad Oberflächendosis.

Auch andere Autoren, die das Korpuscarcinom in gleicher Weise wie das Collumcarcinom mit Spreizkolpostaten bestrahlen, applizieren analog die vaginale Radiummenge (ERNST, ERNST, ERNST, ERNST u. CLELAND).

δ) Die percutane Zusatzbestrahlung der Parametrien und der regionären Lymphknoten

Von jeher hat die percutane Zusatzbestrahlung des Korpuscarcinoms als besonders problematisch gegolten, da es sich in der Mehrzahl der Fälle um Patientinnen mit zum Teil erheblicher Adipositas handelt. Auch das Alter und der reduzierte Kräftezustand der Patientinnen veranlassen dazu, die Percutanbestrahlung nicht routinemäßig oder gar starr anzuwenden (KIRCHHOFF, 1962). Allerdings sind diese Standpunkte vielfach noch auf die Möglichkeiten der Orthovoltgeräte begründet und lassen sich heute zum Teil nicht mehr aufrecht erhalten. Aber auch die oben schon diskutierte Ansicht, daß die in erster Linie betroffenen Lymphknotenstationen paraaortal gelegen seien, hat Veranlassung gegeben, von einer Percutanbestrahlung weniger Gebrauch zu machen. Und schließlich ist die Frage noch nicht ausdiskutiert — und das gilt auch für die percutane Zusatzbestrahlung bei der Behandlung des Cervixcarcinoms —, wie weit diese überhaupt an den Erfolgsziffern ursächlich beteiligt ist (HENSCHKE; PATERSON u. RUSSEL; PIERQUIN). Trotzdem legt der relativ hohe Prozentsatz vom Carcinom befallener Lymphknoten im Becken den Gedanken nahe, in jedem Fall sicherheitshalber von außen zu bestrahlen, auch wenn der Palpationsbefund keinen Anhalt für eine über den Uterus hinausgehende Carcinomausbreitung ergeben hat. Daß dieses Kriterium ohnehin sehr problematisch ist, wurde weiter oben schon ausgeführt. Bei positivem lymphographischen Befund wird die Entscheidung aber unbedingt zugunsten einer Zusatzbestrahlung fallen müssen.

Da in keinem Fall eine Ausbreitung über den Uterus hinaus auszuschließen ist, wird an der Universitäts-Frauenklinik Göttingen der Standpunkt vertreten, daß jedes Korpuscarcinom zusätzlich zur Radiumtherapie percutan bestrahlt werden sollte, vorausgesetzt, daß keine Gegenindikation besteht. Als solche wird vor allem das hohe Alter und ein reduzierter Allgemein- und Kräftezustand, eventuell auch zusätzliche Krankheiten angesehen. Die Adipositas wird nach Einführung der Telekobalttherapie nicht mehr so stark bewertet, da es mit entsprechender Felderlage in jedem Fall möglich ist, eine als erforderlich angesehene Herddosis zu applizieren. Höhere Strahlenenergien sind geeignet,

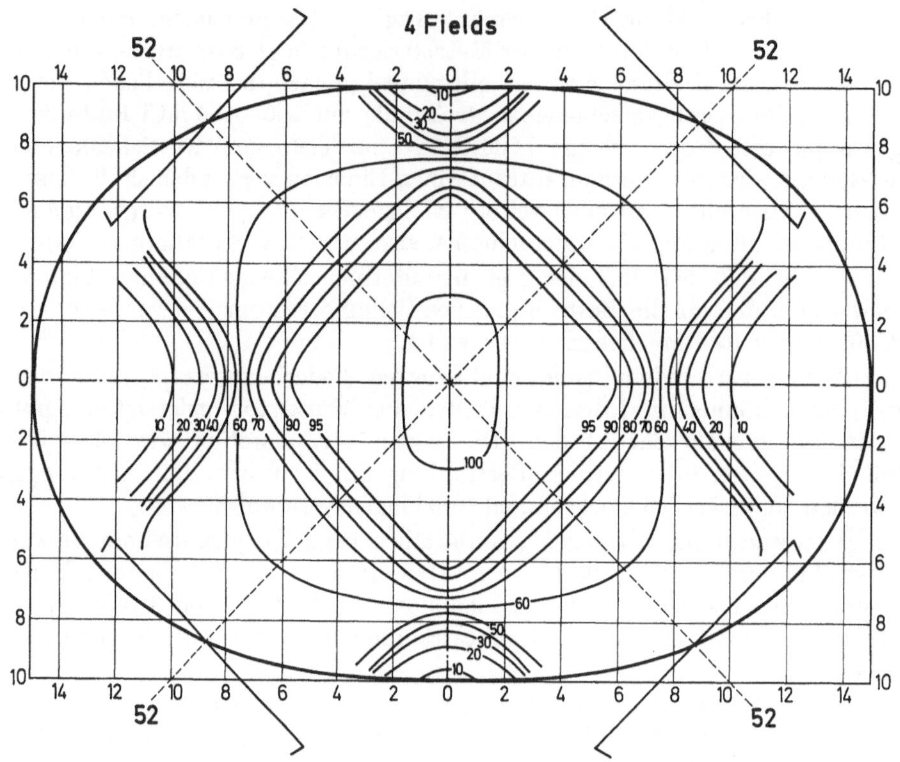

Chart 98 (VII)

Parameter	This chart
Radiation	Cobalt-60 γ-rays
SSD (cm)	100
SCD (cm)	
Number of fields	4
Field arrangement	B, C
Applied dose ratio	1:1:1:1
Field sizes (cm)	10×10
Wedge angle, Φ	—
Θ	90°
S (cm)	0
Axes of body section[a] (cm)	$0 : 30 \times 20$

[a] C = circle, E = ellipse, O = oval, R = real section

Abb. 18a

Abb. 18a u. b. Beispiele für die räumliche Dosisverteilung bei ^{60}Co γ-Strahlung im Vergleich mit einer 20 MV-Röntgenstrahlung. a ^{60}Co γ-Strahlung; b 20 MV-Röntgenstrahlung. (Nach M. Cohen und S. J. Martin, Atlas of Radiation Dose Distributions, Vol. II. Verlag IAEA, Wien 1966)

die Bedingungen weiter zu verbessern. Daß der Unterschied dabei allerdings nicht immer sehr beträchtlich ist, läßt der Vergleich zwischen ^{60}Co- und 20 MV-Röntgenstrahlen erkennen (Abb. 18a und b). Als anzustrebende Dosis wird bei uns bei vollständig durchgeführter Radiumtherapie mit einer Blasen- und/oder Darmbelastung von 6000 R eine Herddosis von 3000 R pro Parametrium bzw. an jeder Beckenwand angesehen. Da nach unseren Messungen vom applizierten Radium bei der Packmethode etwa 1800—2400 R an der Beckenwand eingestrahlt werden, werden bei mittelständigem Uterus insgesamt etwa 4800—5400 R an der Beckenwand appliziert. Muß die Liegezeit des Radiums auf-

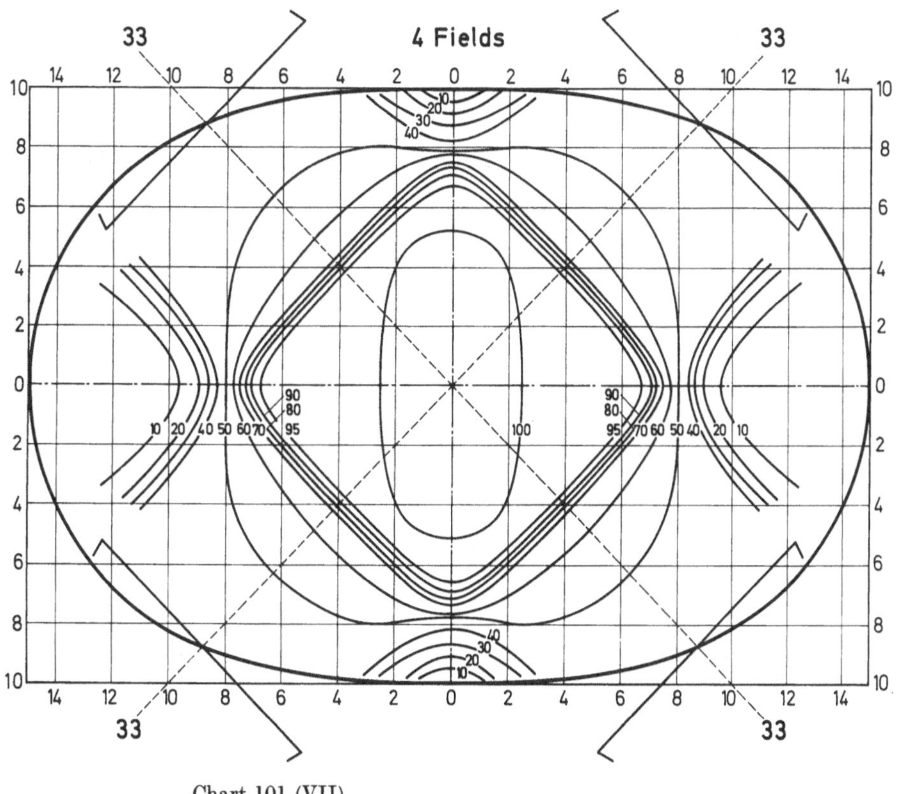

Chart 101 (VII)

Parameter	This chart
Radiation	20 MV X-rays
SSD (cm)	100
SCD (cm)	
Number of fields	4
Field arrangement	B, C
Applied dose ratio	1:1:1:1
Field sizes (cm)	10 × 10
Wedge angle, Φ	—
Θ	90°
S (cm)	0
Axes of body section[a] (cm)	0:30 × 20

[a] C = circle, E = ellipse, O = oval, R = real section

Abb. 18 b

grund zu hoher Blasen- oder Darmbelastung, insbesondere bei sehr muskelschwachen Uteri, reduziert werden, wird die percutane Dosis entsprechend erhöht. Die Dosiskalkulation erfolgt dabei ohne Berücksichtigung eines eventuellen biologischen Wirkungsunterschiedes zwischen der stark protrahierten, wenig fraktionierten Radiumbestrahlung und der hochfraktionierten, nicht protrahierten Percutanbestrahlung.

Die Bestrahlung erfolgt mit Telekobalt („Gammatron I" der Siemens AG, 4000 Ci) seit nunmehr 10 Jahren. Von zwei ventralen und zwei dorsalen Feldern 6 × 14 cm, zwischen denen ein Mittelstreifen von 5 cm Breite ausgespart ist, und bei Patientinnen, die in sagittaler Richtung über 20 cm dick sind, zusätzlich von je einem rechten und linken Seitenfeld 8 × 12 cm aus. Die Felder werden unter Kontrolle durch Lokalisationsaufnahmen in jedem Einzelfall so angesetzt, daß das Foramen obturatum noch vollständig

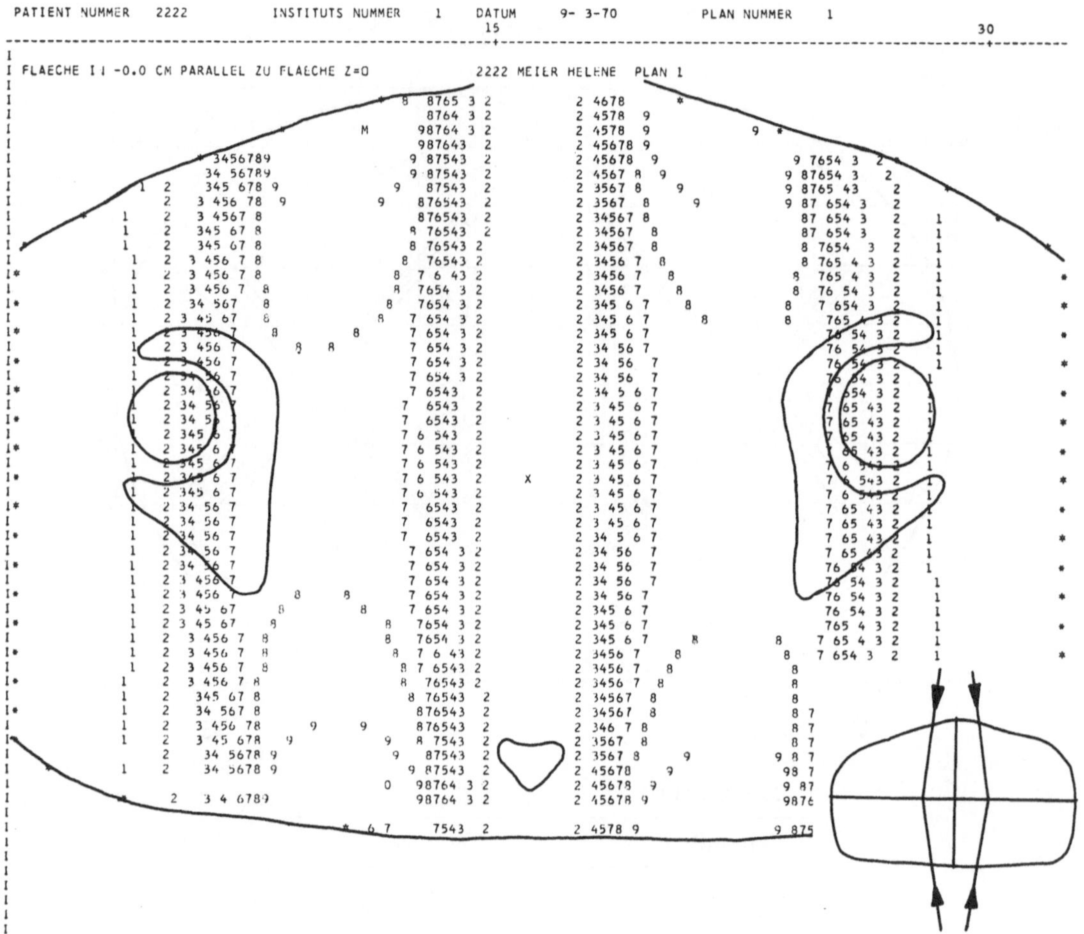

Abb. 19. Bestrahlung der Parametrien und der Beckenwand (^{60}Co-γ-Strahlen) zusätzlich zur intrauterinen Radiumtherapie. Feldgröße 6×14 cm. Berechnung der Dosisverteilung durch Computer. (Strahlenabteilung der Universitäts-Frauenklinik Göttingen)

mit im Strahlengang liegt. Die craniale Feldbegrenzung liegt dann im allgemeinen in Höhe des Promontoriums oder des 5. Lendenwirbels. Die ventralen und dorsalen Felder werden jeweils 5° nach lateral ausgelenkt. Dadurch läuft die mediane Begrenzung des Strahlenkegels parallel zur Sagittalebene. In cranio-caudaler Richtung wird parallel zur Transversalebene eingestellt. Es werden täglich die beiden Bauch- oder die beiden Gluteal-felder bestrahlt. Bei Adipositas wird hiervon unter Umständen Abstand genommen. Um in diesen Fällen die tägliche Dosis ausreichend hoch zu wählen, erfolgt täglich die Be-strahlung einer Seite von drei Feldern aus, so daß also pro Beckenseite ein 48stündiger Rhythmus entsteht.

Der Bestrahlungsplan mündet in jedem Fall in ein elektronisches Rechenprogramm (nach VAN DE GEIJN) mit Ausgabe der Isodosen über einen Schnelldrucker. Die Abb. 19—22 zeigen von ein und derselben Patientin die gerechneten Dosisverteilungen für vier ver-schiedene Bestrahlungspläne. Auch eine biachsiale Pendelbestrahlung kann so dargestellt werden (s.a. Abb. 25). So lassen sich beliebige Bestrahlungspläne zu Optimierungs-zwecken miteinander vergleichen (ROSENOW).

Von einer routinemäßigen Bestrahlung höher gelegener Lymphknotengruppen wird bewußt Abstand genommen. Einmal konnte bisher nicht bewiesen werden, daß eine solche Bestrahlung noch zusätzliche Erfolge bringt, zum anderen ist es bei einer derartigen

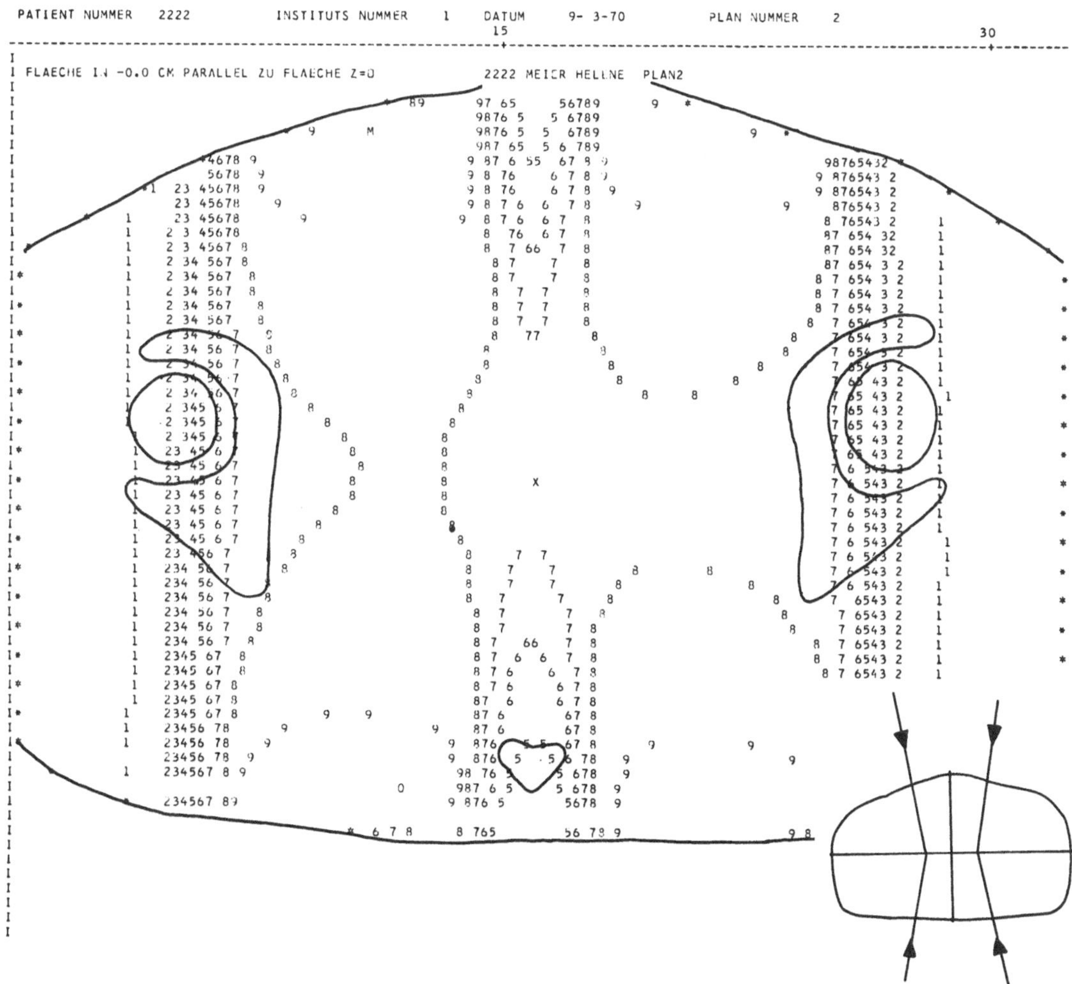

Abb. 20. Bestrahlung des kleinen Beckens von vier Feldern (Feldgröße 8×14 cm, ^{60}Co-γ-Strahlung). Berechnung der Dosisverteilung durch Computer. (Strahlenabteilung der Universitäts-Frauenklinik Göttingen)

Ausbreitung ohnehin unwahrscheinlich, daß noch alle Carcinomausläufer mit der Bestrahlung erreicht werden können. Darüber hinaus kommen, neben weiteren Anteilen des Dünn- und Dickdarms, unvermeidbar Rückenmark und/oder Nieren in den direkten Strahlengang. Da inzwischen feststeht, daß die früher angenommene hohe Strahlentoleranz dieser Organe in keiner Weise besteht und schon bei Strahlendosen von 2000 R an aufwärts mit Komplikationen gerechnet werden muß (BARGON; FEINE; SARRE u. MOSER; SEITZ u. KALM), deren mögliche Schwere im Einzelfall in keiner vertretbaren Relation zu dem erwarteten Nutzen hinsichtlich der Beeinflussung von Lymphknotenmetastasen steht, lehnen wir eine entsprechende Verlängerung der Strahlenfelder nach cranial ab. Auch DU MESNIL DE ROCHEMONT sowie KEPP und HOFMANN versprechen sich von einer prophylaktischen Bestrahlung der paraaortalen Lymphknoten nichts. Von anderer Seite werden die paraaortalen Lymphknoten aber in den Therapieplan mit einbezogen (DIBBELT u. HEINZLER; SCHMERMUND, OBERHEUSER u. KUTTIG u.a.).

Anders ist es natürlich, wenn durch die Lymphographie (gegebenenfalls auch durch die Urographie oder eine Phlebographie) in den paraaortalen oder den cavalen Lymphknoten Metastasen nachgewiesen oder wahrscheinlich gemacht wurden. In den Fällen ist eine Bestrahlung dieser Lymphknotengruppen indiziert. Die Schwierigkeiten, die durch

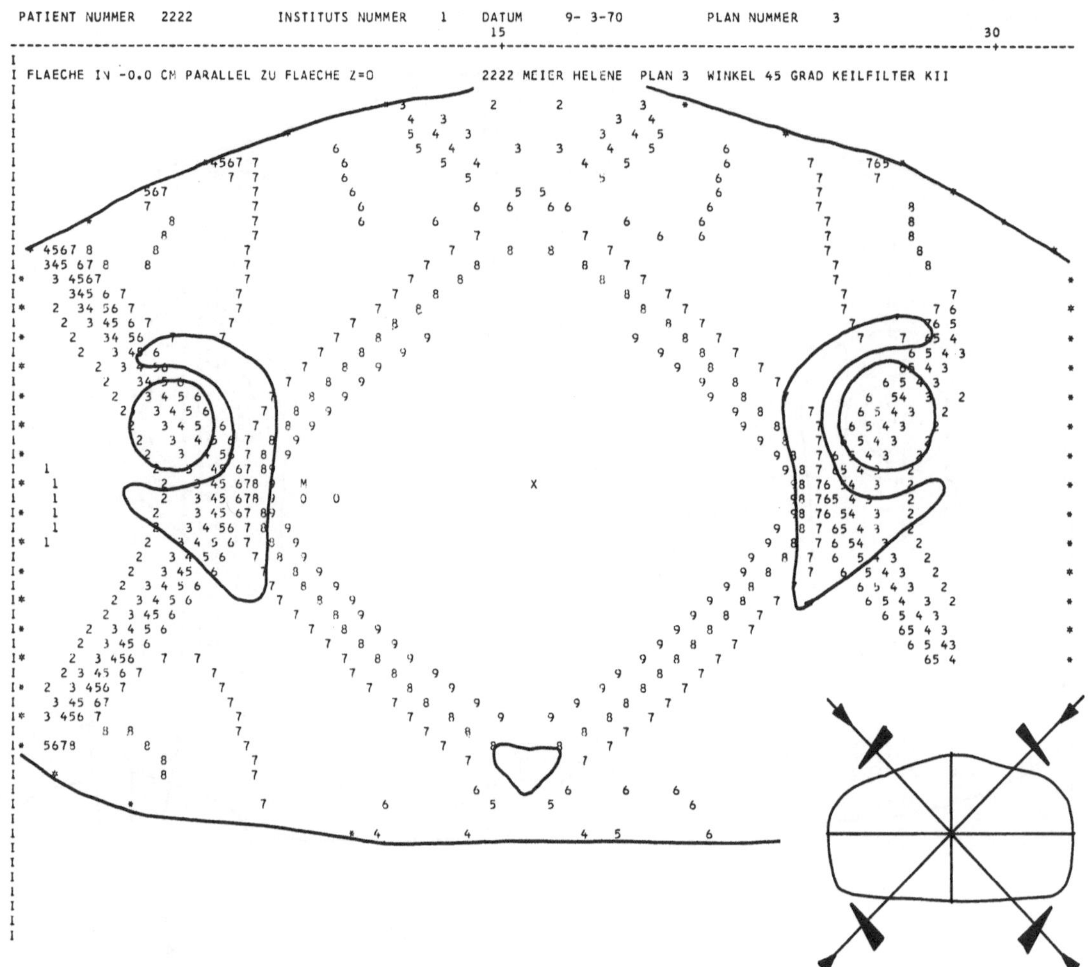

Abb. 21. Bestrahlung des kleinen Beckens von vier Feldern unter Verwendung von Keilfiltern (Feldgröße 10×14 cm, ^{60}Co-γ-Strahlung). (Strahlenabteilung der Universitäts-Frauenklinik Göttingen)

die Notwendigkeit der Schonung der Medulla und der Nieren bestehen, lassen sich nur schwer ausräumen. Es werden daher verschiedene Bestrahlungspläne mit Stehfeldern unter Verwendung von Keilfiltern und auch mit Bewegungsbestrahlung angegeben (Beduhn u. Kuttig).

Die unterschiedlichen Möglichkeiten lassen sich ebenfalls mittels des Computers durchspielen, und die Abb. 23—25 zeigen Beispiele für die Dosisverteilungen bei abgewandelten Bedingungen, wobei die Abb. 25 offenbar die günstigste Möglichkeit darstellt. Die von uns dabei angestrebte Herddosis beträgt 3000 R bei verdächtigen Fällen und 4000 R bei nachgewiesenen Lymphknotenmetastasen. Eine höhere Dosis halten wir wegen der bisher nicht nachgewiesenen Wirksamkeit einer Bestrahlung der lumbalen Lymphknoten auf keinen Fall für verantwortbar (s.a. Frischbier, Strahlenbehandlung des Collumcarcinoms, Seite 137). Auch für diese Rechenprogramme werden bei uns Wirbelsäule bzw. Medulla und Nieren mittels Stereoaufnahmen lokalisiert, wobei die Hautoberfläche mit dargestellt wird.

Die in *Göttingen* analog der zusätzlichen Percutanbestrahlung bei der Therapie des Cervixcarcinoms gewählte Form der Bestrahlung hat ihre entsprechenden Parallelen in anderen Kliniken. So verabfolgt Ries nur bei den weniger adipösen Patientinnen unter

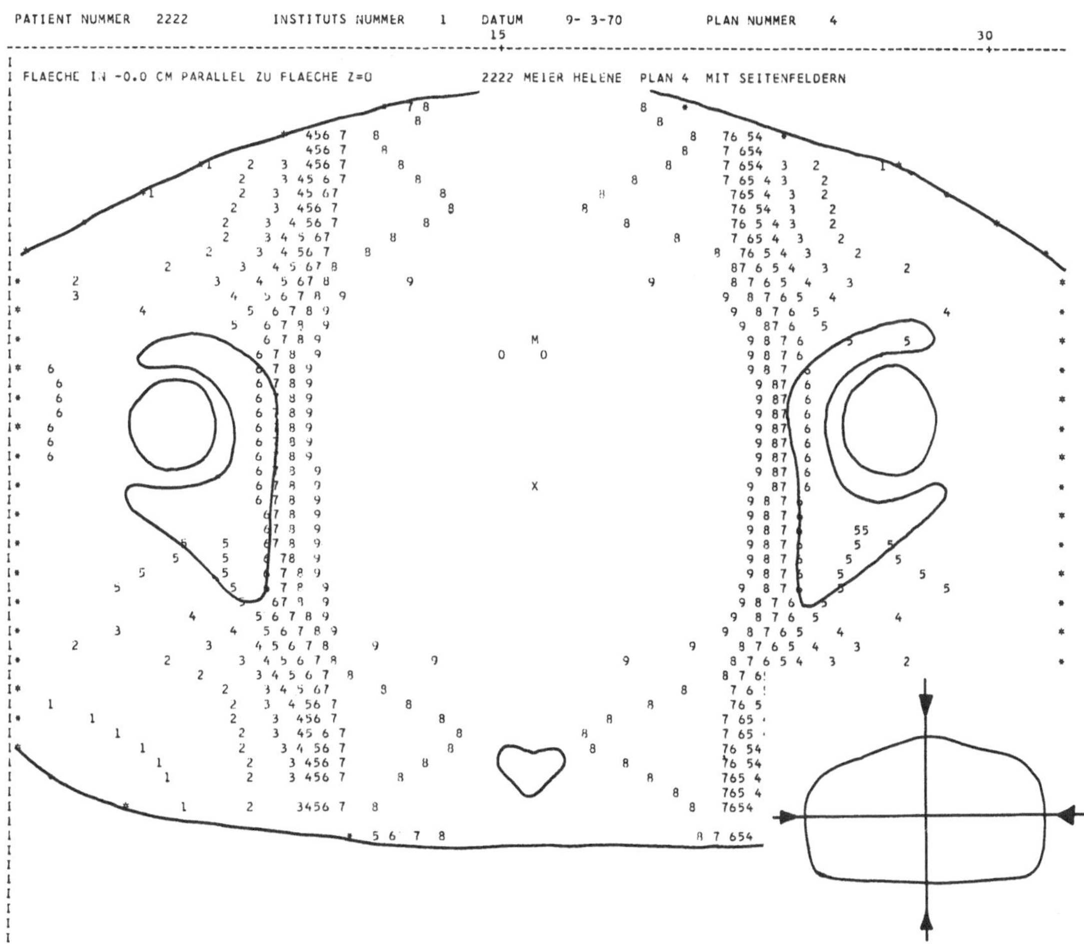

Abb. 22. Bestrahlung des kleinen Beckens von vier Feldern (ventral und dorsal 12 × 14 cm, seitlich 8 × 12 cm, ^{60}Co-γ-Strahlung). (Strahlenabteilung der Universitäts-Frauenklinik Göttingen)

konventionellen Tiefentherapiebedingungen auf 2 Bauch- und 2 Glutealfelder je 8—10mal 200—300 ROD. In fortgeschrittenen Fällen wird unter Umständen auch mittels der Pendelbestrahlung an jeder Beckenwand 4000 RHD appliziert.

Auch J. H. Müller bestrahlte die überwiegende Mehrzahl der Korpuscarcinom-Patientinnen mit der gleichen Methode percutan, wie sie bei der Therapie des Cervix-carcinoms angewendet wird. Mit konventionellen Strahlenqualitäten verabfolgt er auf das Becken von einem ventralen und einem dorsalen Feld von 18 × 18 cm und zusätzlichen Seitenfeldern aus 2400 ROD (Seitenfelder 2000 ROD). Nach Erreichen einer Oberflächendosis von 1000 R wird mit 2 mm Blei ein 5 cm breiter Mittelstreifen ausgespart. Es wird dabei relativ stark gefiltert (Thoraeusfilter) und ein großer Focus-Hautabstand gewählt (ventral und dorsal 80 cm, seitlich 50 cm). Der besondere Zeitplan der Percutanbestrahlung, die mit steigenden Dosen beginnt, wurde von J. H. Müller 1964 ausführlich dargestellt.

Kottmeier bestrahlt nur in fortgeschrittenen Fällen percutan zusätzlich zum Radium und bei Carcinoma corporis et endocervicis. Das letztere wird aber allgemein als Indikation für eine zusätzliche Percutanbestrahlung angesehen.

Fletcher bestrahlt, abgesehen von den beginnenden Fällen, zusätzlich zur Radium-therapie das ganze Becken mit 4000 rad (Tabellen 9, 11—14).

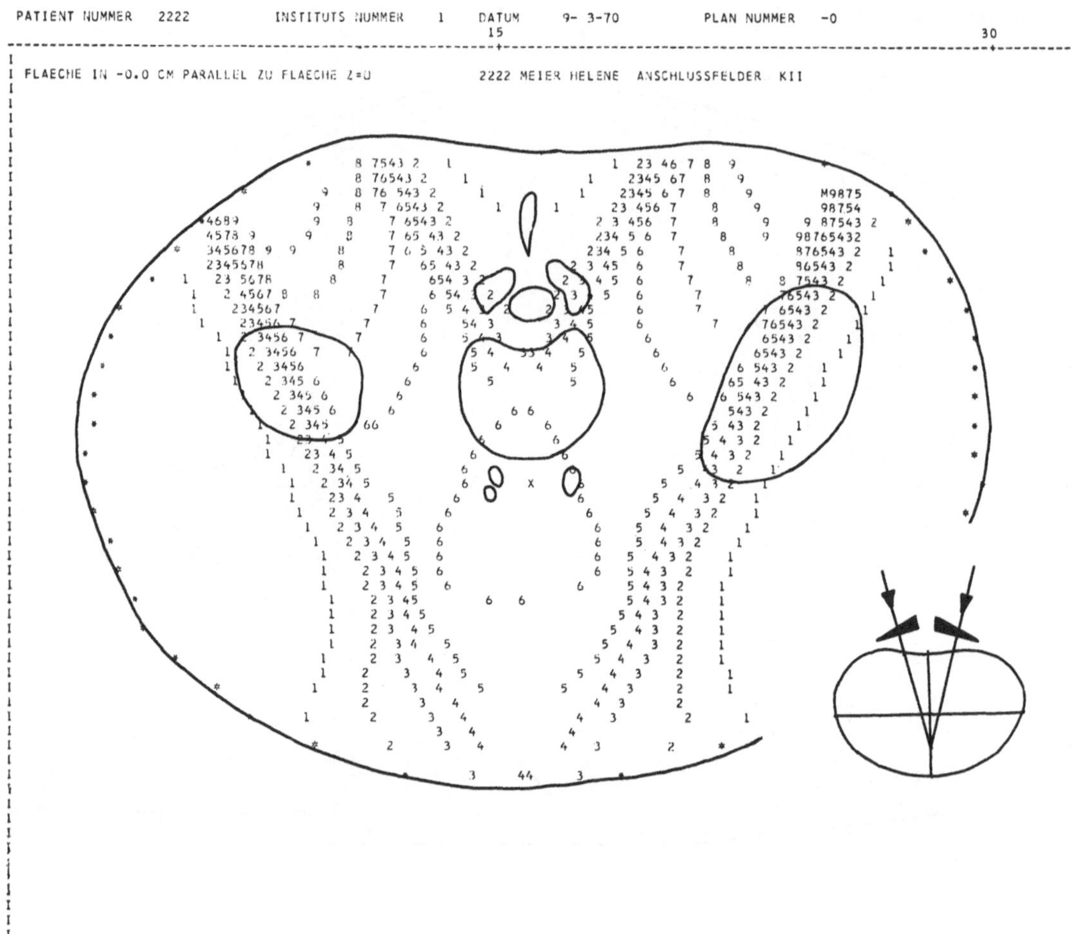

Abb. 23. Bestrahlung der lumbalen Lymphknoten (Feldgröße 5 × 10 cm, ^{60}Co-γ-Strahlung, ∢ 30° nach median, Keilfilter, dicke Seite des Filters nach median). Berechnung der Dosisverteilung durch Computer. (Strahlenabteilung der Universitäts-Frauenklinik Göttingen)

Zusammenfassend halten wir die Feststellung für berechtigt, daß die Prognose des bestrahlten Korpuscarcinoms, soweit sie überhaupt von der Therapie abhängt, steht und fällt mit der Radiumtherapie. Ob und wie weit die zusätzliche Percutanbestrahlung an den Therapieerfolgen beteiligt ist, ist nicht auszusagen. Zumindest dürfte die Problematik ähnlich der beim Cervixcarcinom sein.

b) Die präoperative Bestrahlung

· Es wurde weiter oben schon ausgeführt, daß die operative Behandlung des Korpuscarcinoms allgemein als die wirksamste Therapie angesehen wird. Es finden sich aber zunehmend Stimmen, die eine präoperative Strahlentherapie befürworten, da damit offenbar die Behandlungsergebnisse weiter verbessert werden konnten. Sind schon bei der Operationstechnik bestimmte Regeln zu beachten, um einer Aussaat von Carcinomzellen in Blut- oder Lymphbahnen oder auch in das Wundgebiet vorzubeugen, so soll nach landläufiger Ansicht die vorherige Strahlentherapie die Carcinomzelle so weitgehend devitalisieren, daß verschleppte Zellen nicht mehr angehen können. Diese Auffassung von der Wirkung der Vorbestrahlung ist umstritten, als Arbeitshypothese hat sie sich aber bewährt. Kottmeier (1957) sagt, daß jedenfalls die Möglichkeit, die Krebszellen prä-

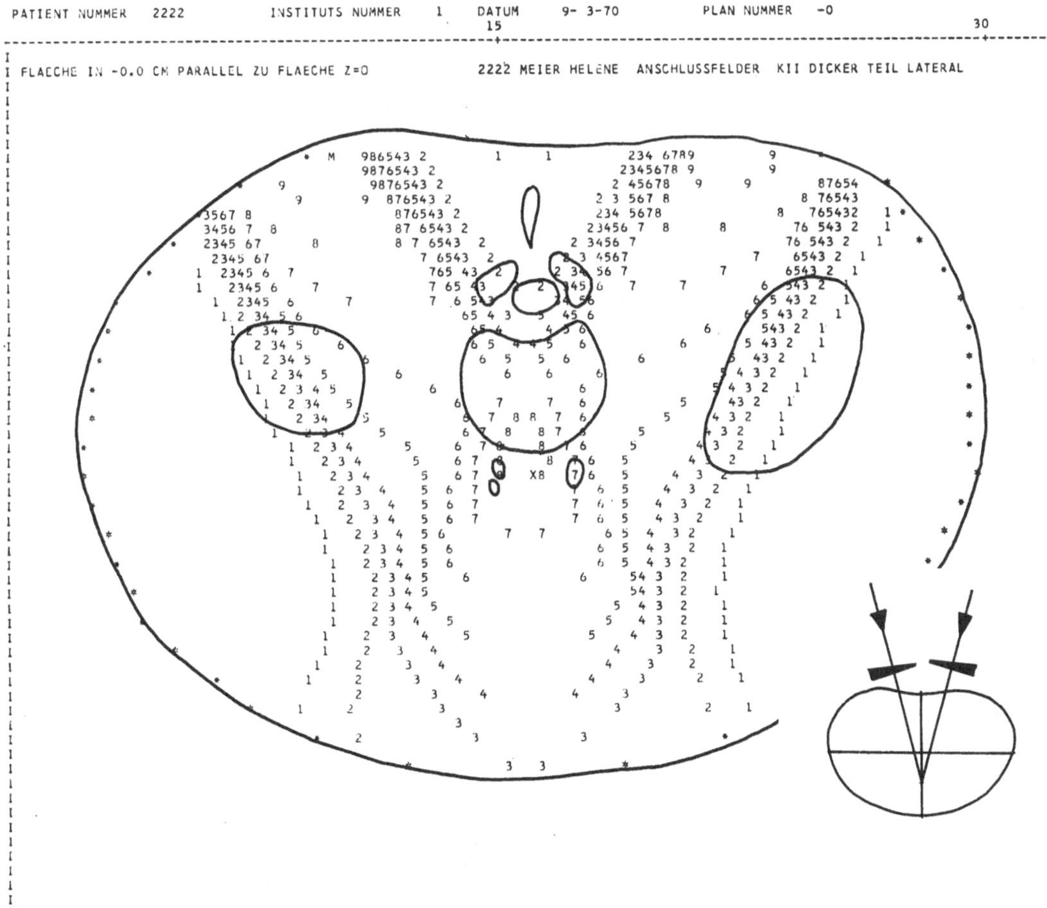

Abb. 24. Bestrahlung der lumbalen Lymphknoten. Bedingungen wie Abb. 23, aber umgekehrte Lage des Keilfilters. Bessere Entlastung der Nieren. (Strahlenabteilung der Universitäts-Frauenklinik Göttingen)

operativ im Lymphknoten durch die Vorbestrahlung wirksam zu beeinflussen, nicht bestritten werden kann.

Ohne auf die Problematik dieses Geschehens hier näher einzugehen, kann jedenfalls festgestellt werden, daß die von manchen Autoren veröffentlichten Ergebnisse es zumindest wahrscheinlich machen, daß durch die Vorbestrahlung die Ergebnisse verbessert werden können (H. G. MÜLLER). So hält DU MESNIL DE ROCHEMONT den Wert der Vorbestrahlung für erwiesen. NOLAN und HARRISON sahen von der Vorbestrahlung einen zwar geringen, aber doch signifikanten Vorteil. Während sich auch MARTIUS für die Vorbestrahlung aussprach, sind RENNING sowie BECK, LATOUR und BOURNE der Ansicht, daß die alleinige Operation mindestens gleich gut, wenn nicht besser sei als die Vorbestrahlung mit nachfolgender Operation. Allerdings räumt RENNING ein, daß vielleicht die verwandte Radiumdosis zu gering gewesen sein könnte. Eindeutig für die Vorbestrahlung sprechen sich weiter DELCLOS, FLETCHER, GUTIERREZ u. RUTLEDGE aus, außerdem GUSBERG, ferner GRIMM sowie MONTGOMERY, LANG, FARELL u. HAHN. ARNESON hält die präoperative Radiumbehandlung insbesondere bei vergrößertem Uterus und bei wenig differenzierten Carcinomen für wertvoll, meint allerdings auch, daß die Komplikationsrate dadurch ansteigt, ebenso wie bei radikalerer Operation. Auf alle Fälle besteht Einigkeit darüber, daß auch bei einer Vorbestrahlung das Hauptgewicht auf die Radiumeinlage in Form der Packmethode zu legen ist. Von den meisten Autoren wird

UMRISSRADIEN GEMAESS DER EINGABE, IN CM

```
   13.8   13.8   12.6   11.4   9.9   9.9   11.6   13.8   14.2   13.6   11.9   10.5   9.4   8.8   8.9   9.6   10.9   12.6
```

```
=============================================================================
INSTITUT  I PATIENT I DIAGNOSE I   DATUM  I PLAN I FLAE I ABSTAND VON   GERAET  I
          I         I          I          I      I      I ZENT.FLAECHEI         I
----------I---------I----------I----------I------I------I------------I----------I
          I         I          I          I      I      I            I          I
    1     I  2222   I   -0     I 9- 3-70 I  -0  I  1 I   -0.0  CM  I    1     I
=============================================================================
```

BEWEGUNGSBESTRAHLUNG
====================

SENKRECHTER STRAHLENEINFALL

FELD 1 KEILFELD, LAGE 2

PENDELFELD NR. 1 TANGENTIAL UM   3.0 GRAD

FELD 2 KEILFELD, LAGE 1

PENDELFELD NR. 2 TANGENTIAL UM -3.0 GRAD

MAXIMUM BEI POS. M = 23.1 RAD, PRO 100 RAD AUF ZENTR.STRAHL MAX.(IN 50.5 CM FOKUSABSTAND)

ZEIT PRO BOGEN 1   2.39 MIN., PRO 100 RAD IN DER 80-PROZENT-LINIE

ZEIT PRO BOGEN 2   2.39 MIN., PRO 100 RAD IN DER 80-PROZENT-LINIE

BOGEN	FELD ABMESS.	GEW. FAKT.	X (CM)	Y (CM)	Z (CM)	PENDEL. WINKEL	VON	BIS	PR CM	INTER VAL	A1	A2	A3	A4	A5
1	3*10	1.00	16.0	10.3	-0.0	110	1	111	65	10	19.2	19.2			
2	3*10	1.00	16.0	10.3	-0.0	110	71	181	65	10	18.8	18.8			
											38.0	38.0			

PENDELACHSE · IPENDEL · BEITRAEGE,PRO 100 RAD IM MAX, AUF

ZONEN-INTEGRALDOSIS, IN RAD PRO 100 IM MAXIMUM

FLAECHEN-ELEMENT 0.094 CM2

PROZ. ZONE	FLAECHE (CM2)	ZONEN-INTEGRAL (RAD·CM2)
20 - 30	46.0	1170.4
30 - 40	60.4	2159.9
40 - 50	83.2	3699.8
50 - 60	55.6	3043.3
60 - 70	45.1	2896.9
70 - 80	25.1	1875.1
80 - 90	24.4	2072.2
90 -100	22.5	2118.5
100 -110	0.2	18.9

PATIENT NUMMER   2222   INSTITUTS NUMMER   1   DATUM   9- 3-70   PLAN NUMMER   -0
                                                      15   30

FLAECHE IN -0.0 CM PARALLEL ZU FLAECHE Z=0   2222 MEIER HELENE ANSCHLUSSFELDER TANGENTIALPENDELUNG KIII

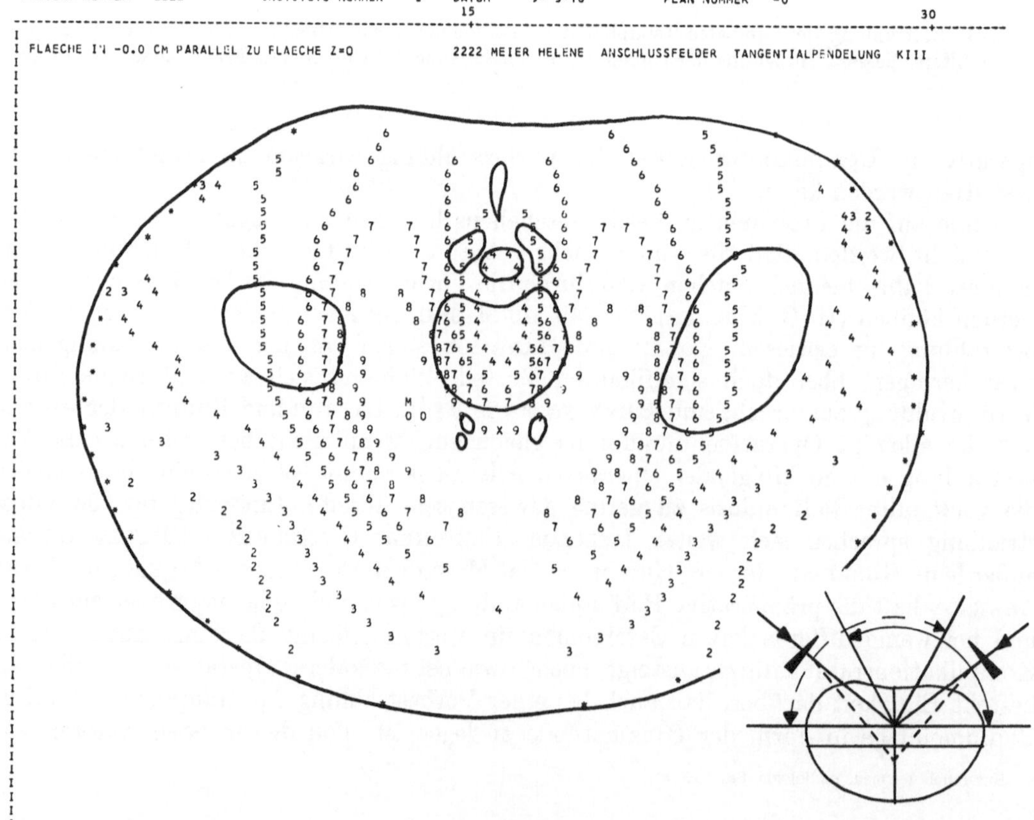

Abb. 25

dazu die prophylaktische Radiumeinlage in die Vagina gefordert (GUSBERG u. YANNO-POULOS). DOBBIE sah nach Vorbestrahlung fast keine Scheidenrezidive mehr und gibt aus der Literatur weitere Beispiele für die dadurch bedingte Verbesserung der Ergebnisse. Im allgemeinen wird dabei eine kurative Dosis angestrebt, wie bei der alleinigen Strahlentherapie.

KOTTMEIER spricht zwar nicht von Vorbestrahlung, er steht aber auf dem Standpunkt, daß eine Totalexstirpation des Uterus 6 Wochen nach der vollständig durchgeführten Radiumtherapie in einer Reihe von Fällen die Ergebnisse weiter verbessern könnte. Etwa 10 % der Korpuscarcinome der Jahre 1951—1960 wurden so im Radiumhemmet nach vorangegangener Bestrahlung operiert. Offensichtlich wird die Operation durch die Vorbestrahlung nicht erschwert. J. H. MÜLLER (1959) sowie HUNT und auch COSTOLOW, NOLAN, BUDENZ und DU SAULT, ferner RANDALL und GODDARD sind der Ansicht, daß sich ihre Ergebnisse durch die Vorbestrahlung gebessert haben. Bei den letztgenannten Autoren stiegen dabei die 5-Jahres-Heilungen von 58,6 auf 75,7 % an.

Während die meisten der vorstehend genannten Autoren vor allem oder ausschließlich dem Radium einen Wert für die Vorbestrahlung zuerkennen, finden sich auch einzelne Stimmen, die die percutane Zusatzbestrahlung auch in diesem Zusammenhang empfehlen, so J. H. MÜLLER (1941) sowie DU MESNIL DE ROCHEMONT, RINGLEB, SCHERER und SCHMITT.

Wie oben erwähnt, ist aus den Zahlen KOTTMEIERS ersichtlich, daß in 10 % der Fälle nach primärer, nicht als Vorbestrahlung gedachter Strahlentherapie später noch der Uterus exstirpiert wurde. Das leitet über zu dem Problem, die ungenügende Wirkung der Strahlentherapie rechtzeitig zu erkennen. Hierfür fordern DYROFF und MICHALZIK, bei jedem ausschließlich strahlenbehandelten Korpuscarcinom, nach einem halben Jahr eine Kontrollabrasio durchzuführen. DU MESNIL DE ROCHEMONT u. Mitarb. schließen sich dieser Auffassung an und führen in jedem Falle, also auch bei völliger Symptomfreiheit, nach 3—12 Monaten eine Kontrollabrasio durch. Daneben sprechen sich eine Reihe weiterer Autoren für die Therapiekontrolle durch Abrasio im ersten Jahr nach der Behandlung aus (GAUWERKY, 1957).

Wird bei einer solchen Kontrollabrasio noch Carcinom gefunden, so ist die Uterusexstirpation die Methode der Wahl, wie es KOTTMEIER praktiziert. Das erhöhte Operationsrisiko bei allgemein schlecht operablen Patientinnen muß in Anbetracht der schlechten Prognose solcher Fälle in Kauf genommen werden. So berichtet ARNESON (1964), daß diejenigen Patientinnen, bei denen im exstirpierten Uterus bei der routinemäßig angeschlossenen Exstirpation nach Vorbestrahlung kein Carcinom mehr gefunden wurde, eine 5-Jahres-Heilungsquote von über 80 % hatten, diejenigen mit Carcinom im Uterus aber weniger als 50 %. ARNESON, STANBRO und NOLAN fanden in 26,3 % der nachträglich exstirpierten Uteri noch Carcinom.

Zusammenfassend kann mit KOTTMEIER gesagt werden, daß vieles dafür spricht, der operativen Behandlung des Korpuscarcinoms den Vorzug zu geben, aber — abgesehen von den Fällen mit kleinem Cavum und gut ausdifferenziertem Tumor (FLETCHER) — nur nach einer Vorbestrahlung, die sich am besten aus intrauteriner, vaginaler und percutaner Strahlentherapie zusammensetzt. D. HOFMANN führt an, daß Hinweise darauf bestehen, daß die präoperative Bestrahlung wirksamer ist als die Nachbestrahlung. Ebenso muß ausgesprochen werden, daß die primäre Strahlentherapie, auch wenn nicht grundsätzlich die spätere Operation beabsichtigt war, von einer sorgfältigen Fallkontrolle gefolgt sein sollte, die auch bei Symptomfreiheit eine Abrasio innerhalb des ersten Jahres

Abb. 25. Bestrahlung der lumbalen Lymphknoten mit zwei Pendelfeldern [Achsenfeld 4×13 cm, Pendelradius 65 cm, ^{60}Co-γ-Strahlung, Auslenkung des Zentralstrahles (gestrichelte Linie) um 3°]. Vollständige Darstellung der Computerberechnung (in den Abb. 19—24 wurde der Tabellenteil aus Platzgründen fortgelassen). (Strahlenabteilung der Universitäts-Frauenklinik Göttingen)

einschließt. Im Falle eines Weiterwachstums oder Rezidivs sollte nach Möglichkeit die Uterusexstirpation unter Mitnahme der Anhänge und einer ausreichend breiten Scheidenmanschette angeschlossen werden. Ob sich eine darüber hinausgehende Radikalität im Einzelfall empfiehlt, wird vom Sitz des Rezidivs, vom Lymphknotenbefall, nicht zuletzt aber vom Allgemeinzustand abhängig zu machen sein.

c) Die postoperative Bestrahlung

Die Frage der Nachbestrahlung einer Patientin nach Totalexstirpation des Uterus und der Anhänge wegen eines Korpuscarcinoms wird im allgemeinen für die Fälle bejaht, in denen keine Vorbestrahlung erfolgt ist. So hält Kirchhoff (1962) eine Radiumeinlage in den Scheidenstumpf in jedem Falle für erforderlich. Dafür werden an der Universitäts-Frauenklinik Göttingen Kunststoffdistanzfilter verwendet (Abb. 26), mit denen 2000 R in 1 cm Gewebstiefe eingestrahlt werden. Kottmeier verwendet hierfür die gleichen Applikatoren wie bei der primären Radiumtherapie und verabfolgt 2500—3000 R/1 cm.

Tabelle 17. *Schwankungsbreite der Meßwerte in Blase und Darm bei 40 postoperativen Einlagen des Filters in Abb. 26 und 27 mit 50 mg Radium für jeweils 16 Std, entsprechend 800 mgeh*

Blase			Rectum		
min. R	max. R	Mittel R	min. R	max. R	Mittel R
384	1280	922	720	2272	1336

Wegen der Häufigkeit der Scheidenmetastasen (s. Tabelle 1 und 2) sprechen sich verständlicherweise für die intravaginale Radiumtherapie eine Reihe weiterer Autoren aus: Dobbie, ferner Fochem und Weghaupt sowie Gauwerky (1957), außerdem Hunt; du Mesnil de Rochemont, Ringleb, Scherer und Schmitt; Ries und Breitner. Dabei werden zum Teil wesentlich höhere Dosen als in Göttingen verabfolgt. Nach Ries und Breitner z.B. zwei- bis dreimal 1200 mgeh im Abstand von 14 Tagen. Es wird dabei eine kleine Platte oder ein „Pilz" (Kork), neuerdings auch ein Röhrenfilter in Hartgummi-Distanzrohr, verwendet. Die Gesamtdosis in Blase und Darm soll dabei 5000 R nicht überschreiten. Der Wert dieser postoperativen vaginalen Radiumeinlage wird allgemein betont. So sah Gauwerky (1957) nach Einführung der vaginalen Radiumapplikation unter 164 Patientinnen kein einziges Scheidengrundrezidiv mehr. Diese Zahl bezieht sich aber auf Uteruscarcinome, enthält also Cervix- und Korpuscarcinome. J.H. Müller verabfolgte in gleicher Weise wie bei der Primärbehandlung mit einem Bügelkolpostaten 2000—2500 mgeh. Er deutete die Tatsache, daß unter den Bestrahlten *Spät*rezidive im Verhältnis 7:2 häufiger sind als unter den nur Operierten dahingehend, daß durch die Bestrahlung das Wachstum verbliebener Carcinomzellkomplexe verlangsamt wird.

Daß bei der postoperativen vaginalen Radiumeinlage die Blasen- und auch die Rectumbelastung ganz besonders zu beachten sind, scheint vielfach nicht klar zu sein. Hier ist zu bedenken, daß die Blase operativ über den Scheidenstumpf herübergezogen wird und daher dem vaginalen Radiumfilter stark angenähert ist, insbesondere, wenn die Scheidennaht postoperativ dehiszent wurde. Als Beispiel werden in Tabelle 17 die Meßwerte in Blase und Darm für das in Abb. 26 (rechts) gezeigte Kunststoffilter gegeben, und zwar für eine Dosis von 800 mgeh, entsprechend etwa 2000 R/1 cm (Isodosen Abb. 27).

Der Wert der *percutanen Nachbestrahlung* wird unabhängig von der verwendeten Quantenenergie sehr unterschiedlich beurteilt. In den Fällen, in denen bereits eine intensive Vorbestrahlung durchgeführt worden ist, wird man die Indikation hierfür zurückhaltender stellen und davon abhängig machen, ob bei der Operation bzw. bei der Untersuchung des Operationspräparates Anhaltspunkte dafür gewonnen wurden, daß das Carcinom sich über den Uterus hinaus ausgebreitet hat und/oder Lymphknotenmetastasen bestanden, die durch die Vorbestrahlung ungenügend beeinflußt waren. Da in diesen Fällen die Prognose schlecht ist, erscheint ein erhöhtes Risiko durch nochmalige Bestrahlung vertretbar.

In den nicht vorbestrahlten Fällen kann man nach übereinstimmender Ansicht auf eine percutane Nachbestrahlung verzichten, wenn das Carcinom vollständig auf die Gebärmutterschleimhaut beschränkt war. RIES und BREITNER bestrahlen nicht nach,

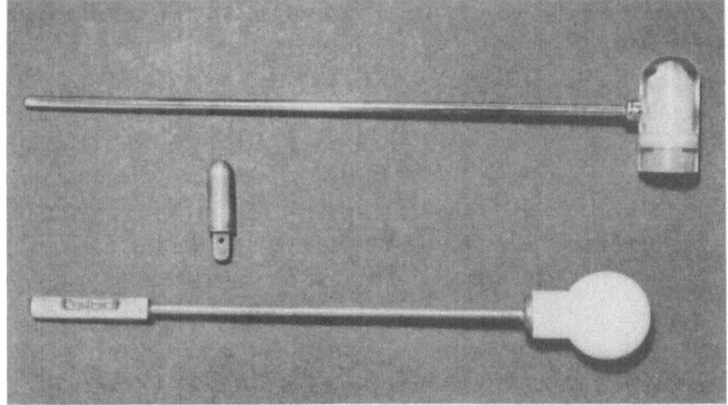

Abb. 26

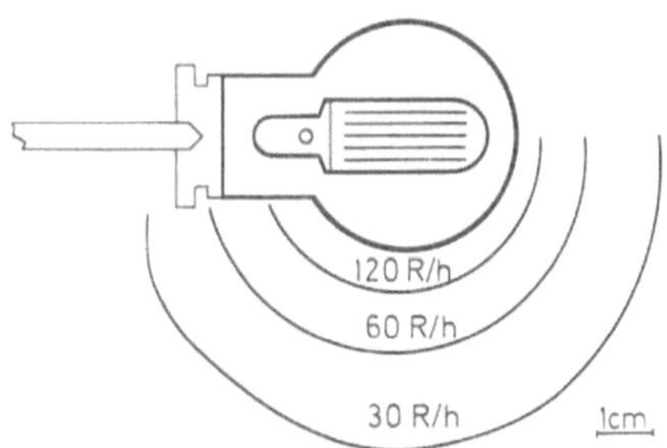

Abb. 26. Kunststoffdistanzfilter zur postoperativen Bestrahlung des Scheidenstumpfes. Die Oberfläche des unteren Filters ist der 250 R/h-Isodose angepaßt (50 mCi Radium) (s. Abb. 27). (Buchler & Co., Braunschweig; Strahlenabteilung der Universitäts-Frauenklinik Göttingen)

Abb. 27. Isodosenbild für 50 mCi Radium. Kunststoffdistanzfilter zur postoperativen Nachbestrahlung des Scheidenstumpfes (s. Abb. 26). Die Oberfläche entspricht der 250 R/h-Isodose

wenn das Carcinom auf den Uterus beschränkt ist. KIRCHHOFF (1962) hält dagegen eine Nachbestrahlung für erforderlich, wenn das Carcinom wenige Millimeter die Uterusmuskulatur infiltriert hat. Während KRAATZ eine Nachbestrahlung percutan im allgemeinen ablehnt, halten DU MESNIL DE ROCHEMONT, RINGLEB, SCHERER und SCHMITT sie ebenso wie GAUWERKY (1957) für erforderlich, wenn das Carcinom nicht auf das Endometrium beschränkt ist, v. MIKULICZ-RADECKI und GANSAU wieder nur dann, wenn es tiefer in die Muskulatur eindringt. Weitere Stimmen lassen sich dafür und dagegen anführen. Wenn aber überhaupt einer percutanen Zusatzbestrahlung, z.B. bei der alleinigen Strahlentherapie oder bei der Vorbestrahlung, eine Bedeutung zuerkannt wird, dann wäre es unseres Erachtens unlogisch, diese Bedeutung bei der Nachbestrahlung zu bestreiten. Es kann die Unterlassung der percutanen Nachbestrahlung nur von den schon genannten Gegenindikationen abhängig gemacht und allenfalls noch für ganz beschränkte Korpuscarcinome befürwortet werden, obwohl auch in letzterem Falle Lymphknotenmetastasen beschrieben worden sind. Auch hier wird ein positiver lymphographischer Befund die Entscheidung erleichtern.

Es ist nicht erforderlich, auf die Technik der percutanen Nachbestrahlung an dieser Stelle sehr ausführlich einzugehen. Sie unterscheidet sich an den einzelnen Kliniken zumeist nicht wesentlich von der Zusatzbestrahlung bei der primären Radiumtherapie und von der Nachbestrahlung des Collumcarcinoms. Als Dosierung wurden im allgemeinen 2 500—3 000 RHD als ausreichend angesehen, wenn es sich um eine prophylaktische Nachbestrahlung mit konventionellen Strahlenqualitäten handelte. Bei Anwendung der Supervolttherapie liegen die Dosen aber vielfach höher und erreichen im allgemeinen zumindest 4 000 R.

Die Bestrahlungstechnik hängt naturgemäß von der verwendeten Energie ab. Bei höheren Energien wird zum Teil mit einem großen ventralen und dorsalen Feld das ganze kleine Becken bestrahlt. Die Telekobalttherapie wird dagegen zumeist von 4 Feldern bzw. bei adipösen Patientinnen von 6 Feldern aus durchgeführt. Auch die Pendelbestrahlung kommt zur Anwendung. Bezüglich der Bestrahlungspläne kann dabei auf die von Frischbier in diesem Handbuch angegebenen Techniken verwiesen werden.

In *Göttingen* wird die Nachbestrahlung mit Telekobalt von 2 ventralen und 2 dorsalen Feldern 8×14 cm, 2,5° aus der Sagittalebene nach median gerichtet, vorgenommen. Dabei wird ventral ein Mittelstreifen von 3 cm, dorsal von 4 cm, ausgespart. Mit dem Telekobaltgerät werden täglich auf 2 Felder etwa 300 ROD (max.) verabfolgt. Die Oberflächendosis variiert, da angestrebt wird, konstante Herddosen, die pro Tag etwa um 200 R liegen, einzustrahlen. Bei adipösen Patientinnen mit einem Sagittaldurchmesser über 20 cm werden zusätzlich Seitenfelder gegeben. Dieser Plan gewährleistet, daß die Mitte nicht zu hoch belastet wird, so daß es mit der intravaginalen Radiumeinlage zusammen hier keine unerwünscht hohe Dosisspitze gibt (Abb. 20).

Dieser Modus der Bestrahlung ändert sich, wenn bei der Operation ein sehr weitgehender Befall des Beckenbindegewebes und der regionären Lymphknoten sowie der Vagina festgestellt wird. Zugleich verliert damit die Bestrahlung ihren prophylaktischen Charakter, und sie wird zur kurativen Maßnahme, die, wenn überhaupt, alleine noch imstande ist, eine Heilung herbeizuführen.

In solchen Fällen wird an der Universitäts-Frauenklinik Göttingen eine Kreuzfeuerbestrahlung vorgenommen, wobei 2 ventrale und 2 dorsale Felder von 10×14 cm auf einen gemeinsamen Konvergenzpunkt so zur Mitte eingekippt werden, daß jedes einzelne Feld das kleine Becken ganz ausleuchtet. Dieser Konvergenzpunkt wird aus der Körperquerschnittszeichnung nach Lokalisationsaufnahmen in 2 Ebenen unter Mitabbildung eines Meßstabes in der Vagina ermittelt (Frischkorn, 1961 und 1963; Lemtis und Frischkorn). Die Bestrahlung erfolgt mit Keilfiltern, die räumliche Dosisverteilung wird mit dem Computer ermittelt (Abb. 21).

Bei Befall der Leistenlymphknoten werden diese in die ventralen Felder, deren Form entsprechend abgeändert wird, mit einbezogen. Da die angestrebte Herddosis im Becken früher erreicht ist, werden die Leisten anschließend bis zu einer Gesamtdosis von 6 000 ROD (max.), entsprechend einer Dosis von etwa 4 500 R/5 cm Tiefe, weiterbestrahlt. Es gelingt so ohne Schwierigkeiten, auch bei adipösen Patientinnen eine Herddosis von 6 000 R im kleinen Becken zu erreichen. Die in jedem Einzelfall für alle Felder in der Vagina vorgenommene Kontrollmessung ergibt im allgemeinen eine gute Übereinstimmung mit dem errechneten Wert. Dieser Bestrahlungsplan wird auch bei inoperablen Fällen angewandt, wenn die Ausdehnung des Carcinoms eine typische Radiumbehandlung nicht zuläßt. Bei guter Rückbildung des Tumors unter der Tiefentherapie wird unter Umständen zu einem späteren Zeitpunkt die Radiumtherapie doch noch durchgeführt. In diesem Falle wird die Herddosis der Percutanbestrahlung für jede Radiumfraktion mit maximal 2 000 R Blasen- oder Darmbelastung um 1 000 R reduziert. Eine Erhöhung der Dosis bei der ausschließlichen Percutanbestrahlung über 6 000 R hinaus halten wir nicht für vertretbar, solange keine befriedigende Abwägung des Nutzens gegenüber den vermehrten Strahlenfolgen möglich ist. Hinzu kommt, daß bei einer Dosis von 6 000 R im ganzen kleinen Becken auch noch mit Dosisspitzen von +10—20% gerechnet werden muß.

Eine zusätzliche intraperitoneale Applikation von kolloidalem [198]Au wurde von J. H. Müller (1966) bei Vorliegen von Ovarialmetastasen empfohlen. An der Universitäts-

Frauenklinik Göttingen wird in vereinzelten derartigen Fällen ebenfalls davon Gebrauch gemacht. Allerdings muß dabei mit einer Erhöhung des Bestrahlungsrisikos gerechnet werden (JOHANNSEN), zumal eine Abschätzung, wie weit sich die einzelnen Bestrahlungsgebiete überschneiden und welche Dosisspitzen sich ergeben, allenfalls größenordnungsmäßig möglich ist. Dabei kann die Radiogoldtherapie (auch andere Betastrahler finden Verwendung) naturgemäß nur auf eine peritoneale Tumoraussaat und allenfalls auf Lymphknotenmetastasen einwirken. Letzteres auch nur, wenn eine wesentliche Aktivität in den betreffenden Lymphknoten gespeichert wird. Eine Bestrahlung größerer Lymphome oder Tumorknoten ist bei der geringen Eindringtiefe der Betastrahlung (im Durchschnitt <1 mm) nicht möglich, zumal die Intensität der Gammakomponente hierfür nicht ausreicht.

6. Die Komplikationen der Strahlentherapie des Korpuscarcinoms

Die Möglichkeit einer Uterusperforation bei der Packmethode und ihre Bedeutung wurde im Zusammenhang mit der Therapie schon besprochen.

Eine relativ häufige Komplikation ist die *Pyometra*, die bekanntlich aber auch schon vor der Behandlung des Korpuscarcinoms gefunden werden kann und die als Befund bei Frauen im Klimakterium dann immer den Verdacht auf Vorliegen eines Korpuscarcinoms erwecken muß. Sie wird mit einer Dilatation des Halskanals und Einlegen eines Fehlingschen Röhrchens für mehrere Tage sowie mit Uterusspülungen und Verabfolgung von kontraktionsfördernden Mitteln behandelt. Falls sie wiederholt rezidiviert, muß man sich zur Uterusexstirpation entschließen.

Zur Vermeidung entzündlicher Komplikationen wird von manchen Autoren eine prophylaktische Antibioticabehandlung vorgeschlagen. Wir lehnen dies ab und halten steriles Arbeiten für ausreichend.

Radiogene Veränderungen am Beckenskelet und am proximalen Oberschenkel kommen ebenso wie bei der Strahlenbehandlung des Cervixcarcinoms vor, sind aber nach besserer Ausblendung (FRISCHKORN, 1960 und 1961) und Einführung energiereicherer Strahlen seltener geworden (GRABIGER; GROSSE-HOLZ, 1964; KIRCHHOFF und IMHOLZ; KLUG; LANDRGOT u. SAUER; REDD. Weitere Literatur bei GROSSE-HOLZ).

Blasenreaktionen und *Ureterschäden* sind bei der Strahlenbehandlung des Korpuscarcinoms offenbar seltener als beim Cervixcarcinom. KOTTMEIER (1964) gibt 1,4% Blasenschäden an und fand in 1% der Fälle einen Ureterverschluß. Seiner Ansicht nach wurde die Verbesserung der Heilungsergebnisse mit einer gewissen Vermehrung der Komplikationen erkauft. Es ist auch an dieser Stelle festzustellen, daß zumindest die Ureterschäden auf keinen Fall gleichsam automatisch auf die Bestrahlung zurückgeführt werden dürfen. Eigene Untersuchungen am Kaninchenureter (CASTAÑO Y ALMENDRAL; NOLTE) machen es wahrscheinlich, daß der Ureter primär gar nicht so strahlenempfindlich ist, sondern daß offenbar andere Einflüsse dazukommen müssen, beim Cervixcarcinom z.B. die Beeinträchtigung der Ureterfunktion durch die Infiltration des umgebenden Bindegewebes im kleinen Becken. Daneben sind sicher zu einem großen Teil auch Harnwegsinfektionen ursächlich mit in Betracht zu ziehen. Handelt es sich doch bei den Korpuscarcinom-Patientinnen um ein Krankengut, bei dem intravesikale Manipulationen sehr häufig sind: Katheterurin, Cystoskopie, Strahlenmessung im Anschluß an jede Radiumeinlage, Dauerkatheter während der Radiumeinlagen. Dazu kommt gegebenenfalls der postoperative Katheterismus, eventuell auch hier noch ein Dauerkatheter. Bis das Gegenteil bewiesen ist, sollte daher immer nur von Folgezuständen gesprochen und das Wort Strahlenschaden, insbesondere bei den Ureterveränderungen, überhaupt vermieden werden. Die Problematik der Diagnose und Behandlung dieser Folgezustände an den Harnwegen ist die gleiche wie beim Collumcarcinom. Abgesehen von der sich aus obiger Feststellung ergebenden Prophylaxe durch möglichst steriles Arbeiten ist es vor allem wichtig, daß Harnwegskomplikationen bei den Nachuntersuchungen rechtzeitig erkannt werden, so daß eine urologische Behandlung zum günstigsten Zeitpunkt gewährleistet ist (Kirchhoff, 1960).

Auch *Darmreaktionen* sind relativ seltener als beim Collumcarcinom. Kottmeier (1964) sah in 2,4 % Rectumschäden. Besonders tragisch wirkt es sich — ebenso wie bei den Harnwegsschäden — naturgemäß aus, wenn die Verschlechterung des Allgemeinzustandes und ein eventueller Ileus oder Subileus automatisch auf das Carcinom bezogen werden und so eventuell der günstigste Zeitpunkt für eine chirurgische Intervention versäumt wird. Insbesondere eine erhebliche Beschleunigung der Blutkörperchensenkungsgeschwindigkeit wird häufig als Zeichen des Carcinomwachstums interpretiert, obwohl bei den hohen Werten eher an eine Harnwegskomplikation gedacht werden sollte.

Die primäre Mortalität der Strahlentherapie beträgt nach Czech, Kepp und Wolthaus 2,4 %. Im Gesamtmaterial der Universitäts-Frauenklinik Göttingen der Jahre 1942—1961 (670 Fälle) beträgt die primäre Mortalität der ausschließlich strahlenbehandelten Patientinnen (391) 4,1 % (16 Frauen). (Primäre Operationsmortalität für den gleichen Zeitraum 4,6 %.)

7. Die Behandlung der Rezidive des Korpuscarcinoms

Vom Rezidiv sprechen wir vereinbarungsgemäß dann, wenn zwischen Abschluß der Behandlung und dem Wiederauftreten ein symptomfreies Intervall liegt. Dieses Intervall wird unterschiedlich angegeben, wir selbst fordern 6 Monate. Ein früherer Rückfall wird als „Weiterwachstum" bezeichnet. Zugegebenermaßen befriedigt eine solche willkürliche zeitliche Festlegung nicht. Es kann ja kein Zweifel sein, daß es sich zumindest bei den Rezidiven der ersten Jahre um ein erneutes Wachstum noch verbliebener Carcinomzellverbände handelt.

Neben der zeitlichen Abgrenzung des Rezidivs ist aber oft auch eine Schwierigkeit hinsichtlich der Unterscheidung der Begriffe „Rezidiv", „Lokalrezidiv" und „Metastase" vorhanden. Auch eine Metastase stellt selbstverständlich nach einem entsprechenden Zeitintervall ein Rezidiv dar und manche Autoren unterscheiden daher das metastatische Rezidiv vom Lokalrezidiv. Als Lokalrezidiv wird dabei im allgemeinen jedes erneute Carcinomwachstum im kleinen Becken, einschließlich Vagina, angesehen. Andere sprechen von Scheiden- oder Beckenwand*metastasen*. Man sollte sich darüber einigen, daß ein Wiederauftreten des Carcinoms nach einem entsprechenden zeitlichen Intervall grundsätzlich als Rezidiv angesprochen wird und daß bei der Angabe der Lokalisation eventuell das Wort Metastase Verwendung findet. Voraussetzung ist, daß mit hinreichender Sicherheit klar ist, daß kein Zweitcarcinom vorliegt.

Nach Amreich sowie Rubin und Gerle u.a. treten $^3/_4$ der Rezidive in den ersten beiden Jahren nach der Behandlung auf. Rezidive im Uterus sollten nach Möglichkeit operiert werden. Entschließt man sich zur Strahlentherapie, dann sollte dies nicht palliativ, sondern kurativ sein, vorausgesetzt, daß Allgemeinzustand und Strahlenvorbelastung dies zulassen.

Die häufigste Lokalisation des Rezidivs ist die Vagina (Schraknepper; du Mesnil de Rochemont, Ringleb, Scherer u. Schmitt; Neuweiler). Insbesondere bei den operierten Patientinnen ohne Vor- oder Nachbestrahlung ist das Scheidenrezidiv relativ häufig, nach Rubin, Gerle, Quick und Greenlaw zehnmal häufiger als nach der Kombination von Operation und Strahlentherapie.

Diese allgemein nicht bestrittene Beobachtung wirft natürlich die Frage nach der Ursache auf, und es liegt nahe, daß diese in der Operation selbst gesehen wird. Dabei ist, abgesehen von der Möglichkeit, daß schon zum Zeitpunkt der Operation eine nicht erkannte Metastase vorhanden ist, zu unterscheiden zwischen Implantationsmetastasen durch Carcinomzellverschleppung unter der Operation und einer retrograden Verschleppung auf dem Lymph- oder Blutweg durch „Massage" des Uterus unter der Operation.

Dieser letztere Weg soll nach RUTLEDGE, TAN und FLETCHER für die Metastasen im unteren Scheidendrittel in erster Linie verantwortlich sein. Die Anatomie der Lymphwege und Venen und entsprechende Beobachtungen an Operationspräparaten unterstreichen diese Ansichten. Die Operationstechnik hat hieraus ihre Konsequenzen gezogen: Es gilt das Corpus uteri so schonend wie möglich anzufassen oder sogar jedes Anfassen durch Anklemmen der Ligamenta rotunda und der Adnexe zu umgehen. Da der Uterus bei der vaginalen Operation mehr alteriert wird, führen diese Gedankengänge auch wieder zu dem Vorschlag, den abdominalen Operationsweg vorzuziehen.

Der Zeitpunkt des Auftretens vaginaler Metastasen liegt in 70% in den ersten beiden und in 90% in den ersten $3^1/_2$ Jahren (PREM). Die Häufigkeit des Befalls der verschiedenen Scheidenabschnitte wird einheitlich dahingehend angegeben, daß im unteren Scheidendrittel höchstens ein Viertel der Scheidenmetastasen lokalisiert sind (s. a. Tabelle 1).

Auffällig und nicht wegzuleugnen ist aber die Verminderung der Metastasenhäufigkeit in der Vagina durch eine Vor- und/oder Nachbestrahlung mittels Radium. KOTTMEIER sah ohne Nachbestrahlung in 15%, mit Nachbestrahlung nur in 6% Scheidenmetastasen.

RUTLEDGE, TAN und FLETCHER berichten von einer Verminderung der Scheidenmetastasen von 20 auf 1,5% bei (kurativer) Vorbestrahlung (korporal und vaginal). Zur Scheidenmetastasierung neigen angeblich vor allem die anaplastischen Tumoren. Ob die Lokalisation in den verschiedenen Scheidenabschnitten unterschiedliche Prognosen bedingen, scheint bisher nicht geklärt. Im übrigen hängt aber die Prognose des Rezidivs sehr wohl von der Lokalisation ab, und hier sind die Scheidenmetastasen, nicht zuletzt wegen ihrer direkten Zugänglichkeit, für die Radiumtherapie mit am aussichtsreichsten.

DU MESNIL DE ROCHEMONT, RINGLEB, SCHERER und SCHMITT halten eine Rezidivbehandlung besonders dann für aussichtsreich, wenn primär bestrahlt wurde, bei den primär Operierten dagegen für schlechter. Während beim Cervixcarcinom die gegenteilige Ansicht vorherrscht, ermöglicht beim Korpuscarcinom die operative Rezidivbehandlung relativ günstige Ergebnisse. Im Gegensatz dazu konnte KOTTMEIER (1959) zeigen, daß auch die Strahlentherapie primär operierter Korpuscarcinom-Patientinnen gute Erfolge haben kann. 41 von insgesamt 102 Rezidivpatientinnen nach primär operativer Behandlung wurden mit Hilfe der Strahlentherapie geheilt (5-Jahres-Überlebenszeit). GROSSE-HOLZ, SCHULZE und VOGELGESANG berichten eine Rezidivheilung in 10,9% der Fälle. PRICE, HAHN und ROMINGER weisen darauf hin, daß sie 28% der Scheidenrezidive heilen konnten. Die Prognose war bei Befall des Scheidengewölbes deutlich besser als bei Befall des unteren Scheidendrittels. BUTTENBERG und ZEITZ berichteten eine absolute 5-Jahres-Heilung bei Scheidenrezidiven von 21,9%. Die Ergebnisse der Rezidivbehandlung liegen nach RUBIN, GERLE, QUICK und GREENLAW unter 30% und nur ausnahmsweise darüber. Das oben von KOTTMEIER berichtete Ergebnis liegt mit etwa 40% absolut an der Spitze. Da es sich dabei ausschließlich um primär operierte, nicht nachbestrahlte Patientinnen handelt, die ja zweifellos nicht als repräsentativ für das gesamte Rezidivkrankengut anzusehen sind, ist diese Zahl mit den anderen Angaben nur bedingt vergleichbar.

Eine *Rezidivdiagnose* allein aufgrund des Tastbefundes halten wir nicht für zulässig. Da die erneute Therapie eine noch größere Schädigungsmöglichkeit hat als die primäre, sollte das Rezidiv in jedem Falle verifiziert sein. Hier bietet sich neben der histologischen Diagnose aus dem Abradat, aus Probeexcisionen oder Punktionszylindern (*Silvermann*-Nadel; FETTIG), aus parametranen Infiltraten die cytologische Untersuchung von Gewebspunktaten (BÖTZELEN u. SCHMIDT-MATTHIESEN) an. Welches Verfahren in Frage kommt, wird in erster Linie von der Lokalisation und damit der Zugänglichkeit abhängen. Dazu kommen die Lymphographie zur Erfassung befallener Lymphknoten oder Feststellung der Verlegung von Lymphwegen, die Arteriographie zur Identifizierung parametraner Infiltrate und die Phlebographie zur Feststellung der Ursache von Abflußbehinderungen. Schließlich ist auch die Urographie in einigen Fällen geeignet, Hinweise zu geben.

Für die Strahlentherapie der Rezidive lassen sich Richtlinien nicht so gut aufstellen wie für die Primärbehandlung. Ist die Frage Operation oder Bestrahlung oder auch die

Kombination beider Verfahren entschieden, kommt das gesamte Spektrum strahlentherapeutischer Möglichkeiten in Betracht. Es ist dabei zu beachten, daß hinsichtlich der Dosierung alle noch verbliebenen Möglichkeiten ausgeschöpft werden, zumal das höhere Erkrankungsrisiko für die Patientin auch ein erhöhtes Risiko bei der Rezidivbestrahlung rechtfertigt. Die anzuwendenden Methoden unterscheiden sich dabei nicht von denen, die bei Rezidiven anderer Ätiologie, aber gleicher Lokalisation zur Anwendung kommen. Am günstigsten liegen die Fälle, die einer Radiumtherapie zugänglich sind und die, wie oben gesagt, noch eine relativ gute Heilungschance haben, die über derjenigen liegt, die wir vom Cervixcarcinom kennen. Ist der Befund im Uterus lokalisiert oder in der Vagina und ist eine Operation ausgeschlossen, ist es erforderlich, mit dem Radium eine Strahlendosis zu verabfolgen, die derjenigen der Erstbehandlung entspricht. Bei Scheidenbefunden streben wir dabei mindestens 6000 R in der Tiefe an, die der größten festgestellten Tiefenausdehnung des Tumors entspricht. Ein Rezidiv im kleinen Becken wird — mit oder ohne vaginales Radium — allgemein einer hochdosierten Supervolttherapie zuzuführen sein, deren anzustrebende Herddosis ebenfalls in der Größenordnung von 6000 R liegen sollte. Von dieser Dosis wird bei erheblicher Vorbelastung nach unten abzuweichen, in anderen Fällen wird nach Ansicht einiger Autoren auch eine höhere Dosis zu vertreten sein.

Gerade für die Strahlentherapie der Rezidive werden streng individualisierte Bestrahlungspläne unter Ausschöpfung aller technischen Möglichkeiten erforderlich. Wie weit sie aber realisiert werden können, wird nicht nur von der Lokalisation des Rezidivs und seiner Ausdehnung, sondern sehr wesentlich von der Vorbelastung bei der Primärbehandlung, von Art und Ausdehnung einer eventuell primär durchgeführten Operation und nicht zuletzt von der Belastbarkeit der Patientin abhängen.

Eine operative Rezidivbehandlung wird im allgemeinen nur in den Fällen in Frage kommen, in denen der Ort des Rezidivs der Uterus und/oder die Vagina ist. Ein Rezidiv mit Blasen- oder Rectumeinbruch wird in Einzelfällen mit besonders guter Allgemeinoperabilität auch noch chirurgisch angegangen werden können. Im allgemeinen wird aber das Alter und der Zustand der Korpuscarcinom-Patientinnen ultraradikale chirurgische Maßnahmen nicht zulassen.

8. Zusatztherapie

Es ist hier nicht der Platz, die Zusatztherapie abzuhandeln, zumal sie sich hinsichtlich der Cytostatika nicht prinzipiell von der bei anderen Carcinomen unterscheidet. Es sei aber erwähnt, daß zurückgehend auf Thiessen (1951), Kaiser (1959) und Kistner (1959) sich die Anwendung von Progesteron, bzw. künstlichen Gestagenen, einen Platz in der Behandlung von Korpuscarcinommetastasen erobert hat. In der Zwischenzeit liegt ein umfangreiches Schrifttum hierüber vor. So berichten neben den genannten Autoren Kottmeier (1962) und Bergsjö (1965) über das Verschwinden von Lungenmetastasen unter dieser Therapie. Bei den letzteren war das in 9 behandelten Fällen viermal der Fall. Auch Kelley und Baker sahen einen Einfluß auf Lungenmetastasen, daneben aber auch Erfolge bei anderen Lokalisationen. Nach ihrer Auffassung reagiert etwa ein Drittel der Fälle. Sie stellten fest, daß nach Wiederauftreten der Metastasen eine zweite Behandlung wirkungslos bleibt. Auch Kennedy sah einen Effekt in 8 von 27 Fällen. Er meint, daß die langsam wachsenden, länger bestehenden Carcinome besser reagieren. Staffan und Nordquist stellten darüber hinaus auch einen Effekt auf das Carcinom in der Gewebekultur fest. Die Wirkungsweise, die gewisse Parallelen zu der natürlichen Wechselbeziehung zwischen Progesteron und Endometrium aufweist, beruht offenbar auf einer cytostatischen Wirkung der Gestagene auf das Endometriumcarcinom. Es kommt zur Reduzierung der Mitosen. Dabei ist auch an den eingangs diskutierten Zusammenhang zwischen hormonalen Funktionen und Endometriumcarcinom zu denken. Eine Ausheilung mit der Gestagentherapie ist nicht zu erwarten. Immerhin liegen aber Berichte mit Überlebenszeiten bis zu 5 Jahren vor (Martz).

9. Ergebnisse

Die Tabelle 18 gibt von einer Reihe von Kliniken aus dem 14. Band des „Annual report on the results of the treatment in carcinoma of the uterus and vagina" die Heilungsergebnisse bei der Behandlung des Korpuscarcinoms wieder. Es sind darunter Kliniken mit vorwiegend operativer, vorwiegend radiologischer und mit selektiver Therapie aufgeführt. Beim Lesen der Tabelle ist zu bedenken, daß für den Berichtszeitraum bis 1961 einschließlich eine andere Stadieneinteilung zugrunde gelegt war, und zwar:

Stadium I: Das Wachstum ist beschränkt auf den Uterus. Gruppe 1: Operation ist ratsam. Gruppe 2: hohes Operationsrisiko.

Stadium II: Ausbreitung des Carcinoms über den Uterus hinaus.

Gleichzeitig wurden die Fälle von Carcinoma corporis et endocervicis, Carcinoma uteri et ovarii und Carcinoma pelvis nicht in die Statistik aufgenommen, sondern lediglich ihre Anzahl angegeben. Der Anteil dieser prognostisch besonders ungünstigen Fälle schwankt von Klinik zu Klinik außerordentlich stark und ist in der Tabelle 18 in der Spalte „nicht in die Statistik einbezogen" angegeben. Diese Schwankungen sind aber wohl kaum echte Häufigkeitsunterschiede, sondern sicher eher durch die unterschiedlich vollständige Erfassung der betreffenden Fälle bedingt. Bei Einbeziehung dieser Fälle könnten sich daher die Erfolgszahlen der betreffenden Kliniken etwas ändern. Diese Schwierigkeiten werden durch die neue Einteilung (Tabelle 4) vermieden.

Beim Studium der Tabelle 18 läßt sich nicht erkennen, daß etwa die vorwiegend operativ tätigen Kliniken prinzipiell anders abschneiden als die Kliniken mit vorwiegender oder ausschließlicher Strahlentherapie. Und auch die Kliniken, die in beiden Gruppen mit ihrem Krankengut etwa gleich stark vertreten sind, die also offenbar eine selektive Therapie treiben, heben sich nicht klar heraus. Den wesentlichsten Einfluß hat offensichtlich die Zusammensetzung des Krankengutes, so daß immer dann die Ergebnisse besonders gut sind, wenn der Anteil des Stadiums I, Gruppe 1, groß ist. Immerhin beantwortet diese Tabelle viele Fragen bezüglich der Behandlungserfolge und gestattet weitere Überlegungen im Hinblick auf ihre Abhängigkeit von Ausbreitung und Therapieform.

Es ließen sich aus der Literatur noch zahlreiche Statistiken herausgreifen mit sehr hohen oder auch sehr niedrigen Heilungsergebnissen (BECK, LATOUR u. BOURNE; BICKENBACH, LOCHMÜLLER u. FLACH; BICKENBACH, LOCHMÜLLER, DIRLICH, RULAND u. THURMAYR; BREITNER u. ADLER; BURR u. ROBERTSON; BUSSE u. SOERGEL; CARMICHAEL u. BEAN; CAROL u. MÜLLER; COPENHAVER u. BARSAMIAN; CZECH, KEPP u. WOLTHAUS; DAVIS JR.; DIBBELT u. GERTEIS; EYMER; GRIMM; GROSSE-HOLZ, SCHULZE u. VOGELGESANG; JANISCH-RASKOVIC; JAVERT u. RENNING; LINZ; METHFESSEL; v. MIKULICZ-RADECKI u. GANSAU; PETERSEN; PHILIPP u. RUMPHORST; PICHA u. WEGHAUPT, 1961, 1965 und 1968; POCKRANDT; PRETTENHOFER; RANDALL u. GODDARD; RANDOW u. KAISER; RUMPHORST, 1961 und 1962; SALA u. DEL REGATO; SCHEELE; STÄUBLE; WADE; WEGHAUPT; WIMHÖFER, ZEITZ u. RUNGE u. a.). Es wird bewußt davon Abstand genommen, da eine Vergleichbarkeit der Zahlenangaben untereinander nicht sicherzustellen ist. Da das Material des „Annual Report" noch am ehesten unter einheitlichen Gesichtspunkten gesammelt wurde und hier die verschiedensten Klinikarten und Einzugsgebiete erfaßt sind, können diese Zahlen wohl noch am besten einen Eindruck vom derzeitigen Stand der Heilungsergebnisse des Carcinoma corporis uteri geben. Nach der allgemeinen Auffassung ist außerdem über längere Zeiträume eine Verbesserung der Heilungsergebnisse festzustellen. Hier ist aber Vorsicht am Platz, denn einmal schwanken die Heilungsergebnisse innerhalb einer Klinik von Jahr zu Jahr unter Umständen erheblich und außerdem ändert sich die Zusammensetzung des Krankengutes. Schließlich sind selbst in den zwanziger Jahren schon sehr gute Ergebnisse berichtet worden. Immerhin scheint es doch berechtigt, zu sagen, daß eine allmähliche Verbesserung der Ergebnisse festzustellen ist.

Tabelle 18. *5-Jahres-Heilung des Korpuscarcinoms von 29 Kliniken in Abhängigkeit von Behandlungsart und Stadium. (Aus* H. L. Kottmeier: *Annual report on the results of treatment in carcinoma of the uterus and vagina, Bd. 14)*

Klinik-Nr. des Annual-Report	Gesamtzahl der untersuchten Patienten	Gesamtzahl der behandelten Patienten	Behandelte Patienten Stadium I Gruppe 1	Behandelte Patienten Stadium I Gruppe 1 %	Uterus-exstirpation	Präoperative Bestrahlung und Uterus-exstirpation	Nur Strahlen-therapie	Nicht in die Statistik einbezogen[a] Anzahl	Relative 5-Jahres-Heilung aller Behandelten %	Relative 5-Jahres-Heilung Stadium I Gruppe 1 %
3	250	240	226	94,2	95	111	34	25	70,8	74,8
5	310	301	258	85,7	249	26	26	17	67,8	75,6
8	261	248	140	56,4	211	1	36	—	60,1	77,1
18	173	168	144	85,7	109	39	20	7	71,4	77,8
20	187	182	139	76,4	131	14	37	—	67,0	83,5
27	397	384	325	84,6	145	193	46	7	72,7	81,2
33	289	285	138	48,4	11	3	271	17	49,8	66,7
34	587	574	150	26,1	7	—	567	45	42,9	74,0
36	698	643	400	62,2	423	17	203	—	65,9	83,3
46	392	391	154	39,4	160	51	180	—	57,3	70,1
48	416	412	126	30,6	134	—	278	67	68,7	86,5
51	720	692	250	36,1	282	5	405	35	58,8	76,4
56	415	411	248	60,3	245	7	159	84	64,7	79,8
58	390	388	152	39,2	50	101	237	5	58,5	85,5
62	306	240	204	69,9	205	—	87	—	55,8	71,1
69	224	223	125	56,1	222	—	1	21	73,1	84,0
76	375	316	107	33,9	33	57	226	77	52,2	80,4
78	935	931	723	77,6	150	158	623	263	74,1	83,0
79	1278	1276	781	61,2	16	273	987	578	68,3	82,1
85	1161	1135	936	82,5	932	69	134	19	67,0	74,8
92	1459	1248	725	58,1	1028	93	127	16	62,1	76,7
104	342	332	267	80,4	210	55	67	41	61,1	71,2
105	386	360	275	76,4	73	217	70	53	60,6	72,0
110	198	198	143	72,2	35	132	31	11	67,7	81,8
111	138	129	105	81,4	25	77	27	25	60,5	67,6
116	222	218	158	72,5	65	100	53	15	68,3	79,1
118	190	182	115	63,2	30	83	69	22	64,3	73,0
119	234	226	183	81,0	107	97	22	6	73,5	83,1
124	270	227	153	67,4	54	132	41	36	53,7	68,6

[a] Alle von den Kliniken gemeldeten Fälle von Carcinoma corporis et endocervicis, Carcinoma uteri et ovarii, Carcinoma pelvis.

10. Das Sarkom des Corpus uteri

Das Sarkom des Corpus uteri ist eine relativ zum Korpuscarcinom seltene Erkrankung. Nach TASCH findet man auf etwa 50 Uteruscarcinome (Collum und Korpus) 1 Sarkom. Insgesamt verhält sich aber die Häufigkeit des Korpussarkoms zu der des Collumsarkoms wie 4:1. Im allgemeinen geht das Sarkom von der Uteruswand aus und nur in einem Zehntel der Fälle von der Schleimhaut. Beim Uterus myomatosus findet sich in 2,8% der Fälle ein Sarkom und in 1,4% ein Sarkom im Myom.

Bezüglich der Symptomatik ist zusätzlich zu den Feststellungen beim Korpuscarcinom kaum etwas zu sagen, außer, daß ein schnell wachsendes Myom den besonderen Verdacht auf ein Sarkom erwecken muß. Die Diagnostik entspricht der des Korpuscarcinoms. Allerdings wird vielfach die Diagnose erst bei einer Laparotomie oder bei der Untersuchung des Operationspräparates gestellt werden.

Damit ist zugleich schon klargestellt, daß sich beim Korpussarkom in vielen Fällen die Frage Operation oder Strahlentherapie nicht mehr stellt. In den durch eine Abrasio diagnostizierten Fällen ist dagegen noch zu überlegen, ob das eine oder das andere Verfahren aussichtsreicher ist. Die Frage der Strahlensensibilität des Uterussarkoms ist mit seinem histologischen Bau verknüpft, aber eigentlich bis heute nicht klar entschieden. So werden im allgemeinen die polymorphzelligen, die Myxo- und die Rundzellsarkome für strahlensensibel, die Spindelzell-, die Fibro-, die Lipo- und Myosarkome dagegen für wenig strahlensensibel gehalten. Die diesbezüglichen Äußerungen sind aber nicht einheitlich. Es wird daher auch für die Korpussarkome allgemein der Operation der Vorzug gegeben (FLETCHER, D. HOFMANN) und im Falle einer Bestrahlung eine höhere Dosierung empfohlen. FLETCHER schlägt vor, sie für praktische klinische Zwecke gleich zu behandeln wie die anaplastischen Korpuscarcinome.

Ist die Diagnose durch Abrasio gestellt und die Patientin allgemein oder lokal inoperabel, wird die Strahlentherapie unter den gleichen Bedingungen durchgeführt wie bei Korpuscarcinomen. Im anderen Fall sollte eine intensive postoperative Bestrahlung erfolgen mit einer Percutanserie und intravaginalem Radium. Die Frage der Vorbestrahlung ist nicht eindeutig zu beantworten, solange nicht klar ist, ob der Tumor strahlensensibel ist. Daher wird man sich im allgemeinen zur primären Uterusexstirpation entschließen, zumal diese zur Abklärung des Befundes oder bei tastbaren Tumoren ohnehin meist indiziert ist. Die angegebenen 5-Jahres-Heilungen liegen im allgemeinen in der Größenordnung zwischen 40 und 50%.

11. Zusammenfassung

Die Strahlentherapie des Korpuscarcinoms wird aufgrund der ansteigenden Frequenz dieser Krankheit eine zunehmende Rolle spielen. Es wurde daher versucht, alle Aspekte der Krankheit selbst, ihrer Symptomatik und ihrer Therapie in dem zur Verfügung stehenden Raum kurz darzustellen.

Es deutet vieles darauf hin, daß die Verfahren

Vorbestrahlung — Totalexstirpation des Uterus unter Mitnahme einer Scheidenmanschette und der Anhänge — eventuell Nachbestrahlung oder aber

primäre Strahlentherapie — routinemäßige Kontrolle des Therapieerfolges durch Abrasio und gegebenenfalls Totalexstirpation — eventuell Nachbestrahlung

zur Zeit die aussichtsreichsten Behandlungsformen darstellen. Für die Indikationsstellung und die optimale Durchführung der Therapie spielt die sorgfältige Abklärung des einzelnen Falles nach Sitz und Ausdehnung der Geschwulst und ihren histologischen Kriterien offenbar eine besondere Rolle.

Die für die Therapie wichtigste Strahlenquelle ist auch heute noch das Radium. Ein völlig neuer und aussichtsreicherer Weg der Behandlung zeichnet sich bisher nicht ab.

Literatur

Abou-Daoud, K. T.: Epidemiology of carcinoma of the cervix uteri in lebanese christians and moslems, Cancer (Philad.) **20**, 1706—1714 (1967).

Albertini, A. v.: Histologische Geschwulstdiagnostik. Systematische Morphologie der menschlichen Geschwülste als Grundlage für die klinische Beurteilung. Epitheliale Geschwülste, S. 468—483. Stuttgart: Georg Thieme 1955.

Alford, Ch. D., Betson, J. R., Di Santi, N.: Wertheim hysterectomy and Pelvic Lymphadenectomy for Carcinoma of the uterine Corpus. Amer. J. Obstet. Gynec. **83**, 1306 (1962).

Amreich, A. I.: In: Biologie und Pathologie des Weibes. Ein Handbuch der Frauenheilkunde und Geburtshilfe, 2. Aufl., Bd. IV. Berlin-Innsbruck-München-Wien: Urban & Schwarzenberg 1955.

Antoine, T.: Neue Gesichtspunkte in der Behandlung der Genitalkarzinome. Wien. med. Wschr. **115**, 687—690 (1965).

Arneson, A. N.: Treatment of benign and malignant diseases of the body of the uterus. In: Clinical therapeutic radiology. Edinburgh-New York-Toronto: Thomas Nelson & Sons 1950.

— An evaluation of the use of radiation in the treatment of endometrial cancer. Bull. N. Y. Acad. Med. **29**, 395—410 (1953).

— Responsibilities of the obstretrician-gynecologist in the treatment of uterine cancer. Amer. J. Obstet. Gynec. **79**, 833—837 (1960).

— Long term follow-up observations in corporeal cancer. Amer. J. Roentgenol. **91**, 3—21 (1964).

— Stanbro, W. W., Nolan, J. F.: Amer. J. Obstet. Gynec. **55**, 64—78 (1948). Zit. nach Hendricks, C. H., Callendine, G. W., Morton, J. L.: A bead packing technique for the application of uniform doses for irradiation to the endometrial cavity. Amer. J. Obstet. Gynec. **69**, 1039—1050 (1955).

Averette, H. E., Hudson, R. C., Viamonte, M. I., Parks, R. E., Ferguson, J. H.: Lymphangioadenography (Lymphography) in the study of female genital cancer. Cancer (Philad.) **15**, 769—775 (1962).

Badib, A. O., Kurohara, S. S., Beitia, A. A., Webster, J. H.: Recurrent cancer of the corpus uteri. Amer. J. Roentgenol. **105**, 596—602 (1969).

Bailar, J. C.: The incidence of independent tumors among uterine cancer patients. Cancer (Philad.) **16**, 842—853 (1963).

Bally, v., K.-E.: Untersuchungen über den Einfluß von Gewebeinhomogenitäten auf die Tiefendosisverteilung bei der Strahlentherapie mit 200 kV Röntgen- und Co 60-Gammastrahlung am Beispiel des Knochens. Diss. Göttingen 1968.

Barter, R. H.: The place of curettage in the diagnosis of carcinoma of the endometrium. Amer. J. Obstet. Gynec. **100**, 696—702 (1968).

Bayer, R.: Die Wirkung von oralen Gestagengaben auf ein Uteruskorpuskarzinom und auf Lungenmetastasen nach Kollum- und Mammakarzinom. Wien. med. Wschr. **116**, 831—835 (1966).

Beck, H.: Erfahrungen mit der Hemipelvektomie bei malignen Tumoren. Münch. med. Wschr. **109**, 126—130 (1967).

Beck, R. P., Latour, J. P. A., Bourne, H. B.: Treatment of endometrial carcinoma reassessed. Comparison of results of 152 cases, 1949 to 1956, with results of 209 cases, 1926 to 1948. Amer. J. Obstet. Gynec. **88**, 178—183 (1964).

Becker, J., Scheer, K. E.: Strahlentherapeutische Anwendung von radioaktivem Kobalt in Form von Perlen. Strahlentherapie **86**, 540—547 (1952).

— — Die radioaktiven Isotope in der Geburtshilfe und Gynäkologie. Basel-New York: S. Karger 1956.

— — Schick, E.: Radiokobaltperlen, offene oder geschlossene Präparate? Strahlentherapie **103**, 158—161 (1957).

Beduhn, D., Kuttig, H.: Die Bewegungsbestrahlung der paraaortalen Lymphknoten mit 60 Co-Gammastrahlen. Strahlentherapie **132**, 481—486 (1967).

Beecham, C. T., Messick, R. R., Wiley, J. H.: Primary surgical therapy for adenocarcinoma of the endometrium. In: Lewis, G. C., Jr., Wentz, W. B., Jaffe, R. M., p. 245—250. Philadelphia: F. A. Davis Company 1966.

Behrens, H.: Follikelhormon und Korpuskarzinom des Uterus. Geburtsh. u. Frauenheilk. **17**, 1126—1135 (1957).

Berger, H.: Ergebnisse rein radiologischer Behandlung von 227 Kollum- und Korpuskarzinomen der Jahre 1950—1956. Strahlentherapie **119**, 607—614 (1962).

Bergsjö, P.: Carcinoma uteri et ovarii. A study from the Norwegian Radium Hospital. Acta obstet. gynec. scand. **41**, 405—411 (1962).

— Progesteron und progestionale Substanzen in der Behandlung des fortgeschrittenen Endometriumkarzinoms. Acta endocr. (Kbh.) **49**, 412—426 (1965).

Bernds, P.: Behandlung und Heilungsergebnisse des Korpuskarzinoms an der Göttinger Universitäts-Frauenklinik aus den Jahren 1942—1961. Diss. Göttingen 1966.

Bickenbach, W.: Vorschläge zur klinischen Einteilung des Carcinoma corporis uteri. Zbl. Gynäk. **77**, 1845—1849 (1955).

— Gärtner, H., Zoeppritz, U.: Die intrauterine Anwendung von Radio-Kobalt-Perlen. Strahlentherapie **97**, 188—193 (1955).

— Lochmüller, H., Dirlich, G., Ruland, G., Thurmayr, R.: Factor analysis of endometrial carcinoma in relation to treatment. Obstet. and Gynec. **29**, 632—636 (1967).

— — Flach, D.: Fünfjährige symptomfreie Überlebenszeit und Übersterblichkeit bei Kranken mit Korpuskarzinom. Geburtsh. u. Frauenheilk. **25**, 580—587 (1965).

Blaikley, J. B., Kottmeier, H. L., Martius, H., Meigs, J. V.: Classification and clinical staging of carcinoma of the uterus. A proposal for modification of the existing international definition. Amer. J. Obstet. Gynec. **75**, 1286—1291 (1958).

Bocci, A., Tetti, A., Barbanti, A., Davitti, L.: Nuovi indirizzi radioterapici nel trattamento del carcinoma corporale uterino. Minerva ginec. **15**, 703—734 (1963).

BÖTZELEN, H. P., SCHMIDT-MATTHIESEN, H.: Ergebnisse der zytologischen Punktionsdiagnostik fraglich karzinomatöser Resistenzen, speziell im Parametrium. 35. Versammlung der Deutschen Gesellschaft für Gynäkologie, München 1965. Arch. Gynäk. **202**, 328—330 (1965).

BOSCHANN, H. W.: Cytologie des Cavumaspirats bei gut- und bösartigen Erkrankungen. Arch. Gynäk. **189**, 376—382 (1957).

BOTELLA LLUSIA, J., NOGALES ORTIZ, F., JIMÉNEZ TEBAR, V., ZAMARRIEGO CRESPO, J.: La accion de la roentgenterapia sobre los ganglios pelvianos estudiada a través de la linfadenectomia pélvica extraperitoneal. Rev. med. Cir. Ginec. Cáncer **26**, 199—214 (1958).

BOUTSELIS, J. G., BAIR, J. R., VORYS, N., ULLERY, J. C.: Carcinoma of the uterine corpus. Amer. J. Obstet. Gynec. **85**, 994—1001 (1963).

— ULLERY, J. C., BAIR, J.: Vaginal metastases following treatment of endometrial carcinoma. Obstet. and Gynec. **21**, 622—626 (1963).

BRAUNBEHRENS, H. v., BUNDE, E., WITTENZELLNER, R.: Schutzfragen bei der Anwendung „bedingt geschlossener" radioaktiver Präparate. Strahlentherapie **103**, 112—114 (1957).

BREIT, A.: Arteriographie vor und nach Tumorbestrahlung. Fortschr. Röntgenstr. **111**, 329—344 (1969).

— Angiographie der Uterustumoren und ihrer Rezidive. Stuttgart: Thieme 1967.

BREITNER, J., ADLER, U.: Die Behandlung des Korpuskarzinoms am Frauenspital Basel von 1943—1953 (mit 5-Jahresergebnissen der Jahre 1935—1948). Geburtsh. u. Frauenheilk. **15**, 113—126 (1955).

BRODERS, A. G.: The grading of carcinoma. Minn. Med. 8, 726 (1925).

BSTEH, P.: Neuer Versuch zur Koordinierung der Radium- und Telekobalttherapie beim Uteruskarzinom. Strahlentherapie **129**, 505—511 (1966).

BUCKOW, I., FLEISCHER, E. M.: Das intra- und extragenitale Doppelkarzinom. Z. Geburtsh. Gynäk. **170**, 21—27 (1969).

BURR, R. C., ROBERTSON, E. M.: Value of radiation therapy in the treatment of cancer of the endometrium. Canad. med. Ass. J. **99**, 206—211 (1968).

BUSSE, O., SOERGEL, W.: Bericht über 800 maligne Erkrankungen des weiblichen Genitales der Jahre 1947—1952. Geburtsh. u. Frauenheilk. **19**, 201—217 (1959).

BUTTENBERG, D., ZEITZ, H.: Vaginalmetastasen beim Kollum- und Korpuskarzinom. Geburtsh. u. Frauenheilk. **17**, 427—434 (1957).

CARMICHAEL, J. A., BEAN, H. A.: Carcinoma of the endometrium in Saskatchewan. A review of 603 cases with a suggest scheme of management for patients with Stage I desease and regarded as good surgical risks. Amer. J. Obstet. Gynec. **97**, 294—307 (1967).

CAROL, W., MÜLLER, W.: Klinik und Behandlungsergebnisse der Genitalkarzinome an der Universitäts-Frauenklinik Jena in den Jahren 1946 bis 1967. Zbl. Gynäk. **90**, 1337—1345 (1968).

CASTAÑO Y ALMENDRAL, A.: Vergleichende Untersuchungen über die Wirkung von 200-kV-Röntgen- und ^{60}Co-Gammastrahlung auf den Kaninchenureter. Habil.-Schr. Göttingen 1966.

— FRISCHKORN, R.: La histerografia en el tratamiento radiologico del carcinoma del cuerpo uterino. Acta Obst. y Ginec. Hisp.-Lus. **16**, 321—330 (1968).

— JOHANNSSEN, H.: Significado e importancia de la medición de la dosis en la vejiga y en el recto para la radiumterapia genecológica. Rev. esp. Obstet. Ginec. **26**, 275—283 (1967).

CASTRO, J. R., LINDBERG, R. D., FLETCHER, G. H.: Clinical application of computer dosimetry in interstitial radium therapy. Amer. J. Roentgenol. **105**, 165—171 (1969).

CHARLES, D.: Endometrial adenoacanthoma. A clinicopathological study of 55 cases. Cancer (Philad.) **18**, 737—750 (1965).

— BELL, E. T., LORAINE, J. A., HARKNESS, R. A.: Endometrial carcinoma — endocrinological and clinical studies. Amer. J. Obstet. Gynec. **91**, 1050—1059 (1965).

CHIARI, H.: Biologie und Pathologie des Weibes. Ein Handbuch der Frauenheilkunde und Geburtshilfe, 2. Aufl., Bd. IV. Berlin-Innsbruck-München-Wien: Urban & Schwarzenberg 1955.

CIANFRANI, T.: Endometrial carcinoma after bilateral oophorectomy. Amer. J. Obstet. Gynec. **69**, 64—71 (1955).

O'CONNOR, K. J.: Mixed mesodermal tumours of the body of the uterus following irradiation therapy for carcinoma of the cervix. A report on four cases. J. Obstet. Gynaec. Brit. Emp. **71**, 281—283 (1964).

COPENHAVER, E. H., BARSAMIAN, M.: Management of stage I adenocarcinoma of the endometrium. Amer. J. Obstet. Gynec. **99**, 864—868 (1967).

CORSCADEN, J. A.: Gynecologic cancer, 3rd ed., p. 341—366. Baltimore: Williams & Wilkins Company 1962.

COSTOLOW, W. E., NOLAN, J. F., BUDENZ, G. C., DU SAULT, L.: Radiation treatment of carcinoma of the corpus uteri. Amer. J. Roentgenol. **71**, 669—673 (1954).

COURETOT, M. F., DOSORETZ, B., DE FELIÚ, A. T. R.: Tratamiento por radiaciones de los tumores malignos genitales. Tratamiento del adenocarcinoma de endomtrio y del carcinoma de ovario. Tecnica de Manchester, Pren. méd. argent. **1957**, 570—574.

CZECH, H.: Die intrauterine Radiumbestrahlung des Gebärmutterkörperkarzinoms an der Universitäts-Frauenklinik Göttingen. Strahlentherapie 84, 524—539 (1951).

— KEPP, R. K., WOLTHAUS, G.: Ergebnisse der Behandlung der bösartigen Genitaltumoren an der Universitäts-Frauenklinik Göttingen in den Jahren 1937—1944. Strahlentherapie 82, 321—354 (1950).

DALLENBACH-HELLWEG, G.: Das Karzinom des Endometriums und seine Vorstufen. Verh. dtsch. Ges. Path. 48, 81 (1964).

— BRÄHLER, H.-J.: Über die Histologie und Lokalisation der Uteruskarzinome mit besonderer Berücksichtigung der drüsig-soliden Mischformen. Z. Krebsforsch. 64, 64 (1960).

DALSACE, J., GARCIA-CALDÉRON, J.: Gynäkologischer Röntgenatlas. Stuttgart-Zürich: Medica-Verlag 1956.

DAVIS, E. W., JR.: Carcinoma of the corpus uteri. A study of 525 cases at the New York Hospital (1932—1961). Amer. J. Obstet. Gynec. 88, 163—170 (1964).

DEBOIS, J. M., DE BAENE, J., VAN DE KERKHOVES, J.: Composite isodose calculation with a digital computer application to total pelvis irradiation in cervical carcinoma with telecobalt radiation. J. belge Radiol. (Brüssel) 52, 190—195 (1969).

DEDE, J. A., PLENTL, A. A., MOORE, J. G.: Recurrent endometrial carcinoma. Surg. Gynec. Obstet. 126, 533—542 (1968).

DELCLOS, L., FLETCHER, G., GUTIERREZ, A. G., RUTLEDGE, F. N.: Adenocarcinoma of the uterus. Amer. J. Roentgenol. 105, 603—608 (1969).

DIBBELT, L., GERTEIS, W.: Behandlungsresultate und Prognose des Uteruskarzinoms unter Berücksichtigung von klinischen und lymphographischen Befunden. Geburtsh. u. Frauenheilk. 27, 1—14 (1967).

— HEINZLER, F.: Die Koordination von Radium- und Supervolttherapie. 35. Verslg der Dtsch. Ges. für Gynäkologie, München 1964. Arch. Gynäk. 202, 312—316 (1965).

— MÜLLER, H. G., EHLERS, F.: Die Häufigkeit konstitutioneller und exogener Faktoren bei Kranken mit einem Karzinom des Corpus uteri. Z. Geburtsh. 160, 1—19 (1963).

— RAHM, G., RENNER, K.: Dosimetrische Untersuchungen zur Gammatronbestrahlung der Lymphwege beim Uteruskarzinom. Strahlentherapie 112, 406—420 (1960).

DIECKHOFF, D.: Schwangerschaft und Tumoren. Diss. Göttingen 1963.

DIECKMANN, J. W., MCCARTNEY, CH. P., CARPENDER, J. W. J.: The treatment of endometrial carcinoma by means of repeated applications of intracavitary radium. Amer. J. Obstet. Gynec. 70, 1258—1270 (1955).

DIETEL, F. G.: Jetzige Methode der Strahlenbehandlung von Uteruskarzinomen an der I. Universitäts-Frauenklinik zu München. Strahlentherapie 63, 614—638 (1938).

DOBBIE, M. W.: Vaginal recurrences in carcinoma of the body of the uterus and their prevention by radium therapy. J. Obstet. Gynaec. Brit. Emp. 60, 702—705 (1953).

DOUGLAS, R. G.: Metástasis vaginales consecutivas al tratamiento del adenocarcinoma del cuerpo del utero (Scheidenmetastasen nach Behandlung des Adenocarcinoma corporis uteri). Rev. Obstet. Ginec. Venez. 25, 491—505 (1965).

DRESCHER, H.: Überseltene Metastasenformen der weiblichen Genitalkarzinome. Strahlentherapie 78, 349—372 (1949).

DYROFF, R., MICHALZIK, K.: Wichtige Gesichtspunkte bei der Nachuntersuchung bestrahlter Genitalkarzinome der Frau. Strahlentherapie 103, 376—382 (1957).

EHRMANN, W.: Untersuchungen über den Gestageneffekt bei der Behandlung des Korpuskarzinoms. Diss. Göttingen 1969.

ERNST, E. C., ERNST, E. C., ERNST, R. P., ERNST, R. E., CLELAND, M.: Radium pelvic measurements for treatment of carcinoma of the cervix and corpus uteri with an expanding type of applicator. Amer. J. Roentgenol. 85, 904—948 (1961).

EVANS, W. G., MABBS, D. V.: Dosage control by direct measurement in the radium treatment of uterine carcinoma. J. Fac. Radiol. (Lond.) 9, 66—67 (1958).

EYMER, H.: In: Biologie und Pathologie des Weibes. Ein Handbuch der Frauenheilkunde und Geburtshilfe, 2. Aufl., Bd. V. Berlin-Innsbruck-München-Wien: Urban & Schwarzenberg 1953.

FEHRENTZ, D., KUTTIG, H., BRAUN, G.: Berechnung von Dosisverteilungen zur ^{60}Co-Teletherapie mit einem digitalen Rechenautomaten. II. Anwendung für koplanare Bestrahlungsmethoden. Strahlentherapie 136, 279—288 (1968).

FEINE, U.: In: Strahlenpathologie der Zelle von E. SCHERER und H. S. STENDER. Stuttgart: Georg Thieme 1963.

FEINER, L. L., GARIN, A.: Cytological response to radiation in noncervical cancer of the female genital tract. Cancer (Philad.) 16, 166—169 (1963).

FERNSTRÖM, I.: Arteriography of the uterine artery. Acta radiol. (Stockh.), Suppl. 122 (1955).

FETTIG, O.: Die Silvermann-Punktionsbiopsie in der Gynäkologie. Zbl. Gynäk. 85, 1257—1268 (1963).

FIEBELKORN, H. J.: In: Lehrbuch der Strahlenheilkunde von R. DU MESNIL DE ROCHEMONT. Stuttgart: Ferdinand Enke 1958.

FLETCHER, G. H.: Textbook of radiotherapy Philadelphia: Lea & Febiger 1966.

— BROWN, TH., RUDLEDGE, F.: Clinical significance of rectal and bladders dose measurements in radium therapy of cancer of the uterine cervix. Amer. J. Roentgenol. 79, 421—450 (1958).

FOCHEM, K., GRÜNBERGER, V.: Zur Frage der Neubildung nach Röntgenkastration. Krebsarzt 18, 175—179 (1963).

FREED, J. H., PENDERGRASS, E. P.: An evaluation on the efficiency of various intrauterine radium techniques in the treatment of cancer of the corpus uteri. Amer. J. Roentgenol. 71, 253—266 (1954).

FRIEBEL, H.-H.: Über Endometriose und Krebs. Zbl. Gynäk. 85, 1710—1717 (1963).

FRISCHBIER, H. J.: Dosimetrische Probleme bei der kombinierten Radium- und Telekobaltbestrahlung. 35. Versammlung der Deutschen Gesellschaft für Gynäkologie, München 1964. Arch. Gynäk. 202, 316—320 (1965).

FRISCHKORN, R.: Unsere Erfahrungen mit der Siebbestrahlung gynäkologischer Karzinome. Strahlenforschung u. Strahlenbehandlung, Bd. II, Sonderbd. Strahlentherapie 46, 128—133 (1960).

— Die Siebbestrahlung im Rahmen der gynäkologischen Strahlentherapie. Strahlentherapie 111, 537—545 (1960).

— Erste Erfahrungen mit der routinemäßigen Anwendung der Kobaltfernbestrahlung in der gynäkologischen Strahlentherapie. Strahlenforschung u. Strahlenbehandlung, Bd. III, Sonderbd. Strahlentherapie 49, 149—156 (1961).

FRISCHKORN, R.: Das Dosierungs- und Lokalisationsproblem in der Radiumtherapie des Kollumkarzinoms. Strahlenforschung u. Strahlenbehandlung, Bd. IV, Sonderbd. Strahlentherapie 52, 107—116 (1963).
— Die ausschließliche Perkutanbestrahlung des Kollumkarzinoms mit Telekobalt. Zbl. Gynäk. 85, 639—644 (1963).
— Untersuchungen über eine ausschließliche Perkutanbestrahlung des Kollumkarzinoms mit Telekobalt. Geburtsh. u. Frauenheilk. 23, 117—130 (1963).
— Der Radium-Isodosenatlas der Universitäts-Frauenklinik Göttingen. Strahlentherapie 125, 39—50 (1964).
— Dosimetrie. Referat IV/B. 35. Verhandlg der Dtsch. Ges. für Gynäkologie, München 1964. Arch. Gynäk. 202, 274—288 (1965).
— Befunde im Arteriogramm beim Kollumkarzinom. Deutscher Röntgenkongr. 1964, Wiesbaden, Teil A. Stuttgart: Georg Thieme 1965.
— Besondere arterio- und phlebographische Befunde beim Collum-Carcinom. Deutscher Röntgenkongr. 1965 Nürnberg, Teil A. Stuttgart: Georg Thieme 1966.
FUCHS, G.: Zum Problem der Krebserzeugung durch Röntgen- und Gammastrahlen. Wien. med. Wschr. 111, 145—148 (1961).
FUCHS, W. A., DAVIDSON, J. W., FISCHER, H. W.: Recent results in cancer research. Lymphography in cancer. Berlin-Heidelberg-New York: Springer 1969.
— ZUPPINGER, A.: Lymphographie und Tumordiagnostik. Berlin-Heidelberg-New York: Springer 1965.
GARNET, J. D.: Constitutional factors in endometrial cancer. In: New concepts in gynecological oncology (G. C. LEWIS JR., W. B. WENTZ, R. M. JAFFE), p. 195—203. Philadelphia: F. A. Davis Company 1966.
GAUWERKY, F.: Ergebnisse und Erfahrungen bei der Behandlung des Uteruskarzinoms. Bericht über die Jahrgänge 1935—1939. Strahlentherapie 77, 325—348 (1948).
— Standardisierung und individuelle Anpassung bei der Strahlenbehandlung der Gebärmutter- und Scheidenkarzinome. Strahlentherapie 103, 16—47 (1957).
GEIJN, J., VAN DE: The computation of two and three dimensional dose distributions in Cobalt 60-therapy. Brit. J. Radiol. 38, 369—377 (1965).
GERTEIS, W.: Die Lymphographie beim Genitalkarzinom der Frau. Übersicht über ihre Möglichkeiten. Arch. Gynäk. 200, 109—130 (1964).
— Die lymphographische Kontrolle der Supervolttherapie des Kollumkarzinoms. 35. Versammlg der Dtsch. Ges. für Gynäkologie, München 1964. Arch. Gynäk. 202, 320—325 (1965).
— Lymphographie und topographische Anatomie des Beckenlymphsystems. Z. Geburtsh., Beilagenheft zu Bd. 165 (1966).
GIBEL, W., BERNDT, H., SCHWARZ, H.: Über multiple primäre Karzinome. Dtsch. Gesundh.-Wes. 17, 1795—1801 (1962).
GIETZELT, F.: Zur Strahlentherapie der „Genitalkarzinome der Frau". Zbl. Gynäk. 80, 456—459 (1958).

GOECKE, P., STÜPER, P.: Statistischer Bericht über bösartige Geschwülste nach Röntgen- oder Radiummenolyse. Zbl. Gynäk. 83, 194—199 (1961).
GOETSCHEL, E.: Untersuchungen über die Beziehungen der glandulär-cystischen Hyperplasie zum Corpuscarcinom des Uterus. Gynaecologia (Basel) 160, 94—104 (1965).
GRABIGER, R.: Osteoradionekrose des Schenkelhalses nach Telekobalttherapie. Strahlentherapie 123, 282—284 (1964).
GRAHAM, J. B.: Evaluation of preoperative and postoperative radiation in cancer of the uterine body. In: G. C. LEWIS JR., W. B. WENTZ, R. M. JAFFE, p. 251—255. Philadelphia: F. A. Davis Company 1966.
GRANONE, G. F., JULIANI, G.: New hysterostat for radium therapy in endometrial carcinoma. Amer. J. Roentgenol. 93, 709—714 (1965).
GRAZIANI, A., CATURANI, F.: Isterosalpingografia e carcinoma del corpo dell'utero. Arch. Obstet. ginec. 66, 766—786 (1961).
GREENBLATT, R. B., STODDARD, L. D., KING, PH. R.: Estrogen in endometrial carcinogenesis. In: G. C. LEWIS JR., W. B. WENTZ, R. M. JAFFE, New concepts in gynecological oncology, p. 211—218. Philadelphia: F. A. Davis Company 1966.
GRIMM, C. A.: Endometrial carcinoma. A thirteen year review. Amer. J. Roentgenol. 85, 497—502 (1961).
GROS, CH. M., KEILING, R.: La curiethérapie des épithéliomas du corps utérin. J. Radiol. Électrol. 47, 629—632 (1966).
— VEILON, A.: Le cancer du corps utérin traité par la packing-method. J. Radiol. Électrol. 34, 667—669 (1954).
GROSSE-HOLZ, K.: Die Osteoradionekrose des Schenkelhalses — ein Dosisproblem? Strahlentherapie 125, 591—598 (1964).
— SCHULZE, E., VOGELGESANG, K. H.: Ergebnisse und Erfahrungen bei der Strahlenbehandlung des Korpuskarzinoms. Strahlentherapie 121, 231—238 (1963).
GRÜNBERGER, V.: Zur Frage der Lymphknotenexstirpation beim Carcinoma corporis uteri. Wien. klin. Wschr. 80, 641—643 (1968).
GUSBERG, S. B.: Adenomatous hyperplasia as a precursor of corpus cancer. La prophylaxie en gynécologie et obstétrique. Genf: Georg & Cie. S.A. 1954.
— COHEN, C. J.: Combination therapy for corpus cancer. In: G. C. LEWIS JR., W. B. WENTZ, R. M. JAFFE, New concepts in gynecological oncology, p. 237—243. Philadelphia: F. A. Davis Company 1966.
— YANNOPOULOS, D.: Therapeutic decisions in corpus cancer. Amer. J. Obstet. Gynec. 88, 157—162 (1964).
HEALY, W. P., BROWN, R. L.: Experience with radiation-therapy alone in carcinoma of the corpus uteri. Amer. J. Roentgenol. 41, 798 und 816 (1939).
— CUTLER, M.: Radiation and surgical treatment of carcinoma of body of the uterus. Amer. J. Obstet. Gynec. 19, 457—489 (1930).

Held, E.: Kritische Bemerkungen zur neuen Einteilung des Korpuskarzinoms. Geburtsh. u. Frauenheilk. **29**, 301—323 (1969).

Hendricks, C. H., Callendine, G. W., Morton, J. L.: A bead packing technique for the application of uniform doses of irradiation to the endometrial cavity. Amer. J. Obstet. Gynec. **69**, 1039—1050 (1955).

Henriksen, E.: Lymphatic spread of carcinoma of the body of the uterus; a study of 420 necropsies. Amer. J. Obstet. Gynec. **58**, 924 (1949).

Henschke, U.: Dosismessungen bei Radiumbestrahlung des Uterus-Ca. Zbl. Gynäk. **63**, 821—827 (1939).

Henschke, U. K., Hilaris, B. S.: Die Zukunft der Strahlentherapie in der Behandlung des Collumcarcinoms. Verhandlungen der Deutschen Gesellschaft für Gynäkologie. Arch. Gynäk. **202**, 289—304 (1965).

Hess, P., Rosendahl, J.: Erfahrungen mit der Radiokobaltperlenbehandlung beim Korpuskarzinom des Uterus. Strahlentherapie **128**, 334—339 (1965).

Heyde, W.: Häufigkeit und Verteilung primärer Zweitkarzinome bei weiblichen Krebskranken. Ärztl. Mitt. (Köln) **65**, 2881 (1968).

Heyman, J.: The so-colled Stockholm method and the results of treatment of uterine cancer at the Radiumhemmet. Acta radiol. (Stockh.) **16**, 129—147 (1935).

— Die sogenannte Stockholmer Methode und die Resultate bei der Behandlung des Uteruskarzinoms am Radiumhemmet. Wien. klin. Wschr. **1935 I**, 129—135.

— The radiumhemmet method of treatment and results in cancer of the corpus of the uterus. J. Obstet. Gynaec. brit. Emp. **43**, 655—666 (1936).

— Annual report on the results of treatment in carcinoma on the uterus and vagina, vol. V. Stockholm 1949.

— Reuterwall, O., Benner, S.: The radiumhemmet experience with radiotherapy in cancer of the corpus of the uterus. Classification, method of treatment and results. Acta radiol. (Stockh.) **22**, 11—98 (1941).

Hilfrich, H.-J., Castaño-Almendral, A., Flaskamp, D., Hofmann, P.: Untersuchungen über die diagnostische Bedeutung der Hysterographie beim Korpuskarzinom. Geburtsh. u. Frauenheilk. **29**, 346—357 (1969).

Hofmann, D.: Klinik der Gynäkologischen Strahlentherapie. München-Berlin: Urban & Schwarzenberg 1963.

— Künzler, E.: Über den Zusammenhang zwischen der Strahlenbehandlung gutartiger gynäkologischer Erkrankungen und der Entstehung bösartiger Geschwülste. Med. Klin. **55**, 68—72 (1960).

Hofmann, P.: Zit. nach H. Simmenroth.

Hofmann, W.-D., Baldus, F.: Dauerheilung eines Korpuskarzinoms durch Kürettage bei einer jungen Frau mit Kinderwunsch. Geburtsh. u. Frauenheilk. **29**, 1072—1075 (1969).

Holzaepfel, J. H., Ezell, H. E.: Sites of metastases of uterine carcinoma. Amer. J. Obstet. Gynec. **69**, 1027—1036 (1955).

Huber, H.: Zur Klinik des Korpuskarzinoms. Z. Geburtsh., Beilageheft zu Bd. 135 (1951).

— Die intra- und extragenitale Tumormultiplizität beim Genitalcarcinom. Ergebnisse einer umfassenden anatomischen, klinischen und statistischen Bearbeitung von über 4000 Genitalcarcinomen. Z. Krebsforsch. **58**, 103—162 (1951).

— Tumorbildung am Genitale nach Röntgenkastration. 32. Tagg der Dtsch. Ges. für Gynäkologie Frankfurt. Arch. Gynäk. **193**, 268—269 (1959).

— du Mesnil de Rochemont, R., Ringleb, D., Roos, H.: Fünfjahresergebnisse der „Marburger Methode" bei Bestrahlung des Kollumkarzinoms. Strahlentherapie **102**, 161—179 (1957).

Hunt, H. B.: Comparative radiotherapeutic results in carcinoma of the endometrium as modified by prior surgery and post-irradiating hysterosalpingooophorectomy. Radiology **66**, 653—665 (1956).

Husslein, H.: Endokrine Gesichtspunkte beim Carcinoma corporis uteri. La prophylaxie en gynécologie et obstétrique. Genf: Georg & Cie. S.A. 1954.

Iklé, F. A.: Radio-active gold seed implants in the treatment of gynaecological cancer. J. Obstet. Gynaec. Brit. Cwlth **71**, 202—213 (1964).

Jameson, D. G., Campion, J. M., Trevelyan, A.: A computer system for interstitial and intracavitary dose calculations. Brit. J. Radiol. **41**, 696—700 (1968).

Janisch, H., Wagenbichler, P.: Lymphographie — diagnostische und therapeutische Hilfsmethode? Wien. klin. Wschr. **80**, 173—176 (1968).

Janisch-Raskovic, W.: Die Therapie des weiblichen Urogenitalcarcinoms in den Frauenkliniken der Berliner Universität in den Jahren 1924 bis 1953. I. Z. ärztl. Fortbild. (Jena) **56**, 633—637 (1962).

Javert, C. T.: The spread of benign and malignant endometrium in the lymphatic system with a note on coexisting vascular involvement. Amer. J. Obstet. Gynec. **64**, 780—802 (1952).

— Renning, E. L.: Endometrial cancer. Survey of 610 cases treated at Woman's Hospital (1919—1960). Cancer (Philad.) **16**, 1057—1064 (1963).

Jensen, P. A., Dockerty, M. B., Symmonds, R. E., Wilson, R. B.: Endometrioid sarcoma ("stromal endometriosis"). Report of 15 cases including 5 with metastases. Amer. J. Obstet. Gynec. **95**, 79—90 (1966).

Joelsson, I., Bäckström, A.: Dose rate measurements in bladder and rectum. Acta radiol. (Stockh.) **8**, 343—359 (1969).

Johannsen, H.: Spätkomplikationen nach intraperitonealer Radiogoldinfusion. Strahlentherapie **127**, 198—205 (1965).

Johannsson, J. M., Lindskoug, B. A. A., Nyström, C. E.: Pelvic dosimetry during radiotherapy of carcinoma of the cervix uteri. Acta radiol. (Stockh.) **8**, 360—372 (1969).

Jones, D. E. A.: A flexible linear gamma ray source (Co^{60}) for treatment of cancer of the uterine body. Acta radiol. (Stockh.) **38**, 41—48 (1952).

Jopp, H.: Über Karzino-Sarkome des Endometriums. Zbl. Gynäk. **87**, 1268—1277 (1965).

— Karzinom und Sarkom des Endometriums als Koinzidenztumoren. Zbl. Gynäk. **87**, 1663 (1965).

KÄSER, O., IKLÉ, F. A.: Atlas der gynäkologischen Operationen. Operationen am Uterus, S. 74—75, 101—102, 268. Stuttgart: Georg Thieme 1965.

KAISER, R.: Der zytostatische Effekt verschiedener gestagener Substanzen. In: Moderne Entwicklungen auf dem Gestagengebiet. 6. Symposion der Dtsch. Ges. für Endokrinologie, Kiel 28. bis 30. 4. 1959. Berlin-Göttingen-Heidelberg: Springer 1960.

— Endokrine Schutzmechanismen gegen Endometrium- und Mammakarzinome. Dtsch. med. Wschr. 94, 2467—2472 (1969).

— Zur Ätiologie und Prophylaxe des Endometriumkarzinoms. Geburtsh. u. Frauenheilk. 29, 431—440 (1969).

KAPP-SCHWOERER, H.: Bereicherung der strahlentherapeutischen Möglichkeiten in der Behandlung der Genitalkarzinome durch Radiogoldseeds-Spickung (Au^{198}). Fortschr. Röntgenstr. 96, 551—557 (1962).

— BUSCH, M.: Über die Anwendung von Radiogoldseeds (Au^{198}) bei der gynäkologischen Strahlentherapie mit Untersuchungen der Isodosenverläufe und Belastung kritischer Organe. Strahlentherapie 120, 481—511 (1963).

KELLEY, R. M., BAKER, W. H.: Progestional agents in the treatment of carcinoma of the endometrium. New Engl. J. Med. 264, 216—222 (1961).

KENNEDY, B. J.: A progestogen for treatment of advanced endometrial cancer. J. Amer. med. Ass. 184, 758—761 (1963).

KEPP, R.: Gynäkologische Strahlentherapie. Stuttgart: Georg Thieme 1952.

— Das Problem des Zusammenhanges der Strahlentherapie gutartiger Erkrankungen mit der Entstehung von bösartigen Tumoren in der Gynäkologie. Zbl. Gynäk. 83, 1—5 (1961).

— HOFMANN, D.: In: Klinik der Frauenheilkunde und Geburtshilfe. Ein Handbuch für die Praxis, Bd. II. München-Berlin: Urban & Schwarzenberg 1964.

KIRCHHOFF, H.: Zur postoperativen Nachbestrahlung gynäkologischer Karzinome. Strahlentherapie 102, 425—434 (1957).

— Die Behandlung der Harnwegskomplikationen als Folge der Therapie des Kollumkarzinoms. Begründung und Zeitpunkt. Strahlentherapie 113, 356—368 (1960).

— Die Strahlentherapie des Korpus-Karzinoms. Dtsch. med. Wschr. 87, 1227—1231 (1962).

— — Frühe Diagnose des Genital-Karzinoms einschließlich des Mamma-Karzinoms. Therapiewoche 14, 311—315 (1964).

— FRISCHKORN, R.: Die Kobaltfernbestrahlung in der gynäkologischen Strahlentherapie. Münch. med. Wschr. 103, 1905—1909 (1961).

— IMHOLZ, G.: Spontanfrakturen des Schenkelhalses nach Röntgenbestrahlung wegen Genitalcarcinom. Strahlentherapie 90, 199—207 (1953).

KISTNER, R. W.: Histological effects of progestins on hyperplasia and carcinoma in situ of the endometrium. Cancer (Philad.) 12, 1106—1122 (1959).

— Hormonal treatment of premalignant lesions. In: G. C. LEWIS JR., W. B. WENTZ, R. M. JAFFE, New concepts in gynecological oncology, p. 287—299. Philadelphia: F. A. Davis Company 1966.

KISTNER, R.W., GRIFFITHS, C. TH., CRAIG, J. M.: Use of progestational agents in the management of endometrial cancer. Cancer. (Philad.) 18, 1563—1579 (1965).

KIVINIITTY, K., UNNÉRUS, C.-E.: Die Strahlenbehandlung der Parametrien bei gynäkologischen Tumoren. Strahlentherapie 136, 416—419 (1968).

KLUG, W.: Die Osteoradionekrose des Schenkelhalses. Zbl. Chir. 90, 68—72 (1965).

KOENIG, H.: Maligne Doppeltumoren der Frau. Arch. Geschwulstforsch. 32, 380—390 (1969).

KOLLER, TH., ADLER, U., KUNZ, L.: Regionale gynäkologische Krebsprobleme. Überalterung, Ca-Häufigkeit und Ca-5-Jahres-Heilung. Gynaecologia (Basel) 151, 240—252 (1961).

KOTTMEIER, H. L.: Die Radiumbehandlung in der Gynäkologie. In: Klinische Fortschritte Gynäkologie. Wien-Innsbruck: Urban & Schwarzenberg 1954.

— Die Stellung der Strahlentherapie und der Chirurgie in der Behandlung des Gebärmutterkrebses. Strahlentherapie 103, 194—213 (1957).

— Carcinoma of the corpus uteri: Diagnosis and therapy. Amer. J. Obstet. Gynec. 78, 1127—1140 (1959).

— Erfahrungen mit Progesteron in Fällen von Korpuskarzinom. Geburtsh. u. Frauenheilk. 22, 1070—1071 (1962).

— Annual report on the results of treatment on carcinoma of the uterus and vagina, vol. 13, Statements of results obtained in 1948 to 1957, inclusive (collated in 1963). Stockholm: Editorial office 1960.

— Complications following radiation therapy in carcinoma of the cervix and their treatment. Amer. J. Obstet. Gynec. 88, 854—866 (1964).

— Differentialtherapie des Uteruskarzinoms. Med. Trib. med. News (N.Y.) 2, 28 (1967).

— Some problems relating to classification and staging of malignant tumours in the female pelvis. J. Int. Gynaec. Obstet. 6, 168—181 (1968).

KRAATZ, H.: Elektive Therapie des Uteruskarzinoms. Dtsch. Gesundh.-Wes. 16, 1287—1327 (1961).

KUHN, E.: Dosierungsprobleme bei der Behandlung von Korpuskarzinomen durch Kobalt 60-Perlen. Zbl. Gynäk. 86, 63—67 (1964).

LABORDE, S., MONTAGNON, J.: Emploi des méthodes radiologiques dans le traitement des cancers du corps utérin. J. Radiol. Électrol. 34, 479—483 (1953).

LADDAGA, M., CALDERAZZI, A., SARGENTI, A.: Prospettive ed utilità della sola telecobalto-irradiazione nel trattamento preoperatorio delle neoplasie uterine. Contributo anatomo-clinico. Radiol. med. (Torino) 54, 666—689 (1968).

LAMPE, I.: Endometrial carcinoma. Amer. J. Roentgenol. 90, 1011—1015 (1963).

LANDRGOT, B., SAUER, J.: Schenkelhalsfrakturen als Folge therapeutischer Bestrahlung bei gynäkologischen Geschwülsten (Vorbeugungsmaßnahmen). Zbl. Gynäk. 87, 835—841 (1965).

LANE, JR., F. W., SHAW, R. K., STIBITZ, G. R.: A computer technique for intracavitary radium dosimetry. Amer. J. Roentgenol. 100, 870—877 (1967).

Lemtis, H., Frischkorn, R.: Vaginalmeßstab als Einstellhilfe in der gynäkologischen Strahlentherapie. Strahlentherapie 120, 449—455 (1963).

Levine, S., Scioosci, E. F.: Squamous cell carcinoma of the uterine corpus and its relation to pyometra. Cancer (Philad.) 19, 485—488 (1966).

Lindgren, L.: The prognosis of carcinoma of the endometrium in its defferent stages treated by surgery combined with postoperative radiotherapy. Acta obstetr. gynec. scand. 36, 426—438 (1957).

Lindsay, W. S.: Variations in prognosis of endometrial carcinoma as indicated by histological structure. Surg. Gynec. Obstet. 44, 646—657 (1927).

Linz, O.: Klinische Untersuchungs- und Behandlungsergebnisse bei Korpuskarzinomen. Zbl. Gynäk. 88, 1281 (1966).

Loeffler, R. K.: A system of radium distribution for treatment of cancer of the corpus uteri. Amer. J. Roentgenol. 73, 425—436 (1955).

Louros, N.: Zit. nach v. Mikulicz-Radecki u. Gansau, Über die Behandlung und Heilerfolge beim Carcinoma corporis uteri. Geburtsh. u. Frauenheilk. 22, 1453—1463 (1962).

Ludovici, P. P., Miller, N. F.: In-vitro detection of characteristic differences in radiation sensitivity of female genital cancer. Obstet. and Gynec. 19, 251—256 (1962).

Lynch, H. T., Krush, A. J., Larsen, A. L., Magnuson, Ch. W.: Endometrial carcinoma: multiple primary malignancies constitutional factors and heredity. Amer. J. med. Sci. 252, 381—390 (1966).

Lyon, F. A.: Intrauterine visualization by means of a hysteroscope. Amer. J. Obstet. Gynec. 90, 443—449 (1964).

MacLean, K. S.: An abrasive endometrial cytologic brush. Amer. J. Obstet. Gynec. 69, 452—454 (1955).

Mahle, A. E.: Morphological histology of adenocarcinoma of the body of the uterus in relation to longevity. Surg. Gynec. Obstet. 36, 385—395 (1923).

Marcial, V. A., Tomé, J. M., Ubinas, J.: The combination of external irradiation and curietherapy used preoperatively in adenocarcinoma of the endometrium. Amer. J. Roentgenol. 105, 586—595 (1969).

Martin, Ch. L., Martin, J. A.: Can endometrial carcinoma of the uterine fundus be eradicated with radium therapy ? Amer. J. Roentgenol. 89, 491—499 (1963).

— — Wilson, R. A.: Can cancer really be cured with radiation therapy ? Amer. J. Roentgenol. 94, 917—923 (1965).

Martius, H.: Über die elektive Therapie beim Gebärmutterkörperkarzinom. Bull. Soc. roy. belge Gynéc. Obstet. 28, 8—14 (1958).

Martz, G.: Die hormonale Therapie maligner Tumoren. Endokrine Behandlungsmethoden des metastasierenden Mamma-, Prostata- und Uterus-Corpuscarcinoms. Heidelberger Taschenbücher, Bd. 41. Berlin-Heidelberg-New York: Springer 1968.

Mayer, E. G.: Zur Krebsentstehung durch ionisierende Strahlen. Wien. klin. Wschr. 72, 129—136 (1960).

— Zum Problem der Krebserzeugung durch Röntgen- und Gammastrahlen. Wien. med. Wschr. 111, 377—379 (1961).

— Zur Frage der Krebserzeugung durch ionisierende Strahlen. Med. Klin. 55, 1824—1830 (1960).

Mayneord, W. V.: Radiation carcinogenesis. Brit. J. Radiol. 41, 241—250 (1968).

Du Mesnil de Rochemont, R.: Über den sinnvollen Einsatz der verschiedenen Krebsbehandlungsverfahren. Med. Klin. 57, 329—334 (1962).

— Ringleb, D., Scherer, E., Schmitt, H.: Klinische Betrachtungen zur Strahlenbehandlung des Korpuskarzinoms. Strahlentherapie 110, 481—490 (1959).

Methfessel, H. D.: Ergebnisse bei der Behandlung des Korpuskarzinoms 1952 bis 1957. Zbl. Gynäk. 85, 1500—1505 (1963).

Mikulicz-Radecki, F. v., Gansau, H.: Über die Behandlung und die Heilerfolge beim Carcinoma corporis uteri. Geburtsh. u. Frauenheilk. 22, 1453—1463 (1962).

Möbius, W.: Beitrag zur Radiumbehandlung in der Gynäkologie. Zwanglose Abhandlungen auf dem Gebiete der Frauenheilkunde, Bd. 10. Leipzig: Georg Thieme 1951.

Montgomery, J. B., Lang, W. R., Farell, D. M., Hahn, G. A.: End results in adenocarcinoma of the endometrium managed by preoperative irradiation. Amer. J. Obstet. Gynec. 80, 972—983 (1960).

Müller, H. G.: Die Metastasierung des Korpuskarzinoms, besonders in die Vagina. Wege zu ihrer Verhütung. Strahlentherapie 110, 280—286 (1959).

Müller, J. H.: Über die Strahlentherapie des Carcinoma corporis uteri; mit einem Beitrag über den Strahlenschutz in der gynäkologischen Radiumtherapie. Strahlentherapie 70, 243—284 (1941).

— Beiträge zur medizinisch-therapeutischen Verwendung der künstlichen Radioaktivität. Strahlentherapie 85, 87—125 (1951).

— Persönliche Mitteilung, 1966.

— Wachsmann, F., Schuster, D.: Die Zürcher Bestrahlungsmethode des Kollumkarzinoms unter besonderer Berücksichtigung der angewendeten zeitlichen Dosisverteilung. Strahlentherapie 125, 502—523 (1964).

Neuweiler, W.: Zit. nach du Mesnil de Rochemont, Ringleb, Scherer u. Schmitt, Klinische Betrachtungen zur Strahlenbehandlung des Korpuskarzinoms. Strahlentherapie 110, 481—490 (1959).

Nielsen, J. C.: Cancer corporis uteri nach Strahlenbehandlung. Ugeskr. Læg. 122, 1239—1242 (1960).

Nolan, J. F.: Symposium on endometrial cancer. Amer. J. Obstet. Gynec. 81, 1099—1100 (1961).

— Harrison, L. A.: Carcinoma of the endometrium: An evaluation of preoperative radiation therapy. Obstet. and Gynec. 17, 601—604 (1961).

Nolte, L.: Urographische Verlaufskontrollen nach Bestrahlung des operativ freigelegten Kaninchenureters. Diss. Göttingen 1966.

NORDQVIST, B.: Hormone effects on carcinoma of the human uterine body studied in organ culture. Acta obstet. gynec. scand. **43**, 296—307 (1964).

NORIEGA, J., RIOS SAN MARTIN, G., FALCÓ, J.: Intraosseous phlebography and lamphadenography in carcinoma of the cervix and other pelvic neoplasia. Radiology **83**, 219—227 (1964).

NORMAN, O.: Hysterography in cancer of the corpus of the uterus. Acta radiol. (Stockh.), Suppl. LXXIX, Lund 1950.

— L'hystérographie dans le cancer de l'utérus. I. Cancer du col, Gynécologie Pratique, vol. II, p. 463—466 (1951). Paris: Vigot Frères 1952.

— L'hystérographie dans le cancer de l'utérus. II. Cancer du corps, Gynécologie Pratique, vol. III, p. 157—162 (1952). Paris: Vigot Frères 1952.

— L'hystérographie dans le cancer de l'utérus. III. Cancer du corps et du col, Gynécologie Pratique, vol. III, p. 157—162 (1952). Paris: Vigot Frères 1952.

— Hysterographically visualized radionecrosis following intra-uterine radiation of cancer of the corpus of the uterus. Acta radiol. (Stockh.) **37**, 96—102 (1952).

— Hysterography in cancer of the uterus. In: J. W. McLAREN, Modern trends in diagnostic radiology (2. Ser.), Kap. 23. London: Buttworth & Co. 1953.

NORRIS, H. J., TAYLOR, H. B.: Mesenchymal tumors of the uterus. III. A clinical and pathologic study of 31 carcinosarcomas. Cancer (Philad.) **19**, 1459 (1966).

NYSTRÖM, C.: Myometrial blood flow studies in carcinoma of the corpus uteri. Acta radiol. (Stockh.) **8**, 193—198 (1969).

OBOLENSKY, W., ZÜRCHER, W. O.: Der Gefäßinflux bei Hysterographien als verdächtiges Zeichen auf Korpuskarzinom. Geburtsh. u. Frauenheilk. **24**, 28—33 (1964).

OESER, H.: Strahlenbehandlung der Geschwülste. München-Berlin: Urban & Schwarzenberg 1954.

ØSTERGAARD, E.: Estrogens in the etiology of cancer of the corpus uteri. La prophylaxie en gynécologie et obstétrique. Genf: Georg & Cie. S.A. 1954.

PARKER, R. T., NEWTON, Z. B., PEETE, C. H.: Nonhormonal chemotherapy of recurrent endometrial cancer. In: G. C. LEWIS JR., W. B. WENTZ, R. M. JAFFE, New concepts in gynecological oncology, p. 269—273. Philadelphia: F. A. Davis Company 1966.

PAROLI, G. B.: Il trattamento radium endouterine delle metropatie emorragiche del climaterio nel campo delle profilassi del cancro del corpo dell' utero. La prophylacie en gynécologie et obstétrique. Genf: Georg & Cie. S.A. 1954.

PATERSON, R., RUSSEL, M. H.: Clinical trials in malignant disease. Part VI — Cancer of the cervix uteri. Is x-ray therapy more effective given before or after radium? Clin. Radiol. **13**, 313—315 (1962).

PAUL, W.: Röntgenstereophotogrammetrische Untersuchungen über den Einfluß der Lagerungen von Patienten während einer gynäkologischen Strahlentherapie auf die Genauigkeit der angestrebten Dosisverteilung. Diss. Göttingen 1966.

PELLER, S.: Weitere Beiträge zum Prinzip der inversen Assoziation. Krebsarzt **23**, 242—250 (1968).

PETERSEN, F.: Erfahrungen und Ergebnisse der Strahlenbehandlung des Korpuskarzinoms des Uterus. Strahlentherapie **116**, 168—179 (1961).

PFLEIDERER, A., JR.: Histochemische Untersuchungen am Carcinom des Corpus uteri. Die Enzymverteilung im infiltrierend wachsenden Tumorabschnitt. Z. Krebsforsch. **70**, 337—349 (1968).

— Enzymhistochemische Untersuchungen am Karzinom des Corpus uteri. Fortschr. Med. **86**, 195—200 (1968).

PHILIPP, E., HUBER, H.: Die Ausbreitung des Korpuskarzinoms. Ein weiterer Beitrag für die Bedeutung der Tubenendometriose. Zbl. Gynäk. **63**, 2153—2173 (1939).

— RUMPHORST, K.: Die Behandlung des Korpuskarzinoms an der Kieler Klinik. (Bericht über die Ergebnisse der Jahre 1948—1952 mit einem Überblick über die Behandlung in den Jahren 1922—1952.) Geburtsh. u. Frauenheilk. **18**, 1393—1399 (1958).

PICARD, J. D., GONGORA, R., SZIGETI, B.: Considérations techniques et primiers résultats des injections intra-lymphatiques de lipiodol radioactif à doses thérapeutique. Ann. Radiol. **7**, 543—553 (1964).

PICHA, E., WEGHAUPT, K.: Methodik der Radiumbehandlung des Carcinoma corporis uteri in den Jahren 1950—1960 und Heilungsergebnisse aus den Jahren 1950—1955. Wien. klin. Wschr. **73**, 595—597 (1961).

— — Ergebnisse der primären Strahlenbehandlung von 141 Korpuskarzinomen in den Jahren 1956—1959. Wien. med. Wschr. **115**, 622—624 (1965).

— — Heilungsergebnisse bei 345 primär bestrahlten Korpuskarzinomen in der Zeit von 1950—1962. Wien. klin. Wschr. **80**, 946—948 (1968).

PIERQUIN, B.: L'iridium 192 peut-il remplacer le radium? Presse méd. Nr 2, 69 (1962).

PLENTZ, K.: Verlaufsbeobachtungen von 735 Karzinomen des Corpus uteri unter besonderer Berücksichtigung der cytostatischen Nachbehandlung. Diss. Göttingen 1967.

POCKRANDT, H.: Die Behandlungsergebnisse des Korpuskarzinoms in den Jahren 1944—1948 an der Universitäts-Frauenklinik Berlin. Zbl. Gynäk. **77**, 1545—1552 (1955).

POLLACK, J. M.: Das symptomlose Korpuskarzinom. Med. Welt 18, 3108—3109 (1967).

PRATT, J. H.: Surgical treatment of recurrent endometrial carcinoma. In: G. C. LEWIS, JR., W. B. WENTZ, R. M. JAFFE, New concepts in gynecological oncology, p. 261—267. Philadelphia: F. A. Davis Company 1966.

PRETTENHOFER, H.: Beitrag zur operativen Behandlung des Carcinoma corporis uteri. Wien. med. Wschr. **116**, 937—942 (1966).

PRICE, J. J., HAHN, G. A., ROMINGER, C. J.: Vaginal involvement in endometrial carcinoma. Amer. J. Obstet. Gynec. **91**, 1060—1065 (1965).

PÜSCHEL, W., MÖBIUS, G.: Histologischer Typ und Prognose des Korpuskarzinoms. Geburtsh. u. Frauenheilk. **27**, 50—58 (1967).

RANDALL, J. H., GODDARD, W. B.: A study of 531 cases of endometrial carcinoma. Surg. Gynec. Obstet. **103**, 221—226 (1956).

Randow, H., Kaiser, P.: Behandlungsresultate des Korpuskarzinoms. Zbl. Gynäk. **91**, 401—406 (1969).

Reagan, J. W.: Cytology of endometrial neoplasms. In: G. C. Lewis Jr., W. B. Wentz, R. M. Jaffe, New concepts in gynecological oncology, p. 219—224. Philadelphia: F. A. Davis Company 1966.

Redd, B. L., Jr.: Bone changes following radiation therapy for malignant lesions in region of the pelvis. Radiol. clin. (Basel) **33**, 60—71 (1964).

Regato, J. A. del: Radiotherapy in the treatment of recurrences of carcinoma of the endometrium. In: G. C. Lewis Jr., W. B. Wentz, R. M. Jaffe, New concepts in gynecological oncology, p. 257—260. Philadelphia: F. A. Davis Company 1966.

Reiffenstuhl, G.: Das Lymphsystem des weiblichen Genitale. München-Berlin-Wien: Urban & Schwarzenberg 1957.

— Das Lymphknotenproblem beim Carcinoma colli uteri und die Lymphirradiatio pelvis. München: Urban & Schwarzenberg 1967.

Reinermann, Th.: Die Kontrolle des Heilungsverlaufes des Korpuskarzinoms durch Hysterographie. Fortschr. Röntgenstr. **102**, 292—297 (1965).

Renning, E. L., Javert, C. T.: Analysis of a series of cases of carcinoma of the endometrium treated by radium and operation. Amer. J. Obstet. Gynec. **88**, 171—177 (1964).

Reuss, A., Brunner, F.: Phantommessungen mit den Mikroionisationskammern des Bomke-Dosimeters an Radium und Kobalt⁶⁰. Strahlentherapie **103**, 279—288 (1957).

— Plesch, R., Mayer, U., Muschwitz, C. v.: Einige Gesichtspunkte zur Messung von Radium- und Radiokobaltstrahlung mit der Kadmium-Sulfid-Kristallsonde. Strahlentherapie **94**, 385—393 (1954).

Ries, J.: Die Radiumdosimetrie beim Uterus-Carcinom. Strahlentherapie **82**, 23—94 (1950).

— Die Technik der Radium-Röntgenbehandlung. Strahlentherapie **86**, 339—344 (1952).

— Röntgen- und Radiumstrahlen als Krebsursache in der Gynäkologie. Le prophylacie en gynécologie et obstétrique. Genf: Georg & Cie. S.A. 1954.

— Ludwig, H., Appel, W.: Antikoagulantien bei der Strahlenbehandlung weiblicher Genitalkarzinome. Med. Welt **19**, 2042—2047 (1968).

Rosenow, U.: Untersuchungen über Grundlagen und Leistungsfähigkeit einer neuen röntgen-stereophotogrammetrischen Meßmethode. Diss. Göttingen 1969.

— Ein klinisch orientiertes Computerprogramm für die Berechnung räumlicher Dosisverteilungen bei gynäkologischen Radiumeinlagen. Röntgen-Bl. **22**, 206—212 (1969).

— Eine einfache computergerechte Darstellung von Körperoberflächen für die elektronische Berechnung dreidimensionaler Dosisverteilungen in der Tiefentherapie. Röntgen-Bl. **22**, 213—216 (1969).

— Zwehl, D. v.: Investigations in the reliability of the basic computational model in a program for the calculation of three-dimensional dose distributions in radiotherapy. Vortragsmanuskript. Internat. Meeting on the Use of Computers in Radiology, Brüssel 17.—20. 9. 1969.

Rotte, K.: Das Rezidiv beim Karzinom des Collum und Corpus uteri. Strahlentherapie **137**, 637—645 (1969).

Roux, G., Marchal, G.: L'oestrogénie continue ou persistante dans le déterminisme du cancer du corps. La prophylaxie en gynécologie et obstétrique. Genf: Georg & Cie. S.A. 1954.

Rubin, A.: Human resistance to cancer. I. Prognosis in pelvic malignancy: correlation between patient survival and tissue culture growth of tumors. Amer. J. Obstet. Gynec. **85**, 149—155 (1963).

Rubin, P., Gerle, R. D., Quick, R. S., Greenlaw, R. H.: Significance of vaginal recurrence in endometrial carcinoma. Amer. J. Roentgenol. **89**, 91—100 (1963).

— Ryplansky, A., Dutton, A.: Incidence of pelvic malignancies following irradiation for benign gynecologic conditions. Amer. J. Roentgenol. **85**, 503—514 (1961).

Rüttimann, A.: Progress in lymphology. Proceedings of the Internat. Symposium on Lymphology Zurich, Switzerland, July 19—23, 1966. Stuttgart: Georg Thieme 1967.

— del Buono, M. S.: Die Lymphographie. In: Ergebnisse der medizinischen Strahlenforschung, N. F., Bd. I. Hrsg. H. R. Schinz, R. Glauner, A. Rüttimann. Stuttgart: Georg Thieme 1964.

Rumphorst, K.: Die Behandlungsergebnisse des Korpuskarzinoms an der Kieler Universitäts-Frauenklinik. Strahlentherapie **114**, 589—594 (1961).

— Kollum- und Korpuskarzinome 1955 (Jahresbericht der Kieler Universitäts-Frauenklinik). Strahlentherapie **117**, 509—513 (1962).

Runge, H., Lindenschmidt, W.: Zur Hormonbehandlung des Krebses. Ärztl. Forsch. **14**, 65—80 (1960).

Rutledge, F. N., Gutierrez, A. G., Fletcher, G. H.: Management of stage I and II adenocarcinomas of the uterine cervix on intact uterus. Amer. J. Roentgenol. **102**, 161—164 (1968).

Rutledge, L. B., Tan, S. K., Fletcher, G. H.: Vaginalmetastases from adenocarcinoma of the corpus uteri. Amer. J. Obstet. Gynec. **75**, 167—173 (1958).

Sala, J. M., del Regato, J. A.: Treatment of carcinoma of the endometrium. Radiology **79**, 12—17 (1962).

Sarre, H., Moser, F.: Hypertonie, Nephritis und Nephrofibrose (-Zirrhose) nach Bestrahlung der Nieren. Med. Klin. **57**, 1626—1631 (1962).

Scheele, R.: Die Behandlungsergebnisse bösartiger Geschwülste der Jahre 1944—1955. Geburtsh. u. Frauenheilk. **21**, 845—855 (1961).

Scheer, K. E.: Radioaktives Yttrium Y⁹⁰ als Strahlenquelle für intraperitoneale und intrapleurale Applikation. Strahlentherapie **101**, 283—288 (1956).

Scherer, E.: Möglichkeiten und Fortschritte in der Strahlentherapie bösartiger Genitaltumoren. Vortrag Düsseldorf 1962. Zbl. Gynäk. **86**, 457—467 (1964).

Schieferstein, W.: Gedanken zur Therapie des Korpuskarzinoms. Referat. Geburtsh. u. Frauenheilk. **24**, 435 (1964).

SCHLAGKAMP, H.: Die Strahlenbehandlung des Korpuskarzinoms mittels Packmethode. Strahlentherapie **101**, 499—506 (1956).

SCHMERMUND, H. J., OBERHEUSER, F., KUTTIG, H.: In: Die Supervolttherapie. Stuttgart: Georg Thieme 1961.

SCHMID, H. H.: Gebärmutterkörperkrebs nach früherer Strahlenbehandlung. Arch. Geschwulstforsch. **17**, 102—107 (1961).

SCHMIDT-MATTHIESEN, H.: Die Hysteroskopie als klinische Routinemethode. Geburtsh. u. Frauenheilk. **26**, 1498—1501 (1966).

— WELLERS, H.: Zur Gestagentherapie fortgeschrittener Korpuskarzinome. Geburtsh. u. Frauenheilk. **28**, 417—427 (1968).

SCHMITZ, H. E., SMITH, CH. J., FETHERSTON, W. C.: Effects of preoperative irradiation in adenocarcinoma of the uterus. Amer. J. Obstet. Gynec. **78**, 1048—1054 (1959).

— — GAJEWSKI, CH. J.: The effect of preoperative radiation of adenocarcinoma of the endometrium. Amer. J. Obstet. Gynec. **64**, 952—966 (1952).

SCHOKNECHT, G.: Eigene Erfahrungen und Systeme für die Ermittlung von räumlichen Dosisverteilungen. Röntgen-Bl. **22**, 196—198 (1969).

— Die Beschreibung von Strahlenfeldern durch Separierung von Primär- und Streustrahlung. III. Das Gewebe-Luft-Verhältnis und der Tiefendosisverlauf bei Gamma- und Röntgenstrahlungen im Bereich von 0,6 bis 42 MeV. Strahlentherapie **136**, 24—32 (1968).

SCHRAKNEPPER, J.: Über Rezidive bei Korpuskarzinomen. Zbl. Gynäk. **81**, 151—155 (1959).

SCHULTE, J. W., HINMAN, F., LOW-BEER, B. V. A.: J. Urol. (Baltimore) **67**, 916 (1952). Zit. nach BECKER und SCHEER: Die radioaktiven Isotope in der Geburtshilfe und Gynäkologie. Basel-New York: S. Karger 1956.

SCOTT, W. P.: Radium alignment applicator. Amer. J. Roentgenol. **94**, 905—913 (1965).

— Cervicovaginal irradiator — a triple applicator. Amer. J. Roentgenol. **96**, 52—55 (1966).

SEITZ, D., KALM, H.: Zur klinischen Differentialdiagnose spinaler Röntgenschäden und intramedullärer Geschwulstabsiedlungen. Dtsch. Z. Nervenheilk. **182**, 155—175 (1961).

SHERMAN, A. I.: Hormonal aspects of endometrial cancer. In: G. C. LEWIS JR., W. B. WENTZ, R. M. JAFFE, New concepts in gynecological oncology, p. 275—286. Philadelphia: F. A. Davis Company 1966.

SIEBER, F.: Die Lymphographie in der klinischen Praxis. Leipzig: Georg Thieme VEB 1966.

SILANDER, T.: Hysteroscopy through a transparent rubber balloon. Surg. Gynec. Obstet. **114**, 125—127 (1962).

— Hysteroscopy through a transparent rubber balloon in patients with uterine bleeding. Acta obstetr. gynec. scand. **42**, 1—10 (1963).

SILVERSTONE, S. M.: The intra-uterine tandem technique. Amer. J. Roentgenol. **89**, 83—86 (1963).

SIMMENROTH, H.: Korpuskarzinom. Histologische Klassifizierung und Prognose. Diss. Göttingen 1969.

SOERGEL, W.: Therapie und Heilungsergebnisse beim Korpuskarzinom. Zbl. Gynäk. **83**, 993—996 (1961).

SOMMERS, S. C.: The significance of endometrial hyperplasias. In: G. C. LEWIS JR., W. B. WENTZ, R. M. JAFFE, New concepts in gynecological oncology, p. 205—209. Philadelphia: F. A. Davis Company 1966.

SOOST, H.: Vortrag Bayerische Gesellschaft für Geburtshilfe und Frauenheilkunde in Erlangen 1960. Ref. Geburtsh. u. Frauenheilk. **21**, 302 (1961).

SPECHTER, H.-J.: Zur Frage der Krebserzeugung durch ionisierende Strahlen. Med. Klin. **42**, 318—320 (1961).

SPIRA, J., ARAL, I.: Radium dosage patterns in the treatment of uterine carcinoma. Amer. J. Roentgenol. **105**, 110—114 (1969).

STÄUBLE, K.: Die Heilungsziffern der Korpuskarzinomfälle der Frauenklinik Basel in den letzten 25 Jahren. Gynaecologia (Basel) **166**, 114—137 (1968).

STALLWORTHY, J.: The malignant uterus yesterday, today and tomorrow. J. Amer. med. Ass. **195**, 465—470 (1966).

STOCK, W.: Kasuistischer Beitrag zum klinischen Problem des Doppelkarzinoms. Geburtsh. u. Frauenheilk. **28**, 1045—1049 (1968).

STRAUSS, G., HIERSCHE, H.-D.: Zur Frage der Adenokankroide (Adenoakanthome) des Corpus uteri. Geburtsh. u. Frauenheilk. **23**, 736—748 (1963).

STRICKLAND, P.: Carcinoma of the uterine body treated with radioactive cobalt. J. Obstet. Gynaec. Brit. Emp. **60**, 898—900 (1953).

— GREGORY, C.: Rectal dose and rectal damage in the intracavitary treatment of uterine cancer. Acta radiol. (Stockh.) **56**, 289—295 (1961).

SYKES, M.: Panel — Chemotherapy in gynecological cancer. Bull. Sloane Hosp. Women **13**, 156—161 (1967).

SZULMAN, A. E.: Histology of endometrial carcinoma including some cytogenetical considerations. In: G. C. LEWIS JR., W. B. WENTZ, R. M. JAFFE, New concepts in gynecological oncology, p. 225—228. Philadelphia: F. A. Davis Company 1966.

TAKI, J., OKAMURA, Y., KATSUKI, E., ARAKAWA, K.: Unterstützende Therapie bei Carcinoma uteri. Ärztl. Prax. **21**, 1065—1068 (1969).

TASCH, H.: In: Biologie und Pathologie des Weibes. Ein Handbuch der Frauenheilkunde und Geburtshilfe, 2. Aufl., Bd. IV. Berlin-Innsbruck-München-Wien: Urban & Schwarzenberg 1955.

TE LINDE, R. W., JONES, H. W., GALVIN, G. A.: What are the earliest endometrial changes to justify a diagnosis of endometrial cancer. Amer. J. Obstet. Gynec. **66**, 953—969 (1953).

THIESSEN, P.: Diskussionsbemerkung. Geburtsh. u. Frauenheilk. **22**, 1071—1072 (1962).

TOD, M. C., MEREDITH, W. J.: Treatment of cancer of the cervix uteri — revised "Manchester Method". Brit. J. Radiol. **26**, 252—257 (1953).

TOMKINSON, J. S.: The management of cancer of the body of the uterus. Practitioner **196**, 41 (1966).

TREITE, P.: Über die kontinuierliche Ausbreitung des Korpuskarzinoms in den interstitiellen Tubenteil. Zbl. Gynäk. **64**, 504—511 (1940).

UICC: TNM, Classification of malignant tumours. Union Internat. Contre le Cancer, Geneva 1968.

Ullman, S. B.: New vistas of chemotherapy of cancer. Diss. Toronto, Canada, 1967.

Varga, A., Henriksen, E.: Hormonal treatment of endometrial cancer. In: G. C. Lewis Jr., W. B. Wentz, R. M. Jaffe, Nes concepts in gynecological oncology, p. 301—308. Philadelphia: F. A. Davis Company 1966.

Verhagen, A.: Radium-Isodosen. Die Radiumdosierung in „r". Stuttgart: Georg Thieme 1958.

Vieten, H., Heinzler, F.: Die Bedeutung ultraharter Strahlungen für die Therapie gynäkologischer Geschwülste. Geburtsh. u. Frauenheilk. **26**, 1—16 (1966).

Virieux, C.: Untersuchungen über die Häufigkeit und Entstehungsweise von Krebsmetastasen in den Eierstöcken. Gynaecologia (Basel) **153**, 209—224 (1962).

Vogelgesang, K. H., Grosse-Holz, K.: Probleme der räumlichen und zeitlichen Dosisverteilung bei der Röntgenbestrahlung des Uteruskarzinoms. Strahlentherapie **125**, 173—190 (1964).

Wade, M. E.: Adenocarcinoma of the endometrium. Amer. J. Obstet. Gynec. **99**, 869—876 (1967).

Walker, L. A.: Radioactive Yttrium 90. A review of its properties, biological behavior, and clinical uses. Acta radiol. Ther. Phys. Biol. **2**, 302—314 (1964).

Wallace, D. M., Walton, R. J., Sinclair, W. K.: Brit. J. Urol. **21**, 357—364 (1949). Zit. nach Becker und Scheer, Die radioaktiven Isotope in der Geburtshilfe und Gynäkologie. Basel-New York: S. Karger 1956.

Walter, J., Jones, J. C., Fisher, M.: Radioactive colloidal Yttrium silicate in the treatment of malignant effusions. I. Clinical aspects and investigations. Brit. J. Radiol. **34**, 337—346 (1961).

Walther, H. E.: Krebsmetastasen. Basel: Schwabe & Co. 1948.

Weber, E.: Beitrag zur Klinik des Corpuskarzinoms. Gynaecologia (Basel) **151**, 232—239 (1961).

Weghaupt, K.: Die Radiumbehandlung der Karzinome des Corpus uteri. Radiol. Austriaca **5**, 167—175 (1952).

Wenig, H.: Die Zytodiagnostik bösartiger Veränderungen im Bereich des Corpus uteri. Zbl. Gynäk. **81**, 1457—1462 (1959).

Wimhöfer, H., Zeitz, H., Runge, H.: Bericht über 403 Korpuskarzinome (1935—1949). (Ein Beitrag zur Frage der Stadieneinteilung und Therapie.) Geburtsh. u. Frauenheilk. **15**, 209—224 (1955).

Winkelmann, J., Robinson, R.: Adenocarcinoma of endometrium involving adenomyosis. Cancer (Philad.) **19**, 901—908 (1966).

Wodon, L., de Paepe, J., Foucart, J., Maumin, A., Petitfrete, C., Poulin, E., Spehl, B., Delcourt, G.: Résultats de la radiumthérapie du "carcinoma corporois" contrôlés lors de l'hystérectomie. Bull. Soc. roy. belge Gynéc. Obstét. **28**, 365—366 (1958).

Wynder, E. L., Escher, G. C., Mantel, N.: An epidemiological investigation of cancer of the endometrium. Cancer (Philad.) **19**, 489—520 (1966).

Zeitz, H., Buttenberg, D.: Genitalkarzinom und Diabetes mellitus. Zbl. Gynäk. **77**, 1540—1545 (1955).

— Zitzmann, H.: Vergleichende Isodosenmessungen an Radium und Kobalt 60. Strahlentherapie **101**, 405—415 (1956).

Zsolnai, B., Nyirö, L.: Zur Hysterographie bei Korpuskarzinom. Zbl. Gynäk. **90**, 273—279 (1968).

IV. Die Strahlenbehandlung des Collumcarcinoms

Von

H.-J. Frischbier

Mit 69 Abbildungen

1. Einleitung

Die Behandlung des Carcinoma colli uteri ist so eng mit der Strahlentherapie verknüpft, daß man den Begriff „gynäkologische Strahlentherapie" unbewußt mit der Strahlenbehandlung des Collumcarcinoms verbindet. Der Grund hierfür ist nicht nur allein in der Häufigkeit des Collumcarcinoms zu sehen, das etwa 70—80 % aller weiblichen Genitalcarcinome darstellt. Viel entscheidender sind die ausgezeichneten Behandlungsergebnisse, die selbst bei fortgeschrittenen Fällen mit ausschließlicher Strahlentherapie erzielt werden. Vergleicht man die Behandlungsresultate rein radiologisch behandelter Collumcarcinome, die bereits Metastasen in die regionären Lymphknoten gesetzt haben, mit den Heilungsergebnissen anderer menschlicher Organkrebse entsprechender Ausbreitungsstadien, so fällt eine signifikante Diskrepanz auf: Von den Patientinnen mit einem Collumcarcinom lebt nach 5 Jahren rezidivfrei noch jede zweite bis dritte Frau, während bei anderen Tumorlokalisationen eine echte Heilung selten ist. Lediglich auf dermatologischem Sektor können mit der Strahlentherapie vergleichbar gute Ergebnisse bei malignen Tumoren erzielt werden. Darüber hinaus sind mit der Strahlenbehandlung auch bei den operablen Stadien des Collumcarcinoms hervorragende Erfolge zu erreichen. Während bei vielen anderen Tumorlokalisationen die Operation als Methode der Wahl gilt und eine ausschließliche Strahlentherapie vornehmlich palliative Bedeutung bei inoperablen Fällen besitzt, werden beim Collumcarcinom, bei dem der Tumor noch auf das Ursprungsorgan beschränkt ist, mit radiologischen Behandlungsmethoden Ergebnisse erzielt, die denen nach radikalen operativen Eingriffen entsprechen.

Da das Collumcarcinom keineswegs als strahlensensibler Tumor angesehen werden kann, ist ein bedeutsamerer Faktor für die guten Behandlungsergebnisse in den günstigen topographischen Gegebenheiten zu sehen. Optimale topographische Verhältnisse gestatten beim Collumcarcinom, per vaginam die Strahlenquelle direkt an den Primärtumor zu bringen und auf diese Weise eine exzessiv hohe Dosis zur vollständigen und sicheren Devitalisierung des Tumors einzustrahlen. Entgegen allen anderen Hohlorganen, die sich zur Aufnahme von Strahlenquellen anbieten, ist der Uterus ein dickwandiges Organ, dessen Wandschädigung und Funktionsbeeinträchtigung unbedenklich sind. Wenn auch in der unmittelbaren Nachbarschaft relativ strahlensensible Organe liegen, wie beispielsweise Blase, Rectum, Sigma, Ureteren, so müssen schwere Strahlenschäden dieser Organe nicht unbedingt deletär verlaufen. Ein partieller Ersatz der Beckenorgane ist durchaus mit dem Leben zu vereinbaren.

Die guten Behandlungsergebnisse bei der Bestrahlung des Collumcarcinoms, die schon sehr früh einen Wettstreit mit den bewährten operativen Maßnahmen hervorriefen, machen es verständlich, daß die Entwicklung der gynäkologischen Strahlentherapie eng mit der Geschichte der allgemeinen Strahlentherapie verknüpft ist. Die Entwicklung der verschiedenen Bestrahlungsmethoden sowie die strahlenbiologischen Erkenntnisse sind mit Namen vieler Forscher verbunden, die auf dem Sektor der gynäkologischen Strahlentherapie gearbeitet haben. Eine Darstellung der geschichtlichen Entwicklung der Strahlentherapie zeigt, daß der gynäkologischen Strahlentherapie ein sehr großer Anteil am Fortschritt der Erkenntnisse zukommt. Daher hat sich im Laufe der Jahrzehnte ein gewaltiges

Schrifttum angesammelt. Es würde aber den Rahmen dieses Beitrages sprengen, sollte
die geschichtliche Entwicklung lückenlos dargestellt und das gesamte Schrifttum
berücksichtigt werden. Hierbei kann man auf umfangreiche ältere Darstellungen in
Handbuchbeiträgen und Monographien verweisen (Seitz und Wintz, 1920; Voltz, 1930;
Kepp, 1952; Eymer, 1953; Kottmeier, 1953; Dyroff und Siegert, 1955; Corscaden,
1956; Ries und Breitner, 1959; Hofmann, 1963 u.a.). Das Anliegen dieses Beitrages
soll vielmehr sein, die bewährten und heute noch praktizierten Behandlungsmethoden
beim Collumcarcinom darzustellen. Darüber hinaus soll das Schwergewicht auf den im
letzten Jahrzehnt entwickelten Behandlungsverfahren liegen. Durch den therapeutischen
Einsatz verschiedener Radionuclide sowie die Entwicklung ultraharter Strahlen wurden
die über mehrere Jahrzehnte gültigen Prinzipien bei der Behandlung des Collumcarcinoms,
wobei das Schwergewicht auf der Radiumeinlage lag und der Percutanbestrahlung nur
eine untergeordnete Bedeutung zukam, durch zahlreiche Behandlungsmethoden erweitert. Eine Analyse der mit diesen neuartigen Behandlungsmethoden gewonnenen
klinischen Erfahrungen und Behandlungsergebnisse soll zeigen, inwieweit heute ein
routinemäßiger Einsatz gerechtfertigt ist.

Bei der Behandlung des Collumcarcinoms fallen Strahlenfolgen besonders ins Gewicht,
da die Patientinnen wegen der besseren Prognose in höherem Maße die Chance haben,
auch Spätkomplikationen mit deletären Folgen zu erleben. Bei der Beurteilung der
Wertigkeit einer Behandlungsmethode müssen deshalb die möglichen Komplikationen
gegeneinander abgewogen werden.

2. Gesichtspunkte für die Indikationsstellung zur Operation oder Bestrahlung

Während in fortgeschrittenen Stadien des Collumcarcinoms die Domäne der Strahlentherapie von keinem Gynäkologen angezweifelt wird, besteht bei den Stadien, die technisch
durchaus operabel sind, keine Übereinstimmung, welcher der beiden möglichen Behandlungsmethoden der Vorzug zu geben ist. Der Grund hierfür ist darin zu sehen, daß bis
heute nicht eindeutig bewiesen ist, ob beispielsweise beim Stadium I, bei dem der Tumor
auf die Cervix beschränkt ist, die radikale Operation oder die ausschließliche Strahlentherapie die besseren Heilungsergebnisse liefert.

Im Laufe dieses Jahrhunderts hat sich die Ansicht über die erfolgreichste Behandlungsmethode beim Collumcarcinom mehrmals gewandelt; selbst renommierte Kliniker haben
innerhalb ihrer jahrzehntelangen Tätigkeit ihre Meinung mehrfach geändert. Die Erklärung für das auch bis heute noch ungelöste Kernproblem der gynäkologischen Therapie
überhaupt ist in der wechselweisen Entwicklung beider Behandlungsmethoden zu sehen.
Die Frage nach der optimalen Behandlung ist deshalb in den verschiedenen Entwicklungs-
phasen beider Methoden unterschiedlich beantwortet worden.

Noch in der zweiten Hälfte des vorigen Jahrhunderts bestand die Behandlung eines
Collumcarcinoms in einer hohen, vaginalen Portioamputation. Ablauf und Folgezustände
dieser Eingriffe waren schrecklich, da es sich vorwiegend um fortgeschrittene Fälle handelte.

Am 8. 8. 1878 führte Czerny in Heidelberg erstmals vaginal eine operative Entfernung
des Uterus durch. Im gleichen Jahr entfernte Freund einen carcinomatös befallenen
Uterus abdominal. Hierbei ließ er Beckenbindegewebe und Lymphknoten unberücksichtigt. Nach den ersten Erfolgsmitteilungen betrug die primäre Mortalität bei Freund
72%. Czerny konnte die primäre Mortalität bei seinem Eingriff auf 32% reduzieren;
bei 81 operierten Frauen endete der Eingriff nur in 26 Fällen tödlich. Die absolute Heilung
lag zwischen 7 und 14%. Den Mut und die persönliche Hingabe dieser Pioniere müssen
wir heute bewundern. Nur aus der Erfahrung, daß die Patientinnen, die unbehandelt
blieben, ihrem Schicksal erlegen waren, schöpften die damaligen Operateure die Kraft, diese
unter damaligen Umständen heroisch anmutende Behandlungsmethode weiter auszubauen.

Durch den Ausbau von Asepsis, Narkose, Blutstillung und die Kenntnis über die
Ausbreitung des Collumcarcinoms wurden bald die Forderungen nach größerer Radi-

kalität erhoben, so daß schon im Jahre 1895 mehrere Operateure in Europa und in Amerika über gelungene Uterusexstirpationen nach modernen Grundsätzen der Radikalität berichteten. WERTHEIM hat seine erste abdominale erweiterte Uterusexstirpation zur Krebsbehandlung im Jahre 1898 vorgenommen. Er erkannte sehr früh, daß der Erfolg von der möglichst weitgehenden Entfernung des parametranen Bindegewebes abhängt. Ihm kommt ein besonderes Verdienst bei der Entwicklung der abdominalen Operationstechnik sowie der histologischen Bearbeitung des Operationsmaterials und der statistischen Erfassung der Heilungsergebnisse zu. Im Jahre 1900 konnte er über 29 Operationsfälle mit einer Mortalität in 11 Fällen berichten, und schon 1911 lagen seiner Monographie ,,Die erweiterte abdominale Operation bei Carcinoma colli uteri'' 500 Fälle zugrunde. Die primäre Operationsmortalität betrug 19%.

Da bei nachgewiesener Lymphknotenmetastasierung die 5-Jahres-Heilung nur 12,2% betrug, entschloß sich WERTHEIM bald, seine ursprüngliche Forderung nach genereller Ausräumung der Lymphknoten aufzugeben. Er führte nur noch eine selektive Lymphonodektomie durch und konnte dadurch bei Vervollkommnung der Operationstechnik trotz weitreichender Indikationsstellung die primäre Operationsmortalität senken und die 5-Jahres-Heilung erhöhen.

Etwa zur gleichen Zeit hat sich in Wien SCHAUTA, Lehrer von WERTHEIM, mit seiner ganzen Kraft der Entwicklung einer vaginalen Operationsmethode beim Collumcarcinom gewidmet (1891). Er entwickelte eine Methode, bei der vaginal der Uterus in toto exstirpiert wurde, das gesamte Parametrium entfernt und die regionären Lymphknoten ausgeräumt werden konnten. Diese als erweiterte vaginale Totalexstirpation bezeichnete Methode wies entscheidende Vorteile gegenüber der abdominalen Operationsmethode auf. Kürzere Operationsdauer, geringere Schockgefahr, leichterer postoperativer Verlauf führten zu einer wesentlich geringeren primären Mortalität. Die durch die Wertheimsche Methode gegebene obligate Freilegung des pelvinen Ureterabschnittes hatte eine hohe Rate urologischer Komplikationen zur Folge. Bei dem von SCHAUTA angegebenen vaginalen Vorgehen brauchten die Ureteren nur bei pathologischen Veränderungen des Parametriums freigelegt zu werden. Die Frequenz urologischer Komplikationen war dadurch niedriger.

Die später von AMREICH methodisch vervollkommnete vaginale Radikaloperation erbrachte Heilungsergebnisse, die denen nach abdominalem Vorgehen entsprechen. Da anfangs versucht wurde, die Behandlungsergebnisse durch möglichst radikale Entfernung sämtlicher Beckenwandlymphknoten zu verbessern, führten die Anhänger der Wertheimschen Methode die nur abdominell mögliche Lymphonodektomie als gewichtiges Argument gegen die vaginale Operation ins Feld. Es wäre zu erwarten gewesen, daß die vaginale Operation die therapeutische Bedeutung einbüßen würde, die ihr früher beigemessen wurde. Die Anhänger beider operativer Schulen spalteten sich jedoch in zwei Gruppen, als man erkennen mußte, daß durch das radikalere Vorgehen unter damaligen Bedingungen keineswegs mit einer Verbesserung der Heilungsergebnisse zu rechnen war und die Komplikationsrate vielmehr die Spätergebnisse beeinträchtigte.

Wenn auch schon bald nach Entdeckung der Röntgenstrahlen und des Radiums ionisierende Strahlen bei Collumcarcinomen mit Erfolg Anwendung fanden, so stellt doch erst der Kongreß der ,,Deutschen Gesellschaft für Gynäkologie'' in Halle im Jahre 1913 einen Markstein in der geschichtlichen Entwicklung der Behandlung des Collumcarcinoms dar. Auf diesem Kongreß berichteten BUMM sowie DOEDERLEIN, KRÖNIG und GAUSS, KROEMER und KLEIN über so gute Behandlungsergebnisse mit einer ausschließlichen Radiumbestrahlung beim Collumcarcinom, daß ihre Ergebnisse eine Wende in der Therapie der Genitalcarcinome der Frau einleiteten. Wenn auch WERTHEIM auf diesem Kongreß resigniert zugab, daß seine erweiterte Totalexstirpation damit wohl überflüssig geworden sei, mögen diese Äußerungen wohl noch übertrieben gewesen sein. Die weitere Entwicklung zeigte aber, daß die Indikation zur damals bereits perfektionierten Standardoperation durch die günstigen Erfolge mit der Radiumbehandlung immer weiter eingeschränkt wurde. Erst durch die Errungenschaften der modernen Chirurgie in den 40er Jahren eroberten sich die operativen Behandlungsverfahren diesen Indikationsbereich zurück (s. S. 141).

Die stürmische Weiterentwicklung der radiologischen Behandlungsmethoden in den folgenden Jahren an allen größeren gynäkologischen Behandlungszentren brachte es mit sich, daß in den folgenden Jahrzehnten bereits der größte Teil der Patientinnen mit einem Collumcarcinom einer Radiumbestrahlung unterzogen wurde. Es zeigte sich, daß bei operablen Stadien Heilungsergebnisse mit ausschließlicher Radiumbestrahlung von 50% und mehr erzielt werden konnten. Zwischen Operation und Bestrahlung entstand ein echter Wettstreit. Für viele Anhänger operativer Schulen bestand die optimale Behandlung in der sog. „elektiven Therapie". Hierunter verstand man die Bevorzugung der Radikaloperation bei den operablen Fällen. Fälle mit allgemeiner oder lokaler Inoperabilität — hierzu zählten die Fälle mit einer bis zur Beckenwand reichenden Tumorinfiltration — blieben der reinen Strahlentherapie vorbehalten.

Die weitere Verbesserung der Behandlungsergebnisse durch die Fortschritte der Strahlentherapie des Collumcarcinoms wurde auch von Anhängern der operativen Methoden anerkannt. Rein operative Schulen gab es nur noch vereinzelt. Meist waren hierfür äußere Umstände entscheidend: Fehlen jeglicher radioaktiver Substanzen, Kenntnis oder Unkenntnis der einen oder anderen Heilmethode. Die Einstellung, prinzipiell der Operation den Vorzug zu geben, weil sie ein hohes Kulturgut darstellt, wurde allgemein abgelehnt. Die Mitteilungen über statistisch belegte Behandlungsergebnisse, in denen Mortalität und Komplikationen berücksichtigt wurden, häuften sich. Es wurde eine exakte Stadieneinteilung gefordert, um Behandlungsmethoden auch bei unterschiedlich zusammengesetztem Patientengut vergleichen zu können. Wenn es auch vielen Operateuren schwer fiel, sich vom erlernten Vorgehen zu trennen, so konnten sie doch die Erfolge der Radiumbehandlung nicht leugnen. Die elektive Therapie fand die größte Anhängerschaft. Gegen rein radiologisches Vorgehen wurden die bekannten Mißerfolge bei strahlenresistenten Tumoren im operablen Stadium ins Feld geführt. Entscheidend mögen auch häufiger psychologische Momente gewesen sein: am Ende der Operation hat der Operateur das beruhigende Gefühl, den Krebsherd eliminiert zu haben. Nach einer Strahlenbehandlung vergehen oft mehrere Wochen, bis der Behandlungserfolg abgesehen werden kann. Die Operation gibt dem Arzt eher das Gefühl, aktiv in das Krankheitsgeschehen und die Rettung des Lebens eingegriffen zu haben, während der radiologisch arbeitende Arzt eher als Zuschauer die Wirkung der in der Tiefe stattfindenden Ionisationsvorgänge abwartet (Eymer).

Bei der elektiven Therapie standen sich somit Bestrahlung und Operation nicht als rivalisierende Methoden gegenüber, sondern beide sind als sich ergänzende Methoden bei der Behandlung des Collumcarcinoms anzusehen. Stoeckel verstand unter elektiver Therapie ein „Miteinander" von Operation und Bestrahlung mit individualisierendem Vorgehen durch Auswahl und Kombination der Methoden für jeden einzelnen Fall. „Allgemein Inoperable" (Martius) wurden primär von der Operation ausgeschlossen. Hierzu zählten erheblich reduzierter Allgemeinzustand, Erkrankungen des Herz-Kreislaufsystems, Lungen- und Nierenerkrankungen sowie andere schwere Organerkrankungen. Eine lokal, durch das Carcinom gegebene Kontraindikation gegen die klassische Carcinomoperation ergab sich nach Amreich bei einer Krebsinfiltration des Parametriums bis an die Beckenwand, bei einer Infiltration der Blase, des Harnleiters oder des Mastdarms und bei einer Fernmetastasierung.

Während etwa im Jahre 1940 im allgemeinen noch Übereinstimmung über die Behandlungsprinzipien des Collumcarcinoms in den Behandlungszentren der Welt bestand, kam die Diskussion über die optimale Therapie dieser Erkrankung in der Folgezeit wieder erheblich in Fluß. Maßgeblich hierfür waren die Fortschritte durch die Errungenschaften der Chirurgie und auch der Carcinomdiagnostik. Anlaß gab die von Meigs propagierte, sehr ausgedehnte Radikaloperation mit vorangestellter Lymphonodektomie. Moderne

Narkoseverfahren, Blutersatz, Schockbehandlung und Infektionsbekämpfung führten dazu, daß in den folgenden Jahren die zwar schon primär von WERTHEIM geforderte, später aber wegen der hohen Mortalität wieder verlassene Radikalität bessere Behandlungsergebnisse versprach. Im Jahre 1955 berichtete MEIGS über 473 operierte Fälle mit einer primären Mortalität von 1,7% und einer relativen 5-Jahres-Heilung von 64,5%. Eine noch größere Radikalität des operativen Eingriffes gab BRUNSCHWIG 1951 an. Bei fortgeschrittenen Carcinomen mit einer Infiltration der Blase und des Rectums führte er eine Evisceration durch. Die Entfernung der Beckeneingeweide richtet sich nach dem Ausmaß der Lokalisation der Tumorinfiltration. Durch eine vordere Evisceration wird neben dem Uterus, den Anhängen, dem Beckenbindegewebe, der Vagina und der Vulva auch die Blase mit Urethra und den distalen Ureterabschnitten entfernt. Diese Operation macht einen künstlichen Blasenersatz notwendig. Bei der hinteren Evisceration wird neben den Genitalorganen Rectum und Sigma entfernt. Die Blase wird belassen. Bei der kompletten Evisceration wird neben den Genitalorganen sowohl die Blase mit Urethra und dem distalen Ureterabschnitt als auch Rectum und Sigma mit der gesamten Vulva entfernt. Anus praeter und Blasenersatz werden erforderlich. Derart ultraradikale Eingriffe dauern 6—8 Std. Die primäre Mortalität liegt zwischen 10 und 30%. Erhebliche Komplikationen können die Folge sein: schwerste Blutungen, Ileus, Fistelbildungen des Harntraktes und des Darmes.

Wenn auch diese ultraradikalen Eingriffe wegen ihrer gefürchteten Komplikationen und der hohen Anforderung an operative Technik noch keine größere Verbreitung finden konnten, ist nicht zu leugnen, daß sie in der Hand eines erfahrenen Chirurgen Ergebnisse bringen, die mit keiner anderen Behandlungsmethode erzielt werden können. Dieses gilt in besonderem Maße für die von BRICKER eng umgrenzte Indikationsstellung, der derartige ultraradikale Eingriffe nur in jenen Fällen durchführt, bei denen andere Behandlungsmethoden versagt haben. Er nimmt eine Evisceration nur dann vor, wenn es sich um Rezidiverkrankungen nach vorausgegangener Operation oder Bestrahlung handelt und durch eine erneute Strahlenbehandlung infolge Strahlenresistenz mit einer Rückbildung des Tumors nicht mehr zu rechnen ist.

Der Entwicklung zu radikalen Behandlungsmaßnahmen des Collumcarcinoms stehen erstaunlicherweise Bestrebungen entgegen, die eine Einschränkung des operativen Eingriffes verlangen. Die Berechtigung zu dieser Ansicht ergibt sich aus der weiteren Entwicklung der Diagnostik. Durch spezielle Untersuchungsverfahren wie Kolposkopie und Cytologie wurde es möglich, Vorstadien und beginnende kleinste Carcinomherde an der Portio zu diagnostizieren. Die als Präcancerose, Oberflächencarcinom, Carcinoma in situ, präinvasives Carcinom, Portiocarcinom Stadium 0, beginnendes Carcinom oder Mikrocarcinom bezeichneten Veränderungen warfen die Frage auf, welche Behandlungsmethode in diesen Frühfällen angezeigt ist. Da sich nur ein Teil dieser „Vorstadien" in einer im Einzelfall nicht abzusehenden Latenzzeit in ein echtes Carcinom umwandelt, erscheint eine „große Krebstherapie" mit den zu fürchtenden Komplikationen nicht gerechtfertigt. So begnügen sich Gynäkologen vielfach mit der Portioamputation bzw. Konisation oder führen allenfalls bei ausgedehnteren Befunden oder in höherem Lebensalter die einfache vaginale oder abdominale Uterusexstirpation durch.

In den letzten Jahren scheint sich an den Behandlungszentren der Welt hinsichtlich der Beurteilung der Indikationsstellung zur Operation oder Bestrahlung eine Wende anzubahnen. Durch die Möglichkeit, neue Energiequellen für strahlentherapeutische Zwecke auszunutzen, scheint sich das Schwergewicht, das in der vorigen Phase auf dem operativen Sektor lag, bei der Behandlung des Collumcarcinoms wieder zugunsten radiologischer Maßnahmen zu verlagern.

Diese Entwicklung ist bis heute noch keineswegs abgeschlossen. Trotzdem findet man im Schrifttum ausreichend Hinweise mit klinisch belegten Heilungsergebnissen dafür, daß die Einführung ultraharter Strahlenenergien in die Percutanbestrahlung sowie die interstitielle, parametrane und neuerdings auch intralymphatische Radionuclidapplikation

Möglichkeiten schaffen, vor allem fortgeschrittene Collumcarcinome in höherem Prozentsatz zu heilen. Hinzu kommt die Erfahrung, daß die bis zur äußersten Radikalität gehende operative Technik mit subtiler Ausräumung aller erreichbaren pelvinen Lymphknoten keinesfalls die Ergebnisse erbracht hat, die man primär erwartet hatte.

So macht sich hinsichtlich der Indikationsstellung zur erweiterten operativen Tumortherapie bereits wieder eine gewisse rückläufige Tendenz bemerkbar, während sich andererseits die Erfahrungen häufen, daß auch topographisch ungünstig gelegene, früher als strahlenresistent angesehene Tumoren bei Anwendung moderner Bestrahlungsverfahren einer Heilung zugeführt werden können. Wenn sich dadurch auch keineswegs erneut Operation und Bestrahlung als konkurrierende Verfahren gegenüberstehen, scheint sich heute aber die Strahlentherapie den Indikationsbereich — allerdings mit größerem Behandlungserfolg — zurückzuerobern, der ihr in der Phase der elektiven Therapie zuerkannt worden war. Während wir mit gewissem Recht behaupten können, daß die operative Technik die Grenze ihrer Leistungsfähigkeit erreicht hat — denken wir beispielsweise an die bereits mit Erfolg durchgeführte Hemikorporektomie — so befindet sich die Strahlentherapie heute ohne Zweifel wieder in einer Phase stürmischer Entwicklung. Methodische Fortschritte bewährter und neuer Verfahren sowie die zunehmende Kenntnis strahlenbiologischer Vorgänge, die die Strahlentherapie von der Empirie zu einer wissenschaftlich und biologisch untermauerten Behandlungsmethode macht, berechtigen zur Hoffnung auf größere Effektivität radiologischer Behandlungsmethoden, die sich auf die Beurteilung der Indikationsstellung zur Operation oder Bestrahlung auswirken.

Besondere Bedeutung kommt bei der Indikationsstellung zur Operation oder Bestrahlung den mit anderen Genitalerkrankungen kombinierten Collumcarcinomen zu. Bei großen Myomen wird man einer primären Operation den Vorzug geben, da sich unter diesen Umständen ungünstige Lokalverhältnisse für die Strahlentherapie ergeben. Auch bei submukösen oder knolligen intramuralen Myomknoten kann durch die Strahlenbehandlung eine Nekrose oder eitrige Einschmelzung eintreten. Während chronische Adnexentzündungen oder Adnextumoren keine Kontraindikation zu einer Bestrahlung darstellen, kann man aber bei einer akuten, entzündlichen Adnexerkrankung oder Pyosalpinx durch eine Strahlentherapie eine Exacerbation mit peritonealen Reaktionen hervorrufen. Selbst bei subchronischen Pyosalpingen kann es zu einem Aufflackern kommen. Deshalb wird in solchen Fällen der primären Operation mit ausschließlicher Exstirpation des Adnexbefundes oder aber bei lokaler Operabilität einer erweiterten Radikaloperation der Vorzug gegeben. Selbst bei Aufflackern eines Entzündungsherdes unter der Strahlenbehandlung sollte der operative Eingriff vorgenommen werden, der dann lediglich in einer Exstirpation besteht. Die Strahlenbehandlung sollte so bald wie möglich fortgesetzt werden. Ovarialtumoren und Collumcarcinom können unabhängig voneinander vorkommen. Da es sehr selten ist, daß ein Collumcarcinom ins Ovar metastasiert, erscheint es angezeigt, den Ovarialtumor operativ zu entfernen. In 20—25% der Fälle ist mit einem bösartigen Ovarialtumor zu rechnen, der unabhängig vom Collumcarcinom bestehen kann. Bei der Kombination Ovarialtumor und Collumcarcinom ist demnach die radikale operative Entfernung des Genitale die Operation der Wahl. Bei der Kombination eines Collumcarcinoms mit einer akuten fieberhaften Adnexitis sollte zunächst eine intensive antibiotische Therapie versucht und bei Versagen eine Salpingo-Oophorektomie mit nachfolgender Bestrahlung des Collumcarcinoms durchgeführt werden (Darcis, 1961). So konnte Kottmeier (1957) bei Fällen mit akuter oder rezidivierender chronischer Salpingitis durch Entfernung der Adnexe vor der Bestrahlung und Anwendung von Radium ungefähr eine Woche nach dieser Operation befriedigende Resultate erzielen. Eine spezielle Indikation zur Operation ergibt sich weiterhin bei einem Totalprolaps des Uterus, der für die Strahlenbehandlung schlechte topographische Voraussetzungen bietet.

Wir müssen heute bekennen, daß die bei anderen Organkrebsen fester umrissene Indikationsabgrenzung von Operation und Bestrahlung beim Collumcarcinom nicht gegeben ist. Die seit nun mehr als 50 Jahren heftig diskutierte Frage, ob die Operation oder die Bestrahlung als Grundstein der Behandlung des Collumcarcinoms anzusehen ist, bleibt auch bis heute noch ungelöst. Trotzdem soll versucht werden, allgemein anerkannte *Behandlungsrichtlinien* für die Therapie des Collumcarcinoms aufzustellen:

Bei den sog. Vorstadien, dem Stadium 0 der internationalen Klassifizierung, wird auf eine große Carcinomtherapie verzichtet. Handelt es sich um jüngere Frauen, wird der Eingriff auf eine Ringbiopsie, Konisation oder Portioamputation beschränkt. Bei älteren Patientinnen wird der vaginalen Totalexstirpation der Vorzug gegeben.

In den operablen Stadien des Collumcarcinoms, dem Stadium I und teilweise auch II (das sog. II a) empfehlen die meisten Gynäkologen die vaginale oder abdominale erweiterte Totalexstirpation, wodurch die besonders bei Frauen vor dem 6. Lebensjahrzehnt mit Folgen behaftete Kastration vermieden werden kann. Von größeren operativen Schulen wird eine obligate Lymphonodektomie durchgeführt. Wenn auch bisher nicht bewiesen ist, daß die Heilungsergebnisse dadurch zu verbessern sind, gestattet die Lymphonodektomie doch zumindest, den Entschluß zu einer postoperativen Bestrahlung bei nachgewiesener Lymphknotenmetastasierung zu erleichtern. Bei fehlendem Lymphknotenbefall ist der Wert einer Nachbestrahlung nicht erwiesen.

Eine ausschließliche Strahlenbehandlung erreicht bei den operablen Stadien des Collumcarcinoms die gleichen Heilungsergebnisse.

In den Stadien III und IV gilt allgemein die Strahlenbehandlung als Methode der Wahl. Es erscheint als sicher erwiesen, daß eine operative Behandlung die Heilungsergebnisse in diesen Stadien signifikant verschlechtert. Trotzdem wird an vielen Stellen in der Welt, oft aus Mangel an radiologischer Erfahrung oder apparativer Voraussetzung, ein Collumcarcinom mit parametraner Infiltration bis zur Beckenwand operiert. Diese Verhältnisse trifft man vor allem an kleineren Kliniken an. Die signifikant schlechteren Behandlungsergebnisse sind jedoch ein Grund, diese Maßnahmen abzulehnen. Wenn derartige Behandlungsmethoden an größeren Kliniken ausgeführt werden, so sind Fanatismus, besonderer operativer Ehrgeiz oder übertriebene und nicht berechtigte Skepsis gegenüber der Strahlentherapie Beweggründe für diese extreme Einstellung.

Ultraradikale Operationsmethoden sollten auch heute noch, trotz der Fortschritte der allgemeinen Chirurgie, auf jene Fälle beschränkt bleiben, in denen die sonst üblichen Methoden absolut erfolglos bleiben würden. Deshalb muß die Brunschwigsche Exenteration lediglich größeren operativen Behandlungszentren bei Rezidiverkrankungen oder erwiesener Strahlenresistenz vorbehalten bleiben. Eine bis zur Beckenwand reichende Tumorinfiltration stellt eine absolute Kontraindikation zu einer ultraradikalen Operation dar.

3. Allgemeine Grundsätze bei der Strahlenbehandlung des Collumcarcinoms
a) Die Strahlensensibilität des Collumcarcinoms

Die Kenntnis der Faktoren, die in ihrer Gesamtheit die Strahlenheilbarkeit eines Tumors bestimmen, ist bis heute noch sehr lückenhaft. Wenn wir auch zahlreiche Faktoren angeben können, die die Strahlensensibilität eines Tumors beeinflussen, so ist es aber nur sehr grob möglich, im Einzelfall den Grad der Strahlensensibilität zu beurteilen.

Plattenepithelcarcinome werden in einer Zusammenstellung der Strahlensensibilität von Geschwülsten nach PATERSON (1933) als „mäßig strahlensensibel" angesehen, während beispielsweise das Seminom, das Lymphom, das Ewing-Sarkom und andere als strahlensensible Tumoren gelten. Adenocarcinome gelten in dieser Zusammenstellung als „mäßig strahlenresistent".

WARREN (1947) bezeichnet das Collumcarcinom als radioresponsiv, da 5000 R als wirksame Strahlendosis gelten, wobei nur wenig Schaden am Normalgewebe entsteht. Eine solche schematische Einteilung besitzt aber nur geringen klinischen Wert; denn wir wissen, daß die Strahlensensibilität der Collumcarcinome stark differieren kann. Eine höhere Ausdifferenzierung der Tumorzellen beispielsweise bedeutet eine herabgesetzte Strahlenempfindlichkeit. Sie wird durch verminderten Stoffwechsel und eine geringere

Zellteilungstätigkeit bedingt sein. In biochemischer Hinsicht ist eine gesteigerte Strahlensensibilität oft mit einem intensiveren Nucleoproteidstoffwechsel verbunden. Reife Plattenepithelcarcinome sind viel strahlenresistenter als die unreiferen Formen. Andererseits erbringen ausgereifte Tumoren günstigere Heilungsresultate als anaplastische. Verhornende Plattenepithelcarcinome haben bei einer Strahlenbehandlung eine bessere Prognose und weisen damit eine größere Strahlensensibilität auf als unreife anaplastische Tumoren. Weiterhin wird die Mitoserate als Index für den Grad der Strahlensensibilität angegeben.

Einen zusätzlichen Einfluß üben Größe des Tumors sowie die dadurch gegebene Gefäßversorgung aus. Es ist bekannt, daß größere Tumoren meist eine schlechtere Vascularisation besitzen. Dadurch verringert sich die Durchblutung und auch die Strahlenempfindlichkeit des Tumors. Durch eine hypoxische Situation kann die Strahlensensibilität erheblich vermindert werden. FLETCHER (1966) nimmt sogar an, daß die differente Sauerstoffversorgung ausschließlich für den Grad der Strahlensensibilität verantwortlich gemacht werden muß. Die Erfahrung, daß die Strahlensensibilität des Tumors bei anämischen Patientinnen verringert war, wurde durch EVANS und BERGSJØ (1965) eindeutig belegt. Sie ermittelten eine signifikant schlechtere Heilungsrate bei Patientinnen mit einer Anämie. Im Stadium II und III waren strahlenresistente Collumcarcinome bei Patientinnen mit einer Anämie besonders häufig. Um die dadurch bedingte Tumoranoxie zu beheben, führen sie in solchen Fällen vor einer Radiumeinlage Bluttransfusionen durch.

Darüber hinaus können auch allgemeine Faktoren die Strahlensensibilität beeinflussen. Eine Infektion des Tumors oder der Tumorumgebung verringert die Strahlensensibilität beträchtlich. Der Allgemeinzustand und das Alter der Patientinnen verändern ebenfalls die Strahlenwirksamkeit. Sie ist bei kachektischen Patientinnen erheblich herabgesetzt. Jüngere Patientinnen haben bessere Heilungschancen. Dieser Unterschied wird durch eine humorale Abwehrfunktion des Organismus erklärt.

Ein besonderes Problem in der gynäkologischen Strahlentherapie stellt die Strahlensensibilität des Adenocarcinoms des Collum uteri dar. Im Schrifttum findet sich die allgemein übereinstimmende Erfahrung, daß das Adenocarcinom eine schlechtere Heilungsprognose hat (LIMBURG und THOMSEN, 1949; DOEDERLEIN, 1953; BUTTENBERG, 1960). In den operablen Stadien ist die Heilungschance die gleiche wie beim Plattenepithelcarcinom. Lediglich bei den radiologisch behandelten, fortgeschrittenen Fällen von Adenocarcinom sind die Heilungsaussichten wesentlich schlechter als beim Plattenepithelcarcinom. Daraus folgert man, daß die Strahlensensibilität beim Adenocarcinom geringer ist. Die schlechtere Prognose beim radiologisch behandelten Adenocarcinom wird aber auch damit begründet, daß es rascher metastasiert. Weiterhin wird das Durchschnittsalter der Patientinnen um 10—15 Jahre älter als das bei den Patientinnen mit Plattenepithelcarcinomen angegeben (DOEDERLEIN, 1953). Wenn andererseits behauptet wird, daß der Beweis noch nicht erbracht wäre, daß das Adenocarcinom strahlenrefraktär sei (KOTTMEIER, 1952; EYMER, 1953; RIES, 1959), muß berücksichtigt werden, daß von vielen Autoren bei Adenocarcinomen eine um 20—25% höhere Strahlendosis gegenüber dem Plattenepithelcarcinom verabreicht wird. Am Patientengut der Universitäts-Frauenklinik Hamburg konnte gezeigt werden, daß beim Adenocarcinom der Cervix die 5-Jahres-Heilung um 20% niedriger liegt, wenn bei der radiologischen Behandlung die gleiche Herddosis wie beim Plattenepithelcarcinom eingestrahlt wird.

Die Strahlenempfindlichkeit der seltenen Collumsarkome soll der bei Plattenepithelcarcinomen etwa entsprechen. RIES und BREITNER (1959) empfehlen die gleiche Strahlendosis wie beim Collumcarcinom, beginnen jedoch mit höheren Einzelfraktionen. Sie warnen vor einer operativen Behandlung des Collumsarkoms, da die Behandlungsergebnisse dann trotz Nachbestrahlung schlechter sind als die der primären Strahlentherapie. Jede Manipulation soll die Gefahr der Metastasierung erhöhen. Einer Gewebsentnahme soll eine unmittelbare Radiumbehandlung angeschlossen werden.

Im Einzelfall ist es trotz Berücksichtigung aller die Strahlensensibilität beeinflussenden Faktoren nicht möglich, einen exakten Hinweis für die Prognose eines Tumors zu geben. Daher wird seit langem versucht, die empirischen Regeln der Strahlensensibilität durch eine spezielle histologische Beurteilung des Anaplasiegrades, der Mitosehäufigkeit und der Plasmabasophilie am Tumor sowie der Bindegewebs- und Gefäßreaktionen am Stroma zu erweitern. Ein anfangs erfolgversprechender Versuch der histologischen Beurteilung der Strahlungsempfindlichkeit wurde von GLUCKSMANN (1945) ausgearbeitet. Beim Collumcarcinom wird hierbei an Hand fortlaufender histologischer Kontrollen während und nach der Strahlenbehandlung aus dem Verhältnis lebensfähiger (ruhender und mitotischer) zu nicht lebensfähigen (differenzierten und degenerativen) Zellen die Ansprechbarkeit der Geschwulst auf die Bestrahlung beurteilt. Bei einer hohen Strahlensensibilität kommt es vor allem zu einem kontinuierlichen Abfall der Ruhezellzahl und einem entsprechenden Anstieg degenerativer Zellen. Auf diese Weise soll in etwa 75 % der Fälle eine Aussage über die die Prognose beeinflussende Strahlensensibilität möglich sein. Andere Autoren konnten diese Ergebnisse aber nicht bestätigen; zwischen Tumormorphologie und dem Ansprechen auf die Bestrahlung brauchen keine engen Beziehungen zu bestehen (HERTIG und GORE, 1962). Andererseits liegen Mitteilungen vor, daß sich die Heilungsergebnisse nach Überschreiten einer bestimmten Dosis wieder verschlechtern (NOLAN und DU SAULT, 1952).

Von GRAHAM und GRAHAM (1953) wurde die Cytodiagnostik des Vaginalepithels zur Beurteilung der Strahlensensibilität beim Collumcarcinom herangezogen. Aus dem Persistieren von Tumorzellen und durch qualitative Erfassung der Strahlenreaktionen an normalen Vaginalepithelien glauben sie, Hinweise auf die Prognose geben zu können. Sie haben diese Testmöglichkeit an Normalepithelien zu einem quantitativen Verfahren ausgebaut. Bei einer guten allgemeinen Strahlensensibilität sollen bereits vor einer Bestrahlung bei mindestens 10 % der Zellen eine distinkte Vacuolisierung, rote Granula und ein verdichtetes Plasma nachweisbar sein. Eine hinreichend gute Ansprechbarkeit des Tumors nach einer Probebestrahlung kann angenommen werden, wenn bei mindestens 75 % der Zellen Vacuolisierung, eine eindeutige quantitativ feststellbare Vergrößerung der Zellen, Kernvergrößerung, Kernveränderungen und Chromatinkondensation beobachtet werden können.

Auch diese cytologischen Veränderungen konnten von anderen Autoren bei Kontrolluntersuchungen nicht eindeutig bestätigt werden. Insbesondere die Untersuchungen von LIMBURG et al. (1952), BUTTENBERG et al. (1960) sowie RUBIO et al. (1965) haben ergeben, daß mit der Vaginalcytologie sowohl bei Berücksichtigung der Reaktionen normaler Zellen als auch bei Beurteilung von Tumorzellveränderungen für die Klinik keine hinreichend sichere Testung der Strahlensensibilität beim Collumcarcinom gegeben ist.

Auf ähnlicher Basis liegen die Untersuchungen von GUSBERG und HERMAN (1962). Sie untersuchten cytologisch und cytochemisch die Wirkung einer Testdosis von 2mal 800 R im Abstand von 24 Std bei Patientinnen mit Cervixcarcinom. Nach H.-E.-Färbung, Methylgrün-Pyroninfärbung und Orcein-Lichtgrünfärbung unterscheiden sie 3 Typen von Tumorzellreaktionen: Tod und Auflösung der Zellen, stärkere Differenzierung der Zellen sowie Vergrößerung der Zellen, der Zellkerne und Nucleolen mit Veränderungen des Chromatinmaterials. Diese Untersuchungen wurden 1966 durch YANAGITA, HERMAN und GUSBERG auch auf autoradiographische Untersuchungen vor und nach einer Testdosis erweitert. Sie versuchen, die autoradiographische Beurteilung der Synthese der Nucleinsäuren DNA und RNA zum Grading der Strahlensensibilität heranzuziehen.

Eng verbunden mit dem Problem der Strahlensensibilität ist die klinisch genau so wichtige Frage nach der optimalen Strahlendosis, die zur sicheren Devitalisierung eines Tumors notwendig ist. Nach Entwicklung der Apparaturen zur Erzeugung von Megavoltenergien, die eine konzentrierte Einstrahlung auch höchster Strahlendosen ermöglichen, findet dieses Problem wieder in zunehmendem Maße im Schrifttum Beachtung. So glaubt man heute schon vielfach, daß das Maß der Strahlensensibilität bzw. Strahlenresistenz ausschließlich ein Problem der Dosishöhe ist. Hierfür sprechen beispielsweise die Erfahrungen von Fletcher u. Mitarb. (1962), die selbst bei den strahlenresistent geltenden Adenocarcinomen nach Einstrahlung einer höheren Dosis eine wesentliche Verbesserung der Heilungsergebnisse erzielen konnten.

Beim Collumcarcinom ist die Schwankungsbreite der von den einzelnen Autoren geforderten Dosishöhe besonders groß, da beim Collumcarcinom durch die intrakavitäre Radiumapplikation mit dem steilen Dosisabfall Strahlendosen von 10000—20000, ja selbst 30000 R ohne Schädigung der Nachbargewebe eingestrahlt werden können. Als erforderliche Dosis werden im allgemeinen aber etwa 10000 R angesehen (Mitra, 1952). Ob die oft höheren Strahlendosen unbedingt zur Tumordevitalisierung notwendig sind, ist bis heute nicht entschieden. So konnte bereits Baclesse 1954 zeigen, daß bei sehr strahlensensiblen Tumoren nach einer ausschließlichen percutanen Röntgenbestrahlung schon Herddosen bis zu 7000 R zu einer Heilung geführt haben. Die Erfahrungen der letzten Jahre unterstützen diese Beobachtungen, nachdem in größerem Umfang insbesondere bei fortgeschrittenen Tumoren auf eine lokale Radiumapplikation verzichtet wird. In derartigen Fällen sah man (Mellor, 1960; Giezelt u. Mitarb., 1962; Frischbier, 1967), daß die gleichen Frühreaktionen an der Portio nach Dosen von etwa 7000—8000 R auftreten wie nach einer lokalen Radiumbehandlung von etwa 5000 mgeh. Kottmeier (1953) hält sogar eine Dosis von 5000—6000 R für den Lokaltumor an der Portio für ausreichend.

Vergleicht man die Behandlungsmethoden und insbesondere die applizierte Dosishöhe in den verschiedenen großen Behandlungszentren der Welt, so erkennt man nur schwer einen Zusammenhang zwischen Heilungsquote und Dosishöhe an der Portio. Trotzdem werden im Schrifttum Radiumdosen empfohlen, die zwischen 3000 und 12000 mgeh liegen (s. Kap. „Intrakavitäre Curietherapie", s. S. 182).

Eine größere Beachtung findet die Strahlendosis in der Umgebung der Portio. Hierbei interessieren einmal die vom Tumor befallenen Organe, Parametrien und Beckenwandlymphknoten, sowie die umliegenden gesunden Organe, Blase, Rectum und Ureteren. Die Gewebstoleranz dieser Organe bewegt sich in wesentlich kleineren Grenzen. Ries (1953) hebt hervor, daß die Gewebsbelastbarkeit von verschiedenen Faktoren abhängt: Feldgröße, Strahlenqualität, Zeitfaktor, Individualität des Gewebes, lokale Veränderungen wie Entzündung und Operationsfolgen sowie Konstitutionstyp der Patienten. Aber auch hier ist es unmöglich, scharfe Grenzen der Gewebstoleranz zu ziehen. So wird in der gynäkologischen Strahlentherapie die Belastbarkeit von Blase und Rectum je nach der Fraktionierung zwischen 4000 und 8000 R angenommen.

Nicht zu unterschätzen ist die bestehende Toleranzdosis des lockeren, gefäßführenden Bindegewebes, des Parametriums, das von der Cervix zur Beckenwand zieht. Noch 1958 gab Ries auf Grund seiner umfangreichen Beobachtungen für das Parametrium eine Toleranzdosis von 4000—4500 R an, wenn nicht das ganze Parametrium, insbesondere der beckenwandnahe Anteil, von dieser hohen Dosis erfaßt wird. Die intensive Mitbestrahlung auch des beckenwandnahen Anteils, von dem die Gefäßversorgung ausgeht, führt zur Gewebssklerosierung mit Ureterstenosen und Blasenschrumpfung. Ries strebt deshalb eine Belastung des Bindegewebes an der Beckenwand von nicht mehr als 3000—3200 R an. Er diskutiert ebenfalls, ob bereits niedrigere Dosen zur Tumorrückbildung genügen.

Während eine Dosis von 3000—4000 R im Parametrium in der Ära der konventionellen Röntgentherapie als allgemein gültige Richtdosis angesehen werden konnte, mehren sich in den letzten Jahren bei Anwendung von Megavoltenergien Stimmen, die zur Devitalisierung der parametranen Infiltration und insbesondere von den Beckenwandlymphknotenmetastasen eine Herddosis von mindestens 4000—6000 R und teilweise sogar mehr als notwendig erachten (Fletcher et al., 1962). Wenn auch bis heute die Heilungsergebnisse durch die Erhöhung der Strahlendosis nicht signifikant verbessert werden konnten, so wurden die Strahlenschäden dadurch keinesfalls erhöht (Nolan, 1965; Fletcher, 1966; Frischbier, 1967.) Die ersten Erfahrungen zeigen aber doch, daß die Zahl der nicht auf ionisierende Strahlen ansprechenden Fälle geringer zu sein scheint. NOLAN (1959) glaubt deshalb, daß eine weitere Dosiserhöhung an der seitlichen Beckenwand ohne Erhöhung der Dosis an den proximalen Anteilen des Parametriums geeignet ist, die Ausbreitung der Krebserkrankung günstig zu beeinflussen. Ähnliche Beobachtungen machte PORTER bereits 1952, obwohl er häufiger Scheidenfisteln sah. Ein Extrem in bezug auf die Dosishöhe stellen zweifellos die von ISCHTSCHENKO (1960) verabfolgten Dosen bei der Behandlung von weiblichen Genitaltumoren mit dem 25-MeV-Betatron dar. Er appliziert bis zu 20000 R Gesamtdosis im Herd, ohne allerdings nähere Angaben über Strahlenfolgen zu machen.

b) Das Lymphknotenproblem

Nachdem in der ersten Hälfte dieses Jahrhunderts das Schwergewicht bei der Behandlung des Collumcarcinoms auf den Primärtumor und die Parametrien gelegt worden war, wurde in den letzten Jahren das Interesse vor allem auf die regionären Lymphknoten gelenkt. Umfangreiche histologische Untersuchungen der Operationspräparate nach Radikaloperation mit obligater Lymphonodektomie haben gezeigt, daß bereits bei klinisch frühen Stadien in einem beachtlichen Prozentsatz mit einer Metastasierung in die Beckenwandlymphknoten zu rechnen ist. Wie aus einer tabellarischen Zusammenstellung aus dem Weltschrifttum (Tabelle 1) zu entnehmen ist, muß im Stadium I mit einer Lymphknotenmetastasierung in 10—40%, im Stadium II in 25—50% und im Stadium III in 40—70% der Fälle gerechnet werden. Danach kann schon in den Fällen, bei denen der Tumor klinisch auf den Uterus oder die uterusnahen parametranen Anteile beschränkt zu sein scheint, eine klinisch nicht nachweisbare Metastasierung in das regionäre Lymphsystem bestehen. Diese Befunde bestätigen die früheren Beobachtungen, daß sich das Collumcarcinom entweder kontinuierlich oder diskontinuierlich ausbreiten kann.

Tabelle 1. *Die Häufigkeit der Lymphknotenmetastasierung beim Collumcarcinom nach Operation.*
(Nach REIFFENSTUHL)

	Zahl der Fälle	Stadium			
		I	II	III	IV
ANTOINE (1959) (FROEWIS u. ULM)	544	8,49%	27,93%		
DEBIASI (1954) (PAPADIA)	135	20,7%	31,9%	70%	
BRUNSCHWIG u. ROESLER (1957)	74	14%	34%	44%	67%
CARTER et al. (1953)	79	16,66%	25,92%		
CATTANEO (1954) (MARZIALE)	66	20%		52,4%	
CHRISTENSEN et al. (1955)	100	21,3%	41%		
CURRIE (1962)	339	16%	38%		
GRAY (1958)	61	11%	35%		
GUSBERG et al. (1953)	64	10%	31%		
KIMBROUGH (1959)	84	34%	51%		
LANGE (1960)	178	28,8%	43,8%		
LIU u. MEIGS (1955)	258	17%	40%		
MARTINEZ et al. (1953)	442	23%	41%		
MEDINA et al. (1959)	60	20%	40%		
MEIGS u. MORTON (1958)	130	18%	37%		
MITANI et al. (1956)	182	39,9%	33,6%	62%	
MITRA (1959)	192	18%	29%	40%	
MORTON et al. (1952)	89	15%	24%		
NAVRATIL (1955)	180	20%	29%	47,3%	
PARSON (1962)	80	13%	22%		
SHERMAN et al. (1952)	176	12%	29%		
TACHIBANA (1956)	416	12%	23,7%		
WELCH et al. (1961)	383	12%	24%		
	4390	18,79%	33,26%	52,61%	

Bei einer Durchwachsung des Tumors durch die Muscularis der Cervix und einem Eindringen in das parametrane Bindegewebe spricht man von kontinuierlicher Ausbreitung. Eine diskontinuierliche Ausbreitung liegt vor, wenn sich schon relativ früh Tumorzellverbände vom Tumor lösen, über die abführenden Lymphgefäße zu den regionären Filterstationen transportiert werden und dort eine Metastase aufbauen.

Die diskontinuierliche Metastasierungsform beim Collumcarcinom rückte in den Brennpunkt des Interesses, als Ober und Huhn 1962 über sorgfältig durchgeführte histologische Untersuchungen von Operationspräparaten berichteten. Sie konnten zeigen, daß Cervix und Parametrium nicht scharf gegeneinander abgegrenzt sind, sondern von einer etwa 5 mm tiefen Grenzzone getrennt sind. Erst wenn diese Zone zur Beckenwand hin vom Tumor überschritten ist, sollte von einer parametranen Beteiligung gesprochen werden. Bedeutungsvoll erscheint der von ihnen geführte Nachweis, daß bei den klinisch operabel erschienenen Collumcarcinomen die Grenzzone zwar relativ selten überschritten wurde, daß aber in einem schon hohen Prozentsatz durch eine diskontinuierliche Metastasierung die Beckenwandlymphknoten befallen waren. Ähnliche Untersuchungsergebnisse wurden mitgeteilt von Cosbie (1960), Lange (1960), Ahrens und Tschoke (1961), Henriksen (1961) und Mitani et al. (1962).

Wenn somit nach den neueren Untersuchungen feststeht, daß der diskontinuierlichen Metastasierung eine wesentlich größere Bedeutung als früher angenommen zukommt, müssen die über mehrere Jahrzehnte geübten und anerkannten Behandlungsmethoden in ihrer Konzeption neu durchdacht werden. Aufgrund der Erkenntnisse über die Tumorausbreitung können wir mit Recht annehmen, daß eine Verbesserung der Heilungsergebnisse nur dann zu erwarten ist, wenn auch das gesamte Lymphabflußgebiet in ausreichendem Maße in den Behandlungsplan eingeschlossen wird.

Die Behandlung von Lymphknotenmetastasen wirft zahlreiche Fragen auf. Zu Beginn muß die Frage gestellt werden: wo können sich Lymphknotenmetastasen beim Collumcarcinom manifestieren? Wenn ein klinisch als Stadium I imponierendes Collumcarcinom bereits in einer Häufigkeit von durchschnittlich 15—20% Lymphknotenmetastasen gesetzt hat — und wir wissen heute, daß selbst frühinvasive Carcinome in seltenen Fällen schon Lymphknotenmetastasen setzen können (Lachs, 1953; Decker, 1956; Schiller, 1958; Friedell et al., 1959; Lock, 1961; Ober, 1962) — dann müßte bei einer sinnvollen operativen Methode nicht nur das gesamte Parametrium entfernt, sondern eine obligate Lymphonodektomie angeschlossen werden. Eine obligate Lymphonodektomie aber ist mit erheblichen Nachteilen verbunden. Sie erfordert eine Verlängerung der Operation mit Zunahme der intra- und postoperativen Komplikationen. Da heute die Kenntnis über die Funktion des lymphatischen Gewebes bei den natürlichen Abwehrvorgängen und insbesondere der Abwehrfunktion von Tumorzellverbänden noch gering ist, besteht bei einer obligaten Lymphonodektomie theoretisch die Möglichkeit, diese natürlichen Abwehrkräfte zu verringern. Andererseits ist es unmöglich, alle regionären Lymphknoten zu exstirpieren. Darüber hinaus besteht die Möglichkeit, daß neben den regionären Lymphknoten auch höher liegende Tumorabsiedelungen beispielsweise in den aortalen Lymphknoten bestehen, so daß damit eine regionäre Lymphonodektomie illusorisch wäre.

Demgegenüber steht die entmutigende Erfahrungstatsache, daß Lymphknotenmetastasen als weitgehend strahlenresistent gelten und es nur gelegentlich gelingt, durch die Strahlenbehandlung eine histologisch nachweisbare Tumorzelldevitalisierung zu erreichen. Im jüngeren Schrifttum, insbesondere durch Anwendung von Megavoltenergien mit ausreichend hohen Herddosen, sind aber viele Mitteilungen zu finden, die diese Ansicht widerlegen (s. S. 156).

Den gesamten Fragenkomplex bei der Behandlung der Lymphknotenmetastasierung fassen wir unter dem Begriff „Lymphknotenproblem" zusammen, das bereits ausführlich von Amreich (1955) und Reiffenstuhl (1967) abgehandelt ist. Wenn wir auch heute bekennen müssen, daß die einzelnen Fragen des Lymphknotenproblems keineswegs gelöst sind, sondern eher neue Fragen hinzukommen, erscheint eine eingehende Erörterung des Lymphknotenproblems bei der Darstellung der Strahlenbehandlung des Collumcarcinoms unerläßlich. In der Hoffnung, daß die entscheidenden Fragen in den nächsten Jahren durch grundlegende Untersuchungen abgeklärt werden können, ist es heute nur möglich, den derzeitigen Wissensstand aus dem Weltschrifttum zusammenzutragen.

Durch die umfangreichen Untersuchungen von REIFFENSTUHL (1957) an Leichen von Neugeborenen sind uns die zahlreichen Abflußwege von der Cervix uteri bekannt. Seine Untersuchungen bestätigen die klinische Erfahrung, daß die Cervix uteri ein weit verzweigtes Lymphsystem besitzt. Dadurch können sich an zahlreichen Lymphknoten im Becken und Retroperitonealraum primär Lymphknotenmetastasen manifestieren. In

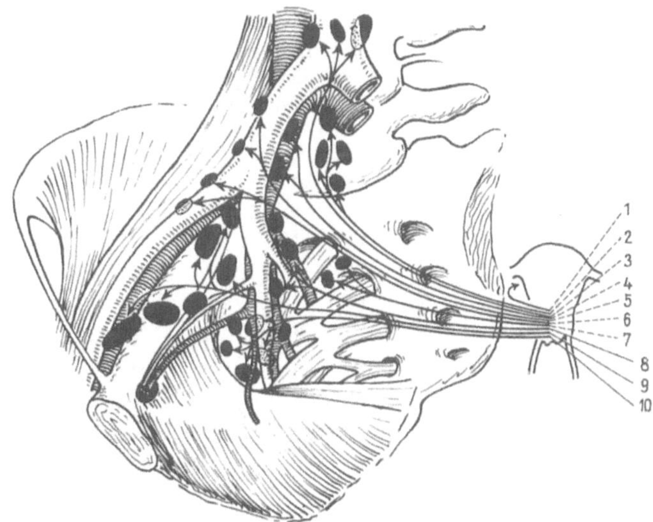

Abb. 1. Die regionären Lymphknotenstationen der Cervix uteri (REIFFENSTUHL). *1* Lnn. rectales; *2* Lnn. subaortici (promontorii); *3* Lnn. aortici; *4* Lnn. iliaci communes mediales; *5* Lnn. iliaci communes laterales; *6* Lnn. iliaci externi laterales; *7* Lnn. sacrales; *8* Lnn. glutei superiores; *9* Lnn. interiliaci; *10* Lnn. glutei inferiores

Abb. 1 sind die verschiedenen regionären Lymphknotenstationen der Cervix uteri wiedergegeben. Die am häufigsten befallenen Lymphonodi iliaci interni et externi sowie die Lnn. obturatorii faßt REIFFENSTUHL unter dem Begriff der Lnn. interiliaci zusammen.

Während früher die Meinung vertreten wurde, daß lediglich die Beckenwandlymphknoten durch direkte Verbindungen mit der Cervix uteri als regionäres Lymphsystem anzusehen sind, konnte REIFFENSTUHL ebenfalls direkte Lymphverbindungen zu den subaortalen Lymphknoten aufzeigen. Daß auch außerhalb des Beckens, oberhalb der Linea terminalis, primäre Lymphknotenmetastasen vorkommen können, konnte schon 1902 SCHAUTA zeigen. Er untersuchte sämtliche Becken- und retroperitonealen Lymphknoten von 60 an Uteruskrebs verstorbenen Patientinnen. Dabei unterschied er Lymphknoten der ersten und der zweiten Etappe. Die Lymphknoten der ersten Etappe sind bei der Operation zugänglich (Lnn. interiliaci, Lnn. iliaci externi et communes laterales, Lnn. sacrales), während die Lymphknoten der zweiten Etappe (Lnn. aortici, Lnn. inguinales) aus technischen Gründen bei der Operation nicht entfernt werden können. SCHAUTA fand nun, daß in 43,3 % der Verstorbenen histologisch keine Lymphknotenmetastasen nachweisbar waren. In 13,3 % waren nur die Lymphknoten der ersten Etappe befallen, in 8,3 % nur die Lymphknoten der zweiten Etappe, in 35 % waren die Lymphknoten

150 H.-J. Frischbier: Die Strahlenbehandlung des Collumcarcinoms

beider Etappen carcinomatös verändert. Die Untersuchungen von Reiffenstuhl erklären die Schautaschen Befunde, bei denen er von einem sprunghaften und inkonstanten Auftreten der Lymphknotenmetastasen spricht.

Es erscheint verständlich, daß in fortgeschrittenen Stadien relativ häufig aortale Lymphknotenmetastasen zu finden sind. Im Schrifttum existieren aber besonders aus den letzten Jahren mehrere Mitteilungen, in denen über eine aortale Metastasierung ohne Befall der Beckenlymphknoten berichtet wird. Diese anscheinend „irregulären" Carcinommetastasen sind durch die zahlreichen Lymphabflußwege von der Cervix durchaus erklärbar. So berichtet Way (1959) über 4 Fälle, bei denen lediglich die Lnn. iliaci communes et aortales befallen waren. Ruch (1957) teilt ebenfalls 2 Fälle von ausschließlicher aortaler Lymphknotenmetastasierung mit.

Tabelle 2. *Lokalisation der Lymphknotenmetastasen beim Collumcarcinom.* (Nach Reiffenstuhl)

Autor	Zahl der Fälle	Lnn. hypogastrici	Lnn. iliaci ext.	Lnn. obturatorii	Lnn. iliaci comm.	Lnn. parametranes	Lnn. glutei sup.	Lnn. glutei inf.	Lnn. aortici	Lnn. sacrales	Lnn. pararectales
Gorton (1964)	87	10,3%	13,8%	52,8%	13,8%	3,4%					
Way (Cherry u. Glucksmann 1955)	91	7%	47%	20%	14%	2%	7%		10%		
Remotti (1962)	71	43,6%	21,1%				25,3%				
Lange (1960)	56	42,3%	20%	37,7%							
Reiffenstuhl	96	44,1%	26,2%	20,7%	4,1%	1,4%	1,4%	0,7%		0,7%	0,7%
Javert (1954)	76	44,4%	33,3%	38,9%			22,2%		22,2%		
	477	*31,9%*	*26,9%*	*34,0%*							
Henriksen (1954)	41 *Autopsiefälle*	36%	39%	39%			*44%*				

Die Häufigkeit des metastatischen Befalls der Lymphonodi iliaci interni, externi und obturatorii wird im Schrifttum bei operierten Fällen mit 25—35 % angegeben (Tabelle 2). Die übrigen Lymphknoten zeigen einen wesentlich selteneren Befall. Hierbei ist allerdings zu berücksichtigen, daß die Möglichkeit, die einzelnen Lymphknoten zu gewinnen von der Radikalität des Eingriffes abhängt. So werden beispielsweise selbst bei „radikaler" Lymphonodektomie die Lymphonodi glutei inferiores wegen technischer Schwierigkeiten zurückgelassen. Die angegebene Häufigkeit des metastatischen Befalls kann somit nur eine Mindestzahl darstellen. Javert (1954) fand in 10 Fällen des Stadiums III und IV bei einer palliativen Operation in etwa 50 % der Fälle einen Befall der paraaortalen Lymphknoten. Andererseits berichtet Henriksen (1954) über autoptische Befunde, bei denen er in den parametranen Lymphknoten wesentlich häufiger einen Befall fand als in den Lnn. interiliaci. An Hand von Obduktionsbefunden stellten Fischer (1956) und von Massenbach (1957) fest, daß die lumbalen Lymphknoten weitaus öfter von Metastasen durchsetzt sind als die Beckenlymphknoten (s. S. 154 und 265).

Die Frequenz der Lymphknotenmetastasierung ist somit weitgehend von Patientengut und Untersuchungsmethoden abhängig. Das angeführte Schrifttum soll nur zeigen, daß praktisch in allen Lymphknotengruppen Metastasen vorliegen können, oft selbst in einem frühen Stadium, und nur *die* Behandlungsmethode zur Beseitigung von möglichen Lymphknotenmetastasen einen Erfolg haben wird, die *sämtliche* Lymphknotenstationen entfernt. Daß eine solche Forderung an eine operative Maßnahme nicht gestellt werden kann, braucht nicht hervorgehoben zu werden.

Besonderes Augenmerk richteten Nogales und Botella-Llusiá (1965) auf die Zusammenhänge zwischen Befall der Lymphknoten und histologischen Charakteristika des Tumors. Sie fanden in 312 Fällen von Collumcarcinom, bei denen eine Ausräumung der Lymphknoten ohne vorhergehende Bestrahlung durchgeführt worden war, daß das basalzellige Carcinom des Plattenepithels eine geringe Neigung zur Metastasierung in die Lymphknoten zeigt (6,5% beim Stadium I, 9,5% beim Stadium III). Dagegen wurde beim spindelzelligen Carcinom eine Invasion der Lymphknoten in 25% des Stadiums I und sogar in 60% des Stadiums III gefunden. Beim Adenocarcinom der Endocervix betrug der Befall im Stadium I 50% und im Stadium II 93%. Da die Autoren in der Quote des Lymphknotenbefalls keinen großen Unterschied zwischen den Stadien II und III fanden, schlossen sie, daß beim Spindelzell- und Adenocarcinom die Infiltrationstendenz sprunghaft ansteigt, sobald die Grenzen der Cervix überschritten sind. Für die unterschiedliche infiltrative Fähigkeit der histologischen Typen des Collumcarcinoms

Tabelle 3. *Relative Dauerheilung bei 315 Collumcarcinompatientinnen ohne oder mit obligater Lymphonodektomie.* (Rauscher und Spurny)

Stadien	Ohne obligate Lymphadenektomie, operiert zwischen Mai 1947 und Mai 1950			Mit obligater Lymphadenektomie, operiert zwischen Mai 1950 und Mai 1953		
	operiert	5-Jahre-geheilt	in %	operiert	5-Jahre-geheilt	in %
I	88	72	81,81	95	83	87,37
II	68	45	66,17	62	36	58,03
III	2	—	—	—	—	—
	158	117	74,05	157	119	75,79
			Unterschied: 1,74%			

werden Unterschiede der bindegewebigen Komponenten der Tumoren verantwortlich gemacht. Die geringe Virulenz des Basalzellcarcinoms wird als Folge der guten bindegewebigen Abgrenzung gegen die Umgebung gedeutet. Aus diesen Untersuchungen folgern sie, daß in Fällen von Basalzellcarcinom die Lymphonodektomie eine geringere Bedeutung als beim Spindelzell- und Adenocarcinom besitzt.

Wenn von einzelnen Autoren die *obligate* Lymphonodektomie empfohlen und gefordert wird, geschieht es in der Annahme, daß theoretisch durchaus die Möglichkeit besteht, einzelne Fälle mit einer Frühabsiedlung auf diese Weise zu heilen. Hierbei ergibt sich nun die wichtige Frage, ob es überhaupt möglich ist, die Behandlungsergebnisse durch die Lymphonodektomie zu verbessern. Da man seit etwa 20 Jahren wieder bestrebt ist, den operativen Eingriff und damit auch die Lymphonodektomie radikaler zu gestalten, nachdem die operativen Komplikationen durch technische Fortschritte gering gehalten werden können, müßten heute im Schrifttum ausreichend Mitteilungen zu finden sein, die aufgrund der Verbesserung der Heilungsergebnisse mit obligater Lymphonodektomie diese operative Erweiterung rechtfertigen.

Derartige statistisch belegte Angaben fehlen aber gänzlich. Vielmehr sprechen die Behandlungsergebnisse der I. Universitäts-Frauenklinik Wien gegen die Wirksamkeit der obligaten Lymphonodektomie (Rauscher u. Spurny, 1959). Innerhalb eines Zeitraumes von 6 Jahren wurde bei 315 Patientinnen mit Collumcarcinom der Stadien I und II eine Wertheimsche Radikaloperation mit Nachbestrahlung durchgeführt, bei der alternierend nur vergrößerte carcinomverdächtige Lymphknoten entfernt wurden oder eine obligate, radikale Lymphonodektomie vorgenommen wurde. Die relative 5-Jahres-Heilung beträgt in der Gruppe ohne obligate Lymphonodektomie 74%, in der Gruppe mit obligater Lymphknotenausräumung 75,8% (Tabelle 3).

Auch Rutledge (1962) konnte bei 440 Patientinnen nach Wertheimscher Radikaloperation mit oder ohne obligater Lymphonodektomie keine unterschiedlichen Heilungsergebnisse erzielen. Er führte an einem Teil seines Patientengutes alternierende Reihen durch. Nach 5—7 Jahren wiesen die Resultate mit und ohne Lymphonodektomie keine Differenzen auf (Gray u. Frick, 1965).

Welchen Einfluß die Zahl der positiven Lymphknoten auf die Heilungsergebnisse ausübt, wiesen Mitani et al. (1962) bei 172 Patientinnen nach: war nur ein Lymphknoten metastatisch befallen, betrug die 5-Jahres-Heilung 51 %, im Vergleich dazu stieg die Heilungsquote auf 76 % bei fehlendem Metastasenbefund; waren 2 und mehr Lymphknoten befallen, wurden nur noch 22 % der Patientinnen geheilt. Bei 5 und mehr positiven Lymphknoten überlebte keine der Patientinnen die Operation mehr als 3 Jahre (Tabelle 4).

Tabelle 4. *Der Einfluß der Lymphknotenmetastasen auf die Prognose* (Mitani et al.)

Zahl der metastatischen Lymphknoten	Prognose			
	Zahl der Fälle	Zahl der 5-Jahre-geheilten Fälle	Zahl der Gestorbenen	5-Jahres-Heilungsrate %
0	110	84	26	76,4
1	31	16	15	51,6
2	11	3	8	27,3
3	6	3	3	50,0
4	4	1	3	25,0
5	2		2	0
6	4		4	0
7				
8				
9	2		2	0
>10	2		2	0
	172	107	65	62,2

Für die Zeilen 2 bis >10 ist zusätzlich eine zusammengefaßte Heilungsrate von 22,6 (Zeilen 2–>10) bzw. 37,1 angegeben.

Schon 1954 hatte Javert durch eine Übersicht aus der Literatur nachweisen können, daß es operativ bei positiven Lymphknoten möglich ist, noch in etwa 20 % eine 5-Jahres-Heilung zu erzielen. Tabelle 5 zeigt eine Zusammenstellung neuerer Mitteilungen aus dem Schrifttum. Eine kritische Durchmusterung der Erfolgsmeldungen bei Lymphonodektomie ergibt allerdings, daß der weitaus größte Teil der Patientinnen, bei denen operativ positive Lymphknoten entfernt wurden, einer Nachbestrahlung unterzogen wurde, so daß die erzielte Heilung keinesfalls Folge der Lymphonodektomie sein muß.

Über die Heilungsaussichten bei einer Lymphknotenmetastasierung nach ausschließlich operativem Eingriff berichten Christensen, Lange und Nielsen (1964). Sie führten in den Stadien I und II eine abdominale radikale Hysterektomie mit beidseitiger Lymphonodektomie durch. Bei 139 Patientinnen im Stadium I wurde ohne Nachweis einer Lymphknotenmetastasierung eine 5-Jahres-Heilung von 92 %, bei 29 Patientinnen des Stadiums II von 86,3 % erzielt; waren die Lymphknoten metastatisch befallen, so betrug die 5-Jahres-Heilung bei 28 Patientinnen des Stadiums I nur 39,3 % und bei 23 des Stadiums II 14,8 %. 61 % der Patientinnen waren jünger als 45 Jahre. Yagi (1961) konnte bei gleicher Operationstechnik durch zusätzliche postoperative Bestrahlung im Stadium I bei einem Befall der Lymphknoten eine Heilung von 50 % und im Stadium II von 29,6 % erzielen. Andererseits berichtet Brunschwig (1955) nach Exenteration ohne Nachbestrahlung bei nachgewiesener Lymphknotenmetastasierung im Stadium I über eine 5-Jahres-Heilung von 52 % und im Stadium II von 31 %. Andere Autoren erreichen bei einer Lymphknotenmetastasierung ohne Nachbestrahlung schlechtere Heilungsergebnisse.

Selbst bei ultraradikalen Eingriffen werden die Heilungsaussichten bei Befall der Beckenwandlymphknoten erheblich vermindert, so daß eine Lymphknotenmetastasierung bereits
als Kontraindikation zur Exenteration angesehen wird (BRICKER, 1966).

Die Berechtigung zur obligaten Lymphonodektomie leiten die Operateure aber aus
einer anderen Indikationsstellung ab. Bei negativem Lymphknotenbefund wird immer
wieder die Ansicht vertreten, daß in diesen Fällen mit gutem Gewissen eine Nachbestrahlung entfallen kann, um so beispielsweise den Patientinnen die Kastration zu
ersparen. Es erscheint aber höchst zweifelhaft, vom Ergebnis der histologischen Untersuchung der entfernten Lymphknoten den Entschluß zur postoperativen, zusätzlichen

Tabelle 5. *5-Jahres-Heilung beim Collumcarcinom nach Lymphonodektomie bei histologisch nachgewiesener
Lymphknotenmetastasierung* (REIFFENSTUHL)

Autor	%		
BONNEY (1941)	23%		
TAUSSIG (1943)	21%		
DOEDERLEIN (1955)	30%		
LIU und MEIGS (1955)	35,0%		
BRUNTSCH (1956)	27,6%		
KÖHLER (HARTL) (1956)	40,3%		
BRUNSCHWIG u. ROESSLER (1957)	20%		
DARGENT (1957)	11—24%	Strahlensensible Fälle	24%
		Strahlenresistente Fälle	11%
ZACHERL (BRANDSTETTER) (1957)	18,2%		
GORTON (1957)	37%		
MITRA (1959)	44,0%	9 Fälle	
WELCH et al. (1959)	49%		
SCHLINK et al. (1960)	29%		
SWEENEY et al. (1962)	35,2%		
BRUNSCHWIG u. DANIEL (1962)	32%		
PARSON (1962)	20—50%	im Stadium I	50%
		im Stadium II	20%
CURRIE (1963)	49,2%	im Stadium I (16 Fälle)	62,5%
		im Stadium IIa (26 Fälle)	65%
		im Stadium IIb (20 Fälle)	35%
		im Stadium III (7 Fälle)	0%
NAVRATIL (1965)	37,9%	im Stadium II (11 Fälle)	
BRUNTSCH (1956) Sammelstatistik 1921—1956	22,2%	891 Fälle	
JAVERT (1954) Sammelstatistik 1912—1953	20,9%	306 Fälle	

Bestrahlung abhängig machen zu können. Die heutigen Kenntnisse über die möglichen Metastasierungswege und der trotz größter Radikalität auch lymphographisch
bewiesene beträchtliche Anteil von zurückgelassenen Lymphknoten nach radikaler
Lymphonodektomie sollte die Gefahr aufzeigen, die ein falscher Rückschluß aufgrund
unzureichender Befunde zur Folge hat. So können einzelne regionäre Lymphknotenstationen beim Collumcarcinom operativ kaum oder nur unvollständig angegangen werden.
Hierzu zählen die Lymphonodi glutei inferiores, sacrales, pararectales, aortici und andere.
Wie wäre sonst die Verschlechterung der Heilungsergebnisse bei Befall nur eines Lymph-
knotens, der zudem noch entfernt wurde, von 76 auf 51% bei den Untersuchungen von
MITANI et al. (1962) zu erklären?

Die zahlreichen technischen Fragen in bezug auf die Lymphonodektomie und die
mögliche Radikalität bei diesem Eingriff können in diesem Rahmen nicht näher beleuchtet
werden. Es wird auf die einschlägige Literatur verwiesen (OKABAYASHI, 1921; NATHANSON,
1946; MEIGS, 1950; ANTOINE, 1952; GORTON, 1953; MITRA, 1955; NAVRATIL, 1955;
BRICKER, 1960; BRUNSCHWIG, 1961; INGIULLA, 1961; LOUROS, 1961; YAGI, 1962).

Nachdem sich in den letzten Jahren aufgrund der angedeuteten Bedenken über den Nutzen der obligaten Lymphonodektomie zahlreiche Mitteilungen finden, gewinnt die Strahlenbehandlung bei der Therapie der Lymphknotenmetastasen erneut an Bedeutung. In diesem Fragenkomplex steht als Kernfrage die oft und mit Recht angezweifelte Wirksamkeit der Strahlentherapie auf die Lymphknotenmetastasen. Da die Frage, ob es überhaupt möglich ist, durch ionisierende Strahlen eine Lymphknotenmetastasierung beim Collumcarcinom zu heilen, im Schrifttum in kaum zu überbietender Weise widersprüchlich und oft mit erheblichen Ressentiments beantwortet worden ist, soll dieses Problem ausführlicher erörtert werden; denn von der Beantwortung dieser Frage hängen Indikation, Technik und Dosierung der Strahlenbehandlung des Collumcarcinoms ab.

SWEENEY und DOUGLAS (1962) führten eine Lymphonodektomie bei 102 Fällen nach einer kombinierten Radium-Röntgen-Therapie durch, bei denen am Punkt B, der etwa der Beckenwand entspricht, 2055 R (!) appliziert wurden. JAVERT untersuchte die Lymphknoten histologisch und fand keinen Effekt durch die ionisierenden Strahlen. Derartige Befunde sind wohl nicht geeignet, eine Aussage über die Strahlenwirkung auf Lymphknotenmetastasen zu machen, da die Dosen viel zu gering waren. Daß nach alleiniger Radiumapplikation auf die Cervix der Primärtumor zwar zerstört werden kann, die Beckenwandlymphknoten aber unbeeinflußt bleiben, wie auch andere Autoren berichten (CHERRY, GLUCKSMANN, DEARING, WAY, 1953), erscheint bei der unter diesen Bedingungen auf die Lymphknoten eingestrahlten Dosis nicht verwunderlich.

„SCHLINK (1950) und MEIGS (1951) sind überzeugt, daß die Strahlentherapie keinen Effekt auf die Lymphknoten besitzt (REIFFENSTUHL, 1967)". Demgegenüber fand aber KOTTMEIER (1953) bei 4000 R bereits deutliche histologische Veränderungen an den Beckenwandlymphknoten, die auf die Strahleneinwirkung zurückzuführen sind.

GLUCKSMANN (1956) vertritt die Ansicht, daß sich die Lymphknotenmetastasen und der Primärtumor hinsichtlich ihrer Strahlensensibilität gleich verhalten und von der Tumorart abhängig sind. RUNGE (1956) sah bei 1242 bestrahlten Collumcarcinomen in 35% Beckenwandmetastasen. Hieraus leitet er die nur mäßige Wirkung der bisher geübten Strahlentherapie auf die Lymphknotenmetastasierung ab.

BROWN et al. (1951) geben an, daß 5000—6000 R die Mindestdosis sind, mit der strahlensensible Lymphknotenmetastasen vernichtet werden können. DARGENT (1965) glaubt, nur bei kleinen Tumorzellkomplexen einen Erfolg der Strahlenbehandlung auf Lymphknotenmetastasen zu finden.

VON MASSENBACH (1957) hat bei 119 Autopsien in 43% paraaortale Lymphknotenmetastasen gesehen. Er fand, daß diese Lymphknotenregion häufiger befallen war als die tiefer gelegenen Lnn. iliaci interni, externi und sacrales und erklärt den isolierten Krebsbefall der aortalen Lymphknoten in 14% damit, daß durch eine vorangegangene Strahlenbehandlung die Beckenwandlymphknoten zerstört worden seien. Gleiche Beobachtungen finden sich auch bei BRUNSCHWIG und PIERCE (1948), HENRIKSEN (1949) und BRUNTSCH (1956). FISCHER (s. Tabelle 20) konnte 1956 an Hand eines Sektionsgutes von 467 Fällen von Collumcarcinom der Jahre 1930—1954 zeigen, daß nach einer Radium-Röntgen-Therapie in 50% der Fälle aortale und nur in 28% pelvine Lymphknotenmetastasen gefunden wurden, während bei unbehandelten Fällen die Zahl der aortalen und pelvinen Lymphknotenmetastasierung 46,1% betrug.

Die Schwierigkeit, die Strahlenwirkung auf die Lymphknotenmetastasierung zu beurteilen, beruht vor allem darauf, daß die Wirkung histologisch nur schwer bestimmt werden kann. Es ist nicht möglich, den histologischen Befund vor der Bestrahlung mit den Befunden nach der Bestrahlung zu vergleichen. Meist werden die histologischen Untersuchungen im Anschluß an die Strahlenbehandlung durchgeführt. Bei einer präoperativen Bestrahlung sind die verabfolgten Dosen stets relativ niedrig. Weiterhin ergibt ein Vergleich der Häufigkeit von positiven Lymphknoten nach einer Vorbestrahlung kein eindeutiges Bild, da nie exakt angegeben werden kann, in welchem Prozentsatz bereits vor der Bestrahlung positive Lymphknoten bestanden. Hinzu kommt die Schwierigkeit, daß es bis heute noch nicht eindeutig gelingt, durch die morphologischen Kriterien der histologischen Untersuchung die Vitalität von Tumorzellen zu bestimmen. Wenn nach einem relativ kurzen Intervall zwischen Strahlenbehandlung und histologischer Untersuchung in den Lymphknoten noch Tumorzellverbände gefunden werden, reichen die morphologischen Befunde wahrscheinlich nicht aus, um ein Maß für die Tumoraktivität zu finden. Diesem Fragenkomplex ist vor allem von pathologisch-anatomischer Seite ein umfangreiches Schrifttum gewidmet.

KOTTMEIER berichtete 1957, daß von 19 Patientinnen, bei denen histologisch eine Lymphknotenmetastasierung bioptisch diagnostiziert worden war, 6 eine Strahlenbehandlung 3—12 Jahre überlebt hatten. Nach seiner Ansicht ist die zur Devitalisierung der Lymphknotenmetastasen nötige Dosis niedriger als die des Primärtumors, die zwischen 5000 und 6000 R liegt. Nach KOTTMEIER ist die Heilungsquote nicht proportional der verabfolgten Strahlendosis.

Tabelle 6. *Die Wirkung unterschiedlicher Strahlendosis auf die Häufigkeit von Lymphknotenmetastasen beim Collumcarcinom Stadium III* (BOTELLA LLUSIÁ et al., 1964)

Fälle	Herddosis	Histologisch gesicherte Lymphknotenmetastasen nach Therapie
44	0	31,8%
15	bis 2000 R	33,3%
15	bis 4000 R	20,0%
15	bis 6000 R	13,3%
15	bis 8000 R	6,7%

MORTON (1947) führte in 2 Behandlungsgruppen eine transperitoneale Lymphonodektomie durch. Er fand in 45 Fällen 35% Lymphknotenmetastasen, in 35 fortgeschrittenen Fällen fand er nach einer Vorbestrahlung nur in 11% Lymphknotenmetastasen. An einem Patientengut von 346 Patientinnen führte GORTON (1957) nach einer Vorbestrahlung eine extraperitoneale Lymphonodektomie durch. Er fand nur in 13,6% Lymphknotenmetastasen, davon entfielen auf das Stadium I (118 Fälle) 8,5% und auf das Stadium II (228 Fälle) 16,2% Lymphknotenmetastasen. GRAY et al. (1958) diagnostizierten bei 61 Patientinnen (Stadium I: 44; Stadium II: 17) Lymphknotenmetastasen und verglichen diese Befunde mit denen von 15 vorbestrahlten Fällen (Stadium I: 28; Stadium II: 23). Bei den vorbestrahlten Patientinnen fanden sie nur in einem Fall Lymphknotenmetastasen. Demgegenüber fanden WELCH et al. (1959) bei einer Lymphonodektomie in den Stadien I und II keinen nennenswerten Unterschied im Vergleich zu einer Patientengruppe, bei der eine Vorbestrahlung durchgeführt worden war.

Bedeutungsvoll erscheinen die Arbeiten von NOGALES et al. (1962). Sie konnten an einem Patientengut von 75 Frauen mit Collumcarcinom des Stadiums III nachweisen, daß bei nicht bestrahlten Patientinnen und bei nur mit Radium (10000—11000 mgeh) behandelten Patientinnen eine Lymphknotenmetastasierung von 33% bestand. Nach einer Strahleneinwirkung von 3000—4000 R an den Lymphknoten nach einer kombinierten Radium-Röntgen-Tiefentherapie sahen sie nur in 20% Lymphknotenmetastasen, bei einer Dosis von 4000—6000 R durch kombinierte Radium- und Bewegungsbestrahlung in 13% und nach alleiniger Telekobalttherapie bei einer Dosierung von 6000—7000 R in nur 6,6% Lymphknotenmetastasen. BOTELLA LLUSIÁ et al. (1964) sicherten diese Ergebnisse an einem größeren Patientengut (Tabelle 6). Gegen derartige Untersuchungen wird der Einwand erhoben, daß nach einer Strahlenbehandlung eine Lymphonodektomie mit beträchtlichen technischen Schwierigkeiten verbunden ist und die Zahl der operativ entfernbaren Lymphknoten stark abnimmt. Dieser Einwand ist aber nur teilweise berechtigt. Zweifellos werden die postradiologischen Narbenbildungen den Eingriff erschweren. Alle Lymphknoten, die metastatisch befallen waren und auf die Bestrahlung durch Einschmelzen angesprochen haben, werden sich später nur noch als narbiger, fibrotischer Strang darstellen. Wird somit die Zahl der Lymphknoten, die excidiert werden können, verringert, so könnte dies bereits eher als strahlentherapeutischer Erfolg angesehen werden. Es wäre geradezu unwahrscheinlich, daß nach Einwirkung ionisierender Strahlen die gleiche Zahl von Lymphknoten gewonnen werden könnte. Keinesfalls würde sich dadurch der prozentuale Anteil der befallenen zu den nicht befallenen Lymphknoten verschieben.

Einen entscheidenden Beitrag zum Problem der Strahlenbehandlung bei Lymphknotenmetastasen leisteten RUTLEDGE und FLETCHER (1958) sowie RUTLEDGE, FLETCHER und McDONALD (1965). Zur Untersuchung der Frage, was die Supervolttherapie bei der Behandlung von Lymphknotenmetastasen leistet, führten sie an 100 Patientinnen des Stadiums III eine Bestrahlung mit 22-MeV-Röntgenstrahlen (Herddosis 6000 R im gesamten kleinen Becken) und bei fortgeschritteneren Fällen eine zusätzliche Radiumapplikation (3000—5000 mgeh) durch, so daß etwa Herddosen von 6000—8000 R an den Lymphknoten wirksam wurden. 3 Monate nach Beendigung der Strahlenbehandlung wurde eine Lymphonodektomie angeschlossen. Eine gründliche histologische Untersuchung zeigte, daß 22 Patientinnen Lymphknotenmetastasen aufwiesen. Von diesen waren die Lymphknotenmetastasen aber bei 8 Patientinnen nur außerhalb des Bestrahlungsfeldes lokalisiert. 5 Patientinnen wiesen *nur* Metastasen *innerhalb* des Beckens auf, obwohl diese Lymphknoten eine volle Tumordosis erhalten hatten. Die weiteren 9 Patientinnen hatten positive Lymphknoten sowohl innerhalb als auch außerhalb der bestrahlten Region. Hieraus folgern sie, daß bei 14 Patientinnen (14 %) die Strahlenbehandlung keine Devitalisierung vermocht hatte. Vergleicht man diese Ergebnisse mit der durchschnittlichen Häufigkeit eines metastatischen Befalls in den einzelnen Stadien (Tabelle 1), so liegt die Quote von 14 % beim Stadium III der Untersuchungen von RUTLEDGE und FLETCHER wesentlich niedriger. Wenngleich nicht unbedingt angenommen werden kann, daß auch in diesem Patientengut bei etwa 50 % vor der Bestrahlung Lymphknotenmetastasen vorgelegen haben müssen, läßt sich aus einer Reduzierung der Frequenz auf 14 % doch ein gewisser Rückschluß auf eine Wirksamkeit der relativ hoch dosierten Strahlenbehandlung ziehen.

Histologisch zeigte sich bei den entfernten und bestrahlten Lymphknoten, daß nach einem Intervall von 3 Monaten nur wenige Lymphonodi deutliche Strahlenreaktionen an den Krebszellen erkennen ließen. In 2 Fällen wiesen innerhalb des Bestrahlungsfeldes liegende Lymphknoten Strahlenreaktionen auf, in anderen Knoten waren aber noch lebende Carcinomzellen zu beobachten. Bei 4 Patientinnen wurden Reste von zerstörten Tumorzellen gesehen, die die Autoren als „ghost cells" bezeichnen. In 4 weiteren Fällen ergaben die histologischen Untersuchungen nekrotische Bezirke, die von einer Fibrose und Fremdkörperreaktion umgeben waren.

Zu gleichen Ergebnissen kommt CHAKRAVORTY (1965) bei 50 Patientinnen mit einem Collumcarcinom Stadium III. Er fand bei einer Lymphonodektomie nach Bestrahlung in 13 Fällen histologisch Lymphknotenmetastasen, von denen bei 7 Fällen die Lymphknoten innerhalb und bei 6 Fällen außerhalb des Bestrahlungsfeldes lagen. Somit war wie bei RUTLEDGE et al. (1965) die Strahlenbehandlung ebenfalls in 14 % erfolglos.

Im Jahre 1965 berichteten RUTLEDGE, FLETCHER und McDONALD über eine zweite, randomisierte Untersuchungsserie, die etwas über den Wert der Lymphonodektomie nach einer vorausgegangenen Strahlenbehandlung aussagen sollte. Die Serie umfaßte 142 Patientinnen der verschiedenen Stadien (Stadium I: 30, Stadium II a: 39, Stadium II b: 25, Stadium III a: 23 und Stadium III b: 25 Patientinnen). Bei diesen Patientinnen wurde eine Lymphonodektomie in gleicher Weise nach einer vollen Strahlenbehandlung durchgeführt. Von den 142 Patientinnen wiesen 11,3 % positive Lymphknoten auf, im Stadium I: 3,3 %, II: 14,1 % und III: 12,5 %. Vergleicht man diese Zahlen wiederum mit den ermittelten Durchschnittswerten (s. Tabelle 1), so ist eine Wirksamkeit der Bestrahlung auf eine Lymphknotenmetastasierung nicht zu leugnen. Bei 8 von den 16 Patientinnen mit positiven Lymphknoten wurden wiederum Lymphknoten in der Paraaortalregion und somit außerhalb des Bestrahlungsfeldes nachgewiesen. Der Vergleich der Behandlungsergebnisse dieser Untersuchungsserie mit einer Kontrollgruppe von 169 Patientinnen nach ausschließlicher Strahlenbehandlung gleicher Stadienverteilung zeigt in den einzelnen Stadien keine größeren Abweichungen. Es fällt allerdings auf, daß die Behandlungsergebnisse in der Kontrollgruppe größtenteils einige Prozent besser sind als in der Untersuchungsgruppe. Die zusätzliche Lymphonodektomie verbessert somit die Behandlungsergebnisse nicht. Vielmehr müssen die zahlreichen postoperativen und teilweise sehr schweren Komplikationen nach der Lymphonodektomie erwähnt werden: große Lymphcysten, Beinödeme, Obstruktion des Ureters, Infektion der Lymphcysten mit Abszeßbildungen, Nierenschäden.

Zu ähnlichen Untersuchungsergebnissen kam GUTTMANN (1965). Eine Patientengruppe, vorwiegend Stadium I und II, wurde operativ durch radikale Hysterektomie und Lymphonodektomie behandelt. Bei einer zweiten Patientengruppe wurde eine kombinierte Radium-Percutanbestrahlung durchgeführt: Corscaden-Applikator 6000 mgeh, 12000 R am Punkt A, zusätzlich 5000 rad, 2-MeV-Röntgen- oder Kobalt-60-γ-Strahlen. Die zweite Gruppe umfaßte 72 Patientinnen. Bei 55 von diesen Patientinnen wurde 3 Monate nach der Strahlenbehandlung eine Lymphonodektomie durchgeführt; es handelte sich um 28 Patientinnen des Stadiums I, 23 des Stadiums II und 4 des Stadiums III. Bei keinem der Patienten des Stadiums I wurden Lymphknotenmetastasen gefunden. Im Stadium II wurden bei einer Patientin (= 3,8 %) Lymphknotenmetastasen diagnostiziert. Von den 4 Patientinnen des Stadiums III wurden in 2 Fällen Lymphknotenmetastasen nachgewiesen. Während 5 Patientinnen einen operativen Eingriff ablehnten und bei weiteren 6 Fällen aus medizinischen Gründen Inoperabilität bestand, konnte nach 3 Monaten bei 6 Patientinnen eine Tumorprogredienz nachgewiesen werden. Eine Operation bei diesen Patientinnen ergab in 3 Fällen positive Lymphknoten bei einem als strahlenresistent geltenden Primärtumor. In den anderen 3 Fällen wurden trotz Tumorprogredienz keine Lymphknotenmetastasen gefunden. Die andere, primär operierte Untersuchungsgruppe umfaßte 61 Patientinnen. Bei diesen Patientinnen fand man bei 44 Fällen des Stadiums I 5mal (11,3 %) und bei 17 Patientinnen des Stadiums II 6mal (35,2 %) Lymphknotenmetastasen. Die Metastasenhäufigkeit entsprach somit in etwa den im Schrifttum angegebenen Durchschnittswerten. Bei einer Patientin der operativen Gruppe konnte wegen multipler Lymphknotenmetastasen nur eine Explorativlaparotomie vorgenommen werden. Die Patientin wurde in der beschriebenen Weise bestrahlt, nach 6 Monaten ergab eine Lymphonodektomie keinen Anhalt mehr für Lymphknotenmetastasen. Die Patientin lebt seitdem 11 Jahre rezidivfrei. Aus diesen Untersuchungsergebnissen folgert GUTTMANN, daß nach einer vollen Strahlenbehandlung keine Indikation zu einer zusätzlichen Lymphonodektomie besteht. Wenn nach der Strahlenbehandlung noch positive Lymphknoten bestehen bleiben, kann das Schicksal der Patientin auch durch keinen operativen Eingriff mehr gewendet werden.

Auch GREISS (1965) konnte zeigen, daß eine zusätzliche Operation mit Lymphonodektomie keine signifikant besseren Resultate erbringt als die Bestrahlung allein. Er sieht die kombinierte Therapie als einen experimentellen Versuch an, der nur zum Zweck gut kontrollierter Studien durchgeführt werden sollte.

Nach einer vollen Strahlenbehandlung durch kombinierte Radium- und Röntgentherapie führte KOTTMEIER (1964) bei 53 Patientinnen eine Lymphonodektomie durch. Bei 24 Patientinnen wurden histologisch keine Lymphknotenmetastasen nachgewiesen. Von diesen blieben 19 Patientinnen (79,2 %) 5 Jahre lang rezidivfrei. In 7 Fällen fand man histologisch noch Lymphknotenmetastasen, die aber deutliche Strahlenveränderungen aufwiesen. Von diesen 7 Patientinnen waren nach 5 Jahren noch 4 (57,1 %) rezidivfrei. Bei 22 Patientinnen wurden Lymphknotenmetastasen ohne jegliche Strahlenschäden gefunden; bei diesen wurde nur in einem Fall (4,5 %) eine 5-Jahres-Heilung erreicht.

Über 10jährige Erfahrungen mit der transperitonealen und extraperitonealen Lymphadenektomie nach einer Strahlentherapie bei 440 Patientinnen der Stadien I und II berichtet Gorton (1964). Eine Lymphonodektomie wurde 4 Monate nach der kombinierten Radium-Röntgentherapie vorgenommen. Über die an den Lymphknoten wirksam gewordene Strahlendosis finden sich keine exakten Angaben. Die histologische Untersuchung der gewonnenen Lymphknoten ergab bei 166 Patientinnen des Stadiums I in 12,6% eine Metastasierung und bei 273 Patientinnen des Stadiums II in 21,6%. Diese Ergebnisse werden mit früher gewonnenen Befunden, bei denen eine Strahlentherapie nicht vorangegangen war, verglichen. In diesen Fällen fand er in 30% Lymphknotenmetastasen (Gorton, 1945). Aus einem Vergleich mit Behandlungsergebnissen aus den Jahren 1943 bis 1947 ist zu entnehmen, daß nach ausschließlicher Strahlenbehandlung in den Stadien I und II die Resultate um etwa 15% niedriger liegen. Hieraus glaubt Gorton die Rechtfertigung für die Durchführung der zusätzlichen Lymphonodektomie ablesen zu können. Insgesamt lebten 13 Patientinnen mit einer Lymphknotenmetastasierung 5 Jahre und länger. Somit ist es in einigen Fällen möglich, trotz Lymphknotenmetastasierung eine Heilung herbeizuführen. Die Aufgabe der Strahlentherapie soll es nach seiner Auffassung sein, den Primärtumor zu heilen, die Zahl der Lymphknotenmetastasen zu verringern und dann die regionalen Lymphknoten durch die Lymphonodektomie zu beseitigen.

Aufgrund des Weltschrifttums kommt Reiffenstuhl (1966) zu dem Schluß, „daß das Problem, ob die Strahlentherapie einen Effekt auf die Lymphknotenmetastasen hat, bis jetzt noch nicht gelöst ist". Hierbei führt er die Behandlungsergebnisse der Universitäts-Frauenklinik Hamburg-Eppendorf an, aus denen er ablesen will, daß ionisierende Strahlen lediglich eine Wirkung auf den Primärtumor an der Cervix ausüben, aber die vorhandenen Lymphknotenmetastasen unbeeinflußt lassen. Diese Folgerung darf nicht unwidersprochen bleiben, da aus den Hamburger Ergebnissen eher ein Effekt der Strahlen auf eine Lymphknotenmetastasierung abgeleitet werden kann. Die von Reiffenstuhl angeführten Zahlen entsprechen nicht den von Schubert et al. (1962) in der zitierten Arbeit mitgeteilten Ergebnissen.

Vielmehr konnte am Patientengut der Universitäts-Frauenklinik Hamburg gezeigt werden, daß eine Heilung bei histologisch nachgewiesener Lymphknotenmetastasierung möglich ist. Von 6 Patientinnen mit einem Collumcarcinom, bei denen durch eine Laparotomie die Lymphknotenmetastasierung bioptisch verifiziert worden war, lebten nach einer Strahlenbehandlung (Herddosis etwa 4000 R) nach 5 Jahren noch 2 Frauen rezidivfrei (Leven, 1967).

Als kasuistischer Beitrag zur Frage der Dosishöhe sollen die Lymphographien einer Patientin mit Collumcarcinom Stadium III angeführt werden. Die vor der Behandlung durchgeführte Lymphographie erbrachte typische Zeichen einer Lymphknotenmetastasierung an der Beckenwand links und im unteren Lumbalbereich (Abb. 2a). Bei der Strahlenbehandlung wurde durch kombinierte Radium-Telekobalttherapie an die Beckenwand 6000 R innerhalb von 5 Wochen appliziert. Die paraaortale Metastasierung wurde durch ein zusätzliches, dorsales Stehfeld (Telekobalt) erfaßt; diese Bestrahlung wurde nach einer Herddosis von etwa 2000 R abgebrochen. Eine Kontrollaufnahme des Beckens und der Lumbalregion ohne erneute Kontrastmittelinjektion zeigte nach 2 Monaten, daß sich die pelvinen Lymphknotenmetastasen fast vollständig zurückgebildet haben. Die Füllungsdefekte wurden weitgehend durch Markierungsreste von erhaltenem Lymphgewebe ersetzt (Abb. 2b). Die mit nur 2000 R belasteten aortalen Lymphknoten in Höhe des 4. und 5. Lendenwirbelkörpers links sind im Vergleich zur Voraufnahme deutlich größer geworden. Man erkennt hier nur noch geringe Reste von markiertem Lymphgewebe.

Für eine Indikation zur Bestrahlung des Lymphsystems und insbesondere für die Wahl der Dosishöhe ist die Frage entscheidend, ob aus einer hochdosierten Strahlenbehandlung schwere Schäden am Lymphsystem resultieren können. Hierbei wird neben den radiologisch bedingten Stauungsödemen in den letzten Jahren vor allem die mögliche Funktionsbeeinträchtigung des lymphatischen Gewebes diskutiert.

Noch im Jahre 1960 glaubte KNOPP aus klinischen Beobachtungen schließen zu können, daß Röntgenbestrahlungen zu Lymphbahnveränderungen mit Stauungsödemen führen. Aufgrund von Lymphadenographien, bei denen nach einer Röntgenbestrahlung keine Markierung der Lymphknoten mehr gelang, glaubt KNOPP, diese Rückschlüsse ziehen zu können. Auch HILLEMANNS (1957) beschreibt einen ähnlichen Effekt der ionisierenden Strahlen auf die Lymphknoten. Nach 3000—3500 R kommt es zu einer ausgedehnten Zerstörung des lymphatischen Gewebes der regionären Lymphknoten. Als Frühreaktion beobachtete er Zerfall der kleinen Lymphocyten und Zerstörung der Sekundärknötchen

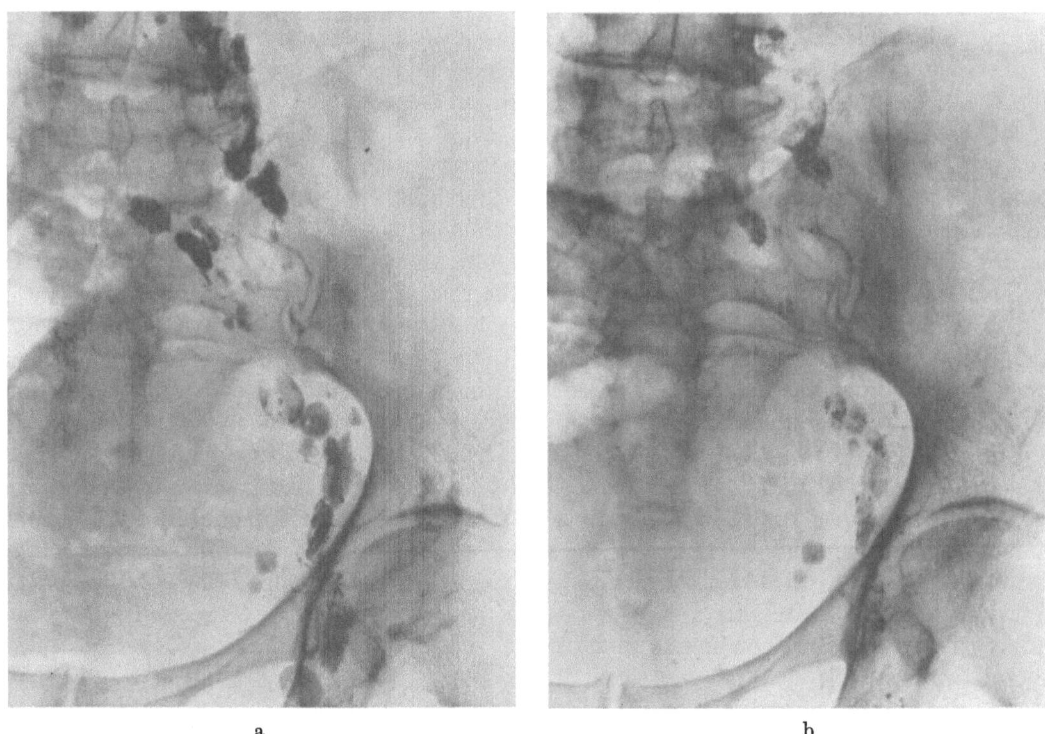

a   b

Abb. 2. a Iliacale und aortale Metastasierung im Lymphogramm bei Collumcarcinom Stadium III. b Kontrollaufnahme 2 Monate nach Bestrahlung

mit unspezifischer akuter Lymphadenitis. Nach Abklingen der unspezifischen Reaktion des Gefäßbindegewebes ist das Grundgerüst von Lymphocyten entblößt. Nach Atrophie des reticulo-histiocytären Gewebes erscheint das Gitterwerk leer, das grobe Stützgerüst und Gefäßbindegewebe zeigen noch keine Zeichen der Degeneration. Als Spätschäden (3.—5. Monat bis zu 5 Jahren) bezeichnet HILLEMANNS die fortschreitenden degenerativen Veränderungen am reticulo-vasculären System des Lymphknotens mit Gefäßobliteration, Hyalinose und Sklerose, die zur sekundären Atrophie und Verschwielung des ganzen Lymphknotens führen, durch die die Funktion des Lymphknotens weitgehend aufgehoben ist.

In den letzten Jahren wurden zu diesem Fragenkomplex weitere experimentelle und klinische Erfahrungen mitgeteilt. Von besonderem Wert sind die eingehenden Untersuchungen von ENGESET (1964). Am Lymphsystem der Ratte führte er umfangreiche Untersuchungen nach einer Strahlendosis von 3000 R/Herd durch. Innerhalb der ersten 2 Wochen nach der Strahlenbehandlung sah er eine sekundäre Atrophie des lymphatischen Gewebes. Lymphangiographische Untersuchungen zeigten, daß das Gefäßsystem innerhalb der ersten 6—9 Monate nach der Bestrahlung nicht alteriert war.

Nach mehr als einem Jahr sah man allerdings ausgeprägte Anastomosen-Kreisläufe der Lymphgefäße, durch die die bestrahlte Lymphknotenregion umflossen wurde. Bedeutungsvoll sind seine Untersuchungen, weil er an den bestrahlten Lymphknoten der Ratte eine Funktionsbeeinträchtigung des lymphatischen Gewebes nachweisen konnte. Die Barrierenfunktion des Lymphknotens prüfte er, indem er verschiedene Stoffe in periphere Lymphgefäße injizierte. Nach einer Röntgenbestrahlung passierten menschliche Erythrocyten und Zellen des Walker-Carcinoms die Lymphknoten leichter als bei nicht bestrahlten Kontrolltieren. Ebenfalls erschien die Barrierenfunktion gegenüber einer Infektion mit DTP-Vaccine vermindert. Durch lymphographische Kontrollen fand ENGESET die Ursache für die innerhalb eines Jahres zunehmende Funktionsbeeinträchtigung in der Ausbildung von Shunts, durch die die Lymphe die Lymphknoten ungefiltert passieren konnte. Diese Veränderungen waren besonders ausgeprägt nach Strahlendosen von 6000 R. Aufgrund dieser Untersuchungsergebnisse sieht ENGESET in der „prophylaktischen" Bestrahlung große Gefahren. Nach einer solchen Bestrahlung könnte es im weiteren Verlauf des Krankheitsgeschehens relativ rasch zu einer Fernmetastasierung kommen, wenn die tumorösen Zellverbände ungehindert das Lymphsystem passieren können. Eine Bestrahlung des Lymphsystems erscheint nach seinen Untersuchungen nur dann gerechtfertigt, wenn bereits mit einer Lymphknotenmetastasierung zu rechnen ist.

Den Effekt der Bestrahlung auf die Lymphe und auf die Lymphgefäße untersuchten LENZI und BASSANI (1963). Sie führten ihre Untersuchungen an Meerschweinchen und Kaninchen durch. Die Tiere erhielten 3000, 6000 oder 8000 R Röntgenstrahlen. Nach einer Woche wurden nach 3000 R keine Veränderungen im lymphatischen Netzwerk gesehen. Nach 6000 R traten einige Erweiterungen und varicöse Auftreibungen, aber keine Unterbrechung auf. Nach 8000 R erschienen die Lymphgefäße gewunden, starr und stark varicös. Nirgends waren sie unterbrochen. Gleiche Erfahrungen machten diese Autoren bei Untersuchungen von Uteri bestrahlter Frauen nach einer intrakavitären Radiumeinlage. Im überlebenden Uterusgewebe sahen sie auch hier keine Unterbrechung der Lymphgefäße. Nur in nekrotischen Arealen, in denen Dosen von 25000—30000 R zur Wirkung kamen, wurde eine völlige Zerstörung der Lymphgefäße festgestellt. Dort, wo eine Dosis von 15000 R eingewirkt hat, waren die Gefäße gewunden und varicös, aber überall durchgängig.

Um die Lymphknotenfunktion nach Bestrahlung oder Operation beurteilen zu können, führten DETTMAN, KING und ZIMBERG (1966) an Hunden Untersuchungen durch. Nach einer subcutanen Radiogoldkolloid-Injektion ist die Radioaktivität normalerweise in den Knielymphknoten lokalisiert. Entfernten sie die Knielymphknoten, so war in dieser Region keine radioaktive Speicherung nachzuweisen. Nach 1 Monat war die Kontinuität des Lymphflusses wieder gewährleistet, und das Radiogold konnte in den abdominellen Lymphknoten nachgewiesen werden. Nach fraktionierter Gabe von 2000 R konventioneller Röntgenstrahlen auf die Region der Knielymphknoten war das Radiokolloid weiter ungehindert in den Knielymphknoten lokalisiert. Nach 6000 R zeigten 3 von 4 Tieren, beginnend 2 Monate nach der Bestrahlung, einen Abtransport des Radiogoldkolloids bis zu den abdominellen Lymphknoten. Nach 10000 R war die Verteilung von Radiogold dieselbe wie bei den Kontrolltieren. Diesen Befund erklären sie durch die entstehende Fibrose. Eine wesentliche Beeinträchtigung der Speicherfunktion durch ionisierende Strahlen in diesem Dosisbereich konnte somit nicht bewiesen werden.

Klinische Erfahrungen über die Wirkung ionisierender Strahlen auf die Lymphgefäße und die Lymphknoten konnten in den letzten Jahren in umfangreichem Maße durch die Lymphographie gesammelt werden. Hierbei zeigte es sich, daß wesentlich seltener als früher vermutet nach einer Strahlenbehandlung mit Gefäßveränderungen oder makroskopischen Veränderungen an den Lymphknoten zu rechnen ist. In etwa $^3/_4$ der Fälle erkennt man nach einem Intervall bis zu mehreren Jahren zwischen Strahlenbehandlung und Lymphographie bei der heute üblichen Lymphangiographie nach KINMONTH einen unauffälligen Lymphgefäßverlauf mit üblicher Markierung der Lymphknoten im Beckenbereich. Als typische Veränderungen im Gefäß- und Speicherbild nach einer Strahlenbehandlung gelten: sehr dünne, kleinkalibrige Lymphgefäße, die die typische perlschnurartige Anordnung vermissen lassen, kleine geschrumpfte Lymphknoten, die oft zahlenmäßig verringert sind. Diese Veränderungen findet man aber fast ausschließlich nur dann, wenn zur Zeit der Strahlenbehandlung Lymphknotenmetastasen vorlagen. Durch Kontrollymphographien konnte gezeigt werden, daß sich das Gefäß- und Speicherbild nach einem Intervall von 1—2 Jahren nach einer Strahlenbehandlung mit einer Herddosis von etwa 5000 R an den Lymphknoten in den Fällen nicht ändert, in denen das primäre Lymphogramm keinen Anhalt für eine Lymphknotenmetastasierung ergab (FRISCHBIER, 1966). Da sich nach der Strahlenbehandlung die Lymphknoten in gleicher Zahl und Form erneut markieren, sind gröbere makroskopische Veränderungen, wie Narbenbildungen, Kollateralkreisläufe, unwahrscheinlich. Diese Untersuchungen wurden vorwiegend durchgeführt, um eine Funktionsbeeinträchtigung des Lymphsystems durch das ölige Kontrastmittel nach Lymphographie zu untersuchen. Selbstverständlich müssen diese Beobachtungen mit der Einschränkung gedeutet werden, daß eine erneute Markierung der Lymphgefäße und Lymphknoten nach einer Strahlenbehandlung über die feinere Funktion nichts aussagt. Würde es aber nach Dosen von 5000 R zu dem von ENGESET (1964) beobachteten Shunt-Mechanismus kommen, so müßte auch das ölige Kontrastmittel ungehindert die Lymphgefäße passieren, indem es die Filterstationen durch Shunts umfließt. Es ist unwahrscheinlich, daß das ölige Kontrastmittel das Lymphsystem auf einem anderen Wege passiert als die Tumorzellverbände. Die direkte Lymphographie speziell unter Verwendung von Radionucliden könnte uns aber in den nächsten Jahren die Möglichkeit geben, nähere Aufschlüsse über die Funktion des lymphatischen Gewebes, insbesondere nach Einwirkung von ionisierenden Strahlen, zu erhalten.

Wenn auch heute unsere Kenntnis über das Lymphknotenproblem noch lückenhaft und nur durch teilweise sich widersprechende Ergebnisse im Schrifttum belegt ist, ist es doch möglich, einzelne Fakten als gesichert anzusehen:

1. Operativ ist es nicht möglich, bei einem Collumcarcinom sämtliche regionären Lymphknotenmetastasen zu entfernen.
2. Eine obligate, radikale Lymphonodektomie erhöht die Mortalität und die Operationskomplikationen. Es ist bisher nicht gelungen, durch obligate Lymphonodektomie beim Collumcarcinom die Behandlungsergebnisse signifikant zu verbessern.
3. Durch eine Strahlenbehandlung ist es möglich, Collumcarcinome mit einer Lymphknotenmetastasierung zu heilen. Die Heilung von Lymphknotenmetastasen durch ionisierende Strahlen ist dosisabhängig. Es ist nicht erwiesen, daß sich die zur Devitalisierung notwendigen Strahlendosen am Primärtumor und am Lymphknoten unterscheiden.
4. Die heute üblichen morphologischen Kriterien reichen zur Beurteilung der Vitalität einer Lymphknotenmetastase nicht aus.
5. Es liegen bis heute keine klinischen Kriterien dafür vor, daß aus einer (prophylaktischen) Sicherheits-Bestrahlung eine erhebliche Funktionsbeeinträchtigung des Lymphsystems resultieren könnte, wodurch die Behandlungsergebnisse verschlechtert würden.

c) Anpassung des Bestrahlungsfeldes an die Tumorausbreitung

Eine Strahlenbehandlung kann nur dann erfolgreich sein, wenn der gesamte Tumor mit seinen Ausläufern und Metastasen vom Strahlenkegel erfaßt wird. Daher ist es vor Beginn einer Strahlenbehandlung unbedingt notwendig, die Tumorausbreitung mit allen zur Verfügung stehenden Methoden festzustellen.

Verglichen mit anderen Tumorlokalisationen ist es beim Collumcarcinom relativ leicht, die Größe des Primärtumors sowie mögliche Infiltrationen in die umgebenden Organe zu bestimmen. Die bimanuelle Palpation, die Speculumeinstellung, die Kolposkopie, die getrennte Cervix-Corpus-Abrasio, die Cystoskopie und die Rectoskopie gestatten es, ohne größeren Aufwand eine Stadieneinteilung beim Collumcarcinom vorzunehmen. Da im allgemeinen Teil dieses Handbuches der Stadieneinteilung ein spezielles Kapitel gewidmet ist, soll an dieser Stelle lediglich die heute international gültige Stadieneinteilung beim Collumcarcinom (Cancer Committee of the International Federation of Gynecology and Obstetrics) angeführt werden:

Stadium 0: Carcinoma *in situ* — auch bekannt als präinvasives Carcinom, intraepitheliales Carcinom usw.

Stadium I: Das Carcinom ist streng auf die Cervix beschränkt.

1a: Präklinisches Carcinom. Das Carcinom kann durch klinische Untersuchungen nicht diagnostiziert werden.

Ib: Alle anderen Fälle von Stadium I.

Stadium II: Das Carcinom überschreitet die Cervix, hat aber die Beckenwand nicht erreicht. Das Carcinom befällt die Vagina, aber nicht das untere Drittel.

IIa: Das Carcinom greift auf die Vaginalwand über, infiltriert aber offensichtlich das Parametrium nicht.

IIb: Das Carcinom infiltriert das Parametrium.

Stadium III: Das Carcinom hat die Beckenwand erreicht (bei rectaler Untersuchung findet sich kein krebsfreier Raum zwischen dem Tumor und der Beckenwand). Das Carcinom befällt das untere Drittel der Vagina.

Stadium IV: Das Carcinom befällt die Blase oder das Rectum oder beides. Oder es hat sich über die oben beschriebenen Grenzen hinaus ausgebreitet.

Die Stadieneinteilung nach dem TNM-System hat bis heute in der Gynäkologie keine größere Verbreitung gefunden.

Mit den erwähnten Untersuchungsmethoden ist es nur recht grob möglich, die Tumorausbreitung zu ermitteln. Deshalb werden vielfach weitere Untersuchungsmethoden wie intravenöses Pyelogramm und Colon-Kontrasteinlauf zur Stadieneinteilung angewandt.

Nachdem in den vergangenen Jahren ausreichend Erfahrungen mit neueren angiographischen Untersuchungen bei Genitalcarcinomen gesammelt werden konnten, erhob sich die Frage, ob sich die Lymphographie, Cavographie oder Arteriographie dazu eignen, die Stadieneinteilung beim Collumcarcinom zu verbessern.

Von den erwähnten angiographischen Untersuchungen gilt die Lymphographie nach intralymphatischer Injektion eines öligen Kontrastmittels (Lipiodol ultrafluid) als die wertvollste Methode, um im Becken- oder Retroperitonealbereich Lymphknotenmetastasen aufzudecken. Der klinische Wert der Lymphographie beim Collumcarcinom ist aber dadurch begrenzt, daß die wichtigsten regionären Lymphknoten der Cervix, die Lymphonodi iliaci interni und parauterini, pararectales sowie präsacrales, nicht oder nur gelegentlich dargestellt werden. Die lymphographisch nachweisbaren Lymphonodi iliaci externi und communes sowie die Lymphonodi aortales sind aber nicht von geringerem Interesse. Sie entziehen sich gerade vollends der bimanuellen Palpation und damit der Beurteilung des Ausbreitungsstadiums. Andererseits wird der klinische Wert der Lymphographie dadurch begrenzt, daß sich Füllungsdefekte in der Speicherstruktur eines Lymphknotens, die als „klassische" Zeichen einer Metastasierung angesehen werden, histologisch als Fibrose oder Lipomatose erweisen können. Deshalb wurde noch vor wenigen Jahren die Bedeutung der Lymphographie für die Metastasensuche sehr unterschiedlich angegeben. Man fand im Schrifttum auf der einen Seite enthusiastische Mitteilungen, in denen die Autoren durch histologische Kontrolluntersuchungen die lymphographischen Befunde in über 90% der Fälle bestätigt sahen. Demgegenüber waren wesentlich häufiger Mitteilungen zu finden, in denen vor einer Überbewertung der Lymphographie gewarnt wird. Teilweise wurde die diagnostische Fehlerquote von einigen Autoren so hoch angegeben,

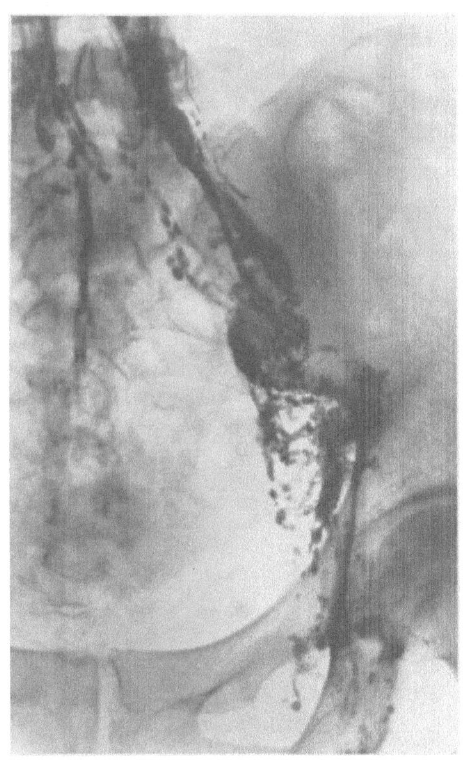

a

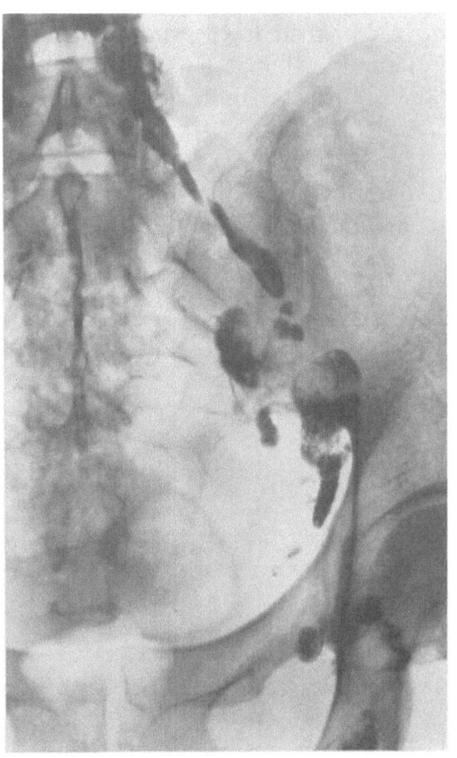

b

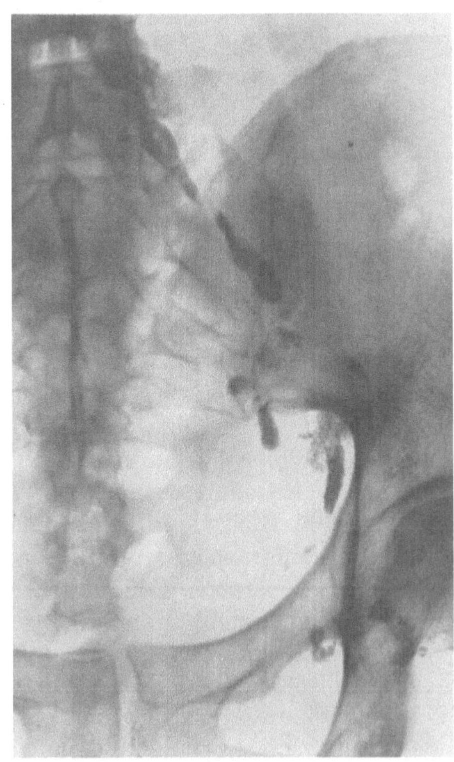

c

Abb. 3 a—c. Lymphographie bei einem Collumcarcinom
Stadium I. a Unauffälliges Lymphangiogramm. b Auf
dem Speicherbild erkennt man unregelmäßig begrenzte
Füllungsdefekte an einem linksseitigen iliacalen
Lymphknoten. Der Befund ergibt größten Verdacht
auf eine Lymphknotenmetastasierung. c Speicherbild
nach Wertheimscher Radikaloperation. Der verdäch-
tige Lymphknoten wurde bei der Operation entfernt.
Die histologische Untersuchung ergab eine Lymphknotenmetastasierung eines Plattenepithelcarcinoms

daß die Lymphographie als Routineuntersuchung abgelehnt wurde. Heute herrscht allgemein die Ansicht vor, daß es mit der Lymphographie bei ausreichender Erfahrung in der Befunderhebung, genauer Kenntnis der individuellen Varianz im Verlauf der Lymphgefäße und in der Anordnung der Lymphknoten und bei guter Aufnahmetechnik möglich ist, eine Treffsicherheit von etwa 90 % bei der Metastasensuche zu erreichen. Wenn sich die Lymphographie auch nicht generell zur Früherfassung von Lymphknotenmetastasen und damit zur Stadieneinteilung eignet, so verbessert sie die gynäkologische Tumordiagnostik doch bedeutend insofern, als über die meist nur palpablen, regionären Lymph-

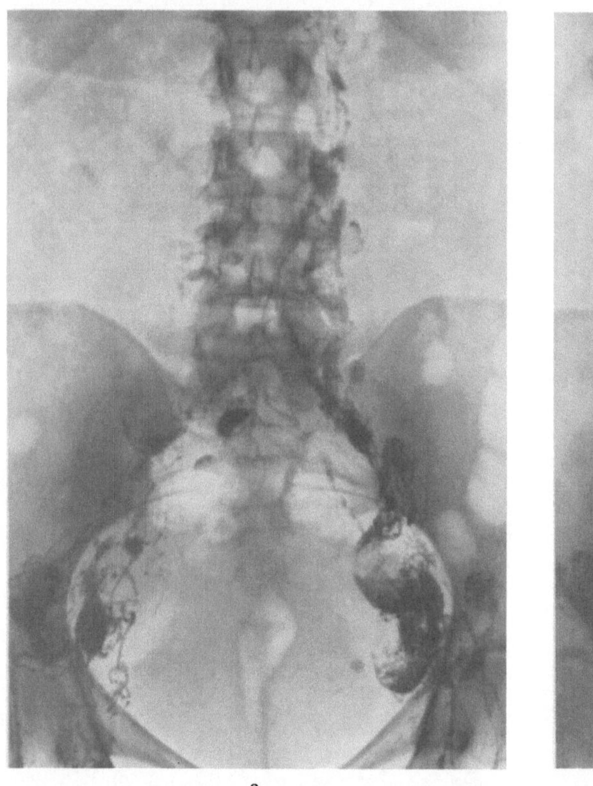 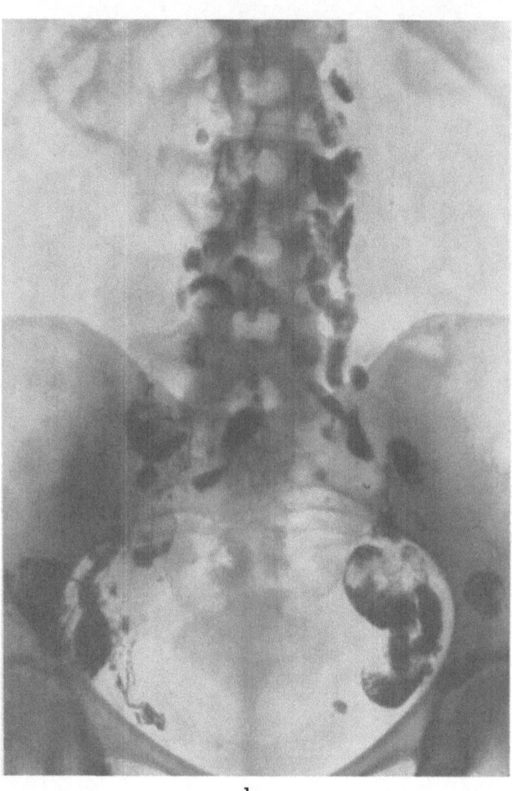

a   b

Abb. 4a u. b. Lymphographie bei einem Collumcarcinom Stadium III mit beidseitiger parametraner Infiltration bis zur Beckenwand. a Gefäßbild; b das Speicherbild ergibt eine bis zum 4. Lendenwirbel reichende beidseitige Lymphknotenmetastasierung mit zahlreichen Füllungsdefekten in vergrößerten Lymphknoten

knotenstationen hinaus mit der Lymphographie auch die zweiten und dritten Lymphknotenstationen makroskopisch beurteilt werden können. In therapeutischer Hinsicht erlangen diese Befunde eine große Bedeutung, da sie die operative oder radiologische Behandlung weitgehend beeinflussen. Durch eine routinemäßige Anwendung der Lymphographie bei allen Collumcarcinomen ist es einmal möglich, Beckenwandmetastasen bei einem klinisch als Stadium I imponierenden Fall aufzudecken (Abb. 3). Klinisch wertvoller erscheint uns aufgrund unserer Erfahrungen aber die Lymphographie bei den fortgeschritteneren, inoperablen Collumcarcinomen (Abb. 4). So konnte am Patientengut der Universitäts-Frauenklinik Hamburg bei den inoperablen Collumcarcinomen in 15—20 % mit der Lymphographie eine Lymphknotenmetastasierung außerhalb der üblichen parametranen, percutanen Bestrahlungsfelder aufgedeckt werden.

Während von uns die Lymphographie als routinemäßige Untersuchung zur Festlegung des Bestrahlungsplanes und Anpassung des Bestrahlungsfeldes an die Tumorausbreitung angesehen wird, wird von anderen Autoren wie Fuchs und Kottmeier (1964) der Phlebographie oder Cavographie der Vorzug gegeben. Mit diesen Untersuchungsmethoden ist es indirekt möglich, infiltrierte, vergrößerte Lymphknoten durch randständige und unregelmäßig begrenzte Eindellungen in die Venenwand zu erkennen. Zweifellos kann der Aussagewert einer Lymphographie durch eine zusätzliche Cavographie erhöht werden (Abb. 5).

Mit der transfemoralen Arteriographie gelingt es, parametrane Tumorinfiltrationen zu diagnostizieren (BREIT, 1967). Der Aussagewert der Arteriographie beim Collumcarcinom ist aber wohl zu begrenzt, um diese Untersuchungsmethode als Routineverfahren zur Stadieneinteilung durchzuführen.

Die Kenntnis der Ausbreitungswege des Collumcarcinoms ist die wichtigste Voraussetzung, um das Bestrahlungsfeld der Tumorausbreitung anpassen und vor allem eine Sicherheitszone um den Tumor herum einschließen zu können.

Das Collumcarcinom kann sich endophytisch oder exophytisch an der Portio entwickeln oder aber innerhalb des Cervicalkanals als sog. Cervixhöhlencarcinom entstehen. In etwa 95% der Fälle finden wir es als Plattenepithelcarcinom der Portio und in 5% als Adenocarcinom, das vom drüsigen Epithel des Cervixkanals ausgeht. Es werden drei Ausbreitungsrichtungen bevorzugt: Das Carcinom wächst kontinuierlich in das parametrane Bindegewebe, breitet sich über die Cervix hinaus auf das Scheidengewölbe und die Scheide aus oder dringt in Richtung auf das Uteruscavum vor. Diese Eigenschaften bestimmen die Form des Bestrahlungsfeldes bei den Frühfällen des Collumcarcinoms, die klinisch als Stadium I imponieren. Der zu bestrahlende Herd besitzt die Form eines Kegels; die Kegelspitze liegt im Fundus uteri und die Basis schließt die Portio, das Scheidengewölbe und den cervixnahen Abschnitt des Parametriums ein.

Ohne große technische Schwierigkeiten kann dieses Volumen durch die lokale Einlage bei einer Strahlenquelle erfaßt werden. Diese günstigen topographischen Bedingungen führten zur Entwicklung der Radiumtherapie beim Collumcarcinom, die über mehrere Jahrzehnte bis heute als Domäne der intrakavitären Radiumtherapie anzusehen ist. Das kegelförmige Bestrahlungsvolumen wird durch die Kombination einer intrauterinen mit einer intravaginalen Einlage erreicht. Während bei einer exophytischen Entwicklung des Collumcarcinoms das Schwergewicht der Radiumapplikation auf dem intravaginalen Radiumträger liegen wird, besitzt bei einem Cervixhöhlenneoplasma der intrauterine Radiumträger die größere Bedeutung.

Da der Uterus ein sehr strahlenresistentes Organ ist und auch die Vagina relativ hohe Strahlendosen verträgt, waren der Radiumdosierung weite Grenzen gesetzt. Man erkannte jedoch schon bald, daß eine gute Tumorrückbildung durch hohe Dosierung nur mit schweren Früh- und Spätreaktionen an Blase und Rectum erreicht werden konnte. Erst die Möglichkeit, exakte Dosismessungen an Blase und Rectum durchführen zu können, erbrachte die Grundlage für die Kenntnis der Strahlentoleranz dieser beiden Nachbarorgane. Der Lage der Radiumpräparate in Uterus und Vagina wurde größte Bedeutung beigemessen. Genormte Präparatekombinationen und sorgfältig durchgeführte Scheidentamponade dienten dazu, Blase und Rectum möglichst weit von der Strahlenquelle zu distanzieren.

Die Radiumbehandlung wurde über mehrere Jahrzehnte als einzige Methode der radiologischen Therapie des Collumcarcinoms durchgeführt. Erst nach etwa 2—3 Jahrzehnten erkannte man, daß insbesondere bei fortgeschrittenen Stadien die beckenwandnahen Anteile der Tumorinfiltration keine ausreichende Dosis erhalten. Hierzu wurden zwei Wege beschritten. Besonders von SEITZ und WINTZ (1920) wurde die konventionelle Röntgentherapie zur Bestrahlung der Parametrien über Bauch- und Rückenfelder entwickelt. Bei der hohen Strahlensensibilität der Haut war aber der Dosisgewinn am Parametrium und an den Beckenwandlymphknoten nur gering. Während in der weiteren Entwicklung die zusätzliche Percutanbestrahlung bei inoperablen Stadien von vielen radiologisch eingestellten Gynäkologen gefordert wurde, zweifelten andere an ihrem Wert und beschränkten sich ausschließlich auf die Radiumtherapie. Sie entwickelten hierzu besondere Applikatoren, die im seitlichen Scheidengewölbe liegen, wodurch die Distanz zur Beckenwand verringert werden kann. Eine weitere Möglichkeit wurde in der Anwendung des Körperhöhlenrohrs gesehen, wodurch die Beckenwand ebenfalls ohne Hautbelastung bestrahlt werden konnte.

Die ablehnende Haltung vieler Gynäkologen gegenüber der Percutanbestrahlung ist aus dem damaligen Entwicklungsstand zu verstehen; denn es war technisch nicht möglich, ohne stärkere Reaktionen eine tumorwirksame Dosis an die Beckenwand zu applizieren. Heute erscheint es selbstverständlich, daß bei einer Strahlenbehandlung des

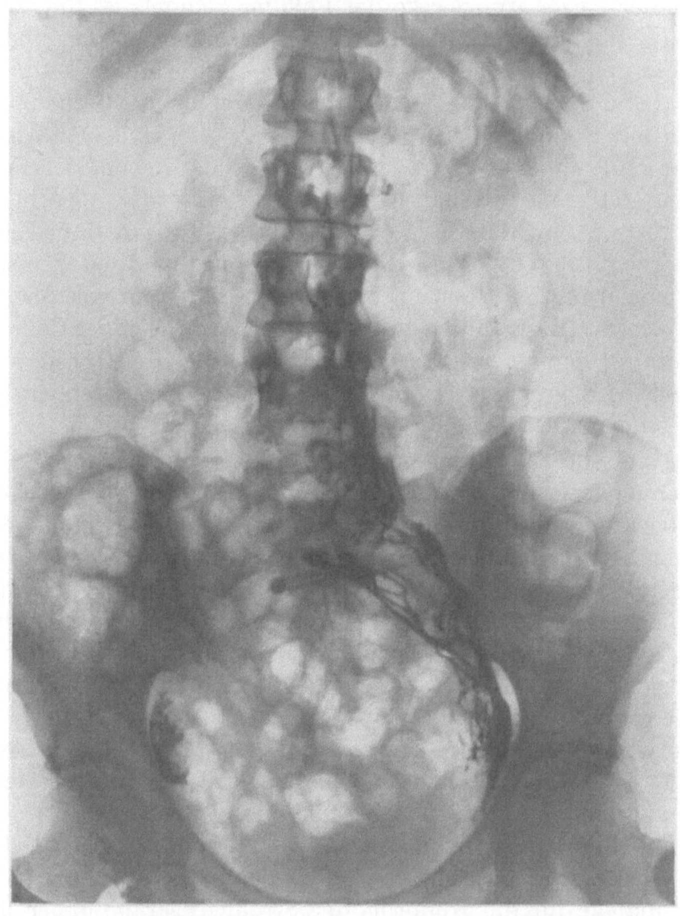

Abb. 5a u. b. Collumcarcinom Stadium III. a Die Lymphographie ergibt eine tumorbedingte komplette Lymphblockade rechts iliacal. Es markiert sich ein vergrößerter iliacaler Lymphknoten mit deutlichen randständigen Füllungsdefekten. Auf der rechten Seite proximal der Blockade keine Lymphknotenmarkierungen. b Die transfemorale Phlebographie ergibt rechts an der Teilung der Vena iliaca communis eine komplette Blockade. Das Kontrastmittel wird vorwiegend über die Vena lumbalis ascendens abtransportiert. Die nur schwach markierte Vena cava ist von medial her verdrängt und eingeengt. Der Tumorprozeß reicht somit bis zum zweiten Lendenwirbel

Collumcarcinoms das Bestrahlungsfeld über die Cervix hinaus bis zur Beckenwand reichen muß. Dies gilt bis auf wenige Ausnahmen für alle Stadien. Die Erkenntnis, daß es selbst in frühen Stadien durch eine diskontinuierliche Metastasierung zu Tumorabsiedelungen an der Beckenwand kommen kann, unterstreicht die Bedeutung der Bestrahlungsmethoden, durch die die Dosis an der Beckenwand ergänzt wird. Wie bereits ausgeführt, können die Tumorabsiedelungen an zahlreichen Lymphknoten im Becken lokalisiert sein. Die einzelnen Lymphknotengruppen können aber in sehr unterschiedlicher Entfernung zum Radiumträger liegen. Bei der üblichen Radiumdosierung schwankt die an die Lymph-

knoten gelangende Dosis gewaltig. Sie reicht von wenigen 100 R bis maximal 1 500 R.
Wenn wir mit gewisser Berechtigung annehmen können, daß die zur Zerstörung der
Metastasen notwendige Dosis an den Lymphknoten in der Größenordnung von etwa
5 000—6 000 R liegt, muß die durch die Percutanbestrahlung verabfolgte Dosis mindestens
4 000 R betragen.

Da die Dosisverteilung bei der intrakavitären Radiumapplikation weitgehend stan-
dardisiert ist, muß der Dosisverlauf der zusätzlichen Percutanbestrahlung dieser angepaßt werden. Hierbei gilt es, Dosisspitzen und unterdosierte Regionen im Bereich des

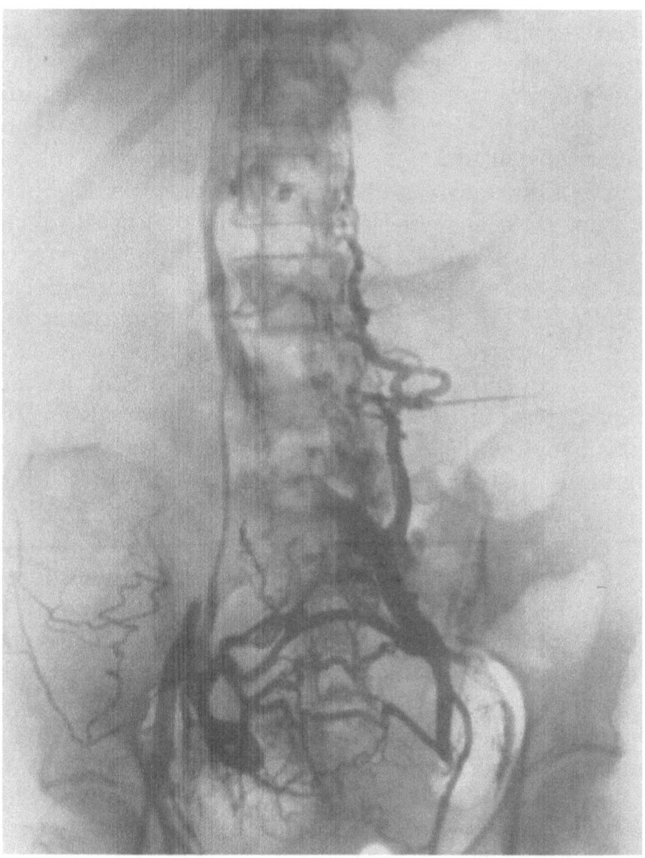

Abb. 5 b

Parametriums zu vermeiden. Die Dosis innerhalb des gesamten Parametriums soll homogen sein. An der Beckenwand wäre ein erneuter Dosisanstieg erstrebenswert. Fast alle
Lymphknoten können von einem rechteckigen Bestrahlungsfeld erfaßt werden. Lediglich
die präsacralen Lymphknoten liegen nahe der Mittellinie, die bei der Percutanbestrahlung
ausgespart werden muß, um nicht die Dosis an Blase und Rectum zu erhöhen.

Die untere Begrenzung der percutanen Felder liegt etwa beim Ligamentum inguinale,
damit die im Foramen obturatorium liegenden Lymphknoten sicher eingeschlossen sind.
Die seitliche Begrenzung muß die knöcherne Beckenwand mit den Lymphonodi iliaci
externi einschließen. Keinesfalls sollte der Schenkelhals im Bestrahlungsfeld liegen, da
bereits nach 3 000—4 000 R Schenkelhalsfrakturen gesehen wurden. Der größte Teil der
Lymphknoten liegt entlang der Vasa iliaca, einer nach cranial konvergierend verlaufenden
Achse. In Höhe des 4. und 5. Lendenwirbelkörpers vereinigen sich die beidseitigen Lymphwege. Wollte man somit die percutanen Bestrahlungsfelder ideal der Lymphknoten-
lokalisation anpassen, müßte die Achse der Percutanfelder ebenfalls cranial konvergieren.

Hierzu wurden von mehreren Autoren spezielle Bestrahlungsmethoden zur optimalen Anpassung an das Lymphsystem entwickelt (Surmont, 1957; Dibbelt, Rahm und Renner, 1960; Frischbier u. Würthner, 1971).

Es entspricht schon lange der klinischen Erfahrung, daß man in progredienten Fällen des Collumcarcinoms und vor allem im Finalstadium auch in der Lumbalregion Lymphknotenmetastasen findet. Diese Beobachtungen blieben jedoch für die gynäkologische Tumortherapie ohne therapeutische Konsequenz. Der Grund mag darin zu sehen sein, daß es unter konventionellen Strahlenbedingungen fast unmöglich erschien, das lumbale Lymphsystem ohne Strahlenschäden mit einer vollen Tumordosis zusätzlich erfassen zu können. In den letzten Jahren finden sich im Schrifttum häufig Hinweise, daß man bereits in Frühfällen vereinzelt Metastasen in den aortalen Lymphknoten sehen kann. Diese Beobachtungen werden vor allem durch routinemäßig durchgeführte Lymphographien bestätigt (Frischbier, 1965; Gerteis, 1966). Andererseits scheint die Zahl der Fälle zugenommen zu haben, bei denen man nach einer Tumortherapie eine lumbale Metastasierung findet, obwohl das kleine Becken vom Tumor vollkommen frei ist. So wurde in den letzten Jahren mehrfach die Frage diskutiert, ob die Behandlungsergebnisse durch eine zusätzliche, fälschlicherweise auch „prophylaktisch" genannte Bestrahlung des lumbalen Lymphsystems verbessert werden könnten.

Die Ausweitung des bestrahlten Volumens über das kleine Becken hinaus bis zur Cisterna chyli stellt jedoch an die Bestrahlungsplanung und Durchführung erhebliche Anforderungen, die erst durch Anwendung von Megavoltenergien bewältigt werden können. Das paraaortale Lymphabflußgebiet bietet für die Strahlenbehandlung hinsichtlich seiner Topographie wesentlich ungünstigere Bedingungen als im Beckenbereich, da es von mehreren strahlenempfindlichen und lebenswichtigen Organen umgeben ist: Rückenmark, Nieren, Ureteren und Intestinum. Durch spezielle Bestrahlungsmethoden bei Verwendung von Megavoltenergien ist es durchaus möglich, im Bereich der aortalen Lymphknoten eine volle Tumordosis einzustrahlen und die benachbarten strahlenempfindlichen Organe trotzdem zu schonen. Die ersten Erfahrungen von Weishaar (1967) ergeben, daß es beim Collumcarcinom des Stadiums I und II durch Erweiterung des Bestrahlungsfeldes auf die Lumbalregion nicht möglich ist, die Behandlungsergebnisse zu verbessern. Nach seinen Erfahrungen scheint eine absolute Indikation nur in den Stadien III und IV vorzuliegen. Da bisher aber nur an wenigen Stellen routinemäßig die Lumbalregion beim Collumcarcinom mitbestrahlt wird, fehlt es an Erfahrungen, um über die Bedeutung der zusätzlichen Bestrahlung der Lumbalregion eine Aussage machen zu können. Vielleicht ist es aber möglich, durch die primäre Bestrahlung der Lumbalregion ausgedehnte Formen einer Metastasierung in die aortalen Lymphknoten zu verhindern, die in einem hohen Prozentsatz über den Ductus thoracicus zu einer diffusen Lungenmetastasierung führen. Zwar ist es bis heute statistisch noch nicht erwiesen, daß Lungenmetastasierungen bei einem tumorfreien Befund im kleinen Becken in den letzten Jahren zugenommen haben. Den Strahlentherapeuten erschüttern jedoch jene Fälle, in denen im kleinen Becken ein ausgezeichneter Behandlungserfolg zu verzeichnen ist, eine aber schon zur Zeit der Primärbehandlung in der Lumbalregion bestehende Metastasierung im weiteren Verlauf zu Lungenmetastasen führt, für die es bis heute keine sinnvolle Behandlung gibt. Solange eine Ausdehnung des Bestrahlungsherdes bis zur Cisterna chyli nicht mit einer höheren Komplikationsrate verbunden ist, bestehen keine ernsten Bedenken dagegen, die Sicherheitszone bei der Bestrahlung des Collumcarcinoms über das kleine Becken hinaus nach cranial zu erweitern.

Da bereits im Stadium I des Collumcarcinoms in etwa 10—20 % mit einer Lymphknotenmetastasierung zu rechnen ist, gelten die dargestellten Behandlungsprinzipien der Kombination von lokaler Radiumtherapie und Percutanbestrahlung gleichermaßen für die Stadien I—III. Lediglich ein breites Übergreifen des Portiotumors auf die Scheide sowie die Infiltration des Tumors in die Blase oder in das Rectum erfordern eine Änderung der Bestrahlungsplanung.

Hat der Portiotumor bereits das obere Drittel der Vagina oder mehr befallen, ist eine zusätzliche Radiumapplikation notwendig. Vielfach werden diese Befunde wie primäre Vaginalcarcinome durch größere vaginale Applikatoren behandelt. Auch das Körperhöhlenrohr oder die Verwendung von schnellen Elektronen über einen Vaginaltubus kommen in Betracht.

Einer Änderung des Bestrahlungsplanes bedarf das Stadium IV, wenn der Tumor in die Blase oder das Rectum eingebrochen ist. Wie Abb. 9 zeigt, wird der Tumor in seiner Ausdehnung nach ventral oder dorsal hin durch den steilen Dosisabfall bei kombinierter Radiumapplikation nicht mehr voll belastet. Die Dosis an den äußeren Partien des Tumors kann nur durch eine Erhöhung der gesamten Radiumeinlage erreicht werden. Dabei müssen auch nicht infiltrierte Regionen höher belastet werden, so daß stärkere Strahlenreaktionen unvermeidbar sind. Vor allem kommt es durch die Fraktionierung der Radiumapplikation zu einem schnellen Einschmelzen des in das Hohlorgan vorgedrungenen Tumors. Die Folge hiervon sind Fistelbildungen, die den Behandlungserfolg oft vereiteln.

Seit Einführung von Megavoltenergien ist von verschiedenen Autoren der Versuch unternommen worden, bei derart fortgeschrittenen Tumoren die Radiumdosis insgesamt zu verringern und das Schwergewicht auf eine homogene Durchstrahlung des ganzen kleinen Beckens mit der Percutanbestrahlung zu legen. FLETCHER (1962) führt deshalb in solchen Fällen nur noch eine homogene Bestrahlung mit 22-MeV-Röntgenstrahlen von 4 großen Einfallsfeldern durch. Bei Verwendung von Telekobalt-γ-Strahlen bietet die Bewegungsbestrahlung, meist in Form der biaxialen Pendelbestrahlung (GIETZELT et al., 1962; FRISCHBIER u. KUTTIG, 1964), technisch die Möglichkeit, Dosen von 6000 bis 8000 R unter Vermeidung von stärkeren Hautreaktionen ins kleine Becken einzustrahlen. Die bisherigen Erfahrungen sind erfolgversprechend. Die ersten Behandlungsergebnisse haben gezeigt, daß es auch unter Verzicht auf eine lokale Radiumapplikation möglich ist, ausgedehnte Beckenbefunde mit Einbruch ins Rectum oder in die Blase über mehrere Jahre rezidivfrei zu bekommen. Es erscheint bedeutungsvoll, daß vor allem die Zahl der schweren Rectum-Scheiden- oder Blasen-Scheiden-Fisteln erheblich verringert werden konnte.

d) Kombination von Operation und Bestrahlung

α) Die präoperative Bestrahlung

Die präoperative Strahlentherapie hat auch in der Gynäkologie bei der Behandlung des Collumcarcinoms wenig Anhänger gefunden. Die ursprünglich angegebene Indikation zu einer Vorbestrahlung, durch die eine Peritonitis und die allgemeine Sepsis bei verjauchenden Carcinomen vermieden werden sollte, ist heute weitgehend bedeutungslos. Auch die Devitalisierung der Tumorzellen durch eine reduzierte Strahlendosis bei der Vorbestrahlung erscheint nach unseren heutigen Kenntnissen zweifelhaft. Trotzdem sehen viele Gynäkologen in der Vorbestrahlung eine sinnvolle Ergänzung der Operation, durch die die Behandlungsergebnisse verbessert werden könnten. Als mögliche Vorteile der präoperativen Bestrahlung werden angegeben: Verminderung der Infektionsgefahr, Verringerung einer Tumoraussaat intra operationem, Vermeidung von Stumpfrezidiven, Steigerung der Operabilitätsrate und die Möglichkeit zu intensiver, allgemeiner Vorbehandlung. Als Nachteile werden angesehen: der zweimalige Krankenhausaufenthalt, ein eventuell fortschreitendes Wachstum von nicht genügend bestrahlten Metastasen, die dosisbedingte Erschwerung des operativen Eingriffs sowie die Störung der Wundheilung.

Über die angegebenen Vor- und Nachteile findet man im Schrifttum unterschiedliche Ansichten. CURRIE (1952) bezweifelt, daß der Halskanal des Uterus durch eine präoperative Radiumeinlage gereinigt und die Gefahr der Infektion herabgesetzt wird. SCHMITZER (1961) betont, daß die präoperative Bestrahlung nicht in kurativer Absicht durchgeführt werden soll, sondern nur zur Unterdrückung des Vermehrungs- und Invasionspotentials der Zellen. Als Bestrahlungsmethode wird deshalb vielfach eine intrauterine Radiumeinlage mit etwa 2000—4000 mgeh empfohlen (Currie, 1952; Schubert, 1953; Schmidt-Elmendorff und Dibbelt, 1956; Leb, 1959; Hollenbeck, 1960; Sicard, 1960).

Als bester Operationstermin wird die Zeit von 1—2 Monaten nach der Radiumeinlage angesehen. Zu dieser Zeit soll die örtliche Strahlenreaktion abgeklungen und die „Aktivität" der Carcinomzellen am geringsten sein (Sicard, 1960). Die als Bestrahlungsfolgen auftretenden narbigen Veränderungen sollen sich zu diesem Zeitpunkt noch nicht ausgebildet haben.

Neben der intrauterinen Radiumtherapie werden auch die Kombination mit der Percutanbestrahlung (Dargent, 1957; Dragon und Trestioreano, 1963; Greiss, 1965; Lenzi et al., 1965) oder die ausschließliche Percutanbestrahlung (Liegner et al., 1960; Hai, Held u. Schwarz, 1963) als Methode zur Vorbestrahlung angegeben.

Die Schwierigkeit der präoperativen Bestrahlung des Collumcarcinoms liegt darin, daß der Effekt einer Bestrahlung bei niedriger Dosis ohne Erhöhung des operativen Risikos gering ist und andererseits das Operationsrisiko bei einer kurativen Dosis beträchtlich ansteigt.

Über ein großes Erfahrungsgut verfügen Dragon und Trestioreano (1963). In 94 Fällen des Stadiums I und in 319 Fällen des Stadiums II führten sie eine Vorbestrahlung durch. In 106 Fällen wurden mit dem Körperhöhlenrohr 10000—15000 R appliziert, in 307 Fällen erfolgte eine lokale Radiumbehandlung mit etwa 7200 mgeh, ergänzt durch eine percutane Röntgentherapie. Die operative Behandlung war technisch nicht erschwert. In ihrem Patientengut fanden sie einen örtlichen Erfolg der Vorbestrahlung in 82% der Fälle. Die 5-Jahres-Heilung lag im Stadium I bei 89,3% und im Stadium II bei 74,6%.

Bei 66 Fällen des Stadiums I und 18 Fällen des Stadiums II hatte Hollenbeck (1960) eine einmalige intrakavitäre Kobalt-60-Einlage durchgeführt, wobei auf den Punkt A eine Dosis von etwa 5500 R eingestrahlt wurde. Nach 6—8 Wochen folgte die Radikaloperation nach Wertheim in der Modifizierung nach Meigs. Das operative Vorgehen war durch die Vorbestrahlung in keiner Weise beeinträchtigt. Die Operationsmortalität betrug rund 1%. Ureter- und Blasenfisteln traten bei 6 Patientinnen (= 7,2%) auf. Bei den 84 behandelten Fällen wurde eine 5-Jahres-Heilung im Stadium I von 95,2% und im Stadium II von 85,7% erzielt. Bei 10 Patientinnen fand man positive Lymphknotenmetastasen. In diesen Fällen lag die 5-Jahres-Heilung in beiden Stadien bei 75%.

Dargent, Mayer und Butel (1957) berichten über ihre Erfahrungen mit der Vorbestrahlung an 400 Fällen. Sie fanden, daß der radiologische Effekt in 213 Fällen vollkommen war. Bei 47 Fällen fanden sie im Uterus noch Carcinomnester, bei 85 in den Lymphknoten, bei 55 im Uterus und in den Lymphknoten und bei 3 Fällen in den Ovarien. Die primäre Operationsmortalität betrug 7,2%. In den Fällen, in denen durch die Vorbestrahlung alle Carcinomnester verschwunden waren, betrug die Heilung 80%, bestanden noch Herde im Uterus 67% und bei Befall der Lymphknoten trotz Bestrahlung nur 24%. An Komplikationen wurden 10 Ureterfisteln, 14 Blasen-Scheidenfisteln und 12 Rectum-Scheidenfisteln beobachtet.

Lenzi u. Mitarb. (1965) versuchen, an ausgewählten Patientinnen aus einem Patientengut von 105 Fällen die präoperative Telekobalttherapie mit der präoperativen Radiumtherapie zu vergleichen. Sie bestrahlten 10 Patientinnen des Stadiums I und 10 des Stadiums II präoperativ durch eine intrakavitäre Radiumeinlage. Hierbei wurden 7000 R am Punkt A und 2500—3000 R am Punkt B appliziert. Bei einer gleichen Zahl von Patientinnen führten sie in einer Serie mit 4500 R/Herddosis im kleinen Becken eine Telekobaltbestrahlung über 4 Kreuzfelder (15×8 cm) durch. Bei den 10 mit Radium behandelten Patientinnen des Stadiums I waren mäßige Operationsschwierigkeiten zu verzeichnen (2 vesico-vaginale Fisteln). Im Stadium II waren die Operationsschwierigkeiten größer: in 8 Fällen traten Beckenwandinfiltrationen auf. Bei der Telekobalttherapie bestanden keine Operationsschwierigkeiten. Eine histologische „Sterilisation" wurde bei den Radiumpatientinnen im Stadium I in 8 Fällen und im Stadium II in 5 Fällen, nach der Telekobalttherapie im Stadium I bei 6 Fällen und im Stadium II bei 7 Fällen erreicht. — Auch LIEGNER, BERRY und OAKMAN (1960) führen eine präoperative Telekobalttherapie durch. Sie applizieren innerhalb von 30 Tagen auf das ganze Becken bis zur Aortenbifurkation 4000 R. Die Strahlenreaktionen waren minimal. Das Intervall zwischen der Strahlenbehandlung und der Operation variierte zwischen 4 Tagen und 4 Wochen. In 5 von 8 Fällen wurden bei der Operation noch Tumorreste an der Cervix gefunden. Die Blutstillung machte keine Schwierigkeiten. Der postoperative Verlauf war stets unauffällig.

TOPOL und GROSS (1961) führten eine percutane Vorbestrahlung mit 4200—6200 R im gesamten Beckenbereich innerhalb von 4—5 Wochen durch. Zusätzlich wurden 1200—2000 R intravaginal auf das Collum uteri verabfolgt. An Hand detaillierter histologischer Untersuchungen von 52 Operationspräparaten haben sie gezeigt, daß es durch die percutane Strahlentherapie im Stadium I in 72,4 % möglich war, das Carcinom zum Verschwinden zu bringen. Im Stadium II gelang es nur in 52,6 % der Fälle.

Aus der Tatsache, daß 5-Jahres-Heilungen auch in den Fällen zu erreichen waren, in denen nach der präoperativen Strahlenbehandlung noch Tumorreste zurückgeblieben waren, leiten diese Autoren die Berechtigung zu ihrer Behandlungsmethode ab.

RIECK (1958) glaubt, die Behandlungsresultate durch eine präoperative Bestrahlung mit dem Körperhöhlenrohr verbessern zu können. Er berichtet über die Ergebnisse bei 79 Collumcarcinomen des Stadiums I, bei denen die Portio in 10 Sitzungen 6400 R erhielt; die Dosis entspricht 2000 R in 2 cm Tiefe. Demgegenüber konnte HALTER (1960) zeigen, daß eine Vorbestrahlung mit dem Körperhöhlenrohr (60 kV), bei der versehentlich in 18 Sitzungen insgesamt 20500 R/Oberfläche appliziert worden waren, keinen Therapieerfolg gebracht hatte. 5 Monate später war an der Portio ein großes Krebsgeschwür aufgetreten. Im Operationspräparat wurde histologisch nachgewiesen, daß noch überall Carcinom vorhanden war.

Wenn auch einzelne Autoren mit dieser Methode gute Ergebnisse erzielt haben, wie beispielsweise SCHLINK (1950), der beim Stadium III bei 44 von 99 Patientinnen eine 5-Jahres-Heilung erzielen konnte, so wird doch vielfach der aufgrund der Kombination beider Behandlungsmethoden erzielte Gewinn durch eine Operationsmortalität von 5 bis 8 % zunichte gemacht, ungerechnet der Fisteln und der Verstümmelungen (LABORDE u. REDON, 1954). Deshalb wird die Bedeutung einer präoperativen Strahlenbehandlung von einigen Autoren ausschließlich in der Vermeidung von Lokalrezidiven gesehen (SCHMIDT-ELMENDORFF und DIBBELT, 1956; BURCH, CHALFANT und LAVELY, 1957).

In Ergänzung zu den Ergebnissen von SCHLINK (1950) erscheinen die Untersuchungen von GREISS (1965) aufschlußreich. Nach seiner Ansicht ist die Radiokurabilität beim Collumcarcinom des Stadiums III abhängig von der Radiosensibilität des Primärtumors, von dem hohen Lymphknotenbefall, den Schwierigkeiten bei Befall der unteren Vagina und der geringen Resistenz des Nachbargewebes und einem mikroskopisch nicht nachweisbaren Vergleich von ruhenden Tumorresten nach kurativer Strahlentherapie, die später ein agressives Verhalten wiedergewinnen können. Er zieht es deshalb vor, die Patientinnen nicht erst bei einem Rezidiv (SCHJÖTT-RIVERS und ISTRE, 1959) zu operieren, sondern in einer früheren Phase relativer Tumorruhe. In einer Serie von 93 Fällen der Stadien I—III erhielten die Patientinnen durch eine kombinierte Radium-Röntgentherapie 3600 R am Punkt B und 7200 R am Punkt A (s. S. 178). Schwere Komplikationen nach radikaler Operation wurden in 20 % gesehen, von denen 14 % zu Lasten der Operation gingen. Durch die mangelnde Blutversorgung der Beckenorgane infolge der Bestrahlung und der radikalen Operation, kommt es bei der Kombination von Vorbestrahlung und Operation zu einem Anstieg schwerer Komplikationen, die 2—4mal höher als bei der Strahlenbehandlung allein und 2—3mal höher als nach der primären radikalen Operation sind. Wenn bei der Operation kein Resttumor mehr vorhanden ist, beträgt die Heilung 86%, wenn lokal in der Cervix oder in der benachbarten Vagina Tumor zurückgeblieben ist 48% und beim Vorhandensein von Lymphknotenmetastasen 30—50%. Die Bedeutung der Vorbestrahlung im Stadium III glaubt GREISS an Hand von 25 Fällen ablesen zu können. Bei diesen Patientinnen war in 10 Fällen die Radiosensibilität schlecht. Alle Patienten verstarben während der ersten 2 Jahre. Bei 15 Patientinnen sprach die Vorbestrahlung gut an. In 10 von diesen Fällen wurde eine radikale Operation im Anschluß an die Strahlenbehandlung durchgeführt. Bei 7 dieser Fälle war kein Tumor mehr nachzuweisen. Alle überlebten 5 Jahre. In 2 weiteren Fällen wurde ein Carcinom in der Cervix gefunden, trotzdem überlebten die Patientinnen. Nur eine Patientin mit einer Lymphknotenmetastase bekam nach 8 Monaten ein Rezidiv. Von den 5 nicht operierten Patientinnen sind 2 geheilt, während 3 nach 6—42 Monaten ein Rezidiv bekamen. Von den 25 Patientinnen leben somit nach 5 Jahren noch 44%, davon 13,3% der nicht operierten und 90% der zusätzlich operierten.

Auch CHEN, LOFSTROM und BUDDEN (1963) untersuchten an 87 unausgewählten Patientinnen der Stadien I und II die Wirkung der Bestrahlung auf den Primärtumor. Sie applizierten in der einen Gruppe 10000 R auf Punkt A innerhalb 8—10 Wochen, während die andere Gruppe in 5 Wochen 8000 R auf Punkt A erhielt. Die Dosis wurde durch eine einmalige Radiumeinlage (Paris, Manchester) und durch eine Percutanbestrahlung (250-kV-Röntgen oder Kobalt-60) eingestrahlt. Die Operation (erweiterte Totalexstirpation mit Lymphonodektomie) nahm man nach unterschiedlichen Intervallen von 3 Monaten bis 2 Jahren vor. Handelte es sich um ein Plattenepithelcarcinom, so wurde in 19,6% der Frauen bei der Operation Carcinomgewebe nachgewiesen. Beim Adenocarcinom war noch in 3 von 4 Fällen Carcinomgewebe zu registrieren. Bei 16 von 19 Patientinnen war das Carcinom im Collum, bei 8 Patientinnen in Lymphknoten nachweisbar. Die Patientinnen, die 10000 R in 10 Wochen erhalten hatten, zeigten in 37,4% und diejenigen mit 8000 R in 5 Wochen noch in 9,4% der Fälle Carcinomgewebe.

THEILHEFER und DARGENT haben zusammen 75 Fälle von Collumcarcinom des Stadiums I nach vorausgegangener Strahlentherapie radikal operiert. Bei einer Mortalität von 8,4% fanden sie bis zu 30% Carcinomzellinseln im bestrahlten Collum und in den Lymphknoten.

Die im Schrifttum vorhandenen Angaben reichen keinesfalls aus, um mit statistischer Signifikanz beweisen zu können, daß durch eine Vorbestrahlung die Heilungsergebnisse verbessert werden können. Trotzdem muß als gesichert angesehen werden, daß es durch präoperative Bestrahlung möglich ist, in einem von der Dosis abhängenden Prozentsatz den Tumor zu devitalisieren. Hierbei spielt das Zeitintervall zwischen Bestrahlung und Operation eine wesentliche Rolle. Die Kenntnis über die Wirkung der Vorbestrahlung auf den Tumor ist aber bis heute noch sehr lückenhaft, da die Vitalität eines Tumors mit den vorhandenen Untersuchungsmethoden nur ungenau bestimmt werden kann. Morphologische Kriterien reichen zur Beurteilung keinesfalls aus. So wird von SCHJÖTT-RIVERS und ISTRE (1959) auch darauf hingewiesen, daß eine Vorbestrahlung nur dann eine Bedeutung hat, wenn vorher die Strahlensensibilität bestimmt werden kann.

β) Die postoperative Bestrahlung

Die postoperative Bestrahlung des Collumcarcinoms wird von vielen Gynäkologen als unerläßliche Ergänzung der Operation bei der Behandlung des Collumcarcinoms angesehen. Trotzdem sind im Schrifttum viele kritische Stimmen zu finden, die den Wert einer Bestrahlung nach Radikaloperation bezweifeln. Andererseits ist es nur mit Mühe möglich, im Schrifttum Arbeiten zu finden, die den eindeutigen Wert einer zusätzlichen Nachbestrahlung beweisen.

Überzeugend waren die von SCHINZ (1936) in einer Sammelstatistik mitgeteilten Erfahrungen, daß die nur operierten Collumcarcinome des Stadium I eine 5-Jahres-Heilung von 41% erbracht hatten, während die operierten und nachbestrahlten Fälle mit 55,3% eindeutig bessere Ergebnisse gezeigt hatten.

Derartig überzeugende Behandlungsergebnisse sind in der Folgezeit im Schrifttum nicht wieder zu finden. Es fehlte weitgehend an alternierenden Reihen, die allein eine Aussage über den Wert einer vorsorglichen Nachbestrahlung machen könnten. Es fanden sich viele Gynäkologen, die den Wert mehr aus theoretischen Erörterungen anerkannten: durch eine postoperative Bestrahlung sollte eine Vernichtung von zurückgelassenem Tumorgewebe und vor allem von mikroskopischen Lymphknotenmetastasen erreicht werden. Die Schwierigkeit lag aber vor allem darin, daß die zur Wirkung gelangende Dosis in einer Größenordnung liegen mußte, die keinesfalls die Abwehrkräfte des Körpers ungünstig beeinflussen durfte. Als Toleranzdosis wurden 3000—3200 R angesehen (HOFMANN, 1963). Bei einer höheren Dosis sei mit einer Schädigung der Beckenwandgefäße zu rechnen, woraus sich die Gefahr der Sklerosierung im Bereich der Ureteren und der Blase ergibt. Diese Dosishöhe wurde entscheidend durch die Untersuchungen von HILLEMANNS (1957) beeinflußt, der nach 3000 R eine nahezu vollständige Zerstörung des lymphatischen Gewebes der Beckenwandlymphknoten beobachtete.

Nach unseren heutigen Kenntnissen war zu erwarten, daß eine vorsorgliche Bestrahlung der Beckenwandlymphknoten mit 3000 R in klinischer Hinsicht nicht sehr erfolgreich sein konnte, da zur Devitalisierung von Lymphknotenmetastasen sicher eine weit höhere Dosis notwendig ist. Es erscheint daher nicht verwunderlich, daß die vor etwa 15 Jahren von KIRCHHOFF aufgerufene Arbeitsgemeinschaft deutscher Frauenkliniken zur Klärung der Frage, ob radikal operierte Collumcarcinome prophylaktisch nachbestrahlt werden sollen, praktisch ergebnislos verlaufen war. KIRCHHOFF hatte gefordert, daß 5 Jahre lang alle radikal operierten Fälle des Stadiums I alternierend 1 Jahr lang nachbestrahlt und dann wieder 1 Jahr lang nicht nachbestrahlt werden sollten.

An Hand von 620 operierten Collumcarcinomen von 6 deutschen Frauenkliniken konnte KIRCHHOFF zeigen, daß die Gruppe der vorsorglich nachbestrahlten — wenn auch sehr gering — günstiger abschneidet und die primären Heilungsergebnisse der Rezidivbestrahlungstherapie bei den vorbestrahlten Fällen nicht schlechter sind. HELBING (1961) konnte nachweisen, daß am Patientengut der Universitäts-Frauenklinik Jena im Zeitraum von 1948—1955 bei 242 operierten und nachbestrahlten Patientinnen des Stadium I die 5-Jahres-Heilung 76 % betrug, während bei 262 nur operierten Patientinnen die Heilung bei 74 % lag. HELBING diskutierte auch die Frage ausführlich, warum die Ergebnisse der radikal operierten Fälle durch eine Nachbestrahlung nicht eindeutig verbessert werden konnten. Einmal war die Form der Nachbestrahlung technisch unzureichend gewesen. Als weitere Gründe führt er an: eine Herabsetzung der Strahlenwirkung durch Sauerstoffmangel im Operationsgebiet, eine Verminderung der Strahlenempfindlichkeit der Carcinomzellen durch eine Entzündung im Operationsgebiet sowie die Vermutung, daß der Tumor eine gewisse Mindestgröße erreicht haben muß, um auf die Bestrahlung zu reagieren.

Als günstigster Zeitpunkt für den Beginn der Nachbestrahlung wird ein Intervall von 3 (VONESSEN, 1957) bis 8 Wochen (HOFMANN, 1963) angesehen. HOFMANN glaubt, daß der Beginn einer „prophylaktischen" Nachbestrahlung nicht vor der 6.—8. Woche nach der Operation liegen sollte, da die Patientinnen sich erst dann vom Trauma der Operation erholt haben, daß die Nachbestrahlung keine entscheidende Beeinträchtigung der körpereigenen Abwehrkräfte bedeutet.

Bei Anwendung von konventionellen Röntgenstrahlen war die Technik der Nachbestrahlung relativ einheitlich. Es wurde meist eine lokale Radiumeinlage in den Scheidenstumpf mit einer Dosierung von 1000—3000 mgeh empfohlen. Die höhere Radiumdosis wurde gewählt, wenn der Verdacht bestand, daß das Operationspräparat nicht voll im Gesunden abgesetzt werden konnte. Zusätzlich erfolgte eine Homogenbestrahlung der Beckenwand von 2 ventralen und dorsalen Feldern.

An der Universitäts-Frauenklinik Hamburg wird seit 5 Jahren die postoperative Bestrahlung nach Wertheimscher Radikaloperation mit einer homogenen Telekobalttherapie des ganzen kleinen Beckens durchgeführt, bei der teils über Stehfelder, teils über eine biaxiale Pendelbestrahlung 6000 R innerhalb von 4 Wochen verabfolgt werden.

Die bisherigen Erfahrungen zeigen, daß die 10 Tage post operationem begonnene Strahlenbehandlung ohne lokale Radiumeinlage von den Patientinnen gut vertragen wird.
Der postoperative Verlauf wird nicht gestört. Die bisherigen Beobachtungszeiten reichen
nicht aus, um eine Verbesserung der Heilungsergebnisse durch die Dosis von 6000 R ab-
leiten zu können.

Verständlicherweise wird man von einer Nachbestrahlung nur in den Fällen einen
Erfolg erwarten können, in denen bereits eine Lymphknotenmetastasierung besteht. Da
es ohne wesentliche Erhöhung des Operationsrisikos nicht möglich ist, das gesamte
fakultative Lymphabflußgebiet der Cervix uteri operativ auszuräumen, hängt die Verbesserung der Heilungsergebnisse vom Befall der Lymphknoten ab. Rechnet man im
Stadium I mit etwa 10—20% Lymphknotenmetastasen, so erscheint eine generelle,
routinemäßige Nachbestrahlung schon von Nutzen zu sein. Allerdings wird selbst bei
optimaler Dosierung nicht in allen Fällen einer Lymphknotenmetastasierung eine Heilung
zu erreichen sein, da ein nicht abschätzbarer Prozentsatz von Lymphknotenmetastasen
bei der üblichen Dosierung als radioresistent angesehen werden muß. Die Verbesserung
der Behandlungsergebnisse muß demnach geringer als 10—20% sein. Wenn es auch nur
an großen randomisierten Reihen möglich sein wird, diese Verbesserung der Ergebnisse
zu objektivieren, ergeben sich doch zumindest keine schweren Kontraindikationen gegen
eine Nachbestrahlung, wenn man von der mit Folgen behafteten Kastration junger Frauen
absieht.

Alarmierend waren allerdings die bereits mitgeteilten Untersuchungen (s. S. 159) von
Engeset (1964). Wenn diese Untersuchungsergebnisse auch nicht vorbehaltlos auf den
Menschen übertragen werden können, sollte die Indikation zu einer Sicherheitsbestrahlung
doch eingeengt werden. Die bisherigen klinischen Erfahrungen mit der postoperativen
Behandlung sprechen aber gegen die Befunde von Engeset, da sonst bei den nachbe-
strahlten Patientinnen eine Fernmetastasierung wesentlich häufiger auftreten müßte.
Hierfür findet sich im Weltschrifttum aber kein Anhalt.

γ) Die Bestrahlung nach unvollständiger Operation

Von der vorsorglichen, postoperativen Sicherheitsbestrahlung muß die Bestrahlungs-
indikation streng abgetrennt werden, die sich aus einer nicht radikal möglichen Operation
ergibt. Der in solchen Fällen indizierten Nachbestrahlung kommt die Bedeutung einer
primären Strahlenbehandlung zu. Bestrahlungsmethodik und Dosierung entsprechen
somit denen bei der primären Strahlenbehandlung.

Beim Collumcarcinom stellen sich aber bei inkompletter Entfernung des Tumors
größere technische Schwierigkeiten ein, da meist der als Radiumträger dienende Uterus
entfernt wird. Es kann dann nur noch eine relativ niedrig dosierte Radiumeinlage ins
Scheidengewölbe erfolgen. Die Dosislimitierung ergibt sich infolge der durch die hohe
Blasen- und Rectumbelastung veränderten topographischen Verhältnisse. Der weitaus
größte Teil der Dosis muß über eine percutane Bestrahlung erreicht werden; denn die
Tumorreste befinden sich meist an der Beckenwand in unmittelbarer Nähe der größeren
Gefäße, die eine vollständige Entfernung des Tumors verhindern. Bei Anwendung von
konventionellen Röntgenstrahlen können somit höchstens 3000 oder mit der Bewegungs-
oder Siebbestrahlung 4000—4500 R appliziert werden.

Daher scheint es nicht verwunderlich zu sein, daß die Behandlungsergebnisse wesentlich ungünstiger sind, wenn der Tumor makroskopisch nicht im Gesunden entfernt werden
konnte. So fand Cosbie (1963) in derartigen Fällen nur eine 3-Jahres-Heilung von 24%.
Statistisch ist es aber an Hand des Weltschrifttums sehr schwierig, den Beweis anzu-
treten, daß die Heilungsergebnisse bei unvollständiger Operation mit Nachbestrahlung
beim Collumcarcinom signifikant schlechter als nach ausschließlicher Strahlenbehandlung
sind. Dessen ungeachtet findet man im Schrifttum die einhellige Meinung, daß wegen der
verringerten Heilungschance bei lokaler Inoperabilität der alleinigen Strahlentherapie

der Vorrang zu geben ist. Ungünstig verlaufende Einzelfälle mögen diese Einstellung zu Recht begründet haben. Ob bei Anwendung von Megavoltenergien, mit denen eine homogene, hochdosierte Durchstrahlung des kleinen Beckens auch unter Verzicht auf Radium erfolgen kann, andere Bedingungen gegeben sind, kann bis heute nicht beantwortet werden.

δ) Die intraoperative Bestrahlung

Eine besondere Form der Kombination von Strahlenbehandlung und Operation stellt die intraoperative Bestrahlung dar. Diese Bestrahlungsform findet nur sehr selten Anwendung. Meist soll sie dazu dienen, unter Vermeidung von Hautreaktionen eine Tumordosis an die Beckenwandlymphknoten zu applizieren.

Über Erfahrungen mit einer solchen kombinierten chirurgisch-radiotherapeutischen Behandlungsmethode berichten CENTARO et al. (1958) bei 12 Fällen. Nach einer präoperativen Radiumapplikation führten sie nach einem Intervall von 30 Tagen die transvaginale radikale Hysterektomie durch. Für die intraoperative Zusatzbestrahlung verwendeten sie Kobaltperlen mit einem Durchmesser von 0,5 cm und einer Aktivität von 5,7—6 mCi ^{60}Co, die in die zentrale Bohrung von 2 ovoiden Trägern eingeführt werden. Zur Homogenisierung der Isodosen werden die aktiven Perlen mit inaktiven versetzt. Eine Bestrahlungseinheit von 2 ovoiden Trägern, beziehungsweise 4 aktiven Perlen, wird in eine grob gelochte Schaumgummiplatte versenkt, die die Größe der Operationshöhle hat. Nach vollständiger Peritonealisierung wird beidseits je eine chargierte Schaumgummiplatte in das Operationscavum parallel zur Beckenwand auf Höhe der Spina ischiadica eingelegt und antamponiert. Die Berechnung der Dosisverteilung erfolgt nach Anfertigung einer Beckenaufnahme unter Berücksichtigung der effektiven Lage des Präparates zur Beckentopographie. Bei einer erwünschten mittleren Dosis von 3500 R auf Höhe des Beckenbodens und in 1 cm Abstand beträgt die Liegezeit des Präparates 36—48 Std. Zusammen mit der Vorbelastung von 1500—2000 R wird nach der Meinung der Autoren die notwendige Tumorzerstörungsdosis erreicht. Die Methode ist nicht durch Nachblutungen belastet. Lediglich die Wundheilung soll langsamer erfolgen.

Eine andere Möglichkeit, intraoperativ Radium an die Beckenwand zu applizieren, beschreibt GUSSO (1954). Selbst in fortgeschrittenen Fällen legt er 40—50 Tage nach ultraradikaler Operation durch einen großen Schnitt vom Rippenbogen bis zum Leistenband nach extraperitonealem Freilegen der Arteria iliaca interna an die vordere und seitliche Beckenwand von der Aponeurose des Musculus obturator aufwärts bis zu den aortalen Lymphknoten ein Radiumlängspräparat ein. Es bleiben 110—120 mg Radium für 4—5 Tage liegen. Bei 51 Fällen kam es zu einem Todesfall im postoperativen Verlauf. In der Regel schließt sich die Wunde nach Entfernen des Radiumträgers innerhalb von 14 Tagen.

Eine weitere Anwendungsmöglichkeit ergibt sich durch die intraoperative Injektion oder Implantation von Radionucliden bei umschriebenen, nicht entfernbaren Tumoren (KAPP-SCHWOERER, 1962). Diese Bestrahlungsform ist im Kapitel „Interstitielle Curietherapie" (s. S. 191) näher beschrieben.

4. Bestrahlungsmethoden beim Collumcarcinom

a) Kontakttherapie

α) Intrakavitäre Curietherapie

Die intrakavitäre Radiumbestrahlung ist als klassische Methode der gynäkologischen Strahlentherapie zu bezeichnen. Bei der Behandlung des Collumcarcinoms erfüllt sie optimal die Forderung, eine möglichst hohe Strahlendosis an den Ausgangspunkt des Carcinoms heranzubringen. Zur Erzielung einer therapeutisch wirksamen Dosis am Primärtumor und im Parametrium unter Schonung von Blase, Ureter und Rectum wurden in mehr als 5 Jahrzehnten unzählige Behandlungsmethoden entwickelt.

Bei den Collumcarcinomen war die Möglichkeit einer Standardisierung der Bestrahlungsmethoden schon relativ früh gegeben. Die Voraussetzungen dazu ergaben sich durch die Häufigkeit dieser Tumoren und aus der Forderung nach Zentralisation der Therapie in Schwerpunkten mit großer Patientenzahl. Die Bestrebungen, eine sehr spezialisierte Strahlenbehandlung zentral mit guter ärztlicher Erfahrung und optimaler apparativer Ausstattung durchzuführen, gingen vor allen Dingen von Skandinavien, Frankreich und den angelsächsischen Ländern aus; sie waren die Voraussetzung für die Entwicklung der klassischen Methoden der Strahlenbehandlung des Collumcarcinoms, die von den früheren Zentren in Paris, Stockholm, Manchester, New York, München, Heidelberg und anderen ausgegangen war.

Die entscheidende Vorbedingung für die Entwicklung der klassischen Standardmethoden beim Collumcarcinom war aber durch die Konstanz der Abmessungen des Beckenraumes mit der zentralen Lage des Uterus und der Vagina sowie die typische

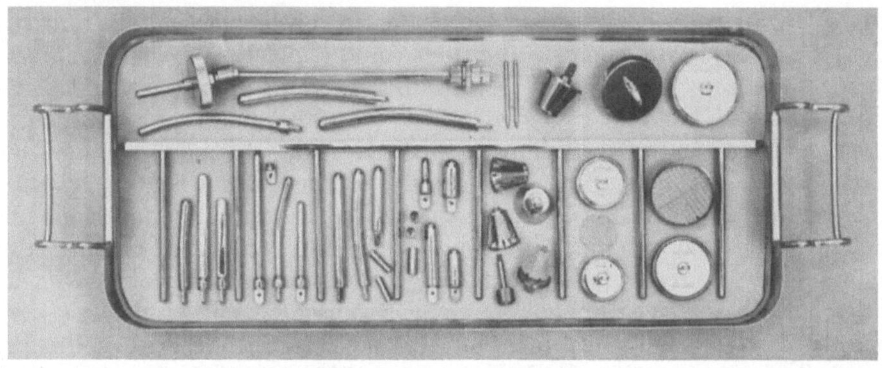

Abb. 6. Verschiedene gerade, gebogene, kraterförmige und runde Radiumträger (Buchler & Co., Braunschweig)

Ausbreitungsweise der Collumcarcinome gegeben. Andererseits wurden die zahlreichen Abweichungen der einzelnen Bestrahlungsmethoden untereinander dadurch beeinflußt und entwickelt, daß die verschiedenen Stadien eine Fülle von Tumorformen und Lokalisationen zuließen, die eine individuelle Anpassung an die topographischen Verhältnisse und damit ein Abweichen vom Grundprinzip der Radiumtherapie notwendig machten.

Die einzelnen Standardmethoden der Radiumtherapie unterscheiden sich durch die jeweilige Art und Weise der Auseinandersetzung mit dem anatomischen Raum. Gauwerky (1957) ordnet die verschiedenen Verfahren der gynäkologischen Curietherapie nach:

1. Raumausnutzungsmethoden,
2. Raumerweiterungsmethoden,
3. Raumanpassungsmethoden.

Unter *Raumausnutzungsmethoden* sind jene Verfahren zusammenzufassen, die die Deformierbarkeit und Dehnungsfähigkeit der Scheide dazu benutzen, eine optimale Verteilung der Radionuclide in Uterus und Scheide anzustreben. Einerseits sollen dadurch Überdosierungen im Bereich der Blase und des Rectums vermieden werden, andererseits soll im Bereich des Lymphabflußgebietes der Cervix uteri eine tumorwirksame Dosis erzielt werden. Das Raumausnutzungsprinzip liegt der klassischen *Pariser Methode* (Regaud) und der davon abgeleiteten *Manchester Methode* (Paterson und Tod) zugrunde. Bei diesen Methoden wird die gesamte Länge des Uteruscavums durch eingelegte Röhrchen oder Stifte zur Aufnahme von Radiumzellen ausgenutzt. Die Dehnbarkeit der Vagina gestattet es, die Strahlenquelle durch Spreizkolpostaten im seitlichen Scheidengewölbe und damit nahe der Beckenwand zu fixieren. Während sich noch bei Regaud der Federbügel des Kolpostaten während der langen Liegedauer verändern konnte, ist er von anderen Autoren (KAHANPÄÄ, 1946; CORSCADEN, 1948; ERNST, 1949; VON HELD, 1951) durch starre Spreizkolpostaten ersetzt worden. Auf diese Weise konnte an die Beckenwand eine Dosis bis zu 3000 R und mehr appliziert werden.

Als *Raumanpassungsmethoden* werden die Methoden bezeichnet, mit denen unter Verzicht auf eine Dehnung der Vagina durch die Kombination einer intrauterinen und intravaginalen Radiumeinlage eine optimale Anpassung und Annäherung an den Primärtumor erzielt wird. Als Standardmethode gehört hierher die weit verbreitete *Stockholmer Methode* (FORSSELL, HEYMAN, KOTTMEIER). Aus dieser Standardmethode haben sich zahlreiche abgewandelte Formen entwickelt, die vor allem in Europa verbreitet sind: Kopenhagen (NIELSEN, TRUELSEN), Heidelberg-München (MENGE, EYMER, RIES), Würzburg (GAUSS, NEEFF), Leipzig (SCHRÖDER, KIRCHHOFF, MÖBIUS), Berlin (STOECKEL), Göttingen (MARTIUS), Hamburg (SCHUBERT), Gießen (KEPP), Hamburg-St. Georg (HOLTHUSEN, GAUWERKY) und viele andere. Generell wird bei diesen Methoden darauf verzichtet, die Beckenwand mit einer ausreichenden Radiumdosis zu bestrahlen; die Methoden werden daher stets mit einer auf das Parametrium gerichteten Percutanbestrahlung ergänzt. Zusätzlich kann aber bei der Raumanpassungsmethode die Strahlendosis an der Beckenwand durch Erhöhung der gesamten applizierten Strahlenmenge des zentralen Strahlers erreicht werden. Um dann die strahlenempfindlichen Nachbarorgane weitgehend schonen zu können, sind hierfür geeignete Schwermetallabschirmungen des zentralen vaginalen Strahlers entwickelt worden (DU MESNIL DE ROCHEMONT, 1938; NEARY, BLOMFYELD, 1947; GAUWERKY, 1957).

Bei den *Raumerweiterungsmethoden* wird auf traumatischem Wege versucht, das Radionuclid möglichst weit im kleinen Becken zu verteilen. Dies ist durch transvaginale Spickmethoden mit Radium- oder Kobalt-60-Nadeln oder durch transvaginale parametrane Infiltration mit radioaktiver Flüssigkeit möglich. Die einzelnen Methoden werden im Kapitel „Interstitielle Curietherapie" ausführlicher behandelt.

Neben der räumlichen Dosisverteilung kommt vor allem der zeitlichen eine entscheidende Bedeutung zu. Die protrahierte Einzeitbestrahlung liegt der *Pariser Methode* zugrunde, bei der das Radium über 5 Tage (120 Std) liegen bleibt. Hingegen wird das Radium bei der *Stockholmer Methode* fraktioniert, meist in Form von 2 Radiumapplikationen mit einem Intervall von 3 Wochen, verabfolgt. Während der Vorteil der Pariser Methode in der erheblichen Steigerung der Elektivität der Strahlung durch die starke Protrahierung besteht, ergeben sich Nachteile durch die erhöhte Infektionsgefahr, die durch Sekretstauung infolge der langen Verweildauer des Radiumpräparates bedingt ist. Bei der *Stockholmer Methode* wird die günstige Protrahierung nicht ausgenutzt.

Das Problem einer exakten Radiumdosierung für klinische Belange hat bereits mehrere Generationen beschäftigt und ist bis heute nicht zufriedenstellend gelöst. Während die Berechnung der Gewebsdosis bei punktförmigen Präparaten und Kenntnis der Dosiskonstanten relativ einfach ist, kann sie bei kompliziert gestalteten Trägern äußerst schwierig und für die Praxis undurchführbar sein (MINDER, 1961). Eine exakte Dosisangabe bei der Radiumbestrahlung wird lediglich durch eine direkte Messung gewährleistet, die wegen des steilen Dosisabfalls in der Nähe eines Radiumpräparates nur unter bestimmten Bedingungen möglich ist.

Das seit langem und am meisten benutzte Maß für die Radiumdosierung ist daher die Milligrammelementstunde (mgeh), die das Produkt aus der applizierten Menge des Radiumelementes und der Liegezeit des Trägers in Stunden darstellt. Es braucht in diesem Zusammenhang nicht hervorgehoben zu werden, daß die Angabe in „mgeh" kein eigentliches Maß für die applizierte Dosis im Gewebe darstellt. So kann beispielsweise bei gleichen mgeh-Werten, aber differenten Radiummengen und dadurch unterschiedlichen Liegezeiten bei verschiedenen Trägerformen der biologische Effekt sehr variieren.

Aufgrund dieser Unzulänglichkeiten wurde versucht, die Radiumdosierung den klinischen Belangen besser anzupassen. Eine ausführliche Darstellung der zahlreichen Möglichkeiten ist bei MÖBIUS (1951), ANDREAS (1959) und MINDER (1961) zu finden. Neben den biologischen und photographischen Methoden wird heute vor allem die Dosierung in „Röntgen" diskutiert. Die Voraussetzung hierzu schufen vor allem das von BOMKE und EBERLE entwickelte Momentandosimeter und das Gammameter. Wegen ihrer kleinen Dimensionen gestatten sie es, eine Direktmessung in den Hohlorganen, Vagina, Blase und Darm vorzunehmen.

Während das Momentandosimeter und das Gammameter sich vorwiegend nur für eine kurzzeitige Messung eignen, wurde von anderen Autoren (WATSON, 1965; BAILY, NORMAN und HILBERT, 1967) auf die Bedeutung der Thermoluminescenz hingewiesen. Mit Hilfe von Lithium-Fluorid ist es möglich, in den Hohlorganen integrierende Messungen durchzuführen. Durch die geringen Dimensionen der Lithium-Fluorid-Kristalle können auf diese Weise auch Messungen im Ureter während der Radiumapplikation vorgenommen werden (HÜLLEMANN, 1964; FRISCHBIER, 1966; HILD, 1967).

Trotz der Direktmessungen in den Hohlorganen haben die Dosisangaben aber doch nur beschränkte Bedeutung, weil kleine Verschiebungen des Meßkörpers wegen des steilen Dosisabfalls die Meßergebnisse beträchtlich beeinflussen können. Da sich die topographischen Verhältnisse durch den Füllungszustand von Blase und Darm und Änderung der Scheidentamponade während der Liegezeit ändern können, sind die Meßergebnisse erheblichen Schwankungen unterworfen, so daß nur bedingt die Voraussetzungen erfüllt sind, die Radiumdosierung auf ermittelte Dosiswerte in der Nachbarschaft zu stellen. Der große klinische Nutzen der Dosismessungen in Blase und Rectum liegt aber darin, die Strahlentoleranz dieser Organe näher bestimmt und durch routinemäßige Messungen die Zahl schwerer Strahlenschäden reduziert zu haben.

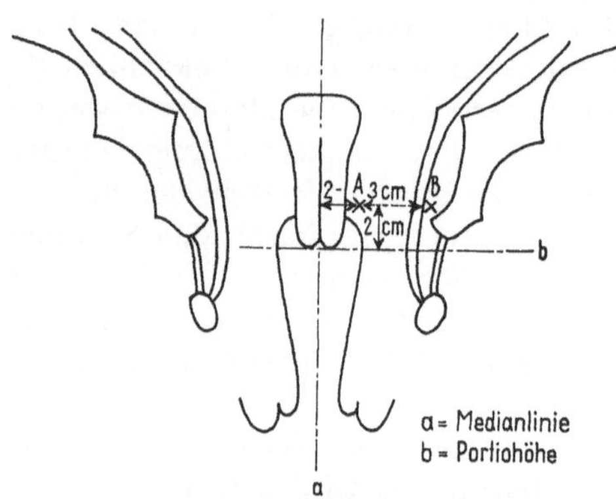

Abb. 7. Die Lage der von TOD und MEREDITH angegebenen Punkte A und B

Für die praktische Durchführung einer Radiumtherapie bei der den individuellen Gegebenheiten Rechnung getragen werden muß, haben sich Isodosenatlanten bewährt, die klare Vorstellung von der räumlichen Dosisverteilung der Gammastrahlen im kleinen Becken in jedem Einzelfall garantieren. Hierbei werden die Summationsisodosen der verschiedenen Strahlerkombinationen zu den topographischen Verhältnissen in Beziehung gesetzt. Um die Isodosenkurven auf die topographischen Verhältnisse beziehen zu können, wurden von TOD und MEREDITH (1938) einige typische Punkte im kleinen Becken definiert (Abb. 7), auf die die Dosisverteilung im kleinen Becken bezogen wird. Diese Punkte wurden von GAUWERKY (1957) und FRISCHKORN (1964) ergänzt.

A Paracervicales Lymphknotengebiet, 2 cm oberhalb und 2 cm seitlich vom äußeren Muttermund. Diese Stelle bezeichnet etwa die Kreuzungsstelle des Ureters mit der Arteria uterina.

B Beckenwand, der Punkt liegt 3 cm lateral vom Punkt A. Er entspricht den Obturatorlymphknoten.

P Äußerer Muttermund.

U Uterusschleimhaut, unmittelbar neben der Mitte des intrauterinen Strahlers, also etwas oberhalb des inneren Muttermundes, gewöhnlich etwa 3 cm oberhalb vom Punkt P gelegen.

H Das Gebiet der sog. hypogastrischen Lymphknotengruppe hingegen der Bifurkation der Arteria iliaca communis. Der Punkt H liegt etwa 4 cm oberhalb von Punkt B.

R Stelle der maximalen Strahlenbelastung der Rectumschleimhaut, in der Regel an der Rectumvorderwand in Höhe der Portio gelegen.

V Stelle der größten Strahlenbelastung der Blasenschleimhaut, in Höhe der Portio am Blasenboden, also ein wenig oberhalb des Trigonum gelegen, aber abhängig vom Füllungszustand der Blase.

X Spitze des Röhrenfilters intrauterin,

K_0 Seitenkante des Scheidenfilters,

K_1 Punkt 1 cm lateral der Seitenkante des Scheidenfilters.

Die ursprünglich von TOD und MEREDITH definierten Punkte „A" und „B" bei der intrakavitären Radiumbehandlung eignen sich zur Dosisangabe in den Fällen, in denen der Uterus mit dem Radiumträger genau in der Medianlinie liegt. Da sich die Punkte auf den Uterus beziehen, verschieben sich diese mit einer Lateralverlagerung oder Verkantung des Uterus. Zum Zweck einer exakten Radiumdosierung schlagen deshalb KAPOOR et al. (1966) vor, daß der Punkt „A", wie ursprünglich, sich auf die Lage des Uterus beziehen soll. Unabhängig von der Lage des Uterus geben sie somit den Punkt 2 cm oberhalb des äußeren Muttermundes und 2 cm lateral an. Der Punkt „B" soll stets der Lage der Obturatorlymphknoten an der Beckenwand entsprechen. Er verschiebt sich nicht mit einer Dislokation des Uterus.

Bis vor wenigen Jahren erfolgte die Dosisberechnung bei den einzelnen linearen Strahlenquellen mit Hilfe graphischer Darstellungen oder Tabellen. Die am häufigsten verwandten stammen von PATERSON und PARKER (1934) sowie QUIMBY (1944). Zur Bestimmung der Dosisverteilung bei der Kombination mehrerer Strahlenquellen müssen für den einzelnen Punkt die Dosisanteile der verschiedenen Strahler aus den Kurven oder Tabellen entnommen und dann addiert werden. Bei einer größeren Anzahl von Strahlenquellen, wie beispielsweise bei der Moulagetechnik, ist dieses Verfahren sehr zeitraubend. Größere Schwierigkeiten ergeben sich bei der Implantation von Nadeln, da ihre Anordnung nicht in vorher bestimmbaren geometrischen Figuren erfolgen kann.

Neue Möglichkeiten wurden durch die Verwendung elektronischer Rechenautomaten erschlossen, durch die relativ schnell und mit einer für die klinischen Belange ausreichende Genauigkeit die Dosen selbst einer größeren Zahl von linearen oder punktförmigen Strahlenquellen an den interessierenden Punkten errechnet werden können. In den letzten Jahren wurden für die intrakavitäre und interstitielle Radiumtherapie zahlreiche Rechenprogramme angegeben (BUSCH, 1965; POWERS et al., 1966; ROSE et al., 1966; ROSENOW, 1967; RICHTER et al., 1967). Wenn derartige Computeranlagen heute auch noch ausschließlich größeren Zentren vorbehalten sind, zeichnet sich doch die Möglichkeit ab, auf diese Weise eine exakte Dosierungsgrundlage bei der Radiumtherapie schaffen zu können.

Eine Verbesserung der klinischen Radiumdosimetrie brachten bereits die Isodosenpläne für die einzelnen Träger und Trägerkombinationen, die nach Schaffung meßtechnischer Voraussetzungen aufgestellt werden konnten. In immer größerem Umfang werden diese Isodosenpläne bei der routinemäßigen Radiumapplikation zu den topographischen Verhältnissen im kleinen Becken in Beziehung gebracht und zur Errechnung der in den interessierenden Punkten verabfolgten Dosis herangezogen. Durch Röntgenaufnahmen in mehreren Ebenen oder Röntgenstereoaufnahmen wird die Strahlendosis mit Hilfe von Isodosenschablonen bestimmt.

Im Göttinger Radiumisodosenatlas hat FRISCHKORN 1964 die Isodosen, die den Wert R pro Stunde angeben, für viele Trägerkombinationen ausgemessen und die Dosis für die verschiedenen Punkte angegeben. Vor Festlegung der Bestrahlungsdauer wird eine obligatorische Strahlenmessung in Blase und Darm durchgeführt, wobei für die einzelne Einlage Dosen von 2000 R nur im Notfall überschritten werden. Bei jeder Radiumeinlage wird die Strahlenbelastung in den einzelnen Punkten neben den üblichen Eintragungen protokolliert, um so die Voraussetzung für eine spätere Erkennung der Zusammenhänge zwischen Methode und Erfolg oder Mißerfolg zu schaffen.

Eine typische Isodosenschar einer Trägerkombination mit den entsprechenden errechneten Dosisangaben für die einzelnen Punkte des Göttinger Radiumisodosenatlas ist
Abb. 8 zu entnehmen.

Zur Veranschaulichung der räumlichen Dosisverteilung bei den Trägerkombinationen
sind derartige Isodosenatlanten von größter Bedeutung. Selbst wenn vor der Radiumeinlage durch verschiedene Röntgenkontrastuntersuchungen die Lage des inneren weiblichen Genitales, der Verlauf der Ureteren und die anatomischen Beziehungen zwischen
Vagina und Uterus sowie Rectum und Blase relativ gut bestimmt werden können, sind

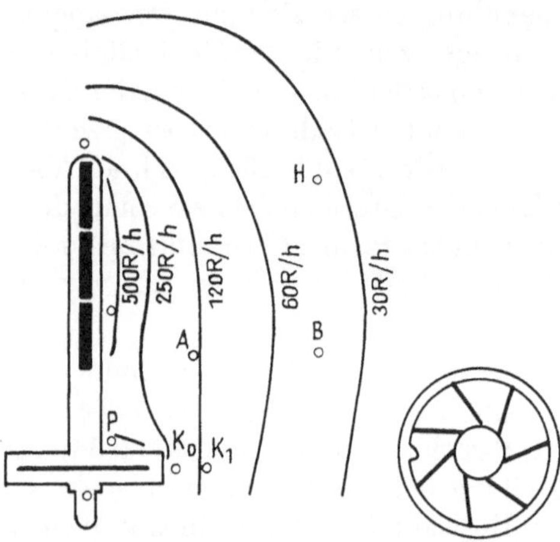

Filter Nr. 52

Röhrenfilter mit 90 mCi Radium, 1. Etage blind
Rundfilter   mit 70 mCi Radium

Röhrenfilter $\varnothing$ 0,8 cm/Rundfilter $\varnothing$ 3,9 cm/Sondenlänge 6,8 cm

mgeh	Bestrahlungs-dauer	mgeh/R-Vergleichsdosis für die Punkte							
		P	U	X	A	B	H	K_0	K_1
1000	6 Std 15 min	4120 R	3370 R	1250 R	812 R	269 R	212 R	1345 R	663 R
2000	12 Std 30 min	8240 R	6740 R	2500 R	1624 R	538 R	424 R	2690 R	1326 R

Abb. 8. Isodosenkurven einer kombinierten intrauterinen und vaginalen Filterkombination des Göttinger
Radiumisodosenatlas mit den für die einzelnen Punkte errechneten Dosisangaben (Frischkorn)

Lageveränderungen durch die Tamponade, die Peristaltik des Darmes und den unterschiedlichen Füllungsgrad der Blase möglich. So kann durch die Isodosenkurven über die
Belastung des Ureters im Einzelfall keine exakte Angabe gemacht werden.

Für alle Dosisberechnungen ist eine exakte Lagebestimmung des Radiumpräparates
im kleinen Becken die wichtigste Voraussetzung. Auf die Bedeutung und Notwendigkeit
einer röntgenologischen Lagekontrolle der Präparateanordnung wurde von zahlreichen
Autoren hingewiesen; sie wird heute fast routinemäßig vorgenommen, insbesondere bei
der Kombination mit einer percutanen Strahlenbehandlung. Als Methoden werden Röntgenaufnahmen in 2 Ebenen (Spechter, 1962, u. a.), stereoskopische Aufnahmen (Dietel
und Volz, 1938, u. a.) oder a.p.-Aufnahmen mit verschiedenen Focus-Film-Abständen
(Wenzel, 1958, u. a.) angegeben.

Die Forderung einer regelmäßigen Lagekontrolle des Radiumträgers durch Röntgenaufnahmen ergibt sich durch den hohen Prozentsatz von Verlagerungen aus der Medianen
(s. S. 188). In etwa der Hälfte der Fälle ist der Träger um mehr als 1 cm verlagert, so daß die

Dosis an der Beckenwand beträchtlich erhöht oder vermindert sein kann. Bei einseitiger parametraner Infiltration bewirkt vor allem die Verkürzung des befallenen Parametriums eine Verziehung des Uterus zur erkrankten Seite hin. Weiterhin verursachen die Scheidentamponade eine Verlagerung des Radiumträgers. So fand SPECHTER (1962), daß die Basis des Präparates wesentlich höher nach rechts als nach links abwich. Die ganze Radiumkombination lag in 29,6 % der Fälle links und in 34,2 % rechts der Medianen. Das häufige Abweichen der Basis nach rechts erklärt SPECHTER durch das rechtshändige Tamponieren. Er weist darauf hin, daß diese Seitenabweichungen einen erheblichen Einfluß auf die Dosis am Ureter haben können, die er bei diesen Verlagerungen in den entsprechenden lateralen Anteilen von Blase und Rectum registrieren konnte. Bedeutungsvoll sind diese Beobachtungen durch die nachgewiesenen Beziehungen zwischen den Seitenverlagerungen des Radiumträgers und den später infolge pathologischer Abflußbehinderung auftretenden Hydronephrosen. Bei 9 nachgewiesenen, nicht durch Carcinom bedingten Hydronephrosen der

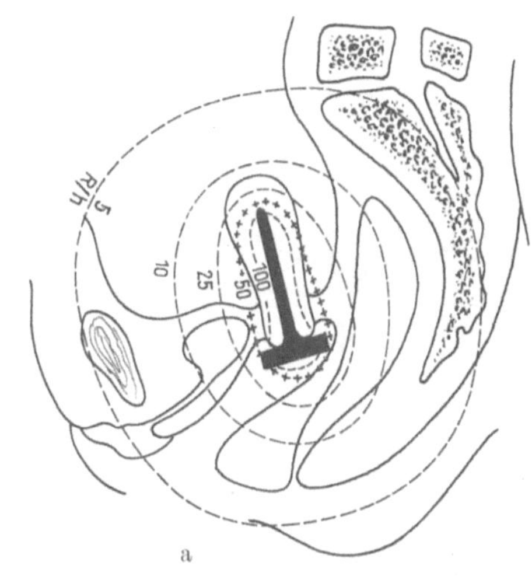

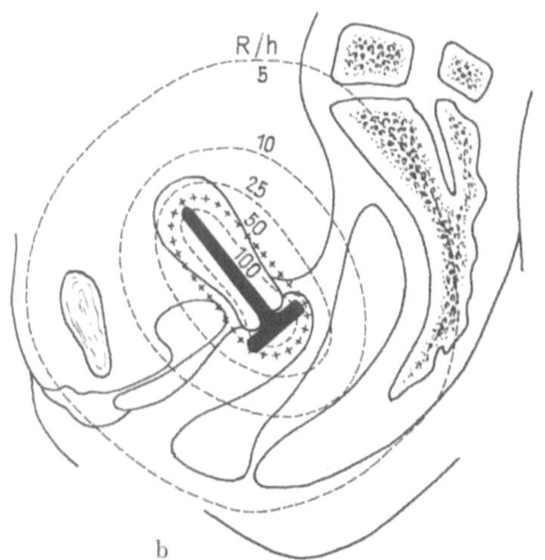

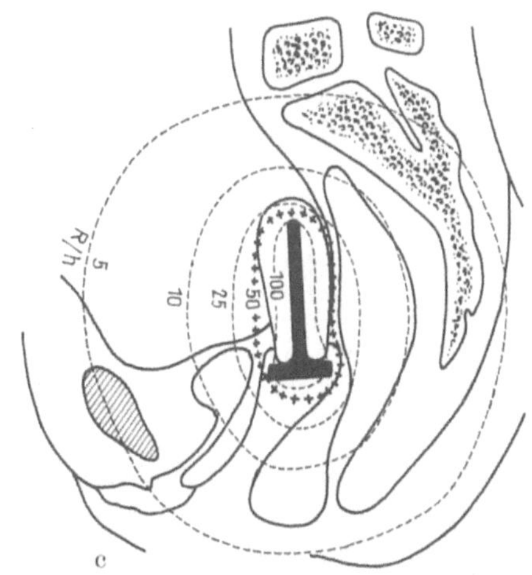

Abb. 9a—c. Lagebeziehungen der Radiumträger zu Blase und Rectum mit Strahlenbelastung bei Mittelstellung (a), Anteversion (b) und Retroversion (c) (RIES und BREITNER)

rechten Seite lag der ganze Radiumträger in 8 Fällen 1—3 cm rechts von der Medianen und einmal schräg gekippt im kleinen Becken, wobei die Basis rechts und die Spitze links der Medianen lag. Bei 3 linksseitigen Hydronephrosen befand sich das Radiumpräparat einmal links im kleinen Becken, einmal von links nach rechts gekippt und einmal 1 cm in toto nach rechts verlagert.

Als unentbehrlich haben sich in der intrakavitären Radiumtherapie auch die Dosismessungen in Blase und Rectum erwiesen. Die routinemäßigen Messungen ermöglichten es, an einem großen Patientengut die Toleranzdosen von Blase und Rectum zu bestimmen. So konnte KOTTMEIER (1964) bei der Stockholmer Methode zeigen, daß die Toleranzdosis am Rectum bei 4200 R und an der Blase bei 5000 R liegt, wenn die Dosis als Mittelwert in einem Bereich von 3 cm gemessen wird. Nach seinen Erfahrungen darf die Dosis im Rectum 2500 R innerhalb von 24 Std nicht überschreiten. Bei Berücksichtigung dieser Toleranzdosen können schwere Strahlenreaktionen an Blase und Rectum vermieden werden. Demgegenüber konnte allerdings FLETCHER (1966) zeigen, daß hohe Blasen- oder Rectumbelastungen nicht unbedingt schwere Reaktionen zur Folge haben müssen. Komplikationen stehen auch nicht in direktem Zusammenhang mit den für die Punkte A und B errechneten Dosiswerten. Vielmehr sind andere Ursachen, wie vorausgegangene Operationen, eine Ureterocele, mitverantwortlich zu machen. Er warnt aber ebenfalls vor Dosen von über 6000 rad am Rectum. Die durchschnittliche Dosis sollte im Rectum bei

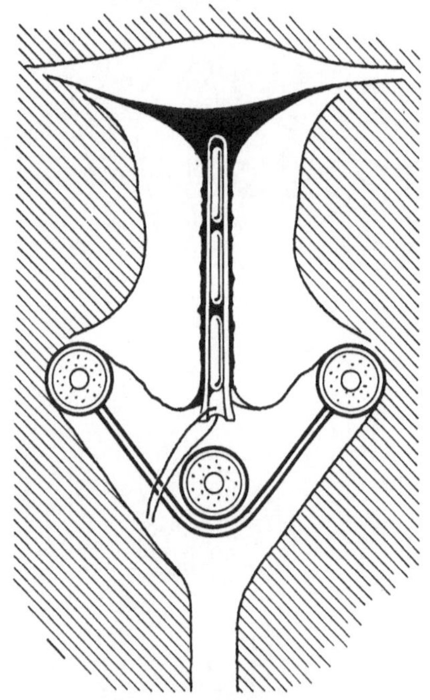

4000 rad innerhalb von 144 Std liegen, bei einer Dosis von mehr als 8000 rad innerhalb von 144 Std ist mit einer Perforation zu rechnen. Nach seinen Erfahrungen sind derartige Dosismengen besonders in fortgeschrittenen Fällen zur Applikation einer individuellen Herddosis bei Variation der Standardtechnik nützlich, während sie bei einer standardisierten Technik in Frühfällen keine Vorteile bringen (FLETCHER, BROWN und RUTLEDGE, 1958).

Die Momentan-Dosimetrie erbrachte für die Kenntnis der Toleranzdosen von Blase und Rectum wichtige Aufschlüsse; das Problem der möglichen und effektiven Dosisbelastung am Ureter besteht aber nach wie vor. Da der Verlauf der Ureteren im Becken erheblichen Schwankungen unterworfen sein kann, ist eine Dosiskalkulation für den Einzelfall bedeutungslos. Eine Dosisermittlung wäre nur nach exakter Bestimmung des Ureterverlaufes während der Radiumeinlage durch Kontrastmittel oder schattengebende Sonden möglich. Von Einzelfällen abgesehen gestattet aber erst die individuelle Dosismessung durch intraureteral liegende Meßkammern eine sichere Aussage über die am Ureter wirksam werdende Dosis. Hierzu eignet sich die Thermoluminescenz mit kleinsten Lithiumfluoridkristallen, die leicht in Uretersonden untergebracht werden

Abb. 10. Lage der Radiumträger bei kombinierter intrauteriner und vaginaler Radiumapplikation bei der Pariser Methode

können. Die ersten Meßergebnisse an 20 Patientinnen zeigten, daß bei einer kombinierten intrauterinen und intravaginalen Radiumapplikation (modifizierte Stockholmer Methode) von 2000 mgeh am Ureter Dosen von 500—4500 R wirksam werden. Das Dosismaximum lag bei diesen Fällen zwischen 4 und 8 cm oberhalb des Ureterostiums (FRISCHBIER, 1966; HILD, 1967).

Zur Behandlung des Collumcarcinoms durch die intrakavitäre Radiumtherapie wurden im Laufe der Jahrzehnte einige *Standardmethoden* entwickelt, mit denen an einem großen Patientengut ausreichende Erfahrungen gesammelt und gute Behandlungsergebnisse erzielt werden konnten. Die wichtigsten sollen in Kürze dargestellt werden.

Pariser Methode. Bei der ursprünglich von REGAUD am Radiuminstitut in Paris entwickelten Bestrahlungsmethode wird eine einzeitige, stark protrahierte Radiumeinlage vorgenommen, bei der 33,33 mg Radium intrauterin und 33,33 mg intravaginal verabfolgt werden. Die intravaginale Radiummenge wird auf 2 Zylinder eines Kolpostaten verteilt. Bei einer Liegezeit von etwa 5 Tagen ergibt sich somit eine Gesamtdosierung von 7900 mgeh. Wenn zusätzlich an der Portio, an der Achse des Kolpostaten, ein weiterer Radiumträger mit 66,66 mg Radium gelegt wird, erhöht sich die Dosierung auf 8700 mgeh. Die Lage der Radiumträger zeigt Abb. 10. Bei einer Infiltration des Parametriums wird eine zusätzliche Percutanbestrahlung in Form von Teleradium- oder Röntgentiefentherapie gegeben. Zwischen Radiumeinlage und der Percutantherapie wird eine Pause von 5—10 Tagen eingelegt.

Manchester Methode. Auch bei der Manchester Methode (PATERSON, TOD und MEREDITH) besteht die Trägerkombination aus einem intrauterinen Stift und aus einem Kolpostaten, durch den in das seitliche Scheidengewölbe Applikatoren, Ovoide genannt, variabler Größe und Ladung gebracht werden. In dem von TOD und MEREDITH angegebenen Punkt A soll die Radiumdosis 8000 R und im Punkt B 3000 R betragen. Sie wird durch 2 Radiumeinlagen von 3tägiger Dauer erreicht. Zwischen beiden Radiumeinlagen liegt eine Pause von 4—7 Tagen.

Bei einer zusätzlichen Röntgenbestrahlung bei den Stadien III und IV wird die Radiumdosis auf 6500 R im Punkt A verringert. Die percutan eingestrahlte Dosis beträgt im Punkt B 3000 R.

Die Manchester Methode wurde im Jahre 1953 revidiert. Seitdem wird das Verhältnis von intrauterinem und vaginalem Dosisbeitrag zum Punkt A, das beim alten Manchester System 1:1 betrug, in Übereinstimmung mit Arbeiten aus dem Radiumhemmet durch Erhöhung der intrauterinen Dosis auf 1,6:1 abgeändert. Die früher vernachlässigte und zu Dosisverlusten bis zu 10% führende wechselseitige Filterwirkung bei Verwendung von 2 oder mehr gebündelten Radiumzellen wird beim neuen Ladungssystem berücksichtigt. Bei enger Scheide oder bei Übergreifen des Collumcarcinoms auf die Scheide werden die vaginalen Ovoide in der sog. Tandemposition hintereinandergeschaltet. Die angestrebte Dosis von 8000 R im Punkt A wird bei alleiniger Radiumbestrahlung mit zwei Einlagen von zusammen 140 Std Liegezeit erreicht.

Hinsichtlich der Dosierung bei der intrakavitären Radiumtherapie konnte PATERSON (1954) zeigen, daß die besten Heilungsergebnisse bei einer Dosierung im Punkt A von 8000 R erzielt werden konnten. Bei einer Dosierung von 6000 R in Punkt A waren die Behandlungsergebnisse etwa 10% schlechter; die Behandlungsergebnisse verschlechterten sich ebenfalls bei einer Dosis von 9000 R in Punkt A.

Stockholmer Methode. Die primär von FORSSELL angegebene und von HEYMAN und KOTTMEIER weiterentwickelte Bestrahlungsmethode beruht auf der fraktionierten, nicht protrahierten Radiumbestrahlung. Hierbei wird eine intrauterine und intravaginale Radiumeinlage kombiniert. Während ursprünglich die Radiumbehandlung in 3 Applikationen erfolgte, wurde sie 1953 von KOTTMEIER insofern modifiziert, als nur noch zwei kombinierte intrauterine und intravaginale Radiumeinlagen in 3wöchigem Abstand vorgenommen wurden. Es lagen 53—88 mg Radium im Uteruscavum und 60—80 mg in der Vagina. Die Dosisleistung in einer Entfernung von 2 cm vom Zentrum des uterinen Applikators betrug etwa 75 R/Std. Die Filterung entsprach 3 mm Blei. Die Liegezeit für jede Applikation schwankte zwischen 22 und 27 Std. Bei der zusätzlichen Röntgenbestrahlung auf die Beckenwand wurde die Herddosis in Beckenmitte von 1500 R nicht überschritten. Bei der Radiumapplikation wurde besonderer Wert darauf gelegt, daß die intrauterine Dosis sich gleichmäßig vom Fundus uteri bis 2 cm oberhalb des äußeren Muttermundes verteilt und die unteren 2 cm des Cervicalkanals freibleiben. Die Dosis in Punkt A betrug durchschnittlich 6250 R. Umfangreiche Dosismessungen am Phantom und an Patientinnen durch WALSTAM erbrachten die Grundlagen für eine individualisierte Radiumtherapie beim Collumcarcinom. Bei ausgedehnteren, in die Parametrien infiltrierten Carcinomen oder bei endocervicalen Carcinomen wurde die intrauterine Radiumdosis auf Kosten der verringerten intravaginalen Radiumdosis erhöht. Die Abb. 11a und b zeigen die Dosisverteilung in R/Std bei der typischen Applikatorkombination der Stockholmer Technik. Während von 1949—1957 die zusätzliche Percutanbestrahlung unter konventionellen Strahlenbedingungen durchgeführt wurde, wird seit 1958 die Percutanbestrahlung mit Megavolttherapie eines 15-MeV-Betatrons und einer Telekobalteinheit vorgenommen.

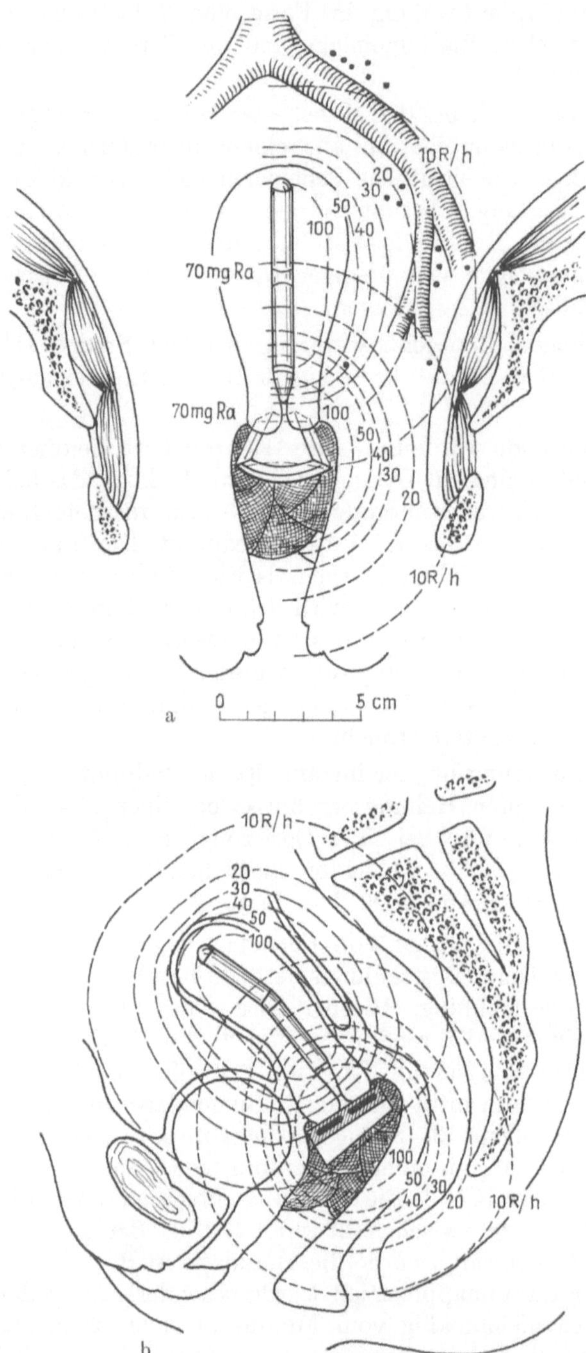

Abb. 11a u. b. Isodosenkurven (in R/Std) bei Kombination eines intrauterinen und eines intravaginalen Radiumapplikators (je 70 mg Radium) bei der Stockholmer Technik (KOTTMEIER)

Bei der Stockholmer Technik wird eine weitgehende Anpassung an die Verhältnisse des Einzelfalles angestrebt. Die in Form und Größe variablen Vaginalapplikatoren sollen grundsätzlich möglichst groß gehalten werden.

New-Yorker Methode. Von CORSCADEN und BUTZ (1952) werden bei der Radiumtherapie ein stabförmiger Träger in den Cervicalkanal und kurze zylindrische oder eiförmige Träger an flexiblen Stäben möglichst weit in das seitliche Scheidengewölbe eingeführt. Hierbei wird besonderer Wert auf eine ausreichende Tamponade gelegt. Bei der Radiumeinlage soll der Uterus zur Vagina möglichst in einem Winkel von 90% stehen, die Lage der Träger wird durch Röntgenaufnahmen kontrolliert. Es werden 7000 mgeh verabfolgt. Es zeigte sich, daß eine stärkere Protrahierung bessere Behandlungsergebnisse erbrachte: die absolute Heilungsziffer betrug bei einer Radiummenge von 70 mg und einer Bestrahlungszeit von 100 Std 43%, bei Verwendung von 175 mg Radium und einer Bestrahlungszeit von 40 Std nur 36%. Die stärkere Protrahierung wirkte sich auch günstiger auf die Behandlungskomplikationen aus. Durch eine Reduzierung der Radiummenge und Verlängerung der Bestrahlungszeit bei gleicher verabfolgter Dosis und sonst gleichen Bestrahlungsbedingungen konnten Blasen- und Darmreaktionen gänzlich vermieden werden.

Münchener Methode. Bis 1942 erfolgte die Radiumtherapie einzeitig bei einer Liegedauer von 60—65 Std und einer Gesamtdosis je nach Länge des Uterus von 3900 bis 8125 mgeh (EYMER). Heute wird die Radiumbestrahlung bei der Münchner Methode fraktioniert durchgeführt. Sie besitzt den Vorteil der größeren Elektivität zugunsten des Bindegewebes. Es wird eine Fraktionierung von 3 Einlagen zu je 24 Std vorgenommen, gewöhnlich im Abstand von 14 Tagen. Der Abstand zwischen den beiden Einlagen soll nicht geringer als 10 Tage und nicht länger als 21 Tage sein. Die Radiumträgerkombinationen bestehen aus einem uterinen Längsfilter und einem Platten- bzw. Kraterfilter. Die Filterkombinationen sind miteinander fest verschraubt. Die Längsfilter werden mit 40—50 mg Radium und die Platten mit 30—40 mg Radium beschickt. Bei jeder Radiumeinlage werden etwa 2360 mgeh appliziert (RIES und BREITNER, 1959).

Die Größe und Form der Radiumträger richtet sich nach Tumorgröße und -ausdehnung. Bei gut zugänglichen Tumoren macht man von der Radiumspickung Gebrauch. Bei Befall tieferer Vaginalabschnitte werden zusätzlich längliche Radiumträger für die Vagina verwendet, die aus Hartgummi oder Holz mit einer zentralen Bohrung bestehen.

Die Radiumtherapie wird mit einer percutanen Röntgenbestrahlung unter Stehfeldbedingungen kombiniert, so daß an der Beckenwand eine Herddosis von mindestens 3000 R angestrebt wird.

Methode Hamburg-St. Georg. Durch eine Modifizierung der Stockholmer Methode gab HOLTHUSEN eine Radiumtherapie an, bei der im Verlaufe von 4—6 Wochen 3mal vaginal Radium vor die Portio gelegt wird. Hierbei werden die Stockholmer Platten von rechteckiger Gestalt quer vor den Tumor antamponiert. Bei einer der 3 Radiumeinlagen wird gleichzeitig ein zylindrischer intrauteriner Träger (Intrauterinstift) gelegt, der die ganze Länge des Uteruscavums ausfüllt. Dieser Stift bleibt einzeitig für 120 Std liegen. Zwischen den Radiumapplikationen wird die Röntgenbestrahlung der Parametrien durchgeführt.

Da die quer gelegten rechteckigen Portioplatten mehr nach lateral ausladen als nach dorsoventral, entsteht ein glocken- oder birnenförmiger Isodosenkörper. Die applizierte Dosis im Punkt A schwankt je nach Größe der Portioplatte zwischen 4800 und 7200 R und im Punkt B von 1600—2300 R.

Nach GAUWERKY besteht folgende Dosisabhängigkeit der verschiedenen Gewebsreaktionen an der Cervix: bis 4000 R keine Tumorvernichtung, 4000—7000 R Tumorvernichtung möglich, 7000—15000 R Tumorvernichtung, keine Nekrose, 15000 bis 30000 R Nekrose möglich.

Im Laufe der vergangenen Jahrzehnte sind zahlreiche Kombinationen und Variationen der beschriebenen Standardmethoden entwickelt worden, die sich teilweise nur durch geringe Änderung der Trägerformen und der verschiedenen Trägerkombinationen unterscheiden. Darüber hinaus sind einzelne methodische und apparative Verbesserungen angegeben, durch die insbesondere bei speziellen Tumorlokalisationen die Dosisverteilung günstiger dem Herd angepaßt werden kann.

NUYTTEN, GIAUX und HERBEAU (1953) beschreiben eine Methode der Radiumapplikation nach einem Vorschlag von SWYNGEDEAUW, bei dem das präcervicale Radiumpräparat in der Mitte der Vagina in einem bestimmten Abstand vor der Portio liegt, wodurch eine homogene Durchstrahlung des Collum uteri und des parametranen Gewebes erzielt wird. Das Präparat ist am Ende einer drehbaren Sonde befestigt. Blase und Rectum werden durch einen U-förmigen, an der Sonde fixierten, metallischen Tubus vor zu starker Strahlung geschützt. Die Vorrichtung wird durch Bänder außen am Unterleib der Patientin fixiert und kann ohne Belästigung je nach Stärke des Präparates (40 bis 50 mgeh) 8—11 Tage getragen werden.

Durch mehrere kleinere vaginale Applikatoren kann die Dosisverteilung günstiger gestaltet werden als bei der Verwendung von ein bzw. zwei größeren vaginalen Trägern, wie Morris, Chang und Page (1965) zeigen konnten (Abb. 12a und b). Deshalb entwickelten diese Autoren spezielle vaginale Träger aus Gummi, die das Präparat in einer zentralen Bohrung enthalten. Derartige vaginale Träger können den lokalen Verhältnissen an der

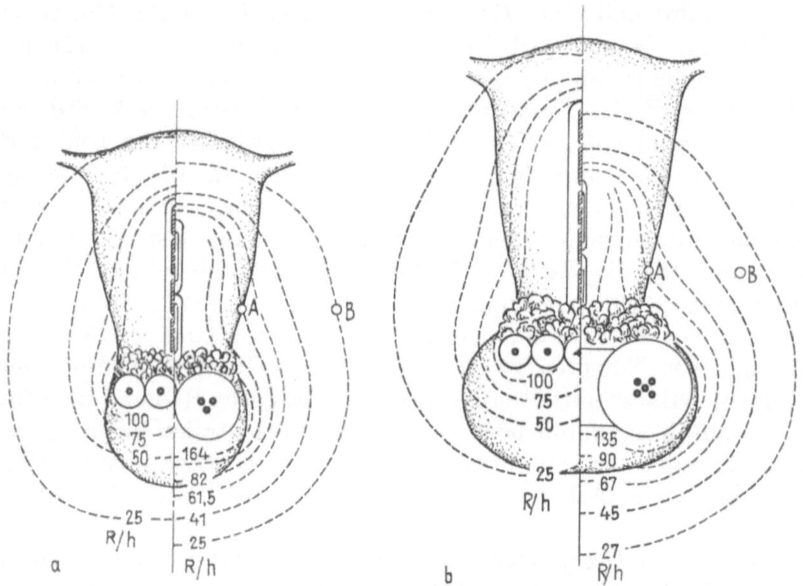

Abb. 12a u. b. Vergleichende Dosisverteilung bei der Verwendung mehrerer kleiner oder eines größeren vaginalen Applikators (Manchester Methode), (Morris et al.)

Portio wesentlich besser angepaßt werden. So zeigt Abb. 12, daß bei einem großen exophytischen Tumor der vorderen Muttermundslippe durch einen festen Kolpostaten die Dosisverteilung wesentlich schlechter ist als bei der Verwendung der flexiblen fünfteiligen Vaginalträger aus Gummi von Morris.

Fletcher u. Mitarb. (1952) verwenden die variable Kombination eines intracervicalen Radiumträgers mit 2 walzenförmigen Ovoiden, die in das seitliche Scheidengewölbe hineinpassen und an 2 Griffen gelenkig miteinander verbunden sind, so daß sie je nach Bedarf mehr oder weniger weit auseinandergespreizt werden können. Die Entfernung der Radiumpräparate von der Scheidenhaut kann durch verschiedene Abstandszylinder reguliert werden, die über die Träger gezogen werden. Bei dieser Technik trägt der intracervicale Träger besonders zur Blasendosis und im Fall eines atrophischen Uterus auch zur Rectumdosis bei, während die Rectumdosis durch die Ovoide relativ wenig erhöht wird. Fletcher variiert die räumliche und zeitliche Dosisverteilung je nach den topographischen Verhältnissen.

So wird bei nicht zu starker Retro- oder Anteflexion des Uterus und mehr infiltrierenden Prozessen die intrauterine Radiummenge erhöht und die vaginale reduziert. Die Gesamtdosis an der Blase wird unter 7000 R und des Rectums unter 6500 R gehalten.

Buttenberg (1964) lehnt eine feste Verbindung zwischen intrauterinem Stift und Portioplatte ab, weil sich so die Portioplatte besser dem Tumor anlegt.

An der Mayo-Klinik (FRICKE und DECKER, 1956) besteht die Radiumbehandlung des Collumcarcinoms in einer im Verlauf von 4—5 Wochen ausgeführten 10—12maligen Einlage je eines einzigen mit 50 mg Radium geladenen Dominici-Röhrchens, das an verschiedenen Stellen des Cervicalkanals, des Uteruscavums und in den Vaginalgewölben so plaziert wird, daß eine sehr individuelle, den anatomischen Gegebenheiten angepaßte Röntgendosisverteilung erreicht wird.

Eine noch bessere Anpassung des vaginalen Trägers an den Portiobefund versuchen TWOMBLY und ROSH (1955) zu erreichen, indem sie in Knie-Ellenbogenlage bei Hochdrücken der hinteren Vaginalwand mittels eines Speculums mit einer zahntechnischen Masse eine Art Gipsausguß der Vagina herstellen. An diesem Präparat können sie die Ausdehnung des Collumcarcinoms deutlich ablesen und entsprechende Radiumträger anbringen.

Als Weiterentwicklung des ursprünglich bei der *Pariser Methode* verwandten Spreizkolpostaten ist der Universalkolpostat von GUTTMANN anzusehen. Das Instrument wird während der Radiumapplikation von einem Stativ gehalten und garantiert dadurch eine gute Fixierung des Trägers an der gewünschten Stelle. Bei der von VON HELD (1951) angegebenen Ausführungsform des Spreizkolpostaten können die beiden Seiten verschieden abgespreizt werden. Da sich bei allen Spreizkolpostaten die Scheide aus verständlichen Gründen bei stärkerer Dehnung zur Seite hin in der Sagittalrichtung zusammenzieht und Blase und Rectum sich damit annähern, wurde von FIEBELKORN ein vierarmiger Kolpostat entwickelt, der es gestattet, die Dehnungsmöglichkeit der Vagina in alle Richtungen maximal auszunutzen.

Einen dreiteiligen starren Spreizkolpostaten zur Behandlung des Collumcarcinoms beschreiben ODDIE und MESCHAN (1955), deren vaginale Strahlenquellen in definierter Weise durch den Einsatz von sog. Spacern voneinander distanziert werden können. Bei der postoperativen Behandlung verwenden RIESS und BREITNER (1959) bei der lokalen Radiumapplikation einen pilzförmigen Kork, der an die Scheidenabschlußnarbe tamponiert werden kann.

Besondere Applikatoren erfordern die großen exophytischen Portiotumoren, die nicht selten mehr als gänseeigroß werden, so daß eine gewölbte Tumorfläche ohne oder mit Übergang auf die vordere Vaginalwand von Handtellergröße zustande kommen kann. Die üblichen vaginalen Träger reichen in ihrer Größe nicht aus, um den ganzen Tumor völlig zu bedecken und vor allem einen guten Kontakt zu gewährleisten. Während früher solche exophytischen Tumoren vor der Radiumeinlage durch eine Elektrokaustik abgetragen wurden, verzichtet man heute meist auf einen solchen Eingriff. Derartige Tumorbefunde erfordern eine individuelle Radiumtherapie und machen die Verwendung von speziellen Radiumträgern notwendig, wenn nicht im zentralen Tumorgebiet eine Radionekrose entstehen und gleichzeitig im Randgebiet eine unzureichende Dosis in Kauf genommen werden soll. Genau wie SCHJÖTT-RIVERS empfiehlt deshalb auch GAUWERKY (1957) für derartige Tumoren eine nach Maß angefertigte Radiummoulage aus Stanzmasse. Auf diese Weise bilden sich große Tumoren in kurzer Zeit zurück, so daß bei einer zweiten oder dritten Radiumeinlage die üblichen Trägerformen verwandt werden können. Technisch einfacher und auch sicherer erscheint es aber, bei großen exophytischen Portiotumoren mit der homogenen Percutanbestrahlung den Tumor zum Schrumpfen zu bringen, um eine bessere Ausgangssituation für die anschließende Radiumtherapie zu schaffen.

Für die vaginalen Tumorausbreitungen beim Collumcarcinom empfiehlt GAUWERKY zylindrische Strahlungsträger mit axialer Anordnung der radioaktiven Substanz, bei denen infolge des größeren Abstandes zwischen Radium und Scheidenhaut der Dosisabfall weniger steil wird, so daß der Tumorgrund und bereits bestehende parakolpische Tumorausbreitungen besser erfaßt werden können. Eine Abschirmung von den strahlenempfindlichen Nachbarorganen bei der Benutzung von Radium oder Radiokobalt ist aber nicht möglich, da bei der hohen Durchdringungsfähigkeit der γ-Strahlung des Radiums auch bei Anwendung wirksamster Schutzstoffe Schichtdicken nötig werden, wie sie in der engen Vagina nicht untergebracht werden können. Durch die Verwendung von Radionucliden mit einer weicheren γ-Strahlung kann die Schichtdicke der benötigten Abschirmung aber beträchtlich reduziert werden.

Deshalb verwendet GAUWERKY (1957) für solche Zwecke Caesium-137. Es eignet sich besonders wegen seiner wesentlich günstigeren Halbwertschicht von 3,9 mm in Wolfram, so daß eineinhalb Halbwertschichten ohne weiteres intrakavitär untergebracht werden können. Hierzu entwickelte er zwei Typen eines Vaginalzylinders von 2,5 bzw. 3 cm Durchmesser, der aus einem kochbaren Kunststoff besteht und axial ganz oder teilweise mit mehreren Monel-Röhrchen zu je 50 mCi Caesium-137 beladen werden kann. Durch Einfügen oder Fortlassen von Abschirmkörpern aus Wolframmetall kann die Strahlung entweder zirkulär austreten oder in verschiedenen Winkelbereichen herabgesetzt werden. Derartige Vaginalzylinder eignen sich vor allem bei den verschiedenen Formen vaginaler oder parakolpischer Tumorinfiltrationen, wodurch jede gewünschte Isodosenmodellierung erreicht wird.

Auch für den von GAUWERKY (1957) verwandten Portioblock wird Caesium-137 benutzt. Dieser Portioblock wurde entwickelt, um beispielsweise bei einer engen Scheide im Bereich der Portio einen zentralen Strahler applizieren zu können. Mit diesem Portioblock kann durch kleine Schwermetalleinsätze die Dosis zur Blase und zum Rectum hin um ein Drittel geschwächt werden. Durch die geringere Belastung von Blase und Rectum ist es möglich, eine höhere Dosis ans Parametrium zu bringen, wie es der Wirkungsweise des Körperhöhlenrohres entspricht. Der Vorteil bei Verwendung von Caesium-γ-Strahlung liegt somit in der größeren Abschirmung, wodurch die Dosisverteilung in wünschenswerter Weise modelliert werden kann.

Welche Bedeutung die Art und Technik der intravaginalen Tamponade für die Dosisverteilung hat, wird im Schrifttum vielfach diskutiert. Bei Anwendung einer festen, rechtwinklig gegeneinander verschraubten intrauterinen und intravaginalen Trägerkombination kann es beispielsweise vorkommen, daß bei einer fixierten Retroflexio uteri die hintere Muttermundslippe nicht von der maximalen Strahlendosis getroffen wird. Andererseits wird bei einer steilen Anteflexio des Corpus uteri die hintere Muttermundslippe von einer Portioplatte nicht bedeckt (SPECHTER und POLLACK, 1965). Durch derartige Unterdosierungen ist das Entstehen von lokalen Rezidiven möglich. Mit Hilfe einer geeigneten Technik beim intravaginalen Tamponieren ist es darüber hinaus möglich, unerwünschte Dosisspitzen an der Rectumvorderwand zu vermeiden. SPECHTER und POLLACK (1965) führten deshalb an einer Reihe von Patientinnen unter Bildverstärkerkontrolle Untersuchungen über die Lage der Radiumträger bei unterschiedlicher Tamponadentechnik durch. Sie konnten deutlich zeigen, daß der Radiumträger, vom Operateur ungewollt, bei der Tamponade unkontrollierbar abweichen kann. Bei Patientinnen mit gut beweglichem Uterus besteht die Gefahr, durch sehr straffes Tamponieren die Träger zu weit nach cranial zu schieben, wodurch höhere Darmabschnitte eine stärkere Belastung erhalten.

Die Frage der optimalen Dosisverteilung untersuchten NOLAN und DU SAULT (1954) anhand von 420 Patientinnen mit einem Collumcarcinom, die in den Jahren 1933—1950 behandelt worden waren. Das Behandlungsergebnis wurde zu der verabfolgten Dosis in Beziehung gesetzt. An graphischen Aufzeichnungen über die Heilungen in Abhängigkeit von der Dosis konnten die Verfasser zeigen, daß es eine optimale Dosis gibt, deren Überschreiten zu einem supraletalen Effekt führt. Die optimale Dosis wird auf 6000 ± 1000 R geschätzt, verabfolgt innerhalb von 8 Wochen. Sie betonen die Wichtigkeit, eine homogene Dosis auf die tumorbefallenen Partien zu applizieren.

RUNGE und WIMHÖFER konnten statistisch eindeutig nachweisen, daß die Behandlungserfolge verschlechtert werden, wenn im Laufe einer Radiumbestrahlung eines Collumcarcinoms Temperaturen auftreten. Deshalb wurde von zahlreichen Autoren eine Prophylaxe mit Sulfonamiden und später mit Antibiotica bei der intrauterinen Radiumeinlage gefordert (THOMSEN, 1950; DOUJAK und PICHA, 1962). Man glaubte, die Temperatursteigerungen, die durch entzündliche Komplikationen zustande kamen, durch eine Prophylaxe verhindern zu können. In den letzten Jahren ist aber die prophylaktische Therapie von vielen Autoren wieder verlassen worden. Man beschränkt sich meist auf eine antibiotische Therapie bei bereits vorliegenden Temperaturerhöhungen.

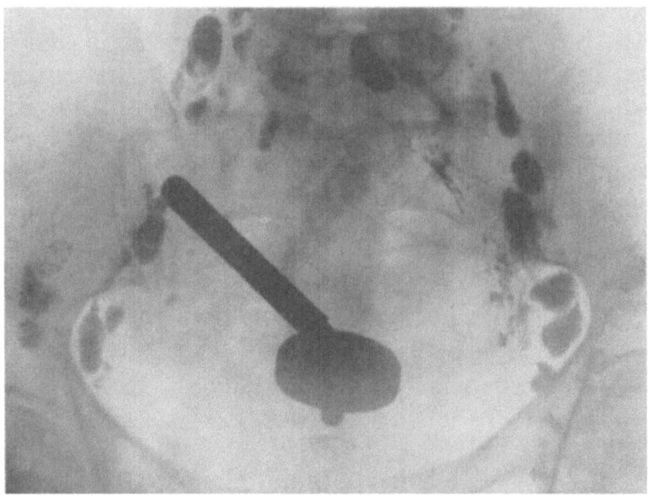

a

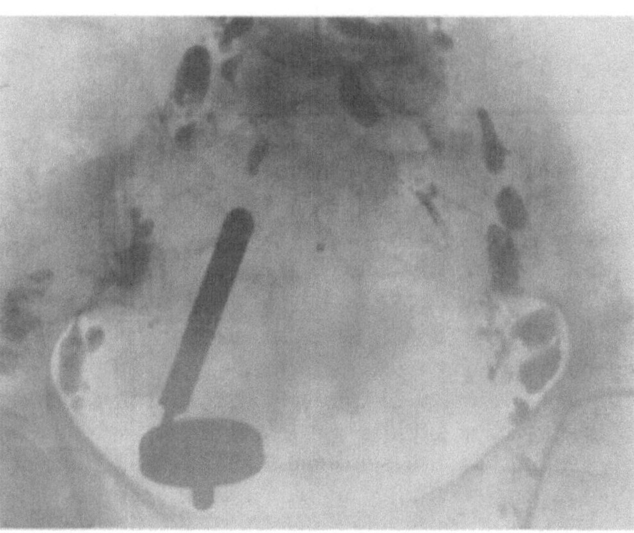

b

Abb. 13a u. b. Hochgradige Abweichung des Radiumträgers aus der Mittellinie bei unterschiedlicher Tamponade

Die intrakavitäre Radiumtherapie wirft allgemein bekannte und schwierig zu lösende *Strahlenschutzprobleme* auf. Deshalb wurde von HENSCHKE, HILARIS und MAHAN (1964, 1966) ein als „afterloading" bezeichnetes Ladungssystem entwickelt. Bei der Behandlung eines Collumcarcinoms wird zunächst der Applikator ohne radioaktives Material in Uterus und Vagina eingeführt. Er besteht aus 2 intravaginalen Ovoiden und einem intracervicalen Stift. Sie münden in 3 Anschlußschläuche, die mit dem Tresor verbunden sind. Über diese Schläuche kann die Strahlenquelle, deren Ende mit langen Drähten armiert ist, durch Fernbedienung elektromotorisch an ihren Ort im Applikator befördert werden. Während die beiden im Scheidengewölbe liegenden Quellen verbleiben, kann die intracervical liegende Strahlenquelle in verschiedenen Bewegungstypen ständig periodisch hin und her bewegt werden, so daß jedes gewünschte Dosis- und Verteilungsmuster erreicht werden kann. Die Bewegung der Quellen geschieht durch einen Motor mit einem doppelten Steuerungssystem für Länge und Geschwindigkeit der Bewegung. Die jeweilige Lage der radioaktiven Quellen ist auf einem Anzeigegerät sichtbar. Bei Beendigung der Bestrahlung werden die Radiumquellen in den Schläuchen durch Fernbedienung hinter eine Bleiwand zurückgezogen, so daß keinerlei Strahlenbelastung für das Personal entsteht (Abb. 14). Als Strahler kommen alle üblichen natürlichen und künstlichen Radioisotope in Betracht. Es können sehr hohe Aktivitäten appliziert werden, so daß durch die daraus resultierende kurze Bestrahlungszeit ambulante Bestrahlungen möglich sind. Als Strahlenquelle werden verwandt: Radium-226, Kobalt-60, Caesium-137, Iridium-192. Henschke bevorzugt vorerst 3 Einlagen in 2wöchigem Abstand, ohne endgültige Empfehlungen geben zu wollen.

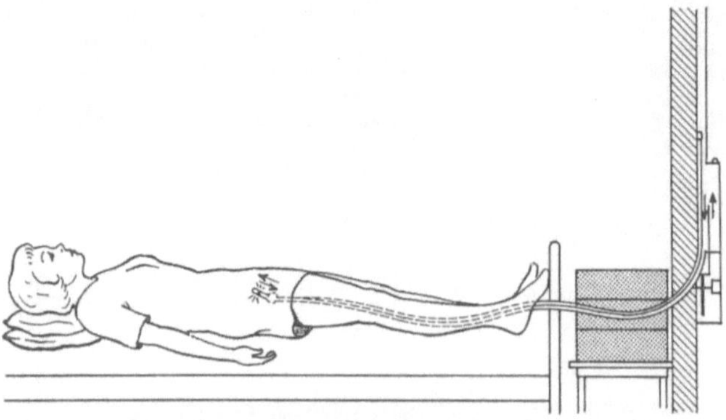

Abb. 14. Prinzip des „afterloading" (Henschke)

Weniger aus Strahlenschutzgründen als vielmehr zur stärkeren Fraktionierung der Radiumbestrahlung legt Ridings (1963) intrauterin ein dünnes Röhrchen von nur 4 mm Dicke in das Uteruscavum, das erst nachträglich mit Radiumzellen gefüllt wird, jederzeit entleert werden kann und so lange liegenbleibt, bis die Bestrahlung beendet ist. Auf diese Weise kann die sonst mehrmals notwendig werdende Anaesthesie vermieden werden. Auch hierbei handelt es sich um einen „afterloading"-Applikator.

Apparaturen für eine einfache nachträgliche Ladung, bei der der Strahler manuell über Führungsleitungen vorgeschoben werden kann, sind heute so weit entwickelt, daß sie selbst kleineren Instituten empfohlen werden können. Diese Verfahren bieten gegenüber den herkömmlichen Methoden wesentliche Vorteile hinsichtlich des Strahlenschutzes. Ferngesteuerte Apparate für eine nachträgliche Ladung bringen noch technische, klinische und strahlenbiologische Probleme mit sich.

Seit etwa 15 Jahren wird versucht, in der intrakavitären Curietherapie des Collumcarcinoms das Radium durch *künstliche Radionuclide* zu ersetzen. Besondere Verwendung fand hierbei das Kobalt-60, das bei gleicher Halbwertschicht eine wesentlich weichere β-Strahlung als das Radium besitzt. Daher werden zur Ausfilterung dieser Strahlung wesentlich dünnere Filter, ein Zwanzigstel des üblichen Wertes, benötigt (Meiling, 1953).

Für die postoperative Bestrahlung der Vagina nach einer Hysterektomie wegen Collumcarcinom entwickelte Ariel (1966) einen speziellen intravaginalen Applikator, dessen dreiteilige Ovoide mit Kobalt-60 beschickt werden. Morton et al. (1953) verwandten radioaktives Kobalt für intrauterine oder intravaginale Applikationen beim Collumcarcinom. Meschan et al. (1955) luden die Spreizkolpostaten mit Kobalt-60. Eine besondere Art der Kobalt-60-Therapie beim Collumcarcinom führten Körbler, Frank und Stojanov (1963) bei fortgeschrittenen Collumcarcinomen durch. Sie legten Kobaltperlen in einem Ring um die Portio und verabreichten 15000—30000 rep. Eine größere

Verbreitung fand das Kobalt-60 in Form des Plastobalts nach den Angaben von BECKER und SCHEER (1956). Das Plastobalt wird vor allem bei den verschiedenen Formen der vaginalen und Portiotumoren angewendet, da es eine individuelle Gestaltung der Strahlenoberfläche ermöglicht.

Ein anderes für die Curietherapie verwandtes Radionuclid ist das Iridium-192. Bei Verwendung von Iridium kann mit Hilfe besonderer intravaginaler Träger eine wesentlich höhere Dosis an die Beckenwand herangebracht werden. Vor allem ist infolge des viel geringeren Penetrationsvermögens von radioaktivem Iridium die Gefahr der Überdosierung an Blase und Rectum viel geringer als bei Verwendung von Radium (TUDWAY, 1953). Dieses Radionuclid ermöglicht es, von der Vagina aus nahezu gleiche Dosen an die Cervix und an die Beckenwand heranzubringen. Auch PIERQUIN (1965) gebraucht Iridium-192 anstelle von Radium. In Form von Drähten kann es durch Stahlschienen oder Führungssonden relativ leicht appliziert werden.

Eine andere Möglichkeit, die Dosis im Parametrium ohne zusätzliche Belastung von Rectum und Blase zu erhöhen, sehen TER-POGOSSIAN und SHERMAN (1955) in der Verwendung von Radiogold, das eine Gammastrahlung von nur 411 keV aussendet. Sie konstruierten einen entsprechenden Schutzkörper aus Blei, dessen Wanddicke 6 mm beträgt. Wenn bei einer mittelweiten Scheide an der Beckenwand eine Dosis von 4500 R in 30 Std erreicht werden soll, muß die Aktivität des Radiogoldpräparates zu Beginn der Behandlung etwa 2 Ci betragen.

Über die Verbreitung von kleinen geschlossenen Strahlenquellen zur Verwendung bei der intrakavitären und interstitiellen Therapie führte eine Sachverständigengruppe der Internationalen Atomenergie-Organisation in den Jahren 1964 und 1965 Untersuchungen durch (Strahlentherapie *132*, 155—157, 1967). Die Sachverständigengruppe wies in ihrem Bericht darauf hin, daß die Hauptgefahr bei Verwendung von Radium nicht die Möglichkeit einer Explosion durch Aufbau eines inneren Gasdruckes ist. Viel gefährlicher ist es, daß die Strahlenquellen während des Gebrauches beschädigt werden können. Aufgrund dieser Überlegungen erscheint es gerechtfertigt, Caesium-137 in unlöslicher Form als Strahlenquelle zu empfehlen. Die weichere Gammastrahlung dieses Isotops erleichtert einerseits die Abschirmung zur Erzielung einer günstigen Dosisverteilung, zum anderen verringert sie die Strahlenbelastung des Personals. Außerdem ist der Kapitalaufwand bei Ankauf eines Vorrats von Caesiumquellen wesentlich geringer als bei den entsprechenden Radiumpräparaten. Diese Vorteile des Caesiums sollten den Nachteil aufwiegen, daß die Aktivität des Präparates im Jahr um etwa 2 % abnimmt.

Es liegen heute bereits genügend Beweise dafür vor, daß zwischen den strahlentherapeutischen Wirkungen des Radiums und jenen der neuen Strahlenquellen mit Ausnahme der weichen γ-Strahler kein Unterschied besteht, so daß diese Strahler gefahrlos angewandt werden könnten (HORSTER, JONES und STACEY, 1964).

β) Interstitielle Curietherapie

Das Bestreben, eine bei der intrakavitären Radiumbehandlung mögliche Dosisverteilung auch bei solchen Tumorlokalisationen zu erreichen, bei denen zur Applikation des Radionuclids kein Cavum vorhanden, der Tumor von außen aber relativ leicht zugänglich ist, führte zur Entwicklung der interstitiellen Curietherapie.

Eine interstitielle Curietherapie beim Collumcarcinom kann in Form einer Spickung mit Nadeln oder in Form einer interstitiellen Injektion eines Kolloids vorgenommen werden. Bei der Implantation fester Strahlenquellen unterscheidet man zeitlich begrenzte Implantationen, bei der nach einer bestimmten Liegezeit das Radionuclid entfernt wird, und interstitielle Dauerimplantationen.

Die interstitielle Applikation fest umschlossener Strahler wird mit Platinnadeln vorgenommen, die in ihrem Innern das Radionuclid enthalten. Sie lassen sich ohne großes Trauma in das Gewebe einstechen. Während früher als Radionuclid ausschließlich Radium verwandt wurde (Donaldson, 1930; Günsel, 1953; Quimby und Castro, 1953; Corscaden, Gusberg und Kosar, 1954; Kleine, 1954; Bloedorn, 1956), werden heute vor allem Kobalt-60 (Barnes, 1954; Ezell und Holzaepfel, 1957) sowie Iridium-192 und Tantal-182 verwendet (Henschke, Hilaris und Mahan, 1963, 1965). Der Vorteil dieser neueren Radionuclide liegt darin, daß man nicht so starr an die Nadellängen gebunden ist, die beim Radium wegen der Notwendigkeit des gasdichten Abschlusses nicht zu verändern sind.

Während in der gynäkologischen Strahlentherapie die interstitielle Spickung vor allem beim Urethral- und Vulvacarcinom Verwendung fand, wird sie bei der Behandlung des Collumcarcinoms nur selten benutzt. Hier wird sie hauptsächlich zur homogenen Bestrahlung größerer Portiotumoren und zur Erhöhung der Dosis bei parametranen Infiltrationen angewandt. Eine besondere Indikation ergibt sich bei parametranen und Beckenwandrezidiven, die nach einer üblichen Strahlenbehandlung aufgetreten sind. Bloedorn (1956) glaubt allerdings, daß die interstitielle Radiumtherapie auch nach Einführung der Megavolttherapie noch einen bedeutenden Platz im Rahmen der Tumortherapie besitzt. Nach seiner Ansicht bietet die interstitielle Therapie Vorteile, die von keiner anderen Methode erreicht werden, wenn die Behandlungsmethode richtig angewandt wird. Es kommt bei der interstitiellen Radiumapplikation zu einer maximalen Strahlenbelastung des malignen Gewebes, während das gesunde umgebende Gewebe weitgehend geschont werden kann. Als Vorteile gelten die genaue Lokalisation des Tumors und seiner Ausdehnung, die Beschränkung der Bestrahlung auf das Tumorvolumen mit der guten Anpassungsmöglichkeit an den Tumor, eine höhere Strahlendosis aufgrund des eng begrenzten räumlichen Volumens und kürzere Behandlungszeiten. Weiterhin werden als Vorteile angesehen: die Schonung des Blasenbodens durch Wegfall massiver, vor der Portio liegender Radiummengen, Bestrahlung der uterusnahen parametranen Infiltrate und geringe Allgemeinreaktion der Patientinnen durch Verzicht auf die Röntgenbestrahlung.

Der unbestreitbaren Wirksamkeit stehen aber auf der anderen Seite erhebliche Nachteile und Gefahren entgegen: Schwierigkeiten in der Dosimetrie, Strahlenbelastung des Personals und des Operateurs sowie die Gefahren bei der unkontrollierbaren Punktion von Gefäßen und der Ureteren. Die ungenaue Dosierungsmöglichkeit bei der Spickung führt zu unvermeidlichen Strahlenreaktionen in den Parametrien und im Darm.

Ezell und Holzaepfel (1957) registrierten bei 99 Patientinnen nach einer Therapie mit radioaktiven Kobalt-Nadeln in die Cervix und Parametrien, bei der die gesamte verabfolgte Strahlendosis 6 000—7 000 R betrug, in 43 Fällen Bestrahlungsproktitiden mit einer starken Darmblutung. Unter diesen Komplikationen fanden sich 11 Recto-Vaginalfisteln, 6 Vesico-Vaginalfisteln, 11 Dickdarmstenosen, die eine Kolostomie erforderten, eine Dünndarm- und eine Ureterstenose.

Corscaden, Gusberg und Kosar (1954) sahen bei 108 Fällen einer interstitiellen Radiumtherapie, bei der 8 Nadeln von 3,2 cm Länge mit je 1,98 mg Radium in 1 cm Entfernung zirkulär in die Cervix und paracervical in das Parametrium eingeführt wurden, nur in 2 Fällen ernste Strahlenschädigungen. In 4 Fällen wurde eine Vene anpunktiert. Kleine (1954) sah bei 87 Patientinnen der Stadien II—IV bei einer applizierten Einzeldosis von 1 680—4 300 mgeh nur in einem Fall eine durch die Strahlung entstandene Blasenfistel, die operativ verschlossen werden konnte. Maliphant (1955) hält aufgrund seiner Erfahrungen die intrauterine Radiumbehandlung sogar für gefährlicher als die Radiumspickung, obwohl er relativ häufig Fisteln beobachtete.

Ezell und Holzaepfel (1957) entwickelten zur Applikation der radioaktiven Kobalt-Nadeln beim Collumcarcinom ein in der Scheide liegendes Zielgerät aus durchsichtigem Kunststoff, durch dessen vorgebohrte Kanäle die Nadeln eingeführt und dann eingestochen werden. Die gesamte verabfolgte Strahlendosis liegt etwa zwischen 6 000 und 7 000 R.

Um eine bessere und vor allem übersichtliche Dosisverteilung zu erhalten, fertigen sich HENSCHKE, HILARIS und MAHAN (1963) vorher zur Berechnung der Strahlendosis ein Modell an. Bei entfernbaren Implantaten applizierten sie in einem ersten Schritt leere Nylonröhrchen in das Gewebe. In einem zweiten Schritt nach ausreichender Fixation und operativer Versorgung werden erst die radioaktiven Seeds oder Drähte, bei denen Iridium-192 bevorzugt wird, eingeführt. Die Nylonfäden mit den Iridium-Seeds werden im äußeren Teil des Nylon-Schlauches durch einen kleinen Klip befestigt. Bei Abschluß der Implantationszeit von etwa 5—8 Tagen werden die Iridiumimplantate mit einem Spezialinstrument herausgezogen. Diese Technik erscheint sicherer, da die optimale Verteilung der radioaktiven Seeds auf der Basis von Messungen geplant werden kann.

Die Berechnung der Dosis des implantierten Volumens wird meist nach den Tabellen von PATERSON und PARKER (1947) oder QUIMBY (1944) vorgenommen. Nähere Einzelheiten sind im Allgemeinen Teil dieses Handbuches ausgeführt, auf die an dieser Stelle verwiesen wird.

Bei vaginalen und paravaginalen Tumorinfiltrationen eines Collumcarcinoms konnte LIEGNER (1964) mit entfernbaren Iridium-192-Nylonfäden und -Drähten bei Verwendung der „Afterloading"-Technik bei einem allerdings kleinen Patientengut in einigen Fällen eine gute Tumorrückbildung beobachten. Schwere Komplikationen wurden nicht registriert.

Gegenüber der zeitlich begrenzten Radionuclidimplantation wird bei einer interstitiellen *Dauerimplantation*, der sog. *parametranen Implantation*, fast ausschließlich das radioaktive Gold-198 verwandt (KRAUSE, 1961; SCHUMACHER, 1961; KAPP-SCHWOERER, 1962; THOMSEN, 1962; LIEGNER, 1964). Darüber hinaus wird von HENSCHKE (1965) und LIEGNER (1964) Xenon-133, Caesium-131, Jod-125 oder Radon benutzt.

Bei der Dauerimplantation fallen die Schwierigkeiten beim Legen und die spätere Entfernung weg. KAPP-SCHWOERER und BUSCH (1964) beschreiben eine ausführliche Technik, bei der sie mit einer handlichen Pistole die 2,5 mm langen Seeds von 0,8 mm Durchmesser gut interstitiell deponieren können. Die Gold-Seeds sind von einem 0,15 mm dicken Platinmantel umgeben, der die β-Strahlung praktisch völlig abschirmt. Die weichere γ-Strahlung von nur 0,4 MeV im Vergleich zu härteren Radium-γ-Strahlung erleichtert den Strahlenschutz. Als Vorteil wird bei der permanenten Implantation neben der besonders günstigen relativen Herdraumdosis mit Schonung des Tumorbettes und der kritischen Nachbarorgane vor allem die exponentiell abfallende Langzeitbestrahlung angesehen. Als Indikation gelten größere Collumtumoren, vor allem strahlenresistente Rezidive und die Möglichkeit einer Implantation intra operationem. Bei Verwendung eines Seeds mit etwa 10 mCi ergibt sich im Abstand von 1 cm eine Gesamtdosis von 2232 R.

KAPP-SCHWOERER verfügt über langjährige Erfahrungen. Er sieht den geringeren Strahlenschutzaufwand, den kleineren Eingriff ohne längere Liegezeit der Patientinnen, die individuellen Anwendungsmöglichkeiten, die hohe Tumordosis bei Schonung der Nachbarschaft und besonders die Möglichkeit einer günstigen Protrahierung als positive Merkmale dieser Bestrahlungsmethode an. In vielen Fällen war eine gute Rückbildung des Tumors ohne Ulcerationen zu erkennen. Die Goldseedspickung wurde fast ausnahmslos ohne zusätzliche Beschwerden vertragen. Bei dem kurzen kleinen Eingriff bestehen praktisch keine Kontraindikationen.

HENSCHKE und LAWRENCE (1965) halten die Verwendung von Caesium-131 für die permanente Implantation für günstiger als Aurum-198 oder Radon-222. Die monochromatische 29,4 keV-Strahlung des Caesium-131 wird im Gewebe in den ersten Zentimetern wegen der fehlenden primären und sekundären β-Strahlung geringer absorbiert als die Strahlung von Radon oder Gold, (Abb. 15). Ebenfalls erscheint die längere Halbwertzeit von 9,7 Tagen beim Caesium-131 auch aus wirtschaftlichen Gründen vorteilhafter. Darüber hinaus wirkt sich die längere Halbwertzeit auch durch den stärkeren selektiven Effekt auf das Tumorgewebe insbesondere bei langsamer Wachstumsgeschwindigkeit günstig aus.

Eine andere Applikationsform stellt die Infiltration des Tumors mit *flüssigen Radionucliden* dar. Die bereits vor mehreren Jahrzehnten mit Thorium-X durchgeführten Untersuchungen wurden im Laufe des vorigen Jahrzehnts durch die zur Verfügung stehenden kurzlebigen Radionuclide erneut zur Therapie verwandt. Für eine solche permanente Implantation kommen ebenfalls nur kurzlebige Strahler in Frage, da sich die injizierte Substanz keinesfalls entfernen läßt, sondern aus dem Tumor ausgeschwemmt und in bestimmten Organen abgelagert werden kann. Daraus können dann schwere Spätschäden entstehen. Andererseits muß man versuchen, eine möglichst lange Retention des Radionuclids zu gewährleisten. Man erreicht es durch Verwendung von Suspensionen unlöslicher radioaktiver Verbindungen. Hierzu besonders geeignet erscheint das radioaktive Gold-198, das durch Schutzkolloide stabilisiert werden kann. Ein Abtransport des Radionuclids auf

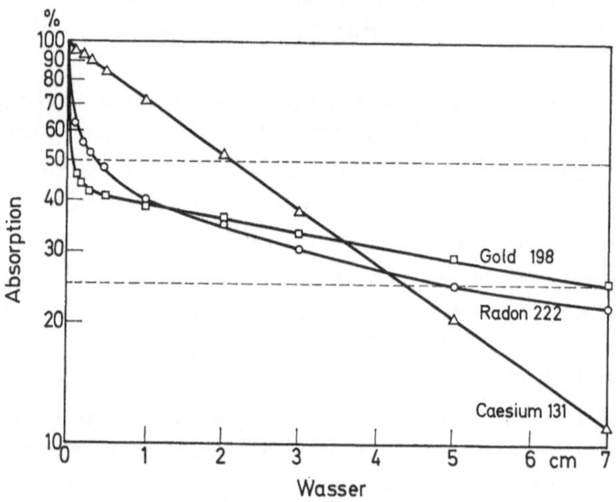

Abb. 15. Absorption von Caesium-131, Radon-222 und Gold-198 in Wasser (Henschke und Lawrence)

dem Lymphwege erscheint nicht ungünstig, da hierdurch möglicherweise kleine Lymphknotenmetastasen devitalisiert werden können (Ruch, Cox, Nurnberger und Trumbull, 1957; Müller, 1958; Barbanti, Bellion und Buchi, 1960; Bellion und Chiarle, 1960).

Bei der Injektion von radioaktivem Gold werden mit einer langen Punktionskanüle in Narkose in das Parametrium 50—120 mCi Aktivität pro Seite injiziert, die in etwa 35 ml Lösungsmittel enthalten sind. Die Goldlösung wird aus einem bleigeschützten Behälter über einen Polyäthylenschlauch angesaugt. Bei 50—75 mCi Aurum-198 wird folgende Dosisverteilung für γ-Strahlung angenommen: Cervix etwa 1 000 R, Parametrium, 3 bis 4 cm seitlich von der Mittellinie, etwa 2 500 R, Beckenwand entlang des Nervus obturatorius etwa 4 000 R (Sherman und Allen, 1957). An den entsprechenden Stellen im Parametrium, an der Beckenwand und in den Lymphknotengebieten soll die β-Strahlung 15 000—30 000 rep entsprechen. Soule (1953) nimmt nach Injektion von 50—75 mCi pro Parametrium an 3 verschiedenen Stellen aufgrund von Messungen mit einem Szintillationszähler eine im Parametrium applizierte Dosis von 75 000 rep hauptsächlich als β-Strahlung an. Durch die gleichzeitige γ-Strahlung werden weitere 2 000—3 000 R im Beckenbereich verabfolgt. Die Lymphknotengruppe im Obturator- und Hypogastrica-Bereich, in denen er einen erheblichen Abtransport von Goldpartikelchen nachweisen konnte, erhalten zwischen 20 000 und 75 000 rep.

Über Erfahrungen an einem größeren Patientengut verfügen Sherman und Allen (1957). Wie aus Tabelle 7 hervorgeht, konnten sie in den Stadien I—III die Behandlungsergebnisse durch eine Kombination von interstitieller Goldtherapie mit einer Radiumapplikation oder einer Wertheimschen Radikaloperation verbessern, verglichen mit einem entsprechenden Patientengut, das nur mit Röntgen-Radium behandelt wurde. Die günstigsten Behandlungsergebnisse erzielten sie durch eine Goldapplikation und erweiterte Radikaloperation nach WERTHEIM einige Wochen später (Tabelle 8). Auch KOTTMEIER (1964) konnte durch eine kolloidale Goldinjektion beim Collumcarcinom gute Behandlungsergebnisse erreichen. Bei klinisch suspekten Fällen mit einem Beckenwandrezidiv registrierte er in 34 von 71 Fällen einen guten palliativen Erfolg.

Über größere Erfahrungen mit einer Radiogoldinjektion bei Beckenwandrezidiven und auch primären Collumcarcinomen verfügen auch VERHAGEN und MUSZYNSKI (1961). Nach ihrer Meinung bleibt die Anwendung der interstitiellen Radiogoldtherapie jedoch auf die Rezidivbehandlung beschränkt. Auch ZERNE, MORRIS und CHANG (1962) empfehlen die

Tabelle 7. *Behandlungsergebnisse nach* ^{198}*Au-Behandlung beim Collumcarcinom* (SHERMAN und ALLEN)

Stadium	Röntgen- und Radiumtherapie			^{198}Au/Radium/Wertheim		
	Zahl der behandelten Fälle	lebend ohne Anhalt für Rezidiv		Zahl der behandelten Fälle	lebend ohne Anhalt für Rezidiv	
		Fälle	%		Fälle	%
I	36	30	83,3	99	90	90,0
II	68	35	51,4	95	83	87,3
III	49	15	30,6	43	30	69,7

Tabelle 8. *Behandlungsergebnisse nach* ^{198}*Au-Behandlung beim Collumcarcinom in Kombination mit anderen Behandlungsmethoden* (SHERMAN und ALLEN)

	Zahl der behandelten Fälle	Lebend ohne Anhalt für Rezidiv	
		Fälle	%
Röntgen- und Radiumtherapie	104	65	62,5
^{198}Au-Applikation und Wertheim	31	28	90,3
^{198}Au-Applikation, Radium und Wertheim	81	72	88,8
^{198}Au-Applikation und Radium	82	71	86,6

Radiogoldapplikation bei Rezidiven. Wegen der sehr schwierigen Dosisberechnung, bei der sich von klinischer Seite zwangsläufig große Fehlermöglichkeiten ergeben können, erscheint eine Bestrahlung eines primären Collumcarcinoms nicht ratsam. Lediglich bei abgrenzbaren Rezidiven ist ein guter Erfolg zu erwarten. Nach ihrer Erfahrung kann bei einem Collumcarcinom der Gruppe III mit einer Tumorinfiltration in beiden Parametrien eine ausschließliche Radium- oder Aurum-198-Therapie nicht zu einer Heilung führen.

Auch andere Autoren schließen aus ihren Beobachtungen, daß diese Methode keinen bemerkenswerten Fortschritt in der Therapie der malignen Genitaltumoren bringt (BARBANTI und TETTI, 1959). SCHULTZ, PECKHAM und KIEKHOFER (1962) kommen aufgrund von Erfahrungen an 152 Frauen zu dem Schluß, daß die Behandlungsresultate durch eine parametrane Goldinstillation als unbefriedigend bezeichnet werden müssen. Sie lehnen daher die kombinierte Behandlung mit Radiogold ab.

Die ablehnende Haltung wird größtenteils auf die nicht seltenen Schädigungen zurückgeführt, die vorwiegend in Strikturen der oberen Harnwege, Ureterfisteln, Blasenfisteln und stärkeren Blasenreaktionen bestehen (SHERMAN und ALLEN, 1957). Als Ergänzungsmaßnahme zur primären Radiumbehandlung beim Collumcarcinom lehnen auch ALLEN, SHERMAN und CAMEL (1958) die Goldinjektion ab. Bei den etwa 4 Wochen nach Goldinjektion durchgeführten Wertheimschen Operationen mit Ausräumung der Beckenlymphknoten beobachteten sie häufiger Komplikationen im Bereich der Ureteren. Sie

13*

glauben allerdings, daß mit ihrer Methode eine stärkere Bestrahlung der Parametrien und Beckenlymphknoten als mit der konventionellen Röntgen- und Radiumbehandlung erreicht wird. Sie registrierten bei einer kombinierten Anwendung von Radiogold und Radium mit nachfolgender Operation häufig Strikturen- und Fistelbildungen im Bereich des Urogenitalsystems (1955). Da Sherman und Allen (1957) die besten Behandlungsergebnisse bei einer Kombination von Radiogoldinstillation und Wertheimscher Radikaloperation fanden und bei dieser Kombination auch die geringste Quote von Behandlungskomplikationen bestand (Tabelle 9), empfehlen sie lediglich die Kombination von Radiogold und Radikaloperation einerseits oder von Radiogold und Radiumbestrahlung andererseits.

Versucht man, die klinischen Erfahrungen der Behandlungsergebnisse und vor allem der Behandlungskomplikationen mit der interstitiellen Curietherapie zusammenfassen, so werden von fast allen Autoren lediglich palliative Behandlungsergebnisse beschrieben. Darüber hinaus limitiert die hohe Komplikationsquote den routinemäßigen Einbau der

Tabelle 9. *Behandlungskomplikationen nach* [198]*Au-Therapie beim Collumcarcinom* (Sherman und Allen)

Stadium	Typ	Fälle	Behandlung
I	Ureterstriktur	3	[198]Au, Radium und Wertheim
	Ureterfistel	1	[198]Au, Radium und Wertheim
II	Ureterfistel	2	[198]Au, Radium und Wertheim
	Vesicovaginale Fistel	1	[198]Au, Radium und Wertheim
	Nierensteine	1	[198]Au und Radium
	Strahlencystitis	1	[198]Au und Radium

interstitiellen Therapie in die Behandlung des Collumcarcinoms. Der weitaus größte Teil der Publikationen stammt aus dem vorigen Jahrzehnt. In den letzten Jahren findet man im Schrifttum nur noch selten Mitteilungen, in denen diese Behandlungsmethode empfohlen wird. Der Grund hierfür dürfte darin zu suchen sein, daß es seit Anwendung von Megavoltenergien in vielen Fällen noch möglich ist, trotz vorausgegangener Röntgentherapie eine nochmalige Percutanbestrahlung zu riskieren. Die Indikationsbreite zur interstitiellen Curietherapie beim Collumcarcinom scheint somit durch die breitere Anwendung der Megavolttherapie zurückzugehen. Da einerseits mit Behandlungserfolgen durch die interstitielle Therapie nur dann zu rechnen ist, wenn der Operateur über größere Erfahrungen mit dieser Therapiemethode verfügt und andererseits auch heute noch große Unsicherheiten in der Dosisberechnung bestehen, aus denen ein erheblicher Teil der Behandlungskomplikationen resultiert, wird die klinische Bedeutung der interstitiellen Curietherapie in der Zukunft zugunsten der Megavolttherapie weiterhin abnehmen.

γ) Intralymphatische Curietherapie

Die endolymphatische Applikation von Radionucliden stellt eine besondere Form der interstitiellen Curietherapie dar. Hierdurch ist der Wunschtraum der Kliniker in Erfüllung gegangen, eine optimale Strahlentherapie der Lymphknotenmetastasen zu ermöglichen.

Die ersten Ansätze einer direkten Kontaktbestrahlung der Lymphknoten sind bereits bei der interstitiellen Radiogoldinfiltration des Uterus und der Parametrien beobachtet worden, bei der es zu einem Abtransport des Radionuclids in die Beckenwandlymphknoten kam (Kottmeier, 1955 u.a.). Allerdings beobachtete man dabei auch schon, daß nur gesundes lymphatisches Gewebe das kolloidale Gold zu speichern vermag, während ein mit Carcinom ausgefüllter Lymphknoten das Radionuclid nicht mehr aufnehmen konnte (Seaman, 1955; Thomas, 1956).

Eine gezielte und direkte endolymphatische Therapie wurde erstmals von Ratti und Chiappa (1962) vorgenommen. Die Technik der endolymphatischen Applikation eines Radionuclids basiert auf der von Kinmonth (1952) angegebenen Technik der direkten

Lymphangiographie. RATTI und CHIAPPA haben die Kinmonthsche Technik der Lymphangiographie verwandt, um radioaktiv markiertes Lipiodol direkt in die Lymphgefäße zu injizieren. Die Speicherung des Jod-131-Lipiodols in den Lymphknoten führte zur Möglichkeit, in den pelvinen und retroperitonealen Lymphknoten eine hohe Strahlenwirkung mit steilem Dosisabfall zu erzielen.

Über ähnliche Untersuchungen berichteten im gleichen Jahr FISCHER (1962) und JANTET (1962), die allerdings Aurum-198 intralymphatisch im Tierversuch und auch bei Patienten injizierten.

Die endolymphatische Therapie mit Jod-131-Lipiodol wurde in den folgenden Jahren hinsichtlich ihrer klinischen Anwendung von zahlreichen anderen Untersuchern erprobt (BORAGEI, 1962; FAVA, 1963; ARIEL, RESNICK, GALEY, 1964; PICARD, GONGORA, SZIGETI, BILSKI-PASQUIER, JAMMET und ARVAY, 1964; FISCHER, 1965; LIEBNER, 1965; SIEGEL und LIEBNER, 1965; VECCHIETTI, ONNIS, BRESADOLA, ROMAGNOLO und COLOMBINI, 1965; ZUM WINKEL, BECKER, JAHNS, SCHEURLEN, HERZFELD, 1967; REIFFENSTUHL, 1967).

Neben Jod-131-Lipiodol fanden bisher zur endolymphatischen Therapie auch folgende Radionuclide Anwendung: kolloidales Aurum-198 (JANTET, 1962; FISCHER, 1962; HORST, 1966; REIFFENSTUHL, 1967), ^{32}P-Chrom-Phosphat (BURGER, ASANO, NAGAMATSU, 1964; REIFFENSTUHL, 1967), ^{32}P-Tri-n-Octylphosphat (VECCHIETTI, ONNIS, BRESADOLA, ROMAGNOLO, COLOMBINI, 1965; DELLEPIANE, TETTI und DAVITTI, 1966), ^{169}Yb-markierte Mikrosphären (HORST, 1966), ^{90}Y- und ^{46}Sc-markierte Mikrosphären (ARIEL, RESNICK, GALEY, 1964) und ^{206}Bi-Phosphat (RATTI, 1962).

Das Phosphor-32 wird dem Jod-131 vorgezogen, weil durch die größere Reichweite der energiereichen β-Strahlen des Phosphors bessere Möglichkeiten für eine lokale Bestrahlung gegeben sind. Andererseits gestattet das Jod-131-Lipiodol wegen seines höheren Anteils von γ-Strahlung, Verteilungsstudien durch externe Messungen und damit auch Dosisberechnungen nach der intralymphatischen Applikation anstellen zu können. Dieser Vorteil besteht auch durch die von HORST (1964) angegebene Doppelmarkierung von Chrom-51 und Phosphor-32 beim Chromphosphat.

Bei dem von den meisten Autoren verwandten Jod-131-Lipiodol werden zwischen 6 und 35 mCi zur Therapie appliziert, im Durchschnitt werden 8—10 mCi verwandt. Schwierigkeiten bereitet vorerst noch die in den Lymphknoten applizierte Dosis. ZUM WINKEL et al. (1967) konnten an Hand umfangreicher Dosismessungen während und nach der Applikation zeigen, daß 39—78% der inkorporierten Radioaktivität in den retroperitonealen Lymphknoten gespeichert wird. Die errechnete absorbierte Dosis in den retroperitonealen Lymphknoten liegt pro 1 mCi Jod-131-Lipiodol zwischen 250 und 1800 rad. Bei einer Applikation von je 10 mCi Jod-131-Lipiodol über beide Fußrücken ergibt sich somit in den Lymphknoten eine Dosis zwischen 5000 und 36000 rad. Die Strahlenbelastung der Lunge reicht von 160—920 rad und die der Injektionsstelle von 3000—13000 rad. SIEGEL und LIEBNER (1965) konnten nach Injektion von 9—22 mCi Jod-131 an Hand histologischer Schnitte eine effektive Dosis für die externen iliakalen Lymphknoten von 14300 rad, für die Obturatorknoten von 14650 rad, für die superfiziellen Inguinalknoten von 10700 rad und für die internen iliakalen Knoten von 11750 rad im Mittel errechnen. Nur 8 der von ihnen excidierten 118 Knoten hatten weniger als 4000 rad absorbiert.

Wenn auch bisher die Untersuchungsergebnisse hinsichtlich der Wirkung des intralymphatisch injizierten Radionuclids an den Lymphknoten und den Metastasen nur sehr beschränkt sind, so konnten die Beobachtungen von LIEBNER an 118 Lymphknoten, die bei Patientinnen mit gynäkologischen Erkrankungen bei einer Operation nach intralymphatischer Therapie gewonnen wurden, zeigen, daß die Tumordosis in den wichtigen Lymphknotenregionen erreicht werden kann. Die Rückbildung ist selbstverständlich weitgehend von der Strahlenempfindlichkeit der Tumorzellen abhängig. Die histologischen Bilder zeigten typische Strahlenfolgen wie Fibrose, Fehlen von Lymphocyten und Gefäßveränderungen.

Im Tierversuch prüften BURGER, ASANO und NAGAMATSU (1964) die Wirksamkeit der intralymphatischen Isotopentherapie bei metastatischem Lymphknotenbefall. Nach nur einseitig durchgeführter Isotopentherapie mit Chrom-Phosphat entfernten sie zu verschiedenen Zeiten nach der Isotopentherapie die Popliteallymphknoten von Kaninchen. Alle unbehandelten Knoten zeigten bei den experimentell durch intralymphatische Tumorinjektion gesetzten Lymphknoten große metastatische Zellnester. Die behandelten ließen eindeutige Bestrahlungseffekte erkennen; die Metastasen waren signifikant kleiner als in den nicht bestrahlten Lymphknoten. In 2 von 9 Fällen ließen sich überhaupt keine lebensfähigen Tumorzellen mehr nachweisen. Die 7 anderen zeigten nur sehr schmale Areale lebensfähig erscheinender Tumorabsiedlungen in der Peripherie und subkapsulär.

Das wichtigste Argument gegen die intralymphatische Curietherapie wird darin gesehen, daß das Radionuclid ausschließlich nur vom lymphatischen Gewebe gespeichert wird und nicht ins Krebsgewebe übergeht. Ein vollständig carcinomatös umgewandelter Knoten erhält somit keine nennenswerte Strahlendosis. Deshalb wird von allen Autoren einstimmig nur bei multiplen Mikrometastasen eine Indikation zur intralymphatischen Therapie gesehen. Eine Injektion nach operativer Lymphonodektomie im Beckenraum erscheint kontraindiziert, da die gleichmäßige und ausgedehnte regionale Ausbreitung des Radionuclids im Lymphsystem infolge von Unwegsamkeit aufgehoben sein kann und durch Aufstauung eine Extravasatbildung in das umliegende Gewebe droht. Kontraindiziert ist eine endolymphatische Therapie außerdem bei einer Tumorblockade des iliacalen oder lumbalen Lymphsystems sowie bei einem lymphatischen Kollateralkreislauf. Hierbei kann im affizierten Lymphgebiet nicht nur eine ausreichende Strahlenwirkung erreicht werden, sondern das vor der Blockade liegende Lymphgewebe wird einer erheblichen Strahlenbelastung ausgesetzt.

Die bisher beobachteten Nebenwirkungen entsprechen denen nach einer diagnostischen Lymphographie. Besonderes Augenmerk muß aber auf die Menge des injizierten Agens gelenkt werden, da bei einer Menge von mehr als 10 ml pro Seite ein höherer Abtransport des Kontrastmittels durch den Ductus thoracicus in die Lungen und das Venensystem erfolgt. Aus der intralymphatischen Therapie kann auf diese Weise eine höhere Strahlenbelastung des Lungenparenchyms mit schweren Folgen resultieren.

Eine besondere Technik der intralymphatischen Curietherapie gibt REIFFENSTUHL (1967) an. Er injiziert unter Lokalanaesthesie das Radionuclid direkt mit einer Punktionsnadel in das Zentrum eines freigelegten Inguinallymphknotens, von wo das Radionuclid über die Vasa efferentia abtransportiert wird. Er nennt seine Methode „Lymphirradiatio pelvis". REIFFENSTUHL glaubt, daß die Beckenwandlymphknoten vollständiger nach Injektion des Kontrastmittels in einen Leistenlymphknoten als nach Injektion über ein frei präpariertes Lymphgefäß am Fußrücken dargestellt werden können. Die von ihm demonstrierten Lymphangiogramme und -adenogramme zeigen jedoch die gleiche Lymphknotenverteilung wie nach der sonst üblichen Technik.

Auch der Aufwand der Methode und die erforderliche Übung des Operateurs scheinen bei beiden Methoden gleich zu sein. Die von ihm erwähnte Möglichkeit einer irrtümlichen intravenösen Verabreichung des Kontrastmittels bei der Technik am dorsum pedis durch Verwechslung einer Lymphcapillare mit einer Blutcapillare wird keiner bestätigen können, der über ausreichende Erfahrungen mit der Kinmonthschen Methode verfügt. Durch die Reiffenstuhlsche Methode kann lediglich der Drainageweg vom Injektionsort bis zu den Beckenwandlymphknoten erheblich verkürzt werden. Bisher liegen allerdings keine Mitteilungen vor, daß sich der Transport des Radionuclids vom Fußrücken bis zur Leiste für den Patienten nachteilig auswirken könnte. Hingegen scheint vielmehr die direkte Injektion in ein fest ligiertes Lymphgefäß sicherer als die Injektion in einen Lymphknoten zu sein. Gerade bei der Verwendung hoher spezifischer Aktivitäten ist der Austritt schon geringer Mengen des Isotops unbedingt zu vermeiden, um schwere Strahlenfolgen an der Injektionsstelle zu verhindern.

b) Percutanbestrahlung

α) Orthovolttherapie

Die in der gynäkologischen Strahlentherapie entwickelten und angewandten Methoden der percutanen Therapie mit konventionellen Orthovolt-Röntgenstrahlen lassen sich hinsichtlich der notwendigen Herddosis nach folgenden Prinzipien einordnen:

1. Die Percutanbestrahlung besitzt nur den Wert einer Zusatztherapie, durch die eine von der Radiumtherapie auf die Parametrien und die Beckenwand applizierte Dosis erhöht werden soll.

2. Durch die Percutanbestrahlung soll eine möglichst hohe Herddosis an der Beckenwand und im Parametrium erreicht werden, weil der vom Radium entfallende Strahlenanteil in dieser Region nur gering ist.

3. Bei der ausschließlichen Röntgenbestrahlung wird eine ausreichende Herddosis im Bereich des Primärtumors und des Lymphabflußgebietes unter Verzicht auf Radium angestrebt.

Noch in der Mitte der ersten Hälfte unseres Jahrhunderts wurde der Wert der Percutanbestrahlung bei der radiologischen Behandlung des Collumcarcinoms von zahlreichen Klinikern überhaupt bestritten. Diese Einstellung erscheint keinesfalls verwunderlich, da mit den damals üblichen Methoden und Apparaturen nur ein geringer Dosisanteil ins kleine Becken eingestrahlt werden konnte, so daß der percutane Dosisanteil im Vergleich zur Radiumdosis minimal war. Die allgemein übliche Methode der percutanen Röntgenbestrahlung bestand in der Technik der Einstrahlung über 2 Bauch- und 2 Rückenfelder unter Stehfeldbedingungen, bei der der Zentralstrahl auf die Beckenwand gerichtet war und die vom Radium belastete mittlere Unterbauchregion ausgespart wurde. Unter diesen Bedingungen lag die erreichte Herddosis im Parametrium zwischen 1200 und 1800 R.

Schon relativ früh erkannte man, daß bei fortgeschrittenen Collumcarcinomen die Rückbildung der beckenwandnahen Tumorinfiltrationen nur durch eine höhere Radiumdosis erreicht werden konnte, die aber mit einer erheblich größeren Komplikationsrate erkauft werden mußte. Daher versuchte man, auf verschiedene Weise die relative Tiefendosis der Percutanbestrahlung zu erhöhen, um den vom Radium an die Beckenwand gelangenden Strahlenanteil verringern zu können. Eine Erhöhung der relativen Tiefendosis war durch Vergrößerung des Bestrahlungsfeldes möglich. Wesentlich günstiger konnte allerdings die Tiefendosis durch Verstärkung der Filterung, Erhöhung des Focus-Haut-Abstandes, Verringerung des Haut-Herd-Abstandes durch Kompression mit einem Tubus und Vermehrung der Strahleneinfallspforten gesteigert werden.

So entwickelte sich aus der Gegenfeldbestrahlung die Mehrfeld- oder Kreuzfeuerbestrahlung, die eine besondere Perfektion bei der *Marburger Methode* (DU MESNIL DE ROCHEMONT, 1950) erlangte. Bei dieser Bestrahlungstechnik wird ein zylindrisches Herdgebiet, das von der einen bis zur anderen Beckenwand reicht, unter möglichst vollständiger Ausnutzung des für den Strahleneintritt geeigneten Oberflächenbereichs mit vielen Kreuzfeuerkegeln angegriffen. Hierzu werden 6—7 quer gestellte 8×15 cm große Felder vom Bauch, vom Gesäß und vom Damm verwandt. Der Zentralstrahl der einzelnen Felder fällt in der Medianebene unter möglichst großen Winkeln ein, bei denen an allen Stellen eine einheitliche Überschneidung der Nachbarkegel in der Tiefe bewirkt wird. Zusätzlich wird die Kompression ausgenutzt, um eine Verkürzung der Herdtiefe und Herausdrängung der Darmschlingen aus dem Strahlenkegel zu erreichen (Abb. 16a u. b).

Eine weitere Möglichkeit, die Dosisverteilung im kleinen Becken zu verbessern, war durch die Sieb- oder Gitterbestrahlung gegeben. Ohne auf die strahlenbiologischen Probleme der Siebbestrahlung eingehen zu können, soll erwähnt werden, daß die Hautverträglichkeit durch die Siebbestrahlung wesentlich stärker erhöht werden konnte als bei der Verminderung der mittleren Dosisleistung am Herd durch die partielle Hautabdeckung. Mit Hilfe der Siebbestrahlung ergibt sich in der gynäkologischen Strahlentherapie die Möglichkeit, selbst adipöse Patientinnen unter Verzicht auf Seiten- und

Vulva-Damm-Felder mit einer ausreichenden Herddosis zu bestrahlen. Da mit der Siebbestrahlung bei guter Allgemeinverträglichkeit vor allem größere Volumina mit einer
relativ hohen und homogenen Dosis bestrahlt werden können, fand sie besonders bei fortgeschrittenen Collumcarcinomen und Rezidiven Anwendung (Freid, Lipman und Jacobson, 1953; Bolognesi, 1954; Becker und Kuttig, 1954; Fochem, 1957; Bistolfi,
1958; Frischkorn, 1960).

Die Siebbestrahlung erlangte in der konventionellen Ära relativ weite Verbreitung.
Es konnten im Becken Herddosen von 3000—4000 R eingestrahlt werden. Der Wert der
Siebbestrahlung konnte insbesondere bei fortgeschrittenen Carcinomen und bei Rezidiverkrankungen in vielen Fällen unter Beweis gestellt werden. Die Verträglichkeit war sehr
gut. Allgemeinreaktionen traten trotz der großen Felder selten auf. Die Hautreaktion in

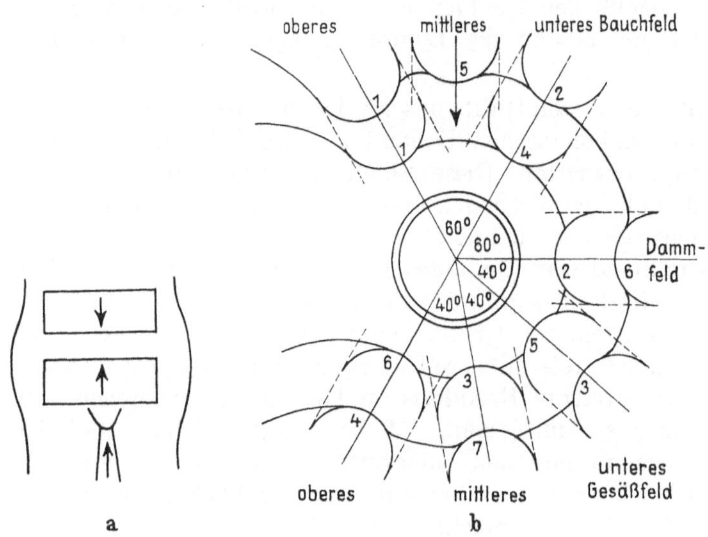

Abb. 16a u. b. Grundgedanke der Marburger Methode zur Röntgenbehandlung von Gebärmutterkrebsen
(Du Mesnil de Rochemont)

Form einer Epidermolyse heilten in relativ kurzer Zeit ab. Der spätere atrophische Zustand der Haut war meist zufriedenstellend. Die Erythemschwelle lag beim ventralen
Feld höher als beim dorsalen.

Die entscheidende Verbesserung der Dosisverteilung und damit der Wirksamkeit der
percutanen Röntgentherapie brachte aber erst die Entwicklung der Bewegungsbestrahlung. Durch sie konnte erstmalig eine wirksame Tumortherapie in der gynäkologischen
Strahlenbehandlung erreicht und das Problem der Erhöhung der relativen Tiefendosis
durch Einführung der verschiedenen Formen der Bewegungsbestrahlung gelöst werden.
Die Volumendosis konnte trotz Zunahme der relativen Herdraumdosis verkleinert werden,
wodurch ein besserer Schutz gesunder Organe erreicht wurde.

Nach umfangreichen Dosismessungen unter den verschiedenen Bestrahlungsbedin-
gungen bei der Rotation- und Pendelbestrahlung (Baeumer, 1952; Wachsman und
Keller, 1952; Koizumi, 1955; Busse, 1956; Spechter, 1956; Goldscheider und
Stern, 1958; Kok, 1958; Ruderman, Šapošnikova und Karibov, 1958; Breit und
Keller, 1959; Keller, 1961 u.a.) sowie bei der Konvergenz- und Pendelkonvergenz-
bestrahlung (Dibbelt, 1954; Siegert, 1954; Maurer, 1955; Eberle und Busse, 1956;
Spechter, 1956; Kallert, 1957; Harbort, 1958; Müller, 1958; Dibbelt und Rahm,
1959 u.a.) fand die Bewegungsbestrahlung auf breiter Ebene Eingang in die gynäkologische
Strahlentherapie.

Die günstigste Dosisverteilung konnte mit der Pendelkonvergenzbestrahlung erzielt werden. WACHSMANN und KELLER (1952) sowie SPECHTER (1956) konnten zeigen, daß bei einer alleinigen Pendelbestrahlung parametraner Herde nicht nur an der Beckenwand ein Dosismaximum auftritt, sondern auch hinter dem Sitzbein und vor dem Schambein. Weiterhin kann ein ungünstiges Tiefendosisverhältnis entstehen, wenn der Pendelwinkel zu klein gewählt wird. Die größte relative Tiefendosis mit konventionellen Röntgenstrahlen kann mit der Pendelkonvergenzbestrahlung erreicht werden, wie SPECHTER (1956) durch seine Untersuchungen zur Dosisverteilung im weiblichen Becken zeigen konnte. Vergleichende Messungen zur Dosisverteilung bei der Konvergenz-, Pendel- sowie Pendelkonvergenzbestrahlung der Parametrien führte MAURER (1955) durch. Die besten Dosisverhältnisse ergaben sich bei der Pendelkonvergenzbestrahlung. Bei einer

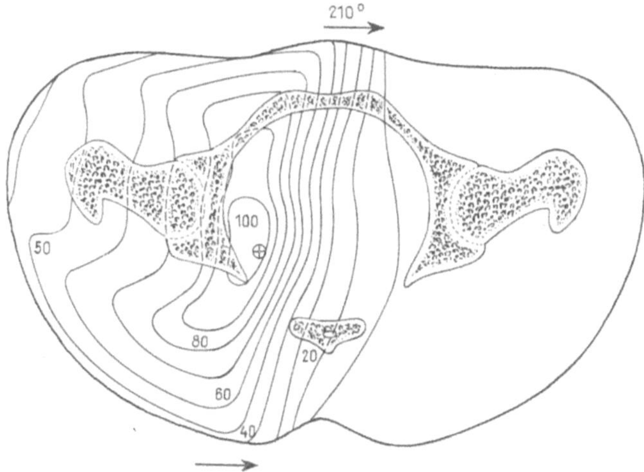

Abb. 17a. Isodosen bei Pendelkonvergenzbestrahlung (210°/60°) über eine Beckenhälfte in der Ebene der Spinae ischiadica. Drehpunkt: 4 cm lateral von der Medianen, Feldgröße 3,5 × 7 cm. HWS: 0,7 mm Cu.

Pendelkonvergenzbestrahlung von 180°/60° und einer Feldgröße von 4,5 × 7 cm erhält man eine relative Tiefendosis von 213 % gegenüber 166 % bei der Pendelbestrahlung um 220° und einer Feldgröße von 4 oder 6 cm. Die Blasenbelastung beträgt bei der Pendelkonvergenzbestrahlung 25 % gegenüber 38 % bei einer Pendelung; durch die zur Schonung des Schenkelhalses erforderliche Bleiabdeckung steigt sie auf 28 und 45 % an. Bei der Pendelkonvergenzbestrahlung ist außerdem die Dosisverteilung innerhalb des Herdfeldes homogener (Abb. 17 a—d).

Die reine Konvergenzbestrahlung bereitet in der gynäkologischen Strahlenbehandlung technische Schwierigkeiten, durch die Krümmung des Beckenumfanges, den im Strahlengang liegenden Knochen und die Gefahr von Dosisüberschneidungen an Haut, Subcutis und Blase. Bei Bestrahlung des Parametriums von zwei Konvergenzgegenfeldern kommt es im Bereich des Herdes zu einer hantelförmigen Eindellung und besonders bei größeren Herdtiefen zu einem stärkeren Auseinanderweichen der Dosismaxima und damit zu unterdosierten Regionen, die HACKENTHAL (1961) durch zusätzliche Stehfelder auszugleichen versucht.

Eine besondere Form der Bewegungsbestrahlung stellt die Schichtbestrahlung oder Stratitherapie (PALMIERI und ZAFFAGNINI, 1959) dar, bei der zur räumlichen Homogenität die chronotope Homogenität hinzukommt. Diese Art der Bewegungsbestrahlung fand in Deutschland keine Verbreitung.

Die Bewegungsbestrahlung und insbesondere die Pendelkonvergenzbestrahlung mit der Möglichkeit, eine Herddosis im Parametrium von 4000—5000 R zu erzielen, warf

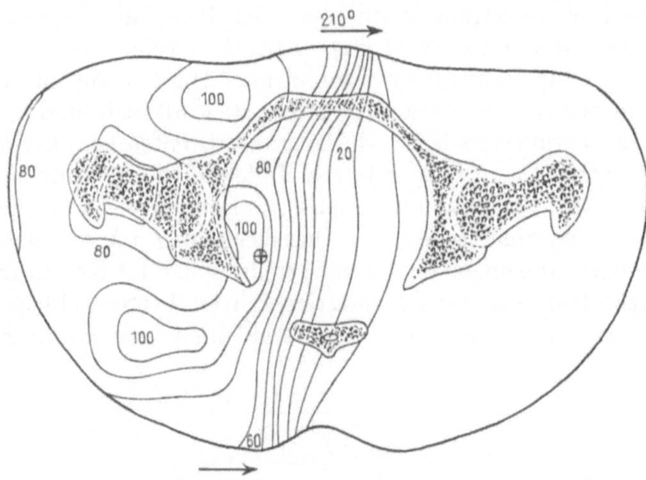

Abb. 17 b. Isodosen bei der Pendelbestrahlung (210°) über eine Beckenhälfte in der Ebene der Spinae ischiadica. Drehpunkt: 4 cm lateral von der Medianen. Feldgröße 3,5 × 9 cm. HWS 0,7 mm Cu.

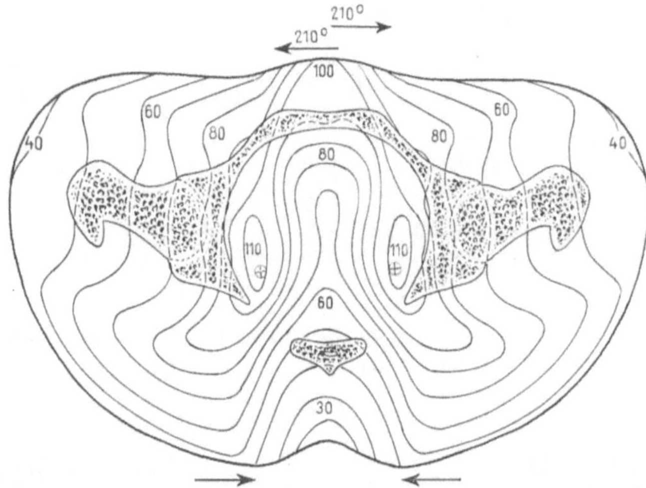

Abb. 17 c. Isodosen bei der Pendelkonvergenzbestrahlung (210°/60°) über beide Beckenhälften in der Ebene der Spinae ischiadicae. Drehpunkt: 4 cm lateral von der Medianen. Feldgröße 3,5 × 7 cm. HWS: 0,7 mm Cu.

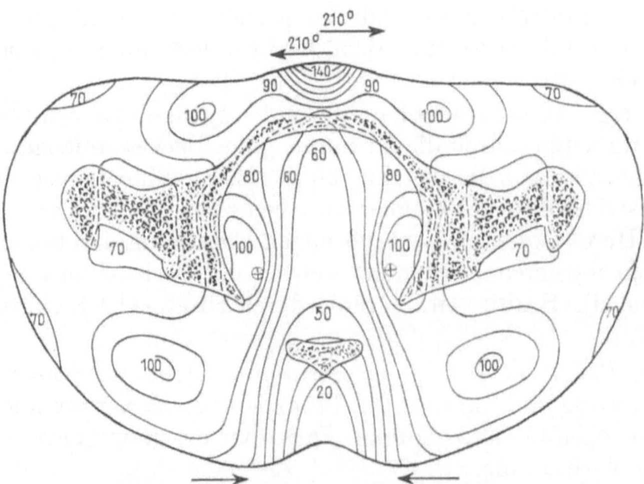

Abb. 17 d. Isodosen bei Pendelbestrahlung (210°) über beide Beckenhälften in der Ebene der Spinae ischiadicae. Drehpunkt: 4 cm lateral von der Medianen. Feldgröße 2,5 × 7 cm. HWS: 0,7 mm Cu

erstmalig das Problem der Dosisangleichung zwischen der Radium-γ-Strahlung und der percutan eingestrahlten Röntgenstrahlung auf. WACHSMANN und KELLER (1952) fanden eine gute Dosisverteilung im kleinen Becken bei der Kombination von 2000 mgeh Radium und doppelseitiger exzentrischer Rotationsbestrahlung. Durch diese Kombination wird im Parametrium eine homogene Dosis von 5000—6000 R erzielt, da sich der steile Dosisabfall des Radiums im Bereich des uterusnahen Anteils gut durch die zur Körpermitte hin abfallende Dosis der Percutanbestrahlung ausgleichen läßt (Abb. 18).

Die Verhältnisse bei einer für die Behandlung des Collumcarcinoms notwendigen Radiumdosis von mindestens 4000 mgeh untersuchten SCHMERMUND und FRANKE (1956). Sie konnten zeigen, daß bei der Kombination einer Radiumeinlage von 4000 mgeh und einer doppelseitigen Pendelkonvergenzbestrahlung mit einer Dosis im Parametrium von 4000 R eine gute Dosisverteilung erreicht werden konnte, wenn der Uterus genau in

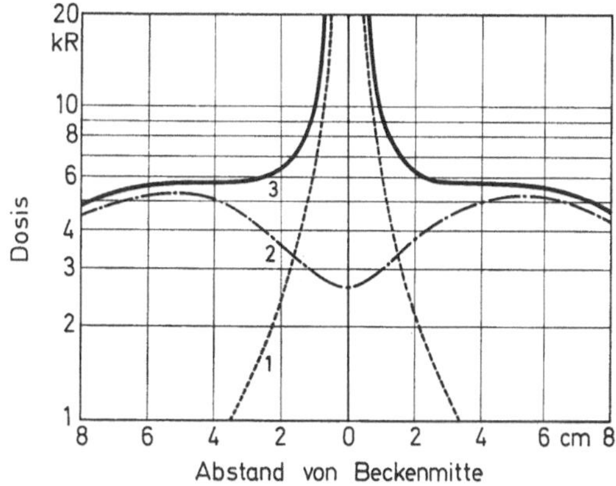

Abb. 18. Dosisverteilung im kleinen Becken in der Frontalebene bei Bestrahlung mit 2000 mgeh Radium (*1*) und mit doppelseitiger exzentrischer Rotationsbestrahlung (*2*). Die Kurve *3* ergibt die Dosissummenkurve. (Nach WACHSMANN und KELLER)

Beckenmitte lag (Abb. 19a). Ist der Uterus aber in der Parametranebene zur Beckenwand hin gekippt (Abb. 19b und c), kommt es innerhalb der einen Parametranhälfte zu einer wünschenswerten Dosiserhöhung; das Parametrium der Gegenseite wird jedoch mit einer Dosis bestrahlt, die unterhalb der notwendigen Herddosis liegt. Diese Untersuchungen ergeben die Notwendigkeit der exakten Lagekontrolle des Uterus als Radiumträger.

Eine weitere Möglichkeit, in das Parametrium und auf die Beckenwand eine ausreichend hohe Herddosis unter Vermeidung einer stärkeren Belastung der Hautoberfläche einzustrahlen, ergab sich durch die Entwicklung der Hohlanodenröhre (SCHÄFER und WITTE; CHAOUL; VAN DER PLAATS). Die Bestrahlung mit der Hohlanodenröhre wurde vor allem in Göttingen unter MARTIUS als fester Bestandteil in die gynäkologische Strahlentherapie eingebaut (KEPP, 1952). Auf diese Weise konnte durch die vaginal einzuführende Hohlanodenröhre bei allerdings stärkerer Belastung der Scheidenhaut, aber unter Schonung von Blase und Rectum eine erhebliche Strahlendosis in das Parametrium und die Beckenwand appliziert werden. Für die Therapie beim Collumcarcinom wurden hierzu vor allem die Schrägtubusse entwickelt.

Durch routinemäßige Verwendung der Hohlanode zur Behandlung des Collumcarcinoms wurde es bei der Göttinger Bestrahlungsmethode möglich, durch Kombination mit Radium und einer Percutanzusatztherapie hohe Dosen an den Ursprungsort des Carcinoms und das Parametrium bis zur Beckenwand zu verabfolgen. Diese Kleinraumbestrahlung sollte eine Mitbestrahlung gesunder Organe vermeiden. So erfolgte bei der Göttinger Bestrahlungsmethode die Lokalbestrahlung der Cervix durch 2 Radiumeinlagen mit einer

Dosierung von 4000 mgeh, durch die in einem Abstand von 3 cm noch etwa 2000 R wirksam wurden. Durch die Hohlanodenröhre wurden in 12 Sitzungen 2400 R in einer Herdtiefe von 5 cm auf die Beckenwand appliziert. Die zusätzliche Percutanbestrahlung bestand in einer Stehfeldbestrahlung von 2 Unterbauch-, 2 Glutäalfeldern und 1 Vulva-Damm-Feld. Der Zentralstrahl der Percutanfelder war nach lateral hin ausgelenkt (Abb. 20).

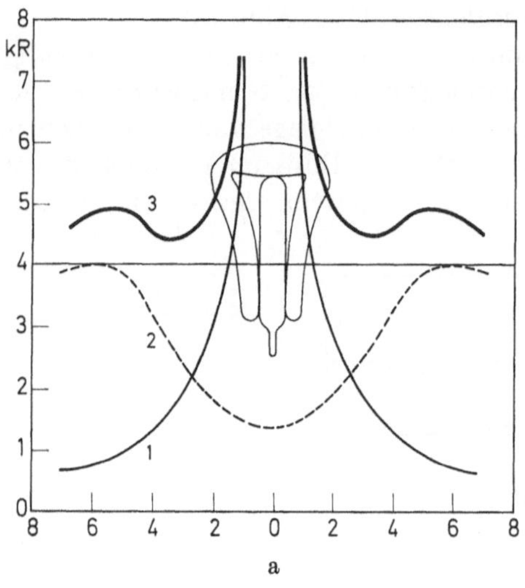

a

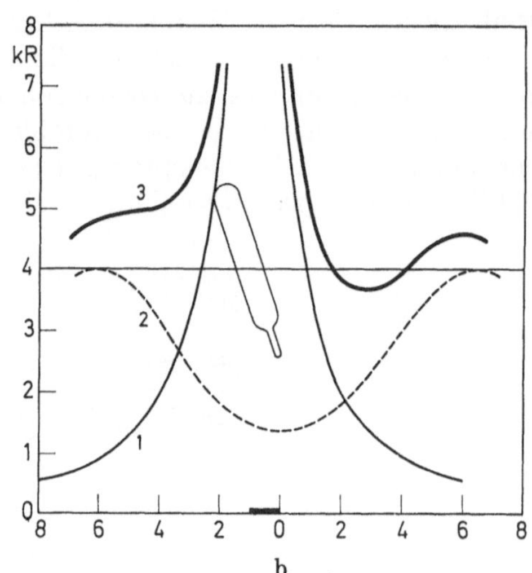

b

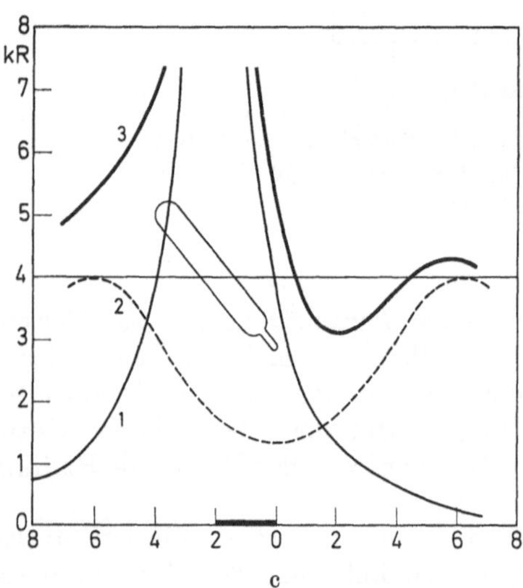

c

Abb. 19a—c. Dosisverteilung in den Parametrien bei Kombination von doppelseitiger Pendelkonvergenzbestrahlung (Drehpunkt 4 cm neben der Mittellinie) mit 4000 mgeh Radium intracervical. Kurve *1*: Radiumdosis; Kurve *2*: Röntgenstrahlendosis; Kurve *3*: Summenkurve. a Der Uterus liegt mit dem Radium in der Mittellinie. b Der Uterus ist in der Parametranebene 1 cm nach rechts gekippt. c Der Uterus ist in der Parametranebene 2 cm nach rechts gekippt. (Schmermund und Franke)

Die intravaginale Bestrahlung geht ursprünglich auf Caldwell zurück, der bereits 1902 Spezialtubusse für diesen Zweck entwickelt hat. Eine besondere Form der transvaginalen Bestrahlung der Portio entwickelte Del Regato (1954), der durch ein die Vagina entfaltendes Röhrchenspeculum eine transvaginale 200-kV-Bestrahlung durchführen konnte.

Die Erfahrungen bei der Benutzung des Körperhöhlenrohres führten zu der Erkenntnis, daß hierbei eine Mitbestrahlung von Teilen des Sigmas mit erheblichen Dosen unvermeidlich ist und zu Strahlenschädigungen des Darmes führen kann (Schmermund, 1955). Weiterhin wurde das Körperhöhlenrohr für die Entstehung von besonders häufigen Ureterstrikturen verantwortlich gemacht (Philipp und Rumphorst, 1958; Hofmann, 1964), da der vom unteren Ureterabschnitt durchzogene Teil des Parametriums durch die Bestrahlung mit dem Körperhöhlenrohr eine hohe Dosis erhält.

Bei der Verwendung des Körperhöhlenrohres muß darauf geachtet werden, daß zur
Erzielung genügend hoher Dosen an den beckenwandnahen Abschnitten eine erhebliche
Belastung der Eintrittspforten an der seitlichen Vaginalwand in Kauf genommen werden
mußte. Auf eine zusätzliche intravaginale Einlage mußte meist verzichtet werden; die
Radiumbestrahlung beschränkte sich auf die intrauterine Applikation. Die oft entstehenden Strahlenulcera der Vaginalhaut pflegten zwar auffallend rasch und komplikationslos
abzuheilen, doch war bei Fehleinstellungen die Gefahr von unterdosierten Zonen gegeben.

Betrachtet man rückschauend die historische Entwicklung der percutanen Strahlentherapie, so sollte man meinen, daß erst in jüngster Vergangenheit der Versuch unternommen werden konnte, eine Therapie des Collumcarcinoms ausschließlich durch eine
percutane Strahlenbehandlung unter Verzicht auf eine lokale Radiumapplikation durchzuführen. Aber bereits vor 1919 entwickelten SEITZ und WINTZ das Prinzip der alleinigen

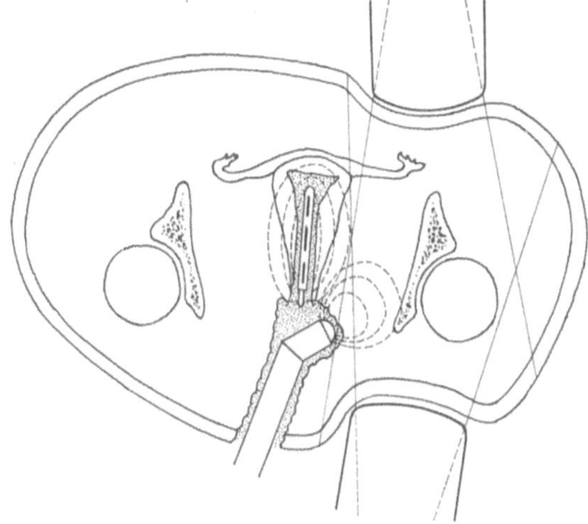

Abb. 20. Göttinger Bestrahlungsmethode des Collumcarcinoms. Kombination von intrauteriner Radiumeinlage,
Hohlanodenröhre und Percutanbestrahlung

Röntgenbestrahlung des Collumcarcinoms, die der *Erlanger* Bestrahlungsmethode zugrunde lag. In den Jahren 1920—1926 behandelte WINTZ das Collumcarcinom prinzipiell
nur mit Röntgenstrahlen. Als carcinolytische Dosis forderte er für das Plattenepithelcarcinom der Cervix eine Dosis von 100% der HED (Haut-Erythem-Dosis) bei einzeitiger
Einstrahlung. Er erreichte diese Dosis durch geeignete Felderwahl und insbesondere durch
Überschneidung der von den verschiedenen Feldern kommenden Strahlenkegel im Bereich
der Portio. Die Technik der „Konzentrationsbestrahlung" war so entwickelt, daß von 6
Feldern aus bei einer Feldbelastung von 80—100% der HED bei normalen Dickenverhältnis-
sen im Überschneidungsbereich eine Dosis von 110% der HED erreicht werden konnte. An
einem Tage wurden 2 ventrale Felder, die mit ihrem Zentralstrahl von oben und seitlich
auf die Cervix gerichtet waren, 2 dorsale Felder, ebenfalls etwas nach innen und unten gekippt, sowie 1 Coccygealfeld angesetzt. In die 4 ersten Felder wurden 90%, ins Coccygealfeld
80% der HED eingestrahlt. Am nächsten Tage wurden von einem Vulva-Damm-Feld aus
noch ein Zusatz von 100% der HED gegeben. Mit dieser 2tägigen Strahlenbehandlung war
die Konzentrationsbestrahlung abgeschlossen. Die Dosis an der Beckenwand und dem
beckenwandnahen Anteil des Parametriums wurde durch eine parametrane Zusatzbehandlung 8 Wochen nach Abschluß der Konzentrationsbestrahlung verabfolgt. Auch diese
Bestrahlung war zeitlich in 2 Tagen beendet.

Ähnliche Versuche der alleinigen Röntgenbestahlung des Collumcarcinoms wurden
auch schon vor WINTZ von Amerikanern durchgeführt: CALDWELL, PENNINGTON, ALLEN,
PUSEY, DUNCAN, STUVER und TONSEY. Im Jahre 1902 versuchte CALDWELL erstmals, die

Cervix uteri von der Vagina aus zu bestrahlen. Howson et al. berichten 1953 über Behandlungsergebnisse von 255 Patientinnen durch die Kombination einer transvaginalen und percutanen Strahlenbehandlung. Durch diese Behandlungsmethode konnte in allen Stadien eine bedeutende Verlängerung der durchschnittlichen Überlebenszeit, beim Stadium III eine absolute Heilung von 20,7% und im Stadium IV von 6,5% erreicht werden. Noch 1953 wird von diesen Autoren die transvaginale Röntgenbestrahlung als zusätzliche Behandlung für jede Bestrahlungsmethode des Collumcarcinoms empfohlen.

In diesem Zusammenhang müssen die Versuche von Coutard genannt werden, der durch starke Fraktionierung und gleichzeitige Protrahierung die Empfindlichkeitsdifferenz zwischen Haut- und Carcinomgewebe zu erhöhen versuchte. Die Protrahierung erreicht Coutard durch eine Steigerung der Filterung konventioneller Röntgenstrahlen auf 2 mm Cu und durch eine Vergrößerung des Focus-Haut-Abstandes auf 60—100 cm. Bei einer Dosisleistung von nur 3—5 R/min waren Bestrahlungszeiten von jeweils 2 Std oder mehr die Folge.

In den dreißiger Jahren gelang es Kirchhoff mit der von ihm modifizierten Coutard-Bestrahlung unter Verzicht auf die starke Protrahierung und unter Belastung der Haut bis zur Toleranzgrenze deutliche Therapieerfolge insbesondere bei fortgeschrittenen Collumcarcinomen zu erzielen.

Durch die rasche Entwicklung der Radiumtherapie verlor die ausschließliche Percutanbestrahlung immer mehr Anhänger. So lehnte selbst Wintz die Radiumbehandlung nicht prinzipiell ab, sondern baute sie sogar 1926 in Form einer Radiumzusatzdosis in seine *Erlanger* Bestrahlungsmethode ein. Er begründete die Einführung des Radiums in die Strahlenbehandlung damit, daß durch die dosismäßige Auslastung bei Anwendung von Radium eine größere Sicherheit zu erzielen sei.

Auch Baclesse, Reverdy und Jammet zeigten an Hand von 23 Heilungen aus einer Gesamtzahl von 100 Fällen, daß bei sehr strahlensensiblen Carcinomen die von den meisten Strahlentherapeuten bezweifelte Heilung mit ausschließlicher percutaner Röntgenbestrahlung möglich ist. Die geheilten Frauen überlebten mindestens 6, meist aber 10 bis 22 Jahre. Die Bestrahlungen wurden mit 180 kV, in einigen Fällen mit 250 kV und 500 kV Röhrenspannung von mehreren Feldern aus durchgeführt. Die Dosis beträgt bis zu 7 000 R an Cervix und Rectum, 6 000 R an der Blase und 4 500 R an der Beckenwand. Die Hautdosis ist erheblich und beträgt auf einzelnen Feldern bis zu 4 500 R. Die Bestrahlungen erfolgten in den letzten Jahren innerhalb von 9—12 Wochen. An Komplikationen wurden Hautveränderungen, Darmreaktionen, Schenkelhalsfrakturen und Blutbildveränderungen beobachtet. Baclesse glaubt, durch Steigerung der Röhrenspannung insbesondere auch bei Anwendung der Bewegungsbestrahlung weitere Fortschritte erzielen zu können.

β) Megavolttherapie
αα) Telecurietherapie

Die erste Telecurietherapie wurde bereits im Jahre 1923 von Lysholm am Radiumhemmet, Schweden, in Form einer Radiumfernbestrahlung vorgenommen. Siewert (1930) und Benner (1947) führten am Radiumhemmet eine Teleradiumtherapie als Halbtiefentherapie durch. Für die Bestrahlung des Collumcarcinoms besaß die Radiumfernbestrahlung wegen des zu geringen Focus-Haut-Abstandes von 5 bis maximal 15 cm eine zu geringe relative Tiefendosis, so daß sie in der Therapie des Collumcarcinoms keine Verwendung fand.

Demgegenüber erlangte die Telecurietherapie eine sehr rasche Verbreitung, als zu Beginn des vorigen Jahrzehnts das radioaktive Isotop Kobalt-60 mit seiner harten γ-Strahlung in ausreichenden Mengen für eine Telecurietherapie zur Verfügung stand. Die Anwendung der Kobalt-60-Teletherapie brachte für die Strahlentherapie des Genitalcarcinoms so entscheidende Vorteile mit sich, daß die konventionelle Röntgentherapie binnen weniger Jahre zumindest in größeren Therapiezentren durch die Telekobalttherapie ersetzt wurde.

Die höhere relative Tiefendosis der Kobalt-60-γ-Strahlung gestattet die Beschränkung auf eine geringere Zahl von Einfallsfeldern zur Erzielung derselben Herddosis. Dadurch wird das Auftreten von „hot spots" an den Überschneidungsstellen der Strahlenkegel vermindert. Weiterhin wirkt sich bei der Telekobalttherapie die Hautschonung vorteilhaft aus, die durch den Aufbaueffekt zustande kommt. Bei der Kobalt-60-γ-Strahlung liegt das Dosismaximum je nach Feldgröße und Focus-Haut-Abstand in etwa 4—5 mm Tiefe. Die die Patientinnen belastende Strahlenreaktion tritt viel seltener und erst nach höheren Strahlendosen auf. Höhere relative Tiefendosis und Aufbaueffekt verbessern bei der Bestrahlung des Collumcarcinoms die Dosisverteilung beträchtlich. Eine Gegenüberstellung der Dosisverhältnisse im Becken bei konventionellen Röntgenstrahlen (HWS 1,0 mm Cu)

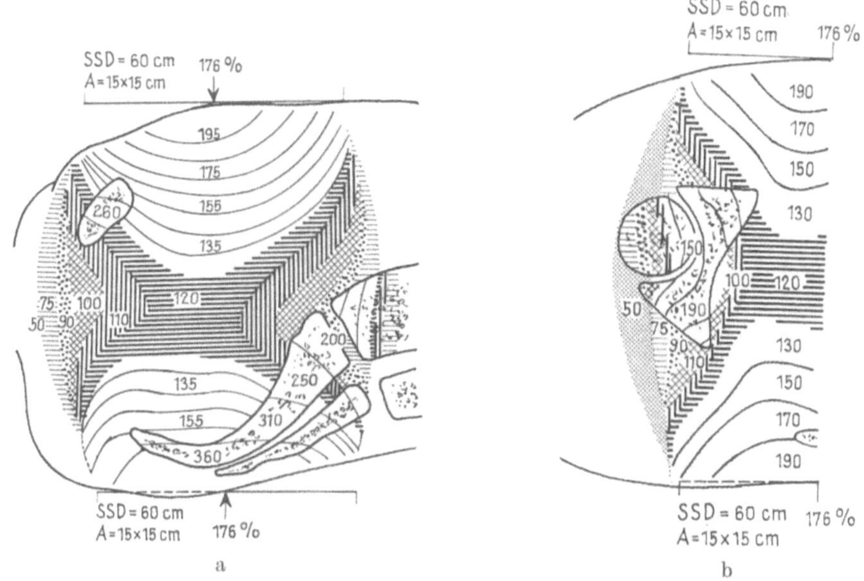

Abb. 21 a u. b. Dosisverteilung bei einem medialen und horizontalen Schnitt 5 cm oberhalb der Symphyse bei Verwendung zweier Gegenfelder (15×15 cm) bei Orthovoltstrahlen (HWS: 1,0 mm Cu) Dosismaximum an der Beckenwand = 100%. (RANUDD)

und Telekobalt-γ-Strahlung (Abb. 21 und 22) zeigt, daß im subcutanen Gewebe ein Dosismaximum von 190% und an der Hautoberfläche von 176% entsteht, wenn die Dosis an der Beckenwand als 100% genommen wird, während unter gleichen Bedingungen bei der Telekobaltbestrahlung die Dosis in der Subcutis 120% und an der Hautoberfläche nur 88% beträgt.

Der bei der Kobalt-60-γ-Strahlung für alle Gewebearten etwa um 1 liegende Massenabsorptionskoeffizient bewirkt, daß die gerade im Beckenbereich bei Bestrahlung mit Orthovoltstrahlen durch Knochen entstehende Dosisverzerrung und Dosisverminderung weniger störend ins Gewicht fallen. Hierdurch wird die Herddosisbestimmung erleichtert und das hinter dem Knochen liegende Gewebe mit einer höheren Dosis belastet.

Ein weiterer Vorteil ist die stärkere Bündelung der Strahlung mit einem am Feldrand steilen Dosisabfall. Hierdurch kommt es zu einer verminderten Raumdosis und damit zu geringerer Strahlenbelastung des Gesamtorganismus. Die Allgemeinreaktionen können auf diese Weise vermindert werden.

Bestrahlungsplanung und Einstelltechnik erfordern allerdings größere Genauigkeit und einen erheblichen Aufwand, da aus Fehleinstellungen schwere Komplikationen resultieren können.

Umfangreiche Dosismengen haben gezeigt, daß die von der Orthovolttherapie her bekannten Methoden der Percutanbestrahlung bei Kombination mit Radium nur bedingt in der Telekobalttherapie Anwendung finden können. So betont Weishaar, daß bei der üblichen Bestrahlung des parametranen Lymphabflußgebietes in Kombination mit Radium durch 2 ventrale und 2 dorsale Stehfelder unter Ausspaarung der Mittellinie Feldbreiten von je 6 cm ausreichen, um im Herdbereich eine optimale Dosisverteilung zu erhalten. Die in der konventionellen Strahlentherapie verwandten 8 und 10 cm breiten Felder erscheinen in der Telekobalttherapie ungeeignet.

Schon bald zeigte sich, daß sich mit der Telekobalt-γ-Strahlung infolge ihrer besonderen physikalischen Eigenschaften durch verschiedene Feldformen und Feldanordnungen Isodosenverläufe modellieren ließen, die dem Lymphausbreitungsgebiet im kleinen Becken

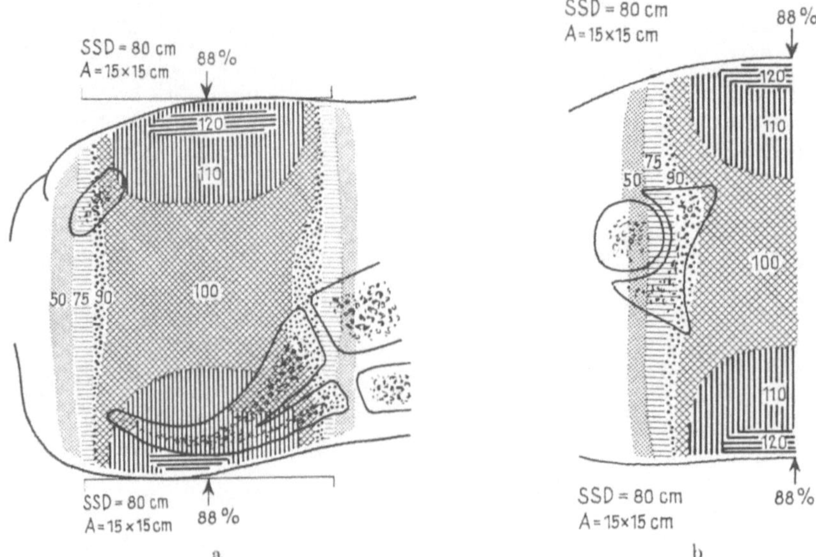

Abb. 22a u. b. Dosisverteilung bei 2 Gegenfeldern bei Verwendung von Kobalt-60 (Feldgröße 15×15 cm) in einem medialen (a) und in einem horizontalen (b) Schnitt 5 cm oberhalb der Symphyse. Dosis an der Beckenwand = 100% (Ranudd)

wesentlich günstiger angepaßt werden konnten. Für die Entwicklung immer neuer und vielfältiger Bestrahlungsmethoden in der Telekobalttherapie waren verschiedene Gründe ausschlaggebend. Bei der üblichen Dosierung von etwa 4000—5000 R im Bereich des Parametriums über Stehfelder konnten zwar Strahlenfrühreaktionen an der Cutis vermieden werden; im Verlauf von 6 Monaten entwickelten sich aber bei den Patientinnen Indurationen im Subcutangewebe, die teilweise schwerste Formen annahmen und das Allgemeinbefinden erheblich beeinträchtigten. Die ersten Mitteilungen hierüber findet man bei Leucutia (1959), Hinz und Renner (1960), Birkner und Hoffmann (1961), Liegner und Michaud (1961). Die anfangs gehegten Hoffnungen, daß die Haut und ihre Anhangsgebilde durch die Verlagerung des Dosismaximums auch nach höheren Dosen völlig verschont würden, erwiesen sich somit nicht als berechtigt. Schon 1958 hat Becker, Gudden und Kuttig vor einer möglichen Induration gewarnt und deshalb die Siebbestrahlung in der Telekobalttherapie empfohlen.

Ausgehend von der Vorstellung, durch höhere Herddosen eine bessere und sichere Rückbildung der Tumorinfiltrationen im Parametrium und an der Beckenwand zu erreichen, wurde von zahlreichen Autoren die Applikation von Herddosen über 4000 bis zu 6000 R und mehr versucht. Hierdurch nahm die Zahl von schweren Strahlenreaktionen in der Tiefe, an Blase, Rectum und Uretern gewaltig zu. Wenn auch Blase und Rectum eine Dosis von 6000 R tolerieren sollten, so ist als Ursache für stärkere Strahlenkomplikationen die Entstehung von Dosisüberschneidungen bei der Kombination mit der intrakavitären Radiumapplikation anzusehen. Der wesentlich steilere Dosisabfall der Telekobalt-γ-Strahlung am Feldrand kann sich bei der Kombination mit Radium eher ungünstig auswirken. Während in der Orthovolttherapie im Herd die Dosis bereits von der Feldmitte gleichmäßig zum Feldrand hin abfällt, entsteht bei der Telekobalttherapie unter gleichen Bedingungen in der Tiefe ein Plateau und erst am Feldrand setzt ein steiler Dosisabfall ein. Daher muß bei Verwendung von Megavoltenergien der Lage des Uterus als Radiumträger eine wesentlich größere Beachtung beigemessen werden. Während beispielsweise bei Medianlage des Uterus unter Aussparung der Mittellinie von einem etwa 4 cm breiten Steg eine gute und homogene Dosisverteilung mit gleichmäßigem Dosisabfall

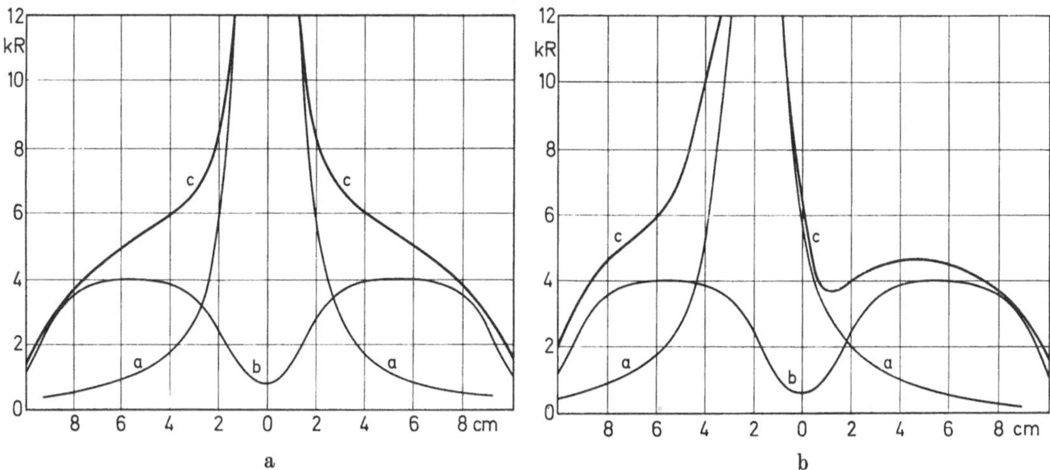

Abb. 23. a Dosisverteilung im kleinen Becken (Frontalebene in Höhe des inneren Muttermundes) bei kombinierter Radium- und Telekobalttherapie. Lage des Uterus in der Mittellinie. Ordinate: Dosisangabe in kR. Abszisse: Abstand von der Beckenmitte in cm. *a* Radiumdosiskurve bei 5000 mgeh in kombiniertem Träger. *b* Telekobalt-Dosiskurve bei Bestrahlung über 2 ventrale und dorsale Felder unter Aussparung der Mittellinie. Dosis im Parametrium 4000 R. *c* Summendosiskurve. b Dosisverteilung im kleinen Becken bei kombinierter Radium- und Telekobalttherapie entsprechend Abb. 23a. Verlagerung des Uterus nach lateral um 2 cm

im Parametrium erreicht wird (Abb. 23a), macht sich bei einer Verlagerung des Uterus um 2 cm zur Beckenwand hin bei gleicher Anordnung der percutanen Stehfelder die Verlagerung wesentlich stärker bemerkbar (Abb. 23b). Auf der einen Seite kommt es durch Summation zu einer Dosis von 7000 R 5 cm lateral der Mittellinie, wobei der Ureter eine noch wesentlich höhere Dosis enthält; auf der Gegenseite kommt es im Parametrium zu einer Unterdosierung, das Parametrium wird teilweise mit weniger als 4000 R belastet. Die Dosisverteilung in der Parametranebene unter gleichen Bestrahlungsbedingungen bei Medianlage des Uterus, Parallelverlagerung zur Beckenwand hin und bei Verkantung des Uterus zeigen die Abb. 24—26.

Während die Dosisverteilung bei der Telekobalttherapie wesentlich übersichtlicher als bei der konventionellen Röntgentherapie und die Dosis bei präziser Feldeinstellung an jedem Punkte des Beckens genau zu ermitteln ist, kann die Dosisverteilung bei der lokalen Radiumapplikation nicht exakt bestimmt werden. Zwar haben die zahlreichen dosimetrischen Untersuchungen bei den verschiedenen Applikatorformen und -kombinationen, die Dosisangabe in R und die Momentanmessungen in Blase und Rectum zur Kenntnis der Radiumdosimetrie erheblich beigetragen, für den Einzelfall sind diese Angaben aber speziell hinsichtlich der zusätzlichen Percutanbestrahlung nicht von ausreichendem Wert. Der Strahlentherapeut benötigt daher bei der Kombination mit der Telekobalttherapie

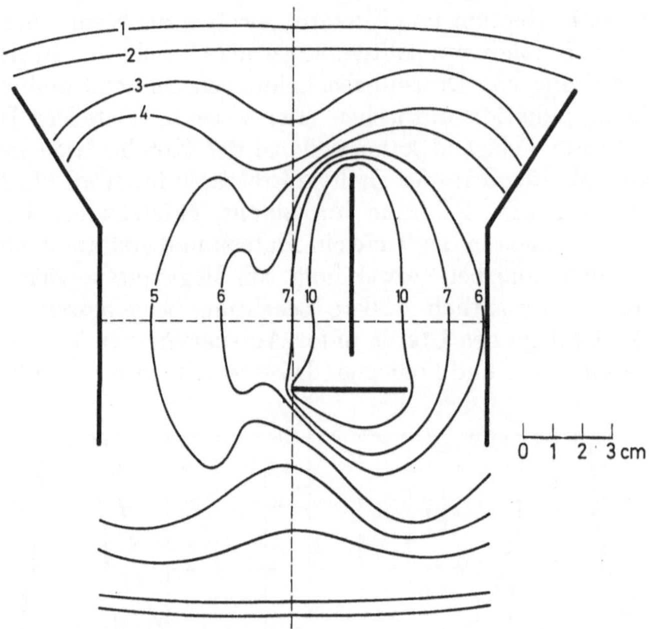

Abb. 24. Dosisverteilung im kleinen Becken in der Parametranebene. Radium 5000 mgeh, 120 mg im Längs-filter, 90 mg als Platte. Seitwärtsverlagerung des Trägers um 2 cm. Telekobalttherapie: 4000 R pro Para-metrium über 2 ventrale, 2 dorsale Stehfelder, Feldgröße 8 × 15 cm, Zentralstrahl um 10° nach lateral gekippt, Herdtiefe 8 cm. Hautfelder medial aneinandergrenzend. Dosisangabe in kR

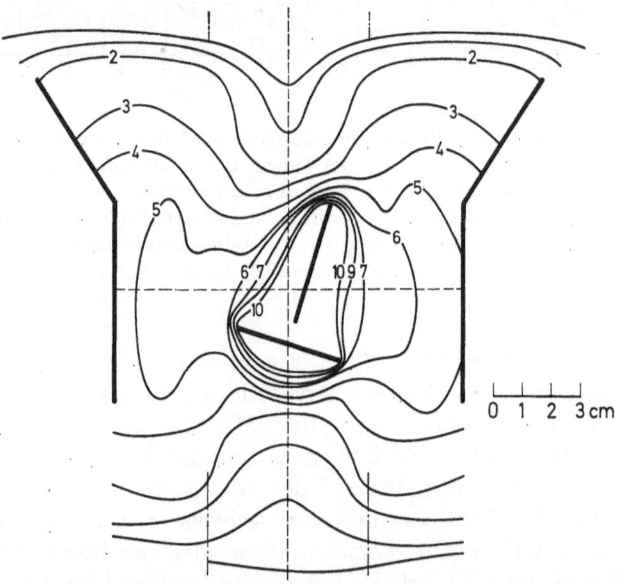

Abb. 25. Dosisverteilung im kleinen Becken in der Parametranebene. Radium: 5000 mgeh, 90 mg im Längs-filter, 130 mg als Platte. Kippung des Trägers mit Verlagerung von Spitze gegenüber Basis um $1^1/_2$ cm. Herd-tiefe 10 cm. Telekobalttherapie: 4000 R pro Parametrium über 2 ventrale, 2 dorsale Stehfelder; Feldgröße 6 × 15 cm, Zentralstrahl um $3^1/_2$° nach lateral gekippt (senkrechter Strahleneinfall am medialen Feldrand). Feldabstand auf der Oberfläche 6 cm. Dosisangabe in kR

genaue Angaben der Lage des Uterus mit der Präparateanordnung. Diese Bestimmung kann ohne größeren Aufwand durch Röntgenaufnahmen vorgenommen werden. Erst nach genauer Lagebestimmung des Radiumträgers darf die Einstellung der Percutanfelder erfolgen, um stärkere, unerwünschte Überschneidungen zu vermeiden.

Sicherer lassen sich Feldüberschneidungen bei Lageabweichungen des Uterus vermeiden, wenn man den bei konventionellen Röntgenstrahlen langsamen Dosisabfall zum Feldrand mit der Kobalt-60-Strahlung nachahmt. Hierzu eignen sich Keilfilter (FRISCHBIER und KUTTIG, 1964), die so in den Strahlengang gebracht werden, daß sie die Strahlung an der medialen Feldbegrenzung stärker schwächen, während der vorteilhaft steile Dosisabfall an der lateralen Feldseite erhalten bleibt (Abb. 27a und b). Die Summation der Radium- und percutan applizierten Dosis bewirkt bei der Anwendung eines harmonischen Keilfilters einen steilen Abfall neben dem Uterus, das ganze Parametrium wird bis zur Beckenwand homogen durchstrahlt (Abb. 27c).

Die Anwendung von Ausgleichsfiltern für die zusätzliche percutane Bestrahlung der Parametrien zur lokalen Radiumbestrahlung in der Megavolttherapie wurde erstmals

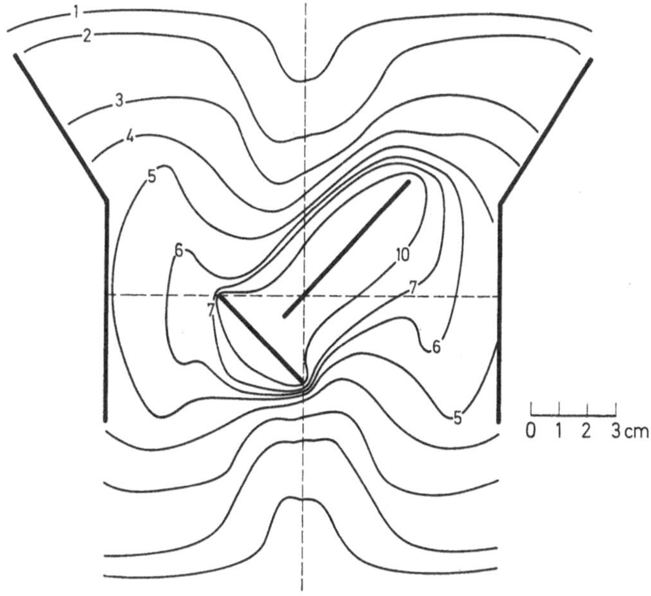

Abb. 26. Dosisverteilung im kleinen Becken in der Parametranebene. Radium 5000 mgeh, 120 mg im Längsfilter, 90 mg als Platte. Kippung des Trägers um 45°, Telekobalttherapie: 4000 R pro Parametrium über 2 ventrale, 2 dorsale Stehfelder; Feldgröße: 6×15 cm, Zentralstrahl um $3^1/_2$° nach lateral gekippt (senkrechter Strahleneinfall am medialen Feldrand). Feldabstand auf der Oberfläche 6 cm. Dosisangabe in kR

von TRANTER (1959) für 4-MeV-Röntgenstrahlen beschrieben und von TAYLOR (1963) für die Telekobalttherapie übernommen. Es wurden bei der split-field-Technik ein zur Aussparung der Beckenmitte dienender Bleiabsorber seitlich so abgeschrägt, daß ein Angleich an die Radiumdosis zustande kommt.

Eine andere Möglichkeit, ungewollte Dosisüberschneidungen zu vermeiden, ist durch eine Reduktion der Radiumdosis gegeben. Durch die mit Megavoltenergien höher einzustrahlende Herddosis ist sie zu rechtfertigen. Die Radiumbehandlung sollte also ihrer Natur gemäß auf die Funktion einer Kontakttherapie beschränkt werden. Dieser Gedanke liegt der *Marburger* Methode zugrunde, die bei einer reduzierten Radiumdosis über 3 Einfallsfelder das ganze Becken homogen durchstrahlen läßt (Abb. 28).

Wenn die Dosisverteilung bei der Telekobalttherapie durch 2 gegenüberliegende Stehfelder im Beckenbereich auch wesentlich günstiger gestaltet ist als unter gleichen Bedingungen der Orthovoltstrahlen, so kann die Dosisverteilung doch keinesfalls als optimal angesehen werden. Bei der Stehfeldtechnik liegt der zu bestrahlende Herd keinesfalls in einem umschriebenen Dosismaximum (Abb. 29). Bei adipösen Patientinnen verschlechtert sich das Dosisverhältnis um 20—40%. Auch durch Kompression ist der anteriorposteriore Durchmesser der Patientinnen nicht so stark zu verringern, daß das subcutane

14*

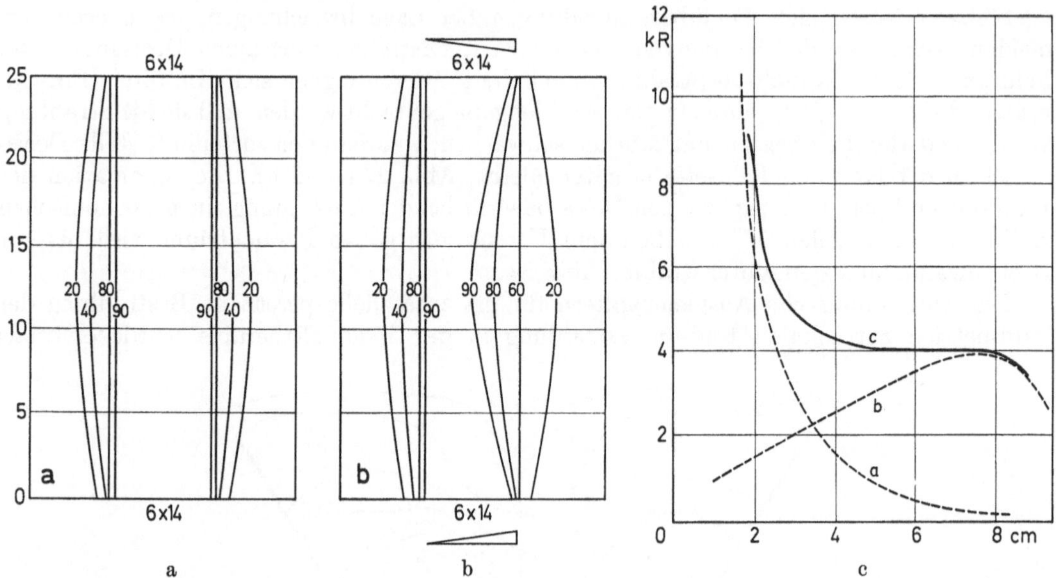

Abb. 27. a Dosisverteilung im Beckenphantom, 25 cm Durchmesser, bei Telekobalttherapie von einem ventralen und dorsalen homogenen Feld, Feldgröße 6 × 14 cm, QHA 50 cm. Dosismaximum in Beckenmitte 100 %. b Dosisverteilung im Beckenphantom bei Telekobalttherapie von einem ventralen und dorsalen Feld mit harmonischem Keilfilter, Feldgröße 6 × 14 cm, QHA 50 cm. c Summendosiskurve bei kombinierter Radium- (5000 mgeh) Telekobalttherapie (ventrales und dorsales Stehfeld mit harmonischem Keilfilter, Feldgröße 6 × 14 cm, Dosis an der Parametranebene 4000 R). a Radiumdosiskurve, b Kobalt-60-Dosiskurve, c Summendosiskurve

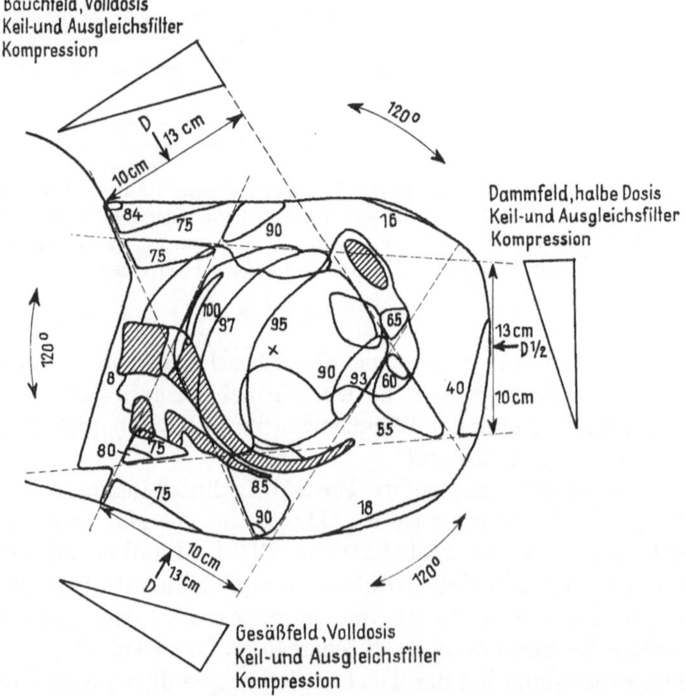

Abb. 28. Telekobaltbestrahlung der Uteruskrebse nach der Marburger Methode (Du Mesnil de Rochemont)

Gewebe die gleiche Dosis wie der parametrane Herd erhält. Die Entwicklung führte daher zu den verschiedenen Methoden der Bewegungsbestrahlung. So entwickelten Brizel, Lanzl und Duthorn (1963) eine allerdings technisch aufwendige Methode der Bewegungs-

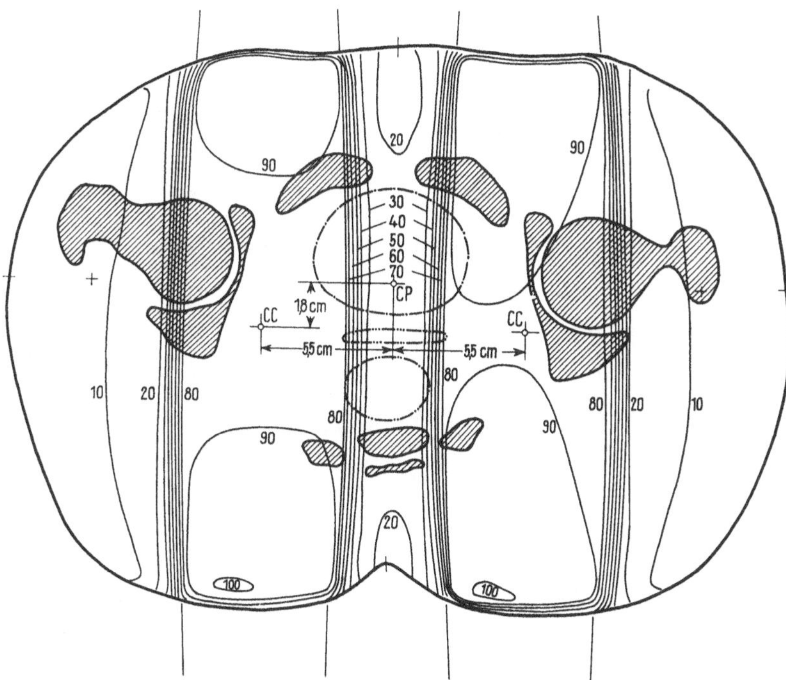

Abb. 29. Dosisverteilung bei der Telekobalttherapie des Parametriums über je zwei gegenüberliegende Stehfelder. Feldgröße 7 × 15 cm (Brizel, Lanzl und Duthorn)

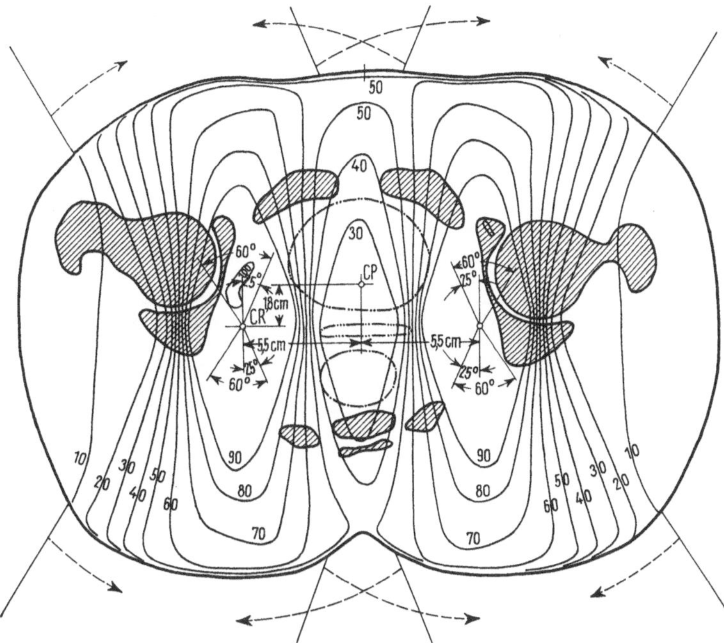

Abb. 30. Dosisverteilung bei der Telekobalt-Pendelbestrahlung des Parametriums über 4 Pendelfelder. Der Sektor beträgt jeweils 60°, die Feldgröße 5 × 15 cm (Brizel et al.)

bestrahlung, bei der über 4 verschiedene Bogen gependelt wird. Das Parametrium und die Beckenwand erhalten ein umschriebenes Dosismaximum mit einem relativ steilen Dosisabfall zur Beckenmitte und vor allem zur Körperoberfläche hin (Abb. 30 und 31).

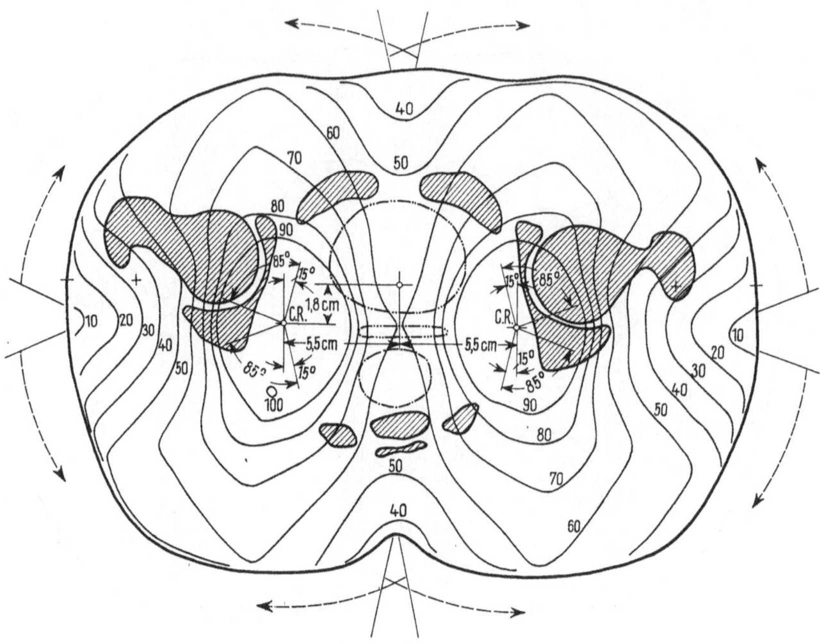

Abb. 31. Telekobalt-Pendelbestrahlung über 4 Felder zur Bestrahlung des Parametriums. Der Pendelsektor
beträgt 85°, Feldgröße 7 × 15 cm (Brizel et al.)

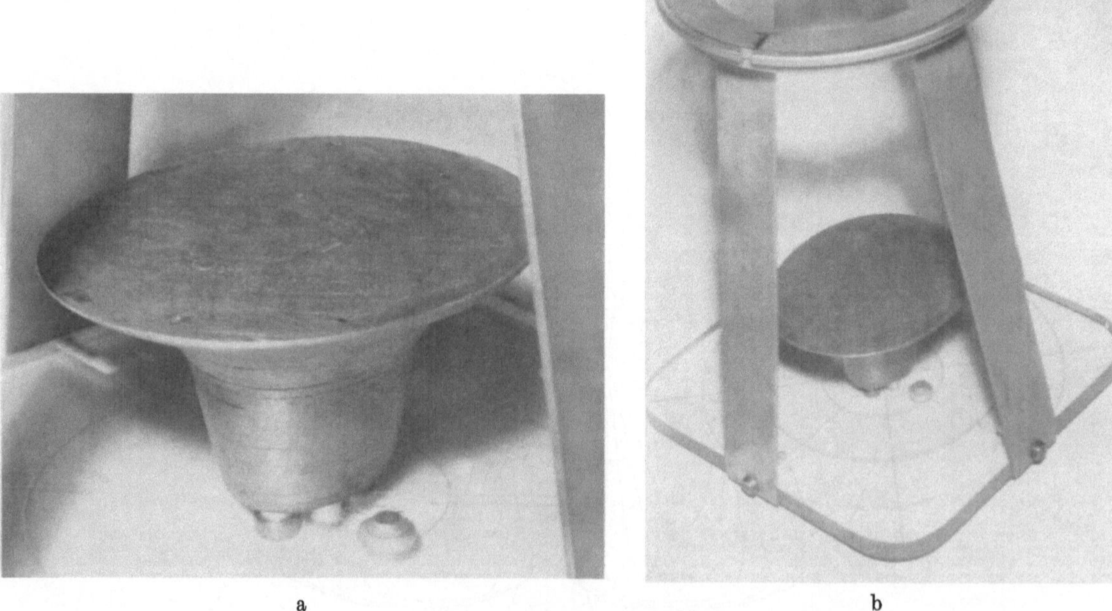

a   b

Abb. 32a u. b. 5 cm dicker glockenförmiger Bleiabsorber zur Entlastung der Beckenmitte bei kombinierter
Radium-Telekobalttherapie

Eine weitere Möglichkeit der Aussparung der Beckenmitte bei der Kombination der
Telekobalttherapie mit der intrakavitären Radiumapplikation ergibt sich durch Verwendung eines Bleiabsorbers, durch den ein großes Bauch- und Rückenfeld in 2 parametrane
Felder geteilt werden kann. Zur ausreichenden Verringerung der Dosis in der Beckenmitte sind Bleistege von etwa 5 cm Dicke notwendig.

Einen runden Bleiabsorber, der sich optimal dem Dosisabfall der lokalen Radiumeinlage nicht nur in parametraner Richtung, sondern auch nach cranial und caudal hin anpaßt, konstruierten Würthner und Harde zum Telekobalt-Bestrahlungsgerät Gammatron 3. Der 5 cm dicke Bleiabsorber wird zur Vermeidung von wirksamen Sekundärelektronen quellennah in einem Kompressionsrahmen angebracht (Abb. 32 a und b). Die Abb. 33 zeigt den Dosisverlauf in 10 cm Tiefe bei 2 gegenüberliegenden (ventral und dorsal) Feldern. Bei einer Herddosis von 4000 R an der Beckenwand wird die vom Radium erfaßte Region mit weniger als 1000 R belastet. Die Summenisodose bei Kombination der lokalen Radiumdosis und der Dosis über 2 gegenüberliegende Telekobalt-Stehfelder zeigt Abb. 34. An

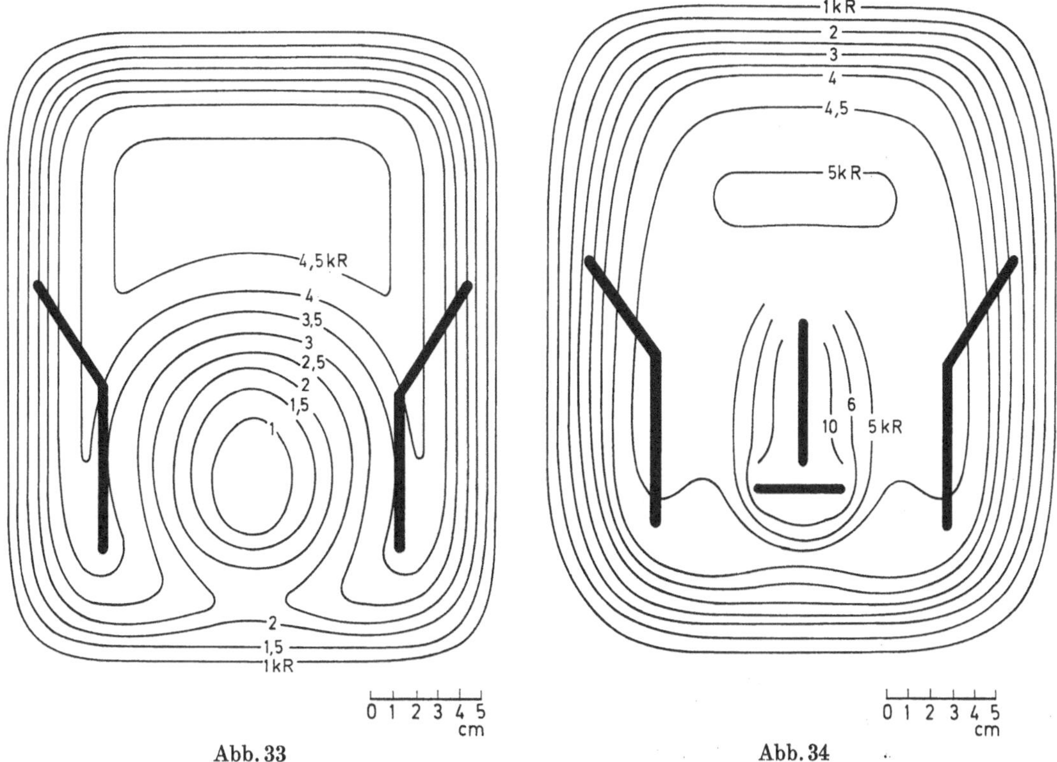

Abb. 33   Abb. 34

Abb. 33. Isodosen in 10 cm Tiefe bei einem 16×21 cm großen Feld unter Verwendung eines zentralen Bleiabsorbers. Herddosis

Abb. 34. Summenisodosen bei lokaler Radiumapplikation (Kombination von Stift und Platte, 90 mg/130 mg, 5000 mgeh) und zwei gegenüberliegenden Feldern (16×21 cm, Dosis in Punkt B 3000 R) bei Verwendung eines Bleiabsorbers

der Universitäts-Frauenklinik Hamburg wird diese Bestrahlungskombination durch eine weitere Telekobalt-Pendelbestrahlung von 1500 R/Herd ergänzt, so daß im ganzen Parametrium bis zur Beckenwand eine Gesamtdosis von 6000 R wirksam wird (Abb. 35 a und b). Der Vorteil dieser Bestrahlungsmethode liegt darin, daß die durch Lokalisationsaufnahmen bei liegendem Radiumträger festgestellte Lageabweichungen aus der Mittellinie relativ einfach und sicher berücksichtigt werden kann und die präsacralen und unteren aortalen Lymphknoten, die außerhalb der Reichweite der Radiumbestrahlung liegen und auch bei den üblichen 4 parametranen Stehfeldern nicht erfaßt werden, eine volle Herddosis erhalten. Die percutan eingestrahlte Herddosis durch die beiden großen Stehfelder mit Bleiabsorber, die aus Gründen der subcutanen Spätreaktionen 4000 R nicht überschreiten sollte, muß allerdings durch eine biaxiale Pendelbestrahlung aufgefüllt werden (Frischbier und Würthner, 1971).

Eine andere Feldanordnung unter Verwendung eines solchen Bleisteges und zusätzlicher Keilfilter wird von Kottmeier (1964) und Ranudd (1966) angegeben. Diese Autoren decken bei der Verwendung eines großen abdominalen Unterbauchfeldes den Uterus durch einen runden kegelförmigen Conus ab und ergänzen die Dosis im Beckenbereich durch 2 seitliche Stehfelder (Abb. 36a—c). Auf diese Weise läßt sich an der Beckenwand eine 100%-Isodose erhalten mit einem Dosisabfall zur Beckenmitte um 25%.

Die Abdeckung des Uterus in Beckenmitte wird ebenfalls durch eine von Dibbelt, Rahm und Renner (1960) angegebene Methode erreicht, bei der die Feldform dem nach cranial konvergierenden Verlauf des Lymphabflußgebietes angepaßt wird. Auf diese Weise

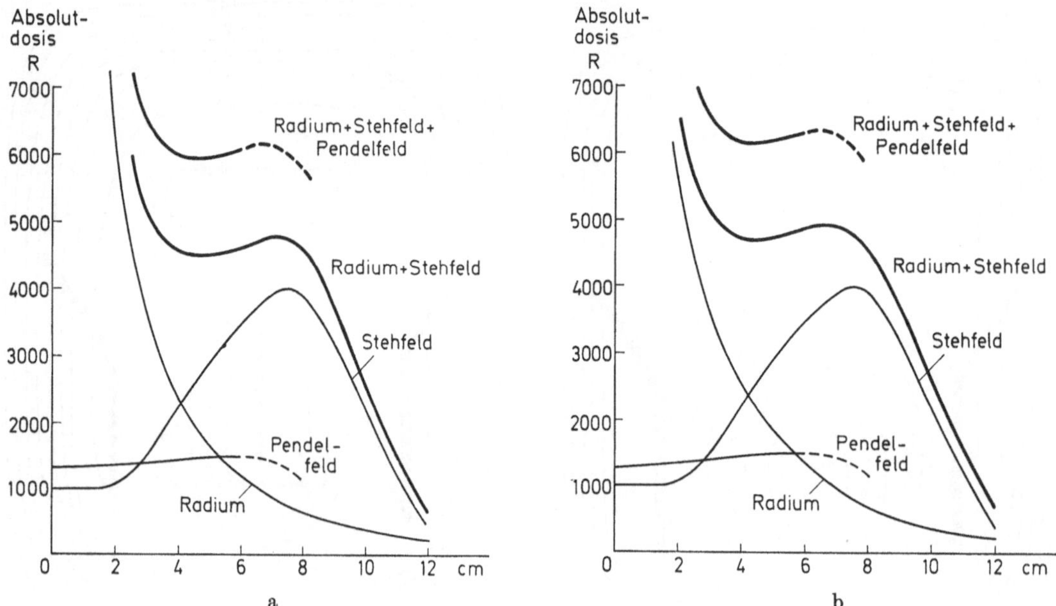

Abb. 35a u. b. Dosisverteilung im kleinen Becken in der Parametranebene bei kombinierter Radium-Telekobalttherapie. Feldgröße des ventralen und dorsalen Stehfeldes 16 × 21 cm. Herddosis in Punkt B 3000 R. Verwendung eines zentralen Bleiabsorbers. Zur Erhöhung der Herddosis Pendelzusatzfeld durch biaxiale Telekobaltpendelbestrahlung (Feldgröße 6 × 18 cm, Achsabstand 10 cm, Herddosis 1500 R). a Dosiskurven bei 5000 mgeh Radium. Filterkombination 90 mg Stift und 130 mg Platte. b Dosiskurven bei 5000 mgeh Radium. Filterkombination 120 mg Stift und 90 mg Platte

lassen sich auch die unteren aortalen Lymphknoten in das Bestrahlungsfeld einschließen. Die Feldform wird durch ein besonderes Blendensystem erreicht, das im Abstand von etwa 45 cm von der Oberfläche bei einem Quellen-Haut-Abstand von 80 cm angebracht wird. Durch eine zusätzliche Wolframblende entsteht die Feldform eines umgekehrten U. Der abgedeckte Uterus erhält noch eine Dosis prozentual zur Beckenwand von 60%. Durch diese oberflächenferne Ausblendung macht sich jedoch der Halbschatten sehr störend bemerkbar. Auch Blase, Rectum und Schenkelhals werden stärker belastet als bei den anderen Methoden.

Auch bei der von Surmont (1958) sowie Buraggi, Romanini und Roncoroni (1959) angegebenen Bestrahlungsmethode paßt sich die Form des Bestrahlungsfeldes dem cranial konvergierenden Verlauf des Lymphabflußgebietes an. Sie geben eine Methode an, mit der durch eine Telekobalt-Pendelbestrahlung über 2 cranial konvergierende Achsen im Winkel von jeweils 200° im caudalen Feldanteil 2 getrennte Dosismaxima an der Beckenwand entstehen, während in Beckenmitte im Bereich des Uterus eine niedriger dosierte Zone gebildet wird. Nach cranial kommt es durch die Konvergenz der Pendelachsen zu einem einzigen Dosismaximum in Höhe des 5. LWK (Abb. 37 a—c).

Zur Verminderung der Integraldosis geben BOTSTEIN, SCHULZ und SIMON (1962) ein rautenförmiges Feld an, bei dem die Achse um 45° gedreht ist. Auf diese Weise kann die Feldgröße auf 12×12 cm reduziert werden. In der Diagonalen besitzt das Feld dann einen Durchmesser von 17 cm, wodurch das Lymphabflußgebiet beim Cervixcarcinom ausreichend erfaßt werden kann. Innerhalb des kleinen Beckens ändert sich die Dosisverteilung nicht. Auf diese Weise läßt sich die Integraldosis um 35 % reduzieren. Auch bei dieser Form kann die Beckenmitte bei einer intrauterinen Radiumapplikation durch einen Bleiblock von 3,5 cm Breite und 5 cm Dicke abgedeckt werden.

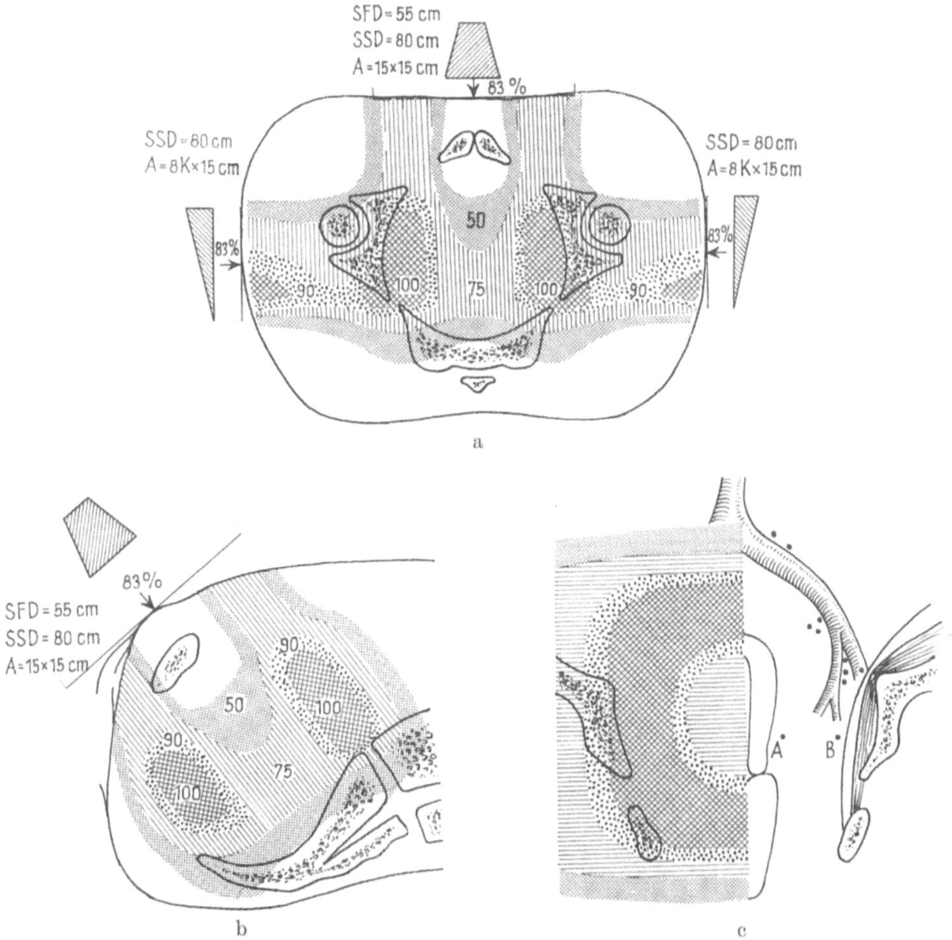

Abb. 36a—c. Telekobalttherapie des kleinen Beckens bei der Kombination mit Radium: Ventrales Stehfeld, 15×15 cm, bei der die Beckenmitte über dem Uterus abgedeckt wird durch einen Bleikonus. Zusätzlich zwei laterale Stehfelder unter Verwendung eines Keilfilters (RANUDD)

Da die Haut in der Telekobalttherapie die Dosis nicht mehr in dem Maße wie bei Orthovoltstrahlen limitiert, versuchen viele, die Organe des Beckens mit einer bis an die Toleranzgrenze gehenden Strahlendosis zu belasten. Wie bereits ausgeführt, kommt der Koordination von intrakavitärer Radiumtherapie und Percutanbestrahlung dann eine große Bedeutung zu, da es möglich ist, fast jede beliebige Isodosenform durch die verschiedenen Bestrahlungsmethoden zu modellieren. Dem Dosisabfall der percutanen Isodosen muß somit bei der Kombination mit Radium größte Beachtung geschenkt werden. Deshalb wurden die gebräuchlichsten Methoden der Telekobalttherapie bei Kombination mit Radium zusammengestellt (Abb. 38). Aus dieser Abbildung läßt sich die prozentuale Dosisbelastung an den interessierenden Punkten im kleinen Becken ablesen.

Während in der konventionellen Röntgentherapie die Verwendung der Kompressionsmöglichkeit große Bedeutung erlangt hatte, fand sie bei der Telekobalttherapie nur geringe Verwendung. Kapp-Schwoerer (1964) weist aber darauf hin, daß die Verwendung der Kompression auch in der Telekobalttherapie bedeutungsvoll ist, da sich bei den z.T. stärker gewölbten Bauchdecken und größeren Fettschürzen ungünstige Oberflächenverhältnisse ergeben. Durch einfache Kompressionsrahmen kann einmal die Herdtiefe ver

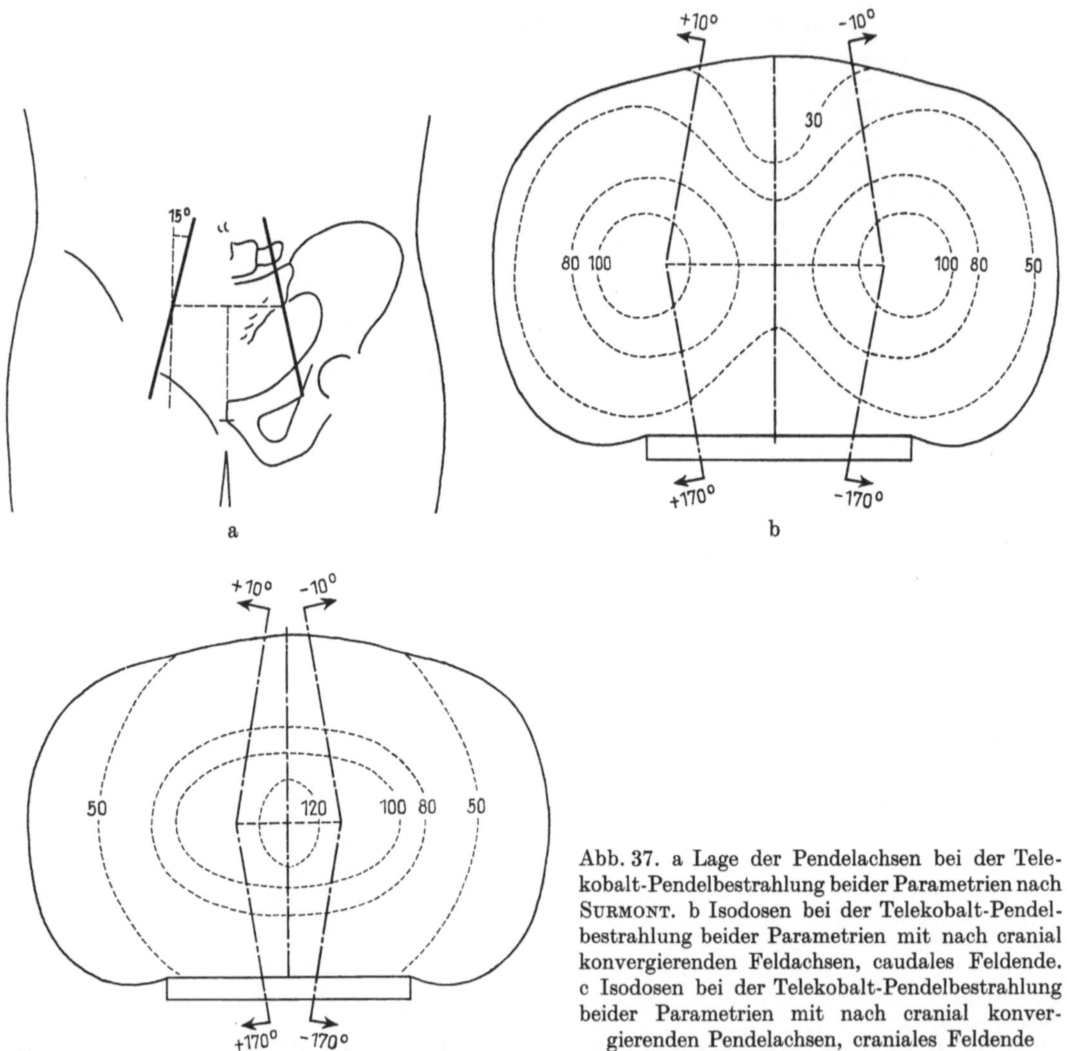

Abb. 37. a Lage der Pendelachsen bei der Telekobalt-Pendelbestrahlung beider Parametrien nach Surmont. b Isodosen bei der Telekobalt-Pendelbestrahlung beider Parametrien mit nach cranial konvergierenden Feldachsen, caudales Feldende. c Isodosen bei der Telekobalt-Pendelbestrahlung beider Parametrien mit nach cranial konvergierenden Pendelachsen, craniales Feldende

mindert werden, zum anderen wirkt sich der Aufbaueffekt nur bei senkrechtem Strahleneintritt aus, während bei stark gewölbter Oberfläche und insbesondere in einer Bauchfalte die Toleranzgrenze der Haut schnell überschritten wird.

Während in der Telekobalttherapie der weiblichen Genitalcarcinome die Keilfilter bisher nur geringe Verbreitung gefunden haben, wird in jüngsten Arbeiten deutlich herausgestellt, daß die Dosisverteilung auch bei der Bestrahlung des Collumcarcinoms durch eine weitere Individualisierung unter Benutzung von Ausgleichsfiltern verbessert werden kann (Frischbier und Kuttig, 1964; Rosenow und Frischkorn, 1965). Sie finden vor allem Verwendung bei der Angleichung der Telekobalt- an die Radiumdosis, zur Begradigung der Isodosen in einer bestimmten Gewebstiefe, zur Kompensation eines schrägen Strahleneinfalls, zur Kompensation unebener Hautfelder und zur Erzeugung von

		Cervix	Punkt A	Becken-wand	Blase	Rec-tum	Collum femoris
A	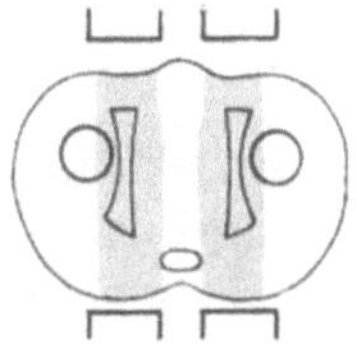 2 ventrale, 2 dorsale Stehfelder (6 × 14 cm)	35	85	100	30	30	20
B	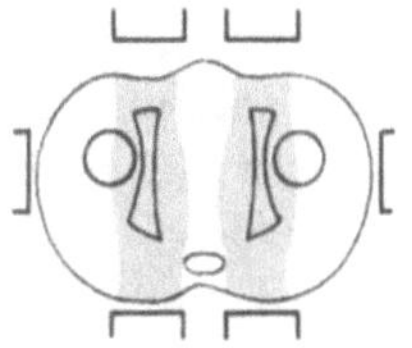 2 ventrale, 2 dorsale, 2 laterale Steh-felder (6 × 14 cm)	65	90	100	55	55	45
C	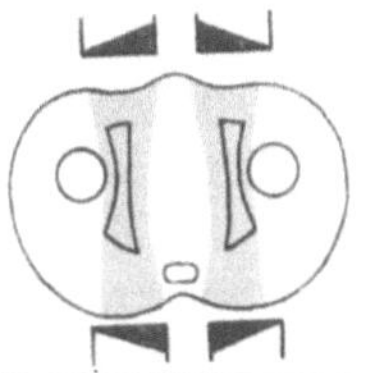 2 ventrale, 2 dorsale Stehlfelder mit Keil-filter (8 × 14 cm) (FRISCHBIER u. KUTTIG)	30	50	100	30	30	20
D	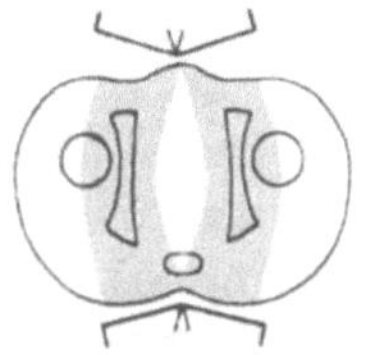 2 ventrale, 2 dorsale Stehfelder, 10° zur Beckenwand gekippt, 8 cm breit (SCHMER-MUND et al.)	50	95	100	50	50	30
E 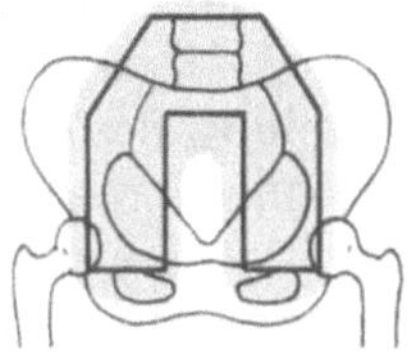	ventrales und dor-sales großes U-för-miges Feld. Ausblen-dung der Beckenmitte (DIBBELT, RAHM u. RENNER)	60	75	100	60	60	55
F	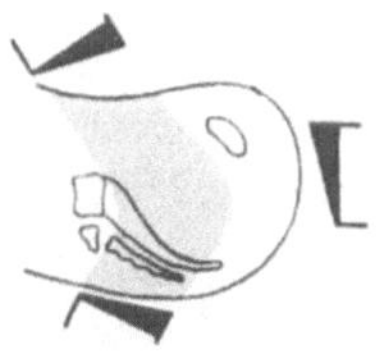 Ventrales und dor-sales Feld (Voll-dosis), Dammfeld (halbe Dosis) mit Keilfilter (10 × 13 cm) (Marburger Methode)	100	100	100	100	100	20
G	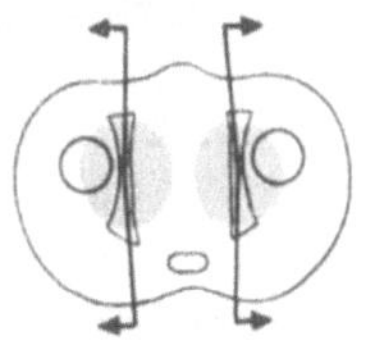 Pendelung über 2 Fel-der, Pendelachse caudal divergierend, PW 200° (8,5 × 16 cm) (SURMONT; BURAGGI et al.)	65	85	100	60	60	60
H	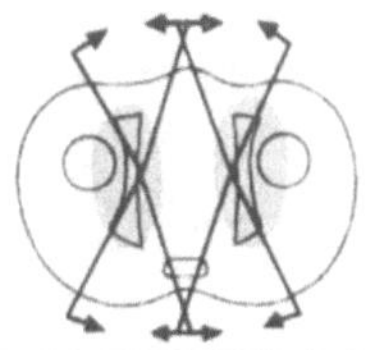 Pendelbestrahlung über 4 Felder, PW je 60° (5 × 15 cm) (BRIZEL et al.)	25	40	100	25	25	15

Abb. 38. Prozentuale Dosisverteilung bei verschiedenen Methoden der Telekobalttherapie des Collumcarcinoms in Kombination mit einer intrakavitären Radiumtherapie

Isodosen, die mit dem Zentralstrahl vorgeschriebene Schnittwinkel bilden (Rosenow und Frischkorn, 1965). Eine weitere Verwendung ergibt sich bei der Pendelbestrahlung, bei der durch die Keilfilter ein Auswandern des Dosismaximums in Richtung der Winkelhalbierenden verhindert werden kann (Welker, 1965, 1967; Rosenow und Frischkorn, 1965; Beduhn und Kuttig, 1967).

In der gynäkologischen Strahlentherapie wurde bisher die Indikation zur Bestrahlung des lumbalen Lymphsystems relativ eng gestellt. Das lumbale Lymphabflußgebiet bietet für die Strahlenbehandlung hinsichtlich seiner Topographie sehr ungünstige Bedingungen, da es von mehreren strahlenempfindlichen und lebenswichtigen Organen umgeben ist. Das Rückenmark, nur wenige Zentimeter von den an der Vorderfläche des Wirbelkörpers liegenden Lymphknoten entfernt, besitzt nur eine begrenzte Strahlentoleranz. Die Häufigkeit von Rückenmarkschäden und insbesondere die zu den Schäden führenden Strahlendosen sind schwer abzuschätzen. Seitlich grenzen die Nieren und die Ureteren an das zylindrisch verlaufende Bestrahlungsfeld. Das Nierenparenchym gilt zwar nicht als besonders strahlenempfindliches Organ, doch sind irreversible Schäden am tubulären und glomerulären Apparat nach einzeitiger Dosisapplikation von 2000—3000 R im Tierversuch beschrieben worden (Mohr, Morgenroth und Schnepper, 1966). Wesentlich ausgeprägter sind die Strahlenreaktionen am Darm. Da es unter konventionellen Strahlenbedingungen fast unmöglich erscheint, ohne Strahlenschäden das lumbale Lymphsystem mit einer vollen Tumordosis zu erfassen, entschloß man sich nur sehr selten zu einer Sicherheitsbestrahlung dieser Region. Lediglich bei einem nachweisbaren metastatischen Befall der aortalen Lymphknoten ergab sich eine absolute Notwendigkeit zur Bestrahlung, wobei dann mögliche Bestrahlungsfolgen in Kauf genommen wurden.

Bei der Behandlung der weiblichen Genitalcarcinome wurde dem Lymphknotenproblem in den letzten Jahren große Beachtung geschenkt, wie bereits ausführlich in Kap. IV/3/b (S. 147) abgehandelt worden ist. Nicht zuletzt durch die Lymphographie häuften sich die Mitteilungen, daß man nicht nur bei fortgeschrittenen Tumoren des Uterus und der Ovarien häufiger als vermutet Lymphknotenmetastasen in der Lumbalregion findet. Diese Untersuchungsergebnisse gaben mehrfach zur Frage Anlaß, ob möglicherweise die Behandlungsergebnisse durch eine zusätzliche Bestrahlung des lumbalen Lymphsystems, zumindest bei fortgeschrittenen Collumcarcinomen, verbessert werden könnten. Langjährige Erfahrungen liegen nur von Weishaar (1967) vor, der in den Stadien I und II keine signifikante Verbesserung der Behandlungsergebnisse erzielen konnte.

Bereits Maurer (1955) versuchte in der Orthovolttherapie zur Erfassung der ileosacralen und unteren paravertebralen Lymphknoten die Dosisverteilung durch Anlegen eines cranial des Parametrienfeldes nach medial verschobenen zweiten Pendelkonvergenzfeldes (180°/20°, Feldgröße 4×9 cm) zu verbessern, um auch in den höheren Lymphknotenstationen eine homogene Ausstrahlung zu ermöglichen.

Bei der Verwendung von 2-MeV-Röntgenstrahlen hat bereits Blomfield (1961) auch die aortalen Lymphknoten in das Bestrahlungsfeld eingeschlossen, wenn es sich um weit fortgeschrittene Fälle handelte.

Für die Telekobalttherapie wurden erstmals von Weishaar und Heller (1962) Phantomuntersuchungen zur Bestrahlung der unteren Lumbalregion durch Anlegung eines zusätzlichen ventralen und dorsalen Stehfeldes durchgeführt. Auf diese Weise konnte ein Dosisgewinn medial in Höhe des Promonturiums und der unteren Lendenwirbelsäule erzielt werden. Mit dieser 6-Felder-Methode läßt sich die untere Lumbalregion ohne technische Schwierigkeiten erfassen. Das gleiche Volumen wird bei der von Dibbelt, Rahm und Renner (1960) angegebenen Methode bestrahlt. Bei dieser Methode können die unteren lumbalen Lymphknoten ebenfalls in das Bestrahlungsfeld eingeschlossen werden. Einen gleichen Effekt erzielen Surmont (1958) sowie Buraggi et al. (1959) mit der von ihnen inaugurierten Pendelbestrahlung, bei der beide Pendelachsen in cranialer Richtung konvergieren, so daß die caudale Lumbalregion mit einer genügend hohen Dosis erfaßt wird.

KAHR (1965) benutzt bei der Bestrahlung eines prävertebralen angenommenen Herdes 2 schräge Felder mit und ohne Keilfilter oder eine Pendelbestrahlung um 180°. DALLA PALMA, RENZI und CAVANI (1964) beschreiben eine technisch komplizierte Bestrahlungsmethode, bei der aber eine optimale Dosisverteilung im paralumbalen Lymphsystem erreicht werden kann. Durch eine exzentrische Pendelbestrahlung über 2 verschiedene Pendelrichtungen kann ein sichelförmiges Dosismaximum bewirkt werden.

Die verschiedenen Möglichkeiten einer optimalen Bestrahlung des lumbalen Lymphsystems mit Kobalt-60-γ-Strahlen untersuchten FRISCHBIER und MÖHLE (1967). Es zeigte sich, daß eine ausreichende Schonung des Rückenmarkes, der Nieren und des Intestinaltraktes bei Einstrahlung über 2 schräge dorsale Felder mit Keilfiltern und einem zusätzlichen homogenen ventralen Stehfeld erreicht werden kann (Abb. 39). Durch die Keilfilter kommt es zu einer oft kaum zumutbaren Verlängerung der Bestrahlungszeiten wegen

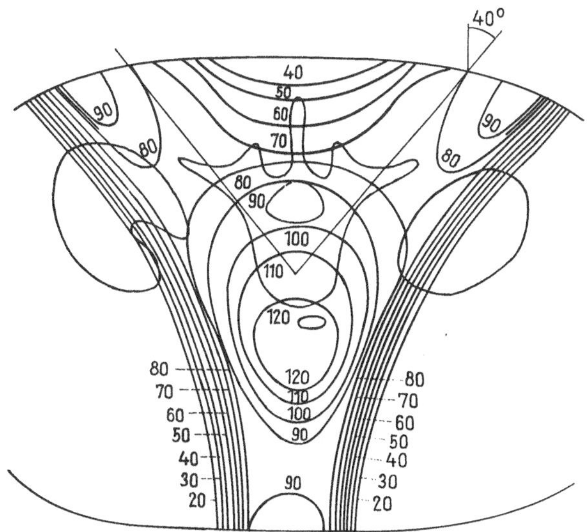

Abb. 39. Isodosen bei Bestrahlung über zwei schräge, dorsale Felder mit Keilfilter (17,5°) und ein zusätzliches Stehfeld von ventral. Feldgröße je 6 × 15 cm, Feldabstand der beiden dorsalen Felder 10 cm, Einstrahlungswinkel 40°, QHA 50 cm, Zentrierung auf 9 cm Tiefe

der Verringerung der Dosisleistung. Um die Bestrahlungszeiten für die Patientinnen in einem erträglichen Maß halten zu können, setzt die Verwendung derart starker Ausgleichsfilter eine Quellenstärke von mindestens 1500 Ci voraus. Bei einer schwächeren Strahlenquelle ist der Pendelbestrahlung der Vorzug zu geben (FRISCHBIER und UBENAUF, 1967), bei der die Dosisverteilung durch die Verwendung von Keilfiltern verbessert werden kann. Die praktische Anwendung und Dosierung wurden von BEDUHN und KUTTIG (1967) ermittelt (Abb. 40).

WELKER (1967) ermittelte die bei der Pendelbestrahlung notwendigen Filterdichten. Er konnte zeigen, daß mit schwächeren Keilfiltern, die nur eine geringe Verlängerung der Bestrahlungszeit bewirken, die gleiche Dosisverteilung zu erhalten ist, wenn nur ein bestimmter medialer Winkelbereich bei der Pendelung ausgespart wird (Abb. 41).

In Anlehnung an eine von ABBATUCCI angegebene biaxiale Pendelbestrahlung entwickelten FRISCHBIER und KARL (1970) eine Bestrahlungsmethode, bei der sich ein nierenförmiges Dosismaximum am günstigsten der Lage und Anordnung der aortalen Lymphknoten anpaßt. Durch die biaxiale Telekobalt-Pendelbestrahlung über 4 Sektoren von je 90° (Abb. 42) wird eine Dosisverteilung erreicht, bei der Nieren und Rückenmark weniger als 50 % der Herddosis erhalten (Abb. 43, 44).

Seit Einführung ultraharter Strahlen wurden von verschiedenen Autoren Bestrahlungsmethoden wieder aufgegriffen, um unter vollständigem *Verzicht auf die Radiumapplikation*

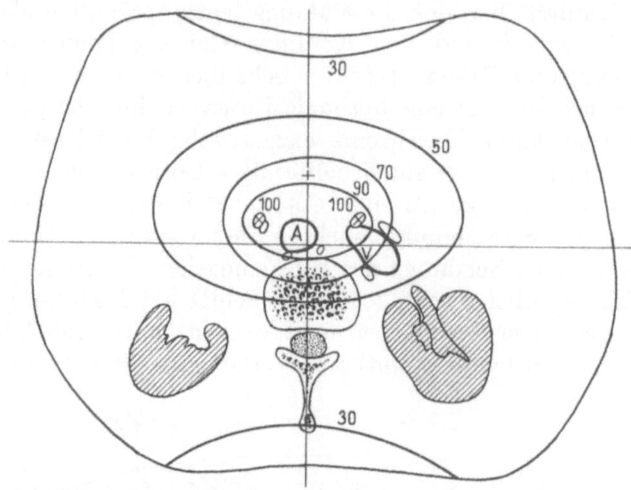

Abb. 40. Isodosen bei Telekobalt-Pendelbestrahlung über zwei Sektoren im Winkel von je 160° (20°/180°) mit 17,5° Keilfilter. Feldgröße 14×6 cm, Pendelradius 65 cm, Keilanordnung: Spitze in 90°-Stellung des Strahlers beidseits nach dorsal gerichtet. Pendelachse 3 cm von Phantommitte nach ventral verlagert (Beduhn und Kuttig)

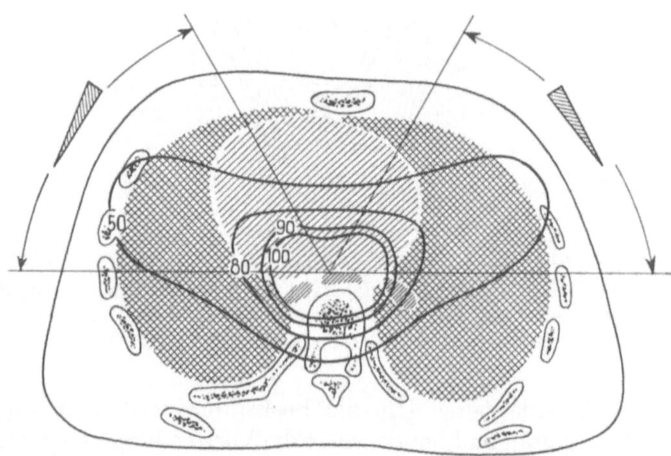

Abb. 41. Dosisverteilung einer 180°-Pendelbestrahlung mit Keilfilter: Feldbreite 6 cm, Keilwinkel 12°, ausgesparter Winkelbereich 60°, Pendelwinkel 180° (Welker)

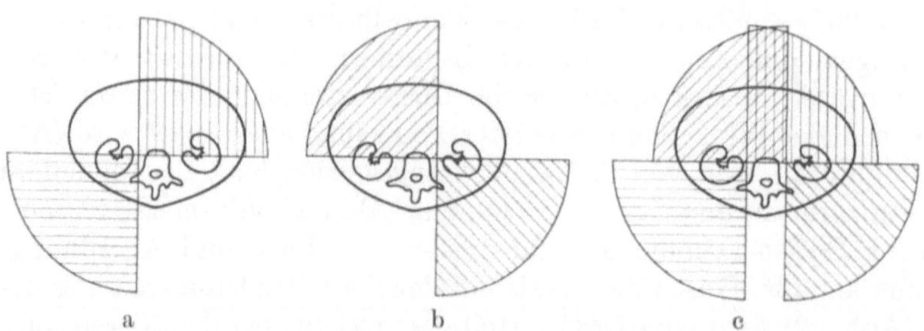

Abb. 42a—c. Schematische Darstellung der biaxialen Pendelbestrahlung über 4 Sektoren von je 90°. a Lage der beiden Sektoren der linken Pendelachse. b Lage der beiden Sektoren der rechten Pendelachse. c Summation der 4 Sektoren über beide Achsen

die Strahlenbehandlung des Collumcarcinoms ausschließlich percutan durchführen zu können (LEENHARDT und POURQUIER, 1957; SURMONT, 1957; KUTTIG und BECKER, 1959; ZANETTI und TOSCA, 1959). Da bei einer Kombination von lokaler Radium- und Telekobalttherapie an den Überschneidungsstellen der Radiumisodosen mit den Isodosen der Percutanbestrahlung Dosisspitzen auftreten können, die zu Dosisüberhöhungen auf der einen Seite und Unterdosierung auf der Gegenseite führen, ist die Kombination von 2 Bestrahlungsmethoden stets mit einem gewissen Unsicherheitsfaktor behaftet. Sie

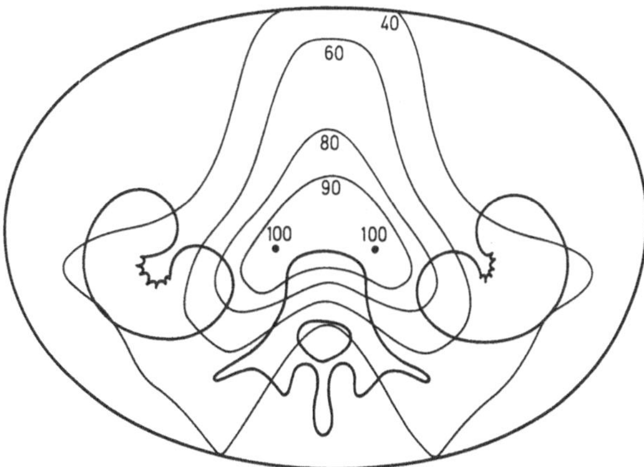

Abb. 43. Dosisverteilung bei biaxialer Telekobalt-Pendelbestrahlung über 4 Sektoren von je 90°, Achsenabstand 6 cm, Feldbreite 4 cm

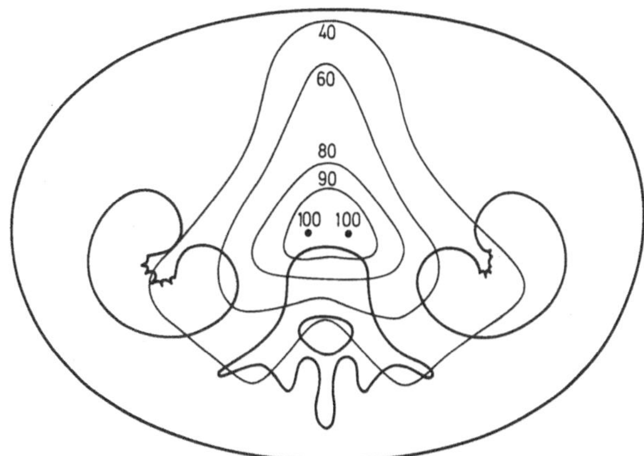

Abb. 44. Dosisverteilung bei biaxialer Telekobalt-Pendelbestrahlung über 4 Sektoren von je 90°, Achsenabstand 4 cm, Feldbreite 4 cm

stellt besondere Anforderungen an die Bestrahlungsplanung. Diese Nachteile mit den daraus resultierenden möglichen Schädigungen und ihren verhängnisvollen Folgen sollten durch Verzicht auf die Lokalbestrahlung mit Radium und Beschränkung auf eine Telekobalttherapie vermieden werden. Neben der Verbesserung der Dosisverteilung innerhalb des kleinen Beckens könnte aber auch eine Verminderung der Strahlenbelastung des Personals durch die Radiumapplikation und bei der Pflege der Patienten während der Radiumbestrahlung erreicht werden. Gerade in Abteilungen mit umfangreicher gynäkologischer Strahlentherapie könnte die auch bei bester Technik und Einhaltung aller Strahlenschutzmaßnahmen nicht zu unterschätzende relativ hohe Strahlenbelastung für den applizierenden Arzt und das Pflegepersonal hierdurch vermieden werden.

Besondere Impulse erhielten diese Bestrebungen durch Mellor, der im Jahre 1960 eine spezielle Methode zur ausschließlichen Percutanbestrahlung des Collumcarcinoms mit Kobalt-60-γ-Strahlen angab. Durch eine biaxiale Pendelbestrahlung mit einem Pendelwinkel von 160° pro Seite und Lage der Pendelachse etwa 3,5 cm seitlich der Medianlinie, gelingt es, das kleine Becken weitgehend homogen zu durchstrahlen (Abb. 45). Bei der von Mellor angegebenen Technik erhält man eine elliptische 80%-Isodose, die das Lymphabflußgebiet der Cervix einschließt. Der Uterus liegt innerhalb der 100%-Isodose, während sich der größte Teil des Rectums und der Blase außerhalb der 80%-Isodose befindet. Insgesamt applizierte Mellor auf die Cervix Dosen von 6500—7000 R, wobei Parametrium und seitliche Beckenwand 6000—6500 R erhielten. Er berichtete bereits über Erfahrungen an 17 Patienten mit einem Collumcarcinom der Stadien II und III, bei denen er in allen Fällen eine ausreichende Strahlenreaktion an Cervix und Vagina und

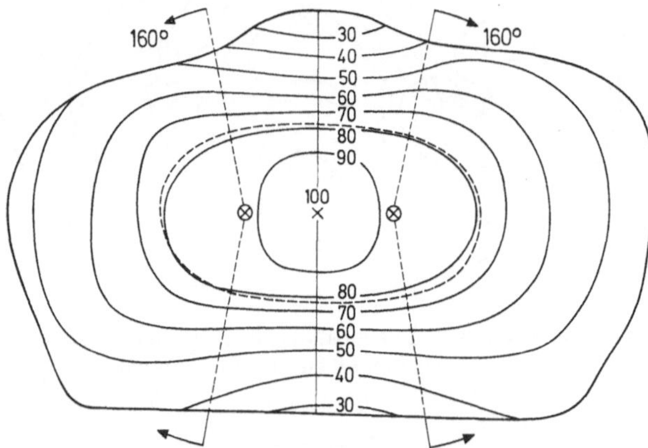

Abb. 45. Dosisverteilung bei biaxialer Telekobalt-Pendelbestrahlung nach Mellor

eine gute klinische Rückbildung des Lokalbefundes und der parametranen Infiltrate beobachtete. Obwohl bei den Patientinnen nur Beobachtungszeiten bis zu 15 Monaten vorlagen, glaubte Mellor, bei der Strahlenbehandlung des Collumcarcinoms mit dieser Methode ohne die zusätzliche Radiumapplikation eine genügende Tumordosis einstrahlen zu können. Blasen- oder Darmreaktionen infolge Dosisüberschneidungen wurden nicht beobachtet.

Die Anwendung der biaxialen Telekobalt-Pendelbestrahlung zur individuellen Anpassung des Dosisverlaufes an die topographisch-anatomischen Gegebenheiten wurden von Matschke und Welker (1963) und ihre dosimetrischen Grundlagen von Frischbier und Hasse (1965) untersucht. Der Vorteil dieser biaxialen Telekobalt-Pendelbestrahlung gegenüber anderen Methoden zur ausschließlichen Telekobaltbestrahlung des Collumcarcinoms wurde darin gesehen, daß durch Veränderung des Pendelachsabstandes, der Feldgröße und des Pendelwinkels der Isodosenverlauf erheblich beeinflußt und den gegebenen Verhältnissen von Fall zu Fall angepaßt werden kann (Abb. 46 und 47).

In den letzten Jahren wurde aus mehreren Zentren über Erfahrungen bei der klinischen Anwendung der ausschließlichen Telekobaltbestrahlung des Collumcarcinoms berichtet: Frischbier und Kuttig (1961), Buttenberg (1962), Gietzelt, Degner, Fürst, zur Horst-Meyer, Schmidt und Roth (1962), Koeck, Jacobson und Hillsinger (1962), Frischkorn (1963), Frischbier und Kuttig (1964), Kuttig (1965), Frischbier und Lohbeck (1967).

Gietzelt u. Mitarb. führten die ausschließliche Percutanbestrahlung bei Collumcarcinomen aller Stadien durch. Möglicherweise bedingt durch Unsicherheiten in der Frage einer optimalen Dosierung waren ihre Behandlungsergebnisse nicht so ermutigend, daß der generelle Verzicht auf Radium Anhänger fand. Besonders von gynäkologischer Seite wurde daher eine eng umgrenzte Indikationsstellung gefordert, um bei der Behandlung des Collumcarcinoms auf die seit Jahrzehnten bewährte Radiumtherapie mit ausgezeichneten Ergebnissen zugunsten einer noch nicht genügend erprobten Methode zu verzichten. So erschien eine homogene Bestrahlung des kleinen Beckens mit Telekobalt-γ-Strahlen nur bei ausgedehnten Carcinomen mit Infiltration in die Blase und das Rectum (FRISCHBIER und LOHBECK, 1967), bei breitem Übergang auf die Scheide (FRISCHKORN, 1963) sowie bei engen anatomischen Verhältnissen und erhöhten Temperaturen (BUTTENBERG, 1962) gerechtfertigt. Auch KUTTIG (1964) hält es für notwendig, erst bei einem allmählichen Übergang Erfahrungen an einem größeren Krankengut sammeln zu können, um eine durch die Megavolttherapie mögliche Methode mit einem kleineren Behandlungsrisiko für den Patienten unter optimaler Anpassung des Dosisverlaufes an das Krankheitsgebiet unter gleichzeitig geringer Strahlenbelastung für das Behandlungs- und Pflegepersonal propagieren zu können.

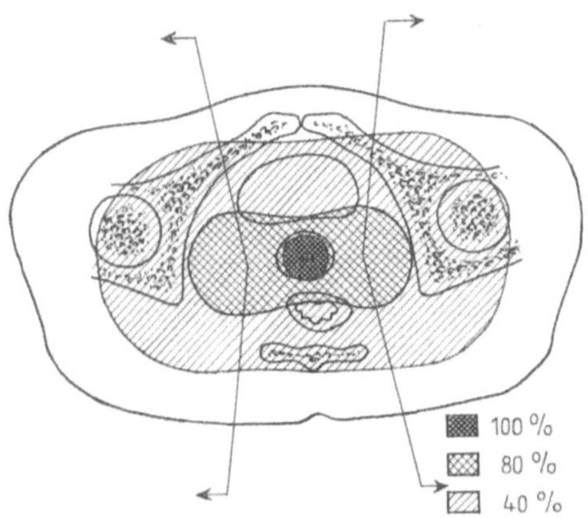

Abb. 46. Dosisverteilung bei biaxialer Telekobalt-Pendelbestrahlung. Pendelwinkel beidseits 160°, Feldgröße 6×16 cm, Pendelachsabstand 6 cm

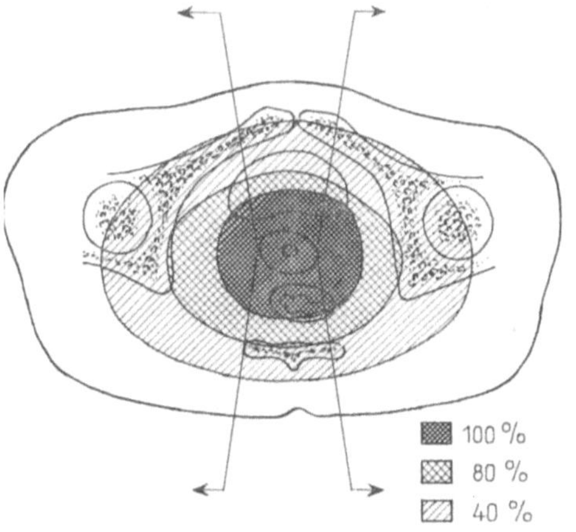

Abb. 47. Dosisverteilung bei biaxialer Telekobalt-Pendelbestrahlung, Pendelwinkel beidseits 160°, Feldgröße 8×16 cm, Pendelachsabstand 4 cm

Die bisherigen Erfahrungen haben gezeigt, daß es bei weit fortgeschrittenen Collumcarcinomen gerechtfertigt ist, auf eine lokale Radiumtherapie zugunsten einer ausschließlichen Telekobaltbestrahlung zu verzichten. In diesen Fällen, in denen durch die bisher übliche Therapie nur in wenigen Prozent eine Heilung erzielt werden konnte, scheint die ausschließliche Telekobalttherapie einige Vorteile zu bringen. Im Stadium IV ist die lokale Radiumtherapie unzureichend, weil der Primärtumor bei einer Infiltration der Blase oder des Rectums die therapeutische Reichweite der vaginalen und intracervicalen Radiumeinlage überragt. Bei einer erheblichen Erhöhung der Radiumdosis entstehen in diesen Fällen große Zerfallshöhlen, Blasen-Scheiden- oder Rectum-Scheidenfisteln, und die Patientinnen erliegen den dadurch gegebenen Komplikationen. Nach der wesentlich stärker fraktionierten Percutanbestrahlung können derartige Zerfallshöhlen, die durch Einschmelzen der großen, bis in die Blase oder das Rectum reichenden Tumoren entstehen, weitgehend vermieden werden. Es kommt nicht zur raschen Nekrose des Tumors wie bei einer hochdosierten Radiumbestrahlung, sondern der Tumor erweicht innerhalb eines Zeitraumes, in dem das Gegengewebe diesen Effekt ersetzen kann. Daher bleiben trotz Tumoreinbruch in Blase und Rectum die gefürchteten Blasen-Rectum-Scheiden-Fisteln aus.

Die vorliegenden Erfahrungen reichen bisher keinesfalls aus, um den klinischen Wert der ausschließlichen Percutanbestrahlung beurteilen zu können. GIETZELT u. Mitarb., die bisher über Erfahrungen an etwa 420 Patientinnen verfügen, konnten im Stadium I eine 3-Jahres-Überlebenszeit von 92% und eine 4-Jahres-Überlebenszeit von 86% finden.

An der Universitäts-Frauenklinik Hamburg wurden von 1964—1968 15 Patientinnen mit einem Stadium IV, bei denen es zu einem histologisch nachgewiesenen Tumoreinbruch in die Blase oder in das Rectum gekommen war, ausschließlich mit einer Telekobalttherapie behandelt. In den ersten beiden Jahren nach der Behandlung verstarben 11 Patientinnen infolge einer Tumorprogredienz. 2 Patientinnen leben jetzt rezidivfrei mehr als 2 Jahre und ebenfalls 2 Patientinnen mehr als 3 Jahre. Bei den 11 verstorbenen Patientinnen kam es in 4 Fällen zu einer diffusen Lungenmetastasierung, ohne daß im kleinen Becken ein Tumorrezidiv nachzuweisen war. Bei 43 Patientinnen wurde eine ausschließliche Telekobalttherapie wegen breiter vaginaler Infiltration vorgenommen. Von diesen Patientinnen lebten nach einem Jahr noch 75% und nach 2 Jahren noch über 50%. Die Nachbeobachtungszeit ist bisher noch zu kurz, um ein endgültiges Urteil über den Wert dieser Bestrahlungsmethode beim Stadium III angeben zu können.

Hinsichtlich der optimalen Dosis bestehen noch erhebliche Unsicherheiten. Es erscheint zwar gesichert, daß die bei einer Radiumbestrahlung erreichte Dosis von 20000 bis 30000 R an der Oberfläche des Präparates zur Tumordevitalisierung nicht notwendig ist. So wurden die besten Ergebnisse bisher nach einer Dosis von etwa 8000 R in Beckenmitte und 6000 R an der Beckenwand erzielt. Nach Dosen von 6000 R sahen Gietzelt u. Mitarb. in einem hohen Prozentsatz Lokalrezidive, wie bereits näher ausgeführt wurde.

Im Laufe der letzten Jahre wurden verschiedenartige Bestrahlungsmethoden angegeben und erprobt, mit denen eine ausschließliche Telekobalttherapie des Collumcarcinoms möglich ist. Einige dieser Methoden sind in Abb. 48 zusammengestellt, von denen die Dosisverhältnisse an den interessierenden Punkten im kleinen Becken unter gleichen Phantombedingungen ermittelt wurden.

Wenn auch in zahlreichen Behandlungszentren der Welt vor mehr als 5 Jahren die Percutanbestrahlung von Orthovolt- auf Telekobalt-γ-Strahlen umgestellt worden ist, reicht das Patientengut, an dem bisher 5-Jahres-Heilungen erzielt werden konnte, noch nicht aus, um den klinischen Wert der Telecurietherapie beurteilen zu können. Trotzdem finden sich im Schrifttum bereits heute Mitteilungen, in denen über verbesserte Heilungsergebnisse bei der kombinierten Radium-Telekobalttherapie berichtet wird.

Cooper und Williams (1962) fanden bei insgesamt 144 Patientinnen mit einem Collumcarcinom nach Kombination einer intrakavitären Radiumapplikation mit percutaner Orthovolt- oder Telekobalttherapie, daß die Behandlungsergebnisse im Stadium I durch die Umstellung von Orthovolt- auf Telekobalttherapie von 72% auf 82%, im Stadium II von 30% auf 56% erhöht werden konnten.

Über 2jährige Behandlungsergebnisse bei 149 Patientinnen mit einem Collumcarcinom der Stadien I—III nach Telekobalttherapie berichtet Weishaar (1965). Nachdem nach Umstellung der Percutanbestrahlung auf Telekobalttherapie die Herddosis um 10% auf 3000—3500 R erhöht worden ist, vergleicht er die 2-Jahres-Überlebensrate mit der eines gleichartigen Patientengutes nach konventioneller Strahlentherapie. Während er in den Stadien I und II gleiche Behandlungsergebnisse fand, konnten die Überlebenszeiten im Stadium III von 51% auf 59% nach Telekobalttherapie erhöht werden.

An der Universitäts-Frauenklinik Hamburg wurde die Percutanbestrahlung im Jahre 1960 auf eine Telekobalttherapie umgestellt. Da seit 1951 die Indikation zur Radikaloperation im Stadium I sowie die Applikationsform und Dosis der intrauterinen Radiumtherapie des Stadiums I—IV nicht verändert wurde, sondern nur die von 1951—1956 mit Orthovoltstrahlen applizierte parametrane Herddosis von 2500—3000 R bei der seit 1957 durchgeführten Megavolttherapie auf 4000—4400 R erhöht wurde (Tabelle 10), lassen sich die Behandlungsergebnisse miteinander vergleichen.

Während sich die 5-Jahres-Heilungsrate (Tabelle 11b) im Stadium I in der Orthovoltära und nach Einführung einer 15-MeV-Röntgenstrahlung oder einer Kobalt-60-γ-Strahlung mit 87% bzw. 86,5% fast entsprechen, konnten in den fortgeschritteneren Stadien nach Anwendung von Megavoltstrahlung bessere Behandlungsergebnisse erzielt

		Cervix	Punkt A	Beckenwand	Blase	Rectum	Collum femoris
A 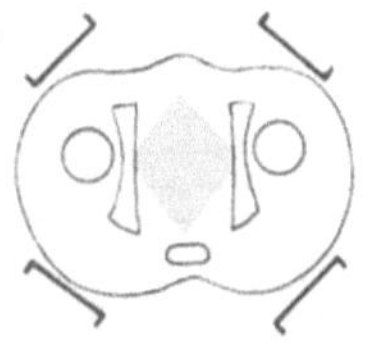	2 ventrale, 2 dorsale schräge Felder, 45—50° Konvergenz (10 × 15 cm) (LEENHARDT; FRISCHKORN)	100	100	90	95	95	45
B 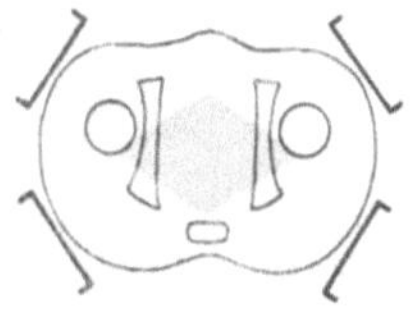	2 ventrale, 2 dorsale schräge Felder, 60° Konvergenz (10 × 15 cm) (LEENHARDT u. POURQUIER)	100	100	95	85	90	55
C 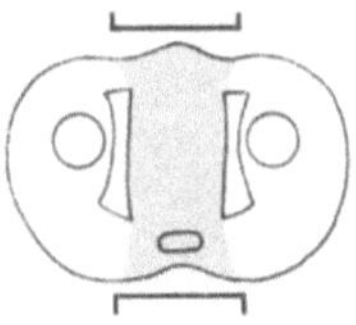	1 ventrales, 1 dorsales Stehfeld (15 × 15 cm)	100	100	80	100	100	20
D 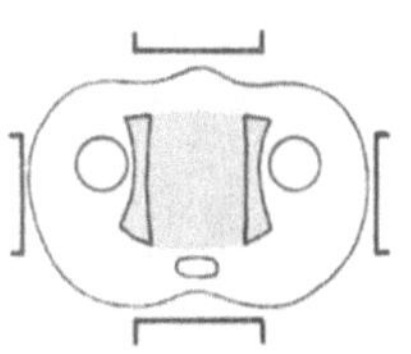	1 ventrales, 1 dorsales, 2 laterale Stehfelder (15 × 15 cm, 10 × 15 cm)	100	100	95	100	100	70
E 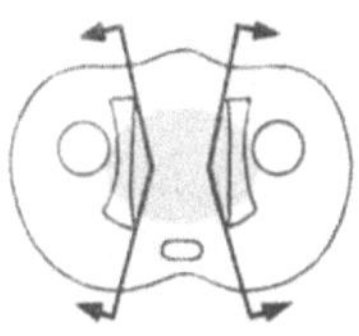	biaxiale Pendelbestrahlung, PW je 160° (9 × 15 cm) (MELLOR)	100	95	80	90	85	40
F 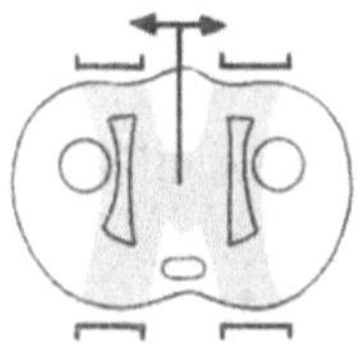	2 ventrale, 2 dorsale Stehfelder und zentrale Pendelbestrahlung, PW 360° (6 × 15 cm) (ZANETTI u. TOSCA)	100	100	90	85	85	45
G 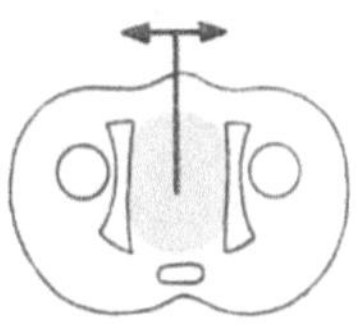	zentrale Pendelbestrahlung, PW 360° (15 × 15 cm u. 8 × 8 cm) (KOECK et al.)	100	100	80	95	95	50
H 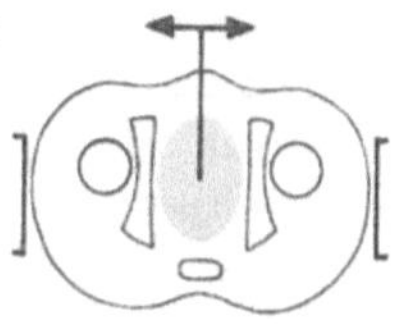	zentrale Pendelbestrahlung, PW 360°, 2 laterale Stehfelder (10 × 15 cm) (LEENHARDT u. POURQUIER)	100	100	60	100	100	45

Abb. 48. Prozentuale Dosisverteilung bei verschiedenen Methoden der ausschließlichen Telekobalttherapie des Collumcarcinoms

Tabelle 10. *Behandlungsmethoden beim Collumcarcinom an der Universitäts-Frauenklinik Hamburg*

Stadium	Operation	Radium	Percutanbestrahlung	
			1951—1956	1957—1963
I (a)	Wertheim-Operation			
I (b)	Wertheim-Operation	1000—1500 mgeh prä- oder post-operativ	2000—2500 R HD 200 kV Röntgen	3000—4000 R HD 15-MV-Röntgen- oder Kobalt-60-Teletherapie
I (inope-rabel) II		4500—5000 mgeh	2800—3000 R Becken-wand 200 kV Röntgen	4000—4400 R HD 15-MV-Röntgen- oder Kobalt-60-Teletherapie
III IV		5000—5500 mgeh	1700 R Beckenwand 200 kV Röntgen und 1500 R Beckenwand Körperhöhlenrohr 60 kV	4000—6400 R HD 15-MV-Röntgen- oder Kobalt-60-Teletherapie

Tabelle 11a. *Anzahl der behandelten Patientinnen mit einem histologisch gesicherten Collumcarcinom an der Universitäts-Frauenklinik Hamburg-Eppendorf in den Berichtszeiträumen von 1951—1956 und von 1957—1963*

Stadium	1951—1956	1957—1963
I	209	127
II	111	73
III	368	497
IV	47	57
I—IV	735	754

Tabelle 11b. *Behandlungsergebnisse beim Collumcarcinom im Berichtszeitraum von 1951-1956, in dem die Percutanbestrahlung in Form einer 200-kV-Röntgentherapie durchgeführt wurde, und von 1957—1963, in dem eine 15-MV-Röntgenstrahlung oder eine Kobalt-60-γ-Strahlung angewandt wurde. Die Prozentzahlen geben die Rate der 5 Jahre rezidivfrei überlebende Patientinnen an. In den Klammern sind die Vertrauensgrenzen für eine Irrtums-wahrscheinlichkeit von 5% angegeben*

Stadium	1951—1956 200-kV-Röntgenstrahlen	1957—1963 15-MV-Röntgenstrahlen (Betatron) Kobalt-60-Teletherapie
I	87,0% $(\pm 4,6\%)$	86,5% $(\pm 6,0\%)$
II	56,8% $(\pm 9,2\%)$ ⎫	76,7% $(\pm 9,7\%)$ ⎫
III	46,1% $(\pm 5,1\%)$ ⎬ 48,8% $(\pm 4,5\%)$	55,7% $(\pm 4,4\%)$ ⎬ 58,5% $(\pm 4,0\%)$
IV	8,5% $(\pm 8,0\%)$ ⎭	12,3% $(\pm 8,5\%)$ ⎭
I—IV	57,0% $(\pm 3,6\%)$	59,7% $(\pm 3,5\%)$

werden. Im Stadium II stieg die 5-Jahres-Heilungsrate um etwa 20% nach Megavolt-therapie an, im Stadium III um etwa 10%. Faßt man beide Stadien zusammen, so zeigt sich, daß in den Stadien II und III nach Megavolttherapie eine Verbesserung der Hei-lungsrate um 10% erreicht werden konnte. Bei dem nur kleinen Patientengut im Stadium IV konnte nur eine geringfügige Erhöhung der Heilungsrate erzielt werden. Bei einer Gegenüberstellung der absoluten Heilungsrate in beiden Berichtsperioden ergibt sich eine Erhöhung der Behandlungsergebnisse nach Megavolttherapie von nur 2,7%. Hierbei ist allerdings zu berücksichtigen, daß in dem Zeitraum von 1957—1963 ein höherer Prozentsatz an Fällen der Stadien III und IV zur Behandlung kamen. Ein Vergleich der Behandlungsergebnisse im Stadium III zwischen beiden Behandlungsgruppen ergibt eine statistische Signifikanz mit einer Irrtumswahrscheinlichkeit von weniger als 0,6%, ein statistischer Vergleich der Behandlungsergebnisse in den Stadien II und III zusammen eine Signifikanz mit einer Irrtumswahrscheinlichkeit von weniger als 0,2%.

Hinsichtlich der notwendigen Dosishöhe besteht bis heute keinesfalls Einigkeit. So werden als optimale Dosis empfohlen: 4000 R von NOLAN et al. (1956), 5000 R von BECKER und SCHUBERT (1961), MACARINI, BESIO und GANDOLFO (1961), GUTTMANN (1962), GARY-BOBO und POURQUIER (1966) und 6000 R von AMBESI IMPIOMBATO, CHELAZZI und MILANESI (1959) und VALDAGNI, CASNATI, MARCHESONI (1959).

Während VALDAGNI et al. nach einer percutanen Dosis im Punkt B von etwa 3500 rad in 20 Tagen und zusätzlich 1900—2500 rad in Punkt B durch das Radium praktisch keine primären- und Spätreaktionen beobachteten, sahen GUZZON und ROMANINI (1963) nach Herddosen von 5000—6000 R innerhalb von 5—8 Wochen schwere proktosigmoiditische Veränderungen.

LALANNE und FAJBISOWICZ (1965) vergleichen die Behandlungskomplikationen nach kombinierter Radium-Telekobalttherapie, bei der 5000—6000 rad innerhalb von 6 Wochen percutan eingestrahlt wurden, mit denen nach kombinierter Radium-Orthovolttherapie von 426 Patientinnen mit einem Collumcarcinom. Sie fanden bei der konventionellen Röntgentherapie 15,5% und nach der Telekobalttherapie 20% Strahlenkomplikationen. Den Unterschied führen sie auf die genauere Überwachung der mit Telekobalt bestrahlten Patientinnen zurück. Obwohl bei der Telekobalttherapie die percutane Herddosis verdoppelt wurde, konnten sie somit eine deutliche Zunahme der Behandlungskomplikationen nicht registrieren.

Die Häufigkeit der am Patientengut der Universitäts-Frauenklinik Hamburg beobachteten Bestrahlungskomplikationen nach Orthovolt- und Megavolttherapie in Kombination mit einer lokalen Radiumtherapie von 4000—5000 mgeh ist aus der Tabelle 12a zu entnehmen. Man erkennt, daß schwerere Strahlenreaktionen an Blase und Ureter in beiden Behandlungsgruppen etwa gleich häufig sind. Lediglich Darmreaktionen mit Ulcera, Stenosen oder Rectum-Scheiden-Fisteln traten nach der Megavolttherapie häufiger auf.

Tabelle 12a. *Behandlungskomplikationen nach Orthovolt- und Megavolttherapie. Die Angaben in Prozent sind auf die Zahl der behandelten Patientinnen bezogen*

	1951—1956 Orthovolttherapie, 520 behandelte Patienten	1957—1963 Megavolttherapie, 446 behandelte Patienten
Blase Ulcus Fistel	2,0%	3,1%
Ureter Hydronephrose stumme Niere	1,4%	1,8%
Darm Ulcus Stenosen Fisteln	3,0%	11,8%
Knochen Fraktur	0,6%	0,2%

Tabelle 12b. *Behandlungskomplikationen nach Megavolttherapie in Abhängigkeit von der percutan eingestrahlten Herddosis an der Beckenwand*

	4000—4500 R Beckenwand, 285 behandelte Patienten		4600—6500R Beckenwand, 161 behandelte Patienten	
Blase Grad II (Ulcus) Grad III (Fistel)	8 1	} 3,1%	4 1	} 3,1%
Ureter (Hydronephrose, stumme Niere)	5	1,7%	3	1,9%
Darm Grad II (Ulcus) Grad III (Stenosen) GradIV (Fisteln)	13 11 —	} 8,0%	18 7 4	} 18,0%
Knochen (Fraktur)	—		1	

Als nach Einführung der Telekobalttherapie für etwa 1 Jahr die Herddosis an der Beckenwand bei Kombination mit Radium auf etwa 4600—6500 R erhöht wurde, trat bei diesen
Patientinnen in 18% der Fälle eine Darmreaktion der Stadien II—IV auf. Es konnten
allein in 4 Fällen Rectum-Scheiden-Fisteln nachgewiesen werden. Bei einer percutan
eingestrahlten Herddosis von 4000—4500 R konnte die Komplikationsrate auf 8% reduziert werden (Tabelle 12b).

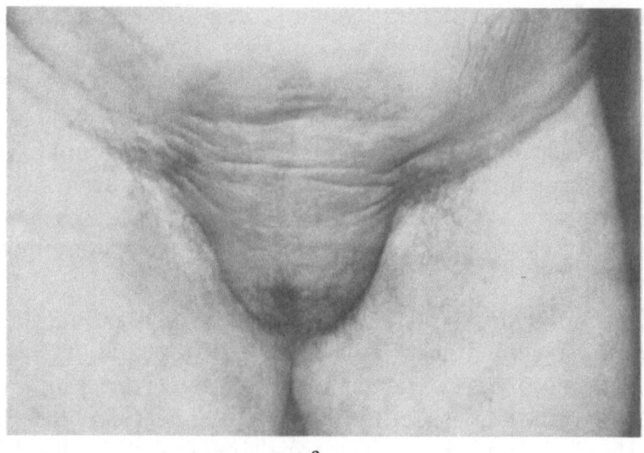

a

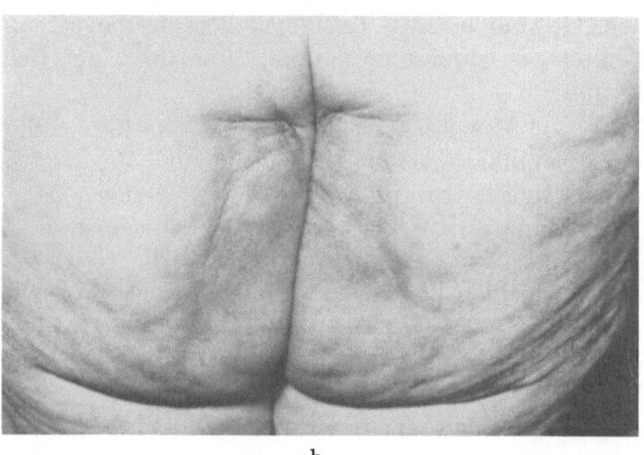

b

Abb. 49a u. b. Subcutane Induration nach Telekobalttherapie

Besonderes Interesse verdienen die nach einer hochdosierten Telekobalttherapie aufgetretenen Hautveränderungen. Bei über der Hälfte der regelmäßig kontrollierten Patientinnen wurden nach einer Herddosis von 4600—6500 R an der Beckenwand subcutane
Indurationen im Bereich der Bestrahlungsfelder gesehen. In 27,7% von 112 Fällen
(Dreyer, 1967) traten stärkere Indurationen in Form dicker, lederartiger und scharf
gegen die Umgebung abgrenzbarer Schwielen oder Narbenplatten der Haut und Subcutis
auf (Abb. 49 a und b). Es bestand eine deutliche Dosisabhängigkeit: in einem Zeitraum
von 8—30 Monaten traten schwere Indurationen bei 27% der Patientinnen mit einer
errechneten Dosis im Dosismaximum (0,5 cm unter der Hautoberfläche) von 4900 bis
5500 R auf, bei 42% lag die Dosis zwischen 5500—6000 R und bei 35% über 6000 R. Unterhalb einer Dosis von 4900 R wurde in keinem Fall eine starke Induration beobachtet.
Bei adipösen Patientinnen bestand eine größere Neigung zur indurativen Umwandlung
des Fettgewebes.

In den letzten Jahren wurde Caesium-137 wegen seiner längeren Halbwertszeit für die Verwendung in Telecuriegeräten empfohlen. Über Erfahrungen mit der Behandlung der Telecaesiumtherapie beim Collumcarcinom sind im Schrifttum bisher keine Angaben zu finden. Da Caesium-137 in physikalischer Hinsicht zwischen der Telekobalt-γ-Strahlung und der 200 kV-Röntgenstrahlung liegt, sind die Vorteile gegenüber der konventionellen Röntgentherapie wesentlich weniger ausgeprägt, so daß der Telekobalttherapie in jedem Fall der Vorzug zu geben ist.

$\beta\beta$) *Therapie mit ultraharten Röntgenstrahlen*

Vor mehr als 2 Jahrzehnten versuchte man schon, bei der Percutanbestrahlung die Dosisverhältnisse durch Verwendung energiereicherer Strahlen zu verbessern. Vor allem im anglo-amerikanischen Schrifttum wurde der Beweis erbracht, daß durch Verwendung von 400—800 kV-Röntgenstrahlen die Heilungsergebnisse in Kombination mit der intrakavitären Radiumtherapie verbessert werden konnten (MURPHY und REINHARD, 1950; RICHARDS, 1950; BAUD und COURTIAL, 1952; GARCIA, 1955). In einigen Zentren wurde sogar die Hochvolttherapie mit Röntgenstrahlen von 800 kV bis 1 MeV durchgeführt (HOLMES und SCHULZ, 1946; BUSCHKE, CANTRIL und PARKER, 1950). Die Voraussetzung für eine Therapie mit Röntgenstrahlen über 1 Million Elektronenvolt wurden erst nach dem zweiten Weltkrieg durch den van-de-Graaff-Generator und den Linearbeschleuniger geschaffen.

Über die ersten Erfahrungen mit Megavoltenergien bei der Behandlung des Collumcarcinoms berichten TRUMP, GRANKE, WRIGHT, EVANS, HARE, EWERT und CONLON (1954), GUTTMANN (1957), HAHN (1957), WINDEYER (1959), BLOMFIELD (1961), McLENNAN, BAGSHAW und McLENNAN (1962), WILLIAMS und KAZEM (1962).

TRUMP u. Mitarb. (1954) berichten über zufriedenstellende Ergebnisse bei 25 Patientinnen mit einem Collumcarcinom bei einer Nachbeobachtungszeit von allerdings nur 2 Jahren. Sie führten eine ausschließliche Percutanbestrahlung mit 2-MeV-Röntgenstrahlen durch, bei der sie mit einer Rotationsbestrahlung 6000 R in 35 Tagen applizierten. Auch GUTTMANN sah in den fortgeschrittenen Stadien nach 2-MeV-Röntgenstrahlen bessere Behandlungsergebnisse als nach konventioneller und Hochvolttherapie.

Eine ausschließliche percutane Strahlenbehandlung mit 1-MeV-Röntgenstrahlen führten WILLIAMS und KAZEM (1962) bei 18 Patientinnen mit fortgeschrittenen Stadien durch. Von diesen Patientinnen starben 4 innerhalb des 1. Jahres, 11 Patientinnen (= 61%) überlebten 3 Jahre oder mehr; 7 Patientinnen lebten länger als 5 Jahre (= 39%). Bei diesen Patientinnen handelte es sich in 62% um ein Stadium III, in 33% um ein Stadium IV. Die applizierte Dosis betrug 5000—6000 R innerhalb von 6 Wochen.

HAHN (1957) konnte nach Behandlung mit 2-MeV-Röntgenstrahlen in Kombination mit der lokalen Radiumtherapie keine besseren Behandlungsergebnisse erzielen. Er beobachtete vor allem in der Anfangszeit, als noch wenig Erfahrungen vorlagen, eine relativ hohe Zahl von behandlungsbedingten Komplikationen: Vulvitis, Urethritis, Vaginitis, Cystitis, Proktitis, Darmverschluß durch Fibrosen, Sacralulcera, Leukopenie oder Femurfrakturen, wovon besonders adipöse Frauen betroffen waren. Er glaubt, daß Energien von mehr als 2 MeV wegen der höheren Austrittsdosen keine wesentlichen Vorteile bringen.

Über größere Erfahrungen mit Röntgenstrahlen eines Linear-Accelerators in Kombination mit der Radiumtherapie berichten McLENNAN et al. (1967). Sie hatten in den Jahren 1956—1965 bei 168 Patientinnen mit einem Collumcarcinom eine Strahlenbehandlung durchgeführt. Es handelte sich in 47% um Stadium I, 33% Stadium II, 15% Stadium III und 5% Stadium IV. Die 5-Jahres-Überlebenszeit betrug 60%, im Stadium I 83%, und im Stadium II nur 41%. Sie beobachteten nach einer Herddosis von 5000 rad in Kombination mit der Radiumtherapie, durch die auf Punkt A etwa 7000 bis 8000 rad innerhalb von zwei Sitzungen appliziert wurden, in einem hohen Prozentsatz Strahlenschäden im Bereich des Intestinums. Ungefähr drei Viertel der Patientinnen klagten während der Behandlung über Durchfälle; in 6% der Fälle mußte im weiteren Verlauf wegen der Strahlenschädigung eine Kolostomie oder eine segmentale Darmresektion vorgenommen werden.

Im Schrifttum finden sich mehrere Angaben, nach denen die physikalischen Eigenschaften der Röntgenstrahlen einer Energie von 15 bis etwa 20 MeV für die Behandlung des Collumcarcinoms vorteilhaft sind (Schinz, 1958; Ischtschenko, 1960; Schmermund und Oberheuser, 1960; Becker und Schubert, 1961; Fletcher, 1962; Fujimori et al., 1963; Takayama, 1964; Dibbelt und Heinzler, 1965).

Als Vorteile der ultraharten Röntgenstrahlen in diesem Energiebereich werden übereinstimmend genannt: die höchstmögliche relative Tiefendosis bei Schonung der Haut, die übersichtliche Dosisverteilung unabhängig von der Feldgröße, die scharfe Begrenzung des Strahlenkegels, geringste Absorptionsunterschiede der verschiedenen Gewebsarten

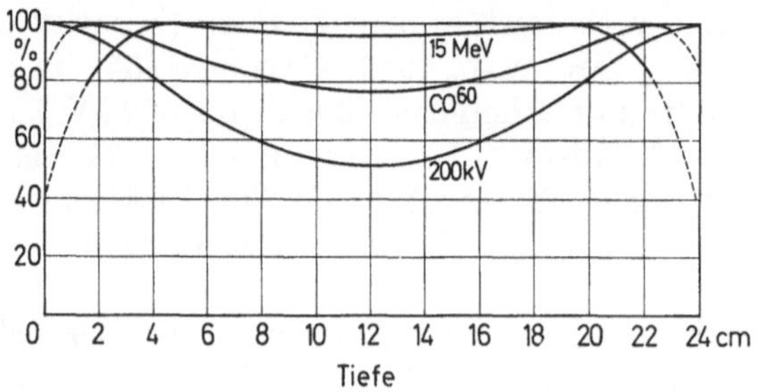

Abb. 50. Relative Tiefendosis bei Bestrahlung von gegenüberliegenden Feldern, bezogen auf 100% in den Dosismaxima (Vieten und Heinzler)

und die kleinstmögliche Integraldosis. Hinsichtlich der Integraldosis und einer optimalen Hautschonung wurde von Schittenhelm (1961) als günstigste Strahlenqualität eine Röntgenstrahlung mit der Energie von 18 MeV angesetzt.

Bei der Bestrahlung des Collumcarcinoms mit ultraharten Röntgenstrahlen erweist sich als besonders vorteilhaft, daß selbst bei adipösen Patientinnen durch die übliche Bestrahlung von zwei genau gegenüberliegenden Einfallsfeldern vom Unterbauch und vom Rücken im Becken ein durchstrahltes Volumen entsteht, das praktisch im Dosismaximum liegt. Die oberflächennahen Schichten werden geschont. Bei der Bestrahlung mit Telekobalt-γ-Strahlen unter gleichen Bedingungen muß man bereits in Körpermitte einen „Durchhang" bis auf die 80%-Isodose in Kauf nehmen. Wesentlich ungünstiger sind die Verhältnisse bei der 200-kV-Röntgenstrahlung, wo der Herd im Körperinnern nur in der 50%-Isodose liegt und das Maximum in die Hautoberfläche verlagert ist (Abb. 50).

Während von Fletcher u. Mitarb. bei der Bestrahlung des Collumcarcinoms mit 22-MeV-Röntgenstrahlen die „whole pelvis technique" (Abb. 51) verwandt wird und lediglich bei der Kombination mit einer lokalen Radiumtherapie die Beckenmitte durch Blei abgedeckt wird, untersuchten Schubert, Schmermund und Oberheuser die Dosisverteilung bei einer 4-Felder-Stehfeldtechnik (Abb. 52).

Eine besondere Form der Bewegungsbestrahlung mit ultraharten Röntgenstrahlen des Betatrons, einer als Schalenbestrahlung bezeichneten Pendelung mit exzentrisch gelegener Pendelachse, wurde durch orientierende Messungen von Becker und Weitzel (1956) sowie Schmermund und Oberheuser (1958) aufgezeigt. Systematische Untersuchungen über die Pendelbestrahlung mit exzentrisch gelegener Pendelachse der ultraharten Röntgenstrahlen wurden von Heinzler (1965) durchgeführt. Er schuf die Voraussetzung zur Errechnung der Herddosis. Durch die Bewegungsbestrahlung ergibt sich die Möglichkeit, eine praktisch beliebig hohe Dosis auf einen verhältnismäßig kleinen Raum zu konzentrieren, was bei der Behandlung des Collumcarcinoms in speziellen Fällen durchaus wünschenswert ist (Vieten und Heinzler, 1966).

Über die größten Erfahrungen mit der Betatronbehandlung des Collumcarcinoms verfügen FLETCHER u. Mitarb. (1962). Sie behandelten in den Jahren 1954—1958 über 750 Collumcarcinome und verglichen die Behandlungsergebnisse mit einem etwa gleichartigen Patientengut der Jahre 1948—1954. Die Behandlungsmethode differiert nur durch die Art der Percutanbestrahlung.

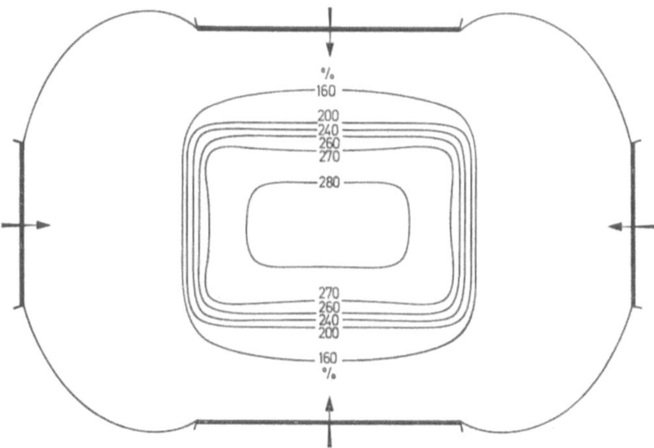

Abb. 51. „Whole Pelvis Technique" bei der Therapie mit 22-MeV-Röntgenstrahlen, je ein anteriores und posteriores Feld (15×15 cm) und 2 laterale Felder (15×9 cm), FHA 100 cm (FLETCHER, RUTLEDGE und CHAU)

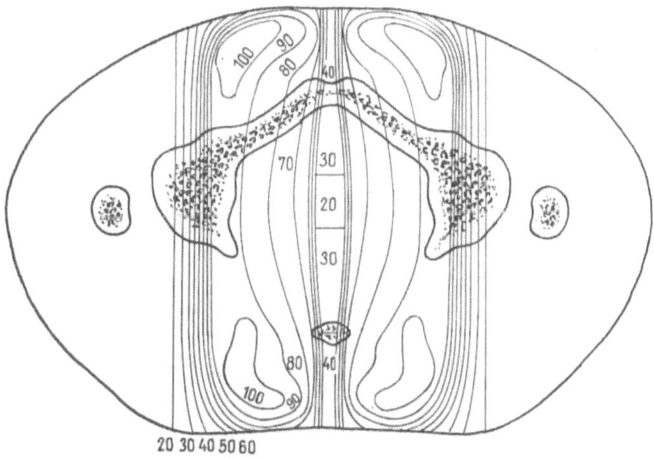

Abb. 52. Isodosen von 15-MeV-Röntgenstrahlen, a.p. Durchmesser 25 cm, 2 Unterbauch- und Glutaealfelder, Feldgröße 6,5×12 cm. Zentralstrahl seitlich zur Beckenwand hin ausgelenkt, Focus-Haut-Abstand 43 cm (SCHMERMUND et al.)

Wegen der wichtigen Aussage der Behandlungsergebnisse bei diesem einmalig großen Patientengut wird die stark individualisierte Strahlenbehandlung in bezug auf das Ausbreitungsstadium des Collumcarcinoms in Tabelle 13 dargestellt. Die percutane Strahlenbehandlung kombinieren FLETCHER u. Mitarb. mit einer lokalen Radiumtherapie bei der es sich um eine modifizierte Manchester-Methode handelt. Bei einer Dosierung von 9000—10000 mgeh (Stadium IB) wird an den Obturatorlymphknoten eine maximale Dosis von etwa 2000 R wirksam, an den externen iliacalen und hypogastrischen Lymphknoten 1000 R. Percutan werden über 15×15 cm große Felder Dosen von 1000 rad pro Woche eingestrahlt, die gut vertragen werden.

Tabelle 13. *Behandlungsmethode des Collumcarcinoms durch 22-MeV-Röntgenstrahlen und intrakavitäre Radiumtherapie* (Fletcher, Rutledge und Chau)

	Lesion	Treatment
Stage I$_A$	≤ 1 cm in diameter	radium only—[a] maximum 10000 mg-h
Stage I$_B$	> 1 cm in diameter or two or more positive quadrant biopsies	radium 9000—10000 mg-h[b]: parametrial irradiation—3000–4000 rads[c]
Stage II$_A$	medial parametrial involvement and or spread to upper two-thirds vagina exceptions: (I$_B$–II$_A$)	treatment same as stage I$_B$
	bulky exophytic lesions, or unfavorable anatomy for radium system-(narrow vault-short uterine canal-asymmetrical fornices)	2000 rads whole pelvis irradiation first: 8000–9000 mg-h[b] radium: then 1000–2000 rads[c] additional to parametria (4 cm central shielding) or 3500 rads whole pelvis irradiation: 500 rads additional to parametria (4 cm central shielding) 5500–6500 mg-h radium[b]
Stage II$_B$	lateral parametrial involvement (with or without upper vaginal extension): or massive involvement of corpus (barrel saphe)[d]	3500 rads whole pelvis irradiation: 500 rads additional parametrial irradiation (with 4 cm central shielding: 5500–6500 mg-h radium[b]
Stage III$_A$	one pelvic wall or lower one-third vagina favorable: one wall involved-not massively-and primary not too massive	4000 rads whole pelvis irradiation-radium 5500–6500 mg-h[b] 1000–1500 rads[c] added on side involved (15 × 6 cm portal)
	unfavorable: more disease than above-still confined to this stage	5000 rads whole pelvis irradiation: radium 4000–5000 mg-h[b] possibly added 1000 rads (15 × 6 cm portal) on side involved
Stage III$_B$	both pelvic walls or one wall plus lower one-third of vagina or	6000 rads[e] whole pelvis irradiation: radium 3000–4000 mg-h[b]
Stage IV	invasion of bladder and or rectum	7000 rads[e] whole pelvis irradiation

[a] Provided there is optimal geometry otherwise external irradiation is used to build up the dose to the paracervical areas. The low incidence of nodal metastases ($< 5\%$) in these early lesions does not warrant routine parametrial irradiation.

[b] The larger figures for radium dose are used in lesions which are more infiltrative, endocervical or have not clinically disappeared at the time of the first radium.

[c] Dose aim for parametrial irradiation depends upon: 1) Extent of disease; 2) Adequacy of the radium system; 3) Location of the radium system within the pelvis. With a moderately high radium system (ovoids superimposed on superior acetabular rims on lateral radiograph) 4000 mg-h contribute 1000 rads to the obturator node at the lateral pelvic wall.

[d] With adenocarcinomas and with large endocervical squamous cell carcinomas regressing slowly, a hysterectomy is performed (10 days to 6 weeks) after completing radiation therapy. A maximum of 5000 mg-h radium is used in cases to be treated by hysterectomy.

[e] After 5000 rads to whole pelvis, the pelvic fields should be reduced to 12 × 12 cm parallel opposing portals and to 10 × 10 cm above 6000 rads.

Die Behandlungsergebnisse zeigen, daß in allen Stadien die 5-Jahres-Überlebenszeit um einige Prozent im Vergleich zur Behandlungsperiode mit konventionellen Röntgenstrahlen verbessert werden konnte (Tabelle 14).

Ähnlich gute Behandlungsergebnisse konnten an der Universitäts-Frauenklinik Hamburg erzielt werden. Nachdem im Jahre 1956 die percutane Strahlenbehandlung von konventionellen Röntgenstrahlen auf ultraharte Röntgenstrahlen eines 15-MeV-Betatrons

Table 14. *Behandlungsergebnisse der Patientinnen mit einem Collumcarcinom nach intrakavitärer Radiumeinlage in Kombination mit Orthovolttherapie oder 22-MeV-Röntgenstrahlen* (FLETCHER, RUTLEDGE und CHAU)

	Stage	Before supervoltage 1948 to september 1954		Supervoltage 1954 to september 1958	
		no treated	survived 5 years %	no treated	survived 5 years %
All squamous cell carcinomas on intact uteri[a]	I	64	90 ($\pm$ 3.6)[a]	117	93 ($\pm$ 2.4)[a]
	II$_A$	129	80 ($\pm$ 3.5)	106	83 ($\pm$ 3.9)
	II$_B$	123	60 ($\pm$ 4.4)	114	73 ($\pm$ 4.2)
	all stages II	252	70 ($\pm$ 2.9)	220	78 ($\pm$ 3.0)
	III$_A$	93	44 ($\pm$ 5.3)	130	56 ($\pm$ 4.7)
	III$_B$	87	31 ($\pm$ 4.9)	148	38 ($\pm$ 4.2)
	all stages III[b]	180	37 ($\pm$ 3.6)	278	46 ($\pm$ 3.2)
	IV	19	5 ($\pm$ 5.1)	37	14 ($\pm$ 6.4)
	all stages	515	59 ($\pm$ 2.2)	652	63 ($\pm$ 2.0)
Pregnancy and up to one year post-partum[c]	all stages	30	40.5 ($\pm$ 9.2)	44	55.5 ($\pm$ 6.4)
Squamous cell carcinomas of stump[d]	all stages	46	61 ($\pm$ 7.2)	51	63 ($\pm$ 8.9)
Adenocarcinomas[e]	all stages	12	50 ($\pm$ 14.4)	27	85 ($\pm$ 7.1)

[a] ($\pm$) Standard error. Prepared, according to Berkson-Gage methol, by MARY C. MACDONALD, Biometrician in the Section of Radiotherapy.

[b] The greatest increase in survival rate is in the Stage III cases. The survival rates for Stage I, II$_A$ and Stage IV cases are relatively unchanged.

About 30% of the Stage IV intact uterus cases in the presupervoltage series were considered worth treating, whereas approximately 45% of the Stage IV cases were treated in the supervoltage series. The absolute survival rate in Stage IV cases with intact uterus is 1.5% in the presupervoltage series and 8% in the supervoltage series.

There are two possible reasons for the apparent discrepancy between the increase in survival rates for each stage and the over-all survival rates: 1) 14.5% of the patients in the presupervoltage series were not treated, compared with 11% in the supermoderately advanced cases, *i.e.*, the Stage II$_B$ and Stage III$_A$ cases, which are most benetited.

[c] The pregnancy and postpartum cases are included in the group of squamous cell carcinomas on intact uteri.

[e] There is no difference in survival rates for all stages of the stump carcinomas. The proportion of Stage III cases is greater in the supervoltage group.

[d] The improvement in survival rates for the small group of adenocarcinomas in the supervoltage group may be partially attributed to the fact that hysterectomies had been performed when possible.

umgestellt wurde, konnten bis 1960 157 Patientinnen mit einem primären Collumcarcinom einer ausschließlichen Strahlenbehandlung in Kombination mit Radium unterzogen werden.

Die Behandlungsergebnisse sind in den in Tabelle 11b aufgeführten Zahlen enthalten. Sie unterscheiden sich von den nach Telekobalttherapie erzielten Ergebnisse nicht.

Im Stadium I ist somit durch die Erhöhung der parametranen Herddosis eine Verbesserung der Behandlungsergebnisse nicht erreicht worden und erscheint auch unwahrscheinlich, da der Tumor durch die lokale Radiumbestrahlung voll erfaßt wird. Die percutane Dosiserhöhung könnte sich nur günstig auf eine möglicherweise diskontinuierlich ausgebreitete Lymphknotenmetastasierung auswirken. Bei den fortgeschrittenen Stadien, bei denen der Tumor nicht mehr ausreichend von der Radium-γ-Strahlung erfaßt wird, wäre theoretisch durch die Dosiserhöhung eine Verbesserung der Resultate zu erwarten, die durch die erzielten Behandlungsergebnisse bestätigt wird.

Bei der Kombination einer lokalen Radiumtherapie und einer hochdosierten percutanen Strahlenbehandlung mit 15-MeV-Röntgenstrahlen ist eine Dosisabstimmung beider Strahlenarten unerläßlich. Schmermund, Oberheuser und Kuttig (1961) untersuchten die Dosisverteilung bei einer Stehfeldbestrahlung über 4 Felder, bei der der Zentralstrahl seitlich zur Beckenwand hin ausgelenkt wird, in Kombination mit einer lokalen, intracervicalen Radiumeinlage von 4000 mgeh. Sie konnten zeigen, daß sowohl bei einer exakten Mittellage des Uterus mit dem Radium (Abb. 53a) als auch bei einer Verlagerung des Uterus um 2 cm zur Beckenwand hin (Abb. 53b) im Parametrium eine wünschenswerte Dosisverteilung erzielt werden kann, bei der Dosisspitzen oder Unterdosierungen vermieden werden. Da bei der von ihnen angegebenen Technik das gesamte kleine Becken fast homogen mit einer Dosis von 4000—5000 R durch die Percutanbestrahlung belastet

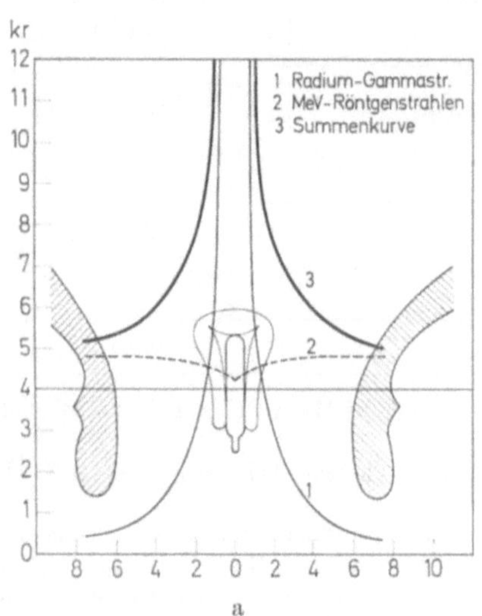
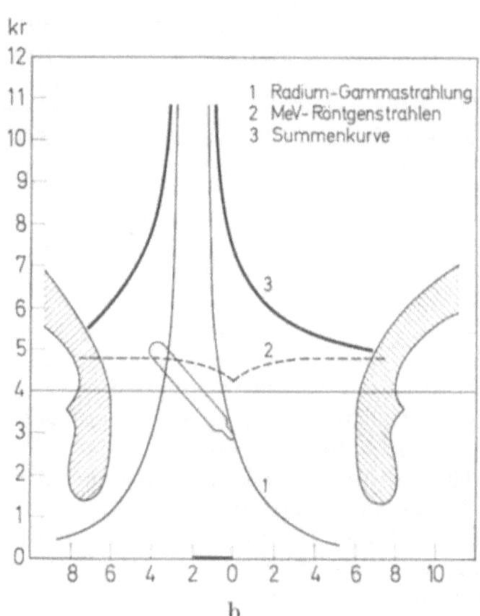

Abb. 53. a Dosisverteilung in den Parametrien bei kombinierter Bestrahlung mit 4600 R Herd, 15-MeV-Röntgenstrahlen und 4000 mgeh Radium intracervical. b Dosisverteilung in den Parametrien unter gleichen Bestrahlungsbedingungen. Verlagerung des Uterus um 2 cm nach rechts (Schmermund und Kuttig)

wird (s. Dosiskurve in Abb. 53a und b), braucht mit über- oder unterdosierten Regionen auch nicht gerechnet zu werden. Es würden sich allerdings andere Dosisverhältnisse ergeben, wenn durch die percutanen Strahlenfelder in Beckenmitte eine einige Zentimeter breite Region ausgespart werden würde, wie es zur Schonung von Blasenhinterwand und Rectumvorderwand notwendig wäre.

Über die beobachteten Komplikationen bei der hochdosierten Beckenbestrahlung beim Collumcarcinom nach 22-MeV-Röntgenstrahlen am M.D. Anderson Hospital and Tumor Institute, Houston, berichten ausführlich Chau, Fletcher, Rutledge und Dodd (1962). Bei den 741 Patientinnen beobachteten sie folgende schweren Strahlenkomplikationen: Proktitis, mit Tenesmen intermittierenden Diarrhöen und rectalen Blutungen 0,8%, Rectumulcerationen 0,6%, Rectosigmoiditis 4,3%, schwere Dysurie 1,4%, Blasenulcera 1,1%, vesicovaginale, ureterovaginale und rectovaginale Fisteln 1,6%. Im Vergleich von Behandlungskomplikationen bei den konventionell bestrahlten Patientinnen ergab sich nur bei der Rectosigmoiditis eine Häufigkeitszunahme. Die Autoren konnten zeigen, daß nach einer „whole pelvis irradiation" von 4000 rad und einer zusätzlichen Radiumdosierung von 5500—6500 mgeh nur selten Komplikationen auftreten und operative Eingriffe nach der Strahlentherapie durchführbar sind. Eine „whole pelvis irradiation" von 6000 rad und in den fortgeschrittenen Fällen von 7000 rad ist ebenfalls gerechtfertigt. In diesen Fällen sollte ein operativer Eingriff nur bei einer Strahlenresistenz oder einem Rezidiv durchgeführt werden, da sonst die Rate der Behandlungskomplikationen auf etwa 20% ansteigt.

Auch am Patientengut der Universitäts-Frauenklinik Hamburg ergab ein Vergleich der Behandlungskomplikationen nach konventioneller Strahlentherapie und Megavolttherapie keine sichere Zunahme schwerer Strahlenfolgen trotz Erhöhung der Herddosis. Eine Gegenüberstellung der Komplikationen an Blase, ableitenden Harnwegen, Darm und Knochen zeigt, daß bei beiden Behandlungsmethoden an der Blase und den ableitenden Harnwegen Behandlungskomplikationen in einer Häufigkeit von etwa 2% auftraten. Lediglich mittelschwere Darmreaktionen, zu denen Stenosen und Ulcera gerechnet wurden, fand man nach konventioneller Röntgentherapie in 3% der Fälle und nach Megavolttherapie in 9%. Die Häufigkeit schwerer Darmreaktionen, hierzu wurden Rectum-Scheiden-Fisteln und operativ zu beseitigende Stenosen gerechnet, betrug bei beiden Patientengruppen etwa 2%. Radiogen bedingte Frakturen wurden bei dem allerdings größeren konventionell bestrahlten Patientengut in 3 Fällen beobachtet; derartige Komplikationen traten nach Megavolttherapie nicht auf.

Auch BECKER u. Mitarb. (1961) konnten nach Strahlendosen von etwa 8000 rad in Beckenmitte und etwa 5000—6000 rad seitlich in den Parametrien nur verhältnismäßig geringe Nebenerscheinungen beobachten. Als Vorteil geben sie an, daß die besonders quälenden Frühreaktionen an Blase und Rectum kaum eine Rolle spielen und die sonst gefürchteten exsudativen Hauterscheinungen mit schlechter Heilungstendenz ausbleiben.

Zu ähnlichen Ergebnissen kommt auch SCHINZ (1958), der deshalb die Betatronquantentherapie als Therapie der Wahl bei Tumoren der weiblichen Genitalorgane in allen Stadien ansieht.

Da ein beträchtlicher Anteil der Collumcarcinome der Stadien I und II ungünstig lokale Voraussetzungen für die primäre intrakavitäre Radiumtherapie bietet und Lokalrezidive Folge von „cold spots" sind (SHERMAN, 1961), halten FLETCHER, WATANAVIT und RUTLEDGE (1966) in solchen Fällen eine „whole pelvis irradiation" mit 4000 rad als primäre Behandlung, der dann erst eine lokale Radiumtherapie mit 4000—7000 mgeh folgt, für angezeigter. Hiermit wollen sie erreichen, daß durch die Percutanbestrahlung der Tumorprozeß bis zur Reichweite der Radiumstrahlung schrumpft. Als Indikation hierzu werden angesehen: conisch verengte, atrophische Vagina, Zustand nach Perforation oder Konisation, exophytische oder asymmetrische Portiotumoren, vaginale Tumorinfiltrationen, parametrane Infiltrationen, massive endocervicale Ausbreitung des Tumors, Collumcarcinom in der Schwangerschaft oder im Verlauf eines Jahres nach der Schwangerschaft und das Cervixstumpfcarcinom. FLETCHER u. Mitarb. übersehen ein Patientengut von 280 auf diese Weise behandelten Collumcarcinomen der Stadien I und II, bei denen sie in etwa 10% der Fälle temporäre Hämaturien, Diarrhöen oder rectale Blutungen sahen. Aufgrund der Behandlungskomplikationen führen sie seit 1964 die „whole pelvis technique" nur bis zu 3500 rad durch und applizieren die letzten 500 rad unter Abdeckung einer 4 cm breiten Region über dem Uterus. In ausgewählten Fällen kann nach einer derartigen Therapie eine konservative Hysterektomie durchgeführt werden. Eine Lymphonodektomie wird wegen schwerer Behandlungsfolgen abgelehnt.

γγ) Therapie mit anderen Strahlenarten

Energiereiche Elektronen fanden bei der Behandlung des Collumcarcinoms bisher nur ganz vereinzelt Anwendung, da hierzu nur selten eine Indikation besteht. Lediglich bei voluminösen, exophytisch wachsenden Portiocarcinomen können durch eine fraktionierte Elektronenbestrahlung bessere Bedingungen für die Zugängigkeit des Cervicalkanals zur Radiumtherapie geschaffen werden.

Eine weitere Indikation kann ein Collumcarcinom in der Schwangerschaft darstellen, wenn beispielsweise von der Patientin eine Interruptio verweigert wird. Unter bestimmten Voraussetzungen (s. Kap. 6, S. 241) kann dann bei Verwendung hoher Elektronenenergien eine Heilung ermöglicht werden.

SCHUBERT, SCHMERMUND und OBERHEUSER (1959) haben in einigen Fällen den Versuch unternommen, das Oberflächencarcinom an der Portio mit schnellen Elektronen zu behandeln. Sie verwandten zur Direktbestrahlung der Portio einen speziellen Scheidentubus. Die Ergebnisse waren zufriedenstellend. Es wird aber darauf hingewiesen, daß in diesen Fällen der kleine operative Eingriff in Form einer Portioamputation nur selten kontraindiziert ist und daß auch eine niedrig dosierte Radiumtherapie ausgezeichnete

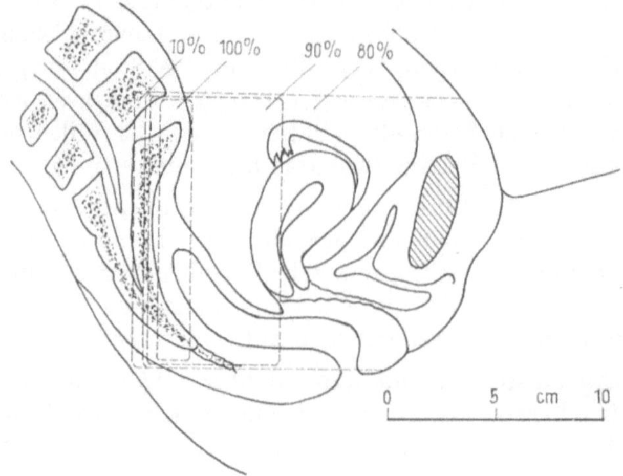

Abb. 54. Dosisverteilung bei einer 185-MeV-Protonenstrahlung (FORS et al.)

Erfolge bringt. Lediglich in Fällen, in denen beispielsweise bei jüngeren Frauen die Ovarialfunktion nicht in Mitleidenschaft gezogen werden soll, kann eine Elektronentherapie angezeigt sein.

Gute Ergebnisse konnte KOTTMEIER (1965) mit einer intravaginalen Elektronenbestrahlung bei Patientinnen mit einem Collumcarcinom und paravaginaler Ausbreitung beobachten. Die an 31 Patientinnen erzielten Behandlungsergebnisse waren nach einer Periode von 3—6 Jahren ermutigend. Die Elektronenbestrahlung wurde mit einer Dosis von 3500 rad in einer Tiefe von 3 cm in 7—10 Einzelsitzungen mit einem Spezialtubus durchgeführt. KOTTMEIER glaubt, daß diese Behandlungsmethode mehr als die früheren zu leisten vermag.

Über erste Erfahrungen mit der Anwendung eines 70-MeV-Synchrotrons bei der Behandlung von Collumcarcinomen berichten STONE und LOUIE (1964). Die Überlebenszeiten unterschieden sich nicht wesentlich von den üblichen Behandlungsergebnissen.

Die erste Mitteilung über die Wirkung hochenergetischer Protonen auf das Genitalcarcinom des Menschen erfolgte von FORS, LARSSON, LINDELL, NAESLUND und STENSON (1964). Sie behandelten 10 fortgeschrittene Fälle von Collumcarcinom mit einer Protonenbestrahlung und bestätigen die schon früher gemachte Erfahrung, daß es durch eine einmalige Dosis von 3000 rad Protonenstrahlung gelingt, ein Plattenepithelcarcinom zur völligen Rückbildung zu bringen. In 2 Fällen konnte ein histologisch verifiziertes Plattenepithelrezidiv nach Radium- und Röntgenbestrahlung geheilt werden, wie sich bei der späteren Obduktion ergab. Die Dosisverteilung bei einer 185-MeV-Protonenstrahlung zeigt Abb. 54. Inwieweit es gelingt, den technischen Aufwand zu überwinden, um die Therapie auf breiter Basis durchführen zu können, bleibt abzuwarten.

5. Bestrahlung des Cervixstumpfcarcinoms

Wenn auch für die Behandlung des Cervixstumpfcarcinoms nach supravaginaler Uterusamputation im allgemeinen die gleichen Gesichtspunkte wie für das Collumcarcinom gelten, sind die topographischen Voraussetzungen für eine Strahlenbehandlung doch wesentlich ungünstiger, weil in vielen Fällen eine intracervicale Radiumeinlage nicht möglich ist. Durch die zur Deckung des Wundgebietes über den Cervixstumpf gezogene Blase oder durch postoperative Darmadhäsionen ist bei einer vaginalen und vor allem intracervicalen Radiumeinlage mit einer starken Dosisbelastung beider Organe zu rechnen.

Die Radiumbehandlung muß beim Cervixstumpfcarcinom den individuellen Verhältnissen angepaßt werden, wobei den Momentandosismessungen in Blase und Rectum hinsichtlich der Wahl der zu applizierenden Dosishöhe eine entscheidende Bedeutung zukommt. HOFMANN (1964) empfiehlt, das obere Ende des Trägers mit Phantomröhrchen zu laden, um eine umschriebene hohe Belastung des Blasenbodens ausschließen zu können. Bei kürzeren Stümpfen gelingt es oft nur knapp, die kürzesten Radiumstifte intracervical einzulegen. In solchen Fällen wird von vielen einem operativen Verfahren der Vorzug gegeben, wobei einfache vaginale oder abdominale Exstirpation, Wertheimsche oder Schautasche erweiterte Radikaloperation durchgeführt werden (JOUNG, 1953; ANZILOTTI und MARTOLINI, 1962; OZSVÁTH, 1965).

CAULK (1954) konnte die Behandlungsergebnisse beim Stumpfcarcinom durch eine transvaginale Röntgenbestrahlung verbessern und eine absolute Heilung von 64 % erzielen. Durch eine kombinierte lokale und percutane Strahlenbehandlung konnte auch BAUD (1952) bei 124 Cervixstumpfcarcinomen (4,6 % bezogen auf alle Collumcarcinome) Behandlungsergebnisse erreichen, die denen der übrigen Collumcarcinome entsprachen. RIES und BREITNER (1959), die nur bei primär hochsitzenden Collumstumpfcarcinomen und besonders beim Adenocarcinom eine cervicale Dosis bis zur äußersten Grenze der Toleranz wählten, heilten von 67 Collumstumpfcarcinomen 52,2 %.

Eine entscheidende Verbesserung der Dosisverteilung ist durch Anwendung von Megavoltenergien zu erwarten, bei der das gesamte kleine Becken durch eine homogene Tumordosis erfaßt werden kann und nur durch eine intravaginale Radiumeinlage eine zusätzliche Dosisspitze am Primärtumor geschaffen wird. An dieser Stelle sei auf die Behandlungsvorschläge von FLETCHER u. Mitarb. (1966) verwiesen, die beim Cervixstumpfcarcinom mit einer ,,whole pelvis irradiation'' 4 000 rad applizieren und die Dosis durch eine spätere Radiumeinlage ergänzen (s. S. 234).

6. Bestrahlung des Collumcarcinoms in der Schwangerschaft und im Wochenbett

Bei der Behandlung des Collumcarcinoms in der Schwangerschaft divergieren die Ansichten über die optimale Methode beträchtlich. Von der primären operativen Behandlung (HUBER und BESSERER, 1952; BEUTHE, 1962; FAUVET, 1966) über die Kombination von Operation und Nachbestrahlung (MAINO und MUSSEY, 1944; STUTZER, 1946; EYMER, 1953; RIES und BREITNER, 1959; BICKENBACH und SOOST, 1960; TWOMBLY, 1963; PRATT und MALKASIAN, 1964; HITTMAIR, 1967) bis zur ausschließlichen Bestrahlung (BAUD und BLANCHET, 1952; McGREE und SALA, 1960; PEAKE, 1960; SCHUBERT, 1960; GUSTAFSSON und KOTTMEIER, 1962; LUCCI, 1962; WALDROP und PALMER, 1963; BOSCH und MARCIAL, 1966; PREM, MAKOWSKI und McKELVEY, 1966; WATANAVIT und RUTLEDGE, 1966) sind alle möglichen Kombinationsformen vertreten.

Selbst ein erfahrener Kliniker verfügt daher nur über geringe eigene Beobachtungen. In jedem Einzelfall ist die schwierige Diskussion nicht zu umgehen, ob das Leben des Kindes geopfert werden muß, um die Überlebens- oder Heilungschance der Mutter zu verbessern. Hinzu kommt, daß durch die schwangerschaftsbedingten Gewebsveränderungen eine palpatorische Erfassung parametraner Carcinominfiltrationen erschwert oder manchmal sogar unmöglich wird, so daß sich oft unter den als lokal operabel beurteilten Befunden bereits fortgeschrittene Prozesse verbergen, für die im Grunde eine operative Behandlung nicht mehr indiziert ist. Andererseits ist die Radikaloperation durch die Schwangerschaftsauflockerung technisch leicht durchführbar, weshalb sie vielfach gegenüber der Strahlentherapie bevorzugt wird. So findet man im deutschsprachigen Schrifttum die Ansicht vorherrschend, daß die primäre Operation in der Schwangerschaft einer Bestrahlung vorzuziehen ist. Die Abwägung der Vor- oder Nachteile der einen oder anderen Behandlungsmethode erscheint müßig, da eine Gegenüberstellung der Behandlungsergebnisse nach Aufgliederung in die verschiedenen Behandlungsmethoden wegen der viel zu kleinen Fallzahl kein klareres Bild erbringt.

Unter dem Eindruck der unterschiedlichen Ansichten über eine optimale Behandlungsmethode des Collumcarcinoms in der Schwangerschaft erscheint es fast unmöglich, Behandlungsgrundsätze und Richtlinien aufzustellen. Trotzdem soll versucht werden, unter Berücksichtigung der von den einzelnen Autoren gesammelten Erfahrungen allgemein anerkannte Richtlinien zusammenzustellen.

Im *ersten Trimester der Schwangerschaft* sollte eine Radikaloperation nach WERTHEIM lediglich in den Fällen durchgeführt werden, die lokal sicher operabel sind. In Zweifelsfällen ist einer ausschließlichen Strahlenbehandlung der Vorzug zu geben, da, wie DU MESNIL DE ROCHEMONT (1958), SCHUBERT (1960) sowie KOTTMEIER (1964) zeigen konnten, die radiologischen Behandlungsmethoden zumindest die gleichen Ergebnisse erzielen wie die operativen Verfahren. Eine supravaginale Uterusamputation bei lokal inoperablen Fällen im ersten Trimester verbessert die Heilungsergebnisse keinesfalls. Die Strahlenbehandlung sollte mit einer intracervicalen Radiumeinlage eingeleitet werden, ohne die Schwangerschaft weiter zu berücksichtigen. Es kommt im Laufe der weiteren Strahlenbehandlung zur Ausstoßung der Frucht, oder der Uterus wird durch Curettage entleert. Wegen der ungünstigen Bedingungen durch den vergrößerten Uterus schlagen deshalb FLETCHER u. Mitarb. (1966) vor, mit der percutanen Strahlenbehandlung zu beginnen. Sie verwenden in diesen Fällen die „whole pelvis technique" mit 22-MeV-Röntgenstrahlen. RIES und BREITNER (1959) sowie BICKENBACH und SOOST (1960) beginnen mit einer vaginalen Radiumeinlage und einer Percutanbestrahlung gleichzeitig. Nachdem es nach 2—4 Wochen zur Spontanausstoßung der Frucht gekommen ist, vervollständigen sie die Radiumapplikation auch durch eine intracervicale Radiumeinlage.

Verfechter der vaginalen Operationsmethode beim Collumcarcinom (FAUVET, 1966) halten die Radikaloperation nach AMREICH unter Belassung der beiden Adnexe für vorteilhafter, da in diesen Fällen, wenn eine postoperative Bestrahlung nach histologischer Beurteilung des Operationspräparates nicht notwendig ist, eine Kastration der Frauen vermeidbar ist.

Für das *zweite Schwangerschaftstrimester* gelten in etwa die gleichen Bedingungen. Von den operativ eingestellten Gynäkologen wird die Frage der Operabilität allerdings in diesem Stadium vorsichtiger und zurückhaltender gestellt. Einer Strahlenbehandlung wird vielfach der Vorzug gegeben. Um bessere Bedingungen für die Radiumtherapie zu bekommen, wird eine supracervicale Uterusamputation gegebenenfalls nach einer Radiumvorbehandlung empfohlen, bei der gleichzeitig auch die Anhänge mitentfernt werden. Die weitere Strahlenbehandlung gestaltet sich nach den gleichen Grundsätzen wie beim Cervixstumpfcarcinom. Ein Hinausschieben der Behandlung in diesem Stadium im Hinblick auf die Lebenserhaltung des Kindes erscheint in keinem Fall gerechtfertigt. Der Arzt sollte von der bestmöglichen Heilungschance für die Mutter ausgehen, die durch ein weiteres Zeitversäumnis erheblich verschlechtert wird. Auch in diesem Stadium ist bei Verwendung von Megavoltenergien ein Behandlungsbeginn mit einer homogenen Percutanbestrahlung des gesamten Beckens ratsam und vorteilhaft.

Schwieriger wird die Situation, wenn im *dritten Schwangerschaftstrimester* das Kind noch nicht lebensfähig ist. Man glaubt, den Behandlungsbeginn um 2 oder 3 Wochen hinausschieben zu können, ohne die Prognose für die kranke Mutter signifikant zu verschlechtern. Darüber hinaus ist eine Verzögerung des Behandlungsbeginns für das Leben der Mutter nicht zu verantworten. Vor dem Versuch, strahlentherapeutische Maßnahmen unter Aufrechterhaltung des kindlichen Lebens zu beginnen, wurde mehrfach gewarnt. Ob es möglich ist, wie RIESCH sowie BICKENBACH und SOOST glauben, eine lokale Radiumbestrahlung mit monelgefiltertem Radium vornehmen zu können und dabei den kindlichen Schädel vor der Behandlung hochzuschieben und durch Bandagen von der Strahlenquelle fernzuhalten, erscheint sehr fraglich; entweder ist die Eindringtiefe der Strahlen zu gering oder aber die Behandlung ist mit erheblichen Gefahren für das Kind verbunden. Wenn auch einzelne Fälle beschrieben worden sind, bei denen gesunde Kinder auf diese Weise geboren wurden, die selbst über mehrere Jahre keine Folgeerscheinungen zeigten, so muß doch an die Untersuchungen von GOLDSTEIN und MURPHY (1929) erinnert werden, die bei 51% der Kinder von Frauen, die in der Schwangerschaft eine Strahlenbehandlung erhalten hatten, Entwicklungs- und Gesundheitsstörungen nachweisen konnten, wie Mikrocephalie, Idiotie, Mikrophthalmie, Katarakt und Skeletschädigungen. Wenn bei solchen Kindern bereits bei der Geburt eine parietale Alopecie infolge der Strahleneinwirkung besteht und diese Alopecie sich auch nach 2 Monaten wieder zurückgebildet hat (DE LEEUW, 1964), so kann selbst durch eine 5jährige Nachbeobachtungszeit bei unauffälliger Entwicklung des Kindes über bereits bestehende und sich erst später manifestierende cerebrale Defekte keine Aussage gemacht werden. Die von KOK (1964) vertretene Ansicht, daß im 3. Schwangerschaftstrimester bei Lebenserhaltung des Kindes mit einer Bestrahlung begonnen werden soll, bei der die Strahlenbelastung des Kindes durch Vergrößerung der räumlichen Entfernung des Kindes von der Bestrahlungsquelle oder durch Wendung in Steißlage verringert werden soll, wird wegen der daraus resultierenden Gefahren entschieden abgelehnt.

Eine ärztlich vertretbare Strahlenbehandlung bei Lebenserhaltung der Frucht ergibt sich nur bei Anwendung einer lokalen Elektronenstrahlung, bei der die Eindringtiefe durch einen starken Dosisabfall sehr begrenzt ist. So berichten 1959 BECKER, KÄRCHER und WEITZEL über die erfolgreiche Elektronenbestrahlung eines exophytisch wachsenden Plattenepithelcarcinoms der Portio in der Schwangerschaft. Da die Patientin die Schwangerschaft (mens VIII) nicht unterbrechen lassen wollte, kam eine übliche Radiumtherapie nicht in Betracht. Sie führten daher eine Elektronentherapie durch, bei der in 9 Sitzungen 5800 rad 8-MeV-Elektronen verabreicht wurden. Die 6 Wochen nach der Bestrahlung durchgeführte Schnittentbindung mit anschließender Radikaloperation nach WERTHEIM ergab eine Heilung. BECKER konnte 1964 mitteilen, daß sich das Kind körperlich und geistig normal entwickelt hatte und die Mutter rezidivfrei geblieben war. Über einen weiteren Fall einer erfolgreichen Elektronenbestrahlung im 4. Schwangerschaftsmonat mit einer Gesamtdosis von 5000 R innerhalb von 24 Tagen berichten COVA und MAESTRO (1964). Trotzdem sollte eine Strahlentherapie in der Schwangerschaft nur auf die seltenen Fälle beschränkt bleiben, in denen von der Mutter eine Interruptio entschieden abgelehnt wird.

Bei Lebensfähigkeit des Kindes sollte die Behandlung durch abdominale Schnittentbindung und supracervicale Uterusamputation nach PORRO beginnen. Die Uterusamputation erscheint schon wegen der möglichen Gefahren einer Infektion ratsam. Die wenige Tage später beginnende Strahlenbehandlung sollte entweder mit der percutanen Bestrahlung oder mit einer lokalen Radiumapplikation eingeleitet werden, wobei der percutanen Strahlenbehandlung der Vorzug gegeben wird, vor allem bei Verwendung von Megavoltenergien. Eine vaginale Entbindung bei Vorliegen eines Collumcarcinoms ist mit Gefahren wie massiver Blutung, Infektion und rascher Dissimination des Tumors verbunden. Wenn möglich, soll eine vaginale Entbindung deshalb vermieden werden.

Bei einer Zusammenstellung der im Schrifttum mitgeteilten Behandlungsergebnisse fällt auf, daß die Heilungsaussichten bei einem Collumcarcinom in der Schwangerschaft etwa denen außerhalb der Schwangerschaft entsprechen. Die 5-Jahres-Heilung liegt zwischen 50 % und 70 %. Hittmair (1967) konnte bei einer Zusammenstellung der Ergebnisse mehrerer Autoren eine 5-Jahres-Heilung von 63,6 % ermitteln. Er konnte ebenfalls zeigen, daß die Heilungsaussichten um so schlechter werden, je höher das Schwangerschaftsalter ist. So betrug die Heilung in dem 1.—4. Schwangerschaftsmonat 71,1 %, im 5.—7. Monat 58,3 und im 8.—10. Monat 53,3 %.

Wesentlich schlechter ist die Prognose bei den post partum behandelten Fällen. Bei 244 Fällen, bei denen das Carcinom erst nach Beendigung der Gravidität erkannt wurde, betrug die Heilung nur 35,6 % (Hittmair, 1967). Bosch und Marcial (1966) erklären diese schlechtere Prognose durch den ungünstigen Einfluß der vaginalen Spontangeburt auf die Tumorausbreitung. Hinzu kommt, daß ein Collumcarcinom unter und nach der Geburt wesentlich schwieriger diagnostiziert wird als in den ersten Schwangerschaftsmonaten, da einer postpartalen Blutung auch von seiten des Arztes wenig Bedeutung beigemessen wird. Obwohl die Carcinome, die post partum diagnostiziert werden, nicht immer einen ausgedehnteren Lokalbefund aufweisen, wird angenommen, daß die Involutionsvorgänge im Puerperium eine diskontinuierliche Ausbreitung zu begünstigen scheinen. Auch an eine Metastasierung auf dem Blutwege wäre zu denken. Unter diesen Umständen sollte die Indikation zu einem radikalen operativen Eingriff wesentlich zurückhaltender gestellt werden und der primären Strahlenbehandlung der Vorzug gegeben werden.

Zusammenfassend läßt sich sagen, daß im Interesse des mütterlichen Lebens das Collumcarcinom in der Schwangerschaft prinzipiell ohne Rücksicht auf die bestehende Schwangerschaft behandelt werden soll. Da sich die Strahlenempfindlichkeit des Collumcarcinoms in der Gravidität nicht von der außerhalb der Schwangerschaft unterscheidet (Baud und Blanchet, 1952), sollte man sich in allen fraglichen Fällen zugunsten einer ausschließlichen Strahlenbehandlung entschließen. Von extremen Einzelfällen abgesehen, soll der Grundsatz bestehen, daß ein Collumcarcinom auch unter Opferung der Schwangerschaft sobald wie möglich mit allen zur Verfügung stehenden Mitteln zu behandeln ist. Das Leben des Kindes sollte nicht durch fakultative Strahlenschäden oder gar eine insuffiziente Behandlung für die Mutter erkauft werden.

7. Beurteilung des Bestrahlungserfolges

Nach einer lokalen Radiumbehandlung des Collumcarcinoms vollziehen sich die makroskopisch sichtbaren Veränderungen an der Portio relativ schnell: die Blutungen sistieren durch die kaustische Wirkung, es stellen sich eitrige oder jauchende Sekretabgänge ein, noch längere Zeit wird der „Radiumschorf" in Form eines dünnflüssigen Fluors ausgeschieden. Selbst große Portiokrater reinigen sich oft rasch, und schon wenige Wochen nach der Behandlung haben sie sich durch sklerosierende Narbenbildungen vom Rand her verkleinert. Dabei verjüngt sich das Scheidengewölbe so stark, daß es zu einer Verklebung des Scheidenendes kommt. Die Verklebungen des Scheidenrohres lassen sich meistens nur unter minimaler Blutung durch den tastenden Finger lösen. Parametrane Tumorinfiltrationen bilden sich relativ langsam zurück. Sie erscheinen aber schon wenige Wochen nach der Behandlung glatter. Oft bleiben parametrane Narbenspangen nach einer Strahlenbehandlung erhalten.

Die subjektive Beurteilung der Tumorrückbildung durch Palpation und Inspektion ergibt leider keinen sicheren Anhalt dafür, ob eine volle Rückbildung des Tumorprozesses und insbesondere eine Dauerheilung erreicht worden ist. Seit langem versucht man daher, den Bestrahlungserfolg durch geeignete objektive Kriterien zu beurteilen.

Auf die verschiedenen mikroskopischen Veränderungen nach der Strahlenbehandlung eines Collumcarcinoms, denen ein breites Schrifttum gewidmet ist, kann in diesem Rahmen nicht eingegangen werden. Es sei auf die diesbezügliche Spezialliteratur verwiesen (siehe Chiari, in: Seitz und Amreich, Biologie und Pathologie des Weibes. Urban & Schwarzenberg, 1955).

Auf die Versuche, durch Serienbiopsien vor, während und nach der Strahlenbehandlung ein objektives Maß für die Reaktion des Cervixcarcinoms auf die Strahlenbehandlung und damit auf die Strahlensensibilität zu erhalten, wurde bereits bei der Besprechung der Strahlensensibilität der Collumcarcinome (s. S. 145) hingewiesen. Während einzelne Autoren glauben, die Ansprechbarkeit des Carcinoms auf die Strahleneinwirkung beurteilen zu können (GRÜNBERGER, 1952; WALTER et al., 1964), wiesen HERTIG und GORE (1962) darauf hin, daß zwischen der Tumormorphologie und der Reaktion auf die Bestrahlung nicht unbedingt Beziehungen bestehen. Strahlensensibilität bedeutet keinesfalls Radiokurabilität. HERTIG und GORE (1962) konnten allerdings feststellen, daß die Strahlenschädigung der Zellen bei guter Ansprechbarkeit 3mal so häufig wie bei schlechter Prognose ist.

Starke Beachtung fanden die cytologischen Untersuchungen von GRAHAM und GRAHAM bei der Beurteilung der Reaktion des Carcinoms auf die Strahlenbehandlung. Auch auf diese Untersuchungen wurde bereits bei der Besprechung der Strahlensensibilität des Collumcarcinoms hingewiesen. Neben der von ihnen angegebenen „sensitisation response" zur Beurteilung der Strahlensensibilität wurde von ihnen eine cytologische Methode zur Beurteilung der „radiation reaction" (RR) angegeben. Eine gute „radiation reaction" liegt nach ihren Angaben vor, wenn nach einer Probebestrahlung bei mindestens 75% der Vaginalepithelien Vacuolisierung, eine eindeutige quantitativ feststellbare Vergrößerung der Zellen, Kernvergrößerung, Kernveränderungen und Chromatinkondensation zu registrieren sind. Diese Untersuchungen wurden relativ schnell in die klinische Routine eingesetzt (MEIGS, 1956; INGIULLA und CENTARO, 1957), da man auf diese Weise glaubte, strahlenrefraktäre Fälle der Operation schon relativ früh zuführen und somit retten zu können. Weil mit einer solchen Untersuchungsmethode ein Wunschtraum der Strahlentherapeuten in Erfüllung gegangen wäre, bereits kurz nach der Strahlenbehandlung die erfolgreich bestrahlten Patientinnen von den strahlenresistenten Fällen trennen zu können, wurde die Methode in zahlreichen größeren Zentren angewandt. Aber schon bald zeigte sich, daß die Methode viel zu unsicher ist, um eine für klinische Belange genügend sichere prognostische Aussage zu erlangen (LIMBURG, NAPP und WILBRAND, 1952; BUTTENBERG, SCHÖNFELDER und STOLL, 1960). Andere Autoren fanden eine gute Übereinstimmung zwischen der direkten Strahlenreaktion und der klinischen Rückbildung und bestätigten auch durch spätere Behandlungsergebnisse den Wert dieses Tests (INGIULLA und CENTARO, 1957; MOORE, CHANG, SCOTT und MORTON, 1962).

Den entscheidenden Schlag versetzten RUBIO, HERTZBERG, KOTTMEIER, OLSSON und ZAJICEK (1965) der von GRAHAM und GRAHAM angegebenen Untersuchungsmethode. Sie untersuchten die Strahlenempfindlichkeit an 720 am Radiumhemmet behandelten Patientinnen mit einem Collumcarcinom. Nachdem vor Beginn dieser Untersuchungsreihen die mit der Durchführung betrauten Mitarbeiter für ein halbes Jahr an das Laboratorium von GRAHAM und GRAHAM geschickt wurden, um sich mit den Originalmethoden vollständig vertraut zu machen, kamen sie zu dem Ergebnis, daß sich zwischen der nach GRAHAM und GRAHAM geprüften Strahlenempfindlichkeit und der Prognose der bestrahlten Patientinnen kein Zusammenhang ergibt. Sie fanden auch keine Übereinstimmung zwischen Strahlenreaktion und Überlebensdauer. Eine gewisse bessere Übereinstimmung besteht lediglich bei den Patientinnen jenseits der Menopause.

Durch Serienbiopsien von der Cervix nach der ersten Radiumapplikation einen Monat lang wöchentlich und später monatlich, versuchten OSHITA, TAKEUCHI und ENDO (1964) die Strahlenansprechbarkeit beurteilen zu können. Meistens waren die Krebszellen innerhalb von 4 Wochen nach Beginn der Strahlentherapie vollständig zerstört. Der destruktive Prozeß begann gewöhnlich eine Woche nach der Therapie, wobei Keratinisierung, Pyknose und Schwellung der hyperchromatischen Kerne beobachtet werden konnten. Als strahlenresistent bezeichneten die Autoren ein Carcinom, wenn 3 Monate nach Ende der Therapie noch lebendes carcinomatöses Gewebe nachweisbar war. Ein Rezidiv wurde angenommen, wenn 6 Monate oder später nach ursprünglicher Ausheilung wieder Carcinomgewebe

16*

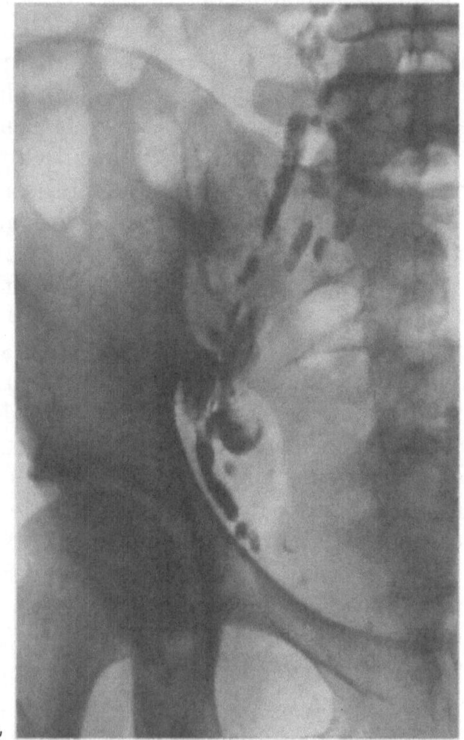
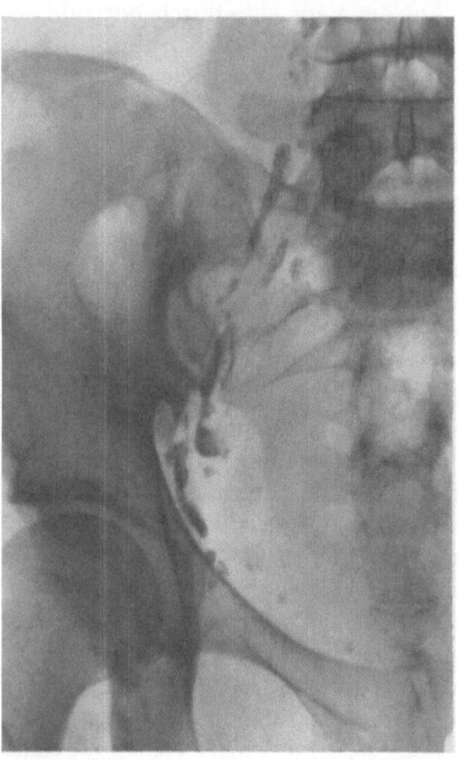

a

b

Abb. 55a u. b. Lymphographie bei einem Collumcarcinom Stadium III mit rechtsseitiger parametraner Infiltration bis zur Beckenwand. a Das Speicherbild vor Behandlungsbeginn ergibt eine iliacale Lymphknotenmetastasierung rechts. b Nach kombinierter Radium-Telekobalttherapie zeigt der metastatische Lymphknoten
eine Schrumpfung der Defektbildung

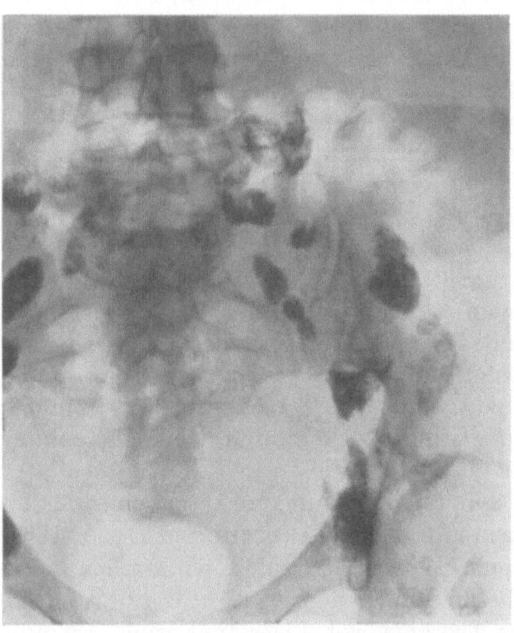
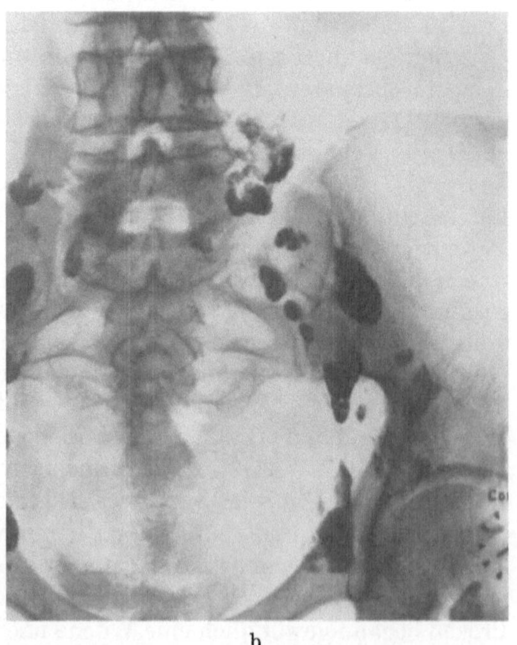

a

b

Abb. 56a u. b. Lymphographie bei einem Collumcarcinom Stadium III mit beidseitiger parametraner Infiltration. a Das Speicherbild ergibt eine ausgedehnte iliacale Lymphknotenmetastasierung links. b Kontrollaufnahme nach Beendigung einer biaxialen Telekobalt-Pendelbestrahlung. Herddosis im Bereich der linken
Beckenwand 5800 R. Es ist eine deutliche Rückbildung der Metastasierung zu erkennen

nachweisbar war. Durch diese Serienbiopsien wurden strahlenresistente Carcinome in 15,5% und Rezidive in 10% aller Fälle aufgedeckt. Aufgrund der ersten 4 Biopsien im 1. Behandlungsmonat hatten sie histologische Prognosen gestellt, die sich bei Patientinnen mit guter Prognose in 91,9% der Fälle und bei denen mit schlechter Prognose in 66,7% bewahrheiteten.

Eine weitere Möglichkeit zur Beurteilung des Behandlungserfolges ergibt sich durch eine lymphographische Verlaufskontrolle. Bei Vorliegen einer lymphographisch nachweisbaren Metastasierung mit Füllungsdefekt erkennt man nach einer wirkungsvollen Strahlenbehandlung eine Schrumpfungstendenz der Defektbildung und des ganzen Lymphknotens. Derartige Befunde sind den Abb. 55 und 56 zu entnehmen. Wenn auch an allen durch die Lymphographie markierten Lymphknoten innerhalb der ersten Tage und Wochen durch eine Entquellung eine Verkleinerung zu sehen ist, so sind doch Rückbildungen an bestrahlten Lymphknotenmetastasen deutlich davon zu unterscheiden. GERTEIS (1964) mißt der lymphographischen Kontrollmöglichkeit zur Beurteilung des Behandlungserfolges eine entscheidende Bedeutung bei. Er konnte an seinem Patientengut exakte Angaben über den Behandlungserfolg machen: in 64,3% der bestrahlten Fälle mit Lymphknotenmetastasen registrierte er eine Regression und in 35,7% eine Progression der Metastasierung.

8. Strahlenreaktionen und Strahlenfolgezustände

Aus didaktischen Gründen wäre es sinnvoll und notwendig, die möglichen Strahlenreaktionen an den verschiedenen Organen und die Strahlenfolgezustände nach Bestrahlung eines weiblichen Genitalcarcinoms durch Unterteilung in Früh- und Spätreaktionen getrennt abzuhandeln. Die Frühreaktionen unterscheiden sich von den Spätveränderungen wesentlich. Ihr Auftreten läßt sich typischen Phasen nach der Behandlung zuordnen. Die Frühreaktionen, die einen geringeren Schweregrad besitzen, sind oft reversibel, während die Strahlenspätreaktionen häufig irreversiblen Folgezuständen entsprechen. Eine scharfe Trennung der Früh- und Spätreaktionen läßt sich aber nicht generell durchführen. Wenn auch die meisten Strahlenfrühreaktionen innerhalb der ersten 3 Monate nach Beendigung der Strahlenbehandlung klinisch manifest werden, so können alle später auftretenden Reaktionen nicht als Spätkomplikationen aufgefaßt werden. Aber nicht nur in zeitlicher Hinsicht, sondern vor allem in bezug auf den Schweregrad und ihre Irreversibilität gibt es zwischen den Früh- und Spätreaktionen fließende Übergänge, die eine exakte Unterteilung unmöglich machen. Darüber hinaus entwickeln sich die Strahlenfolgezustände oft im Verlaufe eines längeren Intervalls aus einer Strahlenfrühreaktion. Die Spätreaktionen übertreffen aber meist die Intensität der Frühreaktion, um erst 1—2 Jahre später als Strahlenfolgezustände zu imponieren. Aus diesen Gründen soll in dieser Abhandlung lediglich eine Unterteilung der Strahlenreaktionen nach Organen vorgenommen werden.

Die nach einer speziellen Behandlung entstehenden Reaktionen sind bei der Besprechung der verschiedenen Bestrahlungsmethoden erwähnt.

a) Haut

Die bei der Percutanbestrahlung des Collumcarcinoms beobachteten Hautreaktionen entsprechen in ihrem Ablauf und Schweregrad den bekannten üblichen Reaktionen nach einer percutanen Strahlenbehandlung, die in einem speziellen Kapitel dieses Handbuches ausführlich abgehandelt sind. Es erübrigt sich daher, näher auf die Früh- und Spätreaktionen der Haut einzugehen.

b) Blase und ableitende Harnwege

Die subjektiven Beschwerden bei der Strahlenfrühreaktion an der *Blase* bestehen in Pollakisurie, Dysurie und Tenesmen. Sie werden durch eine mehr oder weniger ausgeprägte Cystitis hervorgerufen, die nur selten eine Therapie notwendig macht. Gelegentlich muß die Strahlenbehandlung unterbrochen werden. Die radiogene Cystitis ist meist eine Folge der Radiumapplikation, seltener der Percutanbestrahlung. Nach etwa 2 Monaten sind die cystitischen Beschwerden abgeklungen.

Bei der Cystoskopie findet man im akuten Stadium einer Frühreaktion eine hämorrhagische Entzündung. Neben der Rötung besteht ein subepitheliales Ödem vor allem im Trigonumbereich und am Blasenausgang.

Die Strahlenspätreaktionen übertreffen hinsichtlich ihrer klinischen Symptomatik an der Blase die Frühreaktionen. Wesentlich häufiger werden Blasenblutungen angegeben. Bei der Cystoskopie erkennt man meist im Bereich des Blasenbodens starke Ödembildungen mit ulcerösen, auf Berührung blutenden Prozessen. Es bestehen Fibrinauflagerungen, die teilweise zu Konkrementbildungen und Inkrustationen führen. Im weiteren Verlauf

Tabelle 15. *Strahlenveränderungen bzw. Strahlenfolgezustände an der Blase* (Ries)

1. Hämorrhagische Cystitis, eventuell mit Epitheldesquamation und fibrinöser Ausschwitzung
   a) akut
   b) chronisch

2. Bullöses Ödem mit mehr oder minder starker, chronisch entzündlicher Induration des Blasenbodens bzw. der Blasenwand, eventuell grobe breite Querfaltenbildung

3. Himbeerwärzchenbildung (ohne Ulcus)
   (Himbeerwärzchen = hypertrophierte frische Teleangiektasenbildung)

4. Ulcusbildung

5. Teleangiektasenbildung üblicher Art

6. Primäre Blasen-Scheiden-Fistel

7. Ulcusbildung infolge eines Kombinationsschadens
   Spätschäden — Spätulcera (Strahlennarbe + schwere infektiöse Cystitis, geplatzte Teleangiektasen + Infekt)

8. Dauerschäden am Schließmuskelapparat (narbige Schrumpfung und Sklerose, Harnaustreibungsschwäche [Incontinentia urinae]) auf dem Wege über die Stationen 2, 4, 7

kommt es zu umschriebenen Nekrosen und Ulcerationen, in deren Folge Blasen-Scheiden-Fisteln oder Narbenbildungen mit Schrumpfung der Blase auftreten. Den Spätreaktionen geht nicht generell eine Frühreaktion voraus, doch werden zumindest Frühreaktionen an anderen Organen beobachtet (Hofmann, 1963). Den Ablauf der Veränderungen an der Blase stellte Ries (1961) an Hand über 400 beobachteter Fälle zusammen (Tabelle 15). Die Spätreaktionen treten nach Monaten oder erst nach Jahren auf. Kottmeier (1964) konnte zeigen, daß die Strahlenveränderungen an der Blase später als am Rectum auftreten (Abb. 57).

Der Wert einer Gradeinteilung der Strahlenschäden wird immer wieder bezweifelt. Um jedoch Strahlenschäden vergleichen zu können, ist unter Vorbehalt eine Stadieneinteilung von Nutzen. So bezeichnet Kottmeier (1964) als Grad I jene Spätreaktionen, die nur mäßige subjektive Beschwerden und geringgradige objektive Veränderungen der Schleimhaut verursachen. Größere Bedeutung erlangen erst die Schweregrade II und III, die Kottmeier als Strahlenschäden zusammenfaßt. Als Stadium II bezeichnet er eine mehr oder weniger ausgedehnte Nekrosenbildung, die mit Blutungen oder Schmerzen einhergeht und eine stationäre Behandlung notwendig macht. In Gruppe III sind die mit Fistelbildungen einhergehenden Strahlenschäden enthalten. Der Zeitpunkt des Auftretens von Strahlenschäden am Patientengut des Radiumhemmet ist in Abb. 58 und die Häufigkeit in Abhängingkeit der in der Blase gemessenen Dosis in Tabelle 16 wiedergegeben.

Im Gegensatz zu den Blasenreaktionen verursachen ionisierende Strahlen am *Ureter* keine klinisch faßbaren Frühveränderungen. Trotzdem kommt es zu histologisch nachweisbaren Gefäßschädigungen, die einen Plasmaaustritt in den perivasalen Raum und das umgebende Bindegewebe hervorrufen (HOHENFELLNER, 1965). Dieses Strahlenfrühödem soll durch eine Schädigung der nervalen Gefäßreceptoren bedingt sein, die eine

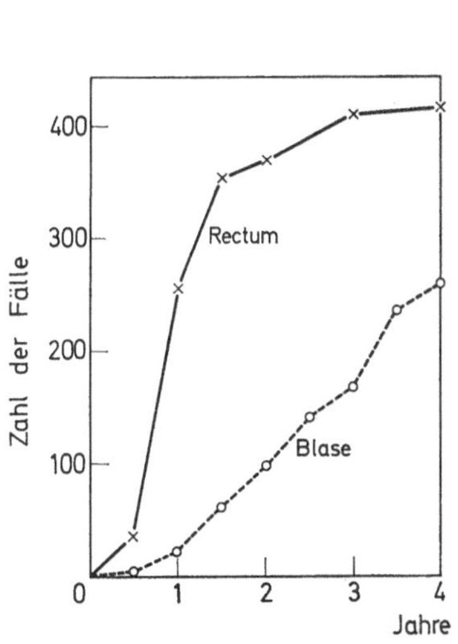

Abb. 57. Strahlenspätreaktion und Strahlenschäden am Rectum und in der Blase bei 3484 Patientinnen mit Collumcarcinom des Radiumhemmet 1949—1957

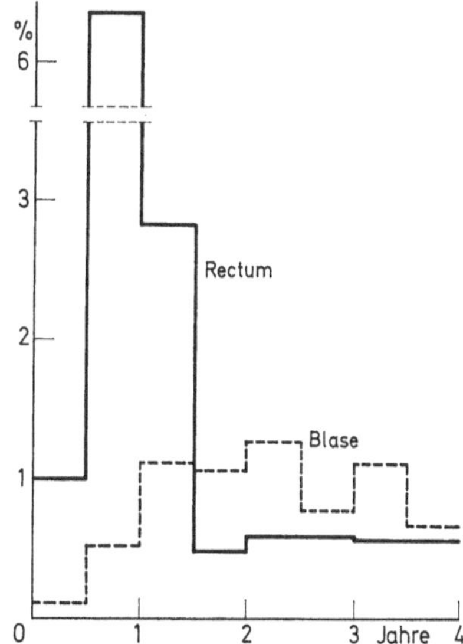

Abb. 58. Zeitliches Auftreten von Strahlenschäden nach Strahlenbehandlung bei 3484 behandelten Cervixcarcinomen des Radiumhemmet von 1949—1957

Tabelle 16. *Blasenkomplikationen in Abhängigkeit von der in der Blase gemessenen Strahlendosis* (KOTTMEIER)

γ-R	Zahl der Patienten	Grad I %	Grad II und III %
0—1999	54	11,1	3,7
2000—2999	102	15,6	3,9
3000—3999	93	11,8	6,4
4000—4999	57	22,8	10,5
5000—5999	40	17,5	2,5
6000 und mehr	16	6,2	31,2

Vasomotorenparese und Vasodilatation zur Folge hat. Dadurch kommt es besonders im distalen Ureterabschnitt zu einer mechanischen Behinderung des Peristaltikablaufes, wobei der Ureter selbst frei sondierbar ist.

Diese Veränderungen können im Verlauf mehrerer Jahre langsam in die Strahlenspätschäden übergehen. Hierbei stehen die fortschreitenden Gefäßveränderungen in Form der Endangitis obliterans und die vicariierende Bindegewebsbildung im Vordergrund (HOHENFELLNER, 1965). Neben diesen sich in der Muscularis abspielenden fibrösen Veränderungen macht KLOSTERHALFEN (1960) die Degeneration der intramuralen nervösen Substanz für den Verlust der Harnleiterperistaltik und Harnleitermotilität verantwortlich. Auch CHIARI (1961) fand neben mechanischen Narbenstenosen schwere degenerative Veränderungen der autonomen Ganglien. Hierfür sprechen auch die oft noch für Sonden glatt durchgängigen Ureteren, obwohl eine deutliche Abflußbehinderung besteht.

Neben den direkten kommen aber auch indirekte Ursachen für die an den Ureteren auftretenden Spätveränderungen in Betracht. Die Bestrahlung führt zu einer bindegewebigen Induration des Parametriums, die das Ergebnis von Strahlenwirkung, Tumorzerfall und perifokaler Entzündung ist. Die Vernarbung der Parametrien kann eine Strikturierung des Ureters hervorrufen. MUTH (1957) konnte zeigen, daß eine aufsteigende Infektion die Abflußdynamik des Harns durch Beeinträchtigung der Ventilwirkung an den Ostien schädigt. Daneben kann das Carcinom selbst eine Obliteration des Ureters

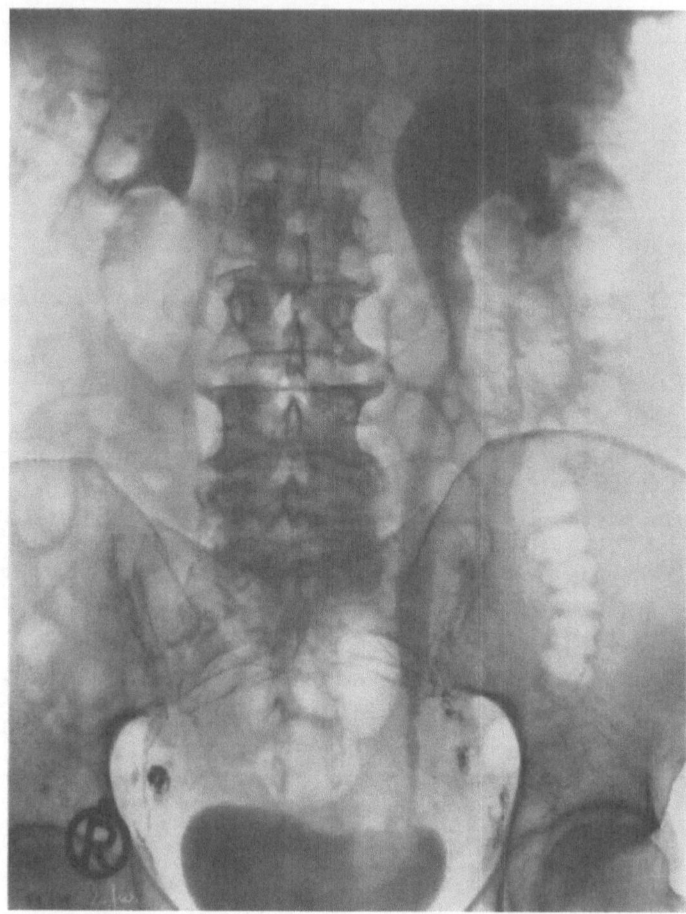

Abb. 59. Stauungsniere und Stauungsureter links 2 Jahre nach kombinierter Radium-Telekobalttherapie. Palpatorisch waren beide Parametrien strangförmig, narbig

bewirken, wie bereits die vor Behandlung bestehenden Harnstauungen zeigen (KIRCHHOFF, 1960; MUTH, 1957). Eingehende Untersuchungen des Krankengutes vor Behandlungsbeginn zeigten aber, daß nur ein verhältnismäßig kleiner Teil der Patientinnen Harnstauungen aufweist. HOFMANN (1963) und FRISCHBIER (1965) fanden Harnstauungen vor Behandlungsbeginn in weniger als 10% der Fälle.

Von großer Bedeutung für die Entstehung urologischer Komplikationen ist die Strahlentoleranz. Das Problem der Gewebstoleranz schien durch die Momentanmessungen in Urethra und Blase gelöst. So fand RIES (1961) unter gewissen Voraussetzungen der örtlichen und zeitlichen Dosisverteilung eine mittlere Gewebstoleranz zwischen 6000 und 7000 R. Bei dieser Dosierung sind akute Strahlenläsionen praktisch vermeidbar. In etwa 10—15% der Fälle muß aber mit einer erhöhten Strahlensensibilität gerechnet werden, die konstitutionell bedingt und vor der Behandlung nicht festzustellen ist. Daher sollte eine Überschreitung der Toleranzdosis von 5500 R vermieden werden. Trotzdem können Dosen von 4000—4500 R zu Urämietod infolge Schrumpfung des Beckenzellgewebes mit Harnstauung führen (RIES, 1961). Er fordert deshalb ein ausgesprochenes Dosisgefälle von der hohen Dosisspitze der Radium-γ-Strahlung in Beckenmitte zur Beckenwand hin, um eine Schrumpfung des lateral vom Ureter gelegenen Paragewebes zu verhindern, wodurch mangelnde Ernährung und Sklerose des gesamten Hüllgewebes des Ureters die Folge wären.

Alarmierend waren die Mitteilungen von BÖCKLER und PRINZ (1959), die in 19,5% bei den an Urämie nach Behandlung eines Collumcarcinoms verstorbenen Frauen lediglich eine Harnstauung, aber keinen Anhalt für ein Rezidiv als Todesursache fanden. KIRCH-HOFF (1960) sah bei 18 von 68 Patientinnen, bei denen die Urämie die Todesursache war, kein Carcinom mehr.

HELLER und KÄSER (1966) konnten an Hand von Sektionen nachweisen, daß bei 214 obduzierten Patientinnen mit einem Collumcarcinom 9,6% an urologischen Komplikationen verstorben waren, bei denen bei der Obduktion kein Carcinom mehr zu finden war. Nur in wenigen Fällen sah man lediglich kleine Carcinominseln an der Portio oder in Lymphknoten. Mehr als zwei Drittel dieser Frauen waren wegen eines Rezidivs zum zweiten Mal bestrahlt worden. Ähnliche Beobachtungen wurden auch von anderen Autoren gemacht, die etwa die gleiche Anzahl urologischer Komplikationen ohne nach-weisbares Carcinom fanden: ALTVATER und IMHOLZ (1960) 11%, FISCHER, E. (1955) 11%, FISCHER, H. (1956) 10%, HARTL (1961) 12%, MÜLLER (1957) 8,4%.

Wesentlich häufiger können stenosierende Veränderungen *röntgenologisch* an den ab-leitenden Harnwegen nach Bestrahlung eines Collumcarcinoms diagnostiziert werden. Die Zahl schwankt zwischen 20 und 50% (EVERETT et al., 1949; OEHLERT und BUSS, 1955; GANSAU, 1960; KIRCHHOFF, 1960; POCKRANDT, 1960; KÄSER und IKLÉ, 1961; GÜNTHER, 1962).

An dieser Stelle sei darauf hingewiesen, daß es urologische Komplikationen ebenfalls nach Radikaloperationen des Collumcarcinoms gibt. HOHENFELLNER (1965) gibt folgende typische Lokalisationen für postoperative Harnabflußhindernisse an: intramuraler Harn-leiterabschnitt, Harnleiterostium, innerer Blasenmund und prävesikaler Harnleiter-abschnitt. Ureterscheidenfisteln und Blasenscheidenfisteln kommen nach Wertheimscher Radikaloperation heute in einer Häufigkeit von 4—6% vor (LANGREDER, 1961). Beim radikalen vaginalen Vorgehen nach SCHAUTA u. AMREICH liegt die Fistelfrequenz deutlich niedriger (0,8—2,4%).

Da die Harnwegskomplikationen oft symptomarm verlaufen, kommt den Unter-suchungen der oberen Harnwege bei den routinemäßigen Nachkontrollen eine große Bedeutung zu, worauf besonders KIRCHHOFF hingewiesen hat. Regelmäßige Durchführung einer Chromocystoskopie, Urographie oder eines Isotopennephrogramms ist eine wichtige Voraussetzung, um frühzeitig eine Abflußbehinderung aufdecken und rechtzeitig eine Wiederherstellungsoperation am distalen Harnleiter vornehmen zu können.

Hinsichtlich der Therapie urologischer Komplikationen sei auf die Monographien von LANGREDER (1961) und HOHENFELLNER (1965) verwiesen.

c) Darm

Die Strahlenfrühreaktionen am Darm imponieren klinisch durch Stuhldrang, Tenesmen mit Abgang blutigen Schleims und gelegentlichen Durchfällen. Ähnliche, jedoch schwerere Beschwerden machen die Spätveränderungen, die im Vergleich zu den Blasenkomplika-tionen schon früher einsetzen, wie KOTTMEIER (1964) nachweisen konnte (Abb. 58). Sie treten meist nach einem freien Intervall von mehreren Monaten auf. Wie Abb. 58 zeigt, sind die Strahlenschäden am Rectum häufiger als in der Blase.

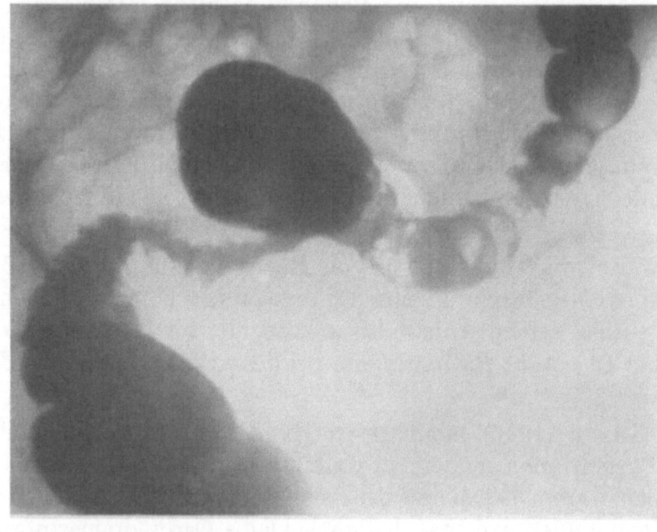

a

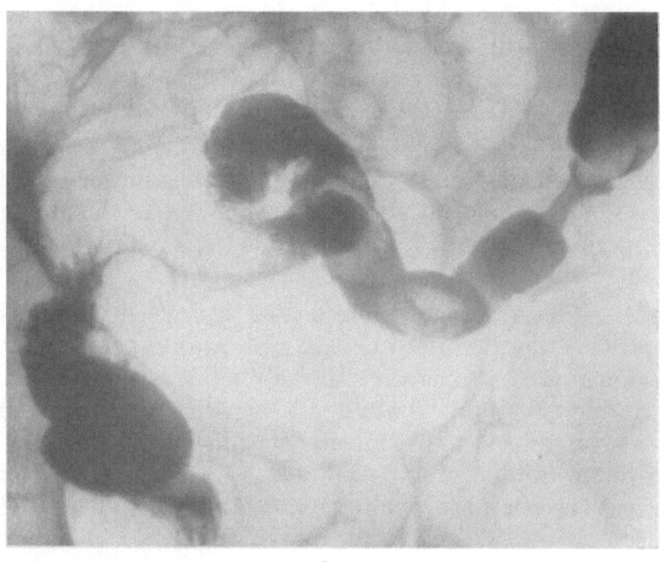

b

Abb. 60a u. b. Ulceröse und stenosierende Sigmaveränderungen nach Rezidivbestrahlung eines
Collumcarcinoms Stadium III

Die Darmkomplikationen werden folgendermaßen eingeteilt: im Grad I sind lediglich geringgradige Schleimhautveränderungen nachweisbar, Grad II zeigt Nekrosen und Ulcerationen oder mäßige Stenosierungen des Darmlumens, im Stadium III ist die Stenose so schwer, daß eine Kolostomie erforderlich wird, oder es besteht eine Fistel. Stärkere Früh- und Spätreaktionen treten in den Fällen auf, in denen Darmschlingen am Uterus adhärent sind. Das obere Rectum und die untere Sigmaschlinge sind die am häufigsten befallenen Darmabschnitte. Wesentlich seltener sind Dünndarmveränderungen beschrieben worden (TWOMBLY, 1954; CORSCADEN, 1956), die nur bei Verwachsungen zwischen Dünndarmschlingen und Uterus auftreten können. Rectumscheidenfisteln sind oft Folge einer Radiumüberdosierung durch die Portioplatte (HOFMANN, 1963). Aber auch das Körperhöhlenrohr kann insbesondere bei adhärenten Darmschlingen zu schweren Darmstenosen führen.

Histologisch findet man bei den Spätveränderungen Schleimhautulcerationen auf dem Boden einer mächtigen Verdickung der Submucosa; röntgenologisch imponieren diese Partien durch verwaschene Schleimhautkonturen. Weiterhin kann es zu einer mehr oder minder starken, narbig bedingten Einschnürung kommen, die zum Subileus oder Ileus führen kann.

RIES und BREITNER (1959) ermittelten bei der Münchener Bestrahlungsmethode für das Rectum eine Toleranzdosis zwischen 6000 und 8000 R. Auch KOTTMEIER und GRAY (1961) konnten eine ähnliche Dosisabhängigkeit bei den Darmreaktionen finden (Tabelle 17). FLETCHER (1966) warnt vor Dosen im Rectum über 8000 R innerhalb von 144 Std, weil dann Perforationen entstehen können. Die Dosis sollte 4000—6000 R nicht überschreiten.

Tabelle 17. *Rectumkomplikationen in Abhängigkeit von der im Rectum gemessenen Strahlendosis* (KOTTMEIER)

γ-R	Zahl der Patienten	Grad I %	Grad II und III %
0—1999	23	17,3	4,3
2000—2999	91	19,7	4,3
3000—3999	122	15,5	9,8
4000—4999	71	12,6	14,0
5000—5999	47	17,0	21,0
6000 und mehr	14	14,2	21,0

d) Knochen

Der erste Fall einer Schenkelhalsfraktur nach Bestrahlung eines Collumcarcinoms wurde 1927 von BAENSCH beschrieben, nachdem bereits von REGAUD 1922 anläßlich einer Veröffentlichung einer Nekrose im Kieferknochen nach Röntgenbestrahlung eines intraoralen Carcinoms der Begriff der *Osteoradionekrose* geprägt wurde. Seitdem sind zahlreiche Publikationen über Beobachtungen von Osteoradionekrosen des coxalen Femurendes nach einer Strahlenbehandlung weiblicher Genitalcarcinome im Schrifttum zu finden, so daß heute Schenkelhalsfrakturen als typische Bestrahlungskomplikationen vor allem nach einer Percutanbestrahlung eines Collumcarcinoms angesehen werden müssen. Im Jahre 1966 konnte FRIES aus dem internationalen Schrifttum 403 Fälle einer Osteoradionekrose im Oberschenkelhals anführen, denen er 12 eigene hinzufügte.

Die Angaben über die Häufigkeit einer Osteoradionekrose nach Bestrahlung eines Genitalcarcinoms schwanken; sie liegen meist um 1%. FOCHEM (1965) konnte bei 3694 bestrahlten Patientinnen 19 Schenkelhalsfrakturen (0,5%) finden. KIRCHHOFF und IMHOLZ (1953) beobachteten unter 1500 Patientinnen 14 Frakturen im Schenkelhalsbereich. Eine Häufigkeit von 2,75% geben OELSSNER, PFEIFFER und BUTTENBERG (1959) an.

Das Durchschnittsalter der Patientinnen, bei denen sich eine Osteoradionekrose entwickelte, war zum Zeitpunkt der Bestrahlung deutlich höher als es dem Durchschnittsalter der Collumcarcinompatientinnen entspricht. KIRCHHOFF und IMHOLZ (1953), SCHNAPPAUF (1957) und FRIES (1966) geben ein Durchschnittsalter von etwa 60 Jahren an.

Die Beschwerden, die auf eine Osteoradionekrose im Hüftbereich deuten, traten meist erst nach 1—4 Jahren nach der Bestrahlung auf. HIRAMAYA (1962) beschreibt einen Fall, bei dem es erst 9 Jahre nach der Bestrahlung zu einer Osteoradionekrose beider Femurköpfe gekommen war.

Eine untere Dosisgrenze für die Entstehung von Schenkelhalsfrakturen kann nicht angegeben werden. FOCHEM (1965) nimmt eine Dosis von 3000—4000 R an, erwähnt aber, daß Frakturen schon nach 1500—2000 R gesehen wurden.

Die Einführung der Megavoltstrahlen, die die Gefahr von Osteoradionekrosen durch den günstigeren Massenabsorptionskoeffizienten verringern sollte, hat bei der Behandlung des weiblichen Genitalcarcinoms die Gefahr nicht ganz gebannt. So konnten in der Universitäts-Frauenklinik Hamburg bei bisher 800 Patientinnen mit einem mit Megavolttherapie behandelten Cervixcarcinom in 4 Fällen radiogene Frakturen beobachtet werden. Bei diesen wurden Dosen von etwa 4000—5000 R an die betroffene Knochenregion appliziert. In einem Fall, bei dem zusätzlich eine Rezidivbestrahlung erfolgt war, kam es zu einer

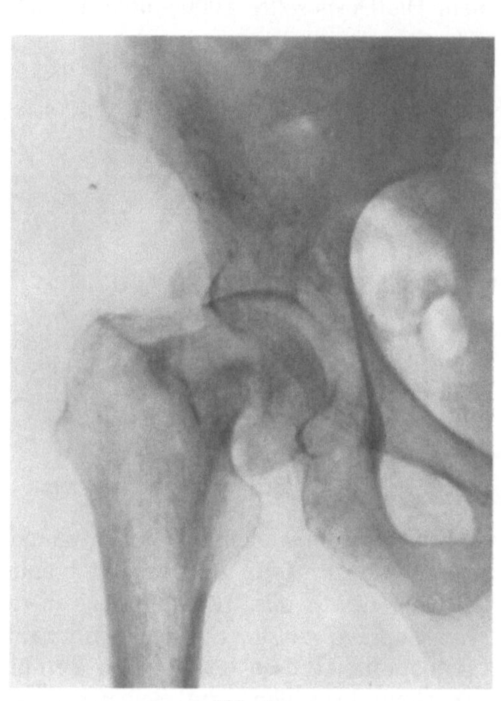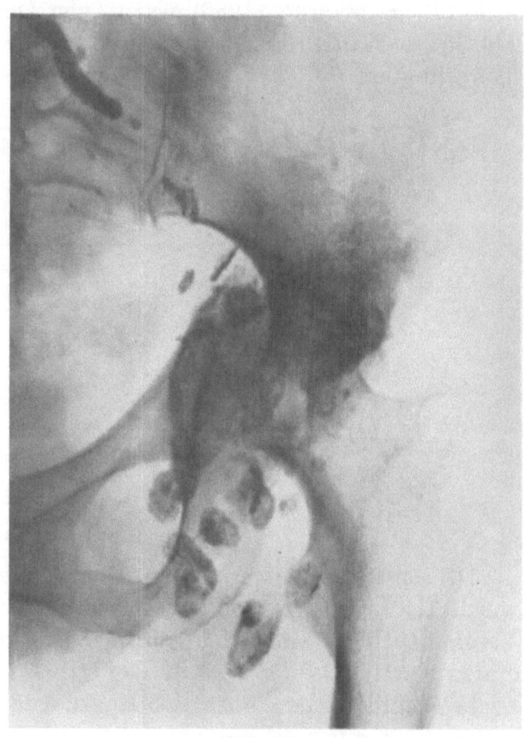

Abb. 61Abb. 62

Abb. 61. Mediale Schenkelhalsfraktur 4 Jahre nach Telekobalttherapie eines Collumcarcinoms Stadium III. Herddosis 5500 R auf die Beckenwand

Abb. 62. Beckenfraktur, ein Jahr nach Telekobalt-Pendelbestrahlung einer Beckenwandmetastasierung mit 5000 R Herd. Primärbestrahlung 10 Jahre vorher mit konventionellen Röntgenstrahlen von 3000 R auf die Beckenwand

kompletten Beckenringfraktur. LALANNE und FAJBISOWICZ (1965) sahen nach Telekobalttherapie bei einer Herddosis an der Beckenwand von 5000—6000 rad in 1,6% der Fälle Schenkelhalsfrakturen.

OELSSNER et al. (1959) unterscheiden je nach Art und Lokalisation der beobachteten Veränderungen reine Umbauzonen vorzugsweise am Schenkelhals, seltener am Scham- und Sitzbein, die Schenkelhalsfraktur, die Schenkelkopfnekrose und die Pfannennekrose mit und ohne Protrusio acetabuli. Alle Veränderungen können ein- oder doppelseitig sein. Die Schenkelhalsfrakturen werden von allen Autoren am häufigsten gefunden. Dabei fällt auf, daß die subkapitale Fraktur, direkt an der Schenkelhals-Kopfgrenze, die häufigste Lokalisation ist (SCHNAPPAUF, 1957; FRIES, 1966). In etwa einem Drittel der Fälle sind Schenkelhalsfrakturen doppelseitig.

In den meisten Fällen treten die Frakturen allmählich in Erscheinung. FRIES weist darauf hin, daß im Vergleich mit einer akuten traumatischen Fraktur die Beschwerden in allen Stadien des Osteoradionekroseprozesses relativ gering sind. Die stärkeren Bewegungsschmerzen, die für eine frische Schenkelhalsfraktur typisch sind, fehlen weitgehend. Oft stehen die geringen subjektiven Beschwerden in keinem Verhältnis zu den röntgenologischen Befunden.

FRIES konnte zeigen, daß bei allen von ihm beobachteten Osteoradionekrosen zu Beginn der Strahlenbehandlung bereits eine mehr oder weniger ausgeprägte, z.T. sogar sehr starke allgemeine Osteoporose, insbesondere der Wirbelsäule und des Beckens bestand. Er mißt der Osteoporose bei der Pathogenese der Osteoradionekrose maßgebliche Bedeutung bei.

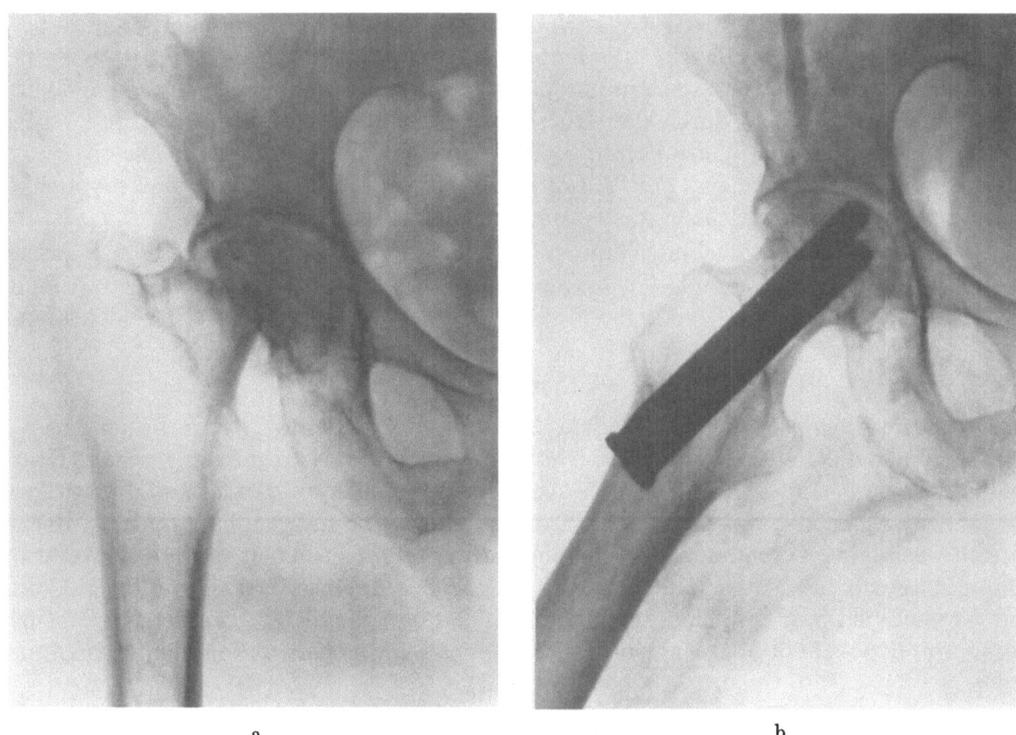

a   b

Abb. 63. a Mediale Schenkelhalsfraktur 2 Jahre nach Telekobaltbestrahlung von 5000 R auf die Beckenwand wegen eines Cervixhöhlencarcinoms. b Zustand nach Schenkelhalsnagelung

KIRCHHOFF und IMHOLZ (1953) sehen bei der Entstehung der Schenkelhalsfrakturen das Primäre in Veränderungen der Knochengefäße mit ausgedehnten Sklerosierungen. Die Entkalkungen und die Osteoporose sind nach ihrer Meinung sekundär.

BIRKNER, FREY und ÜBERSCHÄR (1956) versuchten, die Pathogenese durch tierexperimentelle Untersuchungen aufzudecken. Nach Bestrahlung des Meerschweinchenröhrenknochens konnten sie zeigen, daß durch die Bestrahlung eine Osteocytennekrose auftritt und im Bereich des Periost Nekrosen bei den Osteoblasten zu finden sind. Osteocytennekrose und Periostfibrose entstehen, bevor an den Gefäßen Schädigungsfolgen nachweisbar sind.

Im Röntgenbild können sich erste Veränderungen in Form von Umbauzonen darstellen, wenn die vom gesunden Knochen her vordringenden Umbauprozesse den nekrotischen Bezirk demarkiert haben. Wenn die Kontinuität zwischen totem und gesundem Knochen noch besteht, kann sich die Nekrose an der statischen Belastung beteiligen. Osteolytische Prozesse überwiegen, wenn die latenten Infraktionen die reparativen Vorgänge nicht ausreichend anregen. Durch eine Verringerung der Stabilität kommt es dann mit Erreichen der Belastungsgrenze ohne traumatische Einwirkung zur Fraktur. Dabei sind die Patientinnen besonders gefährdet, bei denen bereits eine allgemeine Osteoporose besteht.

Spontanheilungen einer Osteoradionekrose werden beschrieben (Birkner, Fries). Bei den von Fries beobachteten Spontanheilungen waren aber in allen Fällen starke Coxa-vara-Deformierungen die Folge. Von orthopädischer Seite wird aber gefordert, daß alle Schenkelhalsveränderungen unter Erhaltung optimaler Gelenkverhältnisse ausheilen sollen. Eine abwartende, konservative Behandlung mit Ruhigstellung erscheint wegen der Komplikationen durch die Bettlägerigkeit nicht angezeigt, da vor allem auch der osteoporotische Knochen durch die Inaktivitätsatrophie weiter geschädigt werden kann. Von Kirchhoff und Imholz (1953) wird deshalb eine aktiv chirurgische Behandlung als Methode der Wahl angegeben. Fries empfiehlt in allen frühen Fällen, in denen es noch nicht zur völligen Kontinuitätstrennung des Knochens gekommen ist, eine Schenkelhalsnagelung. Sie verhindert durch den stützenden Effekt eine Deformierung und regt die Reparationsvorgänge an. Gute Erfahrungen konnte er mit der Alloarthroplastik mit der Spezialendoprothese machen. Zur Wiederherstellung der Gelenkkongruenz empfiehlt er die intertrochantere Aufrichtungsosteotomie nach Pauwels.

Da die Behandlungsergebnisse um so besser sind, je früher Osteoradionekrosen zur Behandlung kommen, kommt der nachgehenden Fürsorge mit regelmäßigen Röntgenkontrollen insbesondere bei geringsten subjektiven Beschwerden größte Bedeutung zu.

e) Lymphstauung

Das postradiologische Stauungsödem der unteren Extremität wurde bisher meist als direkte Strahlenfolge durch radiogene Obliteration der Lymphbahnen angesehen (Knopp, 1960). Umfangreiche lymphangiographische Untersuchungen in den letzten Jahren konnten jedoch zeigen, daß es nur in den Fällen zu einer echten Lymphstauung im Beckenbereich nach einer percutanen Strahlenbehandlung kam, in denen primär Beckenwandlymphknotenmetastasen bestanden hatten. Bei primär unauffälligem Lymphangiogramm und Speicherbild war es innerhalb der ersten 2 Jahre nach der Strahlentherapie nach Dosen von 5000—6000 R in keinem Fall zu einem Lymphödem gekommen (Frischbier, 1966).

Diese Beobachtungen decken sich mit den experimentellen Untersuchungen von Lenzi und Bassani (1963), die nach 6000 R an den Lymphgefäßen keine signifikanten Veränderungen registrieren konnten. Erst nach 8000 R erscheinen die Gefäße gewunden und starr, jedoch nicht unterbrochen. In nekrotischen Bezirken von 20000 R wiesen sie Gefäßunterbrechungen auf.

Exakte Angaben über die Häufigkeit eines radiologischen Lymphödems findet man im Schrifttum nicht, da die Unterscheidung von einem durch Tumorprogredienz bedingten Lymphödem oft schwierig ist. Früher wurde fast ausschließlich eine Unterscheidung durch klinische Untersuchungen getroffen: Bei einem fehlenden Palpationsbefund im kleinen Becken und insbesondere bei einem doppelseitigen Ödem der unteren Extremität wurde meist eine radiogene Ursache angenommen. Seit routinemäßiger Anwendung der Lymphographie wissen wir aber, daß sich nicht selten hinter einem Lymphödem trotz Fehlens eines rezidivverdächtigen Palpationsbefundes eine ausgedehnte, hochsitzende Lymphknotenmetastasierung verbergen kann. Bei doppelseitigen Beinödemen sind ausgedehnte metastatische Befunde in der Lumbalregion möglich, die zur Lymphblockade führen, sich aber der Palpation vollends entziehen. Wenn auch die Durchführung einer Lymphographie bei einem Lymphödem oft technisch schwierig sein kann und nicht selten die Beurteilung der Bilder erschwert ist, sollte jedes Lymphödem nach Bestrahlung eines Collumcarcinoms eine absolute Indikation zur Durchführung einer Lymphographie sein.

Nach unseren Erfahrungen sind auf den Lymphangiogrammen bei einem radiogen bedingten Lymphödem typische Befunde zu erkennen, die sich von einer Metastasierung deutlich unterscheiden. Die Lymphgefäße sind in ihrem Kaliber erheblich reduziert. Einzelne Gefäße sind so dünn, daß sie nur noch auf eine Länge von wenigen Millimetern verfolgt werden können. Die sonst übliche Kontinuität der Gefäßmarkierungen ist aufgehoben. Der Gefäßverlauf erscheint unregelmäßig, Gefäßklappen sind nicht mehr sichtbar. Gelegentlich wird eine komplette Blockade vorgetäuscht. Die stets spitz zulaufenden Gefäßbündel sind von den bogigen Gefäßverläufen bei metastatischen Befunden meist zu differenzieren. Typische Befunde zeigt die Abb. 64.

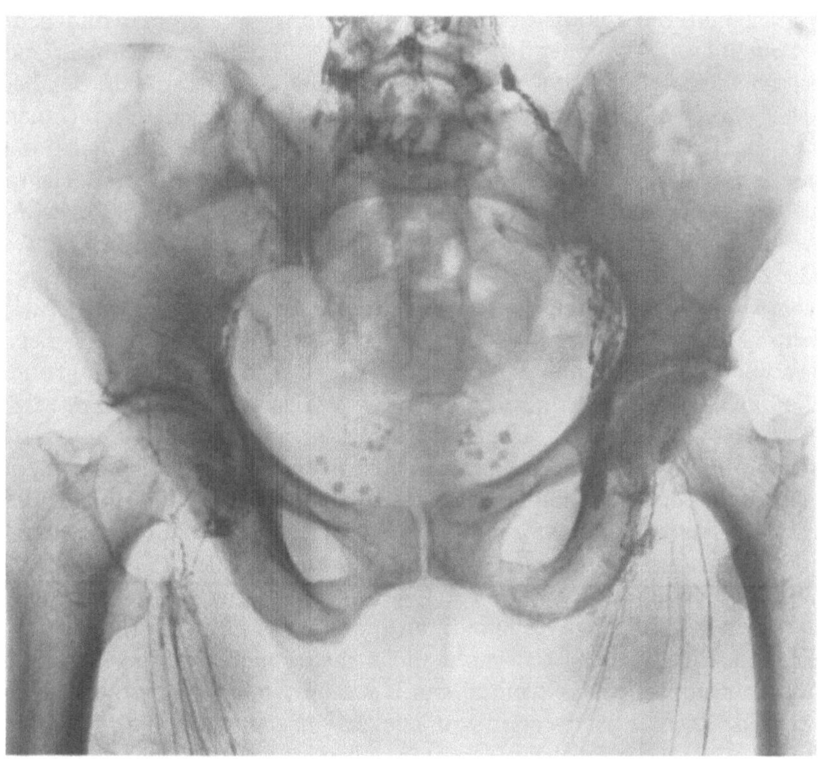

Abb. 64. Lymphangiogramm bei einem 1960 bestrahlten Collumcarcinom Stadium III. Dosis an der rechten Beckenwand 4500 R. 1962 Beckenwandrezidiv rechts. Telekobaltbestrahlung auf die rechte Beckenwand mit 4000 R Herddosis. Im Lymphangiogramm erkennt man auf der linken Seite einen unauffälligen Lymphgefäßverlauf. An der rechten Beckenwand sind nur wenige dünne, klappenlose Lymphgefäße zu erkennen. Im Bereich der Lumbalregion, außerhalb des Bestrahlungsfeldes, zeigen die Lymphgefäße wieder die typische perlschnurartige Anordnung

9. Behandlungsergebnisse

Beim Collumcarcinom kann man sich wie bei keiner anderen Tumorlokalisation über die Behandlungsergebnisse der verschiedenen Behandlungsarten ein klares Bild verschaffen. Der Grund hierfür ist darin zu sehen, daß das Collumcarcinom relativ häufig ist und in der gesamten Welt nach einheitlichen Richtlinien eine exakte Stadieneinteilung vorgenommen wird, die überhaupt erst den Vergleich verschiedener Methoden ermöglicht. Wenn auch die Stadieneinteilung mit erheblichen subjektiven Unsicherheiten behaftet ist, weil sie ausschließlich auf der klinischen Untersuchung basiert, schafft sie aber doch gewisse Voraussetzungen für einen Vergleich der Behandlungsergebnisse. Nachdem HEYMAN für die Zusammenstellung der Jahresberichte, des Annual Report on the Results of Treatment in Carcinoma of the Uterus, allgemein bindende Richtlinien für die Heilungsergebnisse entwickelte, wurden bessere Voraussetzungen für einen Vergleich der Behandlungsresultate geschaffen. Die jährliche zahlenmäßige Zusammenstellung der Behandlungserfolge und Mißerfolge gestattet selbstverständlich nicht, eine optimale Behandlungsmethode zu ermitteln. Aus den Jahresberichten sind auch nicht ohne weiteres Rückschlüsse auf die Zusammensetzung des jeweiligen Patientengutes und die Leistungsfähigkeit einzelner Behandlungsmethoden zu ziehen. Wenn man auch den Wert der Jahresberichte in dieser Hinsicht schmälern könnte, so dienen die jährlichen Zusammenstellungen der Behandlungserfolge der Selbstkontrolle und vor allem der Weiterentwicklung der Bestrahlungstechnik. Man ist gezwungen, sich an Hand des Zahlenmaterials Rechenschaft über die Brauchbarkeit seiner Methoden abzulegen.

Das Ausgangsmaterial für die statistischen Zusammenstellungen bilden *alle* in einer Klinik zur Beobachtung kommenden Patientinnen mit einem Collumcarcinom, gleichgültig, ob sie nachher behandelt worden sind oder nicht. Aus der Zahl der beobachteten und der nach Ablauf von 5 Jahren rezidiv- und metastasenfreien Patientinnen errechnet man die *absolute Heilungsziffer*. Bei der *absoluten Leistungsziffer* werden nur die behandelten Patientinnen berücksichtigt und zu der Zahl der geheilten in Beziehung gesetzt. Von einer relativen Heilungs- oder Leistungsziffer spricht man bei Berücksichtigung der einzelnen Ausbreitungsstadien der Collumcarcinome. So ergibt sich die *relative Heilungsziffer* aus der Zahl der beobachteten Patientinnen eines Stadiums im Verhältnis zu der Zahl der nach 5 Jahren geheilten dieses Stadiums. Bei ausschließlicher Berücksichtigung der behandelten Patientinnen ergibt sich dann in gleicher Weise die *relative Leistungsziffer*.

Voraussetzung für die Stadieneinteilung ist die Eingruppierung aufgrund des Tastbefundes, die auch nach einer Laparotomie nicht korrigiert werden darf, selbst wenn in einem klinisch als Stadium I angesehenen Casus carcinomatöse Lymphknoten bei der Laparotomie gefunden werden. Eine spätere Umgruppierung ist deshalb unzulässig, weil diese Möglichkeit bei den ausschließlich strahlenbehandelten Patientinnen nicht gegeben ist. Weiterhin verlangte Heyman, daß die interkurrent Verstorbenen den Rezidiven zugerechnet werden müssen und nicht von der Gesamtzahl der beobachteten Carcinome abgezogen werden können. Diese Forderung ist allgemein anerkannt bei der Bekanntgabe von Heilungsresultaten nach der Behandlung maligner Geschwülste. Selbst wenn durch eine Autopsie ein Rezidiv oder Carcinom nicht mehr nachzuweisen ist und somit eine interkurrente Todesursache objektiviert werden kann, müssen diese Fälle als Rezidive gerechnet werden. Diese Strenge wird von vielen Untersuchern für nicht gerechtfertigt angesehen.

Die Quote der Patientinnen, die interkurrent verstirbt, ohne daß sich bei Autopsie ein Anhalt für Carcinomgewebe ergibt, ist nicht unbeträchtlich. So fanden Heller und Käser (1966) bei 214 Obduktionen bei Collumcarcinomträgerinnen, daß 23,5% der Frauen nicht am Carcinom verstorben waren. Bei 39 Frauen war Carcinomgewebe überhaupt nicht mehr nachweisbar, bei 11 weiteren bestanden nur noch kleine Inseln an der Portio und den Lymphknoten.

Vom Annual Report ist im Jahre 1964 der letzte Berichtsband erschienen, der als 13. Band die Ergebnisse von 1948—1957, gesammelt im Jahre 1963, enthält. In diesem Band sind die Behandlungsergebnisse von 116 Kliniken der Welt zusammengestellt. Tabelle 18 gibt einen Auszug der Tabellen wieder, die die relative und absolute Leistungsziffer ergeben. Diese Behandlungsergebnisse wurden in den Jahren 1953—1957 erzielt.

Es ist unmöglich, in diesem Rahmen die Behandlungsergebnisse nach Behandlungsmethoden gegenüberzustellen. Die in den einzelnen Kliniken angewandten Behandlungsmethoden sind im mitgeteilten Berichtszeitraum nicht einheitlich. Oft kamen mehrere Behandlungsformen zur Anwendung, oder die Methoden wichen in den einzelnen Ausbreitungsstadien stark voneinander ab. Soweit die Heilungsergebnisse durch spezielle Behandlungsmethoden gewonnen wurden, fanden sie bei der Beschreibung der Methoden Erwähnung.

Einen Versuch, die Behandlungsergebnisse nach Operation oder Bestrahlung miteinander zu vergleichen, hat Kottmeier aufgrund der im 12. Annual Report zusammengestellten Ergebnisse unternommen. In Tabelle 19 stellt er die Behandlungsergebnisse der

Tabelle 18. *Relative und absolute Leistungsziffer bei der Behandlung des Collumcarcinoms 1953—1957.*
(Annual Report, 1964)

Stadium	I	II	III	IV	I—IV
1. Buenos Aires, Argentine	62.9	42.9	18.5	4.3	37.9
3. Melbourne, Royal Women's	70.0	47.1	17.3		52.6
4. Sydney, Royal Hospital	73.3	25.0			38.3
5. Sydney, Royal Prince Alfred	71.9	41.0	25.0	0	52.8
6. Sydney, St. Vincent	73.9	30.4	11.8		43.2
7. Sydney, Women's Hospital	60.0	47.6			46.2
8. Graz, Austria	76.6	44.5	15.8	3.8	44.2
9. Innsbruck	78.8	70.6	33.5		48.9
10. Vienna	79.9	61.5	33.3		57.9
11. Brussels, Belgium	86.8	62.3	30.0		60.5
12. Gand	75.0	46.0	13.2		37.1
13. Liège	71.0	39.5	7.7		38.6
14. Louvain, Acad. Ziekenhuis and Inst. Cancer	68.8	59.7	31.1		51.0
15. Belo Horizonte, Brazil	52.4	31.5	10.1	0	31.1
16. São Paulo	76.5	48.6	28.4	13.5	36.8
17. Halifax, Canada	78.4	47.0	25.0		52.4
18. Montreal, Inst. Cancer	72.1	44.9	30.8	12.9	53.8
19. Montreal, Inst. Radium	83.3	48.8	19.5	0	36.1
20. Montreal, Royal Victoria	88.7	42.4	29.0		64.9
21. Ontario Ca. Found., Hamilton	68.4	55.5	25.0		53.5
22. Ontario Ca. Found., Kingston	68.1	44.7	25.0		48.0
23. Ontario Ca. Found., London	74.8	56.7	28.6		54.5
24. Ontario Ca., Found., Ottawa	77.6	46.2	19.4	11.1	51.5
25. Ontario Ca. Found., Windsor	81.6	69.2	21.7		60.8
26. Saint John	81.4	64.9	40.2	13.3	60.2
27. Saskatoon	80.4	49.4	17.6	5.6	53.7
28. Vancouver	71.2	52.8	34.8	5.3	54.2
29. Winnipeg	66.0	44.4	9.1		45.0
30. Brno, Onkologický Ústav	77.5	67.0	46.1	6.7	54.6
31. Brno, II. Por. Gyn. Klin.	62.2	67.8	29.2		61.1
32. Prague	74.2	53.8	36.0		55.9
33. Aarhus, Denmark	76.4	65.1	36.9	9.3	54.3
34. Copenhagen	75.0	53.5	29.1	12.5	52.3
35. Odense	76.1	53.6	29.7	4.0	52.5
36. Helsinki, Finland	75.0	45.0	16.4		49.4
37. Bordeaux, France	52.9	40.0	26.2	3.8	33.9
38. Lille	66.1	48.8	20.6	9.9	35.4
39. Lyons	60.5	39.8	18.8	2.3	36.3
40. Montpellier		52.5	38.3	14.3	36.5
41. Paris, Inst. G. Roussy	79.3	61.9	30.7	15.2	47.8
42. Paris, Inst. Radium	78.9	54.3	18.4	0	41.7
43. Bremerhaven, Germany	80.6	34.4			57.3
44. Erlangen	80.4	66.1	42.9	15.4	56.5
45. Frankfurt a. M.	80.8	64.9	53.1		63.6
46. Göttingen	72.9	59.8	38.5	5.9	54.3
47. Hamburg	87.9	74.1	52.4	16.3	58.7
48. Heidelberg	80.4	57.6	29.1	0	53.6
49. Jena	72.1	56.5	26.2	3.8	54.0
50. Kiel	88.0	59.8	32.4	5.7	53.8
51. Leipzig	72.2	45.0	33.4	8.6	51.3
52. Lübeck	69.0	47.6	31.9		46.2
53. München, I. Frauenklinik	83.8	69.9	44.9	5.6	58.5
54. München, II. Frauenklinik	93.8	66.3	39.7	7.8	50.4
56. Tübingen	79.9	63.5	42.7	5.3	59.0

Tabelle 18 (Fortsetzung)

Stadium	I	II	III	IV	I—IV
57. Wuppertal-Elberfeld	82.1	58.2	36.6	0	59.1
58. Würzburg	79.0	67.5	48.2		57.4
59. Calcutta, India	52.7	42.9	15.7	0	23.0
60. Bologna, Italy	71.9	59.2	26.5	0	52.1
61. Brescia	67.4	48.0	36.0	9.7	41.4
62. Milan	67.6	46.2	19.3		44.7
63. Padua	66.7	55.2	35.7	14.6	40.0
64. Kumamoto, Japan	83.8	59.3	31.2	12.5	53.9
65. Nagasaki	86.0	70.1	40.9	6.9	54.9
66. Okayama	85.6	68.4	38.1	0	65.8
67. Tokyo	85.0	69.6	46.7	19.7	63.2
68. Amsterdam, Leuwenhoekhuis	64.7	57.4	38.6		49.6
69. Amsterdam, Vrouwenkliniek	78.0	62.2	11.9		63.5
70. Rotterdam	70.0	64.4	51.0	25.0	58.0
71. Utrecht	65.3	55.7	17.4		50.7
73. Oslo, Norway	75.1	51.8	30.4	13.9	55.4
74. Gliwice, Poland	62.9	47.2	23.0	12.2	39.7
75. Krakow	75.2	59.4	42.8	11.1	51.1
76. Warsaw	80.7	57.2	35.5	0	53.3
77. Bucharest, Roumania	81.3	54.5	14.3	2.9	42.1
78. Gothenburg, Sweden	72.8	56.5	21.4	0	52.6
79. Stockholm	86.4	60.0	26.3	8.8	56.8
80. Basel, Switzerland	86.7	49.1	27.5	12.5	56.5
81. Lausanne	80.0	45.2	22.0		46.4
82. St. Gallen	66.7	43.2	16.7		46.5
83. Zurich	88.0	63.8	38.3	35.0	64.9
84. Cape Town, Union of S. Africa	61.7	35.9	16.1	6.0	30.9
85. Birmingham, United Kingdom	70.8	42.4	21.8	2.3	43.0
86. Bristol	76.0	45.5	11.5	8.6	38.4
87. Cambridge	73.8	45.0	29.1	11.5	43.6
88. Cardiff	73.0	42.2	25.2		43.6
89. Coventry	88.5	40.5	27.3	3.4	48.0
90. Edinburgh	75.0	44.5	22.7	0	45.5
91. Glasgow	59.7	42.6	30.1	6.4	37.6
92. Liverpool	69.4	47.1	32.5	11.5	42.0
93. London, Marie Curie	56.4	36.1	20.8	0	37.0
94. London, Middlesex	72.4	53.2	25.0	20.0	49.2
95. London, Royal Marsden	63.1	42.4	14.7		41.4
96. London, Univ. College	67.6	40.8	24.0		41.5
97. Manchester	69.5	46.6	26.3	6.1	42.4
98. Newcastle	74.2	48.6	26.0	14.3	47.5
99. Northwood	57.5	36.7	15.1	10.8	33.2
100. Sheffield	71.7	46.8	30.9	7.7	43.5
101. Southampton	77.3	42.4	24.0		44.2
102. Baltimore, Johns Hopkins, USA	71.0	43.4	15.2		49.0
103. Baltimore, Univ. of Maryland	71.0	52.9	21.4		50.6
104. Boston	80.3	46.9	20.0	2.6	50.0
105. Buffalo	63.1	51.8	22.8	7.0	48.6
106. Columbia	60.0	50.7	41.4	9.7	42.7
107. Houston	86.6	69.9	42.5	12.8	60.6
108. Los Angeles	88.3	64.3	28.0		65.8
109. Madison	80.5	41.0	23.9	4.3	45.0
110. New Haven	85.4	42.6	6.3	19.2	57.3
112. New York, Col.-Presbyterian	80.6	48.8	23.9	3.8	53.2
113. New York, Cornell Univ.	81.6	63.9	20.8		54.6
114. New York, Woman's	57.8	38.2	0.0		39.7

Tabelle 18 (Fortsetzung)

Stadium	I	II	III	IV	I—IV
116. Philadelphia, Univ. Penn.	83.1	54.4	44.4		63.3
117. Providence	70.0	47.8	29.3		48.9
118. Saint Louis	72.5	50.0	30.4		52.1
119. San Francisco	83.9	48.3	28.6		62.9
120. Seattle	71.0	54.5	34.5		57.3
121. Leningrad, U.S.S.R.	82.6	53.2	34.3		60.3
122. Moscow	90.6	71.3	39.9		68.0
123. Ljubljana, Yugoslavia	84.2	50.3	27.2	4.5	56.0
124. Zagreb	80.8	62.2	29.7	5.0	43.8

Tabelle 19. *Gegenüberstellung der Behandlungsergebnisse des Collumcarcinoms nach Operation oder Bestrahlung von 1950—1954* (KOTTMEIER)

Behandlungsmethode	Stadium I			Stadium II		
	Zahl der Fälle	Zahl der 5-Jahres-Heilungen	%	Zahl der Fälle	Zahl der 5-Jahres-Heilungen	%
Operation	4 868	3 590	73,7	6 839	3 437	50,3
Bestrahlung	1 591	1 224	76,9	3 780	2 030	53,7

mehr operativ eingestellten Kliniken denen einer ausschließlichen Strahlentherapie gegenüber. Als operative Klinik wurden jene angesehen, bei denen die primäre radikale Hysterektomie in mehr als 50% der Fälle des Stadiums I durchgeführt wird. Bei dieser Zusammenstellung wurden nur die Institutionen berücksichtigt, die mindestens 50 Fälle von Stadium I behandelt hatten. Die Gegenüberstellung der Behandlungsergebnisse nach vorwiegend operativer oder ausschließlich radiologischer Therapie zeigt, daß keine signifikanten Unterschiede in den Heilungsergebnissen zwischen beiden Behandlungsmethoden bestehen.

10. Bestrahlung der Rezidive und Metastasen

a) Häufigkeit und Lokalisation

Unter einem Rezidiv versteht man im allgemeinen das Wiederauftreten eines Carcinoms an der Stelle seiner primären Lokalisation, nachdem der Tumor als Folge der Therapie für eine bestimmte Zeit nicht nachweisbar war. Zwischen einem Rezidiv und einem Weiterwachstum bzw. einer Tumorpersistenz, bei der es nach der Behandlung gar nicht erst oder nur kurzfristig zu einer Rückbildung der Geschwulst gekommen ist, sollte streng unterschieden werden. Während RIES und BREITNER (1959) für ein Rezidiv ein freies Intervall von 4 Monaten annehmen, versteht man heute unter einem Rezidiv allgemein ein neu aufgetretenes Tumorwachstum am Ort des Primärtumors oder in seiner unmittelbaren Umgebung nach einer objektiv und subjektiv erscheinungsfreien Beobachtungszeit von mindestens 6 Monaten, wenn nach der Behandlung die primären Geschwulstinfiltrate nicht mehr nachweisbar waren (KEPP, 1952; HERIK und FRICKE, 1955). KÄSER und SCHIEFERSTEIN (1966) weisen darauf hin, daß biologisch betrachtet das Carcinomrezidiv nur eine Sonderform der Tumorpersistenz ist, da es durch Nachwachsen bei der Operation zurückgelassener Krebszellen oder durch Aktivierung der durch die Bestrahlung nicht devitalisierten Carcinomherde entsteht.

Während man den Begriff Rezidiv für das Wiederauftreten am Ort des Tumorursprungs oder seiner unmittelbaren Umgebung benutzt, wird der Begriff Metastase für ein räumlich getrenntes Auftreten vom Primärtumor verwandt. Diese beiden Begriffe werden aber in der Gynäkologie nicht scharf getrennt. So bezeichnet man beispielsweise eine Lymphknotenmetastasierung an der Beckenwand meist als Beckenwandrezidiv.

Zuppinger empfiehlt deshalb, nur zwischen einem Rezidiv und einer Metastase einerseits und einer Fernmetastasierung andererseits eine Unterscheidung zu treffen. Unter einem Rezidiv (oder Lokalmetastasierung) sollte man das Wiederauftreten am primären Sitz oder im Lymphabflußgebiet innerhalb des kleinen Beckens verstehen. Hiervon

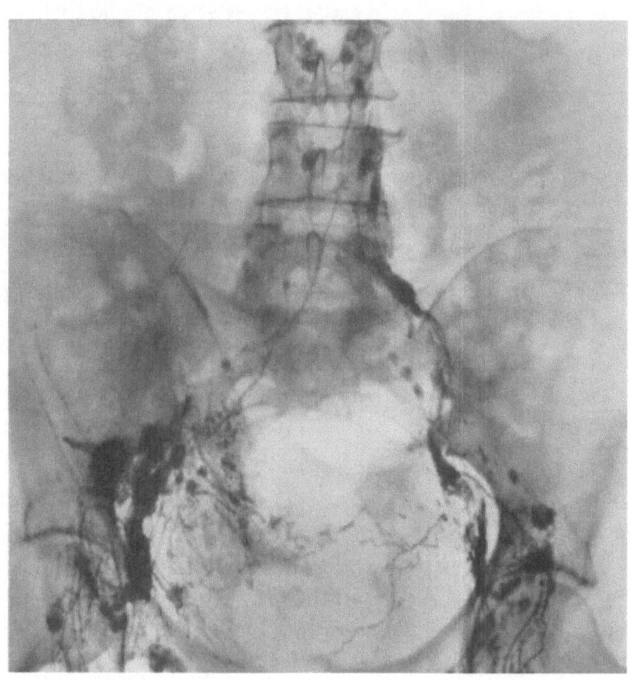

Abb. 65. Lymphangiogramm bei einem rechtsseitigen Beinödem eines operierten und bestrahlten Collumcarcinoms Stadium I. Palpatorisch kein Anhalt für ein Rezidiv im kleinen Becken. Die Lymphographie deckt durch eine komplette Lymphblockade im Bereich der Vasa iliaca communes eine hochsitzende, nicht palpable Beckenwandmetastasierung auf

sollten die Fernmetastasen außerhalb des Beckenbereichs streng unterschieden werden. Diese Differenzierung eignet sich für die klinischen Belange und insbesondere für die Erfolgsbeurteilung am besten.

Über die Häufigkeit der Lokalisation und insbesondere über die bei einem Rezidiv erzielten Behandlungsergebnisse findet man im Schrifttum sehr divergierende Zahlen und Angaben. Die Erklärung hierfür ist in den beträchtlichen Schwierigkeiten der Erkennung eines Rezidivs zu suchen. Ein Lokalrezidiv an der Portio oder in der Vagina ist klinisch relativ leicht zu erkennen und auch histologisch einfach zu sichern. Die parametranen und vor allem die Beckenwandbefunde bereiten dagegen wesentlich größere diagnostische Schwierigkeiten. Insbesondere nach einer Strahlenbehandlung ist es klinisch durch die Palpation oft unmöglich, ein narbiges Parametrium von einer Tumorinfiltration zu unterscheiden. Wenn auch ein Erfahrener einen typischen Befund bei knotiger Infiltration und Progredienz der Veränderungen stets erkennen wird, so sind doch Fehldiagnosen häufiger, als oft angenommen wird. Allgemeine Symptome, wie Gewichtsverlust, erhöhte BSG, Stauungsödeme, ischiasartige Schmerzen, Harnabflußbehinderungen, sind zwar wichtige klinische Kriterien für das Vorliegen eines Rezidivs, doch können sie ebenfalls andere Ursachen haben.

In der Rezidivdiagnostik des Collumcarcinoms haben in den letzten Jahren verschiedene angiographische Untersuchungen größere Verbreitung gefunden. Es zeigte sich, daß bei klinisch unklaren Befunden die Lymphographie, die Phlebographie oder die Arteriographie wichtige Hinweise auf das Vorliegen eines Rezidivs oder einer Metastasierung geben können. Darüber hinaus ist es mit diesen Untersuchungen möglich, die Tumorausbreitung exakter zu bestimmen und damit das Bestrahlungsfeld dem Herd optimal anzupassen (Abb. 65 und 66).

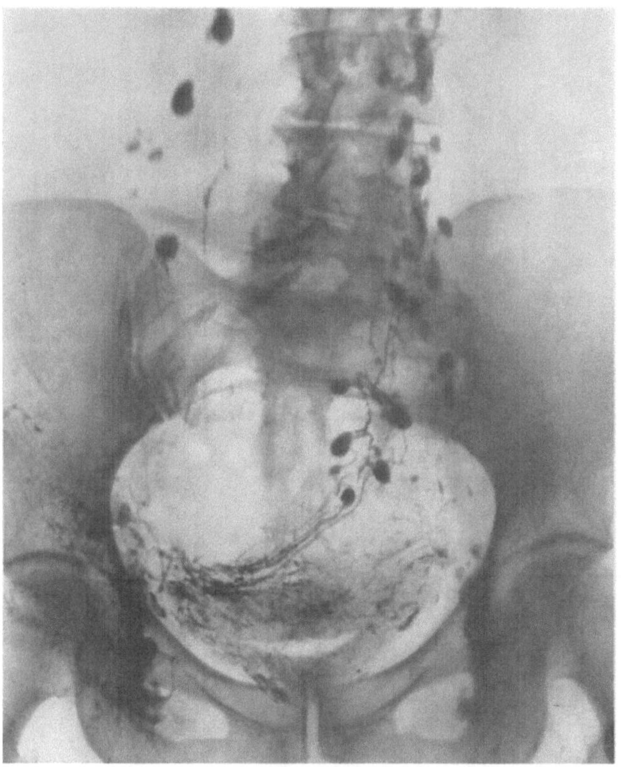

Abb. 66. Lymphangiogramm bei einem rechtsseitigen Beckenwandrezidiv, 2 Jahre nach Radikaloperation wegen Collumcarcinom Stadium I. Es besteht eine komplette Lymphblockade rechts iliacal mit Ausbildung eines Kollateralsystems zur Gegenseite. Die Lymphographie deckt eine bis zur Lumbalregion reichende Lymphknotenmetastasierung auf

Nach unseren Erfahrungen ist die Bedeutung der Lymphographie in der Rezidivdiagnostik von so großem Wert, daß sie routinemäßig bei jedem Rezidivverdacht durchgeführt wird. Bei insgesamt 159 Patientinnen der Universitäts-Frauenklinik Hamburg mit klinisch fraglichen oder gesicherten Rezidiverkrankungen zeigte sich, daß in über einem Drittel aller Fälle durch die Lymphographie die klinische Diagnose entscheidend verbessert werden konnte. In den meisten Fällen wurde durch die Lymphographie eine Metastasierung aufgedeckt ohne daß klinisch ein sicheres Rezidiv nachgewiesen werden konnte. Seltener war lymphographisch die Tumorausdehnung weiter als klinisch vermutet.

Während die Phlebographie in der Rezidivdiagnostik des Collumcarcinoms allein nicht die gleiche Aussagekraft wie die Lymphographie besitzt, kann sie in Kombination mit der Lymphographie den Aussagewert oft steigern (Abb. 67). Eine Kombination beider Untersuchungsmethoden ist insbesondere bei einer kompletten Lymphblockade notwendig, wenn mit der Lymphographie über die proximal der Blockade liegende Tumorausdehnung eine Aussage nicht mehr möglich ist. Weiterhin kann sie bei unklaren lymphographischen Befunden insbesondere in der Lumbalregion überzeugende Bilder liefern (s. Abb. 5).

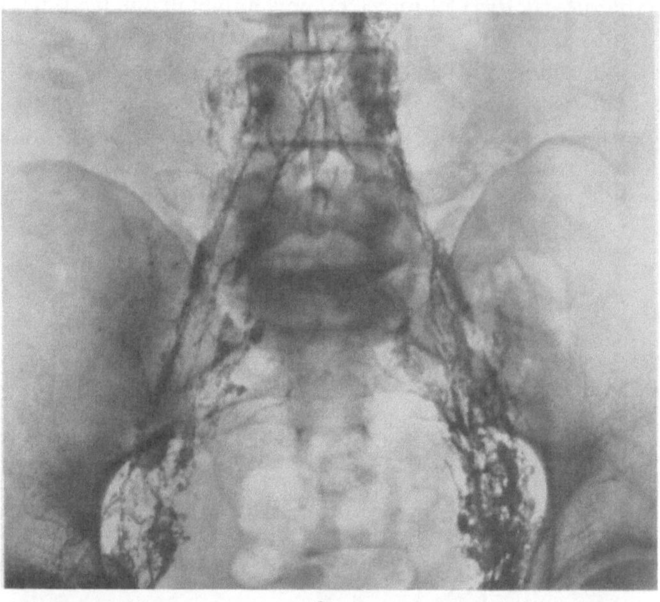

a

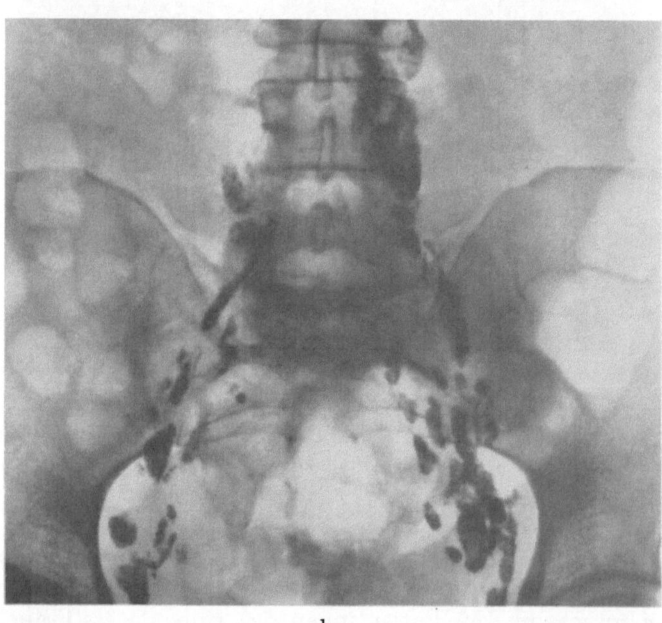

b

Abb. 67a—c. Gewichtsverlust und erhöhte BSG bei Zustand nach Collumcarcinom Stadium I. Palpatorisch kein Anhalt für ein Rezidiv im kleinen Becken. a Lymphangiogramm, keine sicheren Tumorzeichen. b Im Speicherbild unregelmäßige Lymphknotenmarkierung in der Lumbalregion rechts. c Die beidseitige transfemorale Phlebographie ergibt eine komplette Blockade der Vena cava. Das gesamte Kontrastmittel wird über Kollateralen abtransportiert. Eine Explorativlaparotomie bestätigt die ausgedehnte lumbale Metastasierung

Die transfemorale Arteriographie (Abb. 68) wird vor allem von Frischkorn (1964) nnd Breit (1967) empfohlen. Im Gegensatz zur Arteriographie bei Blasentumoren haften der arteriographischen Darstellung eines vom weiblichen Genitale ausgehenden Tumors größere diagnostische Schwierigkeiten an. Lageabweichungen, frühere entzündliche Erkrankungen und viele andere, auch klinisch und anamnestisch nicht auszuschließende Faktoren erschweren die diagnostische Aussage erheblich.

Wenn auch dem Pyelogramm, der Isotopennephrographie, der Lymphangiographie, der Arterio- und Phlebographie sowie den Röntgenuntersuchungsmethoden der Blase und des Dickdarms eine große Bedeutung bei der Diagnostik des Rezidivs zukommt, so vermag erst die histologische Verifizierung eine sichere Diagnose zu ergeben. Eine Gewebsentnahme ist jedoch oft mit großen technischen Schwierigkeiten verbunden. Wenn auch die Verwendung einer Silverman-Punktionsnadel bei nur geringen Gefahren empfohlen

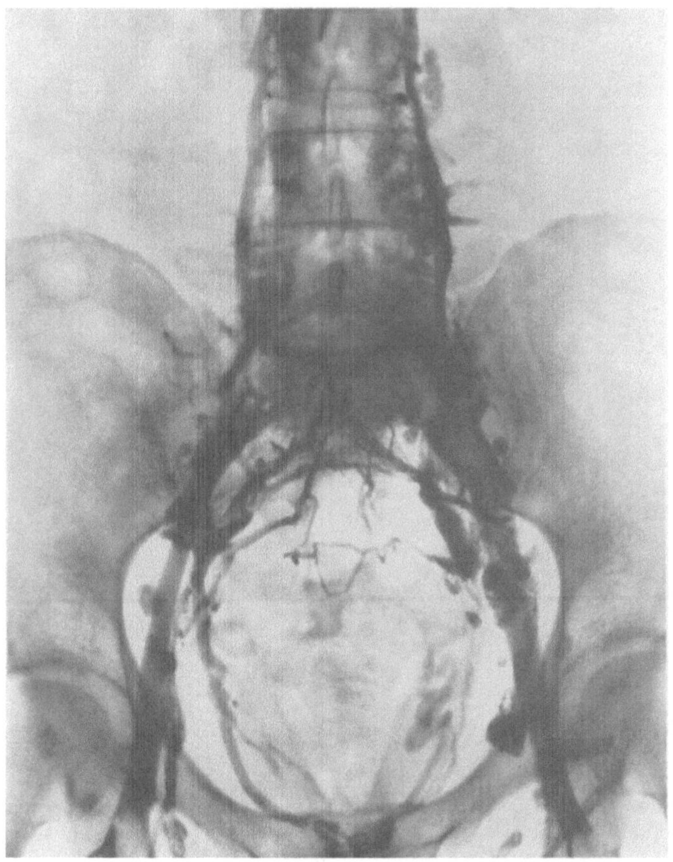

Abb. 67 c

wird, gestattet aber doch selbst eine Probelaparotomie nicht immer eine eindeutige Entscheidung hinsichtlich des Vorliegens eines Rezidivs. So sind die oft widersprüchlichen Angaben im Schrifttum dadurch zu erklären, daß die diagnostizierten Rezidive nur zum kleineren Teil histologisch belegt werden konnten.

Über das zeitliche Auftreten der Rezidive findet man im Schrifttum weitgehend übereinstimmende Angaben. STEGMANN und HANGER (1964) fanden bei 933 Fällen von Collumcarcinom in 54% Rezidive im 1. Jahr, in 28% im 2., in 9,6% im 3., in 6% im 4. und in 2% im 5. Jahr. Auch HERIK und FRICKE (1955) sahen bei 1200 Patientinnen 80% der Rezidive innerhalb von 2 Jahren nach der primären Behandlung. KEPP errechnete 64% Rezidive im 1. Jahr und in den beiden ersten Jahren 85%. HESS und PROPPE (1957) zeigten, daß die Frauen, die das 3. Jahr überlebt hatten, eine Dauerheilungschance von 92% haben. Auch RIES und BREITNER (1959) gelangten zu dem Ergebnis, daß 40% aller Rezidive im 1. Jahr, 25% im 2., 18% im 3. Jahr und nur noch 5% im 4. Jahr auftreten. Damit bestätigen sie die Feststellung, daß die Heilungschance für Frauen, die das 3. Jahr überlebt haben größer als 90% ist.

Nach einer rezidivfreien Zeit von 5 Jahren sind später auftretende, sog. Spätrezidive, relativ selten. Während beispielsweise Nick und Adler (1959) in 2,7% ein Spätrezidiv in ihrem Patientengut fanden, geben Herik und Fricke (1955) eine Häufigkeit von 3,6% an.

Die Rezidivhäufigkeit in den einzelnen Ausbreitungsstadien ist nicht gleich. Stegmann und Hanger (1964) fanden beispielsweise bei den auftretenden Rezidiven im Stadium I 77,2% in den ersten beiden Jahren, im Stadium II 84,2%, im Stadium III 85,5% und im Stadium IV 100%. Hieraus ergibt sich, daß ein prognostisches Urteil in den fortgeschritteneren Stadien früher als in den anderen Stadien möglich ist.

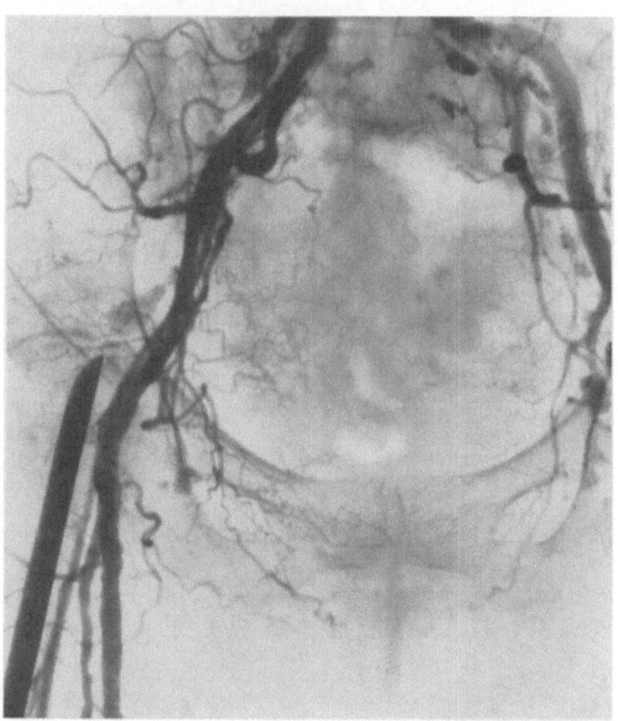

Abb. 68. Beidseitige transfemorale Beckenarteriographie bei einem rechtsseitigen parametranen Rezidiv nach Collumcarcinom Stadium II. In der frühen arteriellen Phase markiert sich ein knäuelartiger Gefäßbezirk im kleinen Becken rechts

Wesentlich stärker unterscheiden sich die Angaben hinsichtlich der Lokalisation der Rezidive, da sie weitgehend von der primären Therapieform abhängen. So fand Schrimpf (1952), daß nach vorangegangener Operation das Rezidiv in der Mehrzahl der Fälle an der Beckenwand und in der Vagina lokalisiert war, während es nach kombinierter Radium-Röntgenbehandlung vorwiegend parametran auftrat. Über die Lokalisation bei 313 Collumcarcinomrezidiven aus den Jahren 1928—1960 berichten Ricci und Bianchi (1966). Lokale Metastasen am Collum uteri und an der Scheide fanden sie in 21,8%, eine Rezidivinfiltration in den Parametrien, in den Ligamenta sacrouterina, den hypogastrischen und Obturatorlymphknoten in 61,3%, Blasen- und Rectumbeteiligung in 3,5% und Metastasen an der Peripherie des Beckens in 13,8%. Nach einer kombinierten Radium-Röntgentherapie sind die parametranen und Beckenwandrezidive wesentlich häufiger als lokale Rezidive an der Portio. Es folgen die Scheidenmetastasen und die Metastasen in Blase und Rectum.

Fernmetastasen sind beim Collumcarcinom relativ selten. Kepp (1952) fand unter sämtlichen Rezidiven nur 17% Fernmetastasen. Da die Fernmetastasen relativ selten klinisch diagnostiziert werden können, gewinnt man nur aufgrund von Sektionen einen

Überblick über die Lokalisation von Fernmetastasen. In klinischer Hinsicht sind diese Angaben von geringem Wert, da sie nur auf die Fälle im Finalstadium bezogen werden können. So findet man die häufigsten Fernmetastasen in der Lunge, der Leber, dem Knochenbaugerüst und in den extraabdominalen Lymphknoten (ALVAREZ, 1953; KELLY et al., 1960; LUCISANO et al., 1960).

Über ein großes Sektionsgut von 460 Fällen von Collumcarcinom berichtet FISCHER (1956). Nur in 48 Fällen konnten keine Metastasen festgestellt werden. Außerhalb des Abdomens fallen neben der thorakalen Lymphknotenmetastasierung von 15,9 % vor allem die Lebermetastasen mit 20,3 %, Knochenmetastasen mit 17,4 % und Lungenmetastasen

Tabelle 20. *Autoptisch festgestellte Metastasenlokalisation bei 467 Fällen von Carcinoma colli uteri* (FISCHER)

	Zahl	%		Zahl	%
Parametrien	240	57,5	Leber	85	20,3
Corpus uteri	120	28,7	Knochen	73	17,4
Beckenbindegewebe	117	27,7	Lungen	68	16,2
Harnblase	114	27,2	Pleura	39	9,3
Vagina	103	24,8	Peritoneum	38	9,1
Rectum	83	19,8	Darm	30	7,1
Douglas	38	9,1	Niere	20	4,8
Ovar	31	7,4	Herz	14	3,3
Vesico vaginal-Fistel	70	16,7	Zwerchfell	12	2,9
Kloake	35	8,4	Muskulatur	11	2,6
Recto vaginal-Fistel	25	6,0	Netz	11	2,6
Lymphknoten, insgesamt	242	57,8	Milz	10	2,4
davon lumbal	187	44,6	Nebenniere	10	2,4
lokal	104	24,8	Pankreas	9	2,1
thorakal	67	15,9	Haut	7	1,6
epigastrisch	43	10,2	Schilddrüse	4	0,9
inguinal	31	7,4	Magen	3	0,7
			Dura mater	2	0,4
			Gehirn	2	0,4

von 16,2 % ins Gewicht (Tabelle 20). Die übrigen Metastasenlokalisationen sind wesentlich seltener. Eine häufigere Metastasierungsfrequenz in diesen Organen fand BAUER (1953). Er sah bei 39 Autopsien in 46,1 % eine Lungenmetastasierung, in 23 % eine Lebermetastasierung, in 41 % eine Knochenmetastasierung und in 53,8 % eine extraabdominelle Lymphknotenmetastasierung. Diese Metastasierungsfrequenzen liegen aber im Schrifttum eindeutig an der Spitze.

Wenn auch immer wieder angenommen wird, daß es sich beim Collumcarcinom um eine hämatogene Metastasierungsform handelt, zeigen die lymphangiographischen Befunde der letzten Jahre deutlich an großen Fallzahlen, daß mit einer extraabdominellen Metastasierung fast stets ein Befall der lumbalen Lymphknoten verbunden ist. Während auch WALTHER (1948) beide Ausbreitungsarten als etwa gleich häufig ansah, scheinen die heutigen Befunde und Erkenntnisse mehr für einen fast ausschließlichen lymphogenen Metastasierungsweg zu sprechen. So ist auch bei fast allen Sektionsbefunden die Rate der lumbalen Metastasierungen stets höher als die anderer Organlokalisationen.

Wesentlich seltener als im Sektionsgut werden klinisch die Knochenmetastasen diagnostiziert. Während im allgemeinen eine Knochenmetastasierung von etwa 1 % angenommen wird (HEISS, 1956), fanden MARQUES, FAILLIÈRES und SANCERNI (1966) bei 1 046 behandelten Patientinnen eine Frequenz von 4 %. Bei 18 Fällen handelte es sich um multiple Knochenmetastasen (Abb. 69).

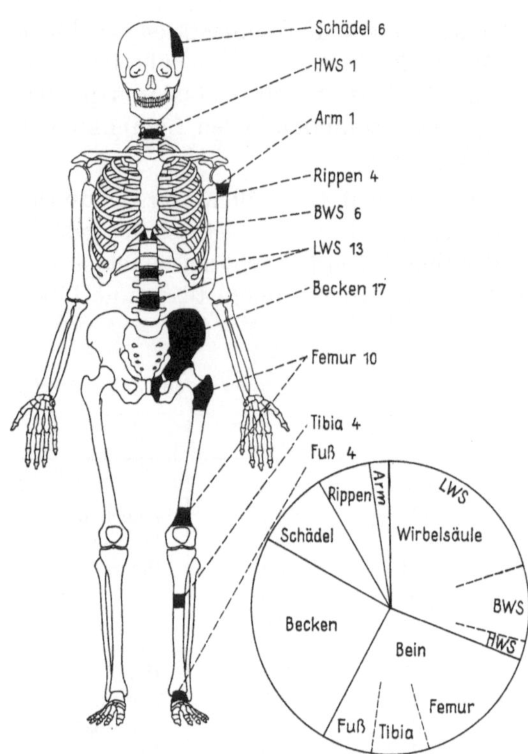

Abb. 69. Lokalisation der Knochenmetastasen (42 Fälle) beim Carcinoma colli uteri (MARQUES, FAILLIÈRES und SANCERNI)

b) Bestrahlungsmethoden

Über die Behandlung der Rezidive finden sich im Schrifttum keine konkreten Behandlungsrichtlinien. Grundsätzlich muß aber unterschieden werden, ob es sich um Rezidive nach einer ausschließlich operativen Behandlung oder aber um bereits bestrahlte Fälle handelt. Bei Rezidiven nach Operation wird die Bestrahlungsmethode und Dosierung weitgehend der einer primären Strahlentherapie entsprechen. Größere Schwierigkeiten ergeben sich bei Rezidiven nach einer Strahlentherapie. Die Bestrahlungsmethode sowie Fraktionierung und Gesamtdosis müssen sich dann nach der vorangegangenen Strahlenbehandlung und vor allem nach dem Intervall zwischen Primärbestrahlung und Rezidiverkrankung richten.

Die lokalen Rezidive sowie die vaginalen Metastasen werden meist durch eine erneute Radiumeinlage angegangen, wobei sich die Filterform nach der Tumorlokalisation und -ausdehnung richtet und ihr optimal angepaßt werden soll. RIES und BREITNER (1959) weisen darauf hin, daß eine intrauterine Radiumeinlage nur im Ausnahmefall vor Ablauf eines Jahres wiederholt werden kann. Sie fordern, daß in einem solchen Fall die primäre Dosis weit unter der Toleranzdosis an Blase und Rectum gelegen haben muß und beide Organe keine Zeichen einer lokalen Strahlenwirkung aufweisen dürfen. Vaginale Einlagen können bereits einige Monate nach der Primärbehandlung gegeben werden.

Die Behandlung vulvanaher Befunde wurde bisher vor allem durch eine Spickung mit Radiumnadeln, durch eine Moulagenbehandlung (BECKER und SCHEER, 1956), mit der Hohlanodenröhre oder durch Elektrocoagulation (KOTTMEIER, 1964) durchgeführt. Wir halten in diesen Fällen eine Bestrahlung mit energiereichen Elektronen für wirkungsvoller und vor allem für schonender.

Größere Schwierigkeiten ergeben sich bei der Behandlung parametraner und beckenwandnaher Befunde. In diesen Fällen wird die erforderliche Herddosis nach vorangegangener Orthovoltpercutanbestrahlung durch die bereits bestehenden Hautveränderungen limitiert. Während bei gut abgrenzbaren Beckenwandlymphknotenmetastasen und vor allem den „Spinarezidiven", den häufig an der Spina ossis ischii lokalisierten Rezidiven, eine intravaginale Bestrahlung mit der Hohlanode möglich ist, können ausgedehntere Befunde ausschließlich percutan erfaßt werden. Unter Orthovoltbedingungen kann eine tumorwirksame Herddosis nur mit der Pendel- oder Pendelkonvergenzbestrahlung erreicht werden.

Um in diesen Fällen die erhebliche Hautbelastung zu umgehen, wurden verschiedene Methoden der lokalen Isotopentherapie angegeben. Während HENSCHKE (1965) für die interstitielle Therapie ein entfernbares Nylonband vorschlug, empfiehlt LIEGNER (1964) eine Spickmethode, um auf diese Weise in ein kleines umschriebenes Volumen eine hohe Strahlendosis applizieren zu können. Hierzu werden empfohlen: Radonkörner, Radiogoldkörner, Radioiridiumkörner, Radioiridiumdraht und Radiokobaltdraht. Als Vorteil der Implantation radioaktiver Körner bei der Behandlung von Rezidivtumoren werden angegeben: die Einfachheit des Eingriffes, das Fehlen hämorrhagischer und entzündlicher Komplikationen, die genaue Lokalisationsmöglichkeit der Körner, die kurze Liegezeit der Patientinnen und das Fehlen von Frühreaktionen. LIEGNER (1964) beschreibt bei 13 Fällen einen zumindest befriedigenden Palliativeffekt. Die Volumendosis lag zwischen 5000 und 8700 γ R. In 10 von 13 Fällen konnte LIEGNER eine rapide Verkleinerung der Metastasen innerhalb weniger Wochen beobachten.

KAPP-SCHWOERER (1962) und THOMSEN (1962) empfehlen für die Behandlung von Collumcarcinomrezidiven die intraoperative Applikation von Radiogoldseeds. Zur Sicherung der histologischen Diagnose kann in vielen Fällen auf eine Laparotomie nicht verzichtet werden, bei der dann in gleicher Sitzung die Seeds in den Tumor appliziert werden können. Die Vorteile der Radiogoldseedsbehandlung erlauben es, bei weitgehender Schonung der Nachbarorgane eine wirksame Dosis an den Tumor zu bringen. Diese Bestrahlungsmethode ist vor allem auch dann noch möglich, wenn die Hautbelastung infolge vorangegangener Bestrahlung eine percutane Therapie nicht mehr zulassen würde. Über die Injektion von kolloidalem Gold liegen bisher keine größeren Erfahrungsberichte vor.

Während der Strahlenbehandlung im allgemeinen nur bei der Behandlung von Rezidiven nach operativer Therapie des Collumcarcinoms ein Erfolg zuerkannt wird, konnte demgegenüber KEPP (1953) zeigen, daß durch die Erhöhung der Strahlendosis bei Anwendung einer kombinierten Strahlenbehandlung unter besonderer Berücksichtigung der intravaginalen Bestrahlung zur größtmöglichen Beschränkung der Raumdosis die Ergebnisse verbessert werden konnten. Dabei läßt sich zwar oft eine schwere Strahlenschädigung von Nachbarorganen bei besonders strahlenresistenten Tumoren nicht vermeiden. Die Rezidivbestrahlung muß im Hinblick auf den Allgemeinzustand der Patientinnen individuell dosiert werden. Es sollen kleinere Einzeldosen bei längerer Bestrahlungszeit appliziert werden.

Bessere Voraussetzungen für eine percutane Rezidivbestrahlung ergeben sich bei Verwendung von Megavoltenergien. So empfehlen FRIEDMAN und PEARLMAN (1965) bei peripheren Lymphknotenmetastasen eine Megavolt-Rotationstherapie, bei der Dosen von 7266 rad innerhalb von 39 Tagen appliziert werden. Das kleine Becken wird in der Regel mit allenfalls 5500 rad belastet. Bei besonders strahlenresistenten Tumoren werden aber auch oft 8000—9000 R notwendig.

Von Megavoltstrahlen wird bei Rezidiven nach Strahlentherapie auch an der Universitäts-Frauenklinik Hamburg Gebrauch gemacht. Nachdem bei der Primärbehandlung die Beckenwand mit etwa 5000 R belastet worden ist, werden bei beckenwandnaher Tumorlokalisation nach einem $^1/_2$ Jahr erneut 6000 R eingestrahlt, die nach einem Intervall von mehr als 1 Jahr und insbesondere funktionsloser Niere auf 8000 R erhöht werden.

HELLER und KÄSER (1966) warnen aufgrund ihrer autoptischen Ergebnisse (s. S. 256) davor, eine erneute Bestrahlung wegen Verdachtes auf ein Rezidiv ohne histologische Sicherung durchzuführen. Sie fordern bei einem Infiltrat im Bereich der Beckenwand oder der Parametrien die Sicherung durch Nadelbiopsie oder Probelaparotomie. Selbst ein falsch negatives Resultat der Punktion oder der Laparotomie erscheint ihnen bei der schlechten Prognose des Rezidivs kein ausreichender Faktor zu sein. Da durch eine unnötige zweite Bestrahlung das Leben der Frau stark gefährdet wird, führen sie ohne histologische Diagnose keine Rezidivbestrahlung durch.

Fernmetastasen, die meist außerhalb des primären Strahlenfeldes liegen, werden unter den sonst üblichen Bedingungen bestrahlt. Da sich aufgrund unserer Erfahrungen nach einer hochdosierten Primärbehandlung solche Fälle zu mehren scheinen, in denen das kleine Becken frei von Tumor ist und lediglich eine isolierte Fernmetastase vorliegt, kommt solchen Bestrahlungsfällen eine größere Bedeutung zu.

Eine Sonderstellung nehmen die Knochenmetastasen am 5. Lendenwirbel oder 1. Sacralwirbel ein. Sie kommen häufig isoliert vor und besitzen nach einer ausreichend hoch dosierten Strahlenbehandlung eine günstige Prognose (ZUPPINGER).

Lediglich bei einer generalisierten Tumoraussaat sollte man sich auf allgemeine palliative Behandlungsmethoden beschränken.

c) Behandlungsergebnisse

Versucht man, die Behandlungsergebnisse nach einem bestrahlten oder operierten Rezidiv zusammenzustellen, erhöhen sich die Heilungsergebnisse um so mehr, je geringer die Quote der histologisch gesicherten Rezidive ist. So konnte FRISCHKORN (1964) nachweisen, daß klinisch diagnostizierte Rezidive nach einem Collumcarcinom ohne histologische Sicherung in 26,2% eine 5-Jahres-Heilung aufwiesen, während die histologisch gesicherten nur eine Heilung von 6,2% zeigten. Ähnlich kraß sind die Beobachtungen von KÄSER und SCHIEFERSTEIN (1966), die bei 108 rezidivbestrahlten Frauen eine Überlebenszeit von 24% erhielten; von den histologisch gesicherten parametranen Beckenwandrezidiven konnte durch eine zweite Bestrahlung aber keines geheilt werden.

Eine weitere Abhängigkeit von der eingestrahlten Dosis in bezug auf die Überlebenschance nach einem Rezidiv konnten NOLAN, VIDAL und ANSON (1957) feststellen. Von 73 bestrahlten Rezidiven wurden mit Hochvolttherapie (Telekobalt bzw. van-de-Graaff-Generator) 27 Patientinnen bestrahlt, von denen 8 überlebten. Von den konventionell bestrahlten Patientinnen überlebten keine. Sie konnten weiter zeigen, daß als Mindestdosis 4500—5000 R innerhalb von 40 Tagen gegeben werden müssen. Bei Verabreichung geringerer Dosen waren alle Frauen verstorben. Auch KEPP (1952) konnte durch Erhöhung der Strahlendosis 5-Jahres-Überlebenszeiten von 18,5% bei den auf das kleine Becken beschränkten Rezidivtumoren beim Collumcarcinom feststellen.

Nach relativ hohen Strahlendosen registrierten FRIEDMANN und PEARLMANN (1965) in einer Serie von 38 Fällen in 42% ein krankheitsfreies Intervall von 5 Jahren. Bei diesen Patientinnen hatte es sich allerdings um Rezidive nach vorangegangener Operation gehandelt, die erfahrungsgemäß wesentlich günstiger auf eine Rezidivbestrahlung ansprechen. In 3 von 11 Fällen vernichteten sie aber sicher eine histologisch nachgewiesene Lymphknotenmetastasierung durch Dosen von 4250—9150 R. Die Patientinnen lebten 5, 6 und 8 Jahre rezidivfrei.

Die meist vorherrschende Ansicht, daß die Heilungsaussichten nach einer kompletten Strahlenbehandlung bei einem histologisch gesicherten Rezidiv durch eine erneute Strahlentherapie gering sind, können durch die Ergebnisse von MURPHY und SCHMITZ (1956) widerlegt werden. Bei 46 Patientinnen mit einem Rezidiv wurde der Befund in 32 Fällen histologisch gesichert. Nach einer intensiven Strahlenbehandlung lebten noch 9 Frauen über 6 Jahre nach Beginn der Wiederbestrahlung; der Befund war histologisch in 7 von diesen 9 Fällen gesichert.

Das Argument, daß die Rezidive nach einer Strahlenbehandlung meist strahlenrefraktär sind, führte dazu, daß man in den letzten Jahren in solchen Fällen von radikalen bzw. ultraradikalen operativen Behandlungsmethoden in zunehmendem Maße Gebrauch machte.

BRUNSCHWIG berichtete 1967 über die Ergebnisse bei 317 Patientinnen mit rezidivierendem oder strahlenrefraktärem Cervix-Carcinom, bei denen in den Jahren 1947 bis 1960 eine vordere (95 Fälle), hintere (5 Fälle) oder totale Exenteration durchgeführt wurde. Von diesen Patientinnen lebten mehr als 5 Jahre 55 Patientinnen (17,6%). Die primäre Mortalität betrug bei der vorderen Exenteration 10,5% und bei der totalen Exenteration 20,0%. Diese hohe Operationsmortalität betraf vor allem Fälle, bei denen bereits die Beckenwand befallen war. Deshalb wird von BRUNSCHWIG wie von BRICKER (1966) eine Beckenwandmetastasierung als Kontraindikation angesehen. Trotzdem beträgt bei BRUNSCHWIG die Operationsmortalität nach Selektion noch 5—10%.

COSBIE (1959) erkennt zwar an, daß die radikale chirurgische Behandlung des Rezidivs zweifellos durch den sehr Erfahrenen Erfolge hat, zeigt aber, daß mit der Wiederholungsbestrahlung ebenfalls in 15% der Fälle 5-Jahres-Heilungen erzielt werden können. Da die Komplikationen bei der erneuten Strahlenbehandlung wesentlich häufiger sind, fordert er, daß eine explorative Laparotomie mit Biopsie durchgeführt werden sollte, wenn ein begründeter Verdacht auf ein Rezidiv besteht.

Durch die Sicherung der Diagnose und das Erkennen der vollen Ausdehnung und Lokalisation des Rezidivtumors wird für die erneute Strahlenbehandlung eine bessere Ausgangsposition geschaffen. Vor allem erscheint es eher gerechtfertigt, in solchen Fällen die durch eine erneute und hoch dosierte Strahlenbehandlung bedingten Komplikationen in Kauf nehmen.

11. Koordination und Durchführung der Behandlung des Collumcarcinoms

Überblickt man heute die Behandlungsergebnisse der letzten Dezennien, so fällt in den einzelnen Jahresberichten des Annual Report das stetige Ansteigen der Heilungsergebnisse auf. Betrug beispielsweise die 5-Jahres-Heilung im Jahre 1937 noch 26,3%, wurden 1951 im Band 7 Ergebnisse von 36,9% mitgeteilt, die heute im 13. Band bei 48% liegen. Diese Verbesserungen sind freilich nicht allein als Folge der Behandlungsfortschritte aufzufassen. Sie sind ebenfalls durch Fortschritte auf diagnostischem Sektor bedingt, bei denen der Kolposkopie und Cytologie die größte Bedeutung zukommen. Andererseits ist auch die Bevölkerung über die Symptome des Krebses stärker aufgeklärt, so daß sich auch hierdurch die zur Behandlung kommenden Stadien verbessert haben.

Seit dem letzten Weltkrieg wurden die diagnostischen und therapeutischen Verfahren immer weiter spezialisiert.

Zur Deutung cytologischer und kolposkopischer Befunde sind spezielle Kenntnisse erforderlich. Eine Gewebsentnahme kann nur dann von Wert sein, wenn sie gezielt aus der richtigen Region entnommen ist. Die histologische Auswertung erfordert gründliche pathologisch-anatomische Erfahrungen. Die Befähigung zur Behandlung eines Carcinoms setzt eine umfassende klinische Ausbildung voraus, um die Diagnose unter Berücksichtigung der Laborwerte und des klinischen Bildes stellen zu können.

Die Einführung ultraradikaler Operationsmethoden fordert nicht nur vom Operateur sondern vom gesamten Operationsteam ein hohes Maß an technischer Qualifikation. Die Narkose und die postoperative Überwachung kann nur einem speziell geschulten Anaesthesieteam übertragen werden.

Bei der Durchführung der strahlentherapeutischen Verfahren kann der Strahlentherapeut heute nicht mehr mit der Kenntnis einiger Bestrahlungsdaten auskommen. Die Anwendung von Megavoltanlagen erfordert umfangreiche physikalische und biologische Kenntnisse; sie setzt technisches Wissen bei der Strahlenerzeugung und praktische Fähigkeiten beim Umgang mit diesen Anlagen voraus. Darüber hinaus erfordert die gynäkologische Strahlentherapie exakte Kenntnisse der topographischen Gegebenheiten im kleinen Becken. Der das Radium applizierende Arzt muß eine gynäkologische Ausbildung besitzen, da die Radiumeinlage ein operativer intrauteriner Eingriff ist.

Es ergibt sich hierdurch zwangsläufig, daß die Carcinomdiagnostik und -therapie heutzutage so spezialisiert ist und Erfahrungen voraussetzt, die kein Kliniker mehr in einer Person besitzen kann. Eine optimale Carcinomtherapie muß heute mehr denn je Aufgabe eines ganzen Teams sein, in dessen Händen nicht nur Diagnostik und Therapie, sondern auch noch die notwendige nachgehende Fürsorge und Überwachung der behandelten Patienten liegen muß.

So erfordert die Trennung von Diagnostik und Therapie einerseits und operativer und radiologischer Therapie andererseits, daß eine ständige gegenseitige Konsultation verschiedener Spezialisten notwendig wird. Hieraus ergibt sich die Konsequenz, daß eine solche Teamarbeit nur in größeren Behandlungszentren möglich ist, die neben der personellen Voraussetzung auch noch über eine optimale apparative Ausstattung verfügen müssen. Leider sind wir in Deutschland hiervon noch weit entfernt.

Literatur

ABBATUCCI, J. S.: Introduction à la radiothérapie des cancers du col utérin au stade III. (Einführung in die Strahlentherapie des Carcinoma colli uteri, Stadium III.) [Soc. Franç. Electroradiol. Méd., 18.—20. X. 1967.] J. Radiol. Électrol. 49, 599—607 (1968).

ADLER, L.: Morphologische Kennzeichen für die Radiumempfindlichkeit der Karzinome des weiblichen Genitales. Zbl. Gynäk. 40, 637—680 (1916).

AHRENS, C. A., TSCHOKE, S.: Lymphknotenbefunde nach Wertheim-Meigsscher Operation. Geburtsh. u. Frauenheilk. 21, 219—224 (1961).

AKASHI, K., KOROKU, Y., TOMITA, H., HASHIMOTO, M., KAWASAKI, I., HORI, C., KOMORI, A., YAMADA, Y.: Studies on the extraperitoneal procedure of lymphonodectomy with ligation of the pelvis vessels and radical vaginal hysterectomy for cancer of the uterine cervix. Jap. J. Obstet. Gynec. 5, 347—355 (1958).

ALDRIDGE, C. W., MASON, J. T.: Ureteral obstruction in carcinoma of the cervix. Amer. J. Obstet. Gynec. 60, 1272—1280 (1950).

ALLEN, W. M., SHERMAN, A. I., ARNESON, A. N.: Cacinoma of the cervix: results obtained from the irradiation of the parametrium with radioactive colloidal gold. Amer. J. Obstet. Gynec. 68, 1433—1446 (1954).

— — — Further results obtained in the treatment of cancer of the cervix with radiogold: a progress report. (Weitere Ergebnisse bei der Behandlung des Cervixcarcinoms mit Radio-Gold: Ein erneuter Bericht.) Amer. J. Obstet. 70, 786—790 (1955).

— — CAMEL, H. M.: Radiogold in the treatment of cancer of the cervix. (Radiogold in der Behandlung des Collum-Carcinom.) Radiology 70, 523—527 (1958).

ALTVATER, G., IMHOLZ, G.: Die Ureterstenosen beim Collumcarcinom. Prognost. Bedeutung u. chirurg. Behandlung. Geburth. u. Frauenheilk. 20, 1214—1229 (1960).

ALVAREZ, R. R. DE: The sites of metastasis in carcinoma of the cervix. West. J. Surg. 61, 623—627 (1953).

AMBESI IMPIOMBATO, G., CHELAZZI, M., MILANESI, R.: Il trattamento del cancro del collo dell'utero con radium e telecobaltoterapia. (Die Behandlung des Collum-Carcinoms mit Radium und der Telekobalttherapie.) Radiol. med. (Torino) 45, 1095—1113 (1959).

AMREICH, A. I.: Klinik und operative Behandlung des Uteruskarzinoms. In: Biologie und Pathologie des Weibes, Bd. IV. Berlin-Innsbruck-München-Wien: Urban & Schwarzenberg 1955.

— — Grenzen und Aussichten der operativen Behandlung des Collumcarcinoms. Geburtsh. u. Frauenheilk. 9, 873—887 (1949).

— Das Lymphknotenproblem bei Operation und Bestrahlung des Kollumkarzinoms. Wien. med. Wsch strahlung des Kollumkarzinoms. Wien. med. Wschr. 107, 6—11 (1957).

ANDERSON, A. F.: Treatment and follow-up of noninvasive cancer of the uterine cervix. Report on 205 cases (1948—1957). (Behandlung und nachgehende Kontrolle des nichtinvasiven Carcinoms der Cervix. Bericht über 205 Fälle [1948—1957].) J. Obstet. Gynaec. Brit. Cwlth 72, 172—177 (1965).

ANDREAS, H.: Dosierungsfragen bei der gynäkologischen Radium-Bestrahlung, 83 S. Leipzig: Georg Thieme 1959.

ANDREWS, R. J.: Dose-time relationships in cancer radiotherapy. A clinical radiobiology study of extremes of dose and time. Amer. J. Roentgenol. 93, 56—74 (1965).

ANSELMINO, K. J.: Lassen sich die Heilungsergebnisse der Schauta- und der Wertheim-Operation beim Kollum-Karzinom durch weitere Radikalisierung verbessern? Geburtsh. u. Frauenheilk. 21, 120—127 (1961).

ANTOINE, T.: Die operative Behandlung des Kollumkarzinoms. Krebsarzt 7, 317—323 (1952).

— Surgical approach to cervical carcinoma and the problem of lymphadenectomy. J. int. Coll. Surg. 29, 620—628 (1958).

— Carcinoma of the cervix. (Das Carcinom der Cervix.) J. int. Coll. Surg. 37, 277—283 (1962).

ANTOINE, T.: Neue Gesichtspunkte in der Behandlung der Genitalkarzinome. Wien. med. Wschr. 115, 687—690 (1965).

ANZILOTTI, A., MARTOLINI, M.: Il cancro del moncone uterino residuo ad isterectomia subtotale. (Das Collum-Stumpf-Carcinom nach subtotaler Hysterektomie.) Riv. Radiol. 2, 1145—1158 (1962).

ARESIN, N., KRAUSS, A.: Kollumkarzinom und Schwangerschaftsfrequenz. Zbl. Gynäk. 89, 1050—1054 (1967).

ARIEL, I. M., RESNICK, M. I., GALEY, D.: The intralymphatic administration of radioactive isotopes and cancer chemotherapeutic drugs. (Die intralymphatische Zuführung von radioaktiven Isotopen und chemotherapeutischen Krebsdrogen.) Surgery 55, 355—363 (1964).

ARNESON, A. N., WILLIAMS, C. F.: Long-term follow-up observations in cervical cancer. (Langfristig nachgehende Untersuchungen beim Cervixcarcinom.) Amer. J. Obstet. Gynec. 80, 775—790 (1960).

ARVAY, N., PICARD, J. D.: La lymphographie. Paris: Masson & Cie. 1963.

ATLEE, H. B., TUPPER, C.: Early diagnosis of deterioration after radiation therapy of carcinoma of the cervix. (Frühdiagnose der Verschlimmerung nach Strahlentherapie des Cervixcarcinoms.) Canad. med. Ass. J. 76, 181—183 (1957).

AVERETTE, H. E., HUDSON, R. C., FERGUSON, J. H.: Lymphangioadenography: Applications in the study and management of gynecologic cancer. Cancer (Philad.) 17, 1093 (1964).

BACH, W., WILLE, P.: Der Einfluß der gynäkologischen Radiumbestrahlung auf die Zerfallsneigung der Thrombozyten. Zbl. Gynäk. 87, 625—630 (1965).

BACLESSE, F., REVERDY, J., JAMMET, H.: Considérations sur la roentgenthérapie transcutanée seule dans le traitement des cancers avancés de l'utérus et du vagin. (Betrachtungen über die ausschließliche percutane Rö-Bestrahlung in der Behandlung des fortgeschrittenen Uterus- und Vaginal-Ca.) J. de Radiol. 35, 57—62 (1954).

BAEUMER, J.: Die Anwendung der Rotationsbestrahlung in der Gynäkologie (Univ.-Frauenkl. Göttingen). Strahlentherapie 87, 290—294 (1952).

BAGNATI, E. P., VILLAMAJOR, R. D.: La linfadenectomia en el carcinoma de cuello uterino. Rev. Asoc. med. argent. 68, 301—303 (1954); Ref. Ber. ges. Gynäk. Geburtsh. 55, 292 (1955).

BAILY, N. A., KRAMER, G.: Lithium-drifted silicon p-i-n junction as x-ray and gamma-ray dosimeter. Radiat. Res. 22, 53—80 (1964).

— NORMAN, A.: Miniature p-i-n junctions for in-vivo dosimetry. Nucleonics 21, 64—65 (1963).

— — HILBERT, J. W.: A direct reading intracavitary dosimeter for use in radium therapy. Amer. J. Roentgenol. 99, 382—386 (1967).

— YODER, V. E.: Isodose curves for certain radium applicators used in treatment of uterine cervical cancer. Amer. J. Roentgenol. 83, 447—454 (1960).

BAKER, W. S., JR.: Carcinoma of the uterine cervix. Interstitial radioactive colloidal gold therapy of the lateral pelvic nodes. (Carcinom des Collum uteri. Interstitielle Behandlung der seitlichen Beckenlymphknoten mit radioaktivem Goldkolloid. Calif. Med. 92, 25—30 (1960).

BARBANTI, A.: Utilizzazione dei radionuclidi in diagnostica e terapia ginecologica. (Die Verwendung der Isotopen in der gynäkologischen Diagnostik und Therapie.) Minerva nucl. 3, 357—366 (1959).

— BELLION, B., BUCHI, G.: Indicazioni e possibilità dell'infiltrazione parametriale mediante radiocolloidi nel trattamento delle neoplasie uterine. (Indikation und Möglichkeiten der parametrialen Infiltration von kolloidalen Radioisotopen in der Behandlung von Uterusmalignomen.) Atti Soc. reg. Ostet. Ginec. 9, 202—204 (1960).

— TETTI, A.: Infiltrazione parametrale con radioisotopi come terapia delle neoplasie. Indicazioni, tecnica e risultati. (Infiltration des Parametriums mit Radioisotopen in der Krebsbehandlung. Indikation, Technik, Resultate.) Atti Soc. Ostet. Ginec. 8, 107—111 (1959).

BARNES, A.: Therapy of the lateral pelvic nodes in cervical carcinoma. (Die Behandlung der seitlichen Becken-Lymphknoten beim Collum-Carcinom.) Amer. J. Obstet. 68, 489—493 (1954).

— Use of cobalt 60 in radiation therapy of gynecologic malignancies. (Die Anwendung von Co^{60} in der Strahlenbehandlung gynäkologischer Tumoren.) Progr. Gynec. 3, 633—642 (1957).

— MORTON, J. L., CALLENDINE, G. W.: The use of radioactive cobalt in the treatment of carcinoma of the cervix. Amer. J. Obstet. Gynec. 60, 1112 (1950).

BARNES, W. E., HOFFMANN, G. W., PICKRELL, K.: Surgical treatment of irradiation injuries of the perineum. Surgery 118, 1067—1072 (1964).

BAŠTECKÝ, J., CHVOJKA, Z.: Modification of the Vinohrady gynecologic radiation technic in telecobalt treatment. (Modifikation der Vinohrady-Bestrahlungsmethode bei der Telekobalttherapie.) Čsl. Radiol. 18, 361—367 mit engl. Zus.fass. (1964) [Tschechisch].

BATTEZATTI, M., DONINI, J., BELARCHI, P., BECCHI, G., MUGGIATI, L.: Die Phlebolymphographie der Leisten-Becken-Region. Fortschr. Röntgenstr. 98, 705 (1963).

— — — — — Association Phlebo-Lymphography dans la region ingenno-plevienne. Presse méd. 27, 537 (1963).

BAUD, J.: Les résultats de la radiothérapie (curiethérapie et roentgenthérapie) de 124 cas d'épithéliomas sur col restant traités dans les services de la fondation Curie de 1919 à 1944 inclus. (Resultate der Strahlenbehandlung [Radium- und Röntgentherapie] bei 124 Collumstumpf-Carcinomen an den Instituten der Curie-Stiftung von 1919 bis 1944 einschließlich.) Bull. Ass. franç. Cancer 39, 100—104 (1952).

— Results of radiotherapy (curietherapy and roentgentherapy) in 124 epithelioma cases of stump of the cervix, treated from 1919 to 1944 at the Curie foundation. (Ergebnisse der Strahlenbehandlung [Radium- und Röntgentherapie] bei 124 Collumstumpfcarcinomen, behandelt zwischen 1919 und 1944 in der Curie-Stiftung.) J. Fac. Radiol. (Lond.) 3, 203—206 (1952).

Baud, J., Blanchet, F.: Évolution clinique de 44 cas d'épithéliomas du col utérin au cours de la gestation, traités par radiothérapie à la fondation Curie de 1929 à 1950. (Verlauf bei 44 Collumcarcinomen während der Schwangerschaft, die in der Fondation Curie zwischen 1929 und 1950 strahlenbehandelt wurden.) Bull. Ass. franç. Cancer 39, 48—62 (1952).

— Courtial, J.: La roentgenthérapie à 500 kV modifie-t-elle les résultats du traitement des cancers du col utérin? Résultats obtenus à la Fondation Curie chez les malades traitées en 1942—43—44 par la roentgenthérapie péripelvienne à 500 kV associée à l'application intracavitaire de radium. (Verändert die Röntgenbehandlung mit 500 kV die Behandlungsergebnisse beim Collumcarcinom? Die Behandlungsergebnisse der Fondation Curie in den Jahren 1942—44 bei den Patientinnen, die neben der intrakavitären Radiumbehandlung mit einer Röntgenbestrahlung von 500 kV des kleinen Beckens behandelt wurden.) Bull. Ass. franç. Cancer 39, 134—140 (1952).

Bauer, K. H.: Fernmetastasen beim weiblichen Genitalcarcinom, insbesondere beim Carcinom des Collum uteri. Geburtsh. u. Frauenheilk. 13, 1096—1105 (1953).

Baum, S., Bron, K. M., Wexler, L., Abrams, H. L.: Lymphangiography, cavography and urography. Radiology 81, 207 (1963).

Beck, H.: Erfahrungen mit der Hemipelvektomie bei malignen Tumoren. Münch. med. Wschr. 109, 126—130 (1967).

Becker, J., Blöch, R., Wachsmann, F.: Dosisverteilung bei Kreuzfeuer- und Bewegungbestrahlung beim Betatron. Strahlentherapie 98, 297—307 (1955).

— Kärcher, H.-K.: Therapeutische Erfahrungen mit schnellen Elektronen. Acta radiol. (Stockh.), Suppl. 188, 32—40 (1959).

— — Weitzel, G.: Elektronentherapie mit Supervolt-Geräten. In: Strahlenbiologie, Strahlentherapie, Nuklearmedizin und Krebsforschung. Ergebnisse 1952—1958, S. 431—510. Stuttgart: Thieme 1959.

— Kuttig, H.: Gezielte Anwendung einiger Bestrahlungsmethoden in der Telekobalttherapie. Radiol. austriaca 13, 7—14 (1962).

— Weitzel, G.: Dreijährige Erfahrungen mit dem 15-MeV-Siemens-Betatron. Strahlentherapie 101, 167—179 (1956).

— — Neue Formen der Bewegungsbestrahlung beim 15-MeV-Betatron der Siemens-Reiniger-Werke. Strahlentherapie 101, 180—196 (1956).

Beduhn, D., Kuttig, H.: Die Bewegungsbestrahlung der paraaortalen Lymphknoten mit Co^{60}-Gammastrahlen. Strahlentherapie 132, 481—486 (1967).

Bellion, B., Chiarle, S.: Indicazioni e considerazioni sulla terapia coi radiocolloidi in ginecologia. (Überlegungen über die Indikationsstellung zur Therapie mit Radiokolloiden in der Gynäkologie.) Atti Soc. Ostet. Ginec. 9, 200—202 (1960).

Belonoschkin, B.: Zur Frage der Dauerheilung des Kollumkarzinoms des Uterus und des Rezidivproblems. Münch. med. Wschr. 1955, 1306—1308.

Benson, R. C., Dotter, C. T., Straube, K. R.: Percutaneous transfemoral aortography in gynecology and obstetrics. Amer. J. Obstet. Gynec. 85, 772 (1963).

Berger, H.: Ergebnisse rein radiologischer Behandlung von 227 Kollum- und Korpuskarzinomen der Jahre 1950—1956. Strahlentherapie 119, 607—614 (1962).

Bergsjø, P., Evans, J. C.: Late radiation reactions in cancer of the cervix. (Spät-Strahlenschäden beim Collum-Carcinom.) Acta obstet. gynec. scand. 43, Suppl. 7, 90—96 (1965).

Bermond, M.: Il problema del trattamento degli infiltrati parametrali del carcinoma della portio. (Das Problem der Behandlung der parametranen Infiltrate beim Portiocarcinom.) Minerva med. 1952, II, 329—331.

Berta, I., Ruzicska, G., Dévényi, I.: Histological examination of the cancer of the cervix of the uterus and clinical experiences in connection with its praeoperative Ra and Co^{60} treatment. (Klinische und histologische Ergebnisse bei präoperativer Behandlung von Cervix-Carcinomen mit Radium oder ^{60}Co.) Magy. Onkol. 9, 1—7 mit engl. Zus.fass. (1965) [Ungarisch].

Birkner, R., Hoffmann, B.: Unterhautindurationen nach Telekobalttherapie. Strahlentherapie 116, 463—477 (1961).

Bistolfi, F., Bolognesi, M.: Considérations sur la roentgenthérapie avec grille des cancers utérins, aux stades III et IV, après trois ans de recul. (Betrachtungen über die Siebbestrahlung des Gebärmutterkrebses Stadium III/IV.) J. Radiol. Électrol. 39, 494—497 (1958).

Bjarngard, B. E., McCall, R. C., Berstein, I.: Lithium fluoride-teflon thermoluminescence dosimeter for radiological dosimetry. First International Conference on Medical Phys., Harrogate, United Kingdom, September 9, 1965.

Blahey, P. R.: Optimum radium distribution in the treatment of cancer of the cervix. I. (Optimale Radiumverteilung bei der Behandlung des Cervix-Carcinoms. I.) Obstet. and Gynec. 16, 679—688 (1960).

— Beique, R. A., Corry, P. M.: Isodose studies of radium patterns suitable for treatment of cervical cancer. II. (Isodosenuntersuchungen bei Radiummodellen, die für die Behandlung des Cervixcarcinoms geeignet sind.) Obstet. and Gynec. 20, 719—725 (1962).

Blaikley, J. B., Lederman, M., Lewis, T. L. T.: Results of treatment of cancer of the cervix. (Resultate der Behandlung des Cervixcarcinoms.) Lancet 1952 II, 950—951.

Bloedorn, F. G.: Application of the Paterson-Parker system in interstitial radium therapy. (Anwendung des Paterson-Parker-Systems bei der interstitiellen Radiumtherapie.) Amer. J. Roentgenol. 75, 457—475 (1956).

— Cuccia, C. A., Mercado, R., Jr.: The place of interstitial gamma-ray emitters in radiation therapy. Indications, technique, examples. (Die Stellung der interstitiellen γ-Strahler in der Strahlenbehandlung. Indikation, Technik, Beispiele.) Amer. J. Roentgenol. 85, 407—447 (1961).

BLOMFIELD, G. W.: Clinical evaluation of results in supervoltage x-ray therapy. J. Fac. Radiol. (Lond.) 7, 260—277 (1956).
— The treatment of cancer of the uterine cervix by radium and X-ray therapy. (Die Behandlung des Carcinoms der Cervix uteri mit Radium- und Röntgen-Therapie.) Brit. J. Radiol. 34, 755—768 (1961).
— CHERRY, C. P., GLUCKSMANN, A.: Biological factors influencing the radiotherapeutic results in carcinoma of the cervix. Brit. J. Radiol. 38, 241—254 (1965).
BÖCKLER, H., PRINZ, D.: Veränderungen der oberen Harnwege nach Bestrahlung und Operation des Kollumkarzinoms. Geburtsh. u. Frauenheilk. 19, 858—867 (1959).
BÖTTGER, H., RUMPHORST, K.: Ergebnisse elektiver Therapie des Kollumkarzinoms 1948—1950. Strahlentherapie 101, 95—100 (1956).
BOLOGNESI, M., BISTOLFI, F.: Primi risultati clinici della roentgenterapia con griglia nel trattamento del cancro dell'utero in stadio avanzato. (Erste klinische Ergebnisse mit der Gitterbestrahlung bei der Behandlung des fortgeschrittenen Uteruscarcinoms.) Ann. Ostet. 76, 427—483 (1954).
BONANNI, G., PISAPIA, M.: Considerazioni sul cancro del collo dell'utero trattato con sola terapia radiologica. (Betrachtungen über die ausschließliche Strahlentherapie des Carcinoma colli uteri.) Nunt. radiol. (Firenze) 31, 275—287 (1965).
BONEBRAKE, M., SHERMAN, A. I., TER-POGOSSIAN, M., ARNESON, A. N.: Clinical results following different methods of radium application used in the treatment of cervical cancer from 1921 to 1947. (Klinische Ergebnisse verschiedener Methoden der Radiumbehandlung des Collumcarcinoms 1921 bis 1947.) Amer. J. Roentgenol. 68, 925—934 (1952).
BONOMINI, B.: Criteri pratici di protezione in radiumterapia. Radiol. med. (Torino) 49, 378—395 (1963).
— VALDAGNI, C.: Telecobaltoterapia del cancro del collo uterino. Tecniche di trattamento e prime osservazioni. (Telekobalttherapie des Gebärmutterhalskrebes. Technik der Behandlung und erste Beobachtungen.) Attual. Ostet. Ginec. 2, 11—28 (1956).
BOSCH, A., MARCIAL, V. A.: Carcinoma of the uterine cervix associated with pregnancy. Amer. J. Roentgenol. 96, 92—99 (1966).
BOTELLA-LLUSIÁ, J.: Das Verhalten der Becken-Lymphknoten beim Carcinoma colli uteri vor und nach Röntgen-Tiefenbestrahlung. Z. Geburtsh. Gynäk. 162, 45—55 (1964).
— GONZALES-MERLO, J., GIMÉNEZ-TÉBAR, V., MARTINEZ-MARTINEZ, M., NOGALES-ORTIZ, F., SILVAN-MARTINEZ, A.: Le metastasi ganglionari nei diversi tipi di carcinoma cervicale uterino. Riv. Ostet. Ginec. 17, 749—752 (1962).
— NOGALES-ORTIZ, F., GIMÉNEZ-TÉBAR, V., ZAMARRIEGO-CRESPO, J.: Effect of radiotherapy on tumor-bearing lymph nodes in carcinoma of the cervix uteri. (Effekt der Strahlenbehandlung auf carcinomatöse Lymphknoten bei Patientinnen mit Collumcarcinom.) Amer. J. Obstet. Gynec. 83, 508—514 (1962).
BOTELLA-LLUSIÁ, J., NOGALES-ORTIZ, F., GIMÉNEZ-TÉBAR, V., ZAMARRIEGO-CRESPO, J.: La acción de la roentgenterapia sobre los ganglios pelvianos estudiada a través de la linfadenectomia pélvica extraperitoneal. (Die Wirkung der Röntgentherapie auf die Beckenlymphknoten, untersucht durch die extraperitoneale Lymphadenektomie.) Rev. mex. Cirurg. Ginec. Cáncer 26, 199—214 (1958).
— — GONZALES-MERLO, J., GIMÉNEZ-TÉBAR, V.: Die Ganglionmetastasen bei verschiedenen histologischen Typen des Cervixcarcinoms. Bol. Soc. ginec. esp. 11, 86—88 (1961); Ref. Ber. ges. Gynäk. Geburtsh. 81, 288 (1963).
BOTSTEIN, CH., SCHULZ, R. J., SIMON, N.: The use of a diamond shaped field in irradiation of pelvic organs, particularly in carcinoma of the cervix uteri. (Ein rautenförmiges Feld zur Bestrahlung der Beckenorgane, insbesondere des Cervix-Carcinoms.) Amer. J. Roentgenol. 87, 44—47 (1962).
BOUWDYK-BASTIAANSE, A. VAN: Treatment of cancer of the cervix uteri. (Behandlung des Carcinoms der Cervix uteri.) Amer. J. Obstet. 72, 100—118 (1956).
— The treatment of carcinoma of the uterine cervix. Acta Un. int. Cancer 15, 410—414 (1959).
BRACK, C. B., EVERETT, H. S., DICKSON, R.: Irradiation therapy for carcinoma of the cervix. Its effect upon the urinary tract. (Die Strahlentherapie des Cervixcarcinoms und ihre Auswirkungen auf den Harntrakt.) Obstet. and Gynec. 7, 196—201 (1956).
BRAESTRUP, C. B., MOONEY, R. T.: Physical aspects of rotating telecobalt equipment. Radiology 64, 17—28 (1955).
BRANDSTETTER, F.: Lymphknotenbefunde bei operiertem Kollumkarzinom. Zbl. Gynäk. 79, 1441—1446 (1957).
BRASCH, J.-P.: Zum Einfluß von Höhe und Verteilung der eingestrahlten Dosis auf die Heilungsziffer von Karzinomen, unter besonderer Berücksichtigung der in den Jahren 1957 und 1950—1952 an der Universitäts-Frauenklinik Erlangen behandelten Kollumkarzinom-Patientinnen. Strahlentherapie 107, 197—233 (1958).
BREDLAND, R.: Uterine cancer. Contribution to the problem of radiological, surgical or combined treatment in carcinoma of the uterus. (Uterusca. Beitrag zum Problem der radiologischen, chirurgischen oder kombinierten Behandlung.) Nord. Med. 50, 1542—1543 u. engl. Zus.fass. 1543 (1953) [Norwegisch].
BREED, J. E.: The radium treatment of recurrent cancer of the uterine cervix. (Die Radiumbehandlung des Carcinomrezidivs beim Collumcarcinom.) Amer. J. Roentgenol. 87, 480—487 (1962).
BREIT, A.: Angiographie der Uterustumoren und ihrer Rezidive. Stuttgart: Georg Thieme 1967.
— KELLER, H. L.: Die Pendelbestrahlung der Parametrien und ihrer Lymphabflußgebiete. Strahlentherapie 110, 83—94 (1959).
BREITNER, J.: Lokalisation und Zeitpunkt des Auftretens der Rezidive beim Collumcarcinom. Oncologia (Basel) 7, 134—140 (1954).

Brezina, K.: Über eine Beobachtung von Osteonekrose und malignem Tumor nach gynäkologischer Röntgenbestrahlung. Krebsarzt **20**, 265—268 (1965).

Brizel, H. E., Lanzl, L. H., Duthorn, E. M.: A comparison of techniques for parametrial irradiation using cobalt 60. (Vergleich der Techniken der Parametriumbestrahlung mit Kobalt-60.) Amer. J. Roentgenol. **89**, 101—107 (1963).

Brown, W. E., Meschan, I., Kerekes, E., Sadler, J. D.: Effect of radiation metastatic pelvic lymph node involvement in carcinoma of the cervix. Amer. J. Obstet. Gynec. **62**, 871—889 (1951).

Brunschwig, A.: Radical surgery for cancer of the cervix metastasized to peripheral lymph nodes (excluding exenterations). Surg. Gynec. Obstet. **100**, 575—582 (1955).

— Pelvic exenteration and advanced carcinoma. J. int. Coll. Surg. **39**, 216—220 (1963).

— Surgical treatment of carcinoma of the cervix, recurrent after irradiation or combination of irradiation and surgery. Amer. J. Med. **42**, 365—370 (1967).

— Daniel, W. W.: Surgical treatment of cancer of the cervix recurrent after previous radiation therapy. (Die chirurgische Behandlung von Rezidiven des Cervixcarcinoms nach vorausgegangener Strahlenbehandlung.) Surg. Gynec. Obstet. **105**, 186—190 (1957).

— — The surgical treatment of cancer of the cervix uteri. Amer. J. Obstet. Gynec. **75**, 875—881 (1958).

— Pierce, A.: Necropsy findings in patients with carcinoma of the cervix. Amer. J. Obstet. Gynec. **56**, 1134—1137 (1948).

— Roesler, E.: Die chirurgische Behandlung des Zervixkarzinoms im Memorial Center New York. Erster Fünfjahresbericht. Geburtsh. u. Frauenheilk. **17**, 1—10 (1957).

Bruntsch, K. H.: Klinische und histologische Untersuchungen zum Lymphknotenproblem beim Gebärmutterhalskrebs. Z. Geburtsh. Gynäk. **146**, 105—166 (1956).

— Die Wertung der histologischen Untersuchung der Parametrien beim operierten Kollumkarzinom im Hinblick auf die Feststellung des Ausbreitungsgrades. Geburtsh. u. Frauenheilk. **17**, 518—523 (1957).

Bruzual, A. D.: La flebografia pelviana. Cirug. Ginec. Urol. **18**, 50 (1964).

Bsteh, P.: Neuer Versuch zur Koordinierung der Radium- und Telekobalttherapie beim Uteruskarzinom. Strahlentherapie **129**, 505—511 (1966).

Buchacker, H. M.: Behandlungsergebnisse beim Kollum- und Korpuskarzinom in den Jahren 1948 bis 1953. Strahlentherapie **111**, 8—13 (1960).

Buchmann, E.: Ureterstenosierung und Hydronephrosenbildung durch Krebsinfiltration und Strahleninduration des Parametriums beim Kollumkarzinom. Strahlentherapie **99**, 20—46 (1956).

Buraggi, G. L.: La terapia radioisotopica dei linfonodi. (Die Radioisotopentherapie der Lymphknoten.) Atti Accad. med. lombarda **17**, 26—29 (1962).

Buraggi, G. L., Carnevali, G., Felci, U., Roncoroni, L.: Telecobaltoterapia di movimento: presentazione di schemi di trattamento. Estrotto da Tumori **14**, 273—295 (1959).

— Romanini, A., Roncoroni, L.: Sul trattamento del carcinoma uterino e delle diffusioni parametrali con la telecobaltoterapia. (Über die Bestrahlung des Uterus-Carcinoms und der Parametrien mit Telekobalttherapie.) Tumori **45**, 507—522 (1959).

Burch, J. C., Chalfant, R. L., Lavely, H. T., Jr.: Preoperative radium irradiation in the treatment of cancer of the cervix. (Die präoperative Radiumbestrahlung in der Behandlung des Cervixcarcinoms.) Progr. Gynec. **3**, 555—564 (1957).

Burger, R. H.: Lymph node response to high-dose intralymphatic injection of radiochromic phosphate. (Lymphknotenveränderungen nach hochdosierter intralymphatischer Injektion von Radiochromphosphat.) Bull. N. Y. Acad. Med. **40**, 142—147 (1964).

— Asano, M., Nagamatsu, G. R.: Intralymphatic isotopes for radiation of node metastases. (Intralymphatische Isotopenanwendung zur Bestrahlung von Lymphknotenmetastasen.) Invest. Urol. **2**, 215—225 (1964).

Burke, E. M.: Metastases in squamous-cell carcinoma. Amer. J. Cancer **30**, 493—503 (1937).

Burnett, H. W.: A vaginal radium applicator. Radiology **84**, 859—860 (1965).

Burns, B. C., Jr., Brack, C. B.: Prognostic factors in radioresistant cervical cancer. (Prognostische Faktoren bei strahlenresistentem Collumcarcinom.) Obstet. and Gynec. **16**, 1—9 (1960).

Burr, R. C., Mandy, J. C., Roberts, D. T.: Radium applicators in the treatment of carcinoma of the cervix. (Radiumapplikatoren bei der Behandlung des Cervixcarcinoms.) J. Canad. Ass. Radiol. **12**, 143—149 (1961).

Busch, M.: Ein Dosierungssystem für die interstitielle Therapie mit radioaktiven Seeds. Strahlentherapie **128**, 351—362 (1965).

Busse, O., Soergel, W.: Bericht über 800 maligne Erkrankungen des weiblichen Genitales der Jahre 1947—1952. Geburtsh. u. Frauenheilk. **19**, 201—217 (1959).

Busse, W.: Einstellung und Dosisbestimmung bei der Pendelbestrahlung der Parametrien. Strahlentherapie **101**, 400—404 (1956).

Buttenberg, D.: Das Adenokarzinom des Collum uteri. Strahlentherapie **112**, 45—53 (1960).

— Die Telekobaltbestrahlung beim Kollumkarzinom. Geburtsh. u. Frauenheilk. **22**, 1107—1111 (1962).

— Die Strahlenbelastung von Blase und Darm durch die lokale Radiumtherapie beim Kollumkarzinom. Strahlentherapie **122**, 511—518 (1963).

— Die Radiumeinlage beim Kollumkarzinom mit Stift und rechteckiger Platte. Radiobiol. Radiother. (Berl.) **5**, 45—50 (1964).

— Kuttig, H.: Telekobaltbestrahlung beim Kollumkarzinom. Zbl. Gynäk. **82**, 1457—1464 (1960).

— Schönfelder, R., Stoll, P.: Zur Prognose der Strahlentherapie des Kollumkarzinoms nach der „Sensitization Response". Strahlentherapie **113**, 538—552 (1960).

CAGNAZZO, G., Ros, A.: Il cobalto[60] nella terapia delle recidive del cancro del collo dell'utero. (^{60}Co-Teletherapie der Collumcarcinom-Rezidive.) Minerva ginec. 14, 806—811 (1962).

CAMERINI, R., MONETTI, C.: Decorso e trattamento delle recidive postradioterapiche di cancro dell'utero. (Verlauf und Behandlung der Rezidive nach Strahlenbehandlung des Gebärmutterkrebses.) Radioter. Radiobiol. Fis. med. 8, 122—137 (1952).

CAMPBELL, E. M., DOUGLAS, M.: The treatment of carcinoma of the uterine cervix using a linear vaginal source and 4 MeV X rays. (Die Behandlung des Cervixcarcinomes mit einer linearen intravaginalen Strahlenquelle und einem 4 MeV-Linearbeschleuniger.) Brit. J. Radiol. 39, 537—546 (1966).

CANALE, G. M.: Artériographie pelvienne en gynécologie. (Die Beckenarteriographie in der Gynäkologie.) Gynaecologia (Basel) 156, 116—124 (1963).

CANDIANI, G. B., REMOTTI, G., MANGIONI, C.: Osservazioni anatomo-cliniche sul materiale operatorio di venti eviscerazioni pelviche per cervicocarcinoma diffuso. Ann. Ostet. Ginec. 84, 359—418 (1962).

CARDIS, R., FLETCHER, G. H., LUCCI, J. A., JR.: Le traitement du cancer invasif du col utérin au cours de la grossesse et du post-partum. (Die Behandlung des invasiven Collumcarcinoms im Verlauf der Schwangerschaft und nach der Geburt.) Ann. Radiol. (Paris) 5, 1—12 (1962).

CARLSSON, E., HOLTZ, S., SHERMAN, A. I.: Demonstration of lymph node metastases by pelvic venography. Amer. J. Roentgenol. 85, 21 (1961).

CARTER, B., PARKER, R. T., THOMAS, W. L., CREADICK, R. N., PEETE, CH., CHERRY, W. B., WILLIAMS, J. B.: The follow up of patients with cancer of the cervix treated by radical hysterectomy and radical pelvic lymphadenectomy. Amer. J. Obstet. Gynec. 76, 1094—1104 (1958).

— THOMAS, W. L., ROSS, R. A., PARKER, R. T., PALUMBO, L.: The place of extensive surgery in cancer of the cervix. The radical hysterectomy (Wertheim) and the radical pelvic lymphadenectomy. Amer. J. Obstet. Gynec. 64 A, 309—323 (1953).

CARULLA-RIERA, V.: Tratamiento radiologico del cancer del cuello uterino en los grados II, III y IV. (Die Strahlenbehandlung des Collumcarcinoms der Gruppen II, III und IV.) Gac. méd. esp. 26, 257—266 (1952).

CAULK, R. M.: Results of radiotherapy in cervical cancer. (Ergebnisse der Strahlenbehandlung des Gebärmutterkrebses.) Med. Ann. D. C. 23, 195—196 (1954).

— Transvaginal roentgen therapy in cancer of the cervical stump. (Transvaginale Röntgentherapie beim Cervixstumpfcarcinom.) Amer. J. Roentgenol. 72, 469—473 (1954).

— Review of seventeen years' experience with transvaginal roentgen therapy in cervical cancer. (Übersicht über 17jährige Erfahrung mit der transvaginalen Röntgen-Therapie des Collumcarcinoms.) Amer. J. Roentgenol. 76, 965—971 (1956).

CAVALLOT, A.: La linfoadenografia nel carcinoma del collo dell'utero. (Die Lymphadenographie beim Carcinoma colli uteri.) J. belge Radiol. 47, 243—252 (1964).

CAVALOT, F., SINISTRERO, G., CARAZZONE, P. F., CORTIS, B.: Valore e limiti della linfoadenografia in ginecologia. (Wertu nd Grenzen der Lymphadenographie in der Gynäkologie.) Minerva radiol. fisioter. radiobiol. (Torino) 10, 67—76 (1965).

— — — TETTONI, E.: La linfoadenografia nel arcinoma dell'utero. (Die Lymphadenographie beim Uteruscarcinom.) Minerva radiol. fisioter. radiobiol. (Torino) 8, 563—594 (1963).

— — TETTONI, E., GHILARDI, F.: Adenografia e flebografia nelle neoplasie dello scavo pelvico. Minerva radiol. fisioter. radiobiol. (Torino) 8, 1—32 (1963).

— — — — Adenografia e flebografia nelle neoplasie dello scavo pelvico. (Adenographie und Phlebographie bei den Tumoren im Becken.) Minerva radiol. fisioter. radiobiol. (Torino) 9, 191—203 (1964).

CENTARO, A., BARACHI, F., BASSANI, G., RUSSO, S.: Possibilità d'irradiazione del pavimento pelvico mediante applicazione intraoperatoria di perle di Co[60] dopo isterectomia radicale vaginale secondo Schauta-Amreich. (Bestrahlung des Beckenbodens durch intraoperative Applikation von Radiokobaltperlen [Co[60]] nach radikaler Hysterektomie. [Technik Schauta-Amreich.]) Riv. Ostet. (Firenze) 13, 76—84 (1958).

CHANTRAINE, H.: Zur Frage der ausreichenden Dosierung bei bösartigen Geschwülsten. Strahlentherapie 93, 400—403 (1954).

CHASSAGNE, D., PIERQUIN, B.: Indications des radioisotopes artificiels en curie-thérapie du cancer du col utérin. Gynéc. Obstét. 61, 617—622 (1962).

CHAU, P. M., FLETCHER, G. H., RUTLEDGE, F. N., DODD, G. D., JR.: Complications in high dose whole pelvis irradiation in female pelvic cancer. (Komplikationen bei hochdosierter Ganzdurchstrahlung des Beckens bei Krebsen der weiblichen Beckenhöhle.) Amer. J. Roentgenol. 87, 22—40 (1962).

CHELAZZI, M., MILANESI, R.: Il trattamento del cancro del collo dell'utero con radium e telecobaltoterapia. Radiol. med. (Torino) 45, 1095—1113 (1959).

CHELIUS, H. H., OHLENROTH, G.: Massenblutungen nach bestrahlten Kollumkarzinomen. Zbl. Gynäk. 89, 934—939 (1967).

CHEN, S. C., LOFSTROM, J. E., BUDDEN, M. A.: Residual disease following radiation therapy of carcinoma of the cervix, stages I and II, as evaluated by postirradiation surgery. (Krebsreste nach Bestrahlungsbehandlung des Collumcarcinoms I. und II., aufgedeckt durch nachfolgende Operation.) Radiology 80, 568—573 (1963).

CHERRY, C. P., FRASER, W. D.: The influence of focal size on local radiocurability of tumors of the uterine cervix. (Der Einfluß der Tumorgröße auf die örtliche Strahlenbehandelbarkeit bei Collumtumoren.) Cancer (Philad.) 13, 951—955 (1960).

— GLUKSMANN, A.: Lymphatic embolism and lymphnode metastasis in cancers of vulva and of uterine cervix. Cancer (Philadelphia) 8, 564-575 (1955).

— — DEARING, R., WAY, S.: Observations on lymph node involvement in carcinoma of the cervix. J. Obstet. Gynaec. Brit. Emp. 60, 368—377 (1953).

Chiappa, S.: Premesse teoriche e primi risultati pratici nell'uso per via linfatica di un mezzo di contrasto radioattivo (Lipiodol „F" [131]I). (Theoretische Voraussetzungen und erste praktische Erfolge bei der intralymphatischen Verabreichung eines radioaktiven Kontrastmittels [Lipiodol „F"-J-131].) Minerva nucl. 7, 460—467 (1963).

— Galli, G., Barbaini, S., Ravasi, G.: La radioterapia endolinfatica: primi risultati di una nuova metodica. (Die intralymphatische Strahlentherapie: Erste Ergebnisse einer neuen Methode.) Radiol. med. (Torino) 48, 663—692 (1962).

— — Guarino, M., Luciani, L., Barbaini, S.: Quelques possibilités de la radiothérapie endolymphatique dans le domaine de la gynécologie. J. Radiol. Électro. 44, 157 (1963).

— Gazzi, G., Barbaini, S., Ravasi, G.: La radioterapia endolinfatica: primi resultati di una nuove metodica. Radiol. med. (Torino) 48, 663—668 (1962).

— — Palmia, C.: Observations on intralymphatic radiotherapy and general chemotherapy. Clin. Rad. 15, 202—209 (1964).

Chiari, H.: Pathologisch-anatomische Grundlagen der urologischen Komplikationen bei bösartigen Gewächsen im kleinen Becken. Krebsforschung und Krebsbekämpfung, Bd. IV, S. 258—267. München-Wien: Urban & Schwarzenberg 1962.

Chiariotti, F.: Sui risultati clinici immediati della telecobaltoterapia. (Klinische Frühergebnisse der Telekobalttherapie.) Minerva med. 51, 1669—1681 (1960).

Christensen, A., Lange, P.: Über Drüsenmetastasen der Beckenregion bei Frühstadien des Cancer colli uteri. Ugeskr. Læg. 290—293 (1955) [Dänisch]; Ref. Ber. ges. Gynäk. Geburtsh. 56, 159 (1955).

— — Nielsen, E.: Surgery and Radiotherapy for invasive cancer of the cervix. Acta obstet. gynec. scand. 43, Suppl. 2, 59—87 (1964).

Christopherson, W. M., Berg, H. F.: A histopathological study of lymph nodes irradiated with colloidal Au 198. Cancer (Philadelphia) 8, 1261—1269 (1955).

Chua, D. T., Iliya, F. A., O'Leary, J. A., Veenema, R. J., Frick, H. C.: Palliative urinary diversion in patients with advanced carcinoma of the cervix. Cancer (Philad.) 20, 93—95 (1967).

Ciambellotti, E., Cugini, A.: Telecobalttoterapia pendolare biassiale simmetrica parallela nel trattamento delle neoplasie della pelvi. (Die biaxiale, symmetrische, parallele Telekobaltpendelbestrahlung zur Behandlung von Tumoren im kleinen Becken.) Radiol. med. (Torino) 47, 249—262 (1961).

Claiborne, H. A., Jr., Thornton, W. N., Jr., Wilson, L. A., Jr.: Pelvic lymphadenectomy for carcinoma of the uterine cervix. Amer. J. Obstet. Gynec. 80, 672—682 (1960).

Clayton, R. S.: Carcinoma of the cervix uteri: ten-year study with comparison of results of irradiation and radical surgery. (Cervix-Carcinom: Vergleich der Ergebnisse nach Bestrahlung und radikaler Chirurgie über einem Zeitraum von 10 Jahren.) Radiology 68, 74—79 (1957).

Clemens, H., Hofmann, D.: Tierexperimentelle und klinische Untersuchungen über die Verwendbarkeit von Thorium X für die Zusatzbehandlung gynäkologischer Karzinome. Strahlentherapie 120, 129—135 (1963).

Coliez, R. T., Loiseau, A. N., Tournier, J.: Étude statistique de 600 cas de cancers du col utérin traités par curiethérapie et rádiothérapie. (Statistische Untersuchungen an Hand von 600 Fällen von Collumcarcinom, die einer Radium- und Strahlentherapie zugeführt wurden.) J. Radiol. Électrol. 46, 735—739 (1965).

Collo, G., Sburlati, L.: I nostri primi risultati nella associazione della terapia radiante e chirurgica nei carcinomi del collo uterino al II. e III. stadio. (Unsere ersten Ergebnisse bei kombinierter Strahlen- und chirurgischer Behandlung des Collumcarcinoms im II. und III. Stadium.) Riv. Ostet. (Milano) 34, 395—401 (1952).

Concannon, J. P., Lake, F. D., Daro, A.: Radium treatment of cancer of the cervix with modified, permanently paired vaginal ovoids. (Radiumbehandlung des Collum-Carcinom mit modifizierten, unverändert paarigen, eiförmigen, vaginalen Radiumträgern.) Obstet. and Gynec. 9, 566—570 (1957).

Cooper, G., Jr., Williams, D. H.: Epidermoid carcinoma of the cervix. Orthovoltage and supervoltage irradiation. (Plattenepithelcarcinom der Cervix. Orthovolt- und Supervoltbestrahlung.) Amer. J. Roentgenol. 88, 971—975 (1962).

Corscaden, J. A.: Gynecologic cancer. Baltimore: William & Wilkins 1956.

— Butz, R. A.: Intracavitary radium technique in the treatment of cancer of the cervix uteri. (Die Technik der intrakavitären Radiumeinlage bei der Behandlung des Gebärmutterhalscarcinoms.) Amer. J. Roentgenol. 68, 47—57 (1952).

— Gusberg, S. B., Donlan, Ch. P.: Precision dosage in interstitial irradiation of cancer of cervix uteri. Amer. J. Roentgenol. 60, 522—534 (1948); Zit. nach Gauwerky, F., Strahlentherapie 103, 16—47 (1957).

— — Kosar, W.: Interstitial radium treatment of cancer of the cervix uteri. Clinical appraisal. (Interstitielle Radiumbehandlung beim Collum-Carcinom.) Amer. J. Roentgenol. 72, 278—283 (1954).

Cosbie, W. G.: The contribution of radiotherapy to the modern treatment of female pelvic cancer. (Der Beitrag der Strahlentherapie zur modernen Behandlung der Krebse des weiblichen Beckens.) J. Obstet. Gynaec. Brit. Emp. 66, 843—856 (1959).

— Radiotherapy following hysterectomy performed for or in the presence of cancer of the cervix. (Strahlenbehandlung nach Hysterektomie in Gegenwart eines Carcinoms der Cervix.) Amer. J. Obstet. Gynec. 85, 332—337 (1963).

Courty, L., Langeron, P., Lamoril, P.: Les phlébites iliaques et ilio-caves. Etio-pathogenie, physiopathologie aspects cliniques. (Die iliacale und ilio-cavale Phlebitis. Ätiopathogenie, Physio-Pathologie und klinische Betrachtungen.) Ann. Chir. (Paris) 16, 1795—1809 (1962).

Coutard, H.: Zusammenfassung der Grundlagen der röntgentherapeutischen Technik der tiefgelegenen Krebse. Strahlentherapie 37, 50—58 (1930).

Cowell, M. A. C.: The hazards of supplementary x-ray therapy in the radiation treatment of carcinoma of the cervix uteri. (Über die Gefahren zusätzlicher Röntgentherapie bei der Strahlenbehandlung des Cervixcarcinoms.) Brit. J. Radiol. **26**, 652—657 (1953).

Crawford, E. J., Jr., Robinson, L. S., Hornbuckle, L. A.: Surgery as an adjunct to irradiation therapy in carcinoma of the cervix. Preliminary report. (Operation als Ergänzung zur Strahlentherapie beim Collumcarcinom. Vorläufiger Bericht.) Amer. J. Obstet. **72**, 125—130 (1956).

Cuccia, C. A., Bloedorn, F. G., Onal, M.: Treatment of primary adenocarcinoma of the cervix. (Die Behandlung des primären Adenocarcinoms des Cervix.) Amer. J. Roentgenol. **99**, 371—375 (1967).

Currie, D. W.: The association of radium and surgery in the treatment of carcinoma of the cervix. (Die Verbindung von Radium und Operation bei der Behandlung des Gebärmutterhalscarcinoms.) Proc. roy. Soc. Med. **45**, 327—331 (1952).

Czech, H., Kepp, R. K.: Rezidive nach der Behandlung von bösartigen Tumoren des weiblichen Genitale. Betrachtungen über das Zustandekommen von Rezidiven und Ergebnisse der Rezidivbehandlung an der Universitäts-Frauenklinik Göttingen. Strahlentherapie **90**, 117—142 (1953).

Čžun-fu, Sja: The results of radiation therapy of cervix uteri carcinoma depending upon the methods of treatment. (Ergebnisse der Strahlentherapie des Gebärmutterhalskrebses in Abhängigkeit von der Behandlungsmethode.) Vop. Onkol. **7**, 29—38 mit engl. Zus.fass. (1961) [Russisch].

Dahle, T.: Combined radiologic-surgical treatment of carcinoma of the cervix. (Die kombinierte radiologisch-chirurgische Behandlung des Cervixcarcinoms.) Surg. Gynec. Obstet. **108**, 600—604 (1959).

Dalla Palma, L., Renzi, R., Cavani, C.: Sulle possibilità d'impiego del movimento pendolare tangenziale in radioterapia. Nota preliminare. (Über die Möglichkeiten mit der tangentialen Pendelbestrahlung in der Strahlentherapie. Vorläufige Mitteilung.) Nunt. radiol. (Firenze) **30**, 265—274 (1964).

Darcis, L.: Cancers du corps et du col de l'utérus. Classification et modes de traitement utilisés au Radiumhemmet (Stockholm). (Das Carcinom des Corpus und Collum uteri. Einteilung und Behandlungsmethoden am Radiumhemmet in Stockholm.) Acta clin. belg. **11**, 59—76 (1956).

— Quelques réflexions au sujet des possibilités de préciser les indications et d'améliorer le rendement de la radiothérapie du cancer cervico-utérin. (Einige Betrachtungen über die Möglichkeiten beim Collum-Ca die Indikation zur Strahlentherapie zu präzisieren und deren Heilungsaussichten zu verbessern.) Bull. Soc. roy. belge Gynéc. Obstét., N. S. **25**, 111—114 (1957).

— Les principes actuels du traitement des cancers cervico-utérins. (Die gegenwärtigen Grundlagen der Behandlung der Cervixcarcinome des Uterus.) J. belge Radiol. **44**, 435—454 (1961).

Dargent, M.: La place de la lymphadénectomie pelvienne dans le traitement du cancer du col de l'utérus. (Die Bedeutung der pelvinen Lymphknotenentfernung für die Behandlung des Gebärmutterhals-Carcinoms.) Mém. Acad. Chir. **78**, 130—132 (1952).

-- Chassard, J. L., Dargent, D.: La lymphographie ilio-pelvienne au lipiodol ultrafluide par voie pédieuse dans le cancer du col utérin. A propos de 33 dossiers avec confrontation anatomoradiologique. (Die Beckenlymphographie mit Lipiodol ultrafluide vom Fußrücken aus beim Collum-Carcinom.) Ann. Chir. (Paris) **17**, 1101—1120 (1963).

— Colon, J., Mayer, M., Motamedi, C.: Valeur de la chirurgie complémentaire de la radiumthérapie dans le traitement des formes opérables de cancer du col utérin. Ann. Chir. **18**, 986—1000 (1964).

— — Motamedi, C.: Valeur pronostique des anomalies de l'urographie intraveineuse dans le cancer du col utérin traité par association radium-chirurgie. (Der prognostische Wert urographischer Veränderungen beim Collumcarcinom nach kombinierter radiologisch-chirurgischer Behandlung.) Ann. Radiol. (Paris) **8**, 445—457 (1965).

— Guillemin, G.: La place de la lmyphadenectomie pelvienne dans le traitment du cancer du col de l'utérus. Lyon chir. **47**, 740—745 (1952).

— — The treatment of operable cancer of the cervix by the combination of radiation and surgery. Report of 250 cases. Cancer (Philad.) **8**, 53—58 (1955).

— Mayer, M., Butel, J.: Résultats d'ensemble de l'association radium-chirurgie dans le traitement du cancer du col utérin (à propos de 400 observations). (Sammelergebnisse der Verbindung Radium-Chirurgie bei der Behandlung des Gebärmutterhalskrebses. [Bericht über 400 Beobachtungen.]) Mém. Acad. Chir. **83**, 479—491 (1957).

Debiasi, E., de Salvia, P.: La radiumterapia parziale pre-operatoria nel carcinoma del collo dell'utero. (Die präoperative partielle Radiumtherapie des Collumcarcinoms.) Riv. Ostet. Ginec. **18**, 421—438 (1963).

Debois, J. M., Roo, M. de, Bonte, J., Baert, A.: Problèmes techniques de l'irradiation par hautes énergies dans le cancer du col utérin. (Technische Probleme bei der Hochvoltbestrahlung des Carcinoma colli uteri.) J. belge Radiol. **48**, 92—108 (1965).

Dedić, St., Marković, M.: Die radiologische Therapie des Kollumkarzinoms. Strahlentherapie **110**, 145—155 (1959).

— Radivojević, S., Marković, M., Kastratović, M.: Sur le traitement du cancer du col de l'utérus et des paramètres. Résultats radiologiques. (Therapeutische Ergebnisse bei Carcinomen des Collum uteri und der Parametrien.) Srpski Arkh. tselok. Lek. **85**, 522—534 mit franz. Zus.fass. (1957) [Serbisch].

Deed, E. P., Barnhard, H. J.: Focused grid tele-cobalt therapy in advanced epidermoid carcinoma of the cervix. (Telekobalttherapie mit fokussiertem Sieb beim fortgeschrittenen Plattenepithel-Ca der Cervix.) Radiology **83**, 228—230 (1964).

Dekker, D. G., Aaro, L. A., Hunt, A. B., Johnson, C. E., Smith, R. A.: Sequential radiation and operation in carcinoma of the uterine cervix. Amer. J. Obstet. Gynec. 92, 35—42 (1965).

Dellepiane, G., Tetti, A., Davitti, L.: Moderni orientamenti della terapia endolinfatica nel trattamento del cancro dell'utero. (Moderne Orientierung über die endolymphatische Therapie bei der Behandlung des Uteruskrebses.) Minerva radiol. fisioter. radiobiol. (Torino) 11, 219—229 (1966).

Denoix, P., Herovici, C.: Die Beziehung zwischen der Tumorbegrenzung und dem Auftreten oder Fehlen von Carcinommetastasen in Beckenlymphknoten. Untersuchung an 100 Fällen von Carcinomen 1. Grades. Mém. Acad. Chir. 88, 590—593 (1962).

De Palo, A., Papadia, S.: Morfologia e significato della reazione linfonodale e radium-irradiazione del territorio tributario. Studio sistematico sui linfonodi satelliti negli epiteliomi della portio sottoposti a radium-irradiazione. (Morphologie und Signifikanz der Lymphknotenreaktion nach Radiumbestrahlung des tributären Gebietes. Systematische Untersuchung der regionären Lymphknoten nach Radiumbestrahlung von Portiocarcinomen.) Quad. Clin. ostetr. 9, 309—374 (1954).

Dettman, P. M., King, E. R., Zimberg, Y. H.: Evaluation of lymphncde function following irradiation or surgery. (Die Bewertung der Lymphknotenfunktion nach Bestrahlung oder Operation.) Amer. J. Roentgenol. 96, 711—718 (1966).

Diaz Bruzual, A., Dominguez Gallegos, A.: Linfangiografia, flebografia y neumografia pélvicas en el diagnóstico de la extensión del cáncer del cervix. (Lymphangiographie, Phlebographie und Pneumographie des Beckens in der Diagnose der Ausdehnung des Cervixcarcinoms.) Acta med. venez. 11, 414—421 (1964).

Dibbelt, L.: Die Bestrahlung gynäkologischer Karzinome mit dem Konvergenz-Strahler. Strahlentherapie 95, 49—58 (1954); Zbl. Radiol. 45, 347 (1954/55).

— Ehlers, F.: Methoden und Ergebnisse der Behandlung des Kollum-Karzinoms an der Akademischen Frauenklinik in Düsseldorf. Geburtsh. u. Frauenheilk. 25, 486—501 (1965).

— Heinzler, F.: Die Koordination von Radium- und Supervolttherapie. Arch. Gynäk. 202, 312—316 (1965).

— Rahm, G.: Untersuchungen über die Anwendung des Konvergenzstrahlers beim gynäkologischen Karzinom. I. Der Einfluß der wechselnden Schichtdicke bei Kreuzfeuerbestrahlung mit Steh- und Konvergenzfehlern. Strahlentherapie 110, 266—279 (1959).

— — Untersuchungen über die Anwendung des Konvergenzstrahlers beim gynäkologischen Karzinom. II. Der Einfluß einer teilweisen Oberflächenabdeckung auf die Isodosen des Konvergenzstrahlers. III. Meßergebnisse bei Bestrahlung eines Beckenphantoms. Strahlentherapie 110, 582—589 (1959).

Dibbelt, L., Rahm, G.: Zur Bewegungsbestrahlung gynäkologischer Tumoren im kleinen Becken. Stellungnahme zur gleichnamigen Arbeit von P. Müller in Bd. 27 dieser Zeitschrift. Radiol. clin. (Basel) 28, 180—187 (1959).

— — Die Technik und Dosimetrie bei der Konvergenzbestrahlung des gynäkologischen Karzinoms. Röntgen- u. Lab.-Prax. 13, R 88—R 98 (1960).

— — Untersuchungen über die Anwendung des Konvergenzstrahlers beim gynäkologischen Karzinom. Strahlentherapie 111, 202—208 (1960).

— — Untersuchungen über die Anwendung des Konvergenzstrahlers beim gynäkologischen Karzinom. Strahlentherapie 116, 131—137 (1961).

— — Renner, K.: Dosimetrische Untersuchungen zur Gammatronbestrahlung der Lymphwege beim Uteruskarzinom. Strahlentherapie 112, 406—420 (1960).

Dick, W.: Die urologischen Komplikationen bei der Behandlung der malignen Tumoren im kleinen Becken. Krebsforschung und Krebsbekämpfung, Bd. IV, S. 276—283. München-Berlin-Wien: Urban & Schwarzenberg 1962.

Dietel, F. G., Volz, E.: Das Raumbild als Grundlage der homogenen Radium-Röntgenbehandlung der Collum-Carcinome. Arch. Gynäk. 166, 488—489 (1938).

Dietz, W.: Strahlentherapie und Heilungsergebnisse beim Kollumkarzinom an der Universitäts-Frauenklinik Freiburg i. Br. 1950 bis 1954. Strahlentherapie 115, 65—71 (1961).

Doederlein, G.: Das Adenokarzinom des Collum uteri. Zbl. Gynäk. 75, 1529—1535 (1953); Arch. Gynäk. 183, 506—511 u. Diskussion 517—518 (1953).

— Wo liegen die Grenzen der operativen Behandlung des Karzinoms am Collum uteri. Strahlentherapie, Sonderbd. 37, 186—190 (1957).

Döpper, T., Jakob, A.: Die Harnstauung beim bestrahlten weiblichen Genitalkarzinom, ihre Häufigkeit und Behandlungsvorschläge. Strahlentherapie 109, 289—294 (1959).

Dolan, P. A., Hughes, R. R.: Lymphography in genital cancer. Surg. Gynec. Obstet. 118, 1286—1290 (1964).

Donaldson, M.: Radiation therapy in gynecology. Brit. J. Radiol. 3, 246—258 (1930).

Doujak, R., Picha, E.: Ist eine Penicillinprophylaxe bei der intrauterinen Radiumeinlage berechtigt? Strahlentherapie 117, 97—102 (1962).

Dragon, V., Herskovits, A., Moldovan, I., Popovici, O., Trancou, A., Chiricutza, I., Trestioreanu, A., Dutzu, R.: Die Grundsätze und Ergebnisse der kombinierten strahlentherapeutisch-operativen Behandlung des Collumcarcinoms Gruppe I und II an der Geschwulstklinik in Bukarest. Ref. Ber. ges. Gynäk. Geburtsh. 69, 30 (1959—1960).

— Trestioreanu, A.: Association radio-chirurgical dans le traitement du cancer du col utérin, stades I et II. (Kombinierte radio-chirurgische Behandlung bei der Therapie des Collumcarcinoms der Stadien I und II. Radiobiol. Radiother. (Berl.) 4, 117—124 (1963).

Dreyer, B.: Indurationen der Subcutis. — Eine Spätfolge nach Telekobalttherapie. Inaug.-Dis. Hamburg 1967.

Ducuing, J., Guilhem, D., Enjalbert, A., Baur, R., Paillé, J.: La phlibographie pelvienne. Paris: Masson & Cie. 1954.

Dunn, J. E., Jr., Buell, P.: Association of cervical cancer with circumcision of sexual partner. (Zusammenhang zwischen Collum-Carcinom und Beschneidung des Sexualpartners.) J. nat. Cancer Inst. **22**, 749—764 (1959).

Durando, C., Scognamiglio, F., Scarzerle, V.: L'arteriografia pelvica nella fisiopatologia ginecologica. (Die Beckenarteriographie in der gynäkologischen Physiopathologie.) Arch. Ist. osped. S. Corona **27**, 401—436 (1962).

Durrance, F. Y., Fletcher, G. H.: Analysis of central recurrent disease in stages I and II squamous all carcinomas of the cervix in intact uterus. Amer. J. Roentgenol. **106**, 831—838 (1969).

Dyroff, R., Siegert, A.: Röntgen- und Radiumbehandlung in der Frauenheilkunde. In: Biologie und Pathologie des Weibes, Bd. III. Berlin-Innsbruck-München-Wien: Urban & Schwarzenberg 1955.

Eberle, H., Busse, W.: Vergleichende Dosismessungen bei den gebräuchlichsten Röntgenbestrahlungsmethoden der parametranen Absiedlungen des Ca. colli uteri. Strahlentherapie **99**, 555—560 (1956).

Eckey, P.: Ergebnisse der Strahlenbehandlung des Kollumkarzinoms in einer kleinen Strahlenabteilung in der Zeit von 1947 bis 1953. Strahlentherapie **110**, 367—373 (1959).

Eichhorn, H.-J., Lessel, A., Richter, E., Rotte, K.-H., Schubert, G., Zühlke, R.: Die 5-Jahres-Ergebnisse in der Krebsbehandlung bei Strahlentherapie als einziger Behandlungsmethode (nach den Berichten der Jahre 1953 bis 1965). Strahlentherapie **131**, 227—254 (1966).

Eiken, M., Madsen, V.: Lymphography in carcinoma of the cervix. Acta obstet. Gynec. scand. **44**, 45 (1965).

Engelking, R. L., Purpón, I., Castañeda, J. de J., Castañeda, F.: La linfografia como metodo de diagnostico, pronostico y tratamiento en metastasis de tumores del aparato genito-urinario. (Die Lymphographie als diagnostische, prognostische und therapeutische Methode bei metastatischen Tumoren des Urogenitaltraktes.) Rev. Urol. (Méx.) **21**, 317—343 (1963).

Engeset, A.: Irradiation of lymph nodes and vessels. Experiments in rats, with reference to cancer therapy. Acta radiol. (Stockh.), Suppl. **229**. (Bestrahlung der Lymphknoten und Lymphgefäße. Experimente bei Ratten mit Berücksichtigung der Krebstherapie.) 125 S. Stockholm: Univ. flg. 1964.

Ernst, E. C.: Dosage measurements in radium therapy. Binghamton, N.Y.: Ansco.

— Probable trends in irradiation treatment of carcinoma of cervix uteri with improved expanding type of radium applicator. Radiology **52**, 46—58 (1949).

— Acta Un. int. cancer. (Brux.) **6**, 1221 (1949); Zit. nach Gauwerky, F.: Strahlentherapy **103**, 16—47 (1957).

— Ernst, E. C., Jr., Ernst, R. P.: Plastic vaginal cylinder. Assessory to the expanding cervico-uterine radium applicator. (Vaginalzylinder aus Plastikmaterial, ein Zusatzgerät zum spreizbaren cervico-uterinen Radiumapplikator.) Radiology **60**, 583—587 (1953).

Esposito, J. M., Zaron, D. M., Zaron, G. S.: Extragenital adenocarcinoma metastatic to the cervix uteri. Amer. J. Obstet. Gynec. **92**, 792—795 (1965).

Eufinger, H.: Zusatzbehandlung operierter und strahlenbehandelter gynäkologischer Karzinome. Strahlentherapie **107**, 371—381 (1958).

Evans, J. C., Bergsjø, P.: The influence of anemia on the results of radiotherapy in carcinoma of the cervix. Radiology **84**, 709—717 (1965).

Everett, H. S., Brack, C. B., Farber, C. J.: Further studies on the effect of irradiation therapy for carcinoma of the cervix upon the urinary tract. Amer. J. Obstet. Gynec. **58**, 908—923 (1949).

Eymer, H.: Die Strahlenbehandlung der Gebärmutterkrebse. In: Biologie und Pathologie des Weibes, Bd. V. Berlin-Innsbruck-München-Wien: Urban & Schwarzenberg 1953.

— Ries, J.: Die Ergebnisse der Strahlenbehandlung des Collum-Karzinoms an der I. Universitäts-Frauenklinik München. Berichtsjahre 1945—1946. Strahlentherapie **90**, 178—182 (1953).

Ezell, H. E., Holzaepfel, J. H.: The use of interstitial radioactive cobalt needles in the treatment of carcinoma of the cervix. (Die Radiumspickung mit radioaktiven Kobaltnadeln bei der Behandlung des Cervixcarcinoms.) Amer. J. Obstet. **73**, 354—358 (1957).

Fauvet, E.: Zur Frage der Therapie des Kollumkarzinoms in der Schwangerschaft. Geburtsh. u. Frauenheilk. **26**, 123—131 (1966).

Fava, G.: Valutazioni dosimetriche nella terapia radioisotopica dei linfonodi con Lipiodol „F" [131]I. (Dosimetrische Abschätzungen bei der Radioisotopentherapie der Lymphknoten mit [131]J-markiertem Lipiodol F.) Minerva nucl. **7**, 467—472 (1963).

— Roncoroni, L.: Body distribution of Lipiodol [131]J following intralymphatic radiotherapy. (Die Verteilung von Lipiodol-[131]J im Körper im Anschluß an eine intralymphatische Strahlenbehandlung.) Nucl.-Med. **5**, 1—11 (1965).

Fernandez-Colmeiro, J. M.: Le traitement des cancers avancés du col de l'utérus par les radiations. (Die Behandlung der fortgeschrittenen Carcinome des Collum uteri mit Bestrahlungen.) Bull. Ass. franç. Cancer **41**, 88—94 (1954).

Ferrari, B., Pipino, G.: Contributo allo studio istochimico del cancro del collo uterino durante la roentgenterapia con griglia. I. (Acidi nucleinici.) (Beitrag zur histochemischen Untersuchung des Collum-Carcinoms während der Röntgentherapie mit Anwendung eines Rasters. I. [Nucleinsäuren.]) Quad. Clin. ostet. **12**, 343a—354 (1957).

Feuerstein, H., Maurer, H.-J.: Zur Frage der Dosisverteilung bei der Strahlenbehandlung des Kollumkarzinoms unter Berücksichtigung der Strahlenbelastung von Blase und Dickdarm. Geburtsh. u. Frauenheilk. **18**, 815—824 (1958).

Fichardt, T.: The Pretoria method in radiotherapy of cancer of the cervix uteri. (Die Pretoriamethode bei der Radiumtherapie des Collumcarcinoms.) S. Afr. med. J. **36**, 303—310 (1962).

Fiebelkorn, H.-J.: Die Strahlentherapie der bösartigen Geschwülste. In: Lehrbuch der Strahlenheilkunde, von R. du Mesnil de Rochement. Stuttgart: Enke 1958.

— Beitrag zur Methodik der Radiumbehandlung des Kollumkarzinoms. Strahlentherapie 117, 238—249 (1962).

Finze, H.: Steigerung der Heilerfolge fortgeschrittener weiblicher Genitalkarzinome durch zusätzliche Teilkörperfernbestrahlung? Strahlentherapie 103, 60—65 (1957).

Fischer, E.: Über Strahlenschäden beim Genitalkarzinom. Zbl. Gynäk. 77, 1192—1197 (1955).

Fischer, H.: Obduktionsbefunde beim Carcinoma colli uteri. Arch. Gynäk. 188, 157—171 (1956/57).

Fischer, H. W.: Intralymphatic introduction of radioactive colloids into the lymph nodes. Prelim. study. (Intralymphatische Applikationen von radioaktiven Colloiden in die Lymphknoten. Vorläufige Untersuchung.) Radiology 79, 297—301 (1962).

— Intralymphatic therapy for lymph node metastases of carcinoma of the cervix. An analysis of the proposition and presentation of pertinent experimental data. (Intralymphatische Therapie von Lymphknotenmetastasen beim Cervixcarcinom. Eine Analyse der Grundlagen und Wiedergabe einschlägiger experimenteller Befunde.) Cancer (Philad.) 18, 1059—1065 (1965).

Fischer, W.: Neuere Erkenntnisse über die Ureterfunktion beim Kollumkarzinom. Zbl. Gynäk. 89, 1112—1121 (1967).

Fletcher, G. H.: Clinical program to evaluate practical significance of higher energy levels than 1—3 Mev. Amer. J. Roentgenol. 76, 866—893 (1956).

— Supervoltage radiotherapy for cancers of the uterine cervix. (Supervolt-Strahlentherapie beim Carcinom des Collum uteri.) Brit. J. Radiol. 35, 5—17 (1962).

— Problems in clinical evaluation of radiotherapeutic methods. (Probleme in der klinischen Bewertung radiotherapeutischer Methoden. J. Amer. med. Ass. 179, 871—877 (1962).

— Brown, T. C., Rutledge, F. N.: Clinical significance of rectal and bladder dose measurements in radium therapy of cancer of the uterine cervix. (Der klinische Wert von Dosismessungen in Blase und Rectum bei der Radiumbestrahlung des Cervixcarcinoms.) Amer. J. Roentgenol. 79, 421—450 (1958).

— Calderon, R.: Positioning of pelvic portals for external irradiation in carcinoma of the uterine cervix. (Die Einstellung der Beckenfelder für die Bestrahlung des Cervixcarcinoms.) Radiology 67, 359—370 (1956).

— Rutledge, F. N., Chau, P. M.: Polices of treatment in cancer of the cervix uteri. (Über die Behandlung des Cervix-Carcinoms.) Amer. J. Roentgenol. 87, 6—21 (1962).

— Shalek, R. J., Wall, J. A., Bloedorn, F. G.: A physical approach to the design of applicators in radium therapy of cancer of the cervix uteri. (Eine physikalische Möglichkeit der Dosisbestimmung bei der Radiumtherapie von Carcinomen der Cervix uteri. Amer. J. Roentgenol. 68, 935—947 u. Diskussion 947—949 (1952).

Fletcher, G. H., Wall, J. A., Bloedorn, F. G., Shalek, R. J., Wootton, P.: Direct measurements and isodose calculations in radium therapy of carcinoma of the cervix. (Direkte Messung und Isodosenberechnung bei der Radiumtherapie des Cervixcarcinoms.) Radiology 61, 885—902 (1953).

— Watanavit, T., Rutledge, F. N.: Whole-pelvis irradiation with 4,000 rads in stage I and stage II cancers of the uterine cervix. Die Beckenganzbestrahlung mit 4000 rad im Std. I und II des Collumcarcinoms.) Radiology 86, 436—443 (1966).

Fochem, K.: Strahlenbiologische Untersuchung der Rasterbestrahlung und ihr Wert für die gynäkologischen Karzinome. Strahlentherapie 102, 451—455 (1957).

— Ergebnisse und Erfahrungen der Bewegungsbestrahlung bei Rezidiven nach gynäkologischen Karzinomen. Radiol. austriaca 12, 147—151 (1961).

— Die Problematik der Osteoradionekrose nach der Bestrahlung weiblicher Genitaltumoren. Wien. klin. Wschr. 77, 802—804 (1965).

— Weghaupt, K.: Zur gynäkologischen Strahlenbehandlung mit der Siebmethode. Wien. med. Wschr. 1957, 96—99.

Fors, B., Larsson, B., Lindell, A., Naeslund, J., Stenson, S.: Effect of high energy protons on human genital carcinoma. (Die Wirkung hochenergetischer Protonen auf das Genital-Carcinom des Menschen.) Acta radiol. (Stockh.), N. S., Ther. Phys. Biol. 2, 384—398 (1964).

Forssell, G.: On permanency of radiological healing in malignant tumours: enquiry based principally on experiences from Radiumhemmet, Stockholm. Acta radiol. (Stockh.), Suppl. II (1928).

Franco, L.: Tecniche telecobaltoterapiche nel trattamento del carcinoma del collo uterino. (Technik der Telekobalt-Therapie bei der Behandlung des Collum-Carcinoms.) Radiaz. alta Energia 5, 51—73 (1966).

Freid, J. R., Lipman, A., Jacobson, L. E.: Roentgen therapy through a grid for advanced carcinoma. (Röntgen-Therapie durch ein Sieb bei fortgeschrittenen Carcinomen.) Amer. J. Roentgenol. 70, 460—476 (1953).

Frick, H. C., Corscaden, J. A., Jacox, H. W., Taylor, H. C., Jr.: Surgical and radiologic treatment of cancer of the cervix in 397 cases. (Operative und radiologische Behandlung des Cervixcarcinoms bei 397 Fällen.) Surg. Gynec. Obstet. 107, 457—468 (1958).

Frick, H. C., II., Taylor, H. C., Jr., Guttmann, R., Jacox, H. W., McKelway, W. P.: A study of complications in the surgical and radiation therapy of cancer of the cervix. (Eine Studie der Komplikationen der chirurgischen und Strahlenbehandlung des Collumcarcinoms.) Surg. Gynec. Obstet. 111, 493—506 (1960).

Fricke, R. E.: Changing concepts in irradiation therapy of cancer of the cervix. (Über die wechselnden Konzeptionen in der Strahlentherapie des Cervixcarcinoms.) West. J. Surg. 67, 173—176 (1959).

FRICKE, R. E., DECKER, D. G.: The intensive divided-dose irradiation therapy of carcinoma of the uterine cervix: rationale and late results. (Die intensiv-fraktionierte Strahlenbehandlung des Collumcarcinoms: Methodische Überlegungen und Spätresultate.) Amer. J. Roentgenol. 75, 502—507 (1956).
— — Late results of radiation therapy for cancer of the cervical stump. (Ergebnisse der Strahlentherapie beim Cervixstumpfcarcinom.) Amer. J. Roentgenol. 79, 32—35 (1958).
FRIEBEL, H.-G.: Klinische Erfahrungen über die Wirkung der oralen Applikation von N-Acetyl-Homocysteinthiolakton auf die Darmreaktion bei der Strahlentherapie gynäkologischer Karzinome. Strahlentherapie 124, 540—546 (1964).
FRIEDELL, G. H., CESARE, F., PARSONS, L.: Surgical treatment of cancer of the cervix recurring after primary irradiation therapy. (Die operative Behandlung des Collum-Carcinoms nach primärer Strahlenbehandlung.) New Engl. J. Med. 264, 781—784 (1961).
— GRAHAM, J. B.: Regional lymph node involvement in small carcinoma of the cervix. Surg. Gynec. Obstet. 108, 513—517 (1959).
FRIEDMAN, M.: Supervoltage (2-Mvp) rotation irradiation of cancer of bladder. Radiology 73, 191—208 (1959).
— HINE, G. J., DRESNER, J.: Principles of supervoltage (2 million volts) rotation therapy. Radiology 64, 1—15 (1955).
— PEARLMAN, A. W.: Carcinoma of the cervix: radiation salvage of surgical failures. (Strahlentherapie des Cervixcarcinoms nach Versagen der operativen Therapie.) Radiology 84, 801—811 (1965).
FRIES, G.: Zur Röntgen-Diagnostik osteoradionekrotischer Hüftveränderungen nach Röntgen-Radiumbestrahlung weiblicher Genitalkarzinome. Strahlentherapie 132, 113—127 (1967).
— Überwachung der Hüftgelenke nach Bestrahlung weiblicher Genitalkarzinome. Münch. med. Wschr. 109, 1499—1502 (1967).
FRISCHBIER, H.-J.: Dosimetrische Probleme bei der kombinierten Radium- und Telekobaltbestrahlung. Arch. Gynäk. 202 316—320 (1964).
— Urologische Komplikationen nach gynäkologischer Strahlentherapie. 7. Tagg der Vereinig. Norddtsch. Urologen, Hamburg 1965.
— Angiographische Untersuchungen zur Rezidivdiagnostik weiblicher Genitalkarzinome. XI. Internat. Kongr. Radiologie, Rom 1965.
— Die Bedeutung der Lymphographie in der gynäkologischen Tumordiagnostik. Deutscher Röntgenkongreß 1964. Stuttgart: Thieme 1965.
— Vergleichende lymphographische, arteriographische und phlebographische Befunde beim weiblichen Genitalkarzinom. Deutscher Röntgenkongreß 1965. Stuttgart: Thieme 1966.
— HASSE, J.: Die biaxiale Telekobalt-Pendelbestrahlung des Kollumkarzinoms. Dosisverteilung, Herddosisberechnung, Einstelltechnik und klinische Erfahrungen. Strahlentherapie 126, 481—494 (1965).
— KARL, B.: Zur Telekobaltbestrahlung der aortalen Lymphknoten. Strahlentherapie 140, 32—36 (1970).

FRISCHBIER, H.-J., KUTTIG, H.: Zur Technik der direkten Feldkontrollaufnahmen mit der Telekobalttherapieeinheit. Strahlentherapie 113, 610—618 (1960).
— — Klinische Erfahrungen in der Therapie mit ultraharten Strahlen. Radiologe 1, 252—263 (1961).
— — Kritische Betrachtungen zur Telekobalttherapie des Kollumkarzinoms. Geburtsh. u. Frauenheilk. 24, 761—770 (1964).
— — Die Anwendung von Ausgleichsfiltern zur Verbesserung der Dosisverteilung bei der Telekobalttherapie des Kollumkarzinoms. Strahlentherapie 125, 161—172 (1964).
— LOHBECK, H. U.: Erste Erfahrungen mit der perkutanen Megavolttherapie des Kollumkarzinoms unter Verzicht auf Radium. 48. Tagg der Dtsch. Röntgenges., Baden-Baden 1967.
— Behandlungsergebnisse und Komplikationen bei der Megavolttherapie des Carcinoma colli uteri. Strahlentherapie 140, 13—19 (1970).
— Möhle, G.: Möglichkeiten zur Telekobalttherapie des lumbalen Lymphsystems. Strahlentherapie. 132, 487—496 (1967).
— SEIFERT, A.: Zur Dosisverteilung bei der kombinierten Radium- und Telekobalttherapie des Kollumkarzinoms. Strahlentherapie 127, 347—357 (1965).
— WÜRTHNER, K.: Dosisverteilung bei der Telekobaltbestrahlung des Kollumkarzinoms unter Verwendung eines zentralen Bleifilters. Strahlentherapie (im Druck).
FRISCHKORN, R.: Unsere Erfahrungen mit der Siebbestrahlung gynäkologischer Karzinome. Röntgen-Kongr. Freudenstadt 1960.
— Die Siebbestrahlung im Rahmen der gynäkologischen Strahlentherapie. Strahlentherapie 111, 537—545 (1960).
— Erste Erfahrungen mit der routinemäßigen Anwendung der Kobaltfernbestrahlung in der gynäkologischen Strahlentherapie. Dtsch. Röntgenkongr. 1961. Strahlenforschung, Bd. III, S. 158—165. München-Berlin-Wien: Urban & Schwarzenberg 1961.
— Das Dosierungs- und Lokalisationsproblem in der Radiumtherapie des Kollumkarzinoms. Röntgenkongr. 1962. Sonderbd. zur Strahlentherapie, 107—116 (1962).
— Erste Erfahrungen mit der routinemäßigen Anwendung der Kobaltfernbestrahlung in der gynäkologischen Strahlentherapie. Strahlenforsch. u. Strahlenbehandl. (Strahlentherapie, Sonderbd. 49) 3, 149—156 (1962).
— Untersuchungen zur Dosisverteilung bei der Bestrahlung des Kollumkarzinoms. Geburtsh. u. Frauenheilk. 22, 1111—1115 (1962).
— Untersuchungen über eine ausschließliche Perkutanbestrahlung des Kollumkarzinoms mit Telekobalt. Geburtsh. u. Frauenheilk. 23, 117—130 (1963).
— Das Dosierungs- und Lokalisationsproblem in der Radiumtherapie des Kollumkarzinoms. [Strahlenforsch. u. Strahlenbehandl. (Strahlentherapie, Sonderbd. 52)] 4, 107—116 (1963).

Frischkorn, R.: Die ausschließliche Perkutanbestrahlung des Kollumkarzinoms mit Telekobalt. Zbl. Gynäk. 85, 639—644 (1963).
— Der Radium-Isodosenatlas der Universitäts-Frauenklinik Göttingen. Strahlentherapie 125, 39—50 (1964).
— Befunde im Arteriogramm beim Kollumkarzinom. Deutscher Röntgenkongreß 1964 Stuttgart: Thieme 1965.
Froewis, J.: Zur Frage der karzinomatösen Lymphknotenbesiedelung beim Collumcarcinom (kasuistischer Beitrag). Wien. klin. Wschr. 74, 357—359 (1962).
— Ulm, R.: Carcinomatöse Lymphknotenbesiedelung beim operierten Collumcarcinom. Gynaecologia (Basel) 148, 234—246 (1959).
Fuchs, G., Hofbauer, J.: Zur Röntgennachbestrahlung des Collumcarcinoms mit besonderer Berücksichtigung des Problems der Strahlenschäden. Krebsarzt 19, 412—422 (1964).
Fuchs, W. A.: Der diagnostische Wert der Cavographie. Radiol. clin. (Basel) 30, 129—149 (1961).
— Lymphographie und Tumordiagnostik. Berlin-Heidelberg-New York: Springer 1965.
Fugazzola, F., Ludovico, N.: La linfografia pelvica in ginecologia. Minerva ginec. 12, 44 (1963).
Fujimori, H., Yamada, F., Sugamoto, I., Kinoshita, H., Kasahara, Y., Kawai, I., Toyoda, N., Goda, S., Hamasaki, H.: Experimental and clinical studies of the treatment of malignant tumors with betatron in the field of gynecology. (Experimentelle und klinische Untersuchungen über die Behandlung maligner Tumoren mit dem Betatron in der Gynäkologie.) J. Jap. obstet. gynaec. Soc. (Engl. Ed.) 10, 247—248 (1963).
Gärtner, F.: Die urologischen Komplikationen bei der Therapie des Uteruskarzinoms. Krebsforschung und Krebsbekämpfung, Bd. IV, S. 294—305. München-Berlin-Wien: Urban & Schwarzenberg 1962.
Ganev, P., Ognjanov, K.: Folgen der Röntgenkastration bei der Frau. Zbl. Gynäk. 87, 1195 (1965).
Gansau, H.: Zur Ureterstenose und deren Folgen beim recidivfreien Kollumkarzinom. Zbl. Gynäk. 82, 1154—1161 (1960).
— Lymphographie im Beckenraum. Geburtsh. u. Frauenheilk. 23, 805—808 (1963).
Ganse, R.: Die Veränderungen der atypischen Gefäße des Portiokarzinoms unter Telecobaltbestrahlung. Geburtsh. u. Frauenheilk. 27, 476—480 (1967).
Garcia, M.: Further observations on tissue dosage in cancer of the cervix uteri. (Weitere Beobachtungen über die Gewebsdosierung beim Collumcarcinom.) Amer. J. Roentgenol. 73, 35—60 (1955).
Garland, L. H.: Radiation therapy of cancer. Current results with megavoltage and orthovoltage. (Strahlenbehandlung des Krebses; derzeitige Resultate mit Megavoltage- und Orthovoltagegeräten.) Amer. J. Roentgenol. 86, 621—639 (1961).
Gary-Bobo, J., Pourquier, H.: Traitement physiothérapique seul (radium télécobalt) du cancer du col utérin. Résultats au-delà de cinq ans d'une série de 163 cas. (Ausschließliche Strahlenbehandlung des Carcinoma colli uteri [mit Radium und Telekobalt]. [Ergebnisse von 163 Fällen aus 5 Jahren.]) J. Radiol. Electrol. 47, 78—81 (1966).
Gatto, A., Rizzuto, E.: Le alterazioni uretero-renali nel carcinoma della portio, prima e dopo trattamento attinico. Attual. Ostet. Ginec. 6, 1—22 (1960).
Gauwerky, F.: Ergebnisse und Erfahrungen bei der Behandlung des Uteruskarzinoms. Bericht über die Jahrgänge 1935—1939. Strahlentherapie 77, 325—348 (1948).
— Die Komplikationen bei der Radiumbehandlung der Kollumkarzinome und ihre Bedeutung für den Behandlungserfolg. Strahlentherapie 80, 51—70 (1949).
— Zur Strahlenbehandlung des Korpuskarzinoms des Uterus unter besonderer Berücksichtigung hysterographischer Befunde. Fortschr. Röntgenstr. 79 (1953), Sonderbd. 36, S. 51—53. Tagungsheft 35. Tagg d. Dtsch. Röntgenges.
— Standardisierung und individuelle Anpassung bei der Strahlenbehandlung der Gebärmutter- und Scheidenkarzinome. Strahlentherapie 103, 16—47 (1957).
Geipel, K.: Der akute Tod bei der Behandlung gynäkologischer Karzinome mit Radium. Zbl. Gynäk. 78, 1538—1546 (1956).
Geller, H.-F., Haller, J.: Ergebnisse der Behandlung des Gebärmutterhalskarzinoms in den Berichtsjahren 1949 — 1951. Strahlentherapie 105, 499—502 (1958).
Gerteis, W.: Die Lymphographie beim Genitalcarcinom der Frau. Übersicht über ihre Möglichkeiten. Arch. Gynäk. 200, 109 (1964).
— Lymphographie und Topographische Anatomie des Beckenlymphsystems. Erg. H. Z. Geburtsh. Gynäk. 165, 1—70 (1966).
Giavelli, S., D'Amico, P., Grattarola, R., Luciani, L., Roncoroni, L.: Risultati preliminari della renographia nelle complicanze urologiche del carcinoma del collo dell'utero. Tumori 51, 39—52 (1965).
Giercke, H.-P.: Zwei Zangen für gynäkologische Radiumeinlagen. Radiobiol. Radiother. (Berl.) 1, 423—425 (1960).
Gietzelt, F., Degner, W., Fürst, G., Zur Horst-Meyer, H., Schmidt, H., Roth, A.: Die biaxiale Pendelbestrahlung des Kollumkarzinoms mit Kobaltgammastrahlung. Radiobiol. Radiother. (Berl.) 3, 521—529 (1962).
— — Schmidt, H., Zur Horst-Meyer, H., Roth, A.: Biaxial supervoltage rotation irradiation of the cervix carcinoma uteri. (Biaxiale Hochvolt-Rotationsbestrahlung beim Collum-Carcinom.) Acta Un. int. Cancr. 20, 1753—1755 (1964).
Gilmour, M., Glucksmann, A., Spear, F. G.: Influence of tumour histology, duration of symptoms and age of patient in radiocurability of cervix tumours. Brit. J. Radiol. 22, 90—95 (1949).
Glocker, K. I.: Zur Frage des Beckenwandrezidivs bei der Strahlenbehandlung des Kollumkarzinoms. Topographische Untersuchungen als Grundlage der Dosisbestimmung an der Spina ossis ischii. Strahlentherapie 90, 191—198 (1953).

GLUCKSMANN, A.: The influence of systemic factors on the differentiation and radiocurability of cervical cancers. Brit. J. Radiol. **29**, 483–487 (1956).

— SPEAR, F. G.: Qualitative and quantitative histological examination of biopsy material from patients treated by radiation for carcinoma of cervix uteri. Brit. J. Radiol. **18**, 313—322 (1945).

— WAY, S.: On the choice of treatment of individual carcinomas of the cervix based on analysis of serial biopsies. J. Obstet. Gynaec. Brit. Emp. **55**, 573—582 (1948).

— — The ten-year results of individualized treatment of carcinoma of the cervix based on the analysis of serial biopsies. J. Obstet. Gynaec. Brit. Cwlth. **71**, 198—201 (1964).

GOEPEL, E.: Hat die operative Therapie beim Kollumkarzinom noch eine Berechtigung? Geburtsh. u. Frauenheilk. **19**, 494—502 (1959).

GOLDSCHEIDER, G., STERN, B. E.: Factors influencing the occurence of reactions during treatment of carcinoma of the cervix uteri by radium. (Faktoren, die das Auftreten von Reaktionen während der Behandlung des Collumcarcinoms mit Radium beeinflussen.) Brit. J. Radiol. **26**, 370—376 (1953).

— — Rotational x-ray therapy planned to complement radium treatment of carcinoma of the cervix uteri. Brit. J. Radiol. **31**, 88—92 (1958).

GOLDSTEIN, L., MURPHY, D. P.: Microcephalic idioty following radium therapy for uterine cancer during pregnancy. Amer. J. Obstet. Gynec. **18**, 189—281 (1929).

GORTON, G.: Post-irradiative prophylactic extraperitoneal lymphadenectomy in carcinoma of the uterine cervix. Acta radiol. (Stockh.) Suppl. **100** (1953).

— Radiation therapy and excision of the lymph nodes in cervical cancer. In MEIGS, J. V., and STURGIS, S. H., Progress in gynecology, vol. 3. New York: Grune & Stratton 1957.

— Radiation therapy and excision of the lymph nodes in cervical cancer. Progr. Gynec. **3**, 594—603 (1957).

— Surgical and radiation treatment of invasive carcinoma of the uterine cervix by H. L. KOTT-MEIER, G. GORTON, A. CHRISTENSEN, P. LANGE, E. NIELSEN. Acta obstet. gynec. scand. **43**, Suppl. **2**, 49—58 (1964).

GRABIGER, R.: Osteoradionekrose des Schenkelhalses nach Telekobalttherapie. Strahlentherapie **123**, 282—284 (1964).

GRAEBER, W.: Das Verhalten verschiedener Blutgerinnungsfaktoren bei der Bestrahlung gynäkologischer Karzinome mit Kobalt 60. Strahlentherapie **124**, 60—68 (1964).

— Die Einwirkung der kombinierten Radium-Telekobalt-Bestrahlung gynäkologischer Karzinome auf das Blutgerinnungssystem. Strahlentherapie **124**, 377—388 (1964).

GRAHAM, J. B.: Effectiveness of radiotherapy in cancer of the uterine cervix. (Über die Wirkung der Strahlenbehandlung beim Cervixcarcinom.) Obstet. gynec. Surv. **9**, 428—431 (1954).

— GRAHAM, R. M.: A method of enhancing the effectiveness of radiotherapy in cancer of the uterine cervix. (Eine Methode der Verbesserung der Wirkung der Strahlenbehandlung beim Collumcarcinom.) Cancer (N.Y.) **6**, 68—76 (1953).

GRAHAM, J. B., GRAHAM, R. M.: The curability of regional lymph node metastases in cancer of the uterine cervix. Surg. Gynec. Obstet. **100**, 149—156 (1955).

— — The sensitization response in patients with cancer of the uterine cervix. Cancer (Philad.) **13**, 5—14 (1960).

— — KOTTMEIER, H.-L.: Potentiation of radiotherapy by supplemental agents in cancer of the uterine cervix (four-year results). (Potenzierung der Strahlentherapie durch zusätzliche Mittel beim Carcinom der Cervix uteri [4-Jahres-Resultate].) Acta Un. int. Cancr. **16**, 1291—1293 (1960).

— SOTTO, L. S. J., PALOUCEK, F.: Carcinoma of cervix. Philadelphia: W. B. Saunders Co. 1962.

GRAHAM, R. M., GRAHAM, J. B.: Cellular index of sensitivity to ionizing radiation; sensitization response. Cancer (Philad.) **6**, 215—223 (1953).

— — Factors in prognosis in cancer of the uterine cervix desquamation of malignant cells. Cancer (Philad.) **13**, 15—19 (1960).

— — Cytologic prognosis in cancer of the cervix. Two year survival rates in a randomized series. (Cytologische Prognose bei Cervix-Carcinom. Zwei-Jahresüberlebensrate bei einer unausgewählten Serie.) Amer. J. Roentgenol. **87**, 56—59 (1962.)

GRANONE, F. G., JULIANI, G.: Applicatore di radium articolato a croce commissa. Isterostato automatico per il fondo. Radiol. med. (Torino) **60**, 283—289 (1965).

GRAY, M. J.: Pelvic lymph node dissections following radiotherapy for carcinoma of the cervix. A preliminary report. Obstet. gynec. Surv. **13**, 265—266 (1958).

— FRICK, H. C.: Pelvic lymph node dissection following radiotherapy for cancer of the cervix. Reevaluation. (Zur Exstirpation der Beckenlymphknoten im Anschluß an die Strahlenbehandlung des Cervixcarcinoms.) Amer. J. Obstet. Gynec. **93**, 110—114 (1965).

— GUSBERG, S. B., GUTTMANN, R.: Pelvic lymph node dissection following radiotherapy. Amer. J. Obstet. Gynec. **76**, 629—633 (1958).

— KOTTMEIER, H. L.: Rectal and bladder injuries following radium therapy for carcinoma of the cervix at the radiumhemmet. Amer. J. Obstet. Gynec. **74**, 1294—1303 (1957).

GREEN, L. S., MUIRHEAD, W.: Improvement in results of treatment of carcinoma of cervix. J. Canad. Ass. Radiol. **14**, 191—199 (1963).

GREENFIELD, M. A., FICHMAN, M., NORMAN, A.: Dosage tables for linear radium sources filtered by 0.5 and 1.0 mm of platinum. Radiology **73**, 418—423 (1959).

GREGORY, C.: Dosage distribution in rotational cobalt 60 therapy; simplified method of computation. Brit. J. Radiol. **30**, 538—543 (1957).

GREISS, F. C., JR.: Can the results be improved by combining radiation and elective radical hysterectomy and lymphadenectomy? (Lassen sich die Heilungsergebnisse der kombinierten Behandlung von Bestrahlung und elektiver radikaler Hysterektomie mit Lymphadenektomie bestätigen?) J. Amer. med. Ass. **193**, 1105—1107 (1965).

GREISS, F. C., BLAKE, D. D., LOCK, F. R.: Complications of intensive radiation therapy for cervical carcinoma. Obstet. Gynec. 18, 417—429 (1961).
— — — Treatment of cancer of cervix by radiation and elective radical hysterectomy. Amer. J. Obstet. Gynec. 82, 1042—1054 (1961).
GROSSE-HOLZ, K.: Die Osteoradionekrose des Schenkelhalses — ein Dosisproblem? Strahlentherapie 125, 591—598 (1964).
— VOGELGESANG, K.-H., SCHULZE, E.: Unsere Ergebnisse bei der Strahlenbehandlung des Kollumkarzinoms im Zeitraum von 1928 bis 1957. Strahlentherapie 122, 501—510 (1963).
GRÜNBERGER, V.: Seltene Metastasenbildung nach operiertem Kollumkarzinom. Ber. allg. spez. Path. 2, 470 (1949).
— Die Prognosestellung der Radiumwirkung auf das Collumcarcinom aus den cytologischen Veränderungen nach GLÜCKSMANN. Arch. Gynäk. 181, 190—209 (1952).
— WEGHAUPT, K.: Die Collumkarzinome an der I. Universitäts-Frauenklinik Wien in den Jahren 1956—1959. Wien. klin. Wschr. 77, 804—809 (1965).
GÜNSEL, E.: Zur Frage der paravaginalen Radiumbehandlung beim Collum-Carcinom. Strahlentherapie 90, 208—212 (1953).
GÜNTHER, H.: Urologische Komplikationen nach radikaloperiertem und strahlenbehandeltem Genitalkarzinom. Zbl. Gynäk. 84, 1283—1292 (1962).
— Die intravenöse Nephropyelographie in der urologischen Diagnostik bei Zervixkarzinompatientinnen. Zbl. Gynäk. 89, 1041—1050 (1967).
GULDBRANDSEN, T., MADSEN, C. B.: Radiation dosimetry by means of semiconductors. Acta radiol. (Stockh.) 58, 226—232 (1962).
GUPTA, S. K., CUNNINGHAM, J. R.: Measurement of tissue-air ratios and scatter functions for large field size, for cobalt 60 gamma radiation. Radiology 39, 7—11 (1966).
GUSBERG, S. B., HERMAN, G. G.: Radiosensitivity testing of cervix cancer by the test dose technique. (Untersuchung der Strahlensensibilität des Cervix-Carcinoms durch die Testdosistechnik.) Amer. J. Roentgenol. 87, 60—68 (1962).
— FISH, S. A., WANG, Y. Y.: The growth pattern of cervical cancer. Obstet. Gynec. N. Y. 2, 557—561 (1953).
— TOVELL, H. M. M., EMERSON, R., ALLINA, H.: Radiosensitivity testing of cervical cancer. A preliminary report. (Ein Test über die Strahlenempfindlichkeit des Cervixkrebses. Ein vorläufiger Bericht.) Amer. J. Obstet. 68, 1464—1471 (1954).
GUSSO, A.: Tentativi di sbarramento all'invasione metastatica del cancro dell'utero mediante Radiumterapia posteriore per via pelvi-extraperitoneale. (Versuche zur Blockierung der metastatischen Invasion des Collumcarcinoms durch extraperitoneale Radiumbehandlung des rückwärtigen Beckenraumes.) Riv. Ostet. (Milano) 36, 113—123 (1954).
GUSTAFSSON, D. C., KOTTMEIER, H. L.: Carcinoma of cervix associated with pregnancy; study of Radiumhemmet's series of invasive carcinoma during period of 1932—1956. Acta obstet. gynec. scand. 41, 1—21 (1962).

GUTTMANN, R.: Effects of radiation on metastatic lymph nodes from various primary carcinomas. Amer. J. Roentgenol. 79, 79—82 (1958).
— Radiation therapy of carcinoma of the cervix uteri. (Strahlenbehandlung des Carcinoms der Cervix uteri.) Bull. N.Y. Acad. Med. 38, 513—526 (1962).
— Which method is better able to cure positive pelvic lymph nodes? (Welche Methode eignet sich besser für die Therapie der Beckenlymphknoten-Metastasen?) J. Amer. med. Ass. 193, 1104 (1965).
— Dose distribution and results in carcinoma of the cervix. A comparison of conventional high voltage therapy including vaginal cone therapy with supervoltage therapy. (Dosisverteilung und Ergebnisse beim Cervixcarcinom. Vergleich der konventionellen Hochvolttherapie mit vaginaler Therapie mit Supervolt.) Amer. J. Roentgenol. 77, 803—814 (1957).
GUZZON, A., ROMANINI, A.: Sulle alterazioni procto-sigmoiditiche secondarie a telecobaltoterapia complementare dei carcinomi uterini. (Proktosigmoiditische Veränderungen als Folge zusätzlicher Telekobalttherapie der Uteruscarcinome.) Minerva radiol. fisioter. radiobiol. (Torino) 8, 314—320 (1963).
HAAM, E. VON, ALBERY, R.: Radiation cell changes in experimentally produced carcinoma of the cervix Symposium. (Celluläre Strahlenveränderungen bei experimentell erzeugtem Cervix-Carcinom.) Acta cytol. (Chic.) 3, 376—379 (1960).
HACKE, W.: Haematogene Knochenmetastasen beim Genitalkarzinom der Frau. Z. Geburtsh. Gynäk. 137, 171—198 (1952).
HACKENTHAL, P.: Klinische Erfahrungen mit einer kombinierten Stehfeld-Konvergenz-Bestrahlung des Kollumkarzinoms. Strahlentherapie 115, 578—585 (1961).
HÄNTSCH, R.: Über die primäre Mortalität bei der Strahlenbehandlung des weiblichen Genitalkarzinoms. Zbl. Gynäk. 77, 2054—2067 (1955).
HAHN, G. A.: An evaluation of supervoltage irradiation therapy in the treatment of pelvic malignancy. (Eine Bewertung der Supervolt-Strahlentherapie bei der Behandlung maligner Beckentumoren.) Amer. J. Obstet. 73, 626—640 (1957).
— WALLACE, S., JACKSON, L., DODD, G.: Lymphangiography in gynecology. (Die Lymphangiographie in der Gynäkologie.) Amer. J. Obstet. 85, 754—771 (1963).
HAI, N. VAN, HELD, F., SCHWARZ, R.: Über die Vorbestrahlung der Parametrien bei operablen Portiokarzinomen mit Bewegungsbestrahlung. Radiobiol. Radiother. (Berl.) 4, 107—111 (1963).
HALDAR, P. K., MITTAL, K. P., AGARWAL, Y. C.: Radiotherapy in cancer of the cervix uteri. An assessment of dosage by radium. (Strahlenbehandlung bei Carcinomen der Cervix uteri; Abschätzung der Dosis bei der Radiumbestrahlung.) Indian J. Radiol. 16, 177—182 (1962).
HALFPAP, E., WITT, H. J.: Behandlungsergebnisse beim Adenokarzinom des Collum uteri an der Universitäts-Frauenklinik Göttingen. Zbl. Gynäk. 77, 1659—1665 (1955).
HALLEY, G.: La curieterapia del carcinoma del cuello uterino por el sistema de Manchester. — Expe-

riencia personal. (Die Radiumtherapie des Carcinoma colli uteri nach dem Manchester-System. Eigene Erfahrungen.) Bol. Liga Cánc. **31**, 111—116 (1956).

HALTER, G.: Zur Vorbestrahlung des Kollum-Karzinoms. Wien. med. Wschr. **110**, 153—156 (1960).

HANKINS, F. D., HOCKIN, J. G.: Radium treatment of cancer of uterine cervix by Manchester system: use of plastic vaginal applicators. Amer. J. Roentgenol. **68**, 272—274 (1952).

HARBORT, G.: Zur gynäkologischen Herdfeineinstellung bei der Bewegungsbestrahlung. Geburtsh. u. Frauenheilk. **18**, 1455—1460 (1958).

HARTL, H.: Harntraktveränderungen beim Kollumkarzinom, ihre Verhütung und Behandlung. Zbl. Gynäk. **83**, 1808—1817 (1961).

— Urologische Komplikationen bei der Behandlung des Kollumkarzinoms. Krebsforschung und Krebsbekämpfung, Bd. IV, S. 267—274. München-Berlin-Wien: Urban & Schwarzenberg 1962.

HARVEY, R. A., HAAS, L. L., LAUGHLIN, J. S.: Betatron cancer therapy. Radiology **58**, 23—34 (1952).

HEINZLER, F.: Untersuchungen mit Ionisationskammern und der Filmschwärzung zur Bestimmung der Isodosen bei der Pendelbestrahlung mit exzentrisch gelegener Pendelachse der ultraharten Röntgenstrahlung einer 17-MeV-Elektronenschleuder (Betatron). Strahlentherapie **128**, 148—183 (1965).

HEISS, H.: Die Vorbestrahlung beim Genitalkarzinom. Medizinische **1955**, 110—113.

— Über Knochenmetastasen beim Kollumkarzinom. Strahlentherapie **101**, 356—370 (1956).

— Experimentelle Untersuchungen über die Strahlenverteilung im kleinen Becken bei der Therapie des Kollumkarzinoms. Strahlentherapie **107**, 234—259 (1958).

— Neue Gesichtspunkte zur Strahlentherapie des Kollumkarzinoms. Krebsarzt **15**, 143—152 (1960).

HELBING, W.: Die Strahlenbehandlung der Kollumkarzinomrezidive. Zbl. Gynäk. **75**, 706—716 (1953).

— Zur Bedeutung der postoperativen Nachbestrahlung beim Kollumkarzinom. Zbl. Gynäk. **83**, 513—518 (1961).

HELD, F., SCHWARZ, R., STEINHOFF, R.: Präoperative biaxiale Bewegungsbestrahlung der Parametrien und der Lymphabflußgebiete des weiblichen Genitale bei operablem Carcinoma colli uteri. Arch. Geschwulstforsch. **20**, 187—198 (1963).

HELD, H. J. v.: Das gynäko-radiologische Kombinations-Applikatorium. (Zur Methodik der Radiumbehandlung der Portio-Kollum-Karzinome.) Z. Geburtsh. Gynäk. **134**, 125 (1951).

— Über die Radiumbestrahlung der Parametrien. Zbl. Gynäk. **75**, 1205—1210 (1953); zit. nach GAUWERKY, F., Strahlentherapie **103**, 16—47 (1957).

HELLER, L., KÄSER, O.: Über Todesursachen beim Kollumkarzinom. Geburtsh. u. Frauenheilk. **26**, 155—164 (1966).

HENDRICKS, C. H., MORTON, J. L., CALLENDINE, G. W., BARNES, A. C.: Irradiation of cancer of the uterine cervix with radioactive Co^{60} in guided aluminum needles and in plastic threads. Amer. J. Roentgenol. **69**, 813 (1953).

HENRIKSEN, E.: Lymphatic spread of carcinoma of cervix and body of uterus: study of 420 necropsies. Amer. J. Obstet. Gynec. **58**, 924—942 (1949).

— Distribution of metastases in stage I carcinoma of the cervix. A study of 66 autopsied cases. Amer. J. Obstet. Gynec. **80**, 919—932 (1960).

HENSCHKE, U. K., HILARIS, B. S.: Die Zukunft der Strahlentherapie in der Behandlung des Collumcarcinoms. Arch. Gynäk. **202**, 289—304 (1965).

— — MAHAN, G. D.: Afterloading in interstitial and intracavitary radiation therapy. (Das nachträgliche Einsetzen radioaktiver Stoffe bei der interstiellen und intrakavitären Strahlentherapie.) Amer. J. Roentgenol. **90**, 386—395 (1963).

— — — Remote afterloading for intracavitary radiation therapy. Progr. clin. Cancer **1**, 127—136 (1965).

— — — Intracavitary radiation therapy of cancer of the uterine cervix by remote afterloading with cycling sources. (Intrakavitäre Strahlentherapie des Cervixcarcinoms im Hinterladerfernverfahren mit bewegter Strahlenquelle.) Amer. J. Roentgenol. **96**, 45—51 (1966).

— LAWRENCE, D. C.: Cesium-131 seeds for permanent implants. Radiology **85**, 1117—1119 (1965).

HERIK, M. VAN: Radiation therapy for carcinoma of the cervix. (Symposium.) (Die Strahlenbehandlung des Cervixcarcinoms.) Proc. Mayo Clin. **35**, 518—522 (1960).

— Fever as a complication of radiation therapy for carcinoma of the cervix. (Fieber als Komplikation der Strahlenbehandlung beim Collum-Carcinom.) Amer. J. Roentgenol. **93**, 104—109 (1965).

— FRICKE, R. E.: The results of radiation therapy for recurrent cancer of the cervix uteri. (Die Ergebnisse der Bestrahlungsbehandlung bei Rezidiven des Collumcarcinoms.) Amer. J. Roentgenol. **73**, 437—441 (1955).

HERTIG, A. T., GORE, H.: Can radiosensitivity and histopathology of cervical cancer be correlated? (Kann Strahlensensibilität und Histopathologie beim Cerivx-Carcinom zueinander in Beziehung gesetzt werden?) Amer. J. Roentgenol. **87**, 48—55 (1962).

HESS, P.: Bestrahlung des Kollumkarzinom-Rezidivs in älterer und neuerer Sicht. Strahlentherapie **103**, 436—443 (1957).

— Umwelteinflüsse auf die Heilung des Kollumkarzinoms. Strahlentherapie **107**, 127—132 (1958).

HEYMAN, J.: Improvement of results in treatment of uterine cancer. J. Amer. med. Ass. **135**, 412—416 (1947).

— Thoughts on forty years of radiation treatment of carcinoma of the uterine cervix. (Gedanken über 40 Jahre Strahlenbehandlung des Gebärmutterhals-Carcinom.) Amer. J. Obstet. **68**, 480—483 (1954).

HIGINBOTHAM, N. L., MARCOVE, R. C., CASSON, P.: Hemipelvectomy: A clinical study of 100 cases with five year follow-up on 60 patients. Surgery **59**, 706—708 (1966).

HILD, J.: Dosisdirektmessungen im Ureter bei der Radiumbehandlung des Kollumkarzinoms. 48. Tagg der Dtsch. Röntgenges., Baden-Baden 1967.

Hilfrich, H. J., Witt, H. J.: Moderne Frühdiagnostik und Verschiebung der Stadienverteilung beim Kollumkarzinom. Geburtsh. u. Frauenheilk. **25**, 1041—1049 (1965).

Hillemanns, H. G.: Die Reaktion des regionären Lymphknotens auf die therapeutische Radium-Röntgen-Bestrahlung beim Collumcarcinom. Z. Geburtsh. Gynäk. **149**, 156—196 (1957).

— Z. Geburtsh. Gynäk. **149**, 156 (1958).

Hillmann, D. C., Tristan, T. A.: Inferior vena cavography in the detection of abdominal extension of pelvic cancer. Radiology **81**, 416 (1963).

Hittmair, A.: Zervix-Karzinom und Schwangerschaft. Geburtsh. u. Frauenheilk. **27**, 513—520 (1967).

Hliniak, A., Darlewski, J., Hliniak, I., Lobodziec, W., Wojcieszek, Z., Petryna, A.: Confrontation of the size of fields of entry of X-ray radiation with the metastatic routes of the carcinoma of the uterine cervix. (Die Vergleichung der Größe der Einfallfelder der X-Strahlung mit den metastatischen Wegen des Cervix-Carcinoms.) Nowotwory **14**, 217—220 mit engl. Zus.fass. (1964) [Polnisch].

Höhne, G., Schubert, G., Uhlmann, G.: Diagnostik und Behandlung des Kollumkarzinoms und seiner Frühstadien. Med. Klin. **59**, 721—727 (1964).

Hofmann, D.: Über den Einfluß der gynäkologischen Bestrahlung auf die Harnwege. Röntgen-Bl. **12**, 321—329 (1959).

— Die Anwendung von radioaktivem Gold in der gynäkologischen Strahlentherapie. Grundlagen und klinische Erfahrungen. Strahlentherapie **111**, 167—181 (1960).

— Klinik der gynäkologischen Strahlentherapie. München-Berlin: Urban & Schwarzenberg 1963.

Hohenfellner, R.: Die urologischen Komplikationen des Kollumkarzinoms. Berlin-Heidelberg-New York: Springer 1965.

— Weghaupt, K.: Urologische Komplikationen als Bestrahlungsfolge des Kollumkarzinoms. Strahlentherapie **122**, 362—372 (1963).

Hollenbeck, Z. J. R.: Carcinoma of the cervix, treatment by radical hysterectomy following central irradiation. (Das Cervixcarcinom, seine Behandlung durch Radikaloperation nach intrakavitärer Strahlentherapie.) Amer. J. Obstet. Gynec. **79**, 944—955 (1960).

Holthusen, H., Gauwerky, F., Mohr, H.: Spezielle Methoden der lokalisierten Curietherapie mit Cobalt⁶⁰. Fortschr. Röntgenstr. **85**, 460—473 (1956); zit. nach Gauwerky, F., Strahlentherapie **103**, 16—47 (1957).

Holtz, S., Powers, W. E., Sherman, A. J.: Effect of radiation on metastatic pelvic lymph nodes judged by pelvic venograms. Radiology **76**, 289 (1961).

Holzaepfel, J. H.: Megavoltage therapy for gynecologic malignancies. Amer. J. Obstet. Gynec. **97**, 625—634 (1967).

Hondo, S.: Responses of silver-activated phosphate glass to α-, β- and γ-rays and neutrons. Hlth Phys. **7**, 25—35 (1961).

Howson, J. Y., Widmann, B. P., Weatherwax, J. L.: Transvaginal cone roentgen irradiation in cancer of the cervix uteri. Report of twelve year's experience. (Bestrahlung des Collumcarcinoms mit transvaginalem Röntgenstrahlenkegel. Erfahrungsbericht über zwölf Jahre.) Amer. J. Roentgenol. **69**, 182—190 (1953).

Hubacher, O.: Erste Erfahrungen bei der Bewegungsbestrahlung mit der Kobaltbombe. Radiol. austriaca **10**, 17—22 (1958).

Huber, H.: Die Behandlungserfolge beim Genitalkarzinom an Hand von 3410 Fällen. Geburtsh. u. Frauenheilk. **13**, 869—881 (1953).

— Du Mesnil de Rochemont, R., Ringleb, D., Roos, H.: Fünfjahresergebnisse der „Marburger Methode" bei Bestrahlung von Kollumkarzinomen. Strahlentherapie **102**, 161—179 (1957).

Hüllemann, R.: Spätveränderungen im Bereich der Kutis und an den ableitenden Harnwegen nach Supervolttherapie des Kollumkarzinoms. Strahlentherapie, Sonderbd. **61**, 272—276 (1965).

— Klinische Erfahrungen bei der Anwendung von Kortikosteroiden während und nach Strahlenbehandlung weiblicher Genitalkarzinome. Geburtsh. u. Frauenheilk. **25**, 514—523 (1965).

— Mauss, H.-J., Adler, H.: Dosisdirektmessungen im Ureter bei der Telekobalttherapie des Collum-Carcinoms. Arch. Gynäk. **202**, 325—328 (1964).

Hurteau, G. D., McLean, M.: Injuries related to radiation treatment of carcinoma of the cervix and complications of supplemental surgery. Amer. J. Obstet. Gynec. **95**, 696—705 (1966).

Il'jašenko, N. A.: Rezidive in der Vaginalnarbe nach kombinierter Therapie und ihre Verhütung. Pediat. Akush. Ginek. **1956**, H. 6, 57—61 [Ukrainisch].

Ingelman-Sundberg, A.: Rectal injuries following Stockholm method of treatment of cancer of cervix uteri. Acta radiol. (Stockh.) **28**, 760—764 (1947).

Ingiulla, W.: Die Entfernung der Vasa iliaca interna in der radikalen Chirurgie. Wien. med. Wschr. **116**, 957—960 (1966).

— Centaro, A.: Irradiazione o chirurgia nel trattamento del cancro del collo dell'utero. Nuovi aspetti del problema. (Strahlen oder chirurgische Behandlung des Carcinoms des Collum uteri. Neue Ansichten des Problems.) Riv. Ostetr. (Firenze) **12**, 53—78 (1957).

Ischtschenko, G. T.: Zur Methodik der Anwendung der Bremsstrahlung eines Betatrons beim Krebs des weiblichen Genitalbereichs. Vestn. Rentgenol. Radiol. (Mosk.) **35**, Nr. 5, 44—49 mit engl. Zus.-fass. (1960) [Russisch].

— Untersuchung der therapeutischen Wirkung der Betatronbestrahlung maligner Tumoren des Genitalbereichs. Med. Radiol. (Mosk.) **5**, Nr 10, 14—18 mit engl. Zus.fass. (1960) [Russisch].

Iwai, S., Saito, T., Shiozawa, K., Itakura, S.: The spreading modus of the uterine cervical cancer and its significance for operative procedure. Gann **50**, Suppl. 161—162 (1960); Ref. Ber. ges. Gynäk. Geburtsh. **73**, 264 (1961).

Iwata, M.: A new procedure for the clearance of intrapelvic lymph nodes at the time of abdominal panhysterectomy. An operative technique for the clearance of intrapelvic lymph nodes preceding uterine excision. Jokohama med. Bull. **12**, 163—167 (1961); Ref. Ber. ges. Gynäk. Geburtsh. **81**, 286 (1963).

JACOBSON, L. E.: Cobalt 60 tumor treatment time and "skin" dosage charts. Amer. J. Roentgenol. **85**, 33—37 (1961).

— KOECK, G. P., HILLSINGER, W. R., SCHWARZ, M. E.: Co⁶⁰ isodose curves for 240° rotation, showing displacement of center of dose from center of rotation. Radiology **77**, 66—76 (1961).

JAEGER, W.: Routinemäßige Anwendung der Siebbestrahlung beim operierten und nicht operierten Kollumkarzinom. Radiobiol. Radiother. (Berl.) **7**, 525—528 (1966).

JANKER, R.: Die Bestrahlung mit dem Betatron. Ärztl. Wschr. **13**, 697—702 (1958).

JANTET, G. H.: Direct intralymphatic injections of radioactive colloidal gold in the treatment of malignant disease. (Direkte intralymphatische Injektion von Radiogoldkolloid in der Behandlung maligner Erkrankungen.) Brit. J. Radiol. **35**, 692—697 (1962).

— EDWARDS, J. M., GOUGH, M. H., KINMONTH, J. B.: Endolymphatic therapy with radioactive gold for malignant melanoma. (Endolymphatische Therapie mit radioaktivem Gold bei malignen Melanomen.) Brit. med. J. **1964 II**, 904—906.

JELIFFE, A. M.: An improved method of introducing the Manchester system "ovoids". (Eine verbesserte Methode zur Applikation der „Manchester System Ovoids".) Brit. J. Radiol. **30**, 106—108 (1957).

JOHANNSSEN, H.: Über die Vermeidbarkeit von Strahlenfolgen am ableitenden Harnsystem und Darm bei der Radiumtherapie. Landarzt **27**, 149—153 (1965).

— Spätkomplikationen nach intraperitonealer Radiogoldinfusionen. Strahlentherapie **127**, 198—205 (1965).

JOHANSSON, J. M., LINDSKONG, B., NYSTRÖM, C. E.: Pelvic dosimetry during radiotherapy of carcinoma of the cervix uteri. Acta radiol. (Stockh.) **8**, 360—372 (1969).

JOHNS, H. E., DARBY, E. K., WATSON, T. A., BURKELL, C. C.: Comparison of dosage distributions obtainable with 400 kVp x-rays and 22 MeVx-rays Brit. J. Radiol. **23**, 290—299 (1950).

— MORRISON, M. T., WATSON, T. A.: Radiation distribution from 1,000 curie cobalt unit using conventional and rotational techniques. Acta radiol. (Stockh.) Suppl. **116**, 550—558 (1954).

— — WHITMORE, G. F.: Dosage calculations for rotation therapy; with special reference to cobalt 60. Amer. J. Roentgenol. **75**, 1105—1116 (1956).

JOHNSON, W. O., WEINFURTNER, B. J.: Carcinoma of cervix associated with pregnancy. Amer. J. Obstet. Gynec. **59**, 1189—1201 (1950).

JOHNSTON, D. O., TREMBLAY, P. A.: Results of radiation therapy in carcinoma of the cervix. (Symposium.) (Ergebnisse der Strahlentherapie bei Cervixcarcinomen.) Surg. Clin. N. Amer. **39**, 815—819 (1959).

JONES, D. E. A., GREGORY, C., BIRCHALL, I.: Dosage distribution in rotational cobalt 60 therapy. Brit. J. Radiol. **20**, 196—201 (1956).

KÄSER, O., IKLÉ, F. A.: Urologische Komplikationen bei der Behandlung des Kollumkarzinoms. Dtsch. med. Wschr. **86**, 2465—2472 u. Bild. 2495—2496 (1961).

— SCHIEFERSTEIN, W.: Diagnose und Therapie der Rezidive gynäkologischer Karzinome. Geburtsh. u. Frauenheilk. **26**, 180—190 (1966).

KAHANPÄÄ, V.: A new simplified radium applicator for intensifying the radiotherapy of the parametria in cancer of the cervix. Acta radiol. (Stockh.) **27**, 495—504 (1946).

— On radiotherapy of cancer colli uteri. (Über die Bestrahlungstherapie beim Collum uteri-Carcinom.) Suom. Lääk.-L. H. **22**, 895—901 (1952) [Finnisch].

— TURTOLA, V.: Ergebnisse bei der Kollumkarzinombehandlung in der Strahlenbehandlungsklinik zu Helsinki in den Jahren 1942—1949. Strahlentherapie **98**, 240—244 (1955).

KAHR, E.: Zur Herdlokalisation am Gammatron 2 und zur Frage der Bewegungsbestrahlung. Sonderbde zur Strahlentherapie **61**, 176—182 (1965).

KAINBERGER, F.: Der Wert der Beckenvenographie in der Rezidivdiagnostik nach Uteruskarzinom. Radiol. austrica **12**, 119—128 (1961).

KALLERT, H.-J.: Die Belastung von Haut, Vagina und Rektum bei der Pendelkonvergenzbestrahlung der Parametrien. Zur Bewegungsbestrahlung gynäkologischer Tumoren im kleinen Becken. IV. Mitt. Radiol. clin. (Basel) **26**, 38—53 (1957).

KAPLAN, A. L., HUDGINS, P. T., WALL, J. A.: Postradiation pelvic fibrosis simulating recurrent carcinoma. (Carcinomrezidiv vortäuschende Strahlenfibrose des Beckenzellgewebes.) Amer. J. Obstet. Gynec. **92**, 117—124 (1965).

KAPOOR, H. K., SAHAI, I., BHARDWAJ, O. P.: Redefinition of point "B" in the treatment of cancer cervix by radiotherapy. (Neue Definition des Punktes „B" bei der Radiumtherapie des Collumcarcinoms.) Indian J. Radiol. **20**, 205—207 (1966).

KAPP-SCHWOERER, H.: Bereicherung der strahlentherapeutischen Möglichkeiten in der Behandlung der Genitalkarzinome durch Radiogoldseeds-Spickung (Au¹⁹⁸). Fortschr. Röntgenstr. **96**, 551—557 (1962).

— Die Radiogoldseeds-Implantation (Au 198) bei der Behandlung gynäkologischer Malignome. Radiobiol. Radiother. (Berl.) **4**, 313—321 (1963).

— Über die Vorteile einer Kompression bei der Telekobalttherapie im kleinen Becken. Strahlentherapie **125**, 395—399 (1964).

— Aktuelle Probleme der Strahlentherapie weiblicher Genitalkarzinome. Med. Welt **17**, 1105—1112 (1966).

— Zum Problem der Kombination einer Radium- und Telekobalt-Therapie beim Kollum-Karzinom. Geburtsh. u. Frauenheilk. **29**, 271 (1969).

— BUSCH, M.: Über die Anwendung von Radiogoldseeds (Au¹⁹⁸) bei der gynäkologischen Strahlentherapie mit Untersuchungen der Isodosenverläufe und Belastung kritischer Organe. Strahlentherapie **120**, 481—511 (1963).

— — Zur optimalen Lokalbestrahlung größerer Kollumtumoren. Geburtsh. u. Frauenheilk. **24**, 114—124 (1964).

Keiser, D. von, Frischbier, H.-J.: Der Wert der Lymphographie bei der Metastasensuche. Fortschr. Röntgenstr. **100**, 299 (1964).

Keller, H. L.: Kriterien der allgemeinen Strahlenbelastung bei verschiedenen Bestrahlungsmethoden, dargelegt am Beispiel verschiedener Bewegungsbestrahlungsmöglichkeiten des Parametriums. Strahlentherapie **108**, 539—542 (1959).

— Die Pendelbestrahlung der Parametrien und ihrer Lymphabflußwege. 9. Int. Congr. Radiol. **1**, 759—761 (1961).

Kepp, R. K.: Neue Gesichtspunkte für die Behandlung von Rezidiven bei gynäkologischen Karzinomen. Wien. med. Wschr. **1952**, 30—36.

— Gynäkologische Strahlentherapie. Stuttgart: Thieme 1952.

— Die Bestrahlungsbehandlung von Rezidiven des Kollumkarzinoms. Dtsch. med. Wschr. **1953**, 1391—1393.

— Methoden und Resultate der Strahlenbehandlung des Collumcarcinoms an der Universitäts-Frauenklinik Göttingen. Arch. Gynäk. **183**, 444—454 (1953).

— Die Hochvolttherapie und ihre Aussichten in der gynäkologischen Strahlenbehandlung. Geburtsh. u. Frauenheilk. **14**, 10—30 (1954).

— Die Therapie mit Radiogold in der Gynäkologie. Geburtsh. u. Frauenheilk. **18**, 10—21 (1958).

— Baeumer, J.: Die Bestrahlung mit wanderndem Strahlenkegel bei der Behandlung bösartiger Tumoren des weiblichen Genitale. Strahlentherapie **90**, 108—116 (1953).

— Clemens, H.: Ergebnisse der postoperativen Radiogoldtherapie bei bösartigen Ovarialtumoren. Strahlentherapie **126**, 65—69 (1965).

— Hartl, H., Müller, K.: Die Bedeutung von Radiogold[198] für die gynäkologische Strahlentherapie. Dtsch. med. Wschr. **80**, 19—21 (1955).

Kihara, Y., Watanabe, E., Wada, M., Fujiwara, A., Mukai, M., Obuchi, T., Ikeda, Y., Tetsuo, F.: Studies on tele-cobalt therapy for uterine cancer. (Beobachtungen bei der Tele-Kobalt-Therapie des Uteruscarcinoms.) J. Jap. obstet. gyneac. Soc. (Engl. ed.) **4**, 171—186 (1957).

Kim, S. K., Jones, W. R.: A pelvic phlebogram. A case report and review of the literature. Amer. J. Roentgenol. **93**, 940 (1965).

Kirchhoff, H.: Die fraktionierte Röntgenbestrahlung fortgeschrittener Kollumkarzinome bei Mitbeteiligung der abführenden Harnwege: Akute Gefahren und primäre Heilungen. Strahlentherapie **65**, 579—594 (1939).

— Zur postoperativen Nachbestrahlung gynäkologischer Karzinome. Strahlentherapie **102**, 425—434 (1957).

— Fortschr. Röntgenstr. **86**, Beiheft 39, 33 (1957).

— Die Behandlung der Harnwegskomplikationen als Folge der Therapie des Kollumkarzinoms. Begründung und Zeitpunkt. Strahlentherapie **113**, 356—368 (1960).

— Komplikationsreiche Veränderungen am Harnsystem nach Strahlentherapie des Kollumkarzinoms. Geburtsh. u. Frauenheilk. **20**, 34—39 (1960).

— Individualisierung Krebskranker. Krebsforsch. **5**, 261—269 (1963).

Kirchhoff, H., Geller, H.-F.: Erfahrungen mit der Zusatztherapie bei 294 Patientinnen mit Kollumkarzinom (1954—1956). Strahlentherapie **105**, 353—356 (1958).

Kistner, R. W., Hertig, A. T.: Correlation of histologic grade clinical stage and radiation response in carcinoma of uterine cervix. Amer. J. Obstet. Gynec. **61**, 1293—1300 (1951).

Kjellgren, O.: Radiation reaction in vaginal smear and its prognostic sifnigicance. Acta radiol. (Stockh.) **1958**, Suppl. 168.

Kleine, H. O.: Die Erfolge der Radiumspickmethode bei der Behandlung der Gebärmutterhalskrebse. Zbl. Gynäk. **76**, 1785—1792 (1954).

Klemm, J.: Ein Beitrag zur Behandlung der Haut- und Schleimhautreaktionen bei therapeutischer Teilkörperbestrahlung in der Megavolttherapie. Strahlentherapie **125**, 536—547 (1964).

Kligerman, M. M., Richmond, J. D.: Volume dosage distribution in the female pelvis in radium therapy. (Räumliche Dosisverteilung im weiblichen Becken bei Radiumbehandlung.) Amer. J. Roentgenol. **70**, 750—758 (1953).

Klosterhalfen, H.: Zur Pathogenese und Therapie der nach Strahlenbehandlung des Genitalkarzinoms auftretenden Harnstauungsnieren. Z. Urol. **53**, 693—700 (1960).

Knoll, H., Bergmann, A.: Muß es das Kollum-Stumpf-Karzinom heute noch geben? Zbl. Gynäk. **88**, 905—909 (1966).

Koeck, G. P., Jacobson, L. E., Hillsinger, W. R.: Cobalt-60 teletherapy of cancer of the cervix by a rotation technic: preliminary report. Radiology **79**, 190—202 (1962).

— — — Results of cobalt 60 rotation therapy in carcinoma of the cervix. (Ergebnisse der Kobalt-60-Bewegungsbestrahlung beim Collumcarcinom.) Amer. J. Roentgenol. **96**, 81—91 (1966).

Köhler, K., Platzbecker, H.: Das gynäkologische Sarkom aus radiologischer Sicht. Strahlentherapie **134**, 181—186 (1967).

König, P. A.: Urologische Komplikationen beim Kollumkarzinom nach Radium- und Röntgenkonvergenzbestrahlung. Zbl. Gynäk. **84**, 1557 (1962).

Körbler, J., Frank, P., Stojanov, E.: Zur Behandlung des Uteruscarcinoms durch Nah- und Fernbestrahlung mit radioaktiven Isotopen. Arch. Geschwulstforsch. **20**, 199—209 (1963).

Koga, K., Yamada, M., Sugimori, H., Takiguchi, Y., Takayama, K., Koga, S., Watanabe, E.: The results of treatment in the cervical cancer for the past 5 years in our clinic. (Die Ergebnisse in der Behandlung des Cervix-Carcinoms in den letzten 5 Jahren an unserer Klinik.) Kyushu J. med. Sci. **15**, 183—187 (1964).

Kohn, H. I., Bailar III, J. C., Zippin, C.: Radiation therapy for cancer of the cervix: its late effect on the lifespan as a function of regional dose. (Strahlentherapie des Collum-Carcinoms: Spätwirkungen auf die Lebensdauer als Funktion der lokal verabreichten Dosis.) J. nat. Cancer Inst. **34**, 345—361 (1965).

Koizumi, Y.: Problems on theoretical distribution of the dose of x-ray in rotatory irradiation in the treatment of carcinoma of the cervix uteri. (Probleme der theoretischen Dosisverteilung der Röntgen-Rotationsbestrahlung bei der Behandlung des Cervixcarcinoms.) J. Jap. obstet. gynaec. Soc. (Engl. ed.) **2**, 371—395 (1955).

KOK, G.: Irradiation of carcinoma of the cervix uteri using a radium colpostat and pendulum therapy (Arc therapy). (Strahlenbehandlung des Cervixcarcinoms mit einem Radium-Kolpostaten und Bewegungsbestrahlung.) J. belge Radiol. **41**, 301—348 (1958).

KOK, P. C.: Zervixkarzinom und Schwangerschaft. (Cervixcarcinoom en graviditeit.) Ned. T. Verlosk. **64**, 45 (1964).

KOLLER, O.: A comparison between the results of irradiation therapy alone and individualized radiological and surgical treatment of cervical carcinoma stage I. (Ein Vergleich zwischen den Ergebnissen nach Strahlenbehandlung allein und individueller Kombination von Bestrahlung und Operation beim Collum-Carcinom Stadium I.) Acta obstet. gynec. scand. **43**, Suppl. 7, 68—74 (1965).

KOLSTAD, P.: The development of the vascular bed in tumors as seen in squamous cell carcinoma of the cervix uteri. Brit. J. Radiol. **38**, 216 (1965).

KOSAREVA, A. N.: Early complications in radiation therapy of cervix uteri cancer. (Frühe Komplikationen bei der Strahlentherapie des Collumcarcinoms des Uterus.) Vop. Oncol. **5**, 202—208 mit engl. Zus.fass. (1959) [Russisch].

KOSTROMINA, K. N.: Die Bedeutung der Verteilung des Dosisfeldes bei der Telegammatherapie des Kollumkarzinoms. Radiobiol. Radiother. (Berl.) **5**, 739—753 (1964).

KOTTMEIER, H. L.: Die Therapie des Collumcarcinoms. Oncologia (Basel) **5**, 243—259 (1952) u. Gynaecologia (Basel) **134**, Suppl. 2, 243—259 (1952).

— Carcinoma of the female genitalia. Baltimore: Williams & Wilkins Company 1953.

— Die Behandlungstechnik und Erfolge der Strahlentherapie des Collumcarcinoms am Radiumhemmet in Stockholm. Arch. Gynäk. **183**, 430—443 (1953).

— Modern trends in the treatment of cancer of the cervix. (Moderne Behandlungsmethoden des Cervixcarcinoms.) Acta radiol. (Stockh.), Suppl. **116**, 405—414 (1954).

— The place of radiation therapy and of surgery in the treatment of uterine cancer. (Die Stellung der Strahlentherapie und Chirurgie bei der Behandlung des Uteruscarcinoms.) J. Obstet. (Lond.), N. S. **62**, 737—773 (1955).

— Erfahrungen mit radioaktivem kolloidalem Gold (Au[198] bei Uteruscarcinom). Arch. Gynäk. **186**, 357—361 (1955).

— Die Stellung der Strahlentherapie und der Chirurgie in der Behandlung des Gebärmutterkrebses. Strahlentherapie **103**, 194—213 (1957); Zbl. ges. Radiol. **57**, 68 (1958).

— Current treatment of carcinoma of cervix. Amer. J. Obstet. Gynec. **76**, 243—251 (1958).

— Malignancy of cervix in puerperium. Clin. Obstet. Gynec. **6**, 975—982 (1963).

— Annual report on the results of treatment in carcinoma of the uterus and vagina, vol. XIII. Stockholm 1964.

KOTTMEIER, H. L.: Modern trends in the treatment of uterine carcinoma. Specially in carcinoma of the cervix uteri. (Moderne Richtungen in der Behandlung des Gebärmutterkrebses, insbesondere des Cervix-Carcinoms.) Arqu. Pat. (Lisboa) **36**, 47—64 (1964).

— Complications following radiation therapy in carcinoma of the cervix and their treatment. Amer. J. Obstet. Gynec. **88**, 854—866 (1964).

— Erfahrungen des Radiumhemmet in Stockholm mit Hochvolttherapie beim Collumcarcinom. Arch. Gynäk. **202**, 305—309 (1965).

— GORTON, G., CHRISTENSEN, A., LANGE, P., NIELSEN, E.: Surgical and radiation treatment of invasive carcinoma of the uterine cervix. (Chirurgische und Strahlenbehandlung des invasiven Carcinoma colli uteri.) Acta obstet. gynec. scand. **43**, Suppl. 2.

— GRAY, M. J.: Rectal and bladder injuries in relation to radiation dosage in carcinoma of the cervix. Amer. J. Obstet. Gynec. **82**, 74—82 (1961).

— MOBERGER, G.: Experience with radioactive colloidal gold as an additional treatment in the radiotherapy of uterine cancer. (Erfahrungen mit radioaktivem Gold als zusätzliche Behandlung bei der Strahlentherapie des Gebärmutterkrebses.) Acta obstet. scand. (Stockh.) **34**, 1—29 (1955).

— VARA, P.: Tumörer i uterus, vagina och vulva. In: Tumör sjukdomar, S. 420—433. Uppsala: Almquist & Wiksell 1963.

— WALSTAM, R.: Intracavitary irradiation in treatment of carcinoma of cervix with paravaginal extension. (Intrakavitäre Bestrahlung bei der Behandlung des Cervixcarcinoms mit paravaginaler Ausbreitung.) Acta radiol. (Stockh.), N. S., Diagn., Ther. Phys. Biol. **3**, 161—168 (1965).

KRANEPUHL, F.: Röntgenschäden nach gynäkologischer Strahlenbehandlung in chirurgischer Sicht. Zbl. Chir. **84**, 104—113 (1959).

KRATOCHWILL, A.: Karzinomatöse oder entzündliche Infiltration der Parametrien? Geburtsh. u. Frauenheilk. **22**, 737—742 (1962).

— SCHÜLER, E.: Objektiver Nachweis von Beckenwandrezidiven nach Kollumkarzinom. Geburtsh. u. Frauenheilk. **22**, 1413—1421 (1962).

KRAUSE, H.: Die Anwendung radioaktiver Stoffe in der Gynäkologie — Indikation und Therapie. Geburtsh. u. Frauenheilk. **21**, 519—520 (1961).

KRAUSSOLD, E.: Lebensalter und Heilungsergebnisse bei 2907 Kollumkarzinomen in der Universitäts-Frauenklinik Berlin in den Jahren 1938 bis 1948. Dtsch. Gesundh.-Wes. **1957**, 36—41.

KREBS, C., BLIXENKRONE-MØLLER, N.: Ovarian function after combined surgical and radiologic treatment of early cervical cancer. (Die Funktion der Ovarien nach einer kombinierten operativen und strahlentherapeutischen Behandlung früher Portiocarcinome.) Acta radiol. (Stockh.) **49**, 128—136 (1958).

KRITTER, H., ARVAY, N., PICARD, J.-D., MANLOT, G.: La lymphographie dans le cancer du col utérin. Ann. Radiol. **5**, 55 (1962).

KUEMMERLE, H.-P., SEYBOLDT, R.: Strahlenfrühreaktionen und Dysbakterieproblem bei der Strahlentherapie des weiblichen Genitalkarzinoms. Eine klinisch-experimentelle Studie zu den Problemen ihrer Prophylaxe und Therapie. Strahlentherapie **115**, 72—89 (1961).

Kundrat, R.: Über die Ausbreitung des Carcinoms im parametranen Gewebe bei Krebs des Collum uteri. Arch. Gynäk. **69**, 355—409 (1903).

Kuttig, H.: Die Telegammatherapie im Rahmen der konventionellen und der Betatronbestrahlung. Röntgen-Bl. **12**, 1—8 (1959).

— Kritische Betrachtungen zur Telekobalttherapie des Kollumkarzinoms. Radiologia Jugoslavia **1**, 49—55 (1965).

— Bedeutung und Möglichkeiten der Megavolttherapie bei gynäkologischen Tumoren. Berl. Med. **16**, 869—874 (1965).

— Supervolttherapie in der Gynäkologie. Arch. Gynäk. **202**, 309—312 (1965).

— Becker, J.: Zur Telekobalttherapie gynäkologischer Karzinome. Vortrag IX. Internat. Congr. Radiol. 1959.

— Frischbier, H.-J.: Zur Herddosisbestimmung und Dosisverteilung bei der Telekobalt-Pendelbestrahlung. Strahlentherapie **112**, 251—261 (1960).

— Piní, M.: Il trattamento del cancro del collo dell'utero secondo la scuola di Heidelberg. Radiazioni di alta energia **5**, 99—107 (1966).

Laborde, S.: Rapport sue le traitement du cancer du col utérin au stade I. (Über die Behandlung des Collumcarcinoms Stad. I.) J. de Radiol. **33**, 109—114 (1952).

— El tratamiento del cancer del cuello del utero en el estadio I. (Die Behandlung des Cervixkrebses im Stadium I.) Gac. méd. esp. **26**, 251—257 (1952).

— Redon, H.: Le traitement du cancer du col utérin au stade I. (Die Behandlung des Uterus-Collumcarcinoms Gruppe I.) J. de Radiol. **35**, 44—47 (1954).

— — Le traitement des cancers du col utérin au stade I. (Die Behandlung der Collumcarcinome Gr. I.) Presse méd. **1954**, 397—398.

Lagrutta, J., Grassi, G., Raimondo, J.: Aspetti della linfangiografia inguino-pelvica associata alla flebografia transpubica nella cancerologia ginecologica. (Die Beckenlymphangiographie kombiniert mit der transpubischen Phlebographie beim gynäkologischen Carcinom.) Acta chir. ital. **19** 977—997 (1963).

Lalanne, C. M., Ascarelli, A. A., Fajbisowicz, S.: La telecobaltoterapia all'istituto Gustave Roussy. V. Tumori del collo dell'utero. (Die Kobalttherapie im Institut Gustave Roussy. V. Geschwülste des Gebärmutterhalses.) Nunt. radiol. (Firenze) **30**, 426—443 (1964).

— Fajbisowicz, S.: Complications post-radiothérapiques dans le cancer du col utérin. Ann. Radiol. **8**, 697—708 (1965).

Lamarque, J. F. P.: Essai critique sur les indications de la télécobaltthérapie. (Kritische Betrachtungen über die Indikationen der Telekobalttherapie.) 9. int. Congr. Radiol. **2**, 811—817 (1961).

Lamarque, P.: La endorroentgenterapia o roentgenterapia endocavitaria. (Die Endoröntgentherapie oder endokavitäre Röntgentherapie.) Acta ibér. radiol.-cancer. **4**, 79—96 (1955).

Landrgot, B., Sauer, J.: Schenkelhalsfrakturen als Folge therapeutischer Bestrahlung bei gynäkologischen Geschwülsten (Vorbeugungsmaßnahmen). Zbl. Gynäk. **87**, 835—841 (1965).

Lane, F. W.: A technic of experimental disometry for intracavitary radium applicators. Radiology **82**, 827—830 (1964).

Langreder, W.: Gynäkologische Urologie. Stuttgart: Thieme 1961.

Laughlin, J. S.: Physical aspects of betatron therapy. Springfield, Ill.: Ch. C. Thomas Publ. 1954.

Lauterwein, C.: Die Morphologie des Kollumkarzinoms und ihre Bedeutung für die Prognose und Therapie. Geburtsh. Gynäk. **128**, 17—106 (1947).

Lax, H.: Die Prognose der Kollumkarzinome auf Grund histologischer Beurteilung. Zbl. Gynäk. **72**, 284—293 (1950).

Leb, A.: Eine „erweiterte Lokalbehandlung" des Gebärmutterhalskarzinoms durch die präoperative Strahlentherapie. Strahlentherapie **109**, 374—385 (1959).

Lederman, M.: The treatment of carcinoma of the cervix. (Die Behandlung des Krebses des Gebärmutterhalses.) Čs. Gynek. **21/35**, 164—167 (1956) [Tschechisch].

Leenhardt, P., Pourquier, H.: La place de la télécobalthérapie dans le traitement du cancer du col utérin. Analyse des possibilités techniques. (Die Stellung der Telekobalttherapie in der Behandlung des Collum-Carcinoms. Untersuchungen der technischen Möglichkeiten.) J. de Radiol. **38**, 924—932 (1957).

Leeuw, J. H. A. de: Zervixkarzinom bei Zwillingsschwangerschaft. (Cervixcarcinoom en tweelingszwangerschap.) Ned. T. Verlosk. **64**, 35 (1964).

Legerlotz, C., Muth, H.: Über die Prognose strahlenbehandelter Kollum-Karzinome nach Prednisolon-Therapie. Geburtsh. u. Frauenheilk. **26**, 1034—1039 (1966).

Lehmacher, K.: Gefahren der Radiumbehandlung des Uteruskarzinoms. Medizinische **1954**, 844—849.

Lehoczky, G., Bartsch, A., Tottossy, B.: Our experiences obtained in connection with the preoperative radiation of collum carcinoma. (Unsere Erfahrungen mit der präoperativen Bestrahlung des Collumcarcinoms.) Acta Un. int. Cancr. (Louvain) **20**, 1751—1752 (1964).

— Vikol, J.: Zwölfjährige Erfahrungen mit der präoperativen Strahlenbehandlung des Kollumkarzinoms. Radiobiol. Radiother. (Berl.) **7**, 517—520 (1966).

Lemke, J.: Ein neuartiger Führungsstab für gynäkologische Radium-Applikatoren. Strahlentherapie **123**, 418—419 (1964).

Lemtis, H., Frischkorn, R.: Vaginalmeßstab als Einstellhilfe in der gynäkologischen Strahlentherapie. Strahlentherapie **120**, 449—455 (1963).

Lenzi, E.: Sull'utilizzazione della via endolinfatica per la diagnosi, la terapia e la prognosi delle neoplasie genitali femminili (con ulteriori osservazioni di linfografia pelvica). Scritt in onore del Prof. Giuseppe Tesauro nel XXV anno del suo insegnamento. Napoli: Montanino editore 1964.

— L'importanza dei fattori tecnici e dosimetrici nelle complicanze della radiumterapia ginecologica. (Die Bedeutung von technischen und dosimetrischen

Problemen mit Bezug auf die Komplikationen der gynäkologischen Radiumtherapie.) Minerva ginec. 14, 43—47 (1962).

LENZI, M., BASSANI, S.: The effect of radiation on the lymph and on the lymph vessels. (Der Effekt der Bestrahlung auf die Lymphe und die Lymphgefäße.) Radiology 80, 814—817 (1963).

— BERGONZINI, R., DE MARIA, D., FEROLLA, G.: Cancer du col de l'utérus: télécobalthérapie préopératoire. Recherches préliminaires. (Carcinoma colli uteri: präoperative Telekobalttherapie. [Vorl. Untersuchungen.]) Ann. Radiol. (Paris) 8, 709—710 (1965).

LEONE, U., GIAMMARIA, G.: Osservazioni sui rapporti tra terapia attinica del carcinoma del collo uterino e complicazioni urologiche. (Beobachtungen über die Beziehungen zwischen der Strahlenbehandlung des Collumcarcinoms und urologischen Komplikationen.) Clin. ostet. ginec. 66, 254—265 (1964).

LEVEN, H.: Die Strahlensensibilität der Lymphknotenmetastasen beim Carcinoma colli uteri. Inaug.-Diss. Hamburg 1967.

LEVEUF, J.: Bull. Soc. Chir. Paris 57, 622 (1931); Zit. nach MEIGS, J. V., LIU, W.: Radical hysterectomy and pelvic lymphadenectomy. Amer. J. Obstet. Gynec. 69, 1—32 (1955).

— GODARD, H.: L'exerese chirurgicale des ganglions pelviens complement de la curie thérapie des cancers du col de l'uterus. J. Chir. (Paris) 43, 177—187 (1934).

LEVITT, S. H., RUBIN, P.: Early invasive carcinoma of the cervix. A problem of definition and treatment. (Das frühe invasive Carcinom der Cervix.) Radiology 85, 711—715 (1965).

LEWIS, G. C., JR., CHAMBERLAIN, R. H., HALE, J., PAYNE, F. L.: Radiation distribution in the treatment of cervical carcinoma. (Strahlendosisverteilung bei der Behandlung des Collumcarcinoms.) Obstet. and Gynec. 1, 378—386 (1953).

— — — — Study of radiation dosimetry in treatment of cervical cancer. Amer. J. Roentgenol. 72, 975—984 (1954).

— PAYNE, F. L.: Symposium on obstetrics and gynecology; advances in control of radium therapy for cervical cancer. Surg. Clin. N. Amer. 34, 1671—1684 (1954).

— RAVENTOS, A., HALE, J.: Space dose relationship for points A and B in the radium therapy of cancer of the uterine cervix. Amer. J. Roentgenol. 83, 432—446 (1960).

LIEBNER, E. J.: An appraisal of radioactive therapeutic lymphography. (Eine Beurteilung der therapeutischen radioaktiven Lymphographie.) Amer. J. Roentgenol. 93, 110—121 (1965).

LIEGNER, L. M.: Radon and radioactive seed volume implants for extensive recurrent vaginal-pelvic cancer. (Über die Implantation von Radon und radioaktiven Körnern bei ausgedehnten rezidivierenden Carcinomen im Bereich der Vagina.) Radiology 82, 786—793 (1964).

— BERRY, W., OAKMAN, C.: Preoperative irradiation of carcinoma of the cervix. Combined radiation-surgical treatment. (Präoperative Bestrahlung des Collum-Carcinoms. Kombinierte Strahlungen und Operationstherapie.) Radiology 74, 92—93 (1960).

LIEGNER, L. M., OLSON, M., NICKSON, J. J.: Postoperative irradiation of 86 cases of carcinoma of the cervix. (Postoperative Bestrahlung von 86 Fällen von Cervix-Carcinom.) Surg. Gynec. Obstet. 108, 313—320 (1959).

LIMBURG, H., NAPP, J.-H., WILBRAND, U.: Die prognostische Beurteilung des Kollumkarzinoms nach Strahlenbehandlung durch Probeentnahme und Scheidenabstrich. Geburtsh. u. Frauenheilk. 12, 723—734 (1952).

— THOMSEN, K.: Das Adenocarcinom des Collum uteri. Stuttgart: Thieme 1949.

LINTNER, L., BENES, J.: Versuch einer standardisierten Methode zur vollständigen Bestrahlung des kleinen Beckens mit verschiedenen Strahlenqualitäten. Strahlentherapie 115, 143—147 (1961).

LIPIN, TH., DAVIDSON, CH.: Metastases of uterine carcinoma to the central nervous systems. A clinico pathologic study. Arch. Neurol. Psychiat. (Chic.) 57, 186—198 (1947).

LITWIN, S. B., FRALEY, E. E., CLOUSE, M. E., ULFELDER, H.: Lymphography in patients with pelvic cancer. (Die Lymphographie bei Patienten mit Beckentumoren.) Obstet. and Gynec. 24, 809—816 (1964).

LIU, W., MEIGS, J. V.: Radical hysterectomy and pelvic lymphadenectomy. A review of 473 cases including 244 for primary invasive carcinoma of the cervix. Amer. J. Obstet. Gynec. 69, 1—32 (1955).

LÖHR, H., HUBER, H.: Mammakarzinom und Genitalkarzinom als Multiplizitätstumoren. Strahlentherapie 115, 257—264 (1961).

LOEW, K.: Die vaginale Radikaloperation im Rahmen der Karzinomtherapie. Geburtsh. u. Frauenheilk. 26, 1012—1014 (1966).

LONDON, D. L., DUNN, L. J.: Radical hysterectomy and pelvic lymphadenectomy following pelvic irradiation. Amer. J. Obstet. Gynec. 93, 1128—1132 (1965).

LOVE, E. J., ALLEN, H. H.: Management of recurrent carcinoma of the cervix. Amer. J. Obstet. Gynec. 77, 539—545 (1959).

LUBE, J.: Die Behandlungsergebnisse der Kollumkarzinome an der Universitäts-Frauenklinik Greifswald von 1940—1950. Zbl. Gynäk. 82, 1740—1749 (1960).

LUCCI, J. A.: Carcinoma of cervix and pregnancy: An analysis of 111 cases of carcinoma of uterine cervix, endometrium and ovary. Chicago: Year Book Medical Publishers, Inc. 1962.

LUCISANO, F., ALEMANNO, L., PICCIONI, V.: Considerazioni su 70 autopsie di pazienti decedute per cancro del collo dell'utero. Scritti ostet. ginec. 13, 251—269 (1960); Ref. Ber. ges. Gynäk. Geburtsh. 76, 37 (1961).

LUKYANOV, V. P.: Tables for estimating the integral absorbed dose during combined radium therapy of malignant neoplasms of the uterine cervix. (Tabellen zur Errechnung der absorbierten integralen Dosis beim Prozeß kombinierter Strahlentherapie der malignen Cervix uteri-Neubildungen.) Med. Radiol. (Mosk.) 7, Nr 12, 13—16 mit engl. Zus.fass. (1962) [Russisch].

Macarini, N., Besio, G. L., Gandolfo, E.: L'associazione radiumterapia-telecobalto-terapia nel trattamento dei tumori dell'utero. (Kombination von Radium- und Telekobalttherapie in der Behandlung der Gebärmuttergeschwülste.) Minerva med. **52**, 2739—2742 (1961).

Mack, H. P., Diehl, W. K., Peck, G. C., Figge, F. H. J.: Evaluation of the combined effects of hematoporphyrin and radiation. I. Treatment of carcinoma of the cervix. (Auswertung über kombinierte Anwendung von Hämatoporphyrin und Radium-Röntgen-Strahlen. I. Collum-Carcinom.) Cancer (Philad.) **10**, 529—539 (1957).

Magara, M.: The technique of the operation of the cancer of cervix, especially systematic and complete removal of pelvic lymphnodes. III. Weltkongr. d. Intern. Feder. f. Gebh. und Gyn., Wien, September 1961.

Magendie, J., Wangermez, Ch.: Curiethérapie préopératoire dans les néoplasmes du col et du corps utérus avec un nouveau colpostat. (Präoperative Radiumtherapie bei Neoplasmen des Collum und Corpus uteri mit einem neuen Kolpostaten.) Presse méd. **68**, 1452 (1960).

Magno, L.: I problemi della irradiazione transcutanea delle neoplasie della pelvi in soggetti obesi. (Probleme der transcutanen Bestrahlung von Beckentumoren bei fettleibigen Patienten.) Tumori **52**, 319—334 (1966).

Maier, E.: Die Strahlenbehandlung des Gebärmutterhalskrebses. Wien. klin. Wschr. **1953**, 412—416.

Maino, C. R., Mussey, R. D.: Carcinoma of cervix coincident with pregnancy. Amer. J. Obstet. Gynec. **47**, 229—244 (1944).

Makowski, E. L., McKelvey, J. L., Flight, G. W., Stenstrom, K. W., Mosser, D. G.: The results of irradiation therapy of carcinoma of the cervix. (Resultate der Strahlenbehandlung des Cervixcarcinoms.) J. Amer. med. Ass. **182**, 637—642 (1962).

Maliphant, R. G.: The results of radium treatment of cancer of the uterine cervix with special reference to glandular and stump cancers. (Die Ergebnisse der Radiumbehandlung des Collumcarcinoms unter besonderer Berücksichtigung der Adenocarcinome und der Stumpfcarcinome.) J. Obstet. (Lond.), N.S., **62**, 367—371 (1955).

Marques, P., Bru, A., Faillières, J., Perret, P., Commanay, L.: Nouvelle technique d'irradiation des tumeurs du pelvis par voie périnéale. (Neue Technik der Bestrahlung von Tumoren des Beckens auf perinealem Wege.) J. belge Radiol. **44**, 519—535 (1961).

— Faillières, J., Sancerni, M.-M.: Les métastases osseuses du cancer du col utérin. J. Radiol. Électrol. **47**, 309—320 (1966).

Martin, Ch. I.: Approximation technique in treatment of cancer of the cervix with irradiation. („Anpassungstechnik" bei der Strahlenbehandlung des Cervixcarcinoms.) Amer. J. Roentgenol. **77**, 388—396 (1957).

Martins, A. F.: Aspekte der Radiumbehandlung des Cervixkrebses. Rev. paul. Med. **40**, 184—198 mit engl. Zus.fass. (1952) [Portugiesisch].

Martius, H.: The radiation treatment of cancer of the uterine cervix. (Die Strahlenbehandlung des Cervixcarcinoms.) Amer. J. Obstet. **68**, 484—488 (1954).

Martius, H.: Chirurgische und Strahlenbehandlung der Genitaltumoren. Congr. internat. de Gynécol. et d'Ostétr. Genève **1954**, 601—607.

Martzloff, K. H.: Carcinoma of the cervix uteri: a pathological and clinical study with particular reference to the relative malignancy of the neoplastic process as indicated by the predominant type of cancer. Bull. Johns Hopk. Hosp. **24**, 141—184 (1923).

Masereeuw, J.: Ureteral stenosis following radiotherapy for cervical cancer. (Ureter-Stenose als Folge der Radiotherapie bei Collum-Carcinom.) Ned. T. Geneesk. **110**, 920—923 mit engl. Zus.fass. (1966) [Holländisch].

Massazza, M.: La telecobaltoterapia dei tumori dell'apparato genitale femminile: contributi clinici ed anatomo-patologici. (Die Telekobalt-Therapie der Tumoren der weiblichen Genitalorgane; klinischer und anatomisch-pathologischer Beitrag.) Ann. Ostet. Ginec. **79**, 933—951 (1957).

Massenbach, W. v.: Obduktionsbefunde an den Lymphknoten beim Carcinoma colli. Strahlentherapie, Sonderbd. **37**, 192—194 (1957).

Mathieu, R.: On the use of bi-axial rotation therapy with cobalt^{60}, physical basis and application in the treatment of carcinoma of the cervix. (Über die doppelseitige Pendelbestrahlung mit ^{60}Co. [Physikalische Grundlagen und Behandlung des Cervixcarcinoms.]) J. Canad. Ass. Radiol. **10**, 47—50 (1959).

Matschke, S., Welker, K.: Die individuelle Isodosenanpassung bei der biaxialen Pendelbestrahlung gynäkologischer Tumoren. Radiobiol. Radiother. (Berl.) **4**, 401—409 (1963).

Maurer, H.-J.: Zur Bewegungsbestrahlung gynäkologischer Tumoren im kleinen Becken. Geburtsh. u. Frauenheilk. **15**, 1006—1012 (1955).

— Praktische Fragen zur Bewegungsbestrahlung der Parametrien. Radiol. clin. (Basel) **24**, 230—239 (1955).

— Die Bewegungsbestrahlung gynäkologischer Tumoren im kleinen Becken. I. Mitt. (36. Tagg Dtsch. Röntgenges. Wiesbaden, 5.—8. IX. 1954). Strahlentherapie **97**, 133—138 (1955).

Maurizio, E., Pescetto, G.: La nostra esperienza in tema di telecobaltoterapia del cancro dell'utero. (Unsere Erfahrungen mit der Telekobalttherapie des Uteruscarcinoms.) Ann. Ostet. Ginec. **79**, 1069—1076 (1957).

Mayer, A.: Kollumkarzinom, Fortpflanzungsvorgänge und Vorbestrahlung. Strahlentherapie **92**, 325—337 (1953).

McGee, J. E., Sala, J. M.: Carcinoma of cervix and pregnancy. J. Iowa St. med. Soc. **50**, 717—721 (1960).

McLennan, C. E., Bagshaw, M. A., McLennan, M.T.: Three sequential experiments in radiation treatment of cervical cancer. (Drei aufeinanderfolgende Versuche der Strahlenbehandlung der Cervix-Carcinome.) Amer. J. Obstet. Gynec. **84**, 1222—1232 (1962).

— McLennan, M. T., Bagshaw, M. A.: The linear accelerator in the treatment of cervical cancer. Amer. J. Obstet. Gynec. **98**, 675—680 (1967).

MEDINA, J., SALVATORE, C. A.: Häufigkeit der Metastasen des Portiokarzinoms I. und II. Grades. An. bras. Ginec. 47, 305—318 (1959) [Portugiesisch]; Ref. Ber. ges. Gynäk. Geburtsh. 69, 307 (1959—1960).

MEIGS, J. V.: Radical hysterectomy with bilateral pelvic lymph node dissections. A report of 100 patients operated on five or more years ago. Amer. J. Obstet. Gynec. 62, 854—870 (1951).

— Surgical treatment of cancer of the cervix. New York: Grune & Stratton 1954.

— Cancer of the cervix, an appraisal. (Krebs der Cervix, ein Rechenschaftsbericht.) Amer. J. Obstet. 72, 467—478 (1956).

— Carcinoma of the cervix—a discussion. (Cervix-Carcinom — eine Diskussion.) Ann. Surg. 143, 744—751 (1956).

— Radical hysterectomy with bilateral lymph-node dissection. Clin. ostet. ginec. 1, 1029—1049 (1958).

— BRUNSCHWIG, A.: A proposed classification for cases of cancer of the cervix treated by surgery. Amer. J. Obstet. Gynec. 64, 413—415 (1952).

— PARSON, L., NATHANSON, I. T.: Retroperitoneal lymph node dissection in cancer of the cervix. Amer. J. Obstet. Gynec. 57, 1087—1097 (1949).

MEINRENKEN, H.: Wandlungen in der operativen Behandlung des Zervixkrebses. Geburtsh. u. Frauenheilk. 26, 191—202 (1966).

MELLGREN, J., KNUTSSON, F., NORIN, T.: Localization and effect of injected radioactive gold (Au^{198}) in the treatment of malignant tumors. Acta path. microbiol. scand. 34, 393—409 (1954).

MEREDITH, W. J.: Dosage distribution and dosage in carcinoma of uterine cervix. Radiology 54, 386—391 (1950).

— Personal communication, March 26, 1957.

MESCHAN, I., EDWARDS, R. R., ROSENBAUM, P. J.: Practical physical aspects in the use of radioactive cobalt 60 as a radium substitute. Amer. J. Roentgenol. 65, 255—264 (1951).

— ODDIE, T. H., REGNIER, G., YOUNG, C. C., JACKSON, C. C.: A method of dosimetry for carcinoma of the cervix utilizing a modified Manchester technic with cobalt 60. (Eine Methode der Dosisbestimmung für die Verwendung einer modifizierten Manchester-Methode mit Kobalt^{60} zur Behandlung des Collumcarcinoms.) Radiology 64, 546—559 (1955).

DU MESNIL DE ROCHEMONT, R.: Lehrbuch der Strahlenheilkunde. Stuttgart: Enke 1958.

— Die Marburger Methode der Bestrahlung des Collumcarcinoms und ihre ersten Fünfjahresergebnisse am Krankengut der Univ.-Frauen- und Strahlenklinik Marburg. Dtsch. med. J. 9, 25—26 (1958).

— Zur Strahlentherapie der Kollumkarzinome. Radiol. austriaca 10, 99—106 (1958).

— BRANDS, K. H., BUSCH, G.: Die Genauigkeit der Herddosisbestimmung bei der Röntgenbestrahlung des Kollum-Karzinoms nach der Marburger Methode. Strahlentherapie 93, 563—566 (1954).

MESSERSCHMIDT, O., MELCHING, H.-J., DINKLOH, H.: Zur Frage der radiologisch-chirurgischen Kombinationsschäden. Med. Klin. 22, 877—882 (1965).

METZGER, M., VALLÉE, G., MICHEL, J. R.: Radiothérapie du cancer du col utérin. (Strahlenbehandlung des Collum-Carcinoms.) France méd. 22, 271—282 (1959).

MIKULICZ-RADECKI, F. v.: Über die Verbesserung der Heilungsresultate beim Carcinoma colli uteri im Laufe der letzten 43 Jahre. Strahlentherapie 111, 1—7 (1960).

— Klinische Erfahrungen bei der Behandlung gynäkologischer Karzinome. Ther. Gegenw. 100, 32—39 (1961).

— Treatment of carcinoma of the uterine cervix. A review of results during forty-five years of progress. (Behandlung des Collumcarcinoms. Erfolgsbericht über die in den letzten 45 Jahren erzielten Fortschritte.) J. int. Coll. Surg. 37, 467—417 (1962).

MILATZ, W.: Die Radiumpunktur und die Moulagentechnik. Strahlentherapie 117, 481—508 (1962).

MILLS, D. C.: Endometrial cancer in patients previously irradiated for cervical cancer. (Das Vorkommen eines Adenocarcinoms des Endometriums bei Patienten nach Bestrahlung wegen Cervixcarcinom.) Obstet. and Gynec. 22, 280—285 (1963).

MITANI, Y., TAKAGI, S., MATSUYAMA, F., YAMAGUCHI, S., YAMURA, M. M., SHIIKI, K., KOYAMA, Y., YAKINARI, S., MATSUMOTO, T., YAMANOUCHI, S.: Studies on histological grading of malignancy of carcinoma of the uterine cervix. Jap. J. Obstet. Gynec. Soc. 3, 277—288 (1956).

— — YAMAGUCHI, S., FUJITA, N., MIYAMURA, M., SHIIKI, K., KOYAMA, Y., TANAKA, M., YAKINARI, S., YAMANOUCHI, S., UEDA, S.: Development of cervical cancer in surgical cases. (Surgical pathology of cervical cancer.) Jap. J. obstet. Gynec. Soc. 3, 324—341 (1956).

MITRA, S.: Symposium on cancer of the cervix uteri. Radiation therapy in cancer of the cervix. (Symposion über das Cervixcarcinom. Die Strahlenbehandlung des Cervixcarcinoms.) Indian J. Radiol. 6, 113—119 (1952).

— BLOMFIELD, G. W.: Discussion on some aspects of surgical and radiological treatment of carcinoma of cervix. Proc. roy. Soc. Med. 40, 907—922 (1947).

MÖBIUS, W.: Die Röntgenintensivbestrahlung in der Gynäkologie. Strahlentherapie 93, 73—83 (1954).

— Die Strahlenbehandlung des Collumcarcinoms. Arch. Geschwulstforsch. 15, 54—69 (1959).

— Komplikationen der Strahlentherapie des Uteruskarzinoms. Radiobiol. Radiother. (Berl.) 2, 215—223 (1961).

— CAROL, W., GALLWAS, K.: Experimentelle Untersuchungen zur Frage der optimalen Fraktionierung bei der Röntgentherapie des Genitalcarcinoms. Arch. Geschwulstforsch. 23, 261—273 (1964).

MÖNCH, L., HOLTORFF, J.: Über die Bedeutung urologischer Spätschäden bei der Behandlung des Uteruskarzinoms. Geburtsh. u. Frauenheilk. 24, 864—881 (1964).

MOHR, H.-J., MORGENROTH, K., Jr., SCHNEPPER, E.: Das morphologische und submikroskopische Verhalten der Meerschweinchenniere bei gezielter einzeitiger und fraktionierter Röntgenbestrahlung. Strahlentherapie 129, 571—585 (1966).

Molnar, G., Berta, J., Szatai, J.: Die nach Behandlung des Uteruskarzinom beobachteten urologischen Spätschäden. Zbl. Gynäk. 88, 333—339 (1966).

Moonen, W. A.: Late ureteral stricture following treatment of cervical cancer. (Spätstriktur des Ureters nach der Behandlung von Cervixcarcinom.) Ned. T. Geneesk. 103, 2492—2495 mit engl. Zus.-fass. (1959) [Holländisch].

Moore, J. G., Chang, N. H., Scott, E., Morton, D. G.: The early assessment of irradiation therapy in cervical cancer. (Die frühzeitige Beurteilung der Strahlentherapie beim Cervixcarcinom.) Amer. J. Obstet. Gynec. 86, 677—692 (1962).

Morczek, A., Neumeister, K.: Die Nebenreaktionen unter der Bestrahlung und ihre Behandlung. Strahlentherapie 121, 349—364 (1963).

Morgan, J. E., Stein, J. J.: Intrapelvic dose distributions from a double crossarm radium applicator. (Dosisverteilung eines Doppelquerarm-Radiumapplikators im kleinen Becken.) Amer. J. Roentgenol. 93, 703—708 (1965).

Morris, J. McL., Chang, Ch. H., Page, V.: A radium technic for treatment of cancer of the cervix. Radiology 84, 849—858 (1965).

Morton, D. G.: Pelvic lymphadenectomy in the treatment of cervical cancer. Amer. J. Obstet. Gynec. 49, 19—31 (1945).

— Dignam, W.: The cause of death in patients treated for cervical cancer. Amer. J. Obstet. Gynec. 64, 999—1010 (1952).

— Kerner, J. A.: Reactions to x-ray and radium therapy in treatment of cancer of uterine cervix. Amer. J. Obstet. Gynec. 57, 625—636 (1949).

— Lagasse, L. D., Moore, J. G., Jacobs, M., Amromin, G. D.: Pelvic lymphnodectomy following radiation in cervical carcinoma. (Beckenlymphknotenentfernung nach Bestrahlung beim Cervixcarcinom.) Amer. J. Obstet. Gynec. 88, 932—943 (1964).

Morton, J. L., Barnes, A. C., Callendine, G. W,. Jr., Myers, W. G.: Individual interstitial irradiation of cancer of the uterine cervix using cobalt 60 in needles. Amer. J. Roentgenol. 65, 737 (1951).

— — Hendricks, Ch. H., Callendine, G. W., Jr.: Irradiation of cancer of the uterine cervix with radioactive cobalt 60 in guided aluminum needles and in plastic threads. (Bestrahlung des Collumcarcinoms mit radioaktivem Kobalt [Co60] in Aluminium-Nadeln und in plastischer Verabfolgung.) Amer. J. Roentgenol. 69, 813—825 (1953).

— Callendine, G. W., Jr., Myers, W. G.: Radioactive cobalt 60 in plastic tubing for interstitial radiation therapy. Radiology 56, 553—559 (1951).

Mossetti, C.: Valore degli esami cito-cariologico ed istologico per la indicazione alla terapia del cancro del collo dell'utero. (Der Wert von cyto-karyologischen und histologischen Untersuchungen für die Indikationsstellung zur Therapie des Collumkrebses des Uterus.) Ann. Radiol. diagn. (Bologna) 26, 384—405 (1953).

Müller, D.: Karzinomrezidiv oder Bestrahlungsfolge? Geburtsh. u. Frauenheilk. 17, 735—741 (1957).

Müller, J. H.: Über die Behandlungserfolge bei Carcinoma colli uteri an der Zürcher Frauenklinik. (Jahrgänge 1939—1946.) Oncologia (Basel) 5, 267—279 (1952); Gynaecologia (Basel) 134, Suppl. 2, 267—279 (1952).

— Über die Verwendungsmöglichkeiten des kolloidalen Radiogoldes für die Bekämpfung der Metastasierung der Uteruskarzinome auf dem Lymphweg. Gynaecologia (Basel) 145, 324—331 (1958).

— Wachsmann, F., Schuster, D.: Die Zürcher Bestrahlungsmethode des Kollumkarzinoms, unter besonderer Berücksichtigung der angewendeten zeitlichen Dosisverteilung. Strahlentherapie 125, 502—523 (1964).

Müller, P.: Zur Bewegungsbestrahlung gynäkologischer Tumoren im kleinen Becken. VI. Zur Anwendung der Konvergenzbestrahlung bei der Bestrahlung der Parametrien, unter besonderer Berücksichtigung der Dosisverteilung im kleinen Becken. Radiol. clin. (Basel) 27, 92—113 (1958).

Muggiati, L.: Linfangiografia inguino-pelvica nel carcinoma della portio. (Die Lymphangiographie im Leisten- und Beckenbereich beim Portiocarcinom.) Minerva cardioangiol. (Torino) 11, 309—313 (1963).

Munnell, E. W., Bonney, W. A., Jr.: Critical points of failure in the therapy of cancer of the cervix. A study of 250 recurrences. Amer. J. Obstet. Gynec. 81, 521—534 (1961).

Murphy, W. T., Schmitz, A.: The results of re-irradiation in cancer of the cervix. (Die Ergebnisse der Rezidiv-Bestrahlung des Collum-Carcinoms.) Radiology 67, 378—385 (1956).

Murrell, D. S.: The results of the Sheffield technique for treating carcinoma of the cervix uteri. (Ergebnisse der Behandlung des Collum-Carcinom mit der Sheffield-Technik.) Clin. Radiol. (Edinb.) 17, 264—273 (1966).

Muth, H.: Über die durch Strahlenbehandlung des Uteruskarzinoms hervorgerufenen Funktionsstörungen der ableitenden Harnwege. Geburtsh. u. Frauenheilk. 17, 983—995 (1957).

— Über Funktionsstörungen der ableitenden Harnwege nach Strahlenbehandlung und Radikaloperation des Kollumkarzinoms. Z. Geburtsh. Gynäk. 151, 267—329 (1958).

Nakamura, I.: Studies on the parametrium in carcinoma of the uterine cervix. I. Histology of the parametrium. Jap. J. Obstet. Gynec. Soc. 1, 23—33 (1954).

Natale, P.: Über die Technik der erweiterten Hysteradnexektomie mit systematischer Lymphadenektomie der lateralen Beckenlymphknotenketten. Attual. Obstet. Ginec. 1, 17—33 (1955); Ref. Ber. ges. Gynäk. Geburtsh. 60, 312 (1956–1957).

— Chiappa, S., Luciani, L.: Il valore della adenolinfografia in rapporto all'intervento di Wertheim allargata. (Symposium.) (Der Wert der Lymphadenographie bei der erweiterten Operationsmethode nach Wertheim.) Atti Soc. Ostet. Ginec. 12, 59—62 (1963).

Nathanson, B. N., Liegner, L. M., Rudolph, J. D., Hodara, M.: Dose verification studies in radium therapy of carcinoma of the cervix. Amer. J. Obstet. Gynec. 97, 808—816 (1967).

NAUJOKS, H.: Zystometrische Befunde während der Strahlentherapie des Kollumkarzinom. Zbl. Gynäk. 81, 573—578 (1959).

NAVRATIL, E.: Die Ergebnisse der Behandlung des Kollumkarzinoms aus dem Jahre 1951 an der Univ.-Frauenklinik Graz. Wien. med. Wschr. 107, 402—404 (1957).

— Beitrag zur Frage der örtlichen Wachstumsschnelligkeit des invasiven Plattenepithelkarzinoms der Portio. Wien. med. Wschr. 110, 494—495 (1960).

— Indications and results of the Schauta-Amreich operation with and without postoperative roentgen treatment in epidermoid carcinoma of the cervix of the uterus. (Indikationen und Ergebnisse der Schauta-Amreich-Operation mit und ohne Röntgenbestrahlung.) Amer. J. Obstet. Gynec. 86, 141—150 (1963).

— Können durch eine zusätzliche obligate Lymphfelderausräumung bei der operativen Behandlung des Gebärmutterhalskrebses des Stadium II die Ergebnisse gebessert werden? Scritti in onore del prof. Giuseppe Tesauro nel XXV anno del Suo insegnamento. Napoli: Montanino editore 1964.

— KASTNER, H.: Unsere Erfahrungen mit 977 Amreichschen Operationen bei der Behandlung des invasiven Zervixkarzinoms. Wien. med. Wschr. 116, 1012—1014 (1966).

NELSON, J. H., ROBERSON, J. O., MASTERSON, J. G.: Regeneration of pelvic lymph nodes after pelvic lymphadenectomy. Amer. J. Obstet. Gynec. 93, 102 (1965).

NEWTON, M.: Carcinoma of the cervix. Use of matched pairs of cases to compare treatment by surgery or radiation. (Collumcarcinom: Vergleich der operativen und der Strahlentherapie bei 15 Patientenpaaren.) Surg. Gynec. Obstet. 99, 29—33 (1954).

NICK, J., ADLER, U.: Spätrezidive und Spätmetastasen bei operativ und radiologisch behandelten Genitalkarzinomen der Frau. Gynaecologia (Basel) 147, 389—396 (1959).

NICOLOV, N.: Über die Strahlenbehandlung der Kollumkarzinome in der Zeit von 1931—1946. Strahlentherapie 91, 161—193 (1953).

NIELSEN, K.: Carcinoma of the cervix following supracervical hysterectomy. (Stumpfcarcinome [Carcinome der Cervix] nach supracervicaler Hysterektomie.) Acta radiol. (Stockh.) 37, 335—340 (1952).

NOGALES, F.: Histogenese der soliden Collumcarcinome des Uterus. Untersuchungen zur Anwendung einer rationelleren Therapie. Acta ginec. (Madr.) 12, 493—501 (1961); Ref. Ber. ges. Gynäk. Geburtsh. 78, 41 (1962).

— BOTELLA-LLUSIÁ, J.: The frequency of invasion of the lymph nodes in cancer of the uterine cervix. A study of the degree of extension in relation to the histological of type tumor. (Häufigkeit des Befalls der Lymphknoten beim Cervixcarcinom. Untersuchung über das Ausmaß der Ausbreitung in Abhängigkeit vom histologischen Typ des Tumors.) Amer. J. Obstet. Gynec. 93, 91—94 (1965).

NOGALES, F., ZAMARRIEGO-CRESPO, J., GIMÉNEZ-TÉBAR, V., BOTELLA-LLUSIÁ, J.: Die Lymphknotenmetastasen des Uteruscarcinoms. An. méd.-quir. Cruz Roja esp. 4, 213—220 (1962); Ref. Ber. ges. Gynäk. u. Geburtsh. 81, 290 (1963).

NOLAN, J. F.: Postoperative radiotherapy for carcinoma of the cervix. A study of 38 cases. (Die postoperative Strahlentherapie des Cervixcarcinoms. Ein Bericht über 38 Fälle.) Amer. J. Obstet. Gynec. 79, 892—898 (1960).

— Response of carcinoma in situ of the cervix to radiation therapy. (Reaktion des Carcinoma in situ der Cervix auf Strahlentherapie.) Amer. J. Obstet. Gynec. 79, 914—920 (1960).

— Late results of treatment of cervical carcinoma with Co^{60} teletherapy and intrauterine radium. (Letzte Ergebnisse der Behandlung von Cervixcarcinom mit ^{60}Co-Teletherapie und intrauterinem Radium.) Amer. J. Obstet. Gynec. 92, 684—693 (1965).

— EMMETT, J. W., ANSON, J. H.: Time-dose relationship in stage I carcinoma of the uterine cervix. (Die zeitliche Dosisverteilung und die Dosishöhe bei der Gruppe I des Cervixcarcinoms.) Amer. J. Roentgenol. 81, 111—114 (1959).

— JONES, E. G., NEIL, R. H.: Parametrial injection of colloidal gold (Au^{198}) in the monkey. Amer. J. Roentgenol. 69, 805—812 (1953).

— DU SAULT, L.: The elimination of untoward radiation sequelae in the treatment of carcinoma of the uterine cervix. (Die Ausschaltung unerwünschter Strahlenfolgen bei der Behandlung des Gebärmutterhalscarcinoms.) Surg. Gynec. Obstet. 94, 539—542 (1952).

— — Optimum dosage studies for radiation therapy of carcinoma of the uterine cervix. (Ermittlungen über eine optimale Dosierung bei der Strahlenbehandlung des Collumcarcinoms.) Radiology 62, 862—867 (1954).

— VIDAL, J. A., ANSON, J. H.: Early experiences in the treatment of carcinoma of the uterine cervix with $cobalt^{60}$ teletherapy and intracavitary radium. (Früherfahrungen in der Behandlung des Cervixcarcinoms mit Co^{60}-Teletherapie und intrakavitären Radiumeinlagen.) Amer. J. Obstet. 72, 789—803 (1956).

— — — Treatment of reccurent carcinoma of the uterine cervix with cobalt 60. (Behandlung rezidivierender Collumcarcinome mit Co^{60}.) West. J. Surg. 65, 358—369 (1957).

NOLAN, J. H., QUIMBY, E. H.: Dosage calculation for various combinations of parametrial needles and intracervical tandems. Radiology 40, 391—402 (1943).

NORIEGA, L. J., LÓPEZ, A.: Comparative study of supervoltage radiotherapy techniques in some pelvic malignancies. (Vergleichende Untersuchung von Supervolttherapie-Techniken bei einigen bösartigen Tumoren im Beckenbereich.) Amer. J. Roentgenol. 87, 488—499 (1962).

— RIOS SAN MARTIN, G., FALCÓ, J.: Intraousseous phlebography and lymphadenography in carcinoma of the cervix and other pelvic neoplasia. (Intraossäre Phlebographie und Lymphadenographie beim Cervixcarcinom und anderen Neoplasmen des Beckens.) Radiology 83, 219—227 (1964).

Novikovová, L. A.: The principles and methods of the treatment of patients with carcinoma of the cervix. (Grundsätze und Methoden der Behandlung der Kranken mit Gebärmutterhalskrebs.) Čs. Gynek. 21/35, 161—164 (1956) [Tschechisch].

Nowosad, K.: The control of the results of irradiation of cancer of uterine cervix with by means of smears. (Kontrolle der Strahlenbehandlungsergebnisse von Collumcarcinomen mit Hilfe von Abstrichen aus Vagina und Portio.) Ginek. pol. 23, 295—302 mit engl. Zus.fass. (1952) [Polnisch].

Nuytten, J., Giaux, G., Herbeau, J.: La curiethérapie vaginale axiale dans le cancer du col. (Die axiale vaginale Radiumtherapie bei Collumcarcinom.) Cancérologie 1, 3—8 (1953).

Ober, K. G., Huhn, F. O.: Die Ausbreitung des Cervixkrebses auf die Parametrien und die Lymphknoten der Beckenwand. Arch. Gynäk. 197, 262—290 (1962).

Oberheuser, F.: Nebenwirkungen der gynäkologischen Supervolttherapie. Geburtsh. u. Frauenheilk. 26, 803—806 (1966).

— Schmermund, H.-J.: Die Anwendung des Betatrons bei der Behandlung gynäkologischer Karzinome. Strahlentherapie 106, 127—129 (1958).

— Schubert, G.: Technik und Dosisverteilung bei der kombinierten Radium-Supervolttherapie gynäkologischer Karzinome nach der Hamburger Methode. Strahlentherapie, Sonderbd. 61, 158—162 (1965).

O'Brien, F. W., Jr., O'Brien, F. W.: Irradiation and surgery in the management of invasive carcinoma of the cervix. (Bestrahlung und Operation bei der Behandlung des invasiven Collumcarcinoms.) Radiology 67, 1—9 (1956).

O'Connor, K. J.: Mixed mesodermal tumours of the body of the uterus following irradiation therapy for carcinoma of the cervix. A report on four cases. (Gemischt mesodermale Tumoren des Corpus uteri nach Bestrahlung von Collum-Carcinomen. Bericht über 4 Fälle.) J. Obstet. Gynaec. Brit. Cwlth 71, 281—283 (1964).

Oddie, T. H., Meschan, I.: The physical aspects of the utilization of the tripartite rigid cobalt 60 applicator for the treatment of carcinoma of the cervix. (Die physikalischen Gesichtspunkte bei der Verwendung eines dreiteiligen starren Kobalt⁶⁰-Applikators zur Behandlung des Collumcarcinoms.) Radiology 64, 560—566 (1955).

Oehlert, G.: Über die Belastung von Blase und Darm bei der Bestrahlungsbehandlung von Gebärmutterhalscarcinomen. Med. Klin. 1958, 495—597.

— Buss, M.: Über die Veränderungen an Blase und Darm nach der Bestrahlungsbehandlung von Gebärmutterhalskarzinomen. Geburtsh. u. Frauenheilk. 15, 462—471 (1955).

Östberg, H., Darcis, L.: Study on sensitization response on 200 patients with carcinoma of the cervix treated at the Radiumhemmet by the current Stockholm technique. (Beobachtung der Sensibilisierungsreaktion bei 200 Patientinnen mit Collumcarcinom, die im Radiumhemmet nach der üblichen Stockholmer Technik behandelt wurden.) Acta obstet. gynec. scand. 35, 25—34 (1956).

Onnis, A., Bertolin, A.: I linfonodi pelvici nel carcinoma del collo uterino. Rilievi istopatologici sui linfonodi pelvici con particolare riguardo alla diffusione metastatica, a precedenti terapie radianti (radiumterapia-telecobaltoterapia-radioisotopoterpia endolinfatica) e ad accertamenti diagnostici (linfografia). (Die Beckenlymphknoten beim Collumcarcinom. Die Histopathologie der Beckenlymphknoten mit besonderer Berücksichtigung metastatischer Infiltrationen, vorangegangener Strahlentherapie und diagnostischer Maßnahmen.) Attual. Ostet. Ginec. 9, 729—760 (1963).

Oshita, M., Takeuchi, K., Endo, K.: The determination of radiosensitivity and recurrence of cancer of the cervix by serial biopsies following radium therapy. (Die Beurteilung der Strahlensensibilität und des Rezidivs beim Cervix-Carcinom durch Serien-Biopsien nach Radium-Therapie.) J. Jap. obstet. gynaec. Soc. (Engl. Ed.) 10, 248 (1964).

Ott, P., Rosteck, K., Wittenbeck, F.: Unsere Behandlung und Fünfjahresergebnisse bei den weiblichen Genitalkarzinomen. Strahlentherapie 106, 538—548 (1958).

— Wittenbeck, F.: Unsere Behandlung und 5-Jahres-Ergebnisse bei den weiblichen Genitalkarzinomen. II. Strahlentherapie 114, 14—18 (1961).

Ozsváth, J.: Über die Behandlung und Prognose des Gebärmutterstumpfkarzinoms. Zbl. Gynäk. 87, 296—301 (1965).

Paepe, J. de: Grossesse, quatre ans après curiethérapie d'un néoplasme cervical. (Schwangerschaft vier Jahre nach Radium-Behandlung eines Collumcarcinoms.) Bull. Soc. roy. belge Gynéc. Obstét., N. S., 26, 595—603 (1956).

Paeschke, K.-D.: Die Kombination der Strahlentherapie des Kollumkarzinoms mit ⁶⁰Kobalt-Radium-γ-Strahlung und dem Zytostatikum SP-I/SP-G. Strahlentherapie 127, 192—197 (1965).

Pahl, R.: Aus dem 9. Jahresbericht der Behandlungsergebnisse von 93541 Uteruskarzinomen aus dem Radiumhemmet Stockholm. (Zugleich Regeln und Voraussetzungen für eine international anerkannte Gültigkeit von Erfolgsstatistiken.) Strahlentherapie 99, 107—120 (1956).

— Die verkürzte Lebensdauer beim Kollumkarzinom in Kombination mit Ureter- oder Nierenstauung und deren Differentialdiagnose. Geburtsh. u. Frauenheilk. 18, 1445—1455 (1958).

Páli, K., Visegrády, L., Sik, J.: Die Phlebographie des kleinen Beckens als gynäkologische diagnostische Methode. Zbl. Gynäk. 85, 224—229 (1963).

Palmieri, G. G., Zaffagnini, E.: Fünfjährige Ergebnisse mit Schichtbestrahlung (Stratitherapie). I. Grundlagen der Methode, Gebärmutterhalskrebs. Strahlentherapie 110, 491—504 (1959).

Palumbo, L., Jr., Talbert, L. M., Brame, R. G., Bream, Ch. A., Dugger, G. S.: Palliation in gynecologic cancer. (Palliativmaßnahmen beim gynäkologischen Krebs.) Amer. J. Obstet. Gynec. 82, 761—776 (1961).

Parker, R. G., Friedman, R. F.: A critical evaluation of the roentgenologic examination of patients with carcinoma of the cervix. (Kritische Auswertung der Röntgenuntersuchung bei Patientinnen mit einem Collum-Carcinom.) Amer. J. Roentgenol. **96**, 100—107 (1966).

PATERSON, R.: Studies in optimum dosage. Brit. J. Radiol. **25**, 505—516 (1952).

— Radiotherapy in cancer of cervix: rising cure rates follow improvement in technique. Acta radiol. (Stockh.), Suppl. 116 (1954).

— PARKER, H. M.: Radium dosage, the Manchester system. Edinburgh: Livingstone Ltd. 1947.

— RUSSELL, M. H.: Clinical trials in malignant disease. VI. Cancer of the cervix uteri. Is X-ray therapy more effective given before or after radium? (Klinische Erfahrungen bei malignen Erkrankungen. VI. Carcinom des Collum uteri. Ist die Röntgenbestrahlung wirksamer, wenn man sie vor oder nach der Radiumbehandlung gibt?) Clin. Radiol. (Edinb.) **8**, 313—315 (1962).

— — Clinical trials in malignant disease. VII. Cancer of the cervix uteri. Evaluation of adjuvant X-ray therapy in stages 1 and 2. Interim report. (Klinische Beobachtungen bei malignen Erkrankungen. VII. Carcinom der Cervix uteri. Auswertung der zusätzlichen Röntgenstrahlentherapie beim Stadium I und II. Vorläufiger Bericht.) Clin. Radiol. (Edinb.) **14**, 17—19 (1963).

PAULLADA, J. J., RUBIO, L. B., MONTAÑO, G. R., PERCHES, R. D., CASTAÑEDA, E., MUNGUIA, H., DURAZO, F.: Combined hormonal and irradiation therapy in advanced cancer of the uterine cervix. (Kombinierte Hormon- und Strahlentherapie beim fortgeschrittenenCollumcarcinom.)Cancer(Philad.) **15**, 437—443 (1962).

PAUNIER, J. P., DELCLOS, L., FLETCHER, G. H.: Causes, time of death, and sites of failure in squamous-cell carcinoma of the uterine cervix on intact uterus. Radiology 88, 555—562 (1967).

PAVLENKO, S. I., KRASTINA, E. M.: Besonderheiten des klinischen Verlaufs des Gebärmutterhalskrebses bei der Behandlung mit radioaktivem Gold (Au[198]). Radiobiol. Radiother. (Berl.) **3**, 345—350 (1962).

— — Complex treatment of cancer of the uterine cervix with the use of radioactive gold. (Kombinationsbehandlung des Cervix-Carcinoms mit Verwendung von radioaktivem Gold.) Acta Un. int. Cancr. **20**, 1774—1775 (1964).

PEAKE, J. D.: Carcinoma of the cervix complicated by pregnancy. (Collum-Carcinom bei Schwangerschaft.) Sth. med. J. **53**, 34—39 (1960).

PEREZ-MESA, C., SPJUT, H. J.: Persistent postirradiation carcinoma of cervix uteri. A pathologic study of 83 pelvic exenteration specimens. Arch. Path. (Chic.) **75**, 462—474 (1963); Ref. Ber. ges. Gynäk. Geburtsh. **83**, 235 (1963).

PEREZ-TAMAYO, R., THORNBURY, J. R., ATKINSON, R. J.: "Second-look" lymphography. Amer. J. Roentgenol. **90**, 1078 (1963).

PERUSSIA, F.: Metodi moderni di radioterapia nel trattamento delle diffusioni pelviche del cancro dell'utero. (Moderne strahlentherapeutische Methoden zur Behandlung der Diffusion des Gebärmutterkrebses im Becken.) Radiol. med. (Torino) **43**, 1101—1109 (1957).

PESCETTO, G.: La ipovitaminosi c nella attinoterapia ginecologica. (C-Hypovitaminose in der gynäkologischen Strahlentherapie.) Ann. Ostet. Ginec. **80**, 960—976 (1958).

PFEIFFER, J., SCHUHKNECHT, H.-J., RÖDER, K.: Zur Strahlenbehandlung des Kollumkarzinoms. Strahlentherapie **132**, 184—189 (1967).

PHILIPP, E., RUMPHORST, K.: Die Therapieresultate des Kollumkarzinoms aus den Jahren 1948—1952. (Im Rahmen der Behandlungsergebnisse eines 30jährigen Zeitraumes.) Strahlentherapie **107**, 78—84 (1958).

PICARD, J. D.: La lymphographie en gynécologie. Ann. Chir. **16**, 1775 (1962).

— GONGORA, R., SZIGETI, B., BILSKI-PASQUIER, G., JAMMET, H., ARVAY, N.: Considérations. techniques et premiers résultats des injections intra lymphatiques de lipiodol radioactifs à doses thérapeutiques. (Technische Überlegungen und erste Resultate der intralymphatischen Injektion von radioaktivem Lipiodol in therapeutischen Dosen.) Ann. Radiol. (Paris) **7**, 543—554 (1964).

PICHA, E.: Über das Sexualleben von Frauen nach Radiumbehandlung gynäkologischer Erkrankungen. Geburtsh. u. Frauenheilk. **17**, 81—90 (1957).

— Die klinische Bedeutung der Strahlensensibilität beim Carcinoma colli uteri. Strahlentherapie **93**, 106—111 (1954).

— Über die Behandlung von Infektionen der ableitenden Harnwege im Rahmen der Strahlentherapie in der Gynäkologie. Strahlentherapie **113**, 281—285 (1960).

PIERQUIN, B.: L'iridium 192 peut-il remplacer de radium? (Kann Iridium-192 das Radium ersetzen?) Presse méd. **73**, 69—72 (1965).

PIPPIG, L., BRAUN, H.: Seltene Lokalisation von Metastasen beim Kollumkarzinom. Zbl. Gynäk. **87**, 1657—1663 (1965).

PISANI, G.: Sul trattamento radioterapico delle metastasi craniche da carcinoma del collo uterino. (Über die Strahlenbehandlung der Schädelmetastasen bei Carcinom des Collum uteri.) Tumori **60**, 296—306 (1954).

PORTER, E. C., SYCAMORE, L. K.: Effect of radiation dosage on the results in carcinoma of the cervix. (Einfluß der Bestrahlungsdosis auf die Behandlungsergebnisse beim Collumcarcinom.) Radiology **59**, 103—106 (1952).

PORTER, E. H.: Dose-rate and survival curves. Brit. J. Radiol. **38**, 607—612 (1965).

POWERS, W. E., SCHNEIDER, A. K., SHUMATE, K., FOTENOS, H., GALLAGHER, T.: Evaluation of methods of computer estimation of interstitial and intracavitary dosimetry. Amer. J. Roentgenol. **96**, 59—65 (1966).

PRATT, J. A., MALKASIAN, G. D.: Treatment of invasive carcinoma of cervix during pregnancy. Ann. N. Y. Acad. Sci. **114**, 868—874 (1964).

PREM, K. A., MAKOWSKI, E. L., McKELVEY, J. L.: Carcinoma of the cervix associated with pregnancy. Amer. J. Obstet. Gynec. **95**, 99—108 (1966).

PRIOLA, I.: Ricerche istologiche sulle linfoghiandole parametrali nel carcinoma del collo dell'utero. Minerva ginec. **9**, 1017—1025 (1957).

PUJOL, H., LAMARQUE, J. L.: Ilio-cavographie et lymphographie dans la recherche des adinopedies rétropéritoniales. Paris: Masson & Cie. 1964.

PUPATO, F.: Die Blasenkomplikationen nach Bestrahlungen im Bereiche des kleinen Beckens. Urol. int. (Basel) **21**, 393 (1966).

QUIMBY, E. H., CASTRO, V.: The calculation of dosage in interstitial radium therapy. (Dosisberechnung bei der Radiumspickung.) Amer. J. Roentgenol. **70**, 739—749 (1953).

RANDOW, H., MOSLER, W., ERKRATH, F. A.: Zur Behandlung des sogenannten Carcinoma in situ. Dtsch. Gesundh.-Wes. **29**, 1362—1366 (1966).

RANUDD, N. E.: Dose distribution studies in external irradiation of carcinoma colli uteri. Acta radiol. (Stockh.) **4**, 353—362 (1966).

RASORI, C.: Valore dell'indagine linfoadenografica nello studio dei carcinomi dell'utero. (Der Wert der Lymphadenogramme beim Studium des Uteruscarcinoms.) Riv. Pat. Clin. **18**, 566—574 (1963).

RATTI, A.: La radioterapia endolinfatica con ^{131}J: primi risultati. (Die endolymphatische Strahlenbehandlung mit ^{131}J. Erste Resultate.) Radiol. clin. (Basel) **31**, 220—228 (1962).

— Die Wiederholung der Strahlenbehandlung von Tumoren mit Telekobalttherapie. Strahlentherapie, Sonderbd., **61**, 82—93 (1965).

RAUSCHER, H., SPURNY, J.: Ergebnisse der Wertheimschen Radikaloperation ohne und mit obligatorischer Lymphadenektomie. Geburtsh. u. Frauenheilk. **19**, 651—655 (1959).

REEVES, J. D.: Radiation therapy of carcinoma of the cervix. A review of fundamental considerations. (Strahlenbehandlung des Cervixcarcinoms. Eine Übersicht über grundsätzliche Erörterungen.) New Engl. J. Med. **246**, 652—661 (1952).

REGATO, J. A. DEL: The role of roentgen therapy in the treatment of cancer of the cervix uteri. (Die Rolle der Röntgentherapie bei der Behandlung des Cervixcarcinoms.) Amer. J. Roentgenol. **68**, 63—71 (1952).

— Integral roentgen therapy for carcinoma of the cervix uteri. (Integralröntgentherapie bei der Behandlung des Cervixcarcinoms.) Amer. J. Roentgenol. **71**, 676—682 (1954).

— COX, J. D.: Transvaginal roentgen therapy in the conservative management of carcinoma in situ of the uterine cervix. Radiology **84**, 1090—1095 (1965).

REICHENMILLER, H., DRESCHER, H.: „Heilung" oder „Rezidiv"? Erfahrungen bei der Überwachung behandelter Collumcarcinome. Strahlentherapie **94**, 191—202 (1954).

REIFFENSTUHL, G.: Das Lymphsystem des weiblichen Genitale. München-Berlin: Urban & Schwarzenberg 1957.

— Zum Lymphknotenproblem des Carcinoma colli uteri. Häufigkeitsbefall der Lymphknoten und Radikalisierung der Lymphonodektomie. Wien. med. Wschr. **109**, 294—295 (1959).

— Über die Lokalisation der lymphogenen Aussaaten des Carcinoma colli uteri. Wien. med. Wschr. **112**, 751—752 (1962).

REIFFENSTUHL, G.: Der Stadien-Index der 1952 bis 1960 nach Schauta-Amreich operierten Kollumkarzinome. Wien. med. Wschr. **116**, 1020—1022 (1966).

— Das Lymphknotenproblem beim Carcinoma colli uteri und die Lymphirradiatio pelvis. München-Berlin-Wien: Urban & Schwarzenberg 1967.

REINOLD, E.: Die Mortalität am Rezidiv bei Carcinoma colli uteri mit und ohne carcinomatösem Drüsenbefall. Geburtsh. u. Frauenheilk. **27**, 311—316 (1967).

REMOLD, F., SIEGERT, A.: Eine Methode zur Ermittlung der Lokalisation intrauteriner Radiumeinlagen in situ. Strahlentherapie **87**, 481—486 (1952).

REMOTTI, G., FRANCINI, M. A.: La telecobaltoterapia nel cervico-carcinoma uterino. (Studio anatomopatologico.) (Die Telekobalttherapie beim Cervixcarcinom [anatomisch-pathologische Studien].) Ann. Ostet. Ginec. **80**, 533—577 (1958).

— — Reperti istologici di linfoghiandole in alcuni casi di cervico-carcinoma dopo radium o telecobaltoterapia. (Histologische Befunde der Lymphdrüsen in Fällen von Cervixcarcinom, behandelt mit Radium oder Telekobalttherapie.) Ann. Ostet. Ginec. **80**, 679—708 (1958).

— MANGIONI, C.: Reperti istologici linfoghiandolari in 131 casi di cervicocarcinoma operati di isterectomia addominale radicale alla Wertheim-Taussig. Ann. Ostet. Ginec. **84**, 803—850 (1962).

REUSS, A., LOHBAUER, R.: Vergleichsmessungen mit dem Bomke-Dosimeter und dem Gammameter in Blase und Rektum bei der Radiumbehandlung des Collum-Carcinoms. Strahlentherapie **98**, 308—319 (1955).

— — Vergleichsmessungen mit dem Bomke-Dosimeter und dem Gammameter in Blase und Rektum bei der Radiumbehandlung des Collum-Carcinoms. II. Mitt. Messungen am Patienten. Strahlentherapie **99**, 147—161 (1956).

RHAMY, R. K., STAUDER, R. W.: Pyelographic analysis of radiation therapy in carcinoma of the cervix. Amer. J. Roentgenol. **87**, 41—43 (1962).

RICCI, S. B., BIANCHI, F.: La terapia radiologica delle recidive vaginali del cancro dell'utero. Presentazione di una casistica di 83 casi. (Radiologische Therapie der Scheidenrezidive des Uteruscarcinoms.) Minerva ginec. **17**, 708—711 (1965).

— — Terapia delle recidive pelviche del carcinoma del collo dell'utero. (Die Behandlung der Beckenrezidive des Carcinoms des Collum uteri.) Minerva ginec. **18**, 603—609 (1966).

RICCIARDI, M.: Die chirurgische Radiumbehandlung des Collumcarcinoms. Clin. ostet. ginec. **60**, 190—201 (1958); Ref. Ber. ges. Gynäk. **67**, 22 (1959).

RICHTER, J., PENTCHEV, P., SCHIRRMEISTER, D.: Die Ermittlung von Dosisverteilungen für lineare Gammastrahlungsquellen mit elektronischen Rechenautomaten. Strahlentherapie **132**, 246—254 (1967).

RIDINGS, G. R.: Fractionated intrauterine radium applications: use of a small-diameter after-loading intrauterine applicator. Prelim. report. (Fraktionierte intrauterine Radiumapplikation: Gebrauch eines dünnen, nachträglich zu ladenden intrauterinen Applikators). Amer. J. Roentgenol. **89**, 500—501 (1963).

RIECK, G.: Über die präoperative Bestrahlung des Kollumkarzinom I mit dem Körperhöhlenrohr. Zbl. Gynäk. **80**, 1242—1250 (1958).

RIEDEN, H.-G., REUSS, A.: Ein Beitrag zur Frage der Einstelltechnik bei der Bewegungsbestrahlung im kleinen Becken. Strahlentherapie **117**, 560—564 (1962).

RIES, J.: Methodik und Ergebnisse der Strahlenbehandlung des Collumcarcinoms an der I. Frauenklinik der Universität München. Arch. Gynäk. **183**, 454—457 (1953).

— Zur Entwicklung der gynäkologischen Strahlentherapie. Münch. med. Wschr. **109**, 3—9 (1967).

— BREITNER, J.: Strahlenbehandlung in der Gynäkologie. Sonderbd. zur Strahlentherapie, Bd. 40. München u. Berlin: Urban & Schwarzenberg 1959.

— MEHRING, W.: Über die histologische Struktur und Prognose des Kollumkarzinoms. Strahlentherapie **123**, 167—176 (1964).

RIES, J. K.: Zur Frage der Gewebstoleranz bei der Strahlentherapie der Karzinome der Frau. Geburtsh. u. Frauenheilk. **18**, 537—540 (1958).

— Die Methoden der Strahlenbehandlung gynäkologischer Krebse an der I. Frauenklinik der Universität München. Strahlentherapie **105**, 485—498 (1958).

— Urologische Komplikationen bei der Strahlenbehandlung von malignen Tumoren des kleinen Beckens. Krebsforschung und Krebsbekämpfung, Bd. IV, S. 283—293. München-Berlin: Urban & Schwarzenberg 1962.

RIESSBECK, K.-H.: Zur Entwicklung der Strahlentherapie gynäkologischer Karzinome. Z. ärztl. Fortbild. **50**, 544—554 (1956).

— Folgerungen aus Dosismessungen in der gynäkologischen Röntgentherapie. Kongreßber. 1. Tagg Med. Wiss. Ges. Röntgenol. DDR v. 24.—26. 3. 1955 in Leipzig, S. 308—325 (1957).

— Betrachtungen zur Bewegungsbestrahlung gynäkologischer Karzinome. Kongreßber. 2. Tagg Med. Wiss. Ges. Röntgenol. DDR, S. 405—414 (1958).

— GEIPEL, K.: Praktische Erfahrungen bei der Bewegungsbestrahlung gynäkologischer Karzinome. Zbl. Gynäk. **78**, 1546—1556 (1956).

RINGLEB, D.: Behandlungsergebnisse der Uteruskarzinome in der Universitäts-Strahlenklinik Marburg 1941 bis 1956. Strahlentherapie **120**, 357—370 (1963).

RODÉ, I., HAJDU, I.: Massive Siebbestrahlung der gynäkologischen Tumoren. Radiobiol. Radiother. (Berl.) **7**, 521—524 (1966).

ROIZ RIVAS, M.: Problemas actuales de la roentgenterapia en el tratamiento del cancer uterino. (Aktuelle Probleme der Röntgentherapie des Uteruscarcinoms.) Acta ginec. (Madr.) **4**, 47—63 (1953).

ROMAN, T. N., LATOUR, J. P. A.: The effect of early diagnosis on survival statistics in carcinoma of the uterine cervix. Amer. J. Obstet. Gynec. **97**, 739—749 (1967).

ROMIEU, C., LEENHARDT, P.: Récidives à évolution lente et fausses récidives des cancers du col utérin, après radiothérapie. (Schleichende und „falsche" Rezidive des Collumcarcinoms nach Strahlenbehandlung.) Bull. Ass. franç. Cancer **42**, 49—56 (1955).

ROSE, J. A., BLOEDORN, F. G., ROBINSON, J. E.: A computer dosimetry system for radium implants. Amer. J. Roentgenol. **97**, 1032—1040 (1966).

ROSENOW, U., BOON-LONG, P.: Möglichkeiten der Berücksichtigung individueller Absorptionsunterschiede bei der Bewegungsbestrahlung des weiblichen Beckens. Strahlentherapie **125**, 29—38 (1964).

ROSENOW, U., FRISCHKORN, R.: Die Verwendung von Keil- nud Ausgleichsfiltern bei der Supervolt-Therapie gynäkologischer Karzinome. Fortschr. Röntgenstr. **102**, 579—585 (1965).

ROSSEL, G.: La lymphadénectomie pelvienne de principe dans le traitement radiochirurgical des cancers du col utérin au stade de début. (Über die prinzipielle Lymphadenektomie des kleinen Beckens bei der Behandlung des beginnenden Collumcarcinoms.) Rev. méd. Suisse rom. **79**, 939—947 (1957).

ROSSMANN, K.: Die Herabsetzung der Dosis im Schenkelhals zur Vermeidung von Spontanfrakturen nach Pendelbestrahlung gynäkologischer Tumoren. Röntgen-Bl. **7**, 107—115 (1954).

ROTH, F.: Bericht über 641 Fälle von Kollum-Karzinom. Strahlentherapie **97**, 161—174 (1955).

— EGGER, G.: Bericht über die Behandlungsergebnisse bei Uteruskarzinomen nach Intensivierung der Strahlentherapie. Schweiz. med. Wschr. **90**, 199—203 (1960).

RUBIN, P., GRISE, W., TERRY, R.: Has postoperative irradiation proved itself? (Hat sich die postoperative Bestrahlung bewährt?) Amer. J. Roentgenol. **88**, 849—866 (1962).

RUBIO, C. A., HERTZBERG, O., KOTTMEIER, H.-L., OLSSON, E., ZAJICEK, J.: Sensitization and radiation response in cases with carcinoma of the uterine cervix. Investigations in 720 cases treated at Radiumhemmet 1954—1961. (Strahlenempfindlichkeit und Strahlenreaktion bei Fällen mit einem Uterushals-Carcinom. Untersuchungen an 720 am Radiumhemmet behandelten Fällen [1954—1961].) Acta radiol. (Stockh.), N. S., Ther. Phys. Biol., **3**, 241—268 (1965).

RUCH, R. M., COX, A. A., NURNBERGER, C. E., TRUMBULL, M. L.: Cervical cancer in aortic lymph nodes treated with radioactive gold. Report of a case. (Metastasen eines Cervixcarcinoms in den aortalen Lymphknoten, behandelt mit radioaktivem Gold. Bericht eines Falles.) Obstet. and Gynec. **10**, 388—392 (1957).

— VAUGHN, H. M., TAYLOR, E. L., CARROLL, D. S.: Decrease in vaginal capacity with radiation therapy. (Schrumpfung der Vagina nach Radium-Therapie.) Obstet. and Gynec. **19**, 499—504 (1962).

RUDERMANN, A. I., ŠAPOŠNIKOVA, N. E., KARIBOV, J.: On rotation roentgen therapy of far-advanced cancer of female genitalia. (Zur Methodik der Rotationsröntgentherapie vernachlässigter Formen von Krebs der weiblichen Geschlechtsorgane.) Vop. Onkol. **4**, 469—475 mit engl. Zus.fass. (1958) [Russisch].

RUMMEL, H. H., WACH, E.: Die primären urologischen Komplikationen bei der Radikaloperation des Kollumkarzinoms nach WERTHEIM. Z. Geburtsh. u. Gynäk. **161**, 305—318 (1963).

Rumphorst, K.: Kollum- und Korpuskarzinome 1955. Strahlentherapie 117, 509—513 (1962).

Runge, H., Wimhöfer, H.: Behandlungsergebnisse beim Carcinoma colli uteri (1936—1941). Geb. Fra. 9, 84—93 (1949).

— Zeitz, H.: Bericht über 2401 Genitalkarzinome (1935—1950). Geburtsh. u. Frauenheilk. 16, 875—890 (1956).

Rutledge, F. N.: Can irradiation destroy metastatic pelvic lymph nodes? (Kann die Bestrahlung Lymphknoten-Metastasen zerstören?) J. Amer. med. Ass. 193, 1102—1103 (1965).

— Burns, B. C.: Pelvic exenteration. Amer. J. Obstet. Gynec. 91, 692—708 (1965).

— Dodd, G. D., Kasilag, F. B.: Lymphocyst: a complication of radical pelvic surgery. Amer. J. Obstet. Gynec. 77, 1165—1175 (1959).

— Fletcher, G. H.: Transperitoneal lymphadenectomy following supervoltage irradiation for squamous-cell carcinoma of the cervix. (Transperitoneale Beckenlymphknotenausräumung nach Supervolttherapie beim Cervixcarcinom.) Amer. J. Obstetr. 76, 321—334 (1958).

— — Radiation therapy in invasive cervical carcinoma. (Die Strahlentherapie des invasiven Cervix-Carcinoms.) Ann. N. Y. Acad. Sci. 97, 821—829 (1962).

— — MacDonald, E. J.: Pelvic lymphadenectomy as an adjunct to radiation therapy in treatment for cancer of the cervix. Amer. J. Roentgenol., 93, 607—614 (1965).

Rüttimann, A., Del Buono, M. S.: Die Lymphographie. In: Ergebnisse der medizinischen Strahlenforschung, Neue Folge, Bd. I. Stuttgart: Thieme 1964.

Sablinska, B.: Investigation on the relation between the age of patients and results of radiation treatment of carcinoma of the uterine cervix. (Untersuchungen über die Abhängigkeit des Alters der Kranken mit einem Cervix-Carcinom von Resultaten der Strahlentherapie.) Nowotwory 15, 309—316 mit engl. Zus.fass. (1965) [Polnisch].

— Relationship of age to survival rate in carcinoma of the cervix (Symposium). (Beziehungen zwischen Alter und Überlebensrate beim Cervixcarcinom.) Radiobiol. Radiother. (Berl.) 7, 677—681 (1966).

Sala, J. M., de Leon, A. Diaz: Treatment of carcinoma of the cervical stump. (Die Behandlung des Cervixcarcinomstumpfes.) Radiology 81, 300—306 (1963).

Savage, D. J., Millin, J. C. B.: Technical aspects of the pretoria approach to the use of radium in the treatment of cancer of the uterus. (Technische Gesichtspunkte der Pretoria-Methode in der Radiumanwendung bei der Behandlung des Uterus-Krebses.) S. Afr. med. J. 37, 703—707 (1963).

Schär, M., Heyden, S.: Kritische Bemerkungen zur Prophylaxe des Kollumkarzinoms. Münch. med. Wschr. 107, 2373—2374 (1965).

Scheer, A. C.: A redefinition of point „A" in radium applications for carcinoma of the cervix. (Eine Neudefinierung des Punktes „A" in der Radiumverabfolgung des Collum-Ca.) Radiology 78, 281—283 (1962).

Scheffey, L. C., Thudium, W. J., Farell, D. M., Hahn, G. A., Lang, W. R.: A twenty-five year evaluation of the treatment of carcinoma of the cervix with irradiation. (Eine 25jährige Entwicklung der Strahlenbehandlung des Collumcarcinoms.) Amer. J. Obstet. 64, 233—247 (1952).

— — — — — A twenty-five year evaluation of the treatment of carcinoma of the cervix with irradiation. (Eine 25-Jahresstatistik der Strahlenbehandlung des Cervixcarcinoms.) Obstetr. a. Gynecol. 8, 250—253 (1953).

Scherer, E.: Möglichkeiten und Fortschritte in der Strahlentherapie bösartiger Genitaltumoren. Zentralbl. für Gyn. 86, 457—467 (1964).

Schewe, E. J., Jr., Sala, J. M.: Bilateral ureteral obstruction complicating the treatment of carcinoma of the cervix. (Doppelseitiger Ureterverschluß als Komplikation in der Behandlung des Cervixcarcinoms.) Amer. J. Roentgenol. 81, 125—129 (1959).

Schindler, A. E., Lewin, H.: Maligne Tumoren des Collum uteri. Zbl. Gynäk. 88, 1643—1649 (1966).

Schinz, H. R.: Neuere Ergebnisse mit dem Zürcher Betatron. Radiol. austriaca 10, 85—98 (1958).

— Fritz-Niggli, H., Schärer, K.: Vier Jahre Züricher Erfahrungen mit dem Betatron. Radiol. Clin. 24, 317—346 (1955).

Schirrmeister, D., Richter, J.: Die Berechnung von Dosisverteilungen mit digitalen Rechenautomaten bei mehraxialer Pendelbestrahlung. Strahlentherapie 125, 211—222 (1964).

Schittenhelm, R.: Physikalischer Vergleich der Therapie mit energiereichen Elektronen und ultraharter Röntgenstrahlung. Strahlentherapie 116, 39—49 (1961).

Schjött-Rivers, E., Istre, B. S.: Pre-operative irradiation in carcinoma of the uterine cervix. (Die präoperative Bestrahlung beim Cervixcarcinom.) Acta obstet. gynec. scand. 38, 681—689 (1959).

Schlink, H. H.: Cancer of cervix uteri; Australian results 1930—1950. J. Obstet. Gynaec. brit. Emp. 57, 714—720 (1950).

Schmermund, H. J.: Moderne Gesichtspunkte bei der Strahlenbehandlung gynäkologischer Carcinome im kleinen Becken. Dtsch. med. J. 1955, 512—519.

— Franke, H.: Die individuelle Dosierung bei der Kombination von Radium- und Röntgen-Pendelbestrahlung des Portiokarzinoms. Sonderbände zur Strahlentherapie Nr. 35, S. 86. München-Berlin: Urban & Schwarzenberg 1956.

— Oberheuser, F.: Die Betatrontherapie gynäkologischer Carcinome, insbesondere des Vulvacarcinoms. In: J. Becker und K.-E. Scheer: Betatron und Telekobalttherapie. Berlin-Göttingen-Heidelberg: Springer 1957.

Schmidt, W., Herrmann, M.: Zur Frage der Nachweisbarkeit eines peroral zugeführten Kolistammes im Stuhl bei Patienten mit Beckenraumbestrahlungen. Strahlentherapie 129, 520—526 (1966).

— Rogge, U.: Fieberhafte Komplikationen bei der Radium- und Röntgentherapie des weiblichen Genitalcarcinom. Zbl. Gynäk. 88, 1120—1126 (1966).

Schmidt-Elmendorff, H. R.: Die Vorbestrahlung von Mamma- und Collum-Carcinom. Med. Klin. 1952, 1344—1346.

SCHMIDT-ELMENDORFF, H. R., DIBBELT, L.: Zur Kombination von Strahlentherapie und Operation bei der Behandlung des Kollumkarzinoms. Geburtsh. u. Frauenheilk. 16, 367—377 (1956).

SCHMIDT-MATTHIESEN, H.: Die Gewebsreaktion bei der Bestrahlung des Kollumkarzinoms. Strahlentherapie 127, 180—191 (1965).

SCHMITZ, H. E.: The management of carcinoma of the cervix with emphasis on the controversial factors in the treatment. Surg. Clin. N. Amer. 30, 249—257 (1950).

— GEIGER, C. J., SMITH, CH. J., BLICHERT, P. A.: Carcinoma of the cervix. Failure of haphazard treatment. (Über das Cervixcarcinom. Das Versagen der schematischen Therapie.) Obstetr. a. Gynecol. 4, 75—81 (1954).

— ISAACS, J. H.: Complications of advanced cervical cancer and their management. (Komplikationen beim fortgeschrittenen Cervixcarcinom und ihre Behandlung.) Radiology 69, 324—329 (1957).

SCHMITZER, GH.: Die prä- und postoperative Bestrahlung des Kollumkarzinoms. Radiobiol. Radiother. (Berl.) 2, 185—190 (1961).

SCHÖNEICH, R.: Siebbestrahlung einer Magenmetastase eines Kollumkarzinoms, zugleich ein Beitrag über erfolgreiche Röntgenbehandlung von sechs weiteren Metastasen bei der gleichen Patientin. Strahlentherapie 110, 110—115 (1959).

SCHOLL, O., WEISHAAR, J.: Die Behandlung unvermeidbarer Strahlenreaktionen in der gynäkologischen Therapie. Z. ärztl. Fortbild. (West-Berl.) 53, 565—574 (1964).

SCHRIMPF, H.: Über Behandlung der Rezidive des Gebärmutterhalskrebses. Zbl. Gynäk. 74, 93—96 (1952).

— Behandlung der Rezidive des Gebärmutterhalskrebses aus dem Quinquennium 1941 bis 1945. Zbl. Gynäk. 75, 500—502 (1953).

— Zur Lymphdrüsenfrage bei der Behandlung des Kollumkarzinoms. Krebsarzt 9, 355—358 (1954).

— Der drüsige Krebs des Gebärmutterhalses. Zbl. Gynäk. 76, 2223—2229 (1954).

— Die erweiterte abdominale Radikaloperation nach WERTHEIM mit besonderer Berücksichtigung der Lymphknotenfrage. Krebsarzt 10, 257—266 (1955).

— Behandlung des Kollumkarzinom aus dem Jahre 1949 an der Universitäts-Frauenklinik in Rostock. Zbl. Gynäk. 77, 961—967 (1955).

— Das Lymphknotenproblem bei der Behandlung des Kollumkarzinoms. Geburtsh. u. Frauenheilk. 16, 519—526 (1956).

— Die Erfolge der Behandlung des Kollumkarzinoms aus dem Jahre 1950 an der Universitäts-Frauenklinik in Rostock. Zbl. Gynäk. 78, 1169—1177 (1956).

SCHUBERT, G.: Moderne Gesichtspunkte bei der Behandlung des Karzinoms am Collum uteri. Dtsch. med. Wschr. 1953, 1005—1008.

— Behandlung und Ergebnisse beim Kollumkarzinom in der Schwangerschaft. Geburtsh. u. Frauenheilk. 20, 1124—1128 (1960).

— Die Beeinflußbarkeit der Strahlenresistenz von Tumorzellen. Deutscher Röntgenkongreß 1961. Strahlenforschung, Bd. III, S. 101—118. München-Berlin: Urban & Schwarzenberg 1961.

SCHUBERT, G.: Die Supervolttherapie gynäkologischer Karzinome mit dem Betatron und dem Gammatron. Dtsch. Med. J. 15, 441—446 (1964).

— Results of the high-voltage radiation treatment of gynecological carcinomata with the use of the betatron and the gammatron. (Ergebnisse der Hochvolt-Strahlentherapie gynäkologischer Carcinome mit Hilfe des Betatrons und des Gammatrons.) Acta Un. int. Cancr. (Louvain) 20, 1747—1750 (1964).

— HÖHNE, G.: Spätergebnisse nach Supervolttherapie gynäkologischer Karzinome. Dtsch. Röntgenkongreß, Sonderbd zur Strahlentherapie 60, 143—146 (1964).

— OBERHEUSER, F.: Neue Behandlungsmethoden und -ergebnisse der Strahlentherapie weiblicher Karzinome mit dem Betatron und Gammatron. Zbl. Gynäk. 84, 1—8 (1962).

— SCHMERMUND, H. J.: Moderne Gesichtspunkte bei der Behandlung des Oberflächenkarzinoms am Collum uteri. Arch. Geschwulstforsch. 6, 333—347 (1954).

— — OBERHEUSER, F.: Die Betatrontherapie gynäkologischer Karzinome. Strahlentherapie 112, 4—16 (1959).

— — UHLMANN, G.: Die Behandlungsergebnisse des Kollum-Karzinoms an der Univ.-Frauenklinik Hamburg-Eppendorf von 1951—1955. Geburtsh. u. Frauenheilk. 22, 1—24 (1962).

SCHULTZ, A., PECKHAM, B., KIEKHOFER, W.: Radioactive colloidal gold in the therapy of cervical carcinoma. (Radioaktives kolloidales Gold bei der Behandlung des Cervixkarzinoms.) Obstet. and Gynec. 20, 567—571 (1962).

SCHULTZ, W.: Bestrahlung und Operation beim Genitalkarzinom. Strahlentherapie 96, 290—292 (1955).

SCHULZ, M., GRAHAM, J. B.: Radiotherapy in the treatment of cancer of the uterine cervix. (Die Strahlentherapie bei der Behandlung des Carcinoms der Cervix uteri.) Progr. Gynec. 3, 656—693 (1957).

SCHUMACHER, W.: Die Anwendung radioaktiver Stoffe in der Gynäkologie. — Dosierung und Behandlungsmöglichkeiten. Geburtsh. u. Frauenheilk. 21, 518—519 (1961).

SCHWARZ, R.: On the treatment of carcinoma of the cervix. (Zur Behandlung des Gebärmutterhalskrebses.) Československ. Gynaekol. 21/35, 168 (1956) [Tschechisch].

SCHWARZ, R.: Probleme der Dosimetrie bei gynäkologischen Radiumeinlagen. Radiobiol. Radiother. (Berl.) 7, 569—572 (1966).

SCHWARZER, R.: Osteoradionekrosen des Schenkelhalses. Dtsch. Gesundh.-Wes. 38, 1767—1771 (1964).

SCHWEIGERT, M.: Betrachtungen über die Meßergebnisse mit dem Momentan-Dosimeter nach Dr. BOMKE während der Radiumeinlage. Strahlentherapie 97, 312—316 (1955).

— REUSS, A., MAURER, H.-J.: Zur Radiumdosimetrie bei der Behandlung gynäkologischer Tumoren hinsichtlich der Blasen- und Rektumbelastung. 1. Mitt. Blase. Strahlentherapie 97, 430—434 (1955).

— — — Zur Radiumdosimetrie bei der Behandlung gynäkologischer Tumoren hinsichtlich der Blasenund Rektumbelastung. 2. Mitt. Rektum. Radiol. clin. (Basel) 25, 12—19 (1956).

Scott, R. M., Brizel, H. E., Wetzelberger, C.: The etiology of treatment failures in early stage carcinoma of the cervix. (Die Ätiologie der Mißerfolge bei der Therapie des Frühstadiums des Cervixcarcinoms.) Amer. J. Roentgenol. 96, 565—569 (1966).

Scott, W. P.: Tumor /air ratio calculators. Radiology 85, 962—964 (1965).

— Radium alignment applicator. Amer. J. Roentgenol. 94, 905—964 (1965).

— Cervicovaginal irradiator—a triple applicator. Amer. J. Roentgenol. 96, 52—55 (1966).

— Modified Manchester system. Adaptation for an alignment applicator. Brit. J. Radiol. 39, 397—398 (1966).

Sedov, V. V., Serebryakov, N. G., Tarasov, N. F.: Prospects of utilizing radioactive colloids for the treatment of malignant affections of lymph nodes. (Die Perspektive der Anwendung von radioaktiven Kolloiden bei der Behandlung der malignen Lymphknoten.) Med. Radiol. (Mosk.) 9, Nr 3, 3—12 mit engl. Zus.fass. (1964) [Russisch].

Seitz, L.: Röntgen- und Radiumbehandlung. In: Biologie und Pathologie des Weibes von Halban-Seitz, Bd. II, S. 291—464. Berlin: Urban & Schwarzenberg 1924.

— Wintz, H.: Unsere Methode der Röntgen-Tiefentherapie und ihre Erfolge. Sonderbände zur Strahlentherapie, Bd. 5. Berlin u. Wien: Urban & Schwarzenberg 1920.

Seitzmann, D. M., Halaby, F. A., Flanagan, R., Wright, R., Freeman, J. H.: Intralymphatic radioisotope therapy. Surg. Gynec. Obstet. 118, 52—58 (1964).

— Wright, R., Halaby, F. A., Freeman, J. H.: Radioactive lymphangiography as a therapeutic adjunct. Amer. J. Roentgenol. 89, 140—149 (1963).

Serra, G. E., Vallerino, V.: Sul centraggio radiografico nella radiumterapia del cancro uterino. (Über die radiographische Zentrierung bei der Radiumtherapie des Gebärmutterkrebses.) Clin. ostet. ginec. 68, 229—239 (1966).

Sherman, A. I.: A study of radiation failures and the role of radioresistance in the treatment of cancer of the cervix. (Eine Studie über Bestrahlungsfehler und über den Einfluß der Strahlenresistenz bei der Behandlung von Collumcarcinomen.) Amer. J. Roentgenol. 85, 466—478 (1961).

— Allen, W. H.: Radioactive colloidal gold in the treatment of cancer of the cervix and cancer of the ovary. (Die Behandlung des Collum- und Ovarialcarcinoms mit kolloidalem radioaktivem Gold.) Progr. Gynec. 3, 620—632 (1957).

— Bonebrake, M., Allen, W. M.: Application of radioactive colloidal gold in treatment of pelvic cancer. Amer. J. Roentgenol. 66, 624—638 (1951).

— Nolan, F., Allen, W. M.: Experimental application of radioactive colloidal gold in treatment of pelvic cancer. Amer. J. Roentgenol. 64, 75—85 (1950); Zit. nach Gauwerky, F., Strahlentherapie 103, 16—47 (1957).

Sherman, A. I., Ruch, R.: The effect of lymph node metastases on prognosis for carcinoma of the cervix and vulva. Sth med. J. 45, 703—707 (1952).

Shimanovsky, R. N.: Enterovaginal fistula following radium therapy of uterine cervix carcinoma. (Dünndarm-Scheidenfistel nach Röntgentherapie bei Carcinoma colli uteri.) Med. Radiol. (Mosk.) 9, Nr 9, 40—42 mit engl. Zus.fass. (1964) Bulgarisch].

Sicard, A.: L'association radium-chirurgie dans le traitement du cancer du col utérin. Essai de cytopronostic. (Kombinierte Radium- und chirurgische Behandlung des Collumcarcinoms. Eine Studie zur Cyto-Prognostik.) Bull. Soc. roy. belge Gynéc. Obstet. ,N.S. 30, 41—51 (1960).

Siegel, P., Liebner, E. J.: Intralymphatic radioactive therapy for pelvic cancer. (Intralymphatische radioaktive Behandlung des Krebses im kleinen Becken.) Amer. J. Obstet. Gynec. 91, 122—131 (1965).

Siegert, A.: Das Problem der Direktmessung im Darm bei intrauterinen und vaginalen Einlagen und dessen Lösung. Strahlentherapie 110, 590—594 (1959).

— Kessler, H.: Die Radiumbehandlung des Kollumkarzinoms. Ein Verteilungsproblem. Strahlentherapie 92, 353—363 (1953).

— Müller, Ph.: Ersatz der Kreuzfeuermethode durch Bewegungsbestrahlung bei der Behandlung des Kollum-Karzinoms. Strahlentherapie 93, 447—453 (1954).

Sievert, R.: Eine Methode zur Messung von Röntgen-, Radium- und Ultrastrahlung nebst einigen Untersuchungen über die Anwendbarkeit derselben in der Physik und der Medizin. Acta radiol. (Stockh.) Suppl. 14 (1932).

Sighinolfi, R.: Importanza dei Parametri — angolo di Tendolazione, Profundità del Focolaio, Ampiezza del Campo — nella Telecobaltoterapia Pendolare. Radiobiol. Radioter. Fis. med. 17, 358—373 (1962).

Silván, A.: Fundamento, sistemática y técnica de las aplicaciones cavitarias de radium en el cáncer del cervix uterino. (Grundlage, Systematik und Technik der kavitären Anwendung von Radium beim Carcinoma cervicis uteri.) Acta oncol. (Madr.) 1, 145—191 (1962).

— Perez-Modrego, S.: Tratamiento del cáncer de cuello de útero con radium endocavitario. Dosimetría pélvica. (Behandlung des Carcinoma colli uteri mit endokavitärem Radium. Dosimetrie des Beckens.) Acta oncol. (Madr.) 3, 1—15 (1964).

Silverstone, S. M.: The intra-uterine tandem technique. Amer. J. Roentgenol. 89, 83—86 (1963).

— Harris, W., Greenberg, M.: Radium therapy for cancer of the cervix uteri with a new type of colpostat. (Radiumtherapie beim Collumcarcinom mit einem neuen Kolpostaten-Modell.) Amer. J. Roentgenol. 67, 294—299 (1952).

— Melamed, J. L.: Effective irradiation with radium for cancer of the cervix. (Über die Radiumbestrahlung des Cervixcarcinoms.) Radiology 69, 360—371 (1957).

Sinclair, W. K.: Dosimetry and relative biologic effectiveness. Amer. J. Roentgenol. 76, 893—894 (1956).

Siracký, J.: The problem of the evaluation of radio-curability of carcinoma colli uteri. (Das Problem der Beurteilung der Strahlenkurabilität des Collum-Carcinoms.) Neoplasma (Bratisl.) 8, 523—529 (1961).

Smith, Ch. J.: Deferred sequelae incident to pelvic irradiation. Amer. J. Obstet. Gynec. 88, 91—96 (1964).

— Cava, J. M., Meyer, J. E.: Lymphovenography in pelvic cancer. Amer. J. Obstet. Gynec. 89, 732—737 (1964).

Smith, J. P., Rutledge, F., Burns, B. C., Soffar, S.: Systemic chemotherapy for carcinoma of the cervix. Amer. J. Obstet. Gynec. 97, 800—807 (1967).

Sørensen, B.: Late results of radium therapy in cervical carcinoma. A clinical-statistical study on 798 patients treated at the radium centre, Copenhagen, during the period 1922—1929. (Spätresultate der Radiumbehandlung beim Cervixcarcinom. Eine klinisch-statistische Untersuchung an 798 Kranken, die im Radium-Zentrum Kopenhagen 1922—1929 behandelt wurden.) Acta radiol. (Stockh.), Suppl. 169, 11—190 (1958).

Sotto, L. S. J., Graham, J. B., Pickren, J. W.: Postmortem findings in cancer of the cervix. An analysis of 108 autopsies in the past 5 years. Amer. J. Obstet. Gynec. 80, 791—794 (1960).

Soule, S. D.: Radioactive colloidal gold in carcinoma of the cervix. (Radioaktives kolloidales Gold bei Cervixcarcinom.) West. J. Surg. 61, 297—300 (1953).

Spechter, H.-J.: Das Dosismaximum bei der Pendel- und Pendelkonvergenzbestrahlung des kleinen Beckens. In: Sonderbd. zur Strahlentherapie 35, 74—80. München-Berlin: Urban & Schwarzenberg 1956.

— Experimentelle Studien über die Bewegungsbestrahlung im kleinen Becken bei gynäkologischen Tumoren. Strahlentherapie 102, 229—269, 629—661 (1957).

— Experimentelle Untersuchungen zur Verlängerung des Dosismaximum entlang der Lymphabflußwege im kleinen Becken. Geburtsh. u. Frauenheilk. 18, 525—531 (1958).

— Die Dosierung während der Bestrahlung von Uteruskarzinomen im Hinblick auf mögliche Rezidive bzw. urologische Komplikationen. Geburtsh. u. Frauenheilk. 22, 1126—1130 (1962).

— Behandlungsergebnisse beim Kollumkarzinom in den Jahren 1954—1958 mit besonderer Berücksichtigung der „Tübinger Radium-Röntgenbewegungs-Bestrahlung". Geburtsh. u. Frauenheilk. 25, 402—409 (1965).

— Pollack, J. M.: Beitrag zur Tamponadentechnik der intrauterinen und intravaginalen Radiumeinlage. Geburtsh. u. Frauenheilk. 164, 102—109 (1965).

Spurny, J., Weghaupt, K.: Die absoluten Heilungsergebnisse bei 312 Kollumkarzinomen (1950 bis 1952). Geburtsh. u. Frauenheilk. 19, 244—252 (1959).

Staffeldt, K.: Zur Frage der multiplen Karzinomentstehung im unteren Genitaltrakt. Geburtsh. u. Frauenheilk. 164, 92—101 (1965).

Stallworthy, J.: Radical surgery following radiation treatment for cervical carcinoma. (Radikaloperation nach Strahlenbehandlung beim Collum-Carcinom.) Ann. roy. Coll. Surg. Engl. 34, 161—178 (1964).

Stegmann, H., Hanger, W.: Über das zeitliche Auftreten von Rezidiven nach erfolgter Behandlung der weiblichen Genital-Karzinome. Med. Klin. 59, 1264—1267 (1964).

Stein, J. J.: Supervoltage radiation therapy of carcinoma. (Supervolt-Strahlentherapie des Carcinoms.) J. int. Coll. Surg. 31, 657—664 (1959).

Stevenson, Ch. S.: The treatment of carcinoma of the cervix with full irradiation therapy followed by radical pelvic surgery. Amer. J. Obstet. Gynec. 75, 888—898 (1958).

— Combined treatment of carcinoma of cervix with full irradiation therapy followed by radical pelvic operation. Amer. J. Obstet. Gynec. 81, 156—165 (1961).

Stone, M. L., Weingold, A. B., Sall, S.: Cervical carcinoma in pregnancy. Amer. J. Obstet. Gynec. 93, 479—485 (1965).

Stone, R. S., Louie, R. V.: The use of a 17-MeV-synchrotron in cancer therapy. II. Clinical aspects. (Die Anwendung eines 17-MeV-Synchrotrons in der Krebstherapie. II. Klinische Gesichtspunkte.) Radiology 83, 797—806 (1964).

Sträuli, P.: Erreichte und erstrebte Ziele der Metastasenforschung. Oncologia (Basel) 15, 123—128 (1962).

Stratev, J.: Über die Applikationstechnik der intravaginalen Röntgentiefentherapie. Strahlentherapie 106, 601—605 (1958).

— Indikationen und Frühergebnisse der intravaginalen Röntgentiefentherapie. Radiobiol. Radiother. (Berl.) 7, 529—531 (1966).

Stüper, P.: Über Beziehungen zwischen histologischer Struktur und Heilung der Kollumkarzinome. 4. Mitt. Untersuchungen zur Frage der „elektiven Therapie". Strahlentherapie 92, 338—352 (1953).

— Über Beziehungen zwischen histologischer Struktur und Heilung der Kollumkarzinome. Strahlentherapie 92, 89—107, 219—236, 237—250 (1953).

— Zur Frage des Malignitätsgrades und der Strahlenresistenz von Kollumkarzinomen. Strahlentherapie 114, 438—445 (1961).

Stütz, G., Maurer, H.-J.: Die Bewegungsbestrahlung gynäkologischer Tumoren im kleinen Becken. III. Mitt. Konvergenz- und Pendelkonvergenzbestrahlung. Strahlentherapie 99, 417—441 (1956).

Stutzer, J. M.: Uteruskarzinom und Gravidität. Strahlentherapie 76, 361—370 (1947).

Surmont, J., Guy, E., Fajbisowicz, S., Dutreix, A.: Possibilités de coordination correcte de la curie et de la roentgenthérapie dans le traitement du cancer du col. (Möglichkeiten der exakten Koordination der Radium- und Röntgentherapie bei der Behandlung des Collumcarcinoms.) J. de Radiol. 37, 252—259 (1956).

Surmont, M.: Résultats de la TCT dans les affections OTR et gynécologiques. (Ergebnisse der Telekobalttherapie in der Gynäkologie und bei Erkrankungen der HNO-Organe.) Ann. Ostet. Ginec. 79, 1061—1068 (1957).

Surmont, M., Fajbisowicz, S.: Méthode pratique de repérage du col et champs á appliquer en harmonie avec la curiethérapie dans la roentgenthérapie du cancer du col utérin. (Praktische Methode zur Markierung des Collums und zu einer mit der Curietherapie harmonierenden Feldeinstellung bei der Röntgenbehandlung des Gebärmutterhalskrebses.) Bull. Ass. franç. Cancer 43, 343—360 (1956).

Sweeney, W. J., Douglas, R. G.: Treatment of carcinoma of the cervix with combined radiation and extensive surgery. (Behandlung des Cervixcarcinoms mit kombinierter Strahlentherapie und umfassender chirurgischer Behandlung.) Amer. J. Obstet. Gynec. 84, 981—991 (1962).

Symmonds, R. E.: Morbidity and complications of radical hysterectomy with pelvic lymph node dissection. Amer. J. Obstet. Gynec. 94, 663—673 (1966).

Tachibana, S.: Lymph node metastasis in cancer of the uterine cervix. Jap. J. Obstet. Gynec. 3, 71—92 (1956).

Täger, F., Buttenberg, D.: Indikationen und Technik der primären Telekobaltpendelbestrahlung bei Patienten mit Kollumkarzinom. Strahlentherapie 121, 239—246 (1963).

Tailhefer, A.: L'envahissement ganglionnaire dans les cancers du col utérin. Conséquences therapeutiques. Presse méd. 1953, 1289—1290.

Takayama, K.: Studies on the dose distribution of rotation therapy with the 15 MeV betatron for cervical cancer. (Untersuchungen zur Dosisverteilung bei Rotationsbestrahlung mit dem 15 MeV-Betatron bei Cervixcarcinom.) Kyushu J. med. Sci. 15, 189—200 (1964).

Talbert, L. M., Palumbo, L., Shingleton, H., Bream, C. A., McGee, J. A.: Urologic complications of radical hysterectomy for carcinoma of the cervix. (Urologische Komplikationen nach radikaler Hysterektomie wegen Cervixcarcinom.) Sth med. J. 58, 11—17 (1965).

Tarlowska, L., Charuk, Ł., Dorociak, R., Jablońska, M., Nowakowski, W.: Comparative results in cases of cancer of the uterine cervix treated at the Institute of Oncology in 1950—1951. (Vergleichende Resultate der Behandlung von Uterus-Carcinom im Onkologischen Institut während der Jahre 1950—1951.) Nowotwory 9, 199—205 mit engl. Zus.fass. (1959) [Polnisch].

Tasch, H.: Über die Behandlung und deren Erfolge beim Kollumkarzinom der Wiener Schule im Wandel der Zeiten. Wien. med. Wschr. 116, 915—917 (1966).

Taussig, F. J.: Iliac lymphadenectomy with irradiation in the treatment of cancer of the cervix. Amer. J. Obstet. Gynec. 28, 650—667 (1934).

— Iliac lymphadenectomy for group II cancer of the cervix. Amer. J. Obstet. Gynec. 45, 733—748 (1943).

Taylor, G. R.: A wedge filter for cobalt 60 supplementation of carcinoma of the cervix uteri previously treated by radium. Acta radiol. (Stockh.) 1, 253—256 (1963).

Taylor, G. W., Nathanson, I. T.: Lymph node metastases. Incidence and surgical treatment in neoplastic disease. New York: Oxford University Press 1942.

Taylor, H. C., Jr.: Controversial points in the treatment of carcinoma of the cervix. (Entgegengesetzte Auffassungen in der Behandlung des Cervix-Carcinoms.) Cancer (N. Y.) 5, 435—441 (1952).

Ter-Pogossian, M., Sherman, A. I.: Radiation dosimetry in the treatment of carcinoma of the cervix uteri by intraparametrial radioactive gold and radium. (Strahlendosimetrie bei der Behandlung des Cervix-Carcinoms mit parametran injiziertem Radio-Gold und mit Radium.) Amer. J. Roentgenol. 74, 116—122 (1955).

— — Radioactive gold for the intracavitary treatment of carcinoma of the cervix. (Radioaktives Gold für die intrakavitäre Behandlung des Collumcarcinoms.) Radiology 65, 779—783 (1955).

Teschendorf, W., Ewald, H. J.: Strahlenbehandlung von Metastasierungen. Strahlentherapie 128, 56—81 (1965).

Tetti, A., Barbanti, A., Notarbartolo, R.: Metodiche radioterapiche nel trattamento del cancro dell'utero. Minerva ginec. 14, 947—991 (1962).

— Chiaudano, G.: Complicanze urologiche nel trattamento radiochirurgico del carcinoma de collo dell' utero. Minerva ginec. 16, 133—167 (1964).

Themann, H., Verhagen, A.: Spätveränderungen an radiumbestrahlten Kollumkarzinomen im elektronenmikroskopischen Bild. Strahlentherapie 115, 427—440 (1961).

Thomas, C. G., Jr.: Lymphatic dissemination of radiogold in the presence of lymph node metastases. Surg. Gynec. Obstet. 103, 51—56 (1956).

Thomsen, K.: Ergebnisse der Sulfonamidprophylaxe bei der Radiumbehandlung des Uteruskarzinoms. Geburtsh. u. Frauenheilk. 10, 816—828 (1950).

— Die Behandlung des Kollumkarzinom-Rezidivs mit Radiogold-Seeds. Geburtsh. u. Frauenheilk. 22, 1116—1120 (1962).

Tobeelaivich, V. P.: Die intrarectale Applikation radioaktiver Präparate bei der Behandlung von Neubildungen der weiblichen Genitalorgane. Vop. Onkol. 4, 66—72 mit engl. Zus.fass. (1958) [Russisch].

— On endorectal radiation methods in cancer of female genitalia (II communication). (Über die Methoden der endorectalen Bestrahlung bei Carcinomen der weiblichen Geschlechtsorgane [2. Mitteilung].) Vop. Onkol. 5, 203—209 mit engl. Zus.fass. (1959) [Russisch].

Tod, M. C.: Optimum dosage in treatment of carcinoma of uterine cervix by radiation. Brit. J. Radiol. 14, 23—29 (1941).

— Meredith, W. J.: Dosage system for use in treatment of cancer of uterine cervix. Brit. J. Radiol. 11, 809—823 (1938).

— — Treatment of cancer of the cervix uteri—a revised "Manchester method". (Die Behandlung des Cervixcarcinoms — eine revidierte „Manchester-Methode".) Brit. J. Radiol. 26, 252—257 (1953).

Topol, O., Gross, K.: Unsere Erfahrungen mit der präoperativen Röntgenbestrahlung des Kollumkarzinoms. Strahlentherapie 115, 441—452 (1961).

TRANTER, F. W.: A wedge filter for use in treatment of carcinoma of the cervix uteri with 4 MV X-rays. (Ein Keilfilter für die Behandlung des Cervixcarcinoms mit 4 MeV-Röntgenstrahlen.) Brit. J. Radiol. **32**, 350—352 (1959).

TRAUTMANN, K., MAURER, H.-J.: Zur Bewegungsbestrahlung gynäkologischer Tumoren unter besonderer Berücksichtigung der Pendelbestrahlung. II. Mitt. Pendelbestrahlung gynäkologischer Tumoren. Strahlentherapie **99**, 400—416 (1956).

TRUELSEN, F.: Cancer of the uterine cervix. Thesis Copenhagen 1949.

TRUMP, J. G., GRANKE, R. C., WRIGHT, K. A., EVANS, W. W., HARE, H. F., EWERT, E. E., CONLON, W. E.: Treatment of tumors of the pelvic cavity with supervoltage radiation. Amer. J. Roentgenol. **72**, 284—292 (1954).

TUBIANA, M.: Nouvelles méthodes de traitement en radiothérapie. (Neue Behandlungsmethoden in der Radiotherapie.) Ann. Radiol. (Paris) **6**, 221—238 (1963).

TUDWAY, R. C.: The use of radio-active isotopes in an applicator for the treatment of carcinoma of the cervix uteri. (Die Verwendung von radioaktivem Iridium in einem Träger zur Behandlung des Carcinoms der Cervix uteri.) Acta radiol. (Stockh.) **39**, 415—422 (1953).

— FREUNDLICH, H. F., MARSHALL, T. S.: An applicator for the treatment of carcinoma of the cervix uteri employing radioactive iridium. (Ein Applikator für die Behandlung des Collumcarcinoms unter Verwendung von radioaktivem Iridium.) Proc. of Radioisotope Conf. **1**, 3—10 (1954).

TURTOLA, V.: Über die Karzinome des Zervixstumpfes. Ann. Chir. Gynaec. Fenn. **42**, 101—108 (1953).

TURUNEN, A., VARA, P.: Results of the surgical and radiological treatment of carcinoma of the cervix at the women's clinic, University of Helsinki, in 1953—1958. Acta obstet. gynec. scand. **43**, 62—67 (1964).

TWOMBLY, G. H.: The anatomy of the female pelvis in relation to cancer of the cervix. Amer. J. Roentgenol. **77**, 796—802 (1957).

— Carcinoma of cervix in second trimester of pregnancy. Clin. Obstet. Gynec. **6**, 949—963 (1963).

— ROSH, R.: A new method for applying radium in the vagina in cases of carcinoma of the uterine cervix. (Eine neue Methode der vaginalen Radiumapplikation beim Collumcarcinom.) Cancer (Philad.) **8**, 1016—1020 (1955).

— TAYLOR, H. C., JR.: The treatment of cancer of the cervix uteri. A comparison of radiation therapy and radical surgery. (Die Behandlung des Collumcarcinoms. Ein Vergleich der Bestrahlungsbehandlung mit der Radikaloperation.) Amer. J. Roentgenol. **71**, 501—508 (1954).

UNNERUS, C.-E., WIDHOLM, O., KIVINIITTY, K.: Measuring ureteral radiation doses. Ann. Radiol. **9**, 741—747 (1966).

VAN VAERENBERGH, M., DEWULF, L., DIERICK, W.: Radio-Cobalt thérapie en gynécologie. (Radio-Kobalt-Therapie in der Gynäkologie.) Strahlentherapie **109**, 233—240 (1959).

VALDAGNI, C.: Cinque anni di telecobaltoterapia. (Fünf Jahre Telekobalttherapie.) Minerva fisioter. **5**, 45—68 (1960).

— CASNATI, E.: Combinazione della radiumterapia endocavitaria con la telegammaterapia nel cancro del collo dell'utero. (Kombination der intrauterinen Radiumtherapie mit γ-Bestrahlung beim Collumcarcinom des Uterus.) Radiol. med. **46**, 65—78 (1960).

— — MARCHESONI, M.: Posizione della telecobaltoterapia nelle tecniche di trattamento del cancro del collo dell'utero. (Stellung der Telekobalttherapie in der Behandlungstechnik des Carcinoma colli uteri.) Ann. Ostet. Ginec. **81**, 740—756 (1959).

VÁNDOR, F., BOZÓKY, L.: New types of radiocobalt sources in gynaecology. (Neue Typen radioaktiver Kobaltträger in der Gynäkologie.) Acta med. Acad. Sci. hung. **14**, 179—187 (1959).

VASTERLING, H.-W., HILFRICH, H.-J.: Über die prognostische Bedeutung der Temperatursteigerung während der Strahlenbehandlung des Kollumkarzinoms. Strahlentherapie **124**, 213—218 (1964).

VECCHIETTI, G., ONNIS, A., BRESADOLA, S., ROMAGNOLO, A., COLOMBINI, C.: Studies and clinical possibilities of intralymphatic isotopic therapy in malignant diseases of the female reproductive system. (Untersuchungen und die klinische Möglichkeit der intralymphatischen Isotopentherapie bei malignen Erkrankungen des weiblichen Genitalsystems.) Acta isotop. (Padova) **5**, 121—139 (1965).

VERHAGEN, A.: Radium-Isodosen. Die Radiumdosierung in „r". Mit einem Geleitwort von K. NORDMEYER. 102 S. Stuttgart: G. Thieme 1958.

— Über die Strahlendosis beim Genitalkarzinom. Z. Geburtsh. **149**, 272—296 (1958).

— MUSZYNSKI, G.: Unsere Erfahrungen mit der interstitiellen Radiogoldtherapie beim Kollumkarzinom. Strahlentherapie **116**, 97—130 (1961).

VOGELGESANG, K. H., GROSSE-HOLZ, K.: Probleme der räumlichen und zeitlichen Dosisverteilung bei der Röntgenbestrahlung des Uteruskarzinoms. Strahlentherapie **125**, 173—190 (1964).

— — Welchen Einfluß hat die Röntgenherddosis auf die Heilungsergebnisse des Kollumkarzinoms? Strahlentherapie **129**, 367—374 (1966).

— — SCHULZE, E.: Das Kollumkarzinom und seine Heilungsaussichten. Strahlentherapie **121**, 46—57 (1963).

VOGT, E.: Über die Grundzüge der elektiven Behandlung des Kollumkarzinoms und ihre Erfolge an der Hand von 616 Beobachtungen. Strahlentherapie **89**, 79—89 (1952).

VOLTZ, F.: Die Strahlenbehandlung der weiblichen Genitalcarcinome, Methoden und Ergebnisse. Sonderbde. zur Strahlentherapie, Bd. 13. Berlin-Wien: Urban & Schwarzenberg 1930.

VONESSEN, A.: Beobachtungen an post operationem bestrahlten Karzinomen des Collum uteri. Strahlentherapie **102**, 448—450 (1957).

WACHSMANN, F.: Über die mit ultraharten Strahlungen erreichbare Dosisverteilung. Radiologe **1**, 245—252 (1961).

WACHSMANN, F., KELLER, L.: Untersuchungen über die Dosisverteilung bei der Rotationsbestrahlung gynäkologischer Tumoren (Med. Univ.-Klinik Erlangen). Strahlentherapie 87, 278—289 (1952).

— SCHUSTER, D.: Die Züricher Bestrahlungsmethode des Kollumkarzinoms, unter besonderer Berücksichtigung der angewendeten zeitlichen Dosisverteilung. Strahlentherapie 125, 502—523 (1964).

WAGNER, H.: Beitrag zur Lymphknotenreaktion beim Kollumkarzinom. Zbl. Gynäk. 81, 1954—1962 (1959).

WALDROP, G. M., PALMER, J. P.: Carcinoma of cervix associated with pregnancy. Amer. J. Obstet. Gynec. 86, 202—212 (1963).

WALLON, É.: Télécabalthérapie et gynécologie. (Telekobalttherapie und Gynäkologie.) Gynéc. prat. 9, 167—178 (1958).

WALTER, L., GLUCKSMANN, A., CHERRY, C. P.: Biological and physical factors in the radiotherapy of carcinoma of the cervix. (Biologische und physikalische Faktoren in der Strahlentherapie des Cervixcarcinoms.) J. Obstet. Gynaec. Brit. Cwlth 72, 575—585 (1965).

— HARRISON, C. V., GLUCKSMANN, A., CHERRY, C. P.: Assessment of response of cervical cancers to irradiation by routine histological methods. (Die Beurteilung der Strahlenwirkung auf Cervixcarcinome mit Hilfe histologischer Routinemethoden.) Brit. med. J. 1964 I, 1673—1675.

WARD, S. V., SELLERS, T. B., DAVIS, J. T., JR.: Causes of the death in carcinoma of the cervix influencing of 248 death from Charity Hospital of Louisiana at New Orleans. Amer. J. Obstet. Gynec. 68, 989—998 (1952).

WARREN, S.: Studies on tumor metastasis. I. Distribution of metastases in carcinoma of the cervix uteri. Surg. Gynec. Obstet. 56, 742—745 (1933).

WARREN, S., zit. nach HÖHNE, G., Grundlagen der praktischen Strahlentherapie. In: Gynäkologie und Geburtshilfe, Bd. III. Stuttgart: Thieme 1968.

WASSERBURGER, K.: Zur Individualisierung der Radiumtherapie des Karzinoms der Cervix uteri. Strahlentherapie 93, 521—527 (1954).

WATERMAN, G. W., DI LOENE, R.: Treatment of carcinoma of the cervix by interstitial radium needles at the Rhode Island Hospital. Amer. J. Obstet. Gynec. 50, 482—488 (1945); Zit. nach GAUWERKY, F., Strahlentherapie 103, 16—47 (1957).

— TRACY, E. M.: Complications following use of low intensity, long radium element needles in treatment of cancer of cervix uteri. Amer. J. Roentgenol. 60, 788—794 (1948).

WATSON, C. R.: Effect of various treatments on thermoluminescence of lithium fluoride exposed to low doses of gamma radiation. Unpublished thesis, University of Washington, 1965.

WATSON, T. A., BURKELL, C. C.: Betatron in cancer therapy. Part II. J. Canad. Ass. Radiol. 3, 25—28 (1952).

WEED, J. C.: Combined irradiation and surgical treatment for carcinoma of the cervix. Analysis of 79 cases of Wertheim hysterectomy and pelvic lymphadenectomy. (Die Kombination der Strahlen- und chirurgischen Behandlung beim Cervixcarcinom.) Eine Analyse von 79 Fällen von Operationen nach WERTHEIM mit Ausräumung der Beckenlymphknoten.) Ann. Surg. 147, 704—713 (1958).

WEBSTER, E. W., SCHULZ, M. D., AGARD, E. TH.: A compact radium safe employing gas sterilization. Amer. J. Roentgenol. 93, 183—189 (1965).

WEGHAUPT, K.: Erfolge der Radiumtherapie weit fortgeschrittener Kollumkarzinome (Colli IV). Wien. med. Wschr. 1953, 134—137.

— Zur Radiogoldtherapie in der Gynäkologie. Radiobiol. Radiother. (Berl.) 3, 351—354 (1962).

— Spezielle Strahlentherapie des weiblichen Genitalkarzinoms. Wien. klin. Wschr. 78, 348—351 (1966).

WEISHAAR, J.: Klinische und physikalische Studien zur Frage der Zweckmäßigkeit der Anwendung von kurzzeitigen Röntgenzusatzbestrahlungen der Parametrien, der Beckenwand und der benachbarten Lymphknotengruppen bei der Strahlenbehandlung des Kollumkarzinoms, unter Zugrundelegung der Ergebnisse bei der Behandlung von über 500 Patientinnen. Strahlentherapie 118, 393—429 (1962).

— Frühergebnisse bei Anwendung der Telekobalttherapie in der Behandlung von Patientinnen mit Kollumkarzinom. Geburtsh. u. Frauenheilk. 25, 3—8 (1965).

— Diskussionsbemerkung Deutscher Röntgenkongr. 1967, Baden-Baden.

— BECK, G., REUSS, A.: Experimentelle Untersuchungen zur Frage der Anwendung und prozentualen Dosisverteilung bei Durchführung von Telekobalt-Bewegungsbestrahlungen mit dem Gerät Theratron junior als Zusatzbehandlung bei Patientinnen mit Uteruskarzinom. Studien am Beckenphantom. Strahlentherapie 133, 484—502 (1964).

— BRÜCKNER, G.: Experimentelle Untersuchungen zur Frage der Feldgröße und prozentualen Dosisverteilung bei der perkutanen Röntgenzusatzbestrahlung des Kollumkarzinoms. Strahlentherapie 119, 250—265 (1962).

— CHRISTAHL, U.: Körpergewicht und 5-Jahres-Überlebensziffern bei vollbestrahlten Patientinnen mit Kollumkarzinom 1949 bis 1958. Strahlentherapie 132, 190—193 (1967).

— DEMLEITNER, H.: Zur Frage der frühzeitigen Feststellbarkeit einer klinischen Strahlenresistenz beim Kollumkarzinom und die sich hieraus ergebenden Konsequenzen. (Ergebnisse aus den Jahren Ende 1948 bis Anfang 1952.) Geburtsh. u. Frauenheilk. 22, 360—372 (1962).

— GRAF, R., REUSS, A.: Experimentelle Studien zur Dosisverteilung bei Anwendung von verschiedenen Filtereinsätzen im Tubus. Strahlentherapie 130, 495—503 (1966).

— HELLER, R.: Experimentelle Untersuchungen zur Frage der Feldgröße und prozentualen Dosisverteilung bei der zusätzlichen perkutanen Röntgen- und Kobaltbestrahlung des Kollumkarzinoms (Messungen am Phantom). II. Strahlentherapie 119, 525—539 (1962).

— LOSGAR, W.: Klinische Beobachtungen bei der Bestrahlung von Patientinnen mit Kollumkarzinom unter besonderer Berücksichtigung von Blutstatus und Gewicht. Strahlentherapie 118, 538—549 (1962).

WEISHAAR, J., LOSGAR, W.: Ergebnisse bei Anwendung von Abschnittsteleröntgentherapie bei Patientinnen mit Abdominalkarzinose. Geburtsh. u. Frauenheilk. **23**, 922—926 (1963).

— MAYER, G.: Strahlenbehandlungsart beim Kollumkarzinom und Nebenerscheinungen. Strahlentherapie **115**, 556—577 (1961).

— RIETZ, G.: Nebenerscheinungen bei Anwendung von Telekobalt- und Röntgenbestrahlungen bei Patientinnen mit Kollumkarzinom 1960—1962 (vergleichende Gegenüberstellung). Strahlentherapie, Sonderbd. **61**, 147—157 (1965).

— SCHINNER, H.: Untersuchungen über Zusammenhangsfragen zwischen histologischem Typ des Kollumkarzinoms und verschiedenen Faktoren sowie Prognose und Therapie, unter Zugrundelegung der Ergebnisse bei primär strahlenbehandelten Patientinnen aus den Jahren 1946 bis 1953. Strahlentherapie **113**, 242—258 (1960).

— SUMYK, J.: Beitrag zum Problem des klinisch strahlenresistenten Kollumkarzinoms. (Nachuntersuchungen der primär bestrahlten Patientinnen aus den Jahren 1949 bis 1952 mit Kollumkarzinomen der Gruppen I und II an der Erlanger Universitäts-Frauenklinik.) Strahlentherapie **106**, 549—566 (1958).

— VOGELSANG, B., REUSS, A.: Spezialtubus zu einem Telekobaltgerät und Untersuchungen der Dosisverteilung bei Anwendung verschiedenartiger Satellitenblenden. Strahlentherapie **132**, 504—515 (1967).

— WÖLFEL, C.: Zur Frage eines Zusammenhanges zwischen der Prognose und der Art des Wachstums (endo- oder exophytisch) beim Kollumkarzinom. Strahlentherapie **113**, 522—537 (1960).

— WUNDER, K., REUSS, A.: Experimentelle Studien zur Dosisverteilung bei Anwendung von Satellitenblenden aus Blei bei der Telekobalttherapie. Strahlentherapie **127**, 53—64 (1965).

— — — Experimentelle Studien zur Dosisverteilung bei der Anwendung von Satellitenblenden aus Blei bei der Telekobalttherapie. Strahlentherapie **127**, 53 (1965).

WELKER, K.: Die Bewegungsbestrahlung mit Keilfiltern in der Co⁶⁰-Teletherapie. Strahlentherapie **128**, 514—524 (1965); **132**, 497—503 (1967).

WENZEL, S.: Beiträge zur Ermittlung der individuellen Dosis an bestimmten Beckenpunkten bei gynäkologischer Radiumbehandlung. 1. Teil: Die Auswertung von a-p-Aufnahmepaaren mit verschiedenem Vergrößerungsmaßstab. Strahlentherapie **107**, 580—596 (1958).

WERTHEIM, E.: Zur Frage der Radikaloperation beim Uteruskrebs. Arch. Gynäk. **61**, 627—668 (1900).

— Kurzer Bericht über eine 3. Serie von 30 Uteruskrebsoperationen. Zbl. Gynäk. **26**, 249—252 (1902).

— Ein neuer Beitrag zur Frage der Radikaloperation beim Uteruskrebs. Arch. Gynäk. **65**, 1—39 (1902).

— Die erweiterte abdominale Operation bei Carcinoma colli uteri. Berlin-Wien: Urban & Schwarzenberg 1911.

— The extended abdominal operation for carcinoma uteri (based on 500 operative cases). Amer. J. Obstet. Gynec. **66**, 169—232 (1912).

WHELTON, J. A., McSWEENEY, D. J.: Successful pregnancy after radiation therapy for carcinoma of the cervix. Amer. J. Obstet. Gynec. **88**, 443—446 (1964).

WICHMANN, H., HEINZEL, F.: Physikalische und methodische Probleme bei der Anwendung der Co⁶⁰-Stehfeld- und Bewegungsbestrahlung. Fortschr. Röntgenstr. **94**, 805—817 (1961).

WIDHOLM, O., UNNÉRUS, C., KIVINITTY, K.: Exact measurement of gamma-ray doses in the ureter. Nature (Lond.) **210**, 1076—1077 (1966).

WILDERMUTH, O., MELHORN, G. I.: The management of adenocarcinoma of the cervix. Amer. J. Roentgenol. **89**, 78—82 (1963).

WILLIAMS, I. G., KAZEM, I.: High voltage X-ray therapy as a primary method of treatment for advanced cancer of the cervix uteri. (Hochvolt-Röntgentherapie als Erstmethode der Behandlung des fortgeschrittenen Carcinoms des Collum uteri.) Brit. J. Radiol. **35**, 18—22 (1962).

WILSON, C. W.: Radiocobalt (Co⁶⁰) as a therapeutic alternative to radium. Amer. J. Roentgenol. **65**, 726—736 (1951).

WIMHÖFER, H.: Behandlungsergebnisse des Kollumkarzinoms in der Heidelberger Klinik (1936 bis 1945). Geburtsh. u. Frauenheilk. **12**, 317—327 (1952).

WINDEYER, B. W.: Radiotherapy in modern treatment of female pelvic cancer. J. Obstet. Gynec. **66**, 849—852 (1959).

WITT, J. H.: Zur parametranen Aussaat des Collumcarcinoms. (Histologische Befunde in den Parametrien von Wertheim-Uteri.) IV. Akad. Tagung deutschsprechender Professoren und Privatdozenten für Geburtsh. u. Gynäkol. Athen, 14.—17. 4. 1965.

WOLFF, J. P., DANON, J.: Onze ans de cancer du col utérin à l'Institut Gustave Roussy. (Elf Jahre Collumcarcinom des Uterus am Institut Gustave Roussy.) C. R. Soc. franç. Gynéc. **35**, 455—465 (1965).

— DOUYON, N: Le traitement au cancer du col utérin au stade I. (Die Behandlung des Collumcarcinom im Stadium I.) C. R. Soc. franç. Gynéc. **33**, 15—26 (1963).

— ROUQUETTE, C., DANON, J.: The value of clinical examination for the prognosis of cancer of the uterine cervix. Amer. J. Obstet. Gynec. **93**, 472—478 (1965).

WOLFRAM, W.: Zur Prognose des Beckenwandrezidivs nach Gebärmutterhalskarzinom. Strahlentherapie **73**, 131—141 (1943).

WÜRTHNER, K., HARDE, E.: Bleifilter zum Dosisausgleich bei der kombinierten Radium-Telekobalt-Therapie des Kollumkarzinoms. Electromedica (im Druck).

YAGI, H., DOSSIBAI, J. R., DADABHOY, R., BOMBAY, S.: Obstetric and gynaecological society's silver jubilee oration. Japanese technique of radical operation for carcinoma of the cervix. J. Obstet. Gynaec. India **12**, 311—317 (1962); Ref. Ber. Gynäk. Geburtsh. **85**, 223—224 (1964).

YANAGITA, T., HERMAN, G. G., GUSBERG, S. B.: Autoradiographic studies in cervical cancer before and after a test dose of irradiation. Amer. J. Obstet. Gynec. **95**, 1051—1058 (1966).

Young, H. A.: Combined surgery and irradiation in the treatment of cancer of the cervical stump. (Kombinierte chirurgische und Strahlentherapie bei der Behandlung des Cervixstumpfcarcinoms.) Surg. Gynec. Obstet. **96**, 288—294 (1953).

Young, M. E. J., Batho, H. F.: Tissue dose due to linear radium sources. J. Canad. Ass. Radiol. **15**, 1—6 (1964).

Zacherl, H.: Therapie inoperabler Genitalkarzinome und Rezidive. Wien. klin. Wschr. **1952**, 228—230.

— Die Behandlung der Rezidive nach Kollumkarzinom. Krebsarzt **7**, 210—218 (1952).

Zacutti, A., Turchetti, G.: Aspetti istologici dei linfonodi pelvici dopo trattamento del cancro del collo dell'utero con infiltrazione parametrale di oro colloidale radioattivo. (Histologische Befunde der Beckenlymphknoten nach Behandlung des Collumcarcinoms des Uterus mittels parametraner Infiltrationen radioaktiven kolloidalen Goldes.) Minerva ginec. **12**, 539—545 (1960).

— — Rilievi scansiometrici della pelvi dopo infiltrazione parametrale con oro coloidale radioattivo nel trattamento del cancro del collo dell'utero. (Scansiometrische Befunde am Becken nach parametraner Infiltration mit kolloidalem Radiogold bei der Behandlung des Collumcarcinoms.) Minerva ginec. **12**, 590—592 (1960).

— — Histologische Befunde der Beckenlymphknoten nach Behandlung des Collum-Carcinoms des Uterus mittels parametraner Infiltrationen radioaktiven kolloidalen Goldes. Minerva ginec. **12**, 539—545 (1960); Ref. Ber. ges. Gynäk. Geburtsh. **73**, 40 (1961).

Zanetti, E., Rossi, G. E.: Alcuni relievi sulla telecobaltoterapia nel trattemento delle diffusioni pelviche del carcinoma della portio. (Zur Telekobalttherapie bei der Behandlung der Lymphabflußgebiete des Portio-Carcinoms.) Ann. Ostet. Ginec. **81**, 905—918 (1959).

— Tosca, L.: Metido di telecobaltoterapia nel trattamento del carcinoma del collo dell'utero. (Telekobalttherapie beim Collumcarcinom.) Mineron med. **50**, 3219—3223 (1959); Ann. Ostet. Ginec. **81**, 731—739 (1959).

— — Rossi, G.: Moderni orientamenti technici e clinical della radiumterapia de carcinoma del collo dell'utero. (Gegenwärtige Stellung der Radium-Therapie in der Klinik des Collum-Carcinom.) Ann. Ostet. Ginec. **85**, 267—310 (1963).

Zdansky, E.: Der heutige Stand der Telekobalttherapie. Radiol. clin. (Basel) **29**, 334—346 (1960).

Zeidman, I.: Experimental studies on the spread of cancer in the lymphatic system. IV. Retrograde spread. (Experimentelle Untersuchungen über die Carcinomausbreitung im Lymphgefäßsystem. IV. Retrograde Ausbreitung.) Cancer Res. **19**, 1114—1117 (1959).

Zeitz, H.: Positive Drüsenbefunde bei der Wertheimschen Radikaloperation. Geburtsh. u. Frauenheilk. **12**, 804—809 (1952).

Zerne, S. R. M., Morris, J. McL., Chang, Chu H.: The significance of pain in cervical cancer and its treatment by interstitial infiltration with colloidal radiogold. (Die Bedeutung der Schmerzen beim Cervixcarcinom und ihre Behandlung mit interstitiellen Infiltrationen mit kolloidalem Radiogold.) Amer. J. Obstet. Gynec. **84**, 992—999 (1962).

Zimmer, K., Schwenzer, A. W.: Bericht über 2601 maligne Genitaltumoren der Jahre 1945—1953. Strahlentherapie **112**, 24—44 (1960).

Zoltán, I., Váczy, L., Molnár, R., Sándor, T., Méhes, G.: Unsere Ergebnisse bei der Behandlung des Porticcarcinoms und über grundsätzliche Fragen der Therapie. Magy. Nöorv. Lap. **19**, 1—15 u. dtsch. Zus.fass. 14—14 (1956) [Ungarisch].

— — — — — Über unsere Resultate in der Behandlung des Portiokarzinoms und über die grundsätzlichen Fragen seiner Therapie. Acta med. (Budapest) **10**, 217—232 (1957).

Zum Winkel, K., Becker, J., Jahns, E., Scheurlen, H., Herzfeld, U.: Indikationsstellung und Dosimetrie bei der endolymphatischen Therapie mit J^{131}-Lipiodol. Strahlentherapie **133**, 481—498 (1967).

Zuppinger, A.: Klinische Erfahrungen mit energiereichen Strahlen. In: Betatron und Telekobalttherapie, S. 50—53. Hrsg. von J. Becker, K. E. Scheer. Berlin-Göttingen-Heidelberg: Springer 1958.

— Indikationsstellung zur Hochvoltbestrahlung. Oncologia (Basel) **13**, 142—164 (1960).

— La thérápie á haute énergie et ses indications. Méd. et Hyg. (Genève) **18**, 268 (1960).

— High speed electron beam therapy. Amer. J. Roentgenol. **99**, 932—938 (1967).

— Poretti, G.: Symposium on high-energy electrons. Berlin-Heidelberg-New York: Springer 1965.

V. Maligne Tumoren der Tuben, Ovarien, Parametrien und der Ligamenta rotunda

Von

W. Dietz

Mit 13 Abbildungen

Für alle malignen Tumoren der Tuben, Ovarien, Parametrien und der Ligamenta rotunda sind chirurgische Maßnahmen die Therapie der Wahl und sollten so früh wie möglich durchgeführt werden. Die Strahlentherapie kann bei den operablen Fällen dieser Erkrankungen immer nur eine Zusatz- oder Ergänzungsbehandlung darstellen. In besonders gelagerten Fällen können darüber hinaus durch präoperative Bestrahlungen und nach den neuen Ergebnissen von SPECHTER u. Mitarb. auch durch präoperative Behandlung mit cytostatischen Substanzen die Voraussetzungen zu operativen Maßnahmen verbessert werden. Grundsätzlich ist aber auch bei den operablen Tumoren der Tuben, Ovarien, Parametrien und Ligamenta rotunda die zusätzliche Strahlentherapie ein wichtiger, u. E. unabdingbarer Bestandteil der Gesamtbehandlung. Weiterhin fällt der Strahlentherapie auch bei den inkurablen Tumoren der Tuben, Ovarien, Parametrien und der Ligamenta rotunda die große Aufgabe zu, noch palliativ wirksam zu werden, — wenn auch oft nur für kurze Zeit — lebensverlängernd zu wirken und vor allen Dingen den Patientinnen die noch verbleibende Lebenszeit einigermaßen lebenswert zu machen.

1. Topographisch-anatomische Vorbemerkungen

Die *Tuben* und *Ligamenta rotunda* sowie die *Ligamenta ovarii propria* sind strangförmige Gebilde, die intraligamentär, extraperitoneal zwischen den *Ligamenta lata* — Bauchfellduplikaturen mit einem vorderen und hinteren Blatt, die sich als Fortsetzung der Uterusserosa zwischen Uterus und Becken ausspannen — liegen.

Die *Tuben* sind runde, aus Mucosa, Muscularis und Serosa bestehende schlauchartige Hohlorgane, die zwischen den Ligamenta rotunda und ovarii propria und etwas höher als diese vom Uterusfundus seitwärts ziehen und sich mit ihrem freien aufgefransten Ende trichterartig in die Bauchhöhle öffnen. Es werden daran drei Abschnitte unterschieden: der interstitielle Abschnitt innerhalb der Uterusmuskulatur, der isthmische Abschnitt = medialer engerer Anteil und der ampulläre Abschnitt = lateraler weiterer Anteil.

Die *Ligamenta rotunda* verlaufen bogenförmig vom Funduswinkel des Uterus an der Innenfläche des vorderen Blattes der Ligamenta lata zur Beckenwand, durch den Leistenkanal und äußeren Leistenring nach außen und spalten sich im subcutanen Gewebe der großen Labien auf. Sie bestehen aus Bindegewebe und glatter, aus dem Uterus in sie übergehender Muskulatur, können außerordentlich verschieden stark sein und verändern sich in der Gravidität.

Die *Ligamenta ovarii propria*, durch die die Ovarien am Uterus aufgehängt sind, zeigen ähnlichen Bau wie die Ligamenta rotunda, sind aber weniger muskulös und verlaufen in der Innenfläche des hinteren Blattes des Ligamentum latum. Entwicklungsgeschichtlich stellen Ligamenta rotunda und ovarii propria Abschnitte des Urnierenleistenbandes dar.

Das *Parametrium* ist das Gewebe, das sich zwischen den beiden Ligamenta lata beiderseits von der Cervix uteri bis zur Beckenwand — nach oben bis zum inneren Mm, nach unten bis zu den seitlichen Scheidengewölben reichend — ausbreitet. Es gehört zum

Beckenbindegewebe, das retroperitoneal von beiden Nieren bis zum Beckenboden reicht und zwischen dem Peritoneum parietale und der seitlichen Bauch- bzw. Beckenwand liegt. Stoeckel vergleicht das Beckenbindegewebe mit dem Kleister, mit dem eine Tapete (Peritoneum) auf eine Wand (Beckenwand) geklebt ist. In diesem Gewebe sind extraperitoneal die Nieren, Ureteren, die inneren Genitalien und teilweise das Rectum eingelagert. Dort, wo Organe von dem Gewebe fixiert werden, verdichtet es sich und trägt besondere Namen, — so — neben dem Uterus gelegenes = parametranes Gewebe. Wichtig ist im Hinblick auf die Ausbreitung von Entzündungen und Tumoren, daß das ganze Beckenbindegewebe eine „Gewebseinheit" bildet. *Intraligamentär* liegen weiterhin die *rudimentären Gebilde* der inneren weiblichen Genitalien, das *Epoophoron* oder *Parovarium.*

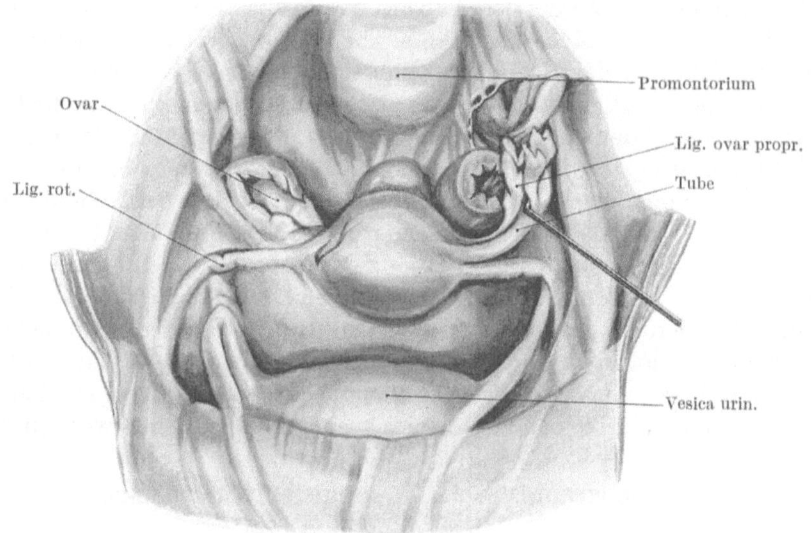

Abb. 1

das dem cranialen Teil, — das *Paroophoron*, das dem kaudalen Teil der Urniere entspricht, und der Wolffsche oder Gartnersche Gang. Dieser bleibt als Rest des Urnierenganges in einzelnen Abschnitten bei ca. 20 % der Frauen erhalten, tritt am Tubenwinkel in den Uterus ein, verläuft in dessen Seitenkante oder intraligamentär neben dem Uterus, tritt in Höhe des inneren Mm in die Cervix ein und verläuft in dieser bis in Höhe des Scheidengewölbes. Alle Reste der Urniere haben einschichtiges Flimmerepithel.

Die normal ausgebildeten *Ovarien* haben Form und Gestalt kleiner Pflaumen (Stoeckel, 1960). Ihre Oberfläche ist um so unregelmäßiger und höckriger, je mehr Follikelnarben bestehen, je älter also die Trägerin ist. Auf dem Schnitt sind die äußere Rindenschicht und die innere Markschicht zu erkennen. Die Ovarien stehen mit der Längsachse sagittal und liegen im allgemeinen in Höhe der Linea terminalis. Sie sind in die hinteren Blätter der Ligamenta lata so eingefügt, daß ein kleiner Abschnitt intraligamentär liegt, der größere Teil über die hintere Ligamentplatte ohne peritoneale Bekleidung in die Bauchhöhle hineinreicht, also intraperitoneal liegt. Das zum intraligamentären Teil — dem Hilus ovarii — ziehende, intraligamentäre, die Ovarialgefäße einscheidende Gewebe ist das Mesovarium. Die Ovarien werden von den ampullären aufgefransten Tubenabschnitten umfaßt und sind am Uterus durch die Ligamenta ovarii propria, an der seitlichen Beckenwand durch die Ligamenta infundibulo pelvica lose und damit verschieblich aufgehängt. Die Ligg. infundibulo pelvica sind in Abb. 1 im Bereich der Ovarien bzw. der Tubenenden gelegen und von diesen überlagert zu denken.

2. Klinik

(Einteilung, Häufigkeit, Histologie, Symptomatologie und Diagnostik, Ausbreitung und Metastasierung, Altersverteilung und Ätiologie)

Im Hinblick auf die außerordentliche Seltenheit der malignen Tumoren der Tuben und noch mehr der malignen Tumoren der Parametrien und Ligamenta rotunda und um einen ganz „zeitnahen" Überblick zu erhalten, habe ich an eine Reihe mir bekannter Strahlentherapeuten von Frauenkliniken des deutschen Sprachgebietes, von denen keine entsprechenden Veröffentlichungen in den letzten Jahren vorlagen, die Bitte gerichtet, mir für diese Abhandlung ihre bezüglichen Beobachtungen zur Verfügung zu stellen. Der Bitte sind eine Reihe von Kollegen nachgekommen, denen ich dafür sehr herzlich danke[1].

a) Die malignen Tumoren der Tuben

Die malignen Geschwülste der Tuben sind sehr seltene Erkrankungen des weiblichen Genitalapparates und machen im Weltschrifttum noch nicht 1% aller bösartigen Geschwülste der weiblichen Genitalorgane aus.

Histologisch werden das primäre Carcinom, das primäre Chorionepitheliom und das primäre Sarkom der Tuben unterschieden. Außerdem werden in seltenen Fällen metastatische Tumoren, insbesondere von primären Ovarialcarcinomen, in den Tuben gefunden.

α) Häufigkeit
αα) Tubencarcinom

Lange Zeit wurde das Vorkommen primärer bösartiger Geschwülste der Tuben überhaupt bestritten. Noch 1899 unterstrich SCHROEDER diese Meinung, obwohl schon 1886 von ORTMANN das erste primäre Carcinom der Tuben beschrieben worden war. In späterer Zeit erfolgten dann laufend neue Veröffentlichungen über primäre Tubencarcinome, so daß bis heute dessen ursprüngliche Seltenheit einer wachsenden Häufigkeit gewichen ist. Im Jahre 1895 führten SÄNGER und BARTH 18 Fälle von Tubencarcinomen aus der Weltliteratur auf, 1902 ZANGEMEISTER 51, 1910 FROMME und HEYNEMANN schon 120 Fälle. In der Zeit von 1952—1958 vergrößerte sich die Zahl der Beobachtungen von primären Tubencarcinomen von 559 Fällen (WIENINGER, 1953) auf 815 Fälle (GUIXA und CEBORELLO, 1959). In der Zwischenzeit sind eine ganze Reihe von weiteren Veröffentlichungen über Tubencarcinome in der Weltliteratur erschienen, unter anderem berichtet ROSS 1962 über 8 eigene Fälle, die er von 1931—1960 beobachtete, KRUGMANN 1960 über 2 eigene Fälle, KRUSCHWITZ 1964 und LOHMEYER 1964 über je 1 Fall. Damit scheint der Schluß erlaubt, daß das primäre Tubencarcinom früher sehr oft nicht diagnostiziert und damit mehr verkannt wurde als selten war.

Tabelle 1 soll, unter Benutzung einer Zusammenstellung von WIENINGER, einer Reihe weiterer Veröffentlichungen, einer persönlichen Mitteilung von ADLER aus dem Jahre 1959 und unserer eigenen Zahlen, einen Eindruck über die prozentuale Häufigkeit des Tubencarcinoms vermitteln.

Der Anhang der Tabelle 1 bringt noch die absoluten Zahlen der Beobachtungen von Tubencarcinomen an einer Reihe deutscher Kliniken (persönliche Mitteilungen), wobei hier die prozentuale Berechnung nicht möglich ist, da die Angaben über die Gesamtzahlen der in entsprechender Zeit beobachteten Genitalcarcinome nicht zur Verfügung stehen.

ββ) Tubenchorionepitheliom

Der Häufigkeit in der Weltliteratur nach folgt auf das Tubencarcinom das primäre Chorionepitheliom mit 63 Fällen (DIETRICH und PETSCH, MUJIKA, HEISS, CRISP und MISELLI). HEISS fand eine Frau mit primärem Chorionepitheliom nach Tubarabort bei 540 Laparotomien (0,18%) wegen Extrauterinschwangerschaften.

---

1 Die Namen der Kollegen und Institute werden an den entsprechenden Stellen genannt.

Tabelle 1. *Häufigkeit des Tubencarcinoms*

Klinik	Zeitraum	Autor	Gesamtzahl Gen.-ca's	Tuben-ca's	(%)
10 Kliniken	5—45 Jahre	Zusammenstellung Wieninger (1952), Graz	24835	70	0,29
UFK Kiel	25 Jahre	Huber (1952)	3410	23	0,6
UFK Leipzig	16 Jahre	Behrens (1954)	6120	29	0,47
UFK Heidelberg	15 Jahre	Runge/Zeitz (1956)	2401	3	0,10
2 amerikanische Kliniken	9 Jahre	Frankel (1956)	1122	10	0,90
UFK Prag	24 Jahre	Dvorák (1958)	6755	12	0,18
Städtische Frauenklinik Dortmund	6 Jahre	Busse/Soergel (1959)	800	1	0,13
Städtische Frauenklinik Aachen	10 Jahre	Kayser (1959)	512	4	0,80
UFK Freiburg	25 Jahre	Dietz/Lohse (1961)	3420	9	0,26
Frauenspital Basel	15 Jahre	Adler (1959)[+] pers. Mitteilung	1141	0	0,0
Summe 19 Kliniken			50516	161	0,32
Weitere (persönliche) Mitteilungen über Tubencarcinome					
UFK Erlangen	30 Jahre	Weisshaar (1960)[+]		3	
FK Med. Ak. Düsseldorf	30 Jahre	Dibbelt (1960)[+]		3	
UFK Tübingen	12 Jahre	Spechter (1960)[+]		6	
UFK Göttingen	7 Jahre	Hosemann (1959)[+]		4	
UFK Heidelberg	8 Jahre	Zeitz (1959)[+]		6	
St. Georg Hamburg	15 Jahre	Gauwerky (1959)[+]		12 + 1 Sarkom + 1 Carcino-sarkom	
Summe				34	

[+] Die Namen der Kollegen und Institute, die mir ihre Zahlen zur Verfügung gestellt haben, sind in der Tabelle mit [+] gekennzeichnet.

Der beobachtete prozentuale Anteil des Tubencarcinoms am Gesamtkrankengut an Genitalcarcinomen überschreitet 1% bei keinem Autor. In der amerikanischen Literatur wird im übrigen die Häufigkeit des Tubencarcinoms mit 0,5—1,09% aller Genitalcarcinome angegeben (Frankel, Johnson, Weekes, Anz und Whiting).

Meine Rundfrage ergab, daß an den 7 Kliniken, die mir ihre Ergebnisse mitteilten, in Zeiträumen bis zu 30 Jahren kein Chorionepitheliom der Tuben beobachtet wurde, und auch an der Universitäts-Frauenklinik Freiburg wurde ein solcher Tumor in den letzten 25 Jahren nicht gesehen.

γγ) Tubensarkom

Das primäre Tubensarkom ist mit 30 Fällen in der Weltliteratur (Abrams, Kasal und Hobbs) der seltenste maligne Tumor der Tuben. Auf meine Umfrage erhielt ich lediglich von Gauwerky (St. Georg-Hamburg) die Mitteilung, daß er außer einem Tubencarcinosarkom (Tabelle 1) auch ein Tubensarkom beobachtet hat. Die anderen 6 Kliniken und auch die Universitäts-Frauenklinik Freiburg beobachteten kein Tubensarkom in den letzten Jahren oder Jahrzehnten.

β) Einteilung nach klinischen Gesichtspunkten

Eine Einteilung der malignen Tubentumoren nach klinischen Gesichtspunkten konnten wir in der Literatur nicht finden. Eine solche Einteilung ist im Hinblick auf die relative Seltenheit dieser Tumoren auch kein dringendes Erfordernis. Zweifellos würde aber die

Zusammenordnung und vergleichende Betrachtung von Einzelmitteilungen durch eine solche Einteilung erleichtert. Man könnte sich — entsprechend einer Anregung von ZUPPINGER (persönliche Mitteilung, 1968) — durchaus einer auf die besonderen Verhältnisse bei den Tubentumoren zugeschnittenen weitgehenden Analogie zur Einteilung der Ovarialtumoren nach klinischen Gesichtspunkten (S. 320) bedienen.

γ) Histologie
αα) Tubencarcinom

In der Mehrzahl der Fälle zeigt das primäre Tubencarcinom histologisch papilläre Gebilde, die aus einem zarten Bindegewebsgerüst bestehen und von zumeist mehrschichtigem atypischem Epithel verschiedener Ausreifung überzogen sind. Es handelt sich dabei meist um papillomatöse Adenome der Tubenschleimhaut, seltener Epitheliome des Wolffschen Ganges, Teratome und undifferenzierte Endotheliome (GUYOMAR, 1961). Infolge der Tatsache, daß die dünne Tubenwand einem raumfordernden Prozeß leicht nachgibt, ist die Tendenz der Carcinomelemente zum Tiefenwachstum anfänglich zumeist nicht sehr ausgeprägt. Solide Tumoren können entstehen, wenn die Epithelmassen an der Oberfläche der papillären Gebilde rasch wachsen und das Stromagerüst zum Schwinden bringen. Dann dringen die Zellmassen zumeist energisch in die Tubenwand ein, substituieren die glatte Muskulatur und bilden alveoläre Herde. An der Peripherie des Herdes kann dann ein endolymphatisches oder ein plexiformes Wachstum einsetzen, wobei die Krebszellen zumeist ihren niederen Reifegrad beibehalten.

Die häufigste Form des Tubencarcinoms ist das Adenocarcinom, aber auch die Entwicklung von Plattenepithelcarcinomen und von schleimbildenden Carcinomen (HASELHORST, 1928; THAISZ, 1940) sowie riesenzellenähnliche Gebilde sind beschrieben worden. Neben den papillären und alveolären Strukturen — wobei häufig Mischformen zu beobachten sind — gibt es auch weitgehend undifferenziertes, auf den ersten Blick sarkomatös anmutendes Geschwulstgewebe mit stärkerer Kernfärbung und häufigeren Mitosen.

Carcinosarkome sind äußerst selten — es wurden bisher 9 Fälle (einschließlich des Falles von GAUWERKY, 1960; Tabelle 1) beschrieben — und zeigen in ihrem Aufbau sowohl sarkomatöse, von der Tubenwand ausgehende, wie auch vom Epithel ausgehende carcinomatöse Elemente (KLOC, CAVALLERO u. RENO ROSSI). Sie werden als Kollisionstumoren aufgefaßt, die unter demselben onkogenetischen Faktor entstehen.

ββ) Tubenchorionepitheliom

Histologisch wird unter primärem Chorionepitheliom der Tube ein lokal primärer Zottenkrebs nach Tubargravidität verstanden. Histogenetisch ist das Chorionepitheliom kein Primärtumor, da es nicht aus Organgewebe besteht, sondern sekundär aus Trophoplastmassen, also fetalen Elementen entstanden ist. So ergibt sich, daß die Ursprünglichkeit des Chorionepithelioms nicht in der Gewebszugehörigkeit zu suchen ist, sondern in der Lokalität. Im histologischen Schnitt finden sich im Stroma der Tubenwand destruierend vorwachsende, atypische Chorionepithelien, z. T. vom Syncytium, z. T. von der Langhansschen Zellschicht abstammend. Diese Epithelien zeigen überall häufig Mitosen und wachsen in den Blutgefäßen vor, die dann „wie mit Epithelien vollgestopft" imponieren. Dadurch kommt es zu Blutungen und Nekrosen in der Tubenwand. Die atypischen, stark proliferierenden Zotten durchbrechen vielfach die Serosa. DE SNOO und HEISS beschreiben allerdings auch Chorionepitheliome der Tuben, die keine Zotten aufweisen, sondern nur atypische Trophoblastelemente.

Beweisend für die Malignität des Wachstums ist die massenhafte choriale Invasion in kleinem Zellverband und das Auftreten von Langhansschen Zellen in Nestern, wobei diese chorialen Zellen grobe Atypien, häufig Mitosen und Polymorphien aufweisen. In manchen Herden ist dabei das Epithel vacuolisiert.

γγ) Tubensarkom

Histologisch ist für das Sarkom die Vielgestaltigkeit der Zellen und der teilweise Reichtum an Riesenzellen charakteristisch. In den meisten Fällen handelt es sich um Rund- oder Spindelzellsarkome. Bei den bis 1946 beschriebenen 22 Fällen handelte es sich nach Scheffey, Lang und Nugent (1946) um 9 Spindelzellsarkome, 4 Rundzellsarkome, 2 Myosarkome, 1 Riesenzellen- und 1 Myxosarkom. 5 Tubensarkome mußten wegen mangelnder histologischer Diagnose in dieser Einteilung unberücksichtigt bleiben.

Das Parenchym besteht aus zahlreichen wirr angeordneten Zellen mit unregelmäßiger, runder, polygonaler, oft auch spindeliger Form, die verschiedene Größe haben und sehr dicht aneinander liegen. Trotz Kernreichtums hat das Parenchym einen lockeren Gesamtaufbau. Nirgends sind alveoläre oder papilläre Bilder zu sehen. Das Cytoplasma kann spärlich entwickelt und die Zellgrenzen können verwischt sein. Die Kerne zeigen reichlich Mitosen, Pyknosen und Chromatinanomalien. Riesenzellen treten beim Tubensarkom nicht so häufig auf wie sonst beim Sarkom. König beschreibt ein fibroplastisches, großzelliges Spindelsarkom mit Inseln von Epitheloidzellensarkom. Die große Vielgestaltigkeit des histologischen Bildes beim Tubensarkom führte dazu, daß eine Vielzahl der als Tubensarkome beschriebenen Fälle nicht ohne weiteres als solche anerkannt wurden. Der Streit der Meinungen ist Folge einmal der Ähnlichkeit epithelialer und mesenchymaler maligner Neoplasmen, zum anderen auch der histogenetisch verschiedenen Deutung (Falge, 1953; König, 1957). Von 23 bis 1953 veröffentlichten Fällen blieben nur 13 ohne Widerspruch (Falge, 1953).

δ) Symptomatologie und Diagnostik

Die Symptomatologie der primären malignen Erkrankungen der Tuben ist außerordentlich vielgestaltig. Die einzelnen Symptome sind weitgehend unspezifisch für eine maligne Erkrankung im Bereich der Adnexe, die klinische Diagnose ist deshalb außerordentlich schwierig. Es liegen aber eine ganze Reihe von Mitteilungen darüber vor, daß die Diagnose vor der Operation gestellt wurde (Islitzer, 1952; Wehner, 1953; Leonhard, 1956; Czipri und Tombor, 1958; Froewis und Kremer, 1958; Israel, Crisp und Adrian, 1954; Wimhöfer u. a.) und vor allem unter Ausnutzung der Möglichkeiten der Cytodiagnostik immer häufiger gestellt wird. So wurden alle drei Fälle von Schwach präoperativ exakt diagnostiziert.

Über die Möglichkeiten der Röntgendiagnostik mit der Hysterosalpingographie bei Tubentumoren liegen lediglich für das Tubencarcinom Mitteilungen vor und werden dort besprochen (S. 315). Die dort angestellten Überlegungen über diagnostische Möglichkeiten mit der Pneumopelvigraphie, Arteriographie und Lymphographie gelten grundsätzlich für alle Tubentumoren.

αα) Tubencarcinom

Als wichtigstes und charakteristischstes Symptom für ein Tubencarcinom beschreibt Latzko einen bernsteingelben, nach Schwach (1961) mehr gelbbraun sanguinolenten Ausfluß, der nach Islitzer (1952) allerdings nur zeitweise im Frühstadium und nach Kremer und Ulm (1955) nur in 28% der Fälle beobachtet wird. Wenn nach einer Abrasio dieser Fluor weiter besteht, ohne daß ein Anhalt für ein Malignom des Uterus gegeben ist, so ist dies ein weitgehend sicherer Hinweis dafür, daß ein Tubencarcinom oder auch ein Ovarialmalignom vorhanden ist, wobei die Tatsache, daß der bernsteingelbe Fluor auch beim Ovarialmalignom vorhanden sein kann, nur differentialdiagnostisch und nicht therapeutisch von Interesse ist. Auch Metro- und Menorrhagien, die nach carcinomnegativer Abrasio weiterbestehen, legen den dringenden Verdacht auf ein Tubencarcinom nahe (Wieninger, Leonhard, Schneider, Boschann, Czipri u. Tombor, Johnson u. a.). Schmerzen können ganz fehlen, werden aber von den meisten Patienten angegeben (Schneider, Wieninger, Boschann, Götz).

Plötzlich auftretendes oder auch langsam sich entwickelndes Druckgefühl im Unterbauch und auch die Zunahme des Leibesumfanges sind späte Symptome, die sich, wie

Johnson und Amos grundsätzlich für alle Symptome annehmen, erst nach Verschluß des Ostiums abdominale tubae entwickeln. Der Palpationsbefund beim Tubencarcinom ist nicht charakteristisch. Zumeist kann nur die Diagnose Adnextumor gestellt werden. An ein Malignom muß aber immer gedacht werden. Bei unklarer Genese des Adnextumors fordern deshalb eine Reihe von Autoren u. a. Pierrot, Götz und Johnson insbesondere bei Patientinnen im klimakterischen Alter eine Probelaparatomie zur endgültigen Klärung. Sicher ist, daß das Tubencarcinom sich lange völlig symptomlos entwickeln kann. Unter diesem Gesichtspunkt ist die Beobachtung von Kruschwitz (1964) besonders interessant, der ein primäres doppelseitiges Tubencarcinom erst histologisch in makroskopisch unverdächtigen Tuben feststellte, wobei der Anlaß zur Exstirpation des Uterus und der Adnexe die Perforation des Uterus im Verlauf einer erneuten, nach zwei vorausgegangenen ergebnislosen Abrasionen wegen blutigen Fluors war.

Antonowitsch, Wieninger, Bret und Legrand betonen den Wert der Hysterosalpingographie für die präoperative Diagnose eines Tubencarcinoms, weisen aber darauf hin, daß durch anatomische Verhältnisse bedingt, auch mit dem Versagen der Hysterosalpingographie gerechnet werden muß. Antonowitsch (1950) stellt als typisch für das Carcinom im Röntgenbild heraus, den gestielten soliden Tumor im Tubenlumen und warzenförmige papilläre Wucherungen. Differentialdiagnostisch sind natürlich benigne Tumoren und die Endometriose in Betracht zu ziehen, während die Tubentuberkulose sich im Röntgenbild grundsätzlich vom Tubencarcinom unterscheidet (Antonowitsch, 1950). Guyomar lehnt die Hysterosalpingographie wegen der Gefahr der Verschleppung von Krebszellen ab und diskutiert die diagnostischen Möglichkeiten der Douglaskopie und Arteriographie. Theoretisch sind u. E. auch mit der Pneumopelvigraphie (= Gynäkographie) und der Lymphographie u. U. wichtige diagnostische Hinweise zu gewinnen. Entsprechende Mitteilungen haben wir aber in der Literatur nicht gefunden.

Den größten diagnostischen Wert hat nach den Erfahrungen der letzten Jahre die cytologische Untersuchung des Vaginalsmears nach Papanicolaou. Damit jedoch ein positiver Befund im Vaginalsmear beim primären Tubencarcinom zustande kommen kann, müssen nach Ennker (1957) 5 Bedingungen erfüllt sein:

1. Ausreichende Sekretbildung und celluläre Desquamationsvorgänge in der befallenen Tube.

2. Verschlossenes Ostium abdominale tubae.

3. Durchgängigkeit der Pars isthmica tubae und Pars interstitialis tubae.

4. Abgang von tubarem Fluor zum Zeitpunkt der Abnahme.

5. Strenge Bettruhe, um optimale Ergebnisse bei vaginaler Entnahme erreichen zu können.

Selbstverständlich schließt ein negativer cytologischer Befund im Vaginalsmear eine carcinomatöse Erkrankung der Tube nicht aus, dagegen ist ein positiver cytologischer Befund bei carcinomnegativer Abrasio eine absolute Indikation zur sofortigen, radikalen, chirurgischen Intervention (Claus, Besserer, Bret und Legrand).

Den Wert der cytologischen Untersuchung unterstreichen auch die Mitteilungen von Freese (1957), der bei 12 Fällen 8mal, Fidler und Lock (1954), die bei 4 Fällen von Tubencarcinomen 3mal einen positiven Vaginalsmear gefunden haben.

Ennker gibt an, daß in den Jahren 1947—1955 26mal präoperativ die Diagnose gestellt worden ist, davon 13mal mit Hilfe der Cytologie.

Eine weitere Möglichkeit der präoperativen Diagnostik des Tubencarcinoms oder überhaupt maligner Tubentumoren ist die Punktion des Adnextumors — die Guyomar (1961) ebenfalls wegen der Gefahr der Verschleppung von Krebszellen ablehnt — und die cytologische Auswertung des Punktates.

Bei carcinompositivem Befund muß das Ovarialcarcinom differentialdiagnostisch in Erwägung gezogen werden, jedoch ist auch hier die exakte Diagnose nicht entscheidend, denn die nachgewiesene Malignität ist eine absolute Indikation zum chirurgischen Handeln (Ennker, Kremer und Ulm). Trotz aller diagnostischen Hilfsmittel der heutigen

Zeit wird doch nur etwa in einem Viertel der Fälle von Tubencarcinomen die Diagnose ante operationem gestellt und das Carcinom wird zumeist intra operationem, oft auch erst später bei der histologischen Aufarbeitung des Operationsmaterials entdeckt. Zur Vermeidung von Relaparotomien ist darum bei jeder Salpingektomie eine genaue makroskopische Untersuchung des Tubeninhaltes zu fordern (Guixa und Cebollero). Wieninger (1953) geht sogar so weit, die Anfertigung von Schnellgefrierschnitten während der Operation bei allen Salpingektomien zu empfehlen.

ββ) Tubenchorionepitheliom

Auch hier fehlt ein typisches Symptombild. Die Symptomatologie entspricht grundsätzlich der einer intakten oder abortierten Tubenschwangerschaft. Wie beim primären Tubencarcinom ist die klinische Diagnose des tubaren Chorionepithelioms sehr schwer, wenn nicht gar unmöglich (Neuweiler). Den ersten Anhaltspunkt für das Bestehen eines Tubenchorionepithelioms muß die Anamnese geben, nämlich eine vorher bestandene Tubargravidität bzw. blutiger Ausfluß nach vorheriger Amenorrhoe.

Weiterhin können genitale Blutungen mäßigen Grades bestehen, heftige krampfartige Schmerzen im Bereich der erkrankten Seite durch Tubenwehen, Kreuzschmerzen, Übelkeit und Brechreiz. Der Tastbefund ergibt eine undeutlich abgrenzbare druckschmerzhafte Resistenz, manchmal auch eine lokale Auftreibung der Tube, ein Befund, wie er jedoch bei den meisten Tubenerkrankungen bestehen kann. Der Uterus aber ist dabei weich wie bei einer jungen Gravidität. Die Abrasio ergibt ein Korpusendometrium wie bei einer Extrauterinschwangerschaft. Von entscheidener Bedeutung sind — wie grundsätzlich beim Chorionepitheliom — die Aschheim-Zondeksche Reaktion und die quantitative Bestimmung des Prolangehaltes im Urin, der beim Chorionepitheliom bedeutend höher ist als bei einer Tubargravidität (Heiss, 1954).

Im fortgeschrittenen Stadium können die Patientinnen mit den Symptomen einer intraabdominalen Blutung in Behandlung kommen. Die Douglas-Punktion ergibt dann zumeist frische Blutkoagel, weil die Blutung im allgemeinen aus dem Tubenende erfolgt. Im Röntgenbild des Thorax können dann schon typische Rundschatten, wie sie als Lungenmetastasen relativ häufig beim uterinen Chorionepitheliom gefunden werden, vorhanden sein. Eine exakte, präoperative klinische Diagnose wird in der uns zugänglichen Literatur nicht mitgeteilt. Zumeist sind es Zufallsbefunde, klinisch wird eine Tubargravidität diagnostiziert und bei der Operation ein Chorionepitheliom der Tube gefunden.

γγ) Tubensarkom

Die Symptomatologie des Tubensarkoms deckt sich weitgehend oder praktisch völlig mit der Symptomatologie insbesondere des Tubencarcinoms. Als Hauptsymptome werden Blutungen oder blutiger Fluor, Schmerzen auf der erkrankten Seite und Zunahme des Leibesumfanges (König, 1957) sowie Miktionsbeschwerden (Scheffey, Lang, Nugent) beschrieben. Der Tastbefund ergibt nach Reiber (1939) einen Tumor von geringer Druckschmerzhaftigkeit oder eine schwer verschiebliche Resistenz im Bereich der erkrankten Adnexe.

Die Möglichkeiten, zu einer weiteren diagnostischen Abklärung zu kommen, decken sich mit den beim Tubencarcinom beschriebenen Maßnahmen.

ε) Ausbreitung und Metastasierung
αα) Tubencarcinom

Das Tubencarcinom ist in der weitaus größten Zahl der Fälle in der Ampulle lokalisiert. Beim Einbruch des Carcinoms in die Tubenwand wächst es in die Lymphbahn ein, so daß es frühzeitig zu lymphogenen Metastasierungen kommt. Dabei kann die Ausbreitung auf drei verschiedenen Wegen erfolgen, entweder entlang den großen Gefäßen, aufsteigend in das große Becken und den Bauchraum oder tief in das kleine Becken hinein und — allerdings sehr selten — über das Ligamentum rotundum in die Leistenbeuge. Auch die Parametrien werden nach Neuweiler bei der lymphogenen Ausbreitung des Carcinoms nur selten befallen, während sich im Ovar und Corpus uteri häufiger Metastasen manifestieren. Das Carcinom kann sich auch intracanaliculär ausbreiten, wenn seine Bildungsstätte nicht vorher durch salpingitische Veränderungen von der freien Bauchhöhle und dem Corpus uteri getrennt wurde. Es können dann Carcinombröckel sowohl in den Bauchraum als in das Cavum uteri gelangen und dort Implantationsmetastasen setzen. Von Vladar (1955) wurden sogar in der Vagina solche Implantationsmetastasen gefunden, ohne daß das Carcinom im Endometrium nachgewiesen werden konnte. Eine weitere Möglichkeit der Ausbreitung des Carcinoms per continuitatem ist die carcinomatöse Infiltration der Tubenwand und das dann mögliche Übergreifen auf die Nachbarschaft.

Das Eindringen des Carcinoms in die Blutgefäße ermöglicht die Aussaat mit dem Blutstrom in die verschiedensten Organe. Am häufigsten werden Metastasierungen in Lunge und Leber gefunden. In einem der von uns beobachteten Fälle — die, wie seit 1950 alle Carcinome an der Universitäts-Frauenklinik Freiburg, systematisch einer Röntgenuntersuchung der Thoraxorgane unterzogen wurden — konnten wir Metastasen an den Rippen und in der Lunge feststellen.

Beiderseitige carcinomatöse Erkrankungen der Tuben kommen in etwa 30 % der Fälle vor (Boschann, 1952, $33^1/_3$ % ; Wieninger, 1953, 25 % ; Nürnberger, 1932, ca. 30 %). Wenn von Huber, Boschann und Götz auch für das doppelseitige Tubencarcinom neuerdings eine multizentrische Genese im Sinne eines Systemcarcinoms diskutiert wird, so ist doch wahrscheinlich für die meisten doppelseitigen Erkrankungen gültig, daß das Carcinom sich primär in einer Tube entwickelte und dann eine Metastasierung in die andere Tube stattgefunden hat. Die These wird gestützt durch die Tatsache, daß sich in der „zweiten" Tube oft Carcinombröckel ohne Zusammenhang mit dem Tubenepithel nachweisen lassen.

Das verschiedene Wachstum des Carcinoms kann zu den verschiedensten Erscheinungsformen führen. Die Tube kann äußerlich vollkommen glatt sein mit einer lokalisierten Auftreibung zumeist in der Ampulle, die Mannskopfgröße erreichen kann. Im Frühstadium kann eine solche Tube zur Bauchhöhle hin geöffnet sein, später ist sie jedoch in der Regel verschlossen, mit markigen Bröckeln und Blut oder einer serös-sanguinolenten Flüssigkeit gefüllt. Das Carcinom kann sich natürlich auch sekundär in einer primär verschlossenen Tube, einer Saktosalpinx, entwickeln. Andererseits kann eine vom Carcinom befallene Tube insgesamt stark gehöckert und mit der Umgebung zu einem Tumorkonglomerat verschmolzen sein. Bei der vaginalen und rectalen Untersuchung ist die Tube in solchen Fällen nur selten noch abzugrenzen. Meistens jedoch imponiert der Tumor als prallelastisches, mehr oder weniger fixiertes Gebilde, so daß — worauf wir schon hingewiesen haben — palpatorisch im allgemeinen nur die Diagnose „Adnextumor" gestellt werden kann.

ββ) Tubenchorionepitheliom

Das Chorionepitheliom der Tube durchbricht das Wandstroma rasch und findet im allgemeinen schnell an die Blutgefäße Anschluß. So kommt es sehr bald zur hämatogenen Aussaat in die verschiedenen Organe, insbesondere in die Lungen, die Leber und das Gehirn.

Andererseits ist die intracanaliculäre Metastasierung in den Uterus und die Vagina sowohl als auch in der anderen Richtung in die freie Bauchhöhle möglich.

Der Primärtumor beschränkt sich im allgemeinen auf die Tube, wobei der Sitz meistens im Isthmus tubae liegt. Er kann Apfelgröße erreichen und ist durch die Eröffnung der Blutgefäße in der Regel durchsetzt von multiplen Hämorrhagien. Er sieht dadurch rötlich bis violett-bräunlich aus und zeigt eine schwammige Konsistenz bei höckeriger Oberfläche.

γγ) Tubensarkom

Infolge des im allgemeinen langsamen Wachstums des Tubensarkoms ist die Tendenz zur Metastasierung nicht so ausgesprochen wie beim Tubencarcinom und Tubenchorionepitheliom. Bevorzugt bei der Metastasierung sind die großen Organe des Thorax- und Bauchraumes. Scheffey, Lang und Nugent geben an, daß von 22 Fällen nur 3 an Metastasen zugrunde gingen. Makroskopisch ähnelt die befallene Tube dem Befund beim Tubencarcinom. In der umschrieben aufgetriebenen Tube — wobei die Auftreibung Kindskopfgröße erreichen kann — werden weiche, grobgekörnte Gewebsteile, teilweise mit blasigem Aussehen (Reiber, König) gefunden. Das Ostium abdominale tubae kann verschlossen sein und das ganze ein retortenähnliches Aussehen haben (Reiber, Scheffey, Lang und Nugent).

ζ) Altersverteilung

Das Prädilektionsalter für das Auftreten des primären *Tubencarcinoms* ist die 5. Lebensdekade, wobei sich aus dem Weltschrifttum ein Durchschnittsalter der befallenen Frauen um 46 Jahre, also um die Zeit des Klimakteriums, errechnen läßt. Allerdings können auch junge Frauen — offenbar aber nie vor der Pubertät — und alte Frauen von Tubencarcinomen befallen werden. In der Literatur liegen Berichte über 18jährige Mädchen und 80jährige Frauen mit Tubencarcinomen vor.

Das *Tubenchorionepitheliom* kam bisher nur im fertilen Alter zur Beobachtung, obwohl, natürlich ein Chorionepithelioma teratosum sich auch früher oder später entwickeln kann. Das *Tubensarkom* wird in gleicher Weise bei jungen wie bei alten Frauen beobachtet. Scheffey, Lang und Nugent fanden bei einer 70jährigen, König bei einer 20jährigen Frau ein Tubensarkom.

η) Ätiologie
αα) Tubencarcinom

Wegen der Seltenheit, mit der das Epithel des Müllerschen Ganges in der Tube gegenüber den anderen Abschnitten des Genitales zur Carcinomentstehung neigt, wurde für die Entstehung des primären Tubencarcinoms nach besonderen auslösenden Faktoren gesucht. Sänger und Barth haben die Ansicht vertreten, daß sich das Tubencarcinom nur auf chronisch-entzündlicher Grundlage entwickeln kann und damit als Fehlregenerat aufzufassen sei. Guyomar weist 1961 erneut auf die ätiologische Bedeutung der chronischen Adnexitis hin. Allerdings wird objektiv beim Tubencarcinom zumeist kein Anhalt für eine vorausgegangene Unterleibserkrankung gefunden, histologisch finden sich nur selten entzündliche Residuen und das Carcinom kann sich auch bei offenem Ostium abdominale entwickeln (Franke), so daß die These von Sänger und Barth doch wenig Wahrscheinlichkeit für sich hat und eine chronische Entzündung lediglich bei allgemeiner Carcinombereitschaft zu einer örtlichen Disposition führen kann. Auch die Kombination von Tuberkulose mit Carcinom ist kein häufiger Befund. Nürnberger (1932) diskutiert als Ursache der Entstehung des Tubencarcinoms versprengte Epithelien in der Tubenwand, die carcinomatös entarten.

Auch die Entstehung von Tubencarcinomen aus gutartigen Papillomen, die immer wieder diskutiert wird, ist nach Franke nicht bewiesen.

In der neuen tschechischen Literatur wird vor allem die Endometriose der Tuben nach Tubentuberkulose für die Carcinomgenese verantwortlich gemacht (Horalek und Kloc, 1958; Vavrik, 1957). Grundsätzlich ist aber auch heute noch die Ätiologie des Tubencarcinoms weitgehend unklar.

ββ) Tubenchorionepitheliom

Die eigentliche Ursache des malignen blastomatösen Wachstums in der Tube ist unbekannt.

Die Grundlage für ein Chorionepitheliom kann neben einer Tubargravidität bzw. Tubenblasenmole, nach DIETRICH und PETSCH (bis jetzt 13mal in der Literatur beschrieben) auch ein Teratom sein, in dem die Abkömmlinge der drei Keimblätter durch den chorionepitheliomatösen Bestandteil überwuchert werden (Chorionepithelioma teratosum).

γγ) Tubensarkom

Auch die Ätiologie des Tubensarkoms ist letzten Endes unbekannt. Zu diskutieren ist die sarkomatöse Entartung von Fibromen, Myofibromen, Adenomyomen oder Adenofibromen der Tuben, die als gutartige Tumoren der Tube öfter beschrieben werden. Selbstverständlich ist auch die primäre Entstehung des Sarkoms aus der Tubenwand möglich.

Als teratoide Bildungen der Tube wurden von OUTERBRIDGE und AMANN Adenocarcinosarkome mit Knochen- und Knorpelanlagen beschrieben.

b) Die malignen Tumoren der Ovarien

α) Häufigkeit

Die malignen Tumoren der Ovarien sind die dritthäufigsten Genitalmalignome der Frau und machten bis vor etwa 10 Jahren noch etwa 10% der Gesamtzahl der Genitalmalignome der Frau aus. Nach ERB haben sie in den letzten Jahren von allen Genitalmalignomen der Frau am stärksten — um das Dreifache — zugenommen, nach amerikanischen Statistiken bei der weißen Bevölkerung stärker als bei der farbigen. PFLEIDERER rechnet damit, daß heute (1967) etwa 20% der Genitalmalignome der Frau die Ovarien betreffen. An der Frauenklinik Basel haben die Ovarialcarcinome nach DA RUGNA von 8% aller gynäkologischer Carcinome im Jahre 1900 auf 17% im Jahre 1965 zugenommen.

RANDALL und GERHARDT (1954) berechnen die Chance einer 40jährigen Frau an einem Eierstockskrebs zu erkranken auf knapp 1%, nach BUTTENBERG und LAU (1959) ist jeder dritte Ovarialtumor bösartig.

Trotz der relativen Häufigkeit lagen im Schrifttum bis vor einigen Jahren (EVA GAEBEL, BEUTEL und ADAM) im Vergleich zu den zahlreichen Mitteilungen über Behandlungsergebnisse beim Collum- und Korpuscarcinom nur wenige Mitteilungen über die Behandlungsergebnisse der malignen Ovarialtumore vor. Auch in umfassenden Arbeiten waren sie oft nur sehr kursorisch abgehandelt. Diese Tatsache war im wesentlichen wohl dadurch bedingt, daß die Ovarialcarcinome soviel schlechtere Heilungsaussichten hatten und haben als das Collum- und Korpuscarcinom. In den letzten Jahren hat nun die Zahl der Veröffentlichungen über die Behandlung und auch über die Behandlungsergebnisse der malignen Ovarialtumoren in der ganzen Welt erheblich zugenommen. Für diese Zunahme dürften neben der schon zitierten absoluten Zunahme zum mindesten der Beobachtungen von Ovarialcarcinomen in den Behandlungszentren, vor allem die neuen therapeutischen Möglichkeiten mit radioaktiven und chemischen Substanzen, für die jetzt eine ausreichende Beobachtungszeit zur Beurteilung abgelaufen ist, die entscheidende Rolle spielen.

β) Einteilung nach klinischen Gesichtspunkten

1964 hat die Internationale Föderation für Gynäkologie und Geburtshilfe (FIGO) eine Stadieneinteilung der malignen Ovarialtumoren beschlossen, die seit 1965 verbindlich ist. Keine der bis dahin gebräuchlichen zahlreichen Einteilungen war international gültig und konnte allen Anforderungen gerecht werden (KOTTMEIER, MARTIUS, MÜLLER). Auch die neue Einteilung kann natürlich, wie jede andere mögliche Einteilung, nicht alle Gesichtspunkte berücksichtigen, ermöglicht aber dann, wenn sie einmal allgemein zur Anwendung kommt, leichter und sicherer die vergleichende Betrachtung von Behandlungsergebnissen.

Tabelle 2. *Stadieneinteilung der Fed. Int. Obst. and Gynec. 1965*

Stadium I	Stadium II		Stadium III	Stadium IV
Ia begrenzt auf 1 Ovar; kein Ascites	Ausdehnung im Becken		ausgedehnte intraperitoneale Metastasen (Netz, Dünndarm)	Fernmetastasen außerhalb der Peritonealhöhle
Ib beide Ovarien; kein Ascites	IIa Infiltration oder Metastasen in Uterus oder Tuben	IIb Befall anderer Beckenorgane		
Ic mit Ascites und Tumorzellen				

Bis zum Beschluß der FIGO 1965 war im deutschen Sprachraum vielfach die Stadieneinteilung von Crainz und Schmiemann gebräuchlich, die sich nur nach den Verhältnissen, wie sie während der Operation oder bei nicht operablen Patientinnen bei der manuellen Untersuchung gefunden werden, richtet. Für den Strahlentherapeuten war schon immer (Beutel) eine mehr anatomische Einteilung günstiger, wie sie z.B. Ries schon vor 10 Jahren angegeben hat.

Stadieneinteilung nach Ries:

1. Das Carcinom ist auf das Ovarium beschränkt (vollständig operabel).

2. Übergreifen auf die nähere und fernere Umgebung — Peritoneum, Netz, Tuben (noch weitgehend operabel).

3. Ausgedehnte Metastasen in der Peritonealhöhle (inoperabler Tumor, gegebenenfalls Teilentfernung möglich).

4. Infiltration in der Vagina, Blase oder Rectum, Fernmetastasen in anderen Organen.

Die Umordnung der Beobachtungen an Ovarialcarcinomen aus den früheren Einteilungen in die neue Einteilung der FIGO ist zu statistischen Vergleichen ohne allzu große Schwierigkeiten möglich.

Da das klinische und makroskopische Bild nicht unbedingt Ausdruck einer bereits bestehenden histologischen Malignität zu sein braucht, können grundsätzlich alle Stadieneinteilungen nach klinischen Gesichtspunkten allein nicht befriedigen.

γ) Einteilung nach anatomischen, histologischen und endokrinen Besonderheiten

Vor fast 100 Jahren (1870) stellte Waldeyer als erster eine Klassifikation der Ovarialtumoren nach histologischen Gesichtspunkten auf. Trotz des intensiven Bemühens vieler Autoren in der Folgezeit (Pfannenstiel, Sternberg, Meyer, Schiller, Müller und Kottmeier, Shanks u.a.) um eine allgemein gültige Klassifikation nach histologischen Gesichtspunkten, hat sich keine der vorgeschlagenen Klassifikationen durchsetzen können. Dieser Umstand ist im wesentlichen darauf zurückzuführen, daß noch eine weitgehende Unkenntnis der histophysiologischen Zusammenhänge der komplexen ovariellen Funktion besteht. Als Glied im komplizierten System der innersekretorischen Drüsen unterliegt der Eierstock mannigfaltigen hormonellen Einflüssen. Die Produktion eigener Hormone und die Reifung der Follikel erfordern den komplizierten Aufbau des Organs. Ist ein Glied des innersekretorischen Cyclus ausgefallen — also die hormonelle Harmonie gestört —, kann sich dies in einem histologischen Umbau des Ovars manifestieren. Die Verschiedenartigkeit der histologischen Struktur, der im Pathologischen eine Fülle unterschiedlicher Geschwülste entspricht, läßt das „Ovar zu einem der komplexesten Organe des menschlichen Körpers" werden (Kottmeier, Koller und Schiller).

αα) Epitheliale Ovarialtumoren

Um die therapeutischen Berichte aus allen Teilen der Welt exakt vergleichen zu können, wurde das Krebskomitee der FIGO aufgefordert, einen Vorschlag zur Einteilung der häufigsten epithelialen Ovarialtumoren zu machen. 1961 fand zu diesem Zweck in Stockholm eine Konferenz statt, an der Vertreter aus Dänemark, Deutschland, England,

Schweden, der Schweiz und den USA teilnahmen. Im Hinblick auf die Bedeutung der gefällten Entscheidungen folgen aus der offiziellen Mitteilung die wesentlichen Ausführungen.

„Es gibt viele ausgezeichnete Einteilungen von Ovarialtumoren, die jeweils auf anatomischen, histologischen oder endokrinen Besonderheiten dieser Tumoren beruhen. Einzelne gut erkennbare Typen von primären Ovarialgeschwülsten gehen z.B. vom spezifischen Gonadenstroma, den Keimzellen, dem sog. Germinalepithel, den angeborenen Geweberesten und vom unspezifischen Bindegewebe aus. Obwohl alle diese Typen von Ovarialtumoren ihr malignes Gegenstück haben, entschloß sich die Konferenz nur zu einer genaueren Einteilung derjenigen Tumoren, die vom Keimepithel herstammen. Sie wurden deshalb gewählt, weil sie die überwiegende Mehrzahl aller Ovarialcarcinome ausmachen.

Histopathologische Bilder und klinische Erfahrungen lassen es in gleicher Weise ratsam erscheinen, hier eine intermediäre Gruppe zwischen den offenkundig gutartigen und offenkundig bösartigen Tumoren einzuführen; sie umfaßt Fälle, die man als Grenzfälle oder „möglicherweise maligne" Neoplasmen bezeichnen könnte. Früher wurden diese derartigen Tumoren als Carcinome mit geringer Malignität aufgefaßt. In diese Gruppe fallen Tumoren, bei welchen differenziertes Cylinderepithel Drüsen sowie cystische Hohlräume auskleidet und Papillen überzieht. Diese epitheliale Struktur ist überall gewahrt, auch wenn das Epithel zu zwei oder mehr Lagen geschichtet ist. Die Epithelzellen zeigen mehr oder weniger deutliche Kernanomalien. Es bestehen jedoch keinerlei Anzeichen eines infiltrativen und destruierenden Wachstums, das gegen das mehr oder weniger reichliche Stroma des Tumors gerichtet wäre. Eine Ausbreitung gleichartigen Geschwulstgewebes auf das Peritoneum und sogar Ascites kann eventuell gelegentlich einer Operation beobachtet werden. Die Tumoren dieser intermediären Gruppe wurden deshalb als proliferierende — seröse, papilläre oder mucinöse — Cystadenome ohne Stromainvasion (möglicherweise maligne) bezeichnet.

Die Konferenz war der Meinung, daß es eine Gruppe von Ovarialtumoren gibt, deren histologischer Bau dem von epithelialen Geschwülsten des Endometriums ähnelt. Der Ursprung dieser Tumoren ist im allgemeinen unbekannt, wenn auch in seltenen Fällen gezeigt werden konnte, daß sie aus einer Endometriose hervorgehen. Für diese Gruppe schlägt die Konferenz die Bezeichnung „endometrioid" vor. In dieser Gruppe gibt es, wie in der oben besprochenen, intermediäre Typen von zweifelhafter Malignität, welche dann ebenfalls als „möglicherweise maligne" bezeichnet werden sollten.

Schließlich kommen immer Ovarialtumoren vor, die so undifferenziert sind, daß man sie nicht mit Sicherheit in eine der angeführten Gruppen einordnen kann. Sie sollten als „undifferenzierte Carcinome" bezeichnet werden. Da sie relativ häufig sind, ist anzunehmen, daß auch sie der großen Gruppe der Tumoren des Keimepithels angehören. Die Konferenz empfiehlt, die häufigsten epithelialen Tumoren des Ovars in folgender Weise einzuteilen:

1. Seröse Cystome.

   a) Benigne seröse papilläre Cystadenome.

   b) Proliferierende seröse papilläre Cystadenome ohne Stromainvasion (möglicherweise maligne).

   c) Seröse Cystadeno-Carcinome (alle Malignitätsgrade).

2. Mucinöse Cystome.

   a) Benigne mucinöse Cystadenome.

   b) Proliferierende mucinöse Cystadenome ohne Stromainvasion (möglicherweise maligne).

   c) Mucinöse Cystadeno-Carcinome (alle Malignitätsgrade).

3. Endometrioide Tumoren.
  a) . . .[1].
  b) Proliferierende, endometrioide Adenome und Cystadenome (möglicherweise maligne).
4. Undifferenzierte Carcinome (Zuordnung zu normalen Zelltypen unmöglich).

Gewöhnlich ist in Ovarialtumoren nur ein Typ von Epithelzellen vorhanden. Wenn eine Mischung von verschiedenen Zelltypen gefunden wird, wie es gelegentlich der Fall sein kann, dann sollte der überwiegende Typ zur Diagnosestellung herangezogen werden.

Die Konferenzmitglieder empfehlen, in Veröffentlichungen diese Einteilung anzuwenden und jede Serie von Fällen in Form der folgenden Tabelle 3 wiederzugeben. Auf diese Weise kann sofort überblickt werden, in welchem Ausmaß jeweils eine Klinik oder ein Laboratorium die beobachteten Fälle als benigne, intermediäre und maligne Formen deutet.

Tabelle 3

	a	b	c
Seröse Cystome	. . .	. . .	. . .
Mucinöse Cystome	. . .	. . .	. . .
Endometrioide Tumoren		. . .	. . .
Undifferenzierte Carcinome			. . .

Die Ovarialcarcinome können primär im Eierstock als solche sich entwickeln, sekundär durch Entartung eines Cystadenoms, oder metastatisch von anderen Primärcarcinomen entstehen.

Der solide Eierstockskrebs ist selten. Er durchsetzt zumeist den ganzen Eierstock und vergrößert ihn. Die Tumoren erreichen selten mehr als Mannskopfgröße und zeigen oft eine grobhöckerige Oberfläche. Auch in diesen soliden Tumoren finden sich oft cystische Anteile, die teils vom Bau der Adenocarcinome, teils durch Nekrose als Erweichungscysten entstanden.

Das carcinomatöse Cystom oder sekundär carcinomatös entartete Cystadenom ist häufiger, gleicht makroskopisch oft durchaus den gutartigen Cystadenomen und kann auch histologisch im wesentlichen gutartige und nur vereinzelt carcinomatöse Teile enthalten.

Ca. 25% (Martius) aller Eierstockscarcinome entstehen metastatisch von primären Carcinomen anderer Organe, wobei nach Maurer neuerdings die Ansicht vertreten wird, daß dieser metastatische Eierstockskrebs häufiger ist als früher angenommen wurde. Die Primärgeschwulst findet sich zumeist im Magen-Darm-Kanal, aber auch Carcinome des Uterus, der Tube, der Gallenblase, der Bronchien und der Mamma können in die Ovarien metastasieren. Die Metastasierung erfolgt zumeist auf dem Lymphweg, selten auf dem Blutweg.

Die metastatischen Ovarialcarcinome sind ebenfalls teils solide, teils cystisch, zumeist doppelseitig. Sie können oft schon mächtige Tumoren bilden, wenn das primäre Carcinom noch klein ist und kaum Erscheinungen macht. Histologisch sieht man in den metastatischen Ovarialtumoren oft auffallend große gequollene Zellen, Siegelringzellen, die das Kennzeichen der sog. Krukenbergtumoren sind.

Alle metastatischen Ovarialtumoren als Krukenbergtumoren zu bezeichnen ist nicht exakt. Die charakteristische Zellform dieser Geschwulst ist die Siegelringform. Wenn sie in einer Eierstocksgeschwulst gefunden wird, dann ist es fast immer möglich, eine histologisch identische Geschwulst im Verdauungstrakt nachzuweisen (Walther, 1948).

---

1 Diese Spalte (3a) wurde frei gelassen, da es bisher nicht gelang, eine Einigung darüber zu erzielen, ob einige Fälle von ovarieller Endometriose als wirkliche Tumoren zu betrachten sind oder versprengtes bzw. ektopisches Endometrium darstellen.

Besondere Formen der Ovarialcarcinome sind:

1. Die Seminome oder Disgerminome, großzellige Carcinome, die aus liegengebliebenem, undifferenziertem Keimepithel entstehen und geschlechtlich indifferentes Gewebe enthalten. Sie gehen mit Anomalien der Geschlechtsorgane einher, haben aber keine hormonalen Auswirkungen. Die Prognose ist meist ungünstig.

2. Der Tumor ovarii Brenner, eine relativ seltene feste Geschwulst oder Pseudomucincyste mit festen Anteilen, die sich aus den Waltardschen Zellnestern entwickeln und nur lokale Erscheinungen macht.

3. Die bösartigen epithelialen Eierstocksgeschwülste, die neben lokalen Erscheinungen auch hormonale Auswirkungen auf den Gesamtorganismus haben. Sie werden im Kapitelabschnitt δδ, die hormonal aktiven Tumoren, besprochen.

ββ) Bösartige Bindegewebstumoren

1. Die nicht häufigen Sarkome des Ovariums sind meist Spindelzellsarkome, die derbe, glatte, dem Fibrom ähnliche Tumoren bilden, seltener weiche Rundzellsarkome, polymorphzellige Sarkome und Myxosarkome.

2. Die von den Blutgefäßen ausgehenden Sarkome (Peritheliome, Hämangioendotheliome und Lymphangioendotheliome) sind zumeist solide, feste markige Tumoren, deren Abgrenzung von den Ovarialcarcinomen auch histologisch Schwierigkeiten machen kann.

3. Die Thecazelltumoren gehören hinsichtlich Genese und Struktur an sich zu den Bindegewebsgeschwülsten, sind aber klinisch hormonal aktiv und werden bei diesen Tumoren besprochen.

γγ) Ovulogene oder embryonale Tumoren

Das Teratoblastom ist klinisch maligne, wächst destruierend und metastasiert, wobei die Metastasen das gleiche embryonale Gewebe wie der Primärtumor, aber oft auch schon sarkomatös bzw. carcinomatös entartete Zellen aufweisen, die dann auf die bereits erfolgte maligne Entartung des Primärtumors hinweisen.

Histologisch finden sich in den Tumoren Abkömmlinge aller drei Keimblätter, die aber, im Gegensatz zu den Verhältnissen bei den fast immer gutartigen Dermoidcysten, ein wirres, regelloses Durcheinander verschiedener unreifer embryonaler Gewebe zeigen.

Die Teratoblastome sind zumeist große kugelige Tumoren von fester Konsistenz. Sie kommen schon im Kindesalter vor und können positive Hypophysenvorderlappenreaktionen im Harn bedingen.

δδ) Hormonal aktive Tumoren

Das klinische Erscheinungsbild der hormonal aktiven Ovarialtumoren ist gekennzeichnet durch das Auftreten lokaler und Fern-Symptome. Die lokalen Symptome entsprechen weitgehend der Symptomatik bei den übrigen Ovarialtumoren. Die Fernsymptome sind durch die Art der von den Tumoren produzierten Hormone geprägt. Im einzelnen wird auf diese Fragen später, im Abschnitt Symptomatologie und Diagnostik, S. 325, eingegangen.

Das *Arrhenoblastom*, ein relativ seltener epithelialer Tumor der Ovarien ist fast stets einseitig entwickelt, produziert männliche Prägungsstoffe und entsteht (wie die Oestroblastome) aus dem Mesenchym bzw. dessen späteren Formationen (NEVINNY-STICKEL, 1962). Er kann von sehr verschiedener Größe sein. Histologisch zeigt er ein Gewebe, das „aus einem unreif gebliebenen männlichen oder männlich gewordenen Keimdrüsenmaterial" entstanden ist und entweder Drüsen oder solide Epithelwucherungen bildet. Klinisch ist das Erkennen eines Arrhenoblastoms kaum möglich. Sogar die histologische Diagnose muß oft doch durch die hormonalen Befunde ergänzt werden.

Die Arrhenoblastome sind — zumindest klinisch — relativ gutartige Neubildungen. Es wurden aber auch Fälle beschrieben, bei denen die Geschwülste zu ausgedehnten

Metastasenbildungen führten. Auch wurden gelegentlich nach Tumorentfernung Rezidive beobachtet. Die Tumoren besitzen in etwa 25 % der Fälle maligne Eigenschaften.

Die *Oestroblastome* (Granulosa- und Thecazelltumoren) entstehen wie das Arrhenoblastom aus dem Mesenchym oder dessen späteren Formationen und bieten histologisch ein vielgestaltiges Bild (Nevinny-Stickel, 1962). So werden reine Granulosa- und reine Thecazelltumoren, zumeist aber eine Kombination beider Tumorarten gefunden. Die Tumoren produzieren Follikel-Hormon, wobei wahrscheinlich die hormonelle Aktivität im wesentlichen an die thecacellulären Formationen gebunden ist.

a) Der Granulosazelltumor ist häufiger als das Arrhenoblastom, tritt im allgemeinen einseitig, gelegentlich aber auch doppelseitig auf. Obwohl die Tumoren Geschwülste der Eierstöcke sind, können sie gelegentlich auch extraovarial im intraligamentären oder retroperitonealen Bindegewebe gefunden werden. Die Größe dieser Tumoren ist sehr variabel. Die mikroskopischen Charakteristika sind sehr vielfältig, doch können verschiedenartige, gut definierbare Strukturen unterschieden werden, die eine Einteilung in 4 Gruppen (Dubrauszky, 1954) ermöglichen.

Die Granulosazellgewächse gelten klinisch als relativ gutartige Neubildungen. Dubrauszky fand in 20 % seiner Fälle klinische Malignität, obwohl nach dem histologischen Bilde 40 % als bösartige Formen anzusprechen waren. Andererseits beobachtete er auch Tumoren, die histologisch durchaus gutartig erschienen, später aber rezidivierten.

b) Die Thecazelltumoren werden heute ebenfalls in die Gruppe der hormonal aktiven Eierstocksgeschwülste eingereiht, während sie früher als eine besondere Form der Fibrome angesehen wurden. Sie sind etwas seltener als die Granulosazelltumoren, vorwiegend einseitig und sehr unterschiedlich groß (erbsgroß bis mehrere Kilogramm schwer), zumeist aber relativ klein.

Histologisch finden sich in den Thecazelltumoren im allgemeinen kleinere und größere, oft bündelförmig angeordnete spindelige Zellen, die eine gewisse Ähnlichkeit mit den Elementen der Theca interna haben und zur Hyalinisierung neigen. Die Thecazelltumoren sind histologisch und klinisch seltener maligne als die Granulosazellneubildungen (nur etwa 3 % bösartig).

Kombinationen der Granulosa- und Thecazelltumoren werden nicht nur miteinander, sondern auch mit andersartigen Geschwülsten (Fibrom, seröses oder pseudomucinöses Cystom, Disgerminom oder Arrhenoblastom etc.) beschrieben.

Das *Gynandroblastom*, eine sehr selten bösartige Geschwulst, enthält Granulosa-Theca- und Arrhenoblastom-Strukturen und kann sowohl weibliche wie männliche Keimdrüsenhormone produzieren.

Die ovariellen Hypernephroide, bzw. adrenalen oder adrenocorticalen Tumoren der Ovarien, können — wie die Arrhenoblastome — bei den Trägerinnen eine „Entweiblichung" oder „Vermännlichung" hervorrufen. Sie sind sehr selten, zumeist nicht sehr groß. Häufig entwickeln sie sich intraligamentär.

Die histologische Struktur der ovariellen Hypernephroide erinnert an den Aufbau der Nebennierenrinde, doch sind auch atypische Bilder zu finden, bei denen eine einwandfreie histologische Diagnose fast nicht zu stellen ist. Die Prognose ist nicht gut. Von wenigen Fällen abgesehen, handelt es sich um bösartige Neubildungen.

Das ovarielle Chorionepitheliom gehört ebenfalls zu den hormonbildenden Eierstocksgeschwülsten. Es sind nicht sehr große, vorwiegend grobhöckerige Tumoren.

Das histologische Präparat zeigt die typische Struktur eines Chorionepithelioms. Wenn der Tumor sich aber auf dem Boden einer teratogenen Geschwulst entwickelt, finden sich meistens auch noch andersartige Strukturen. Das ovarielle Chorionepitheliom ist erfahrungsgemäß bösartig und metastasiert oft schon früh, bevorzugt in die Lunge.

Die Struma ovarii ist eine nur selten bösartige teratogene Geschwulst, die Schilddrüsengewebe enthält und auch zu den hormonbildenden Neubildungen des Ovars zu rechnen ist. Sie entwickelt sich einseitig, wird nicht allzu groß und hat in der Regel eine höckerige, von einer Geschwulstkapsel gebildete Oberfläche.

δ) *Symptomatologie und Diagnostik*

Alle Autoren sind sich darüber einig, daß die malignen Ovarialtumoren, im Gegensatz zu den meisten anderen gynäkologischen Tumoren, keine Frühsymptome aufweisen und oft lange Zeit keine subjektiven Beschwerden machen, so daß die Patientinnen fast immer in einem mehr oder weniger fortgeschrittenen Stadium zum Arzt kommen. Die ersten Beschwerden oder Zeichen sind oft schon keine „Frühsymptome" mehr. Es gibt auch keine speziellen Untersuchungsmethoden, um maligne Geschwülste des Ovars frühzeitig zu erkennen (HESSELTINE und SMITH, 1956; HOFMEISTER und GROTHEY, 1956; H. H. SCHMID, 1953). In den meisten Fällen liegen bei Klinikaufnahme schon die Stadien II, III oder IV vor.

Die statistische Auswertung des Materials der Universitäts-Frauenklinik Freiburg, hinsichtlich der Reihenfolge des Auftretens der Symptome, deckt sich weitgehend mit den Erfahrungen anderer Autoren (MAURER, FROEWIS und BROSCH u.a.). Mehr als die Hälfte der Patientinnen geben Druck und Schmerzen im Unterbauch als erstes Symptom an, etwa $^1/_4$ der Patientinnen Zunahme des Gewichtes und des Leibesumfanges. — Dann folgen als seltenere Erstsymptome Gewichtsabnahme, Druck auf Blase und Darm sowie Blut im Stuhl und Urin. Nur 5% etwa der Patientinnen mit Ovarialtumoren geben als Erstsymptome Blutungen in der Menopause oder Blutungsstörungen an. Nicht ganz selten bemerken die Patientinnen die Geschwulst auch selbst durch Eigeninspektion oder Palpation des Leibes, oder der Tumor wird zufällig anläßlich anderer Untersuchungen entdeckt.

Die Diagnose eines Ovarialtumors wird klinisch auf Grund des Palpationsbefundes gestellt. Die Größe und Erscheinungsform der Tumoren kann sehr verschieden sein, wobei nur äußerst selten von der äußeren Beschaffenheit auf den Charakter und den histologischen Aufbau des Neoplasmas geschlossen werden kann. Die Operation ist eine Grundvoraussetzung, um zu einer eindeutigen Diagnose zu gelangen. Die Entscheidung über histologische Gut- und Bösartigkeit gelingt nur durch die Untersuchung eines — zumeist erst während der Operation gewonnenen — Gewebsanteils. Bei Frauen, die jünger als 50 Jahre sind und vor der Menopause stehen, erweisen sich nach KOTTMEIER Ovarialtumoren, die kleiner als eine Faust sind, in 95% der Fälle als nicht neoplastisch. Er empfiehlt, solche Patientinnen primär nicht zu operieren, sondern streng unter Kontrolle zu halten, Frauen jenseits der Menopause aber sofort zu laparotomieren, um ein bösartiges Wachstum auszuschließen.

Das *Ovarialcarcinom* tritt häufig bilateral auf, und nicht selten zeigt ein bei der Operation zurückgelassenes makroskopisch unauffälliges Ovar früher oder später malignes Wachstum. Den Befall beider Ovarien fand KERMAUNER (1932) in 36,2%, FRANKL (1920) in 36,8% der Fälle.

Die Ovarialcarcinome machen fast immer Ascites, besonders wenn eine peritoneale Aussaat erfolgt ist. Die Ascitesflüssigkeit ist oft blutig tingiert. Wenn Ascites bei *Sarkomen* (wie häufig) vorhanden ist, ballotiert der Tumor oft, während er sonst dem Uterus im allgemeinen dicht anliegt.

Durch Druckwirkung der Tumoren auf die Gefäße kann es zu erheblichen Zirkulationsstörungen, Ödemen der Beine und Thrombosen kommen. In fortgeschrittenem Stadium verwachsen die Tumormassen und Därme oft zu einem unentwirrbaren inoperablen Knäuel.

Das u.U. hochgedrängte Zwerchfell kann zur Verlagerung des Herzens mit entsprechenden Herzbeschwerden und zu Atembeschwerden führen.

Der Appetit ist zumeist vermindert. Diese Tatsache zusammen mit dem starken Verbrauch der körpereigenen Substanzen zum Aufbau des Tumors führen bald zu starker Abmagerung und Entkräftung.

Der Cyclus ist bei den Ovarialtumoren — worauf wir schon hingewiesen haben — zumeist nicht gestört. Postklimakterische Blutungen können auf *Granulosazelltumoren*, seltener auf *Fibrome* oder *Sarkome* des Ovars hinweisen. Eine vorzeitige Menstruation bei Kindern muß daran denken lassen, daß sich ein *hormonaktiver Ovarialtumor* (u. U. auch schon bei sehr kleinen Kindern) entwickelt haben kann.

Die klinischen Symptome der *hormonal aktiven Neubildungen* der Ovarien äußern sich — wir haben schon darauf hingewiesen — in lokalen und Fernerscheinungen. Die ersteren sind die gleichen wie bei sämtlichen Ovarialtumoren. Die Fernwirkungen können — abhängig von der Art der produzierten Hormone — zu einer Änderung des sexuellen Charakters der Patientin führen. Wenn vorwiegend männliche Hormone produziert werden (Arrhenoblastom, Gynandroblastom, ovarielle Hypernephroidtumoren), kommt es in leichteren Fällen zu einer gewissen „Entweiblichung", in ausgeprägteren Fällen auch zur „Vermännlichung", u. U. mit Hirsutismus, Atrophie der Mammae und des Uterus, Amenorrhoe und Sterilität.

Die *Oestroblastome* können zum Hyperoestrinismus und damit zu Blutungsanomalien, Größenzunahme des Uterus, glandulärcystischer Hyperplasie der Uterusschleimhaut und bei Entwicklung des Tumors vor der Pubertät zu isosexueller Frühreife führen. Bei Frauen jenseits des Klimakteriums kann es zu Erscheinungen kommen, die der Geschlechtsreife ähneln. Bei Gynandroblastomen können sowohl Hyperoestrinismus bzw. Maskulinisierung beobachtet werden, als auch endokrine Veränderungen fehlen (Nevinny-Stickel, 1962).

Die *Struma ovarii* kann gelegentlich zu thyreotoxischen Erscheinungen führen, so daß bei allen unklaren hyperthyreotischen Zustandsbildern bei Frauen, bei denen keine Veränderungen am Hals gefunden werden, auch an eine Struma ovarii gedacht werden soll. Theoretisch müßte es möglich sein, mit nuklearmedizinischen Untersuchungen mit ^{131}I eine Struma ovarii nachzuweisen. Entsprechende Mitteilungen liegen aber in der Literatur bis jetzt nicht vor (Zum Winkel, persönliche Mitteilung, Rössler). Es liegen bisher auch keine Berichte vor über hormonaktive Metastasen im Ovarium bei Schilddrüsencarcinomen.

Das *Chorionepitheliom* des Ovars führt zur erhöhten Chorionprolanausscheidung im Urin, im Kindesalter u. U. mit isosexueller Frühreife. Nicht selten gesellen sich zu diesen Symptomen auch noch psychische Störungen.

Nach der Entfernung der hormonal aktiven Tumoren bilden sich die Fernsymptome im allgemeinen zurück, können aber beim Rezidiv wieder auftreten.

Die Kombination von Ovarialtumoren und Gravidität ist ziemlich häufig, so daß differentialdiagnostisch immer an eine Gravidität gedacht werden muß, wenn sich die Patientin im konzeptionsfähigen Alter befindet, wobei natürlich auch immer eine Extrauteringravidität möglich ist. Bezüglich des Tastbefundes kommen differentialdiagnostisch weiterhin in Frage: Uterusmyome, dystope Nieren (s. Abb. 4a und b), eventuell auch Exsudate im oberen Anteil des Ligamentum latum und intraperitoneale Exsudate im Douglasschen Raum.

Auch tumorartige Aufblähungen und Kotstauungen im Coecum oder der Flexur des Sigmoides — sowie natürlich im Becken gelegene echte Darmtumoren — müssen differentialdiagnostisch erwogen werden.

Neben der Inspektion, Palpation und Perkussion des Leibes, der vaginalen und rectalen Untersuchung sowie Laboratoriumsuntersuchungen ist insbesondere auch die *Röntgenuntersuchung* zur Gewinnung von über den Tastbefund hinausgehenden Anhaltspunkten von großer Bedeutung.

Die *Abdomenübersichtsaufnahme* (zweckmäßig in Bauchlage, mit höchstverstärkender Folie, höchstempfindlichem Film und weicher Strahlung) läßt manchmal Ovarialtumoren über den Tastbefund hinaus genauer beurteilen und ermöglicht oft schon vom 3. bis 4. Schwangerschaftsmonat ab die wichtige differentialdiagnostische Abgrenzung einer Frühschwangerschaft oder einer Frühschwangerschaft bei gleichzeitigem Ovarialtumor, wobei natürlich das Fehlen von kindlichen Skeletteilen zu diesem Zeitpunkt eine Gravidität noch nicht mit Sicherheit ausschließt. In den fast immer gutartigen Dermoidcysten

(Abb. 3) ist es oft möglich, mit der Abdomenübersichtsaufnahme Zähne und Knochen-einlagerungen nachzuweisen. Nicht selten sind auch in papillären Cystadenocarcinomen der Ovarien psammomatöse Verkalkungen vorhanden, die auf der Übersichtsaufnahme zur Darstellung kommen können. So sahen CASTRO und KLEITH (1962) in $3^1/_2$ Jahren

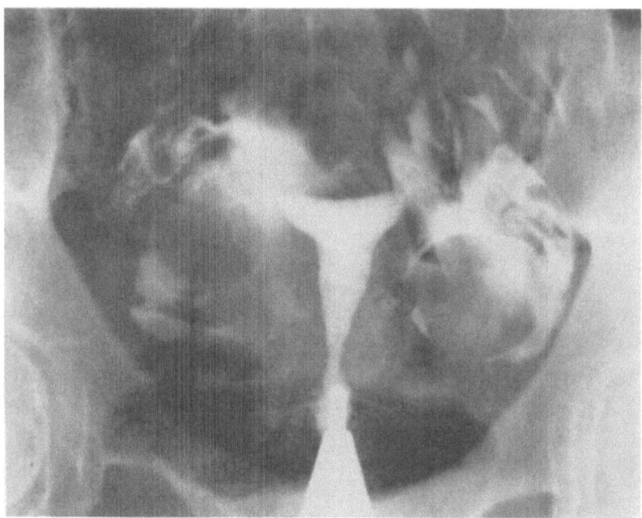

a

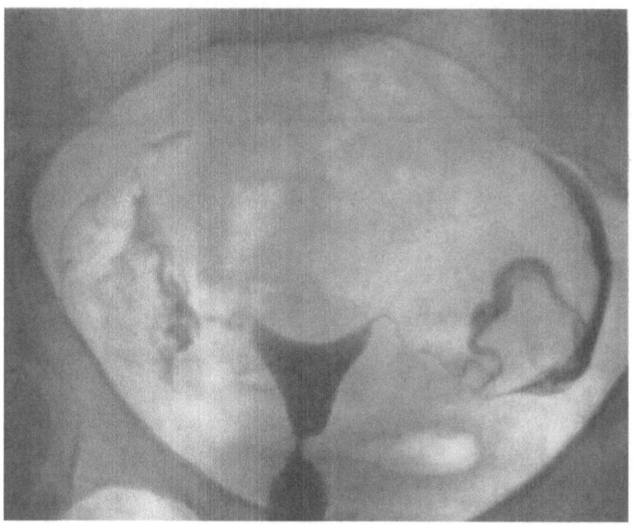

b

Abb. 2a u. b. Hysterosalpingopelvigraphie. a Gute Abgrenzbarkeit, normal großer Ovarien.
b Ovarialtumor links

bei 33 Fällen von papillären Cystadenocarcinomen der Ovarien röntgenologisch verkalkte Tumormetastasen, die als feine granularartige, wenig dichte Kalkschatten meist über das ganze Abdomen diffus verteilt waren.

Mit der *Hysterosalpingopelvigraphie* kann manchmal der Tastbefund durch gute Darstellung der Ovarien und entsprechend auch von Ovarialtumoren (Abb. 2a, b) ergänzt werden.

Das *intravenöse Urogramm*, das wir grundsätzlich bei allen gynäkologischen Tumoren vor der Behandlung und zweckmäßigerweise auch bei Kontrolluntersuchungen nach Behandlung fordern, kann bei den Ovarialtumoren durch Verdrängungserscheinungen und

Druckwirkung auf die Ureteren (mit den entsprechenden Rückwirkungen auf die Nieren-hohlsysteme) und die Blase Hinweise auf Lage und Ausdehnung der Tumoren geben (Abb. 3).

Auf die differentialdiagnostische Bedeutung des Urogramms bei der dystopen Niere (Abb. 4a, b) haben wir bereits hingewiesen.

Die *Magen-Darmpassage* und u.U. auch das *Cholangio-* und *Cholecystogramm* lassen primäre Tumoren im Bereich dieser Organe (Krukenberg-Tumoren) weitgehend ausschließen.

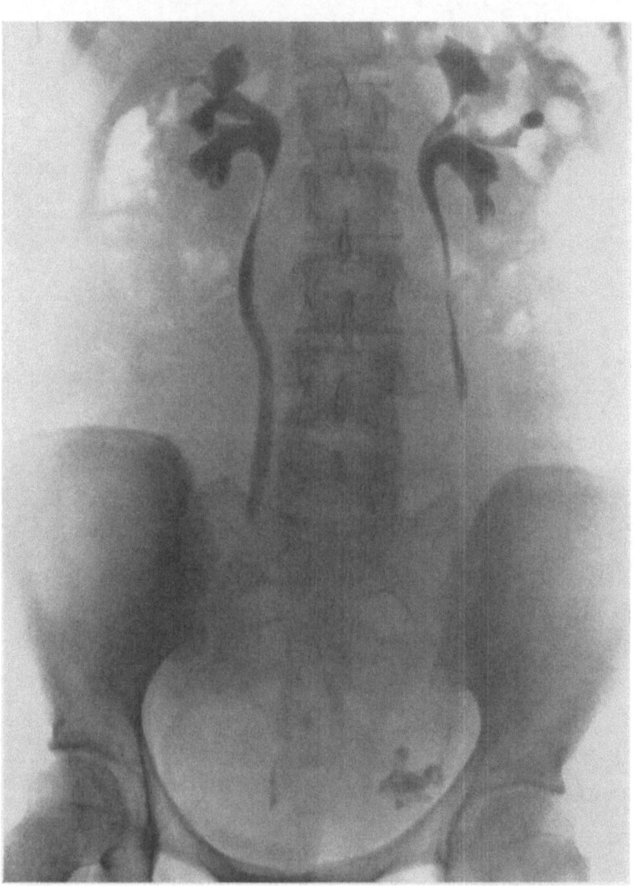

Abb. 3. Dermoidcyste (gutartig), i.v. Urogramm. Druckwirkung auf die Ureteren mit leichter Stauung der Ureteren und Nierenhohlsysteme sowie Verdrängung der Blase

Der *Kontrasteinlauf* kann von Bedeutung sein zur Erfassung der Ausdehnung der Tumoren und der Auswirkung auf die Nachbarorgane durch Verdrängung und Druckwirkung (Abb. 5).

Die Röntgenuntersuchung der *Thoraxorgane* — die wir ebenfalls bei allen malignen Tumoren routinemäßig für unbedingt erforderlich halten — ermöglicht nicht nur die frühzeitige Erfassung von Lungenmetastasen, sondern zeigt gegebenenfalls auch Ver-drängungen der Thoraxorgane durch einen im Bauchraum wachsenden Tumor und kann durch den Nachweis und die differentialdiagnostische Abklärung von Ergußbildungen im Thoraxraum u.U. weitere diagnostische Hinweise liefern. Hier ist das sog. Meigs-syndrom (Meigs und Cass, 1937) von besonderer Bedeutung, bei dem es sich um einen Hydrothorax (Transsudat) bei *benignen* gynäkologischen Tumoren, insbesondere Ovarial-fibromen mit Ascitesbildung handelt. Wahrscheinlich spielen bei der Entstehung dieses Hydrothorax die Lymphgefäße im Zwerchfell die entscheidende Rolle. Differential-

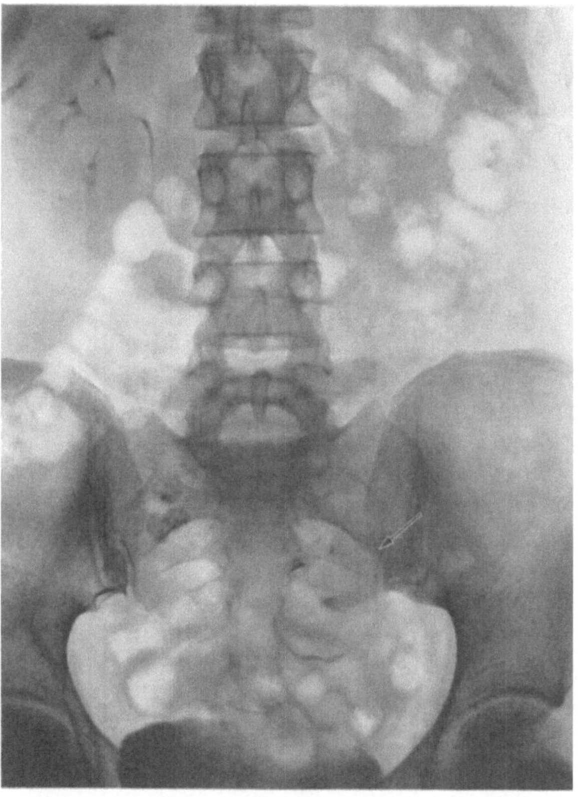

a

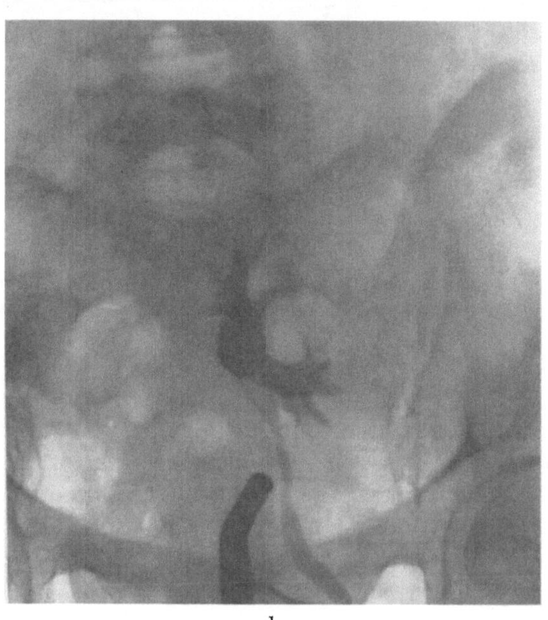

b

Abb. 4a u. b. Beckenniere links. a i.v. Urogramm. b Retrograde Auffüllung des Hohlsystems der dystopen Niere

diagnostisch zur Abklärung gegen andere insbesondere auch krebsspezifische Ergüsse kann neben der Punktion u. U. die Tatsache, daß Tusche dem Ascites beigemengt in der Pleurahöhle erscheint, dienen.

Der Wert der *Lymphographie*, auch zur Erfassung von regionären Metastasen beim Ovarialcarcinom, wurde in den letzten Jahren mehrfach herausgestellt (Little u. Mitarb., Picard u. Mitarb., Fuchs, Marley u. Mitarb.).

Obwohl die Untersuchung erst seit wenigen Jahren an größerem Krankengut durchgeführt wird, hat sich gezeigt, daß die lymphogene Metastasierung viel häufiger ist als man bisher angenommen hat. So fand Frischbier bei 7 von 19, Fuchs (1965) am Berner Material bei 21 von insgesamt 39 lymphographisch untersuchten Patientinnen mit

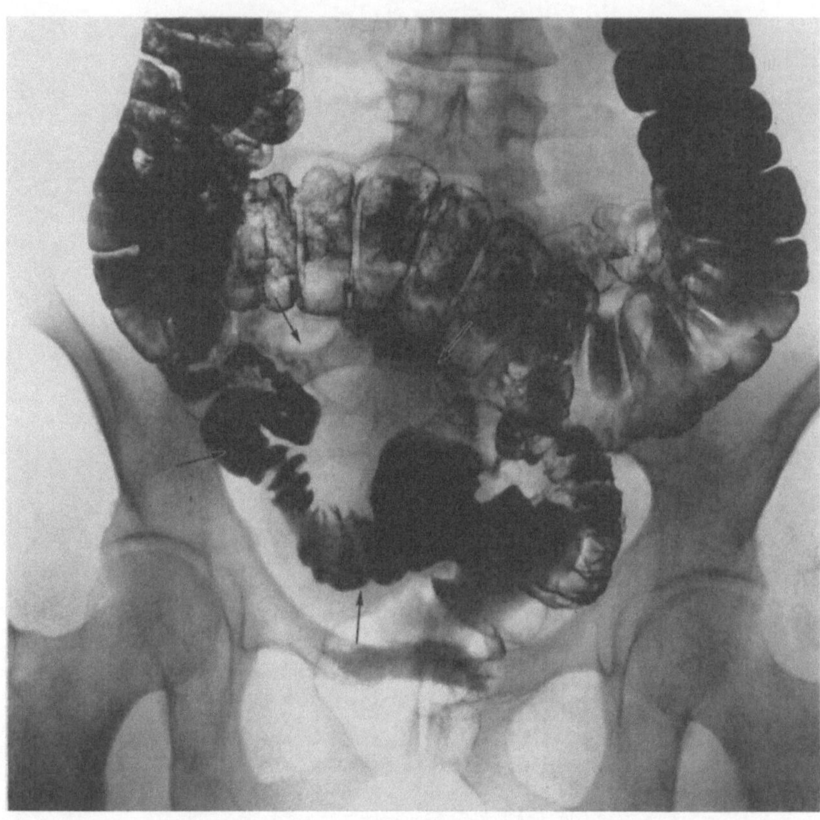

Abb. 5. Kontrasteinlauf und retrograde Auffüllung des terminalen Ileums bei Ovarialtumor rechts. Aufnahme im Stehen, Verdrängung und z. T. Kompression des terminalen Ileums, des Coecums und des Colon transversum

Ovarialcarcinom regionäre Metastasen. Die Aufteilung ergab bei Fuchs regionäre Metastasen beim Stadium I und II in 4 von 13 Fällen, bei den fortgeschrittenen Stadien III und IV bei 17 von 27 Patientinnen. Die aortalen Lymphknoten sind häufiger befallen als die iliacalen. Die Kombination der Lymphographie mit der Cavographie bezeichnet Fuchs (1965) als „wertvolle Untersuchungsmethode, die präoperativ und auch postoperativ dringend angezeigt ist".

Auf die Bedeutung der pelvinen *Pneumographie* und *Arteriographie*, auch für die Diagnostik von Ovarialtumoren gehen u. a. Braband und Bublitz in einer Veröffentlichung 1966 ein. Sie weisen in ihrer Arbeit darauf hin, daß das Beckenangiogramm bei malignen trophoplastischen Tumoren auch normal sein kann und Frühschwangerschaft sowie Missed abortion zu ähnlichen Bildern wie solche Tumoren führen können.

Die pelvine Pneumographie kann dabei u. U. mit der Hysterosalpingographie kombiniert werden, wie die Abb. 6 (eigene Beobachtung) zeigt.

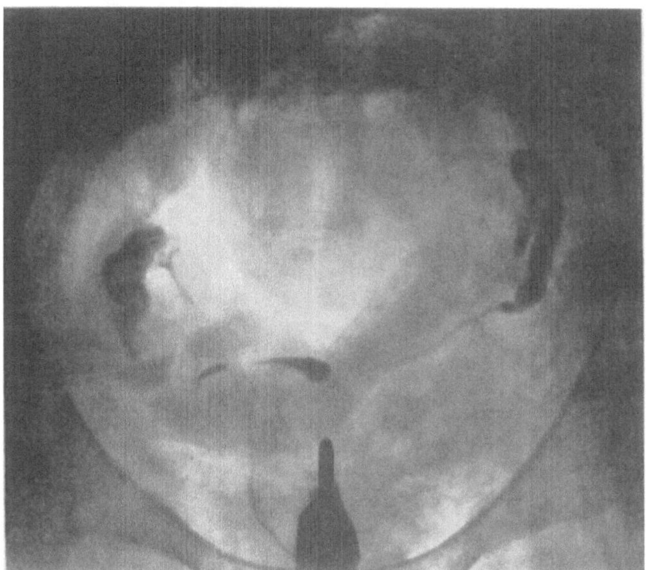

Abb. 6. *Klinischer Befund:* Etwa faustgroßer, nicht sicher abgrenzbarer Tumor im kleinen Becken mehr li. *Pneumopelvigraphie kombiniert mit Hysterosalpingographie:* Tennisballgroßer, glatt begrenzter, gut abgrenzbarer Tumor im Becken, etwas nach li. gelegen — wahrscheinlich cystischer Ovarialtumor. *Histologisch:* Cystischer Ovarialtumor, nicht maligne

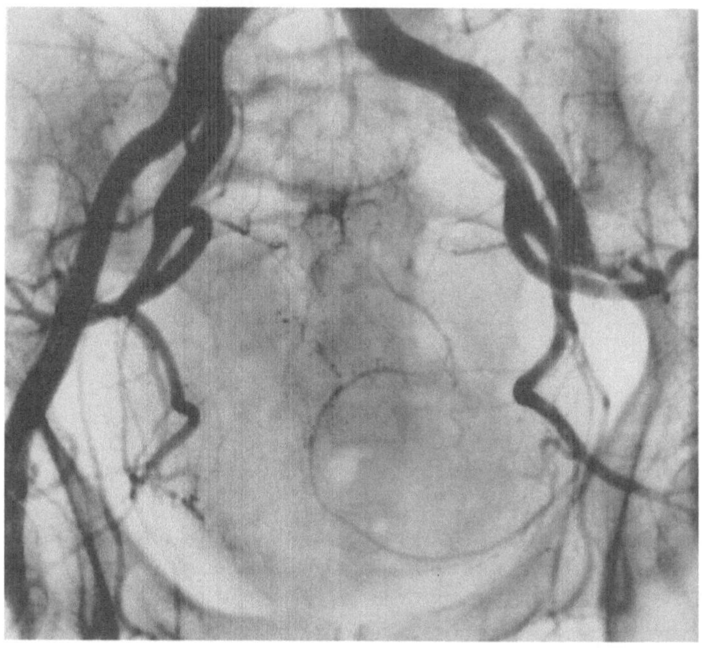

Abb. 7. *Klinischer Befund:* Großer, knolliger Tumor im kleinen Becken li., vom Uterus nicht zu trennen. *Arteriographie:* Gefäßarmes Ovarialcarcinom li. mit deutlicher Verdrängung der A. uterina. *Histologisch:* Gesichertes Ovarialcarcinom

Mit der Arteriographie bei Ovarialtumoren hat sich insbesondere auch BREIT in Passau, der mir die Abb. 7, 8a und b mit Legenden dankenswerterweise für diesen Beitrag zur Verfügung gestellt hat, intensiv und erfolgreich beschäftigt.

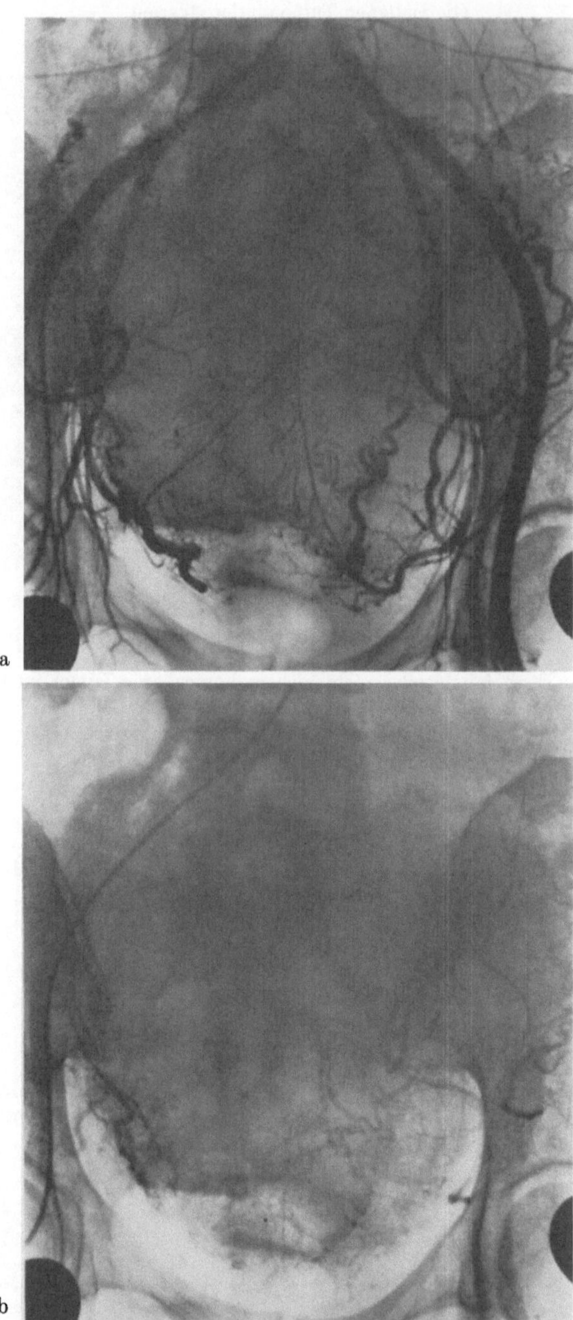

Abb. 8a u. b. *Klinischer Befund:* Das ganze kleine Becken durch knollige Tumoren ausgemauert. *Arterio-graphie:* Gefäßreicher Ovarialtumor mit zahlreichen Gefäßneubildungen und typischer Darstellung beider Aa. ovaricae. a Arterielle, b venöse Phase. *Histologisch:* Gesichertes Ovarialcarcinom

Zur Differentialdiagnose der Ovarialtumoren werden in den letzten Jahren in zunehmendem Umfang und mit wachsendem Erfolg auch Ultraschalluntersuchungen durchgeführt. Damit können in Ergänzung der übrigen Untersuchungsmethoden u. U. Aussagen über Lage, Größe und in gewissem Umfang auch über Form und Konsistenz von Ovarialtumoren erarbeitet werden.

ε) Ausbreitung und Metastasierung

Das Wachstum der Ovarialtumoren vollzieht sich primär tief im kleinen Becken und kann hier relativ lange, d.h. bis zu einer schon relativ bedeutenden Größe praktisch unbemerkt erfolgen. Erst wenn der Tumor eine gewisse Größe erreicht hat, beginnt er

Beschwerden zu machen und die benachbarten Organe zu irritieren. Der Verlauf der Erkrankung ist zumeist langsam, das Wachstum der Tumoren nicht so rasch wie z.B. beim schwangeren Uterus und kann sich über Jahre hinziehen.

Grundsätzlich können die Tumoren sich nach der freien Bauchhöhle oder intraligamentär entwickeln. Bei der Entwicklung zur freien Bauchhöhle hin stielt sich der Tumor. Der Stiel besteht aus dem Ligamentum ovarii proprium, der Tube, dem Ligamentum infundibulo-pelvicum und dem Ligamentum latum. Die Tumoren nehmen je nach Größe verschiedene Lagen ein. Ein kleiner Ovarialtumor bleibt im normalen Bereich des Ovariums liegen, verdrängt erst, wenn er größer wird, den Uterus nach seitlich und vorne, kann infolge seines Gewichtes in den Douglasschen Raum eintreten und u.U. auch im kleinen Becken unterhalb des Promontoriums incarceriert werden. Größere Tumoren haben im Becken keinen Platz mehr und fallen zumeist, wenn der Zustand der Bauchdecken es zuläßt, symptomlos nach vorne.

Die Konsistenz des Tumors entscheidet oft über die Stärke der Symptome. Wenn der Tumor weich ist, kann er oft sehr groß werden, ohne daß Symptome auftreten, während feste Geschwülste zumeist schon früher Symptome machen.

Nicht selten kommt es, wenn der Tumor eine gewisse Größe erreicht hat, nach einer starken Anstrengung zu einer Stieldrehung mit plötzlichen heftigen Symptomen (Kollaps, beschleunigter Puls, Übelkeit, Erbrechen, Schweißausbruch als Ausdruck des peritonealen Schocks). Wenn die Tumoren die Größe eines hochschwangeren Uterus übersteigen, werden u.U. die Funktionen der Bauchorgane erheblich gestört.

Der intraligamentär sich entwickelnde Tumor drängt die Blätter des Ligamentum latum auseinander und kann sich bis zum Beckenboden ausdehnen. Dann kann der Uterus seitlich, nach vorne oder hinten zur Beckenwand gedrängt werden. Der Ureter liegt dem Tumor zumeist medial an, kann aus seiner Verbindung mit dem Ligamentum latum gelöst, u.U. auch weit verdrängt werden und zieht dann als „Strang" über den Tumor. Diese Tatsache ist für den Operateur von großer Bedeutung. Das Sigmoid und Coecum mit Appendix können nach oben, das Rectum nach hinten verdrängt werden. Unter Umständen kann der Tumor sogar das Mesenterium entfalten, so daß Dünndarmschlingen direkt über ihn verlaufen.

Die *Carcinome* brechen früh durch die Oberfläche des Eierstockes durch und können sich dann diffus auf dem Peritoneum in Form kleiner Knötchen oder papillärer Wucherungen ausbreiten. Metastasenbröckel sammeln sich besonders leicht im Douglasschen Raum, wachsen dort fest und bilden kleinhöckerige, harte Geschwülste, die sehr druckempfindlich sein können. Das ganze Becken kann mit einem solchen harten Infiltrat ausgefüllt sein, die Scheidenwand kann durchwachsen werden und das Carcinom in die Scheide einbrechen. Metastasen können sich im Uterus, den Tuben, den aortalen Lymphdrüsen, der Appendix, im Mastdarm, am Nabel, an der vorderen Bauchwand und in der Haut entwickeln, und sogar auch auf dem Stimmband sind metastatische Ovarialcarcinome beschrieben worden.

Sowohl für die häufige Doppelseitigkeit des Carcinoms als die „Metastasen" im Bereich der Genitalorgane muß auch die Möglichkeit der „multizentrischen" Entwicklung der Tumoren (HUBER, KAYSER) diskutiert werden. Auf die Tatsache, daß Doppel- oder Simultancarcinome im Ovar und Corpus uteri relativ häufig vorkommen (FUNK-BRENTANO fand bei 12%, BERGSJØ bei 17% ihrer Patientinnen mit Ovarialcarcinomen Carcinome auch im Corpus uteri), hat KIRCHHOFF auf dem deutschen Röntgenkongreß 1967 in Baden-Baden erneut mit Nachdruck hingewiesen. Dabei ist die Differentialdiagnose Doppelcarcinom oder Metastase histologisch und histochemisch oft unmöglich (HOLZNER u. Mitarb.). Nach KIRCHHOFF ist von besonderer Bedeutung, daß bei einem Drittel der Frauen mit Ovarialcarcinomen, bei denen der Histologe später auch im Corpus uteri Carcinome findet, anamnestisch keine gynäkologische Blutungsstörung zu eruieren ist. Das bedeutet, daß diese Carcinome im Korpus (Metastasen?) lange Zeit latent bleiben können. Deshalb fordert KIRCHHOFF (1967) dann, wenn aus irgendwelchen Gründen bei der Operation eines Ovarialcarcinoms der Uterus belassen werden soll, unter allen Umständen eine Abrasio vor der Operation zum Ausschluß eines Carcinoms im Corpus uteri. Auch die Hysterographie kann unter den geschilderten Gesichtspunkten u. U. aufschlußreich sein.

Sarkome sind offenbar nicht so häufig doppelseitig wie Carcinome und erreichen nur selten Mannskopfgröße. Cystische Tumoren und Kombinationen mit adenomatösen Formen sowie Sarkome bei Kindern können dagegen sehr groß werden. Im Gegensatz zum Carcinom entstehen Metastasen seltener auf dem Peritoneum, sondern entwickeln sich im Magen-Darmkanal, in der Lunge, dem Zwerchfell, den Nieren, der Wirbelsäule und den Beckenlymphdrüsen.

ζ) Altersverteilung

Das *Ovarialcarcinom* tritt mit zunehmendem Alter häufiger auf, kommt aber in jedem Alter vor. Infolge der zunehmenden durchschnittlichen Lebensverlängerung nimmt der

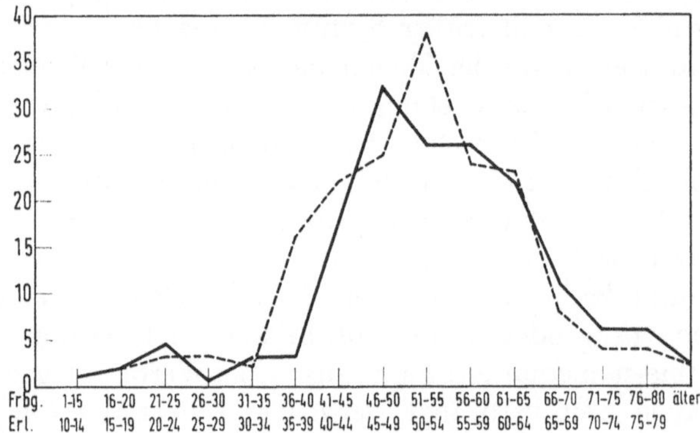

Abb. 9. Die Altersverteilung von 161 Patientinnen Freiburg (———) bzw. von 177 Patientinnen Erlangen (- - - - -) mit Ovarialcarcinomen

Tumor auch absolut zu. Müller gibt an, daß Frauen zwischen dem 41. und 60. Lebensjahr am häufigsten befallen werden, doch seien weder die Greisin noch der Säugling völlig verschont.

Maurer und Thomas werteten das Material an Ovarialcarcinomen der Universitäts-Frauenklinik Erlangen der Jahre 1949—1954 im Hinblick auf das Alter aus, kamen auf ein Durchschnittsalter von 53,3 Jahren und fanden für 177 Patientinnen die im obigen Diagramm (Abb. 9) eingetragene Altersverteilung. Unter etwa den gleichen Gesichtspunkten (die Altersgruppe um je 1 Jahr verschoben) werteten wir unser eigenes Material (Universitäts-Frauenklinik Freiburg) der Jahre 1948—1958 (161 Patientinnen) aus. Wir fanden ein Durchschnittsalter von 54,2 Jahren und die im gleichen Diagramm (Abb. 9) eingetragene Altersverteilung.

Die Altersverteilung ist im vergleichbaren Krankengut der beiden Kliniken bis in Einzelheiten weitgehend gleich und bekräftigt die Aussage Müllers, daß das Ovarialcarcinom sich hauptsächlich zwischen dem 40. und 60. Lebensjahr entwickelt. Die Altersverteilung im Krankengut des Frauenspitals Basel (Da Rugna, 1965) entspricht im wesentlichen ebenfalls der oben dargestellten Altersverteilung.

Das *Disgerminom* kommt bei Jugendlichen, Kindern, Kleinstkindern, aber auch bei völlig normal entwickelten Frauen und Männern vor.

Der *Tumor ovarii Brenner*, entwickelt sich im allgemeinen im höheren Lebensalter zwischen dem 40. und 60. Lebensjahr.

Teratoblastome kommen schon im Säuglings- und Kindesalter, zumeist aber zwischen dem 20. und 30. Lebensjahr vor.

Das *Arrhenoblastom* kann in jedem Lebensalter auftreten, wird aber zumeist zwischen dem 20. und 50. Lebensjahr beobachtet.

Der *Granulosazelltumor* kommt besonders bei alten Frauen vor, ausnahmsweise aber auch bei Kindern und jüngeren Frauen.

Thecazellgewächse fand man bisher bei Frauen unter 16 Jahren nicht. Das Maximum ihrer Häufigkeit fällt in das 6. Dezennium, also etwas später als bei den Granulosagewächsen.

Die *ovariellen Hypernephroide* können in jedem Lebensalter auftreten, doch findet man auch sie meist jenseits des Klimakteriums.

Ovarielle Chorionepitheliome sind in allen Altersstufen zu beobachten. Man findet sie jedoch meistens zwischen dem 20. und 30. Lebensjahr. Ein mit einer normalen oder pathologischen Schwangerschaft verbundenes ovarielles Chorionepitheliom kann natürlich vor der Pubertät nicht auftreten, während ein solches aus liegengebliebenen Chorionelementen auch vor der Geschlechtsreife nicht ausgeschlossen ist.

Eine *Struma ovarii* kann in jedem Lebensalter auftreten, doch findet man sie, wie allgemein die teratoiden Eierstocksneubildungen, zwischen dem 20. und 30. Lebensjahr am häufigsten.

η) Ätiologie

Im Ovar ist eine große Zahl von Gewebstypen zu einer funktionellen Einheit zusammengeschlossen, und jedes dieser Gewebe kann aus nicht bekannten Gründen einen Tumor produzieren. Grundsätzlich kann für die *malignen* Ovarialtumoren, die sich ja vorwiegend bei alten Frauen entwickeln (also die Mehrzahl), die Frage ventiliert werden, ob das atrophische, nicht funktionstüchtige Ovar besonders zur malignen Entartung neigt.

MAURER und THOMAS, MÖBIUS, H. H. SCHMID und CORSCADEN diskutieren die Möglichkeit einer Relation zwischen dem Auftreten von Ovarialcarcinomen und einer besonders geringen Anzahl von Schwangerschaften. So fand MAURER in seinem Krankengut an Ovarialcarcinomen 68% der Patientinnen die Nulli — I oder II — parae waren, also nur 32% der Frauen mit mehr als 2 Kindern. In unserem Krankengut an Ovarialcarcinomen fanden wir sogar 77,6% Nulli — I und II — parae und nur 22,4% Frauen mit mehr als 2 Kindern. Die Auswertung unseres Krankengutes stützt also die Hypothese der oben genannten Autoren. MAURER weist in diesem Zusammenhang darauf hin, daß eine entsprechende Beziehung zwischen Zahl der Schwangerschaften und Entstehung eines Malignoms beim Mammacarcinom vorliegt, während das Collumcarcinom umgekehrt bei Frauen, die mehr als 2 Schwangerschaften hatten, vermehrt auftritt und die Entwicklung des Vulvacarcinoms keine Beziehung zur Kinderzahl erkennen läßt.

Für die *Entstehung der hormonal aktiven Tumoren* sind darüber hinaus noch einige Gesichtspunkte zu diskutieren. Die meisten Autoren sind heute der Meinung, daß die Arrhenoblastome sich aus — infolge einer Fehlentwicklung — männlich determinierten mesenchymalen Resten der fetalen Gonaden, die Granulosazelltumoren und Thecazelltumoren aus embryonalen Mesenchymresten, die bereits eine weibliche Determination besitzen, entwickeln.

Die ovariellen Hypernephroidtumoren werden auf in der Embryonalzeit abgeschnürte und liegengebliebene Nebennierenkeime zurückgeführt.

Für die Entstehung des ovariellen Chorionepithelioms sind folgende Möglichkeiten zu diskutieren:

1. Verschleppung von Chorionepithelzellen bei normaler Placentation oder bei Blasenmole in die Ovarien.

2. Ovarielle Metastasenbildung eines intra- oder extrauterinen Chorionepithelioms.

3. Entwicklung im Anschluß an eine ovarielle Gravidität und

4. Entwicklung aus einer teratogenen Eierstocksgeschwulst.

c) Die malignen Tumoren der Parametrien und der Ligamenta rotunda

α) Häufigkeit

Bösartige, primär extraperitoneale, intraligamentär entstandene Tumoren gehören zu den seltensten bösartigen Geschwülsten überhaupt. H. H. Schmid stellte (1953) insgesamt 267 Fälle aus dem Weltschrifttum zusammen. Breen und Neubecker teilten 1962 mit, daß sie unter 25 Tumoren des Ligamentum rotundum aus den Jahren 1917—1960 zwei mit maligner Entartung gefunden hatten. Lange leugnete man (Sänger) überhaupt, wie bei den malignen Tubentumoren, auch die primäre Entstehung maligner Tumoren der Parametrien oder der Ligamenta rotunda am „Fundort" und ließ sie vom Uterus oder den Ovarien abstammen.

Sänger (zitiert nach Otto) gab schon 1880 folgende (etwas modifizierte) Einteilung aller Tumoren der Ligamenta rotunda:

1. Intraabdominelle Tumoren: von der Haftung des Ligamentes an der Gebärmutter bis zur inneren Öffnung des Leistenkanals.

2. Intracanaliculäre Tumoren: innerhalb des Leistenkanals.

3. Extraabdominelle Tumoren: an außerhalb des Leistenkanals gelegenen Abschnitten des Ligamentes, die sich im weiteren Verlauf auf die großen Schamlippen und unter die Bauchhaut ausbreiten können.

Die Sarkome der Ligamenta rotunda sind besonders selten: mit dem Fall von Navratil lagen bis 1956 nur 17 Mitteilungen vor. Breen und Neubecker fanden 1962 bei der histologischen Aufgliederung einer Zusammenstellung von 227 Tumoren des Ligamentum rotundum in 7—8% Sarkome. Die Sarkome stehen damit in diesem Material an Häufigkeit an 5. Stelle.

Die große Seltenheit der primären intraligamentären bösartigen Geschwülste wird durch das Ergebnis unserer Umfrage (wobei wir in die Betrachtung zusammenfassende Veröffentlichungen der letzten Jahre im deutschen Schrifttum mit einbeziehen) noch einmal besonders unterstrichen: An 9 Frauenkliniken wurde in unterschiedlichen Zeiträumen von 5—30 Jahren kein einziger bösartiger Tumor im Bereich der Parametrien und der Ligamenta rotunda beobachtet.

Ein Retothelsarkom des linken Parametriums und ein Lymphosarkom des rechten Parametriums wurden (beide im Jahre 1954) von Adler an der Strahlenabteilung der Universitäts-Frauenklinik (Frauenspital) Basel (persönliche Mitteilung) in 15 Jahren unter 1141 Genitalcarcinom-Patientinnen, ein Sarkom der linken Beckenwand in 12 Jahren an der Strahlenabteilung der Universitäts-Frauenklinik Tübingen von Spechter beobachtet. In Tübingen wurde in dieser Zeit auch noch ein proliferierendes Leiomyom mit Zeichen von Entdifferenzierung beobachtet (persönliche Mitteilungen).

β) Histologie

Es werden Adenosarkome, Spindelzellsarkome, Fibrosarkome, Fibrommyxosarkome, Myxosarkome, Liposarkome, Fibroliposarkome, Rhapdomyosarkome und Leiomyosarkome (Neumann, Bernstine und Beckinridge, Adler, Spechter) mitgeteilt sowie primäre Chorionepitheliome, sarkomatös entartete Teratome (Neumann), Carcinome in Parovarialcysten und intraligamentäre Carcinome, ausgehend vom Epoophoron (Meyer, Merill).

γ) Symptomatologie und Diagnostik

Die Symptomatologie der primären Geschwülste der Ligamenta rotunda und der Parametrien ist uneinheitlich. Im Anfangsstadium besteht oft verhältnismäßig lange Symptomlosigkeit (Rieck). Im fortgeschrittenen Stadium treten dann bei den intraabdominell lokalisierten Tumoren die für einen raumfordernden Prozeß im Becken typischen Verdrängungserscheinungen auf, und der Tumor kann sowohl von der Vagina als auch vom Rectum aus tastbar werden. Dabei können schon durch relativ kleine

Tumoren im Retroperitonealraum und dadurch relativ geringe Druckwirkungen Reiz-zustände im lumbalen Sympathicusabschnitt ausgelöst werden, die u. U. zu Temperatur-herabsetzungen der unteren Extremitäten führen. Stärkerer Druck dagegen kann zur Lähmung des Sympathicus und damit zu Temperaturerhöhungen der entsprechenden Extremitäten führen (L. SCHMIDT, 1955). Beckenzellgewebssarkome gleichen in Aus-breitung, Sitz und Konsistenz oft ganz außerordentlich harten, alten parametranen Exsudaten (STOECKEL). Symptomatologisch erscheint auch noch die Beobachtung von MERILL (1959) bei seinem Fall eines Adenocarcinoms im Ligamentum latum wichtig. Die Patientin hatte einen pleuralen Erguß, den er trotz der bösartigen Natur des Tumors im Sinne eines Meigs-Syndroms deuten möchte. Der Verfasser weist unter dem Eindruck dieses Befundes auf die Bedeutung einer sorgfältigen Beckenuntersuchung bei ungeklärten Pleuraergüssen hin.

Die Diagnose ist nicht leicht. Der Tastbefund ist von größter Wichtigkeit. Alle Möglich-keiten der vaginalen, rectalen und bimanuellen Untersuchung müssen ausgeschöpft werden, um abzuklären, ob das Neoplasma Beziehung zum Uterus hat. Die Diagnose eines Tumors des Ligamentum rotundum kann (NAVRÁTIL, 1959) ,,leichter gestellt werden, wenn beachtet wird, daß die Tumoren im vorderen seitlichen Quadranten des kleinen Beckens liegen, sehr derb sind und sowohl mit Uterus als mit der Beckenwand in Ver-bindung stehen. Beim Wegdrücken wandern sie sofort in ihre alte Lage zurück, bei Ver-schieben des Tumors nach oben strahlt der Schmerz bis in den Leistenkanal aus". Durch Cysto- und Rectoskopie und die röntgenologischen Untersuchungsmöglichkeiten der ab-leitenden Harnwege sowie der unteren Darmabschnitte und u. E. insbesondere auch die Pneumopelvigraphie, eventuell auch angiographische Untersuchungen können Anhalts-punkte über Lage, Größe der Tumoren und Verdrängungswirkungen auf die Nachbar-organe gewonnen und Neubildungen anderer Organe, insbesondere des Dickdarmes, aus-geschlossen werden. Nach SCHMIDT bleibt im allgemeinen nur die Probelaparotomie zur Identifizierung des Tumors und zur Prüfung der Operabilität.

Differentialdiagnostisch kommen intraligamentär entwickelte Genitalneoplasmen, Knochenblastome und Parovarialcysten, weiterhin nach STOECKEL universelle Lympho-granulomatose und Aktinomykose in Frage. Von grundsätzlicher Bedeutung ist die Tat-sache, daß nach L. SCHMIDT sonderbarer Weise bei den intraligamentär entwickelten Tumoren nicht nur die malignen, sondern gelegentlich auch die benignen Tumoren zu Rezidiven neigen, und dann solche Rezidive oft maligne umgewandelt sind. H. H. SCHMID kommt zu der Feststellung: ,,Wenn man bedenkt, daß ein Teil der Lipome und Myxome bzw. Mischgeschwülste den malignen Tumoren nahe steht, so ergibt sich, daß etwa die Hälfte der retroperitonealen Geschwülste (damit auch der Beckenbindegewebsgeschwülste) als bösartig zu betrachten sind".

δ) Metastasierung und Ausbreitung

Sowohl die gutartigen als die bösartigen extraperitonealen Beckentumoren können sich nach allen Richtungen ausbreiten und dabei allgemeine Verdrängungserscheinungen am Rectum, Sigma, Uterus, Blase und Ureteren verursachen. Das Wachstum der bös-artigen Tumoren ist aber im allgemeinen beschleunigt, und sie können destruierend in die Nachbarschaft einbrechen. Die sarkomatös entarteten Beckenzellgewebsfibrome oder -myome sind im allgemeinen kleinere Tumoren mit geringerer Wachstumstendenz. Die Rundzellensarkome dagegen wachsen schnell und breiten sich rasch infiltrierend aus, so daß der Ursprung des Tumors oft diagnostisch nicht mehr erfaßt werden kann.

ε) Altersverteilung

Grundsätzlich scheinen die intraligamentär entwickelten Tumoren in jedem Lebens-alter auftreten zu können, bevorzugt ist aber offenbar die Zeit nach dem Klimakterium.

ζ) Ätiologie

Die Ursache der Entstehung der Tumoren ist weitgehend unbekannt. Sie entwickeln sich entweder aus den verschiedensten Substraten, die am Aufbau des Beckenbindegewebes beteiligt sind (Bindegewebe, Muskelfasern, Fettgewebe, Blut- oder Lymphgefäße, Nerven), oder aus Resten embryonaler Gebilde in diesem Gewebe (Urniere, Wolffscher oder Gartnerscher Gang, ektopische Nebennierenteile).

3. Therapie

Zur Behandlung der malignen Tumoren der Tuben, Ovarien, Parametrien und Ligamenta rotunda stehen zur Verfügung:

1. Die Operation.
2. Die Bestrahlung.
   a) Intrakavitär mit Radium oder Kobalt.
   α) Intrauterin, wenn Uterus als Träger belassen.
   β) Intravaginal zusätzlich zur intrauterinen Anwendung, oder allein, wenn der Uterus entfernt wurde.
   b) Percutan mit Röntgen- und Supervoltstrahlen[1].
   c) Der Vollständigkeit halber sei die intravaginale Bestrahlung mit der Hohlanodenröhre erwähnt.
   d) Durch intraabdominelle Applikation radioaktiver Substanzen.
3. Die Anwendung chemischer, cytostatisch wirkender Substanzen.

Zumeist kommen Kombinationen von mehreren Behandlungsmöglichkeiten zur Anwendung. Dazu schreibt Meigs 1962: ,,Wesentlich ist, daß bei der Behandlung des Genitalkrebses der Frau Operation und Bestrahlung nicht miteinander rivalisieren, sondern sich ergänzen und daß die Zusatztherapie mit Hormonen und chemischen Stoffen aussichtsreich ist und möglicherweise ein neues Spezialgebiet werden wird.''

a) Operation und Indikation zur Strahlentherapie

α) Die malignen Tumoren der Tuben

αα) Das Tubencarcinom und Tubensarkom

Als Methode der Wahl zur Behandlung der malignen Tumoren der Tuben ist auf Grund der Mitteilungen über die Heilungserfolge in der Weltliteratur heute die abdominale Totalexstirpation des Uterus mit beidseitiger Adnexotomie und Nachbestrahlung mit intravaginaler Radiumapplikation und percutaner Röntgentiefen- oder Supervoltbestrahlung anzusehen. Es darf aber nicht verschwiegen werden, daß auch heute noch einige Autoren der Strahlenbehandlung skeptisch gegenüberstehen. In der amerikanischen Literatur wird von Frankel, Weekes, Anz und Whiting die Röntgennachbestrahlung als von zweifelhaftem Wert erachtet, Horalek und Kloc halten sie sogar grundsätzlich für erfolglos.

Die operative Behandlung sollte bei *allen malignen Tumoren* der *Tuben*, wenn einigermaßen Operabilität besteht, durchgeführt werden. Über die Radikalität des Eingriffes besteht keine Einmütigkeit. Nürnberger fordert die erweiterte abdominale Radikalexstirpation des Uterus mit Adnexen, Ausräumung der Lymphknoten des kleinen Beckens, Resektion des Netzes, nachfolgende intravaginale Radiumapplikation und percutane Nachbestrahlung, während z.B. Ries, Kepp, Huber u.a. mehr strahlentherapeutisch eingestellte Gynäkologen der Auffassung sind, daß die abdominale Totalexstirpation des Uterus mit beidseitiger Adnexotomie und Röntgen- bzw. Supervoltnachbestrahlung ausreicht.

---

1 Unter Supervoltbestrahlung wird im folgenden die Anwendung der Telekobalt-, Betatron- und Linearbeschleunigerstrahlung verstanden. Zumeist wird es sich dabei allerdings um Telekobaltbestrahlung handeln.

Eine einfache und einseitige Adnexotomie ist jedenfalls in Kenntnis der Diagnose oder bei dringendem Verdacht auf malignen Tubentumor unter gar keinen Umständen zu vertreten, wenn auch Berichte über gelegentliche Heilungen nach einfachen Adnexotomien, die in Unkenntnis der Diagnose durchgeführt wurden, vorliegen.

ENGSTRÖM berichtete 1958 über sehr gute Heilungsergebnisse an einem relativ großen Krankengut mit der am Radiumhemmet in Stockholm geübten Behandlungsmethode. Es wurde die beidseitige Adnexotomie unter Belassung des Uterus als Radiumträger durchgeführt und kombiniert mit Radium intrakavitär und Röntgen percutan nachbestrahlt.

Bei inkurablen Fällen wird heute allgemein von einer Palliativoperation Abstand genommen und nur noch mit intrakavitärer Radium- und percutaner Röntgen- bzw. Supervoltbestrahlung behandelt. Sicher können bei diesen Fällen insbesondere auch die intraabdominelle Anwendung von radioaktiven — und die Verabfolgung von cytostatisch wirkenden Substanzen von Vorteil sein. Entsprechende Mitteilungen haben wir in der Literatur nicht gefunden.

ββ) Tubenchorionepitheliom

Als Therapie der Wahl gilt die Totalexstirpation des Uterus mit beiden Adnexen, wobei alle Metastasen, die mit dem Messer erreichbar sind, abgetragen werden, eventuell unter Mitnahme der Parametrien und einer Scheidenmanschette (HEISS). Es sollte unter allen Umständen nachbestrahlt werden. Bei Inoperabilität werden Radium- oder Kobaltintrakavitär und percutane Röntgen- bzw. Supervoltbestrahlung, bei Vaginalmetastasen eine Radium- oder Kobaltkontaktbestrahlung der Metastase und zusätzliche percutane Bestrahlung durchgeführt. Lungenmetastasen bilden sich beim Chorionepitheliom nach *Vernichtung* des Primärtumors oft spontan zurück (u. a. eigene Beobachtungen).

HUBER und HÖRMANN glauben beim Chorionepitheliom des Uterus auch an benigne Formen (Chorionepitheliosis), da sie einige ,,Spontanheilungen", besonders von Metastasen, in der Literatur und in ihrem eigenen Krankengut fanden und nehmen das gleiche für das Tubenchorionepitheliom an.

Solange die bösartigen Fälle von Chorionepitheliomen aber von den gutartigen vor der Behandlung nicht zu differenzieren sind, erfordert jeder Zottenkrebs ein radikales therapeutisches Vorgehen. Während und nach der Behandlung soll die Prolanausscheidung in Kontrolle bleiben, um Rezidive früh genug erkennen und therapeutisch angehen zu können.

β) Die malignen Tumoren der Ovarien

Für alle Ovarialtumoren ist die Laparotomie die primäre Therapie der Wahl. Nur sie ermöglicht es, die räumliche Ausdehnung des Tumors und seine Beziehungen zu den Nachbarorganen zu erkennen. Durch die Inspektion des Tumors und die histologische Untersuchung eines während der Operation gewonnenen Gewebsanteils kann eine exakte Diagnose gestellt werden. Auch die Laparoskopie und bei Metastasen im Douglasschen Raum die Probeexcision aus diesen Absiedlungen können im allgemeinen die Laparotomie nicht ersetzen, sondern stellen zusätzliche, die Patientin oft belastende Eingriffe dar. Da der Laparotomie somit in diagnostischer Hinsicht der Vorrang einzuräumen und außerdem die möglichst vollständige Abtragung des Tumors Voraussetzung für eine dauerhafte Heilung ist, sollte man sich immer gleich zur Laparotomie entschließen (BREITNER und ADLER, 1958; DYROFF und SIEGERT, 1955). Auf die von dieser Vorstellung abweichende Auffassung von SPECHTER und der Tübinger Universitäts-Frauenklinik wird später (S. 359) eingegangen. Eine rasche Laparotomie wird grundsätzlich auch erforderlich, wenn große Tumoren zu Verdrängungserscheinungen führen und Atmung und Kreislauf beeinträchtigen.

Die Notwendigkeit der Laparotomie ist heute zwar von allen Autoren anerkannt, doch bestehen über die Wahl der geeignetsten Operationsmethode Meinungsverschiedenheiten. In Frage kommen:

a) die abdominale Totalexstirpation mit Adnexen,

b) die supravaginale Uterusamputation mit Entfernung der Adnexe,

c) die beidseitige Adnexexstirpation mit Belassung des Uterus als Radiumträger,

d) die einseitige Adnexexstirpation.

Über die Frage, ob der Uterus als Radiumträger belassen werden soll oder nicht, besteht noch keine Einmütigkeit. Es mehren sich aber die Stimmen, die der Radikalität des Eingriffs — abdominale Totalexstirpation des Uterus mit Adnexen — den Vorzug geben. So teilte Rubin 1962 in der Einleitung zu einem Symposion über die Therapie des Eierstockkrebses mit, daß in den Veröffentlichungen von 25 prominenten amerikanischen Kliniken die meisten Autoren die Radikaloperation mit Wegnahme der Gebärmutter durchführen, die Mitnahme des Netzes dagegen wenig üblich sei. Dalley hat 1962 einen Vergleich der Überlebensdauer von zwei vergleichbaren Gruppen von Patientinnen, bei denen die Operation mit bzw. ohne Hysterektomie durchgeführt worden war, mitgeteilt, der eine deutliche Überlegenheit der radikalen Operationsmethode erkennen läßt. Kirchhoff hat sich 1967 fast leidenschaftlich gegen die Belassung des Uterus als Radiumträger ausgesprochen und sich voll hinter eine Äußerung von Hofmann (Münster) gestellt, daß „den Uterus als Radiumträger zurücklassen, heißt, ein Organ erhalten, nur um es nachbestrahlen zu können". Dagegen wird an der ersten Universitäts-Frauenklinik Wien (Fochem und Weghaupt, 1957) das Belassen des Uterus als Radiumträger als Methode der Wahl bezeichnet, und auch an der ersten Universitäts-Frauenklinik München hält man an der Methode der intrauterinen Radiumapplikation als Zusatztherapie fest, um eine höhere Strahlendosis im Becken zu ermöglichen. An der Basler Klinik (Held und Adler) wird der Uterus wegen der Gefahr der Korpusmetastasen supravaginal amputiert, der Cervixstumpf als Radiumträger verwendet. Kirchhoff weist allerdings 1967 darauf hin, daß er im Collum eine Ovarialcarcinommetastase beobachtet hat.

Die Resektion des Omentum majus ist heute eine gebräuchliche vorbeugende Maßnahme, da Metastasen sich frühzeitig im Netz entwickeln können. Kottmeier, Pemberton und Meigs sind der Meinung, daß das große Netz bei maligne entarteten Ovarialtumoren als Routinemaßnahme entfernt werden sollte. Taylor Jr. und Greeley (1942) halten es jedoch für besser, das Netz zu belassen, wenn es unauffällig erscheint.

Die routinemäßige percutane Röntgen- bzw. Supervoltnachbestrahlung wird auch heute noch von den meisten Autoren (Kirchhoff, 1967) als notwendig angesehen, selbst wenn es gelingt, den Tumor in toto zu entfernen. Erstaunlicherweise ist demgegenüber in Stoeckels Lehrbuch der Gynäkologie, Ausgabe 1960, zu lesen: „Eine Röntgennachbestrahlung der radikal operierten Ovarialcarcinome wird besser unterlassen; auch für die unvollständig operierten oder inoperablen Fälle (nur Probelaparotomie!) bringt eine Röntgenbestrahlung nur in seltenen Ausnahmefällen einen Erfolg oder eine Besserung".

Demgegenüber sind sich heute wohl fast alle Autoren darüber einig, daß bei einem malignen Ovarialtumor, der nicht ganz entfernt werden konnte, die Unterlassung der Nachbestrahlung ein Kunstfehler ist (Dyroff und Siegert, 1955). Es wird im allgemeinen vor der Bestrahlung die Entfernung von möglichst viel Tumorgewebe befürwortet, obwohl der Eingriff dadurch — auch infolge der Tatsache, daß die ausgedehnten Tumoren sich meistens schon sehr ungünstig auf den Allgemeinzustand ausgewirkt haben — gefährlicher wird. Die durch die Bestrahlung anfallenden Zerfallsprodukte der Ovarialtumoren werden dadurch vermindert und der Organismus entlastet. Außerdem kann u. U. die notwendige Gesamtbestrahlungsdosis durch die so erreichte räumliche Beschränkung des Tumors verringert werden.

Für einzelne der hormonal aktiven Neubildungen der Ovarien (Arrhenoblastom, Granulosazelltumor) mit „bedingter" Malignität ist die Entscheidung, ob ein radikales Vorgehen angezeigt, oder ein mehr konservatives Vorgehen noch verantwortet werden kann, oft außerordentlich schwierig. Bei klinischer Bösartigkeit sind möglichst Radikaloperation und nachfolgende Strahlenbehandlung durchzuführen. Bei klinisch gutartigen, einseitigen, abgekapselten Tumoren kann bei jungen Frauen im Hinblick auf die Möglichkeit der Erhaltung der Konzeptionsfähigkeit eventuell auf ein radikales operatives Vorgehen verzichtet und primär nur die Entfernung der veränderten Adnexe einer Seite durchgeführt werden. Die Frage der Nachbestrahlung muß dann auf Grund sorgfältiger histologischer Prüfung entschieden werden, wobei, auch trotz nachweisbarer feingeweblicher Malignität des Tumors, gelegentlich einmal unter Würdigung aller Umstände auf eine

Tabelle 4

	Operation und Bestrahlung				Operation allein			
	418 Fälle		Überlebende nach 5 Jahren		74 Fälle		Überlebende nach 5 Jahren	
	Zahl	%	Zahl	%	Zahl	%	Zahl	%
Radikal operierte Fälle	198	47,4	86	43,4	30	40,5	5	16,7
Unvollständig operierte Fälle	127	30,4	11	3,7	19	25,7	0	0
Inoperable Fälle	93	22,2	4	4,3	25	33,8	0	0
Summe	418	100	101	24,2	74	100	5	6,8

KOTTMEIER bezeichnet (zitiert nach MAURER) diejenigen Fälle als radikal operiert, bei denen der Operateur der Ansicht ist, daß das Carcinom insgesamt entfernt und kein Carcinomgewebe zurückgelassen wurde; der Uterus wird als Radiumträger belassen.

postoperative Bestrahlung verzichtet werden kann (DUBRAUSZKY, 1954). So haben MAL-KASIAN und SYMMOND 1964 über 41 Beobachtungen, 26 aus der Literatur und 15 aus den Unterlagen der Mayo-Klinik, bei denen ein konservatives Vorgehen im geschilderten Sinne durchgeführt worden war, berichtet. Die 5-Jahres-Heilung lag dabei bei 82,2 %, die Rezidivquote bei 52,4 %, die Konzeptionsquote bei 37,7 %.

Die grundsätzliche Bedeutung der postoperativen Nachbestrahlungen wird durch die Untersuchungen von KOTTMEIER insbesondere unterstrichen. Er stellt in einer Tabelle (Tabelle 4) die Ergebnisse bei ausschließlich chirurgisch behandelten Ovarialcarcinomen mit sicher invasivem Wachstum den Ergebnissen bei kombiniert chirurgisch-radiologischer Behandlung gegenüber.

Eine ganze Reihe von Autoren (CRAINZ, GAUSS, SCHROEDER und HARTL, RIESS, KOTTMEIER u.a.) befürwortet außerdem die Bestrahlung aller inoperablen Fälle von Ovarialcarcinomen unter dem Gesichtspunkt, daß dadurch — wir haben bereits darauf hingewiesen — u.U. eine Verkleinerung der Tumoren eintritt, die schließlich doch noch zu einer Operabilität führt, und daß sogar Heilungen durch solche Bestrahlungen erzielt werden können. Es liegen Beobachtungen von durch Probelaparotomie histologisch verifizierten, inoperablen malignen Ovarialtumoren vor, die durch alleinige Bestrahlung geheilt (5-Jahres-Heilung) werden konnten (SCHÖMIG, BECKER). SCHÖMIG spricht auch von Spontanheilungen nach alleiniger Probelaparotomie. Solche Ereignisse dürften aber zu den ausgesprochenen Raritäten zählen.

SCHRÖDER vertritt die Auffassung, daß kein Ovarialcarcinom so weit vorgeschritten ist, daß u.U. nicht doch noch durch Strahlentherapie eine Heilung erreicht werden könnte. Unter diesem Gesichtspunkt ist auch die Mitteilung von SCHROEDER und HARTL von Bedeutung, daß sie 5-Jahres-Heilungen nur bei Patientinnen sahen, die nach der Operation noch bestrahlt worden waren.

Von Wichtigkeit ist im Hinblick auf eventuell vorhandene Metastasen, daß diese ihr Wachstum oft einstellen, wenn der Primärtumor entfernt wurde. Selbst Peritoneal-metastasen können dann spontan verschwinden (Kottmeier).

Von grundsätzlicher Bedeutung erscheint im Hinblick auf die Wirksamkeit der percutanen Nachbestrahlung eine Äußerung von Rubin in der schon zitierten Einleitung zu einem Symposion über die Therapie des Eierstockkrebses, in der er unter anderem darauf hinweist, daß bei der Nachbestrahlung oft eine unzureichende Dosis angewendet wird.

Über den Wert der zusätzlichen fakultativen oder routinemäßigen intraabdominellen Verabreichung von radioaktiven Substanzen, die durch Müller 1954 inauguriert wurde, liegen aus den letzten Jahren aus aller Welt eine Flut von Mitteilungen vor. Dabei über-wiegt die Anzahl der positiven Stimmen insbesondere in den letzten Jahren (Müller, Breitner, Rose, Kepp und Clemens, Stanicek, Carazzone, Dörfel und Hai, Økland u.v.a.). Verwendet wird zumeist radioaktives Gold (^{198}Au), selten auch radioaktives Yttrium (^{90}Y) und Chromphosphat (^{32}Cr PO$_4$). Einige andere Radiokolloide haben nach Müller z.Z. nur experimentelles Interesse.

Auch über den Wert der zusätzlichen Behandlung mit cytostatischen Substanzen mehren sich, neben gelegentlichen negativen, die positiven Aussagen (Spechter, Pfleide-rer und Kiyan, Lebherz, Krahe u. Mitarb., Novikova, Lambrethusen, Baksheeva, Bozzo und Cravarezzo, Schwartz, Blinick, Decker u.a.).

γ) Die malignen Tumoren der Parametrien und Ligamenta rotunda

Die primäre therapeutische Konsequenz bei *jedem* Verdacht auf einen intraligamen-tären Tumor ist die sofortige, möglichst radikale Operation, da auch die scheinbar benignen Geschwülste (Lipome, Myxome) ein relativ malignes Verhalten zeigen. Nach L. Schmidt machte bereits 1923 H. H. Schmidt auch den Vorschlag, an jede Radikaloperation maligner und benigner Blastome im Bereich des Beckenbindegewebes eine prophylaktische Röntgennachbestrahlung anzuschließen. L. Schmid selbst dagegen und Laughlin und Sharpe (1938) sprechen der postoperativen Bestrahlung der malignen Fettumoren des Retroperitonealraumes keine Bedeutung zu, während Freund die Strahlenbehandlung besonders bei inoperablen und unvollständig operierten Beckenzellgewebstumoren emp-fiehlt und behauptet, daß auch bei größeren Tumoren Röntgenbestrahlung allein oder auch kombinierte Radium-Röntgentiefentherapie mit Erfolg angewendet werden kann.

Die intraabdominelle Verabreichung radioaktiver Substanzen, wie sie Müller für das Ovarialcarcinom propagiert hat, ist nach theoretischen Überlegungen wenig sinnvoll, da die Tumoren primär retro- bzw. extraperitoneal liegen. Die interstitielle, u.U. auch intra-tumorale Verabreichung radioaktiver Substanzen wäre hier diskutabel. Entsprechende Mitteilungen liegen aber nicht vor.

Für die Anwendung chemischer cytostatischer Substanzen gelten grundsätzlich die gleichen Überlegungen wie wir sie für die malignen Tumoren der Tuben und Ovarien angestellt haben.

b) Spezielle Strahlentherapie

Die Seltenheit der malignen Tumoren der Tuben, Parametrien und Ligamenta rotunda und — wie wir für das relativ häufige Ovarialcarcinom schon ausgeführt haben — die schlechten Heilungsergebnisse führten dazu, daß Röntgenologen und Strahlentherapeuten in zusammenfassenden Veröffentlichungen sich nicht, oder nur am Rande, mit der Strahlen-therapie dieser Tumoren beschäftigt haben. So gehen Vogt und Glauner in ihren Büchern „Diagnostik und Strahlentherapie der Geschwulstkrankheiten" und „Die Indikationen zur Röntgen- und Radiumbestrahlung" nur relativ kurz auf die Behandlung der Ovarial-tumoren und nur hinweisend im Zusammenhang damit auf die Eileitergeschwülste ein. Oeser erwähnt in seinem Buch über die „Strahlenbehandlung der Geschwülste" weder die Ovarialtumoren noch die Tumoren der Tuben, Parametrien und Ligamenta rotunda.

Auch in den Büchern über die gynäkologische Strahlentherapie von KEPP und von RIESS und BREITNER (1959), die ja von Gynäkologen, die sich mit den therapeutischen Möglichkeiten der Strahlenbehandlung auf ihrem Spezialgebiet besonders eingehend beschäftigt haben, geschrieben sind, werden die Ovarialtumoren nur relativ knapp, die malignen Tumoren der Tuben ebenfalls nur ganz hinweisend, und die Behandlung der malignen Tumoren der Parametrien und der Ligamenta rotunda überhaupt nicht abgehandelt.

Die Strahlentherapie, vor allem die ergänzende Strahlentherapie der malignen Ovarialtumoren, aber auch der seltenen bösartigen Tumoren der Tuben, Parametrien und der Ligamenta rotunda gehört aber zweifellos in Zusammenarbeit mit den Gynäkologen zum unabdingbaren Aufgabenbereich des Strahlentherapeuten.

Von grundsätzlicher Bedeutung für den Erfolg der Strahlentherapie ist die Strahlenresistenz der Tumoren. Wie das normale Gewebe haben auch die verschiedenartigen malignen Geschwülste eine verschiedene Strahlensensibilität. Grundsätzlich sind die vom Binde- und Stützgewebe abstammenden bösartigen Tumoren strahlenempfindlicher als die epithelialen Tumoren, wobei außerordentliche individuelle Unterschiede bestehen können, so daß eine Ordnung dieser malignen Geschwülste nach ihrer Strahlenempfindlichkeit nur sehr bedingt gültig wäre.

Die einzelnen von den verschiedenartigen Geweben abstammenden bösartigen Tumoren haben aber auch untereinander wieder eine verschiedene Strahlensensibilität. So zitiert KEPP HOLTHUSEN und führt aus, daß ,,ein Schilddrüsencarcinom z.B. viel strahlensensibler als ein Rectumcarcinom ist, obwohl die normale Rectumschleimhaut eine viel größere Strahlenempfindlichkeit aufweist als das normale Schilddrüsenparenchym".

Die Differenzierung der Zellen, aus denen sich das Malignom entwickelt hat, ist für die Strahlensensibilität von großer Bedeutung, wobei die Tumoren, die sich aus wenig differenzierten Zellen entwickelt haben, im allgemeinen besser auf die Strahlentherapie ansprechen. Die intensiven, insbesondere von gynäkologischer Seite durchgeführten Versuche, aus der histologischen Struktur der bösartigen Tumoren auf die Strahlensensibilität zu schließen, haben bislang nur zu wenig brauchbaren Ergebnissen geführt. Oft lassen auch bösartige Tumoren, die in ihrem histologischen Aufbau Geschwülsten gleichen, bei denen die Strahlentherapie zu Heilungen führt, keine wesentliche Reaktion auf die Strahlentherapie erkennen, sind also strahlenrefraktär.

So sprechen z.B. die Granulosazelltumoren, die Chorionepitheliome und auch die Disgerminome (u.a. neuere Mitteilung von KOLLER und GJØUNAESS, 1964, über 20 Fälle) im allgemeinen auf die Strahlentherapie recht gut an, während die Thecazelltumoren und gemischten Tumoren strahlenresistenter sind.

Für die Strahlentherapie der intraligamentären Tumoren ist von Bedeutung, daß sowohl die Strahlenwirkung auf die Tumoren des lipomatösen Gewebes sehr problematisch ist, als auch über die Strahlenwirkung auf Myxome noch keine endgültigen Aussagen gemacht werden können.

α) *Radium- und Kobaltkontaktbestrahlung (intrakavitär und intratumoral)*

Über die Zweckmäßigkeit der Belassung des Uterus beim operierten Ovarialmalignom als Radiumträger gehen — wir haben schon darauf hingewiesen — die Ansichten z.T. erheblich auseinander.

CRAINZ, GUTHMANN und DÖRR, SCHRÖDER, RUMMEL, KOTTMEIER, FOCHEM und WEGHAUPT u.v.a. haben mit der intrauterinen Radiumapplikation bei malignen Ovarialtumoren gute Erfahrungen gemacht und können mit anderen Autoren (z.B. SCHWARTZ) nicht übereinstimmen, die glauben, daß die Radiumtherapie wegen der Dicke der Uterusmuskulatur von geringem Wert sei. DYROFF und SIEGERT betonen die günstige seitliche Dosisverteilung bei der intrauterinen Radiumapplikation, während KEPP im Gegensatz dazu schon 1952 vor dem Optimismus warnt ,,eine wesentliche Wirkung auf Tumorteile, die in der Umgebung des Uterus zurückblieben, zu erwarten". Kirchhoff hält das bewußte Zurücklassen des Uterus beim Ovarialcarcinom nicht nur für ein unnützes, sondern möglicherweise sogar für ein nicht ungefährliches Verfahren und führt aus, daß mit der Supervolttherapie sowohl eine genügend hoch dosierte homogene Bestrahlung des ganzen Beckenraumes als auch eine den Radium-Isodosen gleichwertige Konzentration an gefahrvollen Punkten möglich ist und deshalb keine Notwendigkeit bestehe, den Uterus für eine zusätzliche Radiumbestrahlung zurückzulassen.

Engström berichtete über günstige Erfolge mit der Belassung des Uterus als Radiumträger beim Tubencarcinom. Unter dem Eindruck dieser Mitteilung erscheint es uns empfehlenswert, nicht nur beim Tubencarcinom sondern auch bei den anderen malignen Tumoren der Tuben, Parametrien und Ligamenta rotunda zumindest dann, wenn unter der Operation klar wird, daß nicht das ganze Tumorgewebe beseitigt werden kann, den Uterus als Radiumträger zu belassen. Wir schließen uns damit der Auffassung von Kremer und Ulm (1955) an, daß der Behandlungsmodus von Engström für diese Tumoren wahrscheinlich eine optimale Therapiemöglichkeit darstellt.

Die Radiumbehandlung wird entweder kombiniert durch intrauterine und intravaginale Radiumeinlagen von insgesamt 5000—7000 mgelh (andere Autoren Runge und Zeitz, 1956, z.B. nur 3000 mgelh), davon ca. $^2/_3$ intrauterin und $^1/_3$ intravaginal oder — wenn der Uterus entfernt wurde — durch alleinige intravaginale Radiumeinlagen (bis 4000 mgelh) durchgeführt. Die Höhe der Dosis richtet sich nach den räumlichen und anatomischen Gegebenheiten — unter Berücksichtigung insbesondere auch der Toleranzdosen an Blase und Rectum. Die intrauterine Radiumeinlage erfolgt zweckmäßigerweise mit den ursprünglich am Radiumhemmet Stockholm entwickelten, dann von verschiedenen Autoren modifizierten intrauterinen eiförmigen und länglichen Radiumträgern für kleine Radiummengen (5—10 mg), mit denen es möglich ist, den Uterus vollzupacken.

Wir haben vergleichende Ausmessungen der Isodosenkurven von intrauterinen Radiumeinlagen einmal mit den von Ries angegebenen eiförmigen Trägern mit kleinen Radiummengen in Stiften und dann mit der gleichen Radiummenge, die gleichen Stifte gebündelt und in Kartuschen in einem dicken Stift hintereinander geordnet, durchgeführt. Der „Uterus" war als Moulage aus reinem Paraffin nach einem Operationspräparat angefertigt worden, die Länge des intrauterinen Stiftes ergab sich aus der Sondenlänge. Die Abb. 10a u. 10b zeigen die Isodosenverläufe und die Anordnung der eiförmigen Träger in der Uterusmoulage in zwei Ebenen. In der Abb. 11 sind die Isodosenverläufe bei Verwendung von „Eiern" und dickem Stift übereinander gezeichnet. Die durchgezogenen Isodosenlinien entsprechen den Ausmessungen bei Füllung der Moulage mit eiförmigen Radiumträgern, die unterbrochenen Linien bei Verwendung des Stiftes. Bei der vergleichenden Betrachtung wird deutlich, daß der Uteruskörper bei Bestrahlung mit den radiumgefüllten Eiern im Zentrum der Strahlenwirkung liegt, während bei Verwendung des dicken Stiftes das Strahlungszentrum etwa in Höhe des inneren Muttermundes gelegen ist.

An Stelle von Radium können zur intrauterinen Einlage auch Kobalt-60-Perlen angewendet werden, die von Becker und Scheer 1952 angegeben wurden. Infolge der kleineren Abmessungen der Perlen, die alternierend mit inaktiven Perlen aus Plexiglas oder anderen Kunststoffen auf Schnüren aufgereiht werden, ist der Uterus oft noch besser „auszutamponieren" als mit den größeren eiförmigen Trägern.

Die intravaginale Radiumeinlage erfolgt bei kombinierter (intrauteriner und intravaginaler) Bestrahlung zumeist mit der Portioplatte, bei alleiniger intravaginaler Radiumeinlage mit phallusähnlichen, verschieden langen Trägern, wie sie z.B. auch von Ries und Kottmeier benutzt werden. Wir haben zu dieser Radiumanwendung eigene Träger konstruiert, die aus mehreren „Etagen" bestehen, die außen kleine Bohrungen für 6—8 Einzelzellen, zentral größere Bohrungen für mehrere, zusammengepackte Zellen haben, so daß eine sehr differenzierte Verteilung der Strahlenquellen und damit Gestaltung der Isodosen möglich ist. Durch Zusammenschrauben von 2 oder 3 „Etagen" ist es außerdem möglich, die Länge des strahlenden Trägers zu variieren. In die zentrale

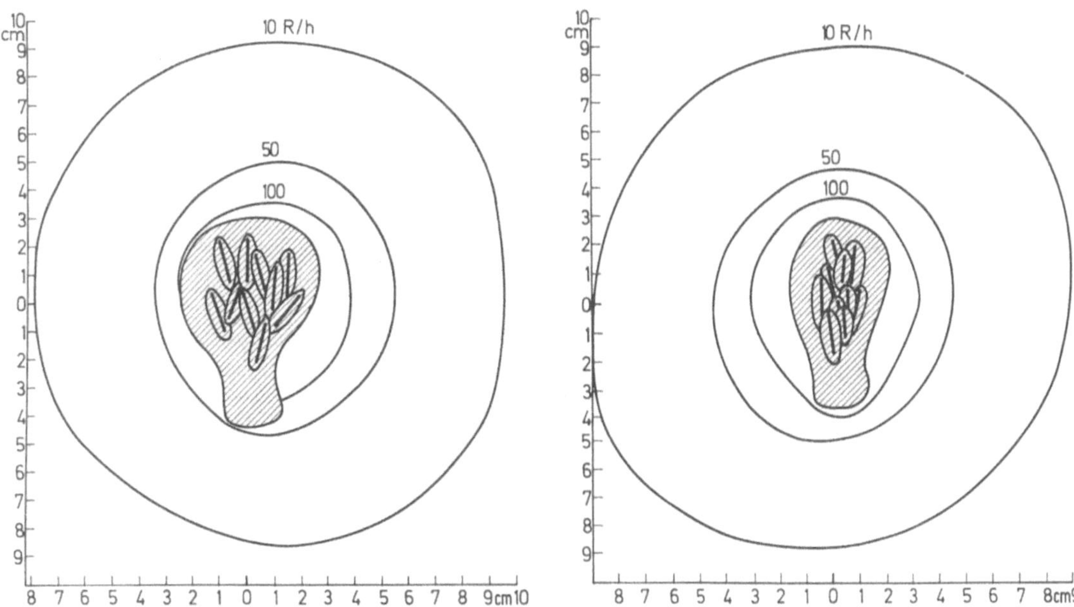

Abb. 10a u. b. Isodosenverläufe bei Austamponieren des Uterus mit eiförmigen Radiumträgern. a Antero-
posterior; b seitlich (Lage der Eier nach Röntgenaufnahmen gezeichnet)

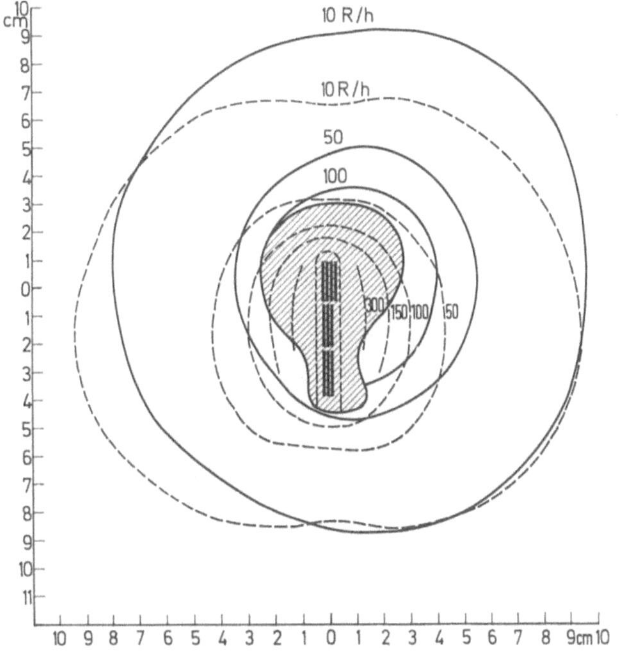

Abb. 11. Isodosenverläufe bei Verwendung von eiförmigen Radiumträgern (----) und dickem Stift (——)
übereinander gezeichnet

Bohrung können an Stelle von Radium auch radioaktive Kobaltperlen als strahlende
Substanz eingebracht werden (Abb. 12).

Die Gesamtdosis wird in 2 oder 3 Einlagen für je 20 oder 24 Std verabreicht. Eigene
vergleichende Untersuchungen über die Reaktionen an Blase und Rectum bei Verabreichung gleicher Gesamtdosen (gleiche Trägerkombination) in 2facher und 3facher
Fraktionierung haben die bekannte bessere Verträglichkeit der Radiumbestrahlung bei
stärkerer Fraktionierung erneut bestätigt.

Die Radiumdosis wird auch heute zumeist noch in mgelh angegeben. Um die Angabe der räumlichen Dosisverteilung — und damit die Berechnung der Dosis in R an jedem beliebigen Punkt — zu ermöglichen, ist die Ausmessung der Isodosenkurven notwendig, die heute insbesondere mit dem Momentandosimeter (Bomke-Eberle) ja sehr einfach durchzuführen ist. Wir haben zu unserem Gebrauch für jede Trägerkombination entsprechende Isodosenkurven ausgemessen (Goette, 1953; Müller-Hummel, 1958).

Die modernen, noch im Ausbau begriffenen Computerverfahren ermöglichen Isodosenberechnungen auch bei der Kombination von percutaner mit intrauteriner Strahlentherapie, wobei man von verschiedenen Möglichkeiten die optimale auswählen kann.

Die Tatsache, daß die Kobalt-60-Strahlung härter ist als die Radiumstrahlung, muß bei Verwendung von Kobalt-60 bei der Dosierung auch im Hinblick auf die verschiedene relative biologische Wirksamkeit (RBW) entsprechend berücksichtigt werden.

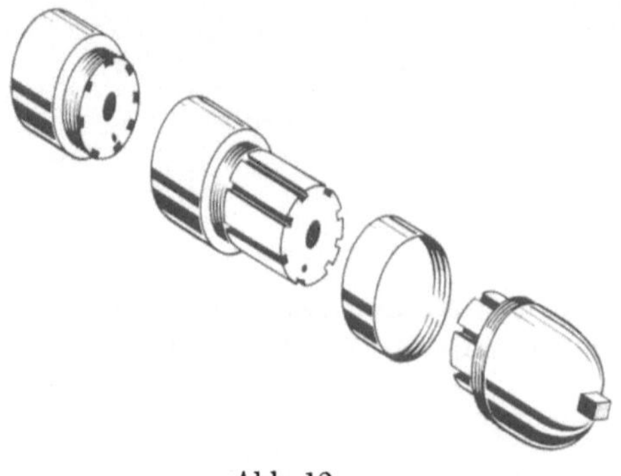

Abb. 12

Der Vollständigkeit halber ist erwähnenswert, daß Stoeckel für die intraligamentären Tumoren die intratumorale Radiumapplikation propagiert, die sicher in Einzelfällen, wenn der Tumor entsprechend gut erreichbar ist, von Vorteil sein kann. Die Radiumapplikation kann mit Spicknadeln disseminiert gleichmäßig über den ganzen Tumor verteilt, oder durch Einlage größerer stiftförmiger Träger, die gewissermaßen in den Tumor „hineingebohrt" werden, erfolgen. Theoretisch ist für diese Behandlungsart der intraligamentären Tumoren auch an Stelle von Radium die insbesondere von Kapp-Schwoerer zur Behandlung anderer gynäkologischer Tumoren empfohlene „individuelle Therapie mittels Radioseeds-Implantation" möglich.

Die Antibiotikaprophylaxe bei der Kontakttherapie mit strahlenden Substanzen hat sich immer mehr eingebürgert und wird heute als unerläßlich angesehen. Für das Collumcarcinom haben Buttenberg und Gutensohn (1964) bei Durchführung der Kontaktbestrahlung mit Radium unter Antibiotikaprophylaxe eine wesentliche Verminderung der fieberhaften Reaktionen und dadurch eine beachtliche Steigerung der 5-Jahres-Heilungen mitgeteilt.

Die enge zeitliche Zuordnung der percutanen und der intrakavitären Radium- bzw. Kobaltbestrahlung ist u. E. für die Auswirkung auf das Tumorgewebe von besonderer Bedeutung.

β) Percutane Bestrahlung (Röntgen, Telekobalt, Elektronenschleuder, Linear-beschleuniger, Hohlanodenrohrbestrahlung)

Bei der postoperativen percutanen Bestrahlung mit Röntgenstrahlen wird bei allen besprochenen Tumoren eine Dosis am Herd — also etwa im Bereich der Parametrien — von 2 500—3 000 R angestrebt. Die Bestrahlung erfolgt im allgemeinen von 2 Unterbauch- und 2 korrespondierenden Glutealfeldern aus, Feldgröße 10 × 15 cm, möglichst harte Strahlung (mindestens 180 kV, 0,5 mm Cu Filter, HWS 0,85 mm Cu, FHA 40 cm und

— soweit möglich — kräftige Kompression). Der Tubus wird etwas in das Becken gekippt und leicht nach innen gerichtet. Durch Unterschieben einer stärkeren Rolle unter die Knie, so daß diese abgestützt werden, kann die Bauchmuskulatur entspannt und damit die Kompressionsmöglichkeit des Leibes verbessert werden.

Zur Verfügung stehen die Vollfeldbestrahlung und die Siebbestrahlung. Im Hinblick auf die wesentlich bessere *Allgemeinverträglichkeit* (u.a. DIETZ und ENSE, 1959; DIETZ und POESCHEL, 1960) und die Möglichkeit der größeren Hautbelastung ist u.E. der *Röntgensiebbestrahlung* gegenüber der Vollfeldbestrahlung der Vorzug zu geben. Die gebräuchlichen Siebe haben ein Öffnungsverhältnis von 60/40 oder 50/50. Der Lochdurchmesser der Siebe sollte nicht kleiner als 5 mm und nicht größer als 10 mm sein (DIETZ und STARCKJOHANN, 1962). Erstaunlicherweise erwähnt KEPP in seinem Buch über die Grundlagen der Strahlentherapie aus dem Jahre 1952 die damals schon bekannte Siebbestrahlung überhaupt nicht. ZUPPINGER glaubt, daß die Siebbestrahlung keinen Vorteil bringt. Wir selbst haben die Siebbestrahlung als Routinebestrahlungsmethode bei gynäkologischen Tumoren 1956 an der Universitäts-Frauenklinik Freiburg eingeführt. Zuvor haben wir (RÖSENER) vergleichende Tiefendosismessungen am Wasserphantom mit Sieb- und Vollfeldbestrahlung durchgeführt, um exakte Unterlagen über die Tiefendosisverhältnisse bei unserer Bestrahlungsmethode zu erhalten.

Über die Anwendung der Siebbestrahlung in der gynäkologischen Strahlentherapie liegen u.a. Mitteilungen von BUTTENBERG und KUTTIG, FOCHEM und WEGHAUPT, MARQUARDT, FRISCHKORN, VAN DER WALL, und zuletzt von RODÉ und HAJDU (1966) vor. VAN DER WALL führte von 1958—1960 bei 214 Patientinnen mit gynäkologischen Tumoren eine Art Blindversuch durch, in dem er die eine Hälfte der Patientinnen mit Sieb-, die andere Hälfte mit Vollfeldbestrahlung behandelte. Er fand beim Vergleich der Überlebensraten und der Veränderungen im roten und weißen Blutbild keinen signifikanten Unterschied und bezeichnet als einzigen Vorteil bei der Siebbestrahlung die bessere Hautverträglichkeit. Im Gegensatz dazu haben wir bei unseren vergleichenden Experimenten mit weißen Ratten bei gleichen Tiefendosen deutliche Unterschiede der Überlebensraten der Tiere und der Regenerationsfähigkeit des weißen Blutbildes zugunsten der Siebbestrahlung gefunden. Die Funktionsdiagnostik der Bildungsstätten der weißen Blutkörperchen haben wir mit dem Leukocytenresistenzwert, einer von uns angegebenen biologischen Größe des Blutes, durchgeführt.

Die Auflage des Siebes oder Siebtubus in exakt gleicher Position bei jeder Bestrahlung halten wir, im Gegensatz zu FRISCHKORN, bei den verabreichten Dosen und den propagierten Sieben nicht für notwendig.

Jedes Feld erhält bei uns 10—15 Einzelbestrahlungen von nicht mehr als 600 R (bei Siebbestrahlung) oder 250 R (Vollfeldbestrahlung). Es werden täglich 2 Felder oder auch, wenn die Allgemeinreaktionen der Patientinnen es zulassen, alle 4 Felder verabreicht, so daß eine Gesamtbestrahlungszeit von 3—6 Wochen resultiert. Durch die zusätzliche Verabreichung eines Vulvadammfeldes (Feldgröße 8 × 10 cm, mindesten 1 mm Cu-Filter, sonst die gleichen Daten) ist es möglich, die Dosis im mittleren Beckenraum weiter zu steigern. Von dieser Möglichkeit machen wir aber nicht routinemäßig Gebrauch.

RODÉ und HAJDU führten ihre Siebbestrahlung mit einem Sieb aus 2 mm dickem Blei, Lochdurchmesser 8 mm bei 50 % Öffnung durch. Sie verabreichten 4 Felder (2 Unterbauch- und 2 parasacrale Felder), je Sitzung 3000 R jeden 2. Tag, innerhalb von 8 Tagen in 4 Sitzungen als 12000 R. Sie weisen auf die gute Verträglichkeit und auf gute Primärerfolge ihrer „massiven Siebbestrahlung der gynäkologischen" Tumoren hin.

Grundsätzlich berechnen wir die Oberflächendosis, die verabreicht werden muß, um die gewünschte Dosis am Herd zu erreichen, aus den Gegebenheiten der Patientin (Dicke, Kompressionsmöglichkeit). Durch kräftige Kompression bei den Bauch- und in gewissem Umfang den Glutealfeldern ist es möglich, das Verhältnis Oberflächen-Herddosis oft erheblich zu verbessern.

Ries verwendet (Vollfeldbestrahlung) beim Ovarialcarcinom (und empfiehlt grundsätzlich die gleiche Therapie bei den malignen Tubentumoren) wie beim Collum- und Korpuscarcinom ebenfalls 2 Unterbauch- und 2 korrespondierende Rückenfelder von 10×15 cm Größe, die nach der Mitte konvergieren. Wurde der Tumor radikal entfernt, so begnügt er sich mit 2400 R Oberflächendosis. Wenn Zweifel an der Radikalität der Operation bestehen, erhöht er die Dosis. Beim Zurückbleiben von Tumorinfiltrationen oder bei peritonealer Aussaat strebt er pro Feld eine Oberflächendosis von 4000 R an, die jedoch wegen der starken Allgemeinbelastung fast nie erreicht wird, besonders wenn — gelegentlich — zusätzliche Oberbauchfelder verabreicht werden.

Andere Autoren, unter ihnen Kottmeier, empfehlen grundsätzlich beim Ovarialcarcinom große Felder, besonders wenn Ascites vorhanden ist, und messen der Bestrahlung des ganzen Abdomens großen Wert bei. Auch Bergmann (1958) hält die Bestrahlung mit Oberbauchfeldern wegen der dort oft auftretenden Metastasen für notwendig. Wir glauben, daß eine Bestrahlung mit großen Feldern, insbesondere auch des Oberbauches, nur als Palliativmaßnahme bei großen inoperablen Tumoren und Ascites gerechtfertigt ist. Als Routinemethode bedeutet doch die Durchstrahlung eines so großen Volumens mit der unvermeidlichen Strahlenbelastung der ganzen Bauchorgane u. E. eine sehr große Belastung, die sich oft negativ auswirkt.

Die Bewegungsbestrahlung mit konventioneller Röntgenbestrahlung bietet bei der rein prophylaktischen Nachbestrahlung, die ja eine homogene Durchstrahlung des Beckenraumes zum Ziel hat, u. E. keinen Vorteil, da die Möglichkeit der Kompression wegfällt und deshalb die Gesamtraumdosis zur Erreichung einer gleichen Herddosis notwendigerweise gesteigert werden muß.

Bei Bestrahlung mit Telekobalt- oder der ultraharten Röntgenstrahlung der Elektronenschleuder und des Linearbeschleunigers sind die Herddosen unter Berücksichtigung der relativen biologischen Wirksamkeit der Strahlung (RBW) zu errechnen. Weisshaar nimmt im Vergleich zur üblichen Röntgenbestrahlung für die RBW der Kobaltstrahlung einen Faktor von 0,9 an, führt aber weiter aus, daß nach seinen bisherigen Erfahrungen (1965) der Faktor wahrscheinlich noch näher bei 1,0 liegt, wie das auch den Beobachtungen z. B. von Kuttig und Schnepper entsprechen würde. Die Allgemeinverträglichkeit dieser Strahlungen ist nach Berichten aller Autoren (Cocchi, Schmermund und Oberheuser, Kirchhoff u. a.) wesentlich besser als die der „klassischen" Röntgentherapie. Ob mit der Supervolttherapie allerdings auch eine Besserung der Heilungsergebnisse bei gynäkologischen Tumoren gegenüber der konventionellen Röntgentherapie zu erreichen ist, ist u. E. noch nicht völlig abgeklärt, obwohl Schubert und Uhlmann schon auf der 35. Tagung der Gesellschaft für Gynäkologie 1964 in München zum Ausdruck brachten, daß auf Grund *besserer Heilungserfolge* die konventionelle Röntgentherapie soweit wie möglich durch die Supervolttherapie ersetzt werden sollte. Demgegenüber schreibt Weisshaar 1965 bezüglich der Behandlung von Patientinnen mit Collumcarcinomen, daß „die bisherigen Überlebensziffern sich bei den beiden Gruppen (übliche Röntgentherapie bzw. Telekobalttherapie) nicht voneinander unterscheiden". Auch bei den Nebenreaktionen fand Weisshaar, abgesehen von den Frühreaktionen der Haut, keine signifikanten Unterschiede. Dabei lagen die Herddosen bei den kobaltbestrahlten Patientinnen jeweils um 10% höher als bei den mit der üblichen Röntgenbestrahlung behandelten Patientinnen. Zweifellos spricht aber schon die bessere Allgemein- und Hautverträglichkeit der Supervoltbestrahlung dafür, daß diese Bestrahlungsmethoden, insbesondere auch bei gynäkologischen Tumorbestrahlungen, soweit wie möglich angewendet werden sollen.

Auch bei Telekobaltbestrahlung empfehlen Buttenberg und Lau (1959) die Anwendung eines Siebes, das Becker, Gudden und Kuttig (1958) angegeben haben.

Die Bewegungsbestrahlung mit der Supervolttherapie ist u. E. gerade auch bei den gynäkologischen Tumoren von besonderem Interesse. So berichtet Kirchhoff 1967 über die an seiner Klinik vor allem zur Anwendung kommende Pendelbestrahlung mit möglichst großem Pendelwinkel, mit der er — wir haben bereits darauf hingewiesen — „auch eine den Radioisodosen gleichwertige Konzentration an gefahrvollen Punkten" erreichen kann, so daß für ihn die Notwendigkeit entfällt, den Uterus für zusätzliche Radium-bestrahlung zurückzulassen. Als Beweis führt er die folgenden vergleichenden Meß-ergebnisse mit Telekobalt-Pendelbestrahlung und Radium an (Abb. 13).

Die intravaginale Bestrahlung mit dem Hohlanodenrohr (SCHAEFER und WITTE, 1932), die insbesondere von KEPP (damals Göttingen) für die Behandlung gynäkologischer Tumoren propagiert und in großem Umfang eingesetzt wurde, ist heute praktisch nur noch von historischem Interesse. Die Methode wurde angewendet zur Bestrahlung von Tumoren oder Resttumoren, die von der Vagina aus gut erreicht werden konnten — also insbesondere bei gut ansprechbaren Infiltrationen im Douglas und seitlich in Uterus-nähe sowie bei entsprechenden Rezidivtumoren. Die Bestrahlung erfolgte im allgemeinen nach der sogenannten Göttinger Methode (KEPP), wobei eine Dosis von ca. 2400 R in 5 cm Tiefe angestrebt und in 12 Einzelsitzungen verabreicht wurde.

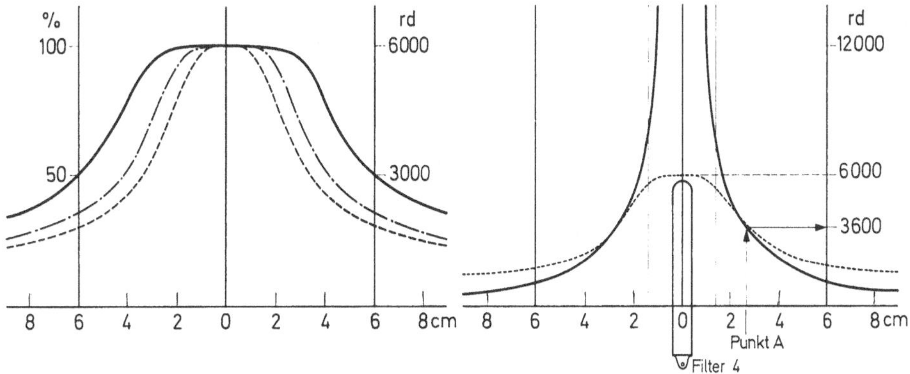

Abb. 13. Telekobalt-Pendelbestrahlungen, Pendelradius 65 cm, Pendelwinkel 360°. Feldgrößen in 50 cm Fokus-abstand: — 6 × 6 cm²; — 4 × 4 cm²; — 3 × 3 cm²; — 120 mg Radium, Filter 4, 3 600 mgeh ≙ 3 600 rad im Punkt A; ····· 6 000 rd im Maximum einer Telekobalt-Pendelbestahlung (nach KIRCHHOFF)

γ) Intraabdominelle Applikation von radioaktiven Substanzen

Die intraabdominelle post-operative Instillation von kolloidalen, radioaktiven Sub-stanzen als Routinemethode zur Behandlung des Ovarialcarcinoms stellt zweifellos einen strahlentherapeutischen Fortschritt dar. Diese Therapie ist nach MÜLLER, der damit 1945 begann, gekennzeichnet durch „Einflußnahmen auf verschiedene Vitalfunktionen des reticuloendothelialen Systems (RES). Es kommt zu einer paraselektiven Konzen-tration der von den histocytären Makrophagen aufgenommenen radioaktiven Partikel um das invasive Carcinom und durch die reticuloendothelialen Makrophagen in den Lymphkanälen und -knoten im Sinne einer radiotherapeutischen Lymphographie". Dabei ist bedeutungsvoll, daß nach KOTTMEIER und MOBERGER nur im gesunden, nicht aber im carcinomatösen Lymphdrüsengewebe die strahlende Substanz gespeichert wird. Da zumeist aber nicht alles lymphatische Gewebe carcinomatös entartet ist, sondern in vielen Lymphknoten neben entartetem noch gesundes Gewebe vorhanden ist, kommt auch hier die Strahlenwirkung therapeutisch zum Tragen. Die chemische Eigenschaft der verwendeten künstlichen radioaktiven Substanzen spielt keine Rolle, entscheidend für die Verwendung sind allein die Qualität der Strahlung, die Halbwertzeit sowie die mechanischen Eigenschaften, d.h., die radioaktive Substanz dient nur noch als Strahler. Das biologische Verhalten wird von dem Kolloid bzw. der Teilchengröße der Suspension bestimmt (KEPP).

Wegen seines biologischen Verhaltens, der günstigen Halbwertzeit und des sehr brauchbaren Emissions-Spektrums ist das Radiogold [198]Au besonders geeignet. Die Halb-wertzeit beträgt 2,69 Tage, das bedeutet, daß die Aktivität nach 10 Tagen unter 10%

und nach 18 Tagen unter 1 % der Anfangsaktivität beträgt. Die Strahlung ist eine Mischstrahlung, die etwa zu 95 % aus β-Strahlen mit einer Energie von max. 0,96 MeV und zu etwa 5 % aus γ-Strahlen von 0,411 MeV besteht. Beim Zerfall der Substanz wird zunächst die β-Strahlung emittiert, nach Erreichen eines Zwischenzustandes kommt es dann zur Aussendung der γ-Strahlung. Mit Beendigung der Strahlung verwandelt sich das Isotop in stabiles Quecksilber. Die bei der therapeutischen Verabreichung von Radiogold verbleibende Menge Quecksilber ist so verschwindend gering, daß ihr keine praktische Bedeutung zukommt. Die β-Strahlung von Radiogold besitzt eine Reichweite von max. 3,8 mm, durchschnittlich 1 mm im Gewebe, so daß bei intrakavitärer Anwendung die Oberflachenwirkung im Vordergrund steht und vor allem bei disseminierter, dünnschichtiger oberflächlicher Carcinomausbreitung eine günstige Auswirkung zu erwarten ist. Nach Kepp ist durch die Anwendung von ^{198}Au zumindest die Zerstörung von Mikrometastasen wahrscheinlich. Ergüsse in den Pleurahöhlen und im Bauchraum bilden sich zurück oder werden eingedämmt. Selbstverständlich müssen bei der Anwendung von Radiogold, im Hinblick auf die γ-Strahlung insbesondere, alle Strahlenschutz-Vorsichtsmaßnahmen ergriffen werden.

Zuppinger u. Mitarb. glauben, daß es günstiger ist, ein Isotop zu verwenden, das eine penetrantere β-Strahlung ohne gleichzeitige γ-Strahlung aussendet, diskutieren ^{32}P, halten aber insbesondere Yttrium-90 für besonders geeignet. Seine Halbwertzeit beträgt 2,54 Tage, die β-Strahlung beträgt max. 2,2 MeV, die Durchdringungstiefe ist damit günstiger als bei Gold und Phosphor (10 mm max., fast 4 mm im Durchschnitt). Besondere Strahlenschutzmaßnahmen sind nicht erforderlich, weil keine γ-Strahlung ausgesendet wird. Größere Erfahrungen mit ^{90}Y haben aber auch Zuppinger u. Mitarb. noch nicht bis zur Veröffentlichung im Jahre 1962 sammeln können. Müller dagegen glaubt, daß ^{90}Y nicht vergleichbar sicher und für die klinische Anwendung ausreichend definiert ist wie ^{198}Au.

Die zahlreichen Arbeiten der letzten 10 Jahre aus aller Welt beweisen, daß zur Behandlung der bösartigen Ovarialtumoren vorwiegend, ja fast ausschließlich ^{198}Au verwendet wird. Die systematische postoperative, auch prophylaktische Radiogoldtherapie soll nach Müller, Kirchhoff, Runge, Buttenberg und Lau u. a. möglichst frühzeitig einsetzen. Zu Beginn der Beschäftigung mit der Radiogoldtherapie wurde die erste Instillation direkt post operationem empfohlen. Dazu mußten Operations- und Beschaffungstermin des Radiogoldes aufeinander abgestimmt werden, so daß direkt post operationem, vor dem endgültigen Schluß der Bauchdecken, das Radiogold instilliert werden konnte.

Bei dieser Art der Anwendung des Radiogoldes ging man von der Vorstellung aus, daß damit eine durch die Operation bedingte Propagation von Tumorzellen möglichst frühzeitig wirkungsvoll bekämpft werden sollte (s. a. Keetel und Elkins, 1956). Die meisten Autoren — auch Müller und Kepp — sind inzwischen dazu übergegangen, die erste intraabdominale Goldverabreichung — die von Müller weniger als „Injektion" denn als „intraabdomineller Eingriff" bezeichnet wird — etwa 3 Wochen nach der Operation durchzuführen. Wenn kein Ascites vorhanden ist, muß ein Hydroperitoneum angelegt werden, um die Verteilung des Radiogoldes im Bauchraum zu gewährleisten. Die Anlage eines Pneumoperitoneums von 300—400 cm^3 Luft oder Co_2, wie sie Cohen u. Mitarb. sowie Ludin (1953) empfehlen, lehnt Müller auf Grund seiner Erfahrungen ab.

Müller hat wohl mit der intraperitonealen Applikation von kolloidalem Radiogold die meisten Erfahrungen, deshalb zitieren wir wörtlich seine Methode der Verabreichung (1967): „Wir nehmen den Eingriff stets in Lokalanaesthesie vor, da wir bei der Paracentese die Mithilfe der Patientin beanspruchen. Die Patientin muß gut vorbereitet (nüchtern, bei gut entleertem Darm), ferner auch, zwecks Vermeidung von Schockreaktionen, adäquat prämediziert sein. Dabei ist dem „hausüblichen" Narkoticum unbedingt $^1/_4$—$^1/_2$ mg Atropin beizufügen.

Vor der Anaesthesie ist das Abdomen nochmals genauestens zu palpieren, weil Stellen mit auch geringen Resistenzen oder Druckschmerzen stets auf Adhäsionen verdächtig sind. Auf diese Weise konnten wir seit nun vielen Jahren Verletzungen des Darmes ausschalten. Vorzugsweise wird neben dem Rectus abdominis links, unterhalb vom Nabel punktiert, gelegentlich auch rechts, seltener in der Mittellinie, jedenfalls immer an einer Stelle, wo die oben betonte sorgfältige Palpation einen freien Zugang zur Bauchhöhle annehmen läßt.

Für die Lokalanaesthesie hat sich seit vielen Jahren 1% Xylocain (mit Epinephrinzusatz) bewährt. Es werden 10—15 ml benötigt. Steriles Vorgehen sollte sich von selbst verstehen.

Die Paracentese erfolgt mit einem Spezialtroicar von 2,8 mm äußerem Durchmesser, mit einem verstellbaren Querstück. Über die vermutlich benötigte Punktionstiefe hat man sich bei der Anaesthesie der Bauchwand ins Bild gesetzt. Während der Punktion wird die Patientin angewiesen, den Bauch nach außen vorzupressen. So wird es möglich, die Bauchdecke Schicht für Schicht zu durchstechen und den Augenblick zu erfassen, in dem man die Bauchhöhle erreicht. Bei immer noch aktiv vorgepreßtem Abdomen wird dann durch das Lumen des Troicars unter Führung durch einen „Klaviersaitenmandrin" mit elastischer Spitze, ein Polythenkatheter sachte eingeführt (ca. 15 cm über die Spitze des Troicars hinaus), und gleich anschließend werden der Troicar und der Mandrin vorsichtig entfernt. Erst jetzt darf die Patientin die Bauchpresse aufgeben. Dann wird über ein mit Pflasterstreifen an der Haut fixiertes Zwischenstück eine intraperitoneale Niederdruckinfusion mit physiologischer Kochsalzlösung angeschlossen; nötigenfalls kann der Polythenkatheter vorsichtig leicht zurückgezogen werden, bis die Flüssigkeit regelmäßig einfließt. Damit ist man zugleich auch sicher in der freien Bauchhöhle. Es hat sich bewährt, zunächst die Hälfte des vorgesehenen Flüssigkeitsvolumens von ca. 400 ml einfließen zu lassen. Dann wird das auf 20 ml verdünnte Radiogoldpräparat mit einer bleigeschützten Spezialspritze eingebracht und unmittelbar anschließend der Rest der physiologischen Kochsalzlösung gegeben. So wird eine rasche Endverdünnung mit gleichmäßiger Verteilung der Radioaktivität erreicht. Hernach wird der Polythenkatheter entfernt und die kleine Wunde versorgt. Nur ausnahmsweise ist es mit unserem Instrumentarium erforderlich, eine Stichincision der Haut durchzuführen.

Diese intraperitoneale Applikation erfolgt bei mäßiger Beckentieflage von ca. 15°. Die Patientin wird angewiesen, sich anschließend während 6—8 Std langsam im Bette zu drehen.

Wenn Adhäsionen bestehen, empfehlen BUTTENBERG und LAU (1959) eine „Laparotomie en miniature": Die Peritonealhöhle wird nach Eröffnung der Bauchhöhle durch einen möglichst kleinen Knopflochschnitt revidiert und ein Katheter eingeführt, wie dies ROMINGER übrigens schon vor vielen Jahren für jede Instillation forderte.

Eine zweite Instillation von Radiogold erfolgt etwa 8 Wochen später. Im allgemeinen werden heute nicht mehr als 150 mCi Radiogold pro Sitzung verabreicht (MÜLLER, KEPP u. v. a.).

Das Radiogold bleibt in der Flüssigkeit des Bauchraumes oder attachiert sich an die serösen Flächen des Darmes und Peritonealraumes. Nur geringe Mengen gelangen resorptiv in Blut- und Lymphwege. Die Ausscheidung in den Exkrementen ist außerordentlich gering, so daß sie auch bei strenger Berücksichtigung des Strahlenschutzes vernachlässigt werden kann.

Die klinische Indikation für die obligate, intraperitoneale Verabreichung des kolloidalen Radiogoldes zur bisherigen vornehmlich chirurgischen Therapie des Ovarialcarcinoms wird davon abgeleitet (MÜLLER), daß es nur auf diese Weise möglich erscheint, die anders nicht erfaßbaren Mikrodisseminationen zu sterilisieren, wie sie bekanntlich auch bei den günstigen, optimal operablen Ovarialcarcinomen in mehr als der Hälfte der Fälle bereits prätherapeutisch vorhanden sind.

Mit dieser Methode haben MÜLLER und auch KEPP ihre Heilungsresultate beim Ovarialcarcinom ganz erheblich verbessern können. Die folgende Tabelle 5 stammt aus dem letzten Bericht von MÜLLER.

Bei der erweiterten Indikationsstellung zur intraperitonealen Applikation von kolloidalem Radiogold fällt der Möglichkeit von Komplikationen erhöhtes Gewicht zu. Solche Komplikationen sind bei klinischer Beherrschung der Methode sehr selten, aber oft doch nicht ganz zu vermeiden (Johannsen, Vulkov und Tzanev u.a.). Nach Müller sind Komplikationen, wie sie im Schrifttum erwähnt werden, wie akute Peritonitis, Nekrosen der Bauchwand und von Darmschlingen etc. ganz einfach auf recht primitive operativtechnische Fehler zurückzuführen. Er führt weiter aus: „Auch das nicht ganz zu ver-

Tabelle 5. *Therapeutic results in true ovarian cancer—colloidal—*[198]*Au-series (from late fall of 1949 to late fall of 1961. Cases operated outside and referred for postoperative therapy are included)* (Müller)

Author's Staging	I	II		I+II		III	IV	Totals		
F.I.G.O's Staging	I_a	$I_{b,c}$	$II_{a,b}$	$I_{a,b,c}$	$II_{a,b}$	*III_a	*III_b IV			
Total number of treated cases										
B	37	47		84 } 99		56 } 70	30	170 } 230		
C	1	14		15		14	31	60		
Alive without symptoms after 5 years										
B	33	28		61 } 63 = 64%		22 31%	0	83 } 85	49% } 37%	
C	1	1		2		0	0	2	3%	
Deceased from Carcinoma before 5 years										
B	1	14		15 } 26 = 26%		34	30	79 } 135	59%	
C	0	11		11		14	31	56		
Deceased from intercurrent disease										
B	3	—		8 } 10 = 10%		0	0	8 } 10	4%	
C	0	—		2		0	0	2		

Potentially curable
Ovarian Cancer cases.
Obtained 5-year cure rate = 50%

B = F.I.G.O. Histological Groups I, II, IIIc; C = F.I.G.O. Histological Group IV.
* Amendment of definition suggested by the author.

meidende akzidentelle Punktieren einer Darmschlinge (auch der Erfahrene wird das bei seltenen Einzelfällen einmal erleben) bleibt bei richtigem Verhalten ohne schädigende Folgen. Ich pflege in einem solchen Fall den Troicar zunächst ja nicht zu bewegen, das anpunktierte Darmlumen sachte abzusaugen und anschließend den Troicar unter dauerndem Nachspritzen von Streptomycinlösung (ca. 1,5 g in 20 ml) ganz allmählich herauszuziehen. Die Radiogoldapplikation muß dann natürlich um ca. 3 Wochen verschoben werden. So haben wir keine primäre Morbidität oder gar Mortalität zu verzeichnen. Trifft man bei eventuell an verschiedenen Stellen durchgeführtem Paracenteseversuchen nicht in die freie Bauchhöhle, so ist auf die Radiokolloidtherapie endgültig zu verzichten".

Neben der intrakavitären Applikation ist für den gynäkologischen Bereich noch die intratumorale Infiltrationsbehandlung mit Radiogold zu erwähnen. Sie hat nach Kepp im wesentlichen drei Indikationen: die Infiltration der Parametrien bei der Behandlung des Collumcarcinoms, die Infiltration von Rezidiven des Collumcarcinoms in den Parametrien und an der Beckenwand und die Infiltration von oberflächlich gelegenen Lymphknotenmetastasen. Entsprechend kann u. E. auch die Infiltration von primären und anderen intraligamentären Tumoren u. U. von Vorteil sein. Entsprechende Mitteilungen liegen nicht vor.

Grundsätzlich ist der intratumoralen Infiltrationsbehandlung mit Radiogold gegenüber Skepsis geboten. VECCHETTI und ONNIS haben 1963 auf Grund eigener Erfahrungen und einer ausgedehnten Literaturübersicht über die parametrane ¹⁹⁸Au Infiltration bei bösartigen Tumoren des weiblichen Genitalapparates festgestellt, daß die Komplikationsrate so hoch ist, daß diese Methode zugunsten anderer sichererer Methoden aufgegeben werden sollte.

δ) Strahlenbehandlung von Rezidiven und Metastasen

Rezidive der besprochenen Tumoren sind strahlentherapeutisch im allgemeinen wie die Primärtumoren anzugehen. Die Behandlung von Rezidiven und Metastasen ist bei allen Tumoren indiziert, auch wenn Heilungen nur zu den Seltenheiten gehören. Der palliative Erfolg ist oft auch nach unseren eigenen Untersuchungen eindeutig. Über den Wert der Strahlenbehandlung bei Rezidiven und weiterwachsenden Primärtumoren des Collumcarcinoms unter besonderer Berücksichtigung der Palliativeffekte haben wir zusammen mit FISCHER sowie HESS auf dem Deutschen Röntgenkongreß 1967 in Baden-Baden berichtet.

Bei Metastasierungen ist grundsätzlich die Lokalisation der Metastase für das besondere strahlentherapeutische Vorgehen entscheidend. Die Strahlenbehandlung, insbesondere von Knochenmetastasen — auch wenn sie multipel auftreten —, bringt palliativ gute und auch relativ dauerhafte Erfolge und verschafft in fast allen Fällen dem Patienten eine zumeist erhebliche subjektive Erleichterung, manchmal sogar für eine gewisse Zeit Beschwerdefreiheit. Sie sollte immer mit Tumordosen — u. U. kombiniert mit hormoneller und chemotherapeutischer Behandlung — durchgeführt werden. In einzelnen Fällen kann so auch eine — lebenswerte — Verlängerung des Lebens erreicht werden.

Die Strahlenbehandlung von Lungenmetastasen — die ja zumeist multipel auftreten — mit Tumordosen bringt u. E. für den Patienten keinen Vorteil, sondern bedeutet zumeist nur eine erhebliche zusätzliche Belastung. Hier ist die Anwendung von Cytostatica und u. U. Hormonen von wesentlich größerer Bedeutung. Wenn allerdings die metastatischen Lungentumoren stärkere Beschwerden machen (heftiger Husten, Schmerzen), ist die Bestrahlung mit kleinen („Entzündungs"-)Dosen von mehrmals 100 R unter Tiefentherapiebedingungen oft subjektiv außerordentlich wirksam.

EVA GAEBEL propagiert als Palliativmaßnahme für Patientinnen, bei denen die Ausdehnung der Tumoren oder der schlechte Allgemeinzustand keine operativen und anderen strahlentherapeutischen Maßnahmen zulassen, die von TESCHENDORF 1927 beschriebene Teleröntgentherapie. Es werden hierbei Röntgendosen angewendet, die noch unter 50 R liegen und in großem Abstand von 1—2 m auf einen Körperabschnitt oder den ganzen Körper gegeben werden. „Hierbei kann die Geschwulstzelle selbst kaum beeinflußt werden. Es muß sich also um eine noch nicht völlig geklärte Allgemeinreaktion des Organismus auf kleine Strahlenmengen bei homogener Durchstrahlung ganzer Körperabschnitte oder Ganzbestrahlung handeln. Bei der Teleröntgenmethode im weiteren Sinne, d. h., eigentlich bei einer Fernbestrahlung mit 50—100 R pro Sitzung in großem Abstand auf ein großes Feld, wie wir sie heute bei bestimmten Krebskranken anwenden, summieren sich die gegebenen Einzeldosen, so daß man mit einer direkten Wirkung auf die Krebszellen rechnen kann. Diese Methode der Fernbestrahlung hat gegenüber der Intensivbestrahlung bei sehr großen Tumoren oder ausgedehnten Prozessen oder bei Metastasierungen über einen ganzen Körperabschnitt den Vorteil, daß man das ganze krebsbefallene Gebiet in jeder Sitzung erfassen kann und dennoch kein so starker Tumorzerfall eintritt, der eine Intoxikation der an sich schon Schwerkranken hervorrufen würde" (EVA GAEBEL, 1961).

Auch wir haben in einzelnen Fällen günstige Auswirkungen der Teleröntgentherapie, insbesondere im Sinne eines analgetischen Effektes gesehen.

ε) Bestrahlungsfolgen und Strahlenschäden

Die Tatsache, daß grundsätzlich bei Anwendung ionisierender Strahlen zur Behandlung bösartiger Tumoren das den Tumor umgebende „gesunde" Gewebe mitbelastet wird, die weitgehende Unkenntnis einer optimalen „Tumordosis", die dazu führt, daß zumeist eine maximale — also ohne stärkere Schädigung des Organismus noch zu verantwortende — Dosis verabreicht wird und der Umstand, daß im Beckenbereich eine Reihe wichtiger Organe oder Teile von Organsystemen räumlich eng beieinander liegen — rücken das Problem der Strahlenfolgen bzw. einer „Strahlenschädigung" in der Gynäkologie immer wieder besonders in den Vordergrund. — Dazu werden durch die zeitlich oft enge Koppelung der Verabreichung verschiedener Strahlungen (Röntgen, evtl. Supervolt, Radium, eventuell Kobalt und Radiogold) mit z.T. verschiedener relativer biologischer Wirksamkeit und durch die Tatsache, daß der Strahlenbehandlung zumeist eine Operation vorausgegangen ist, die Verhältnisse weiter kompliziert.

αα) Haut

Die zur Erreichung des therapeutischen Effektes notwendige Herddosis setzt bei der *percutanen Röntgenbestrahlung* die Belastung der Haut mit einer Oberflächendosis voraus, die — individuell außerordentlich verschieden — zu u.U. stärkeren Hautreaktionen — bis zur Epitheliolyse — führen kann. Als *Siebbestrahlung* wird diese Röntgenstrahlendosis nicht nur allgemein besser vertragen, sondern auch eine u.U. eintretende Epitheliolyse heilt nach Siebbestrahlung wesentlich rascher ab, da von den unter den Siebstegen liegenden abgedeckten, daher relativ wenig belasteten Hautpartien aus, rasch eine Reparation einsetzt. Dabei darf bei kombinierter Behandlung mit Röntgen, Radium oder Kobalt-60 intrakavitär, Gold-198 intraperitoneal nicht außer acht gelassen werden, daß von allen Strahlenquellen aus eine nicht unerhebliche, homogene Strahlung die Haut belastet, die die durch die percutane Strahlung verabreichte Dosis pro Flächeneinheit der Haut erreichen, ja überschreiten kann.

Zur Hautbehandlung unter der Bestrahlung hat sich uns in den letzten Jahren besonders die Puderbehandlung, z.B. mit Azulonpuder oder auch (wie wir dies seit mehr als 10 Jahren durchführen) mit einem antibiotischen Puder bewährt, der u.U. auch mit einem Spray ganz dünn vor der Bestrahlung aufgetragen wird. Bedenken, daß es dadurch, wie bei der prophylaktischen internen Anwendung von Antibiotica zur Züchtung resistenter Stämme kommt, sind dabei nicht berechtigt, da es durch die intakte Haut zu keiner wesentlichen Resorption des Antibioticums kommt. Die Anwendung des antibiotischen Puders führt aber dazu, daß bei Mikroläsionen der Haut Infektionen und Entzündungen, die erfahrungsgemäß ja zu einer schlechteren Hautverträglichkeit der percutanen Bestrahlung führen, vermieden werden. Zur Nachbehandlung hat sich uns, solange keine Epitheliolyse eingetreten ist, ebenfalls die Puderbehandlung, nach Eintritt der Epitheliolyse die Behandlung mit einer modifizierten Zinksalbe oder auch mit Azulon- oder Bepanthensalbe bewährt.

Die Epitheliolyse heilt im allgemeinen — ebenfalls wieder individuell außerordentlich verschieden — in 14 Tagen bis 3 Wochen ab. Als Spätveränderungen der Haut können — ebenfalls wieder individuell außerordentlich verschieden — abhängig von der die Haut von den verschiedenen Strahlenquellen her belastenden Dosis im Bereich der Bestrahlungsfelder Indurationen auftreten, die u.U. auch ulcerieren können. So steht eine Patientin in unserer Beobachtung, die wir im Jahre 1950 (damals 30 Jahre alt) wegen eines Collumcarcinoms, im Jahre 1951 erneut wegen eines Rezidivs mit Radium und percutaner Röntgenbestrahlung behandelt haben und die heute noch ohne jede Zeichen des Wiederauftretens der Erkrankung lebt, bei der sich im Bereich der Bestrahlungsfelder des Unterbauches eine ausgedehnte Induration und seit etwa 10 Jahren eine zentrale, chronische, sich nicht vergrößernde Ulceration entwickelt hat. Die zur Vermeidung einer malignen Entartung der Ulceration von uns vorgeschlagene — und technisch ohne weiteres mögliche — Excision der Induration und Ulceration hat die Patientin bis jetzt immer wieder abgelehnt.

Bei der Durchführung der percutanen Bestrahlung mit Supervolttherapie sind die Hautreaktionen sehr viel geringer als bei normaler Röntgenbestrahlung. WEISSHAAR und GERTRAUD RIETZ haben vergleichende Untersuchungen bei telekobalt- und röntgenbestrahlten Frauen durchgeführt und diese Überlegenheit der Supervolttherapie bestätigen können.

ββ) Rectum, Blase, Ureteren

Die gleiche Problematik der Belastung von verschiedenen Strahlenquellen aus besteht auch für die in nächster Nähe des bestrahlten Herdes liegenden Beckenorgane, Rectum, Blase und Ureteren. Mit der Ermittlung der Toleranzdosis an Blase und Rectum haben sich eine große Zahl von Autoren beschäftigt (NEEFF, DRESCHER, GAUWERKY, RIES u.a.). Die Dosis ist — für das Rectum geringer als für die Blase — bei kombinierter fraktionierter Radium-Röntgenbestrahlung um 7 000 R anzunehmen, wobei die Angaben der einzelnen Autoren z.T. erheblich differieren. Durch Überschreiten dieser Dosis können sich schwer reparable Veränderungen, Ulcerationen und u.U. auch Fistelbildungen entwickeln. TWOMBLY, CACERES und CORSCADEN (1952) beobachteten einen Zusammenhang zwischen steigender Dosis an den Parametrien, bei abnehmender Dosis an der Blase und trotzdem Zunahme von Blasenschädigungen. Es wird daher von ihnen diskutiert ob es sich bei den Blasenreaktionen nicht so sehr um direkte Schädigungen der Blasenschleimhaut, als um trophische Ulcerationen, als Folge der Bestrahlung der Ganglien des Frankenhäuserschen Plexus handeln könnte. H. J. MÜLLER hat 1966 erneut eine entsprechende Stellung eingenommen. Die Blasenschleimhaut scheint (wir haben bereits darauf hingewiesen) strahlenunempfindlicher zu sein als die Rectumschleimhaut. BREITNER, ENDERLE, NICOLOV, LEWIS, CHEMBERLEIN, HALE und PAYNE berichteten über steigende Heilungsaussichten, wenn Blasen- und Rectumläsionen beobachtet wurden. SCHMITZ, GEIGER, SMITH und BLICHERT weisen jedoch darauf hin, daß „Über- und Unterbestrahlung" zu schlechten Resultaten führen.

Durch Routinemessungen der Strahlendosen an Blase und Rectum unter der Bestrahlung kann die Gefahr von Schädigungen vermindert werden, wobei allerdings beim Ovarialcarcinom durch die Tatsache, daß den Bestrahlungen zumeist Operationen vorausgegangen sind, in deren Folgen sich Adhäsionen und Verziehungen entwickelt haben können, die Beurteilung der Verhältnisse erschwert sein kann.

„Über den Wert der Dosismessungen an Blase und Rectum bei der Radiumbehandlung des weiblichen Genitalcarcinoms" haben wir 1958 zusammen mit MÜLLER-HUMMEL ausgedehnte Untersuchungen durchgeführt, wobei auch Ovarialcarcinome, die mit Radium bestrahlt wurden, in die Untersuchungen einbezogen waren. Zumeist handelte es sich aber um Collum-, in geringerem Umfange um Vaginal- und Korpuscarcinome. Aus diesen Untersuchungen ist u.E. wichtig, daß das Verhältnis der Blasenreaktionen zu den Rectumreaktionen sich wie bei anderen Autoren (NEEFF, SRAMENKO u.a.) wie 15:25 verhielt. Wir fanden, daß bei maximalen Effektivdosen von oberhalb 95 R/Std eine Reaktion seitens der Rectumschleimhaut erwartet werden muß. Oberhalb von 100 R/Std ist mit Ulcerationen, über 110 R/Std mit Fistelbildungen zu rechnen. Die Blasenreaktionen treten bei maximalen Effektivdosen auf, die um etwa 5—10 R/Std höher liegen als die, welche zu Rectumreaktionen führen.

Auf Grund der anatomischen Verschiedenheit zwischen männlichem und weiblichem Urogenitalsystem neigen Frauen grundsätzlich wesentlich häufiger zu Blasenerkrankungen als Männer (WILDBOLZ, O'BRIEN, MITCHELL, LAUDA). Dieses Faktum sollte u.E. bei der Beurteilung einer Cystitis berücksichtigt werden, ehe die Diagnose „Strahlencystitis"

23*

gestellt wird. Im Zusammenhang mit der Strahlenbehandlung ist weiterhin die Patientin einer größeren Zahl von intravesicalen Manipulationen (Katheterisieren, Cystoskopieren, intravesicale Dosismessung) ausgesetzt (STOECKEL: ,,Die Cystitis wird häufig ankatheterisiert").

Unter Umständen kann in Zweifelsfällen nicht nur das Effektivdosenprotokoll sondern auch der Zeitpunkt des Auftretens der Reaktionen zur Beurteilung der Frage herangezogen werden, ob es sich bei den Erscheinungen seitens Blase oder Darm um Strahlenfolgen handelt.

Eine Häufung von Strahlenspätreaktionen des Rectums fanden wir um den 6. bis 8. Monat nach der Bestrahlung, KEPP innerhalb der ersten 12 Monate, TWOMBLY, CACERES und CORSCADEN (1952) um den 11,5. Monat. Eine Häufung der Strahlenspätreaktionen an der Blase fanden wir, wie KEPP und TWOMBLY, CACERES und CORSCADEN, zwischen 2 und $2^1/_2$ Jahren nach der Bestrahlung.

Frühreaktionen an Blase und Rectum während und direkt nach der Bestrahlung sind zumeist nur relativ leicht und bedürfen selten einer intensiven Behandlung. Die Spätreaktionen, die, wie wir gesehen haben, am Rectum im allgemeinen wesentlich früher als an der Blase auftreten, sind zumeist ernst zu nehmende Komplikationen, die eine konsequente Behandlung notwendig machen. Bewährt haben sich uns für das Rectum vorsichtige Lebertraneinläufe und auch für die Blase u. a. Instillationen mit gereinigtem Lebertran.

H. J. MÜLLER (1966) empfiehlt dagegen warme Instillationen von anderen — nicht öligen — Präparaten und glaubt, daß die zusätzliche Verabreichung von Ovocyclin über lange Zeit gelegentlich die Heilungstendenz der Blasenläsionen fördern kann. Bei Blutungen ist natürlich die Anwendung von Hämostyptika und gelegentlich auch die punktförmige Elektrokoagulation indiziert.

Von größerer Bedeutung für das Schicksal der Patientinnen ist die Reaktion der Ureteren auf die Bestrahlung. Die abführenden Harnwege können primär schon durch das Tumorwachstum und weiterhin durch die notwendigen operativen Maßnahmen erheblich irritiert und geschädigt worden sein. Die ionisierende Strahlung trifft damit zumeist ein funktionell und organisch nicht mehr normales System und kann sich entsprechend potenziert schädigend auswirken.

WEISSHAAR und RIETZ (1965) fanden bei ihrer schon zitierten vergleichenden Gegenüberstellung der Nebenerscheinungen bei Anwendung von Telekobalt- und Röntgenbestrahlungen bei Patientinnen mit Collumcarcinomen bezüglich der Rectum-, Blasenund Ureterveränderungen keine signifikanten Unterschiede.

Die Therapie der Ureterschädigungen ist konservativ praktisch unmöglich, operative Maßnahmen verstümmeln das System zumeist weitgehend, sind aber im Falle des drohenden völligen Verschlusses der Ureteren die einzige lebensrettende Therapie. Es ist darum — wir haben schon darauf hingewiesen — u. E. unter allen Umständen notwendig, vor Einsatz jeder Therapie und möglichst noch einmal post op. vor Einsatz der Strahlentherapie mit einem intravenösen Urogramm die harnableitenden Wege darzustellen. Diese Untersuchungen erlauben oft prognostische Rückschlüsse und geben therapeutisch wertvolle Hinweise, wie u. a. auch wir dies am Beispiel des Collumcarcinoms zeigen konnten (DIETZ, DIETZ und BEINERT).

γγ) Knochen

Der Vollständigkeit halber ist die Möglichkeit einer Schädigung der Knochen, insbesondere im Bereich des Schenkelhalses, durch die Bestrahlung zu erwähnen, die u. U. zu Schenkelhalsfrakturen führen kann. Wir haben in mehr als 10 Jahren an einem relativ großen gynäkologischen Bestrahlungsgut keine einzige ,,sicher radiogene" Schenkelhalsfraktur beobachtet.

δδ) Knochenmark

Von besonderer Bedeutung ist die Kontrolle des weißen Blutbildes, insbesondere der Leukocyten bei allen strahlentherapeutischen Anwendungen mit größeren Strahlendosen. Das stärkere Absinken der Leukocyten insbesondere macht unter allen Umständen strahlentherapeutische Konsequenzen (Aussetzen der Bestrahlung, stärkere Fraktionierung etc.) notwendig. Die Anwendung von unspezifischen resistenzsteigernden Medikamenten (z.B. Resplant) wirkt sich nach unseren Beobachtungen oft günstig im Sinne einer relativ raschen Erholung der Leukocytenzahlen aus. Auch hier sind die vergleichenden Betrachtungen von WEISSHAAR und RIETZ (1965) nach Röntgen- und Telekobaltbestrahlung von Interesse. Leukopenien beobachteten sie — statistisch wahrscheinlich — bei telekobaltbestrahlten Patientinnen häufiger als bei röntgenbestrahlten.

Bei der intraperitonealen und sicher auch bei der intratumoralen infiltrativen Anwendung von ^{198}Au ist die Gefahr einer Schädigung des Organismus durch stärkere Speicherung der radioaktiven Substanzen in Knochenmark, Leber und Milz nach MÜLLER, HOFMANN-CREDNER, OESER und KEPP relativ gering.

εε) Allgemeinbefinden

Natürlich wird das Allgemeinbefinden insbesondere durch die u.U. großen Raumdosen oft gestört, und es können stärkere „Katerreaktionen" auftreten, zu deren Behandlung eine Fülle von Präparaten angeboten werden. Uns hat sich insbesondere immer wieder Vitamin B_6 bewährt sowie die Anordnung an die Patientinnen, sich soweit wie möglich — bei leichter Bewegung (Spazierengehen) — in frischer Luft aufzuhalten.

WEISSHAAR und RIETZ (1965) fanden bei ihren vergleichenden Betrachtungen, daß die Strahlenverträglichkeit bei den telekobaltbestrahlten Patientinnen nicht besser als bei den röntgenbestrahlten war, obwohl in ihrem Kollektiv die telekobaltbestrahlten Patientinnen statistisch gesichert einen geringeren Prozentsatz von dicken Patientinnen aufwiesen als die röntgenbestrahlten. Diese Beobachtung scheint ihnen um so bemerkenswerter, als die röntgenbestrahlten Patientinnen in der überwiegenden Zahl täglich von 8 Feldern, die Kobalt-60 bestrahlten Patientinnen aber nur von 2 Feldern aus bestrahlt wurden. Sie weisen in diesem Zusammenhang auf L. HENRY GARLAND, St. Franzisko, hin, der in einer Publikation klar dargelegt hat, daß man in den meisten Fällen bei richtiger Anwendung der üblichen Röntgenbestrahlung Ergebnisse erzielen kann, die denen der Telekobaltbestrahlung gleichwertig sind, wobei unter Berücksichtigung des niedrigeren RBW-Faktors bei Kobalt-γ-Strahlung auch die Nebenerscheinungen der Telekobalttherapie nicht geringer wären als bei üblicher Röntgentherapie.

c) Zusatztherapie

α) Hormontherapie

αα) Androgene

Die bösartigen Geschwülste der Tuben und Ovarien gehören zu den Systemkrebsen des weiblichen Genitales (HUBER u. BESSERER, 1952; KAYSER, 1959), deren Entwicklung zumindest zeitweise und deren Wachstumstendenz grundsätzlich einer hormonellen Beeinflussung unterliegen. Während nun das Follikelhormon eine Proliferation aller weiblichen Genitalorgane bewirkt, werden durch Verabreichung von Androgenen nicht nur den Zellen des gesunden Ovars (ELSNER u. TISCHER, 1952), sondern nach K. H. BAUER auch den maligne entarteten Zellen Wachstumsstimulanzen durch Eliminierung des organspezifischen Wuchsstoffes (STAEMMLER, 1958) entzogen, außerdem kommt es zu einer „zentralen" Bremsung der Ausschüttung der adenotropen Hypophysenvorderlappenhormone sowie des allgemeinen Wachstumshormons (ESCHER u. Mitarb., 1958) und damit zu einer allgemeinen Stoffwechselwirkung. Die Stickstoffbilanz wird positiv beeinflußt und der Eiweißanbau gefördert (GORDAN u. Mitarb., JUNKMANN u. UFER,

1955). Graham sowie Weghaupt nehmen auf Grund dieses anabolen Effektes und der dadurch ausgelösten Aktivierung des Bindegewebes eine Sensibilitätssteigerung des Tumorgewebes gegenüber der ionisierenden Strahlung an. Die Auffassung prädestiniert die Androgene grundsätzlich als Zusatztherapeuticum bei der Strahlenbehandlung bösartiger Geschwülste.

Buttenberg und Lau (1959) führen im Rahmen ihrer kombinierten Therapie des Ovarialcarcinoms eine hochdosierte Testovirontherapie durch, die mit 250 mg Testovirondepot begonnen und mit wöchentlichen Gaben von 100 mg „ad infinitum" (Runge) fortgesetzt wird. Hohlweg glaubt, daß damit die Gefahr einer neuen Erhöhung der gonadotropen Funktion des HVL mit daraus resultierender Anregung des Tumorwachstums vermindert werden kann.

Schmauss schlägt ansteigende Hormondosen, Verhagen eine androgene Stoßtherapie mit freien Intervallen vor und beide hoffen so einer „Gewöhnung" der Hypophyse an das Hormon, die zu einer Verminderung der Hemmung der Hypophysenfunktion führen könnte, entgegen zu wirken. Auch bei inkurablen und metastasierenden Tumoren kann sich unter diesen Gesichtspunkten die Androgentherapie günstig auswirken.

Die unvermeidlichen Nebenwirkungen (tiefe Stimme, Heiserkeit, zunehmende „männliche" Behaarung) belästigen die Patientin im allgemeinen erstaunlich wenig. Seltener werden auch einmal Acne und Ödeme unter der Behandlung beobachtet. Buttenberg und Lau (1959) diskutieren bei stärkeren Erscheinungen die Umstellung auf andere Androgene (Notandron oder Durabolin).

K. H. Bauer zitiert eine Reihe von Autoren, die sich mit der Anwendung von Androgenen bei Genitalcarcinomen, u.a. auch bei Ovarialcarcinomen beschäftigt haben (Merz, Prediger, Burger und Drescher, Vasterling, Runge und Lindenschmidt) und kommt abschließend zu der Feststellung, daß: „Im Gegensatz zu den Erfolgen beim Mammacarcinom die Androgentherapie weiblicher Carcinome, selbst wenn sie bewußt bis zur Virilisierung getrieben wird, nicht als zusätzlich effektiv anzusehen ist". Auch der Versuch mit Stilbenen (McInnes, Runge und Lindenschmidt) wurde bei strahlenrefraktären Collumcarcinomen als Vorbehandlung zur Radikaloperation durchgeführt. Die Verfasser geben an, daß mit Cyren durch Erzielung einer starken Hyperämie und damit „Durchsaftung des Bindegewebes" die Strahlensklerosierung des Bindegewebes gebessert werden und dadurch eine nachträgliche Operation ermöglicht werden könne.

ββ) Cortison und ACTH

Die Cortisonanwendung in der Tumortherapie ist noch außerordentlich problematisch. Durch die Behandlung mit Cortison wird nach Walser die ACTH-Produktion des HVL gebremst und damit die andrenogene Oestrogenproduktion vermindert. Dazu kommt die entzündungshemmende und antitoxische Wirkung, die Euphorisierung der Patientin, die Hebung des Allgemeinzustandes, die Anregung des Appetits und günstige Beeinflussung der Schmerzen (Kaiser, 1955). Brandstetter und Heissenberger (1958) geben günstige Auswirkungen der ACTH-Behandlung an. Sie beobachteten Euphorie, Nachlassen der Schmerzen, Gewichtszunahme und Besserung des Allgemeinzustandes.

β) Chemotherapie

Die Ansichten über die Zweckmäßigkeit des Einsatzes cytostatischer Substanzen zur Behandlung von Tumoren des weiblichen Genitales sind auch heute noch außerordentlich verschieden. Während de Moraes die Ergebnisse allgemein noch als schlecht bezeichnete und auch Hillemanns (1958) keine wesentlichen Vorteile durch Anwendung von N-oxyd Lost, Knopp von E 39 sahen, mehren sich die Stimmen, die über positive Ergebnisse mit der cytostatischen Behandlung berichten. Über „erstaunliche objektive und subjektive Besserung" auch beim metastasierenden Ovarialcarcinom mit Trenimon (Trisäthylen-imino-benzochinon — Bayer 231) berichtete Linke schon 1960, Sykes u. Mitarb.

und Rundless u. Mitarb. machten günstige Erfahrungen mit Triäthylenmelamin, Bateman, sowie Shay und Sun mit Thiotriäthylenphosphoramid, Schmermund mit E 39 Bayer, Abbasov sowie Nechaeva mit Sarcolysin bzw. Thiotepa, Bozzo und Cravarezzo mit Citosal, Papavasiliou und Kostouros mit Chlorambucil, etc. etc. Dabei empfehlen die meisten Autoren die Anwendung der Cytostatica zusätzlich in Kombination mit der operativen und Strahlenbehandlung. Wolff und Iconikoff (1963) kommen auf Grund ihrer Erfahrungen zu der Aussage, daß die Radioresistenz und die Resistenz gegen Chemotherapeutica Hand in Hand zu gehen scheinen. Grundsätzlich weisen alle Autoren darauf hin, daß die Chemotherapie ausgesprochen individuell dosiert zur Anwendung kommen muß. Pfleiderer und Kiyan kommen 1967 zu folgender Feststellung: „Die großen Hoffnungen, die man auf die Behandlung des Carcinoms mit Cytostatica gesetzt hatte, haben sich zwar im allgemeinen nicht erfüllt. Eine Ausnahme davon bildet jedoch das Ovarialcarcinom". Die Autoren fahren dann fort: „Mit unseren Beobachtungen überraschender Erfolge bei diesem Carcinom sind wir nicht allein. Die Berichte über erstaunliche Besserung bei scheinbar aussichtslosen Fällen sind in der Literatur so häufig, daß sie kaum aufgeführt werden können. Blinick u. a. (1966) sowie Schwartz u. a. (1966) haben an größeren Fallzahlen mit Thio-Tepa und Decker u. a. (1967) mit Endoxan in vielen Fällen erstaunliche Remissionen beobachtet. Berichte über 3- oder 5-Jahres-Heilungen an ausgedehnten Ovarialcarcinomen, wie sie Spechter (1967) an unserem Beobachtungsgut aufzeigen konnte, fehlen jedoch noch weitgehend".

Spechter hat sich seit 1956 auf der Suche nach weiteren Therapiemöglichkeiten beim ausgedehnten Ovarialcarcinom mit der zusätzlichen Chemotherapie befaßt, aber erst als er die Cytostatica an den Anfang seines Therapieplanes stellte, Erfolge gesehen. Er empfiehlt folgendes Vorgehen: „Bei der Laparotomie wird die Tumorausdehnung festgestellt. Bei unbeweglichen, infiltrierenden, mit der Umgebung verbackenen Tumoren, multiplen Peritonealmetastasen oder rasenartigem Peritonealbefall wird von operativen Manipulationen oder von einem Versuch, diese Carcinome zu mobilisieren, abgesehen und nur eine Probeexcision aus dem Netz, bzw. aus den Peritonealmetastasen, ausgeführt. Instillationen von 10 mg E 39s oder von 200—400 Trenimon verdünnt mit 100—200 cm^3 Periston N in die Bauchhöhle. Sofort beginnen wir mit parenteraler Applikation von Cytostatica. Dabei bevorzugen wir Endoxan 200 mg/täglich i.v. Hat ein Ascites bestanden, geben wir zur vermehrten Diurese täglich Aldactone-A 4mal 25 mg und Saltucin 2mal 5 mg. Aldactone hat als Aldosteron-Antagonist außerdem eine entzündungshemmende Wirkung, die bei Beginn der Carcinom-Therapie günstig ist". Weiter entwickelt Spechter folgende Vorstellungen: „Bei der Devitalisierung von Tumorzellen durch Cytostatica mit dem dann folgenden Abbau bildet sich eine bindegewebige Kapsel. Diese kann die notwendige Medikamentenkonzentration im Tumorzentrum verhindern. Somit werden nach einer gewissen Zeit eingekapselte Tumorreste nicht weiter auf das Cytostaticum reagieren. Hierbei spricht man häufig davon, daß das Neoplasma gegen das Medikament resistent geworden ist. Ich möchte aber in diesen Fällen eine für die Erzielung der örtlich notwendigen Konzentration ungenügende Blutversorgung als wesentliche Ursache annehmen, insbesondere auch deswegen, weil nachgewiesen werden konnte, daß die Resistenz von Tumoren, z.B. gegen alkylierende Substanzen, nicht prinzipiell, sondern quantitativ gegeben ist". Die folgende Tabelle 6 bringt die von Spechter durch die Art seines Vorgehens erzielte erhebliche Verbesserung der Überlebensraten beim fortgeschrittenen Ovarialcarcinom eindrucksvoll zur Darstellung.

Der Folsäure-Antagonist Methotrexat soll sich nach einem Bericht auf dem 16. Internationalen Fortbildungskongreß der BÄK in Davos (März 1968) beim Chorionepitheliom besonders günstig auswirken.

Buttenberg und Lau haben 1959 die Chemotherapie beim Ovarialcarcinom noch abgelehnt, da nach ihrer Ansicht die palliative Wirkung mit der Gefahr einer Schädigung des weißen Blutbildes insbesondere verbunden ist, die sie im Hinblick auf die Beeinflussung insbesondere des leukopoetischen Systems durch die Strahlenbehandlung nicht für vertretbar halten. Armborst vertritt in einer zusammenfassenden Arbeit über die Möglichkeiten der Chemotherapie gynäkologischer Malignome 1967 die Auffassung, daß die Chemotherapie am Ende der therapeutischen Möglichkeiten steht und es sich damit um eine negative Auslese im Hinblick auf den Zustand der Patienten und die Ausbreitung der Tumoren handelt. Er betont die Notwendigkeit einer klaren Indikationsstellung zum Einsatz der cytostatischen Substanzen, sowie einer ausreichenden Leberfunktion, deren Kontrolle und selbstverständlich auch die Kontrolle der Thrombocyten, Leukocyten und der Blutkörperchensenkungsgeschwindigkeit während der Chemotherapie.

Tabelle 6. *Vergleich der Überlebensraten in % beim Ovarialcarcinom Stadium IV* (Spechter)

Beobachtungszeitabschnitt	3 Jahre	4 Jahre	5 Jahre
1944—1956 op. + Rö.[a]	1:144 (0,7%)	1:144	1:144
1957 bis September 1963 Cytostatica (+Rö.)+op.	25:82 (30,5%)	11:53 (21%)	6:36 (17,5%)

[a] 1944—1956 wurden die Ovarialcarcinome bei der ersten Operation so radikal wie möglich entfernt. Anschließend Röntgennachbestrahlung. 1957 begann Spechter mit dem aufgezeichneten Therapieschema. 1959 kristallisierte sich sein jetziges Vorgehen heraus.

γ) Unspezifische Behandlung

Der unspezifischen Behandlung Krebskranker im allgemeinen, also auch der Patientinnen mit malignen Tumoren der Tuben, Ovarien, Parametrien und Ligamenta rotunda kommt „von vorneherein nur der Charakter einer Hilfsmethode für die nur palliative oder gar nur symptomatische Therapie, vor allem bei sogenannten inkurablen Krebsfällen zu (K. H. Bauer, 1956)". Heilungserfolge im Sinne von in Prozenten angebbaren Heilziffern hat die unspezifische Therapie bisher nicht aufzuweisen.

Zur unspezifischen Behandlung Krebskranker gehört auch die *Ernährung*. Die Ernährungsprobleme beim Krebskranken sind die gleichen wie bei allen schwerkranken Patienten und fallen damit in den Bereich der symptomatischen Diätbehandlung als Zusatzmethode bei der Betreuung von Schwerkranken. Eine „Heilkost" oder eine „krebsfeindliche Diät" mit therapeutischem Einfluß auf Remissionen, Lebensverlängerung und Krebsheilung selbst, oder auch auf die Prophylaxe gegenüber Rezidiven und Metastasen gibt es, soweit unsere heutigen Erkenntnisse reichen, nicht. Zusatzbehandlung bei der Betreuung von Krebskranken ist unter den gleichen Gesichtspunkten auch die Verabreichung von *Vitaminen*, *Bluttransfusionen* und *Roborantien*, wie Eisen, Arsen und Leberpräparaten, sowie von Fermentpräparaten als Substitionstherapie.

Die *unspezifische Reizkörpertherapie* ist ebenfalls keine therapeutische Maßnahme gegen das Carcinom, auch ihr kommt nur der Charakter einer Hilfsmethode, die palliativ oder symptomatisch wirkt, zu. K. H. Bauer (1956) führt dazu aus: „Es soll nicht bestritten werden, daß solchen Mitteln (wie Anicin, AF 2, Iscador, beliebigen Impfseren usw.) gelegentlich zeitweise Besserung im Allgemeinzustand und dergleichen zuzuschreiben sind, doch kann keine Rede davon sein, daß ihnen eine krebstherapeutische Wirkung zukommt. Ihr gelegentlicher Effekt ist mit einer unspezifischen Reizwirkung bei Zufuhr körperfremder Proteine ausreichend erklärt". Auch wir, wie u.a. auch Kahr und Weiser, Ries und Blasiu, Prediger, haben bei der Behandlung insbesondere von desolaten „ausbestrahlten" Patientinnen mit solchen Medikamenten günstige Einflußnahmen auf den Allgemeinzustand und die Psyche beobachtet, und konnten gelegentlich auch durch eine dadurch erreichte Linderung von Schmerzen Opiate einsparen.

Selbstverständlich sind die *medikamentöse* Behandlung der Schmerzen, die *Durchführung physikalisch-therapeutischer Maßnahmen* (soweit sie ohne Belästigung und Belastung des Patienten zur Anwendung kommen können) sowie in gewissem Sinne die *pflegerische* und *seelische Betreuung* der unheilbar Krebskranken und die *„nachgehende Fürsorge"* ebenfalls als Möglichkeiten der unspezifischen, damit auch nur symptomatischen und palliativ wirksamen Therapie aufzufassen.

4. Prognose und Heilungsergebnisse

a) Die malignen Tubentumoren

α) Tubencarcinom

Das Tubencarcinom besitzt hochgradige Malignität, wobei die geringe Dicke der Tubenwand und die leichte Ausbreitungsmöglichkeit nach allen Seiten von besonderer Bedeutung sind. Da es auch früh metastasiert, hängt die Prognose ganz besonders von der Frühdiagnose ab. Wenn die Beschwerden die Patientinnen zum Arzt führen, hat das Carcinom sich oft schon stärker ausgebreitet. Ärztlicherseits wird außerdem im Hinblick auf die Seltenheit der Geschwulst oft nicht an das Tubencarcinom gedacht und zu lange konservativ behandelt, so daß die Aussichten auf Heilung dadurch oft noch erheblich verschlechtert werden.

SCHWACH hat in neuester Zeit unter diesem Gesichtspunkt Fälle von 5-Jahres-Heilungen genauer analysiert und gefunden, daß „diese Tubencarcinome meist nicht vor der Operation diagnostiziert werden konnten, sondern bei einer aus anderer Diagnose vorgenommenen Operation am inneren Genitale entdeckt wurden und da oft erst als beginnendes Stadium vom Histopathologen".

Nach KREMER und ULM soll die Prognose günstiger sein, wenn unabhängig vom Stadium das abdominale Ende primär verschlossen ist, nach WIENINGER schlechter, wenn die Pars isthmica tubae erkrankt.

Als dauergeheilt nach 5 Jahren geben BRET und LEGRAND (1955) nur 2,47%, JUNKER 12% und WIENINGER (1953) 13% an. Die besten Resultate hat ENGSTRÖM mit seiner Behandlungsmethode der Belassung des Uterus bei der Operation als Radiumträger und Nachbestrahlung mit Radium-Röntgenstrahlen. Mit dieser Methode wurden am Radiumhemmet in Stockholm 5-Jahres-Heilungen von 35% (insgesamt 39 Patientinnen) erreicht. Sehr gute Ergebnisse gibt auch HUBER (1953) mit 21,7% (5 von 23 Patientinnen geheilt) an.

β) Tubenchorionepitheliom

Die Prognose ist schlecht. Im allgemeinen treten bald starke Blutungen auf, die zu einer erheblichen Anämie führen. Es entwickelt sich dann zumeist rasch eine Kachexie bei multipler Metastasierung. MOHR führte 1939 43 Fälle an, von denen nur 9 Fälle geheilt werden konnten (21%).

HUBER nimmt für das Tubenchorionepitheliom wie für das Uteruschorionepitheliom außer der malignen eine benigne Form (Chorionepitheliosis) an. Die Heilungsziffern dieser „benignen" Form sind nach HUBER beim Uteruschorionepitheliom wesentlich besser (86,4%) als die der (histologisch nicht abgrenzbaren) malignen Form.

HEISS (1954) berichtet von einer Patientin mit einem Tubenchorionepitheliom, die 6 Jahre post op. als geheilt anzusehen ist, obwohl in Unkenntnis der wahren Diagnose nur eine Salpingektomie durchgeführt worden war. Vielleicht ist dieser Fall ein Beweis für die Existenz einer benignen Form beim primären Tubenchorionepitheliom im Sinne von HUBER.

γ) Tubensarkom

Diese Geschwulstform ist so selten und die mitgeteilten Ergebnisse über die Heilungen so vereinzelt, daß eine auch nur einigermaßen gültige allgemeine Stellungnahme zur Prognose nicht möglich ist. Sicher ist die Prognose der Tumoren schon im Hinblick auf die diagnostischen Schwierigkeiten nicht wesentlich von der Prognose des Tubencarcinoms verschieden, die größere Radiosensibilität der Tumoren wird durch die größere Malignität kompensiert.

b) Die malignen Ovarialtumoren

Trotz enormer Anstrengungen konnten die Heilungserfolge beim Ovarialcarcinom in den letzten Jahrzehnten nur unwesentlich verbessert werden. Nach Kirchhoff (1967) ist die Prognose des Ovarialcarcinoms im Vergleich mit anderen Genitalcarcinomen, insbesondere mit dem Collumcarcinom, nach wie vor erschütternd schlecht. Im Weltschrifttum bewegen sich die Heilungserfolge zwischen 12,3% (Forlani) und 40% (Dabney Cerr). In der deutschsprachigen Literatur liegen die Erfolgsberichte von Müller mit 37% „Heilungen" (1967) und von Pfleiderer mit 38% „Überlebenszeit" (1967) an der Spitze. Ries und Breitner errechneten 1959 aus den Angaben von 12 Autoren mit insaesamt 2602 Fällen eine durchschnittliche 5-Jahres-Heilung von 25,3% (12,3—37,6%). Wir selbst haben in der Zeit von 1948—1958 bei 86 Ovarialcarcinomen eine absolute Heilung von 20,9% erzielt.

Eine Zusammenstellung neuerer Heilungsergebnisse bringen Pfleiderer und Kiyan (1967) in der folgenden Tabelle 7.

Tabelle 7. *Ergebnisse der Behandlung des Ovarialcarcinoms in der neueren Literatur*

Autor	Ort	Zahl	5-Jahres-heilung	Besondere Therapie
Adler et al. (1960)	Basel	211	26%	^{198}Au
Aucoin et al. (1960)	New Orleans	226	13%	—
Kent et al. (1960)	Boston	349	36%	—
Dalley (1961)	London	137	24%	—
Kottmeier (1961)	Stockholm	293	23%	^{198}Au
Dockerty (1962)	Rochester	172	54%	—
Lübke (1962)	Berlin	76	20%	Endoxan
Rubin (1962)	Rochester	145	36%	—
Ratzkowski et al. (1963)	Jerusalem	135	21%	Chemotherapie
Raventos et al. (1963)	Philadelphia	275	41%	—
Stone et al. (1963)	New York	131	21%	—
Buka et al. (1964)	Montreal	100	31%	—
Gray et al. (1964)	Louisville	54	41%	—
Koller (1964)	Oslo	?	40%	^{198}Au
Carol et al. (1965)	Jena	275	12%	—
Kepp et al. (1965)	Gießen	130	20%	^{198}Au
Keetel et al. (1966)	Iowa-City	249	25%	^{198}Au, Chemotherapie
Müller (1966)	Zürich	230	37%	^{198}Au
Van Orden et al. (1966)	New Haven	137	23%	—
Pomerance et al. (1966)	Brooklyn	128	27%	—
Da Rugna et al. (1967)	Basel	250	35%	—
Gesamtzahl		3703 = 28%		

Die Tatsache, daß beim Zusammenziehen aller Ergebnisse von 3703 Patienten auch in dieser neuen Zusammenstellung nur 28% 5-Jahres-Heilungen zu verzeichnen sind, unterstreicht noch einmal die auch heute noch schlechte Prognose des Ovarialcarcinoms. Die Hauptschuld an diesen deprimierenden Therapieergebnissen trägt bekanntlich die Symptomarmut dieser Geschwulst, d.h., wenn die ersten, meist völlig uncharakteristischen Erscheinungen von der Kranken beobachtet werden, liegt meist schon ein inoperabler, nicht selten sogar inkurabler Zustand vor.

Bei der vergleichenden Betrachtung der Heilungsergebnisse ist natürlich zu berücksichtigen, daß die Zusammensetzung des Krankengutes an den verschiedenen Kliniken außerordentlich verschieden sein kann. So kommen z.B. die Patientinnen mit Ovarialtumoren in Großstädten im allgemeinen wesentlich früher zur Behandlung als in ländlichen Einzugsbereichen. Weiterhin spielt eine Rolle die Frage, ob die Patientinnen mit malignen Ovarialtumoren in den Kliniken, die die Strahlentherapie oder sonstige Zusatzbehandlung und Nachbehandlung durchführen, selbst operiert wurden, oder „fallweise" nach Operation in oft kleinen Krankenhäusern, der Klinik oder dem Strahleninstitut zur Nach- und Zusatzbehandlung überwiesen werden. Von diesen kleinen Krankenhäusern aus werden im allgemeinen nur die „schlechten" Fälle überwiesen, so daß (RUMMEL) dadurch eine gewisse „negative" Auslese der Nachbestrahlungspatientinnen zustande kommen kann.

Der Vergleich von Heilungsergebnissen unter Berücksichtigung der einzelnen Stadien ist noch wenig sinnvoll, da die meisten Berichte die propagierte einheitliche Stadieneinteilung noch nicht berücksichtigen.

Von der grundsätzlichen, auch heute noch schlechten Prognose der malignen Ovarialtumoren macht lediglich der Granulosazelltumor eine Ausnahme. RUMMEL gibt für diesen Ovarialtumor 83%, RIES 63% 5-Jahres-Heilungen an.

Alle Behandlungsmethoden der malignen Ovarialtumoren zusammen haben also im Verlauf der letzten Jahrzehnte zu einem nur geringen Fortschritt in der Therapie der Ovarialtumoren geführt, wie aus dem nur geringen Anstieg der durchschnittlichen Heilungserfolge (RIES und BREITNER, 1959, 25,3%; PFLEIDERER und KIYAN, 1967, 28%) hervorgeht. Das Problem liegt nach wie vor in der Früherkennung der Erkrankung und damit der frühzeitig einsetzenden Therapie. Hier scheint sich aber trotz der Entwicklung neuer diagnostischer Hilfsmittel noch keine wesentliche Wandlung vollzogen zu haben.

c) Die malignen Tumoren der Parametrien und Ligamenta rotunda

Die Prognose dieser Tumoren hängt ab von der Frühdiagnose, damit von der Operabilität, der Art und Größe des Eingriffes, der Möglichkeit einer Radikaloperation und dem Allgemeinzustand der Patientinnen. Dabei ist zu berücksichtigen, daß nicht nur die primär malignen sondern auch die gutartigen, retroperitonealen Lipome und Myxome zu Rezidiven und Metastasen neigen. Selbst wenn die Metastasen der gutartigen Tumoren — wie zumeist — histologisch wieder gutartig sind (sie können auch sarkomatös umgewandelt sein), kann die Patientin doch am fortlaufenden Wachstum der Geschwulst zugrunde gehen. Grundsätzlich ist also die Prognose der bösartigen Tumoren der Parametrien und Ligamenta rotunda als schlecht, die der gutartigen Tumoren als „nicht sehr günstig" zu bezeichnen (L. SCHMIDT, 1953).

Literatur

ABBASOV, A. T.: The intracavital use of sarcolysin and tiotepa in malignant ovary tumours. Vop. Onkol. 6, 23—30 mit engl. Zus.fass. (1960).

ABRAMS, J., KASAL, H. L., HOBBS, R. E.: Primary sarcoma of the fallopian tube. Review of the literatur and report of one case. Amer. J. Obstet. Gynec. 75, 180 (1958).

ADLER, U.: Pers. Mitteilung.

AMANN: Zit. nach O. FRANKL.

ANTONOWITSCH, E.: Die Diagnose des primären Tubenkarzinoms im Röntgenbild. Fortschr. Röntgenstr. 73, 189 (1950).

ARIEL, I. M.: Results of treating patients with ovarian cancer with radioactive isotopes. N.Y. St. J. Med. 62, 3553—3559 (1962).

— Treatment of ovarian cancer with radioactive isotopes. Amer. J. Roentgenol. 88, 877—885 (1962).

ARMBORST, V.: Möglichkeiten der Chemotherapie gynäkologischer Malignome. Med. Welt Nr 42, 498 (1967).

ARNAL, M. L., HEINZEL, F., RUHRMANN, K.: Die Anwendung kolloidaler Radiogoldlösungen in der Behandlung des Ovarialkarzinoms. Strahlentherapie, Sonderbd. 55, 317—320 (1964).

BAKSHEEVA, A.A.: Chemotherapy in the complex method of treating malignant neoplasms of the ovary. Akush. i Ginek. 40, 14—18 mit engl. Zus.fass. (1964) Russisch]. Ref. Ber. Gynäk. 87, 289 (1965).

BARY, S. v., SCHUCK, J.: Behandlungserg. und andere statistische Daten des weiblichen Genitalcarcinoms unter Verwendung des Krankengutes der Jahre 1933—1944 an der II. U.FKF München. Strahlentherapie 88, 597 (1952).

BASERGA, R., SCHUBIK, P.: The action of cortisone on transplanted and induced tumors in mice. Cancer Res. 14, 12 (1954).

BATEMANN, J. C.: Zit. nach BUTTENBERG u. LAU.

BAUER, K. H.: Das Krebsproblem. Berlin-Göttingen-Heidelberg: Springer 1949.

— Sitzungsbericht 73. Tagg d. Dtsch. Ges. f. Chir. Langenbecks Arch. klin. Chir. 284, 438 (1956).

Becker, J.: Klinische Erfolgsberichte über das stationäre Beobachtungsgut der Jahre 1906—1939 des Heidelberger Krebsinstitutes. Strahlentherapie **72**, 392 (1942/43).

— Gudden, F., Kuttig, H.: Siebbestrahlung mit Co60-Gammastrahlen. Strahlentherapie **105**, 623 (1958).

— Scheer, K. E.: Strahlentherapeutische Anwendung von radioaktivem Kobalt in Form von Perlen. Strahlentherapie **86**, 540 (1952).

Behrens, H.: Das primäre Tuberkarzinom (Erfahrungen aus dem Material der Univ.-Frauenklinik Leipzig in den Jahren 1937—1953) (29 Fälle). Geburtsh. u. Frauenheilk. **14**, 107 (1954).

Bergmann, G.: Über die Behandlung der bösartigen Ovarialtumoren und die Behandlungsergebnisse an der Rostocker Univ.-Frauenklinik im Dezenium 1940—1949. Krebsarzt (Wien) **13**, 310 (1958).

Bernstine, J. B., Beckinridge, R. L.: Sarcoma of the round ligament. Amer. J. Obstet. Gynec. **63**, 1367 (1952).

Besserer, G.: Über das Symptom des Hydrops tubae profluens und seine Bedeutung für die Erkennung des primären Tuberkarzinoms. Geburtsh. u. Frauenheilk. **8**, 610 (1948).

— Über die zytologische Erkennung eines primären Tuberkarzinoms aus dem Scheidenabstrich. Geburtsh. u. Frauenheilk. **11**, 804 (1951).

— Was leistet die Zytodiagnostik bei der Erkennung des primären Tubenkarzinoms? Geburtsh. u. Frauenheilk. **13**, 660 (1953).

Beutel, A., Adam, W. E.: Ergebnisse der Strahlenbehandlung der primären Ovarialkarzinome. Strahlentherapie **109**, 251—256 (1959).

Bianchi, F., Cazzola, D.: Rilievi e considerazioni cliniche e terapeutiche su sinque casi di ca. Primitivo della salpinge. Rev. ital. Ginec. **48**, 167—182 (1964).

Bjersing, L., Skanse, B., Genell, S.: Virilisierender maligner Resttumor des Ovars. Wert des Corticosteroid-Suppressionstests in der Diagnose. Acta obstet. gynec. scand. **40**, 26—39 (1961).

Boschann, H.-W.: Zur Klinik und Pathologie des primären Tubenkarzinoms. Z. Geburtsh. **136**, 58 (1952).

Bozzo, G. B., Cravarezzo, F.: Die cytostatische Chemotherapie in Verbindung mit der chirurgischen und Strahlenbehandlung in 4 Fällen von bösartigen Tumoren der Ovarien im vorgeschrittenen oder Endstadium. Rep. Ostetr. e. Ginecol., Osp. Civ., Asti. Clin. ostet. genic. **63**, 111—124 (1961).

Braband, H., Bublitz, G.: Die pelvine Pneumographie und Arteriographie gynäkologischer Erkrankungen. Röntgenstrahlen H. 15 (1966).

Brandstetter, F., Heissenberger, E.: Symptomatische ACTH-Behandlung Karzinomkranker. Krebsarzt (Wien) **13**, 153—156 (1958).

Brauer, W.: Bewertung strahlentherapeutischer Ergebnisse bei malignen Ovarialtumoren. Münch. med. Wschr. **28**, 1496 (1967).

Breen, J. L., Neubecker, R. D.: Tumoren des Ligamentum rotundum. Eine Literaturübersicht und Bericht über 25 Fälle. Obstet. and Gynec. **19**, 771—780 (1962).

Breit, A.: Persönliche Mitteilung 1970.

Breitner, J.: Die Bedeutung des radioaktiven Goldes (Au198) bei der Behandlung des Ovarialkarzinoms. Dtsch. med. Wschr. **85**, 888—890, 893 (1960).

— Adler, U.: Therapie und Behandlungsergebnisse beim Ovarial-Ca. an der Basler Klinik. Krebsarzt (Wien) **13**, 132 (1958).

Bret, A. J., Legrand, J.: Zit. nach Deimel, H., Das Epithelioma der Tuba Fallopii. [Französisch.] Ber. ges. Gynäk. Geburtsh. **55**, 297 (1955).

Buka, N. J., MacFarlane, K. T.: Bösartige Eierstocktumoren. Amer. J. Obstet. Gynec. **90**, 383—387 (1964).

Busse, O., Soergel, W.: Bericht über 800 maligne Erkrankungen des weiblichen Genitale der Jahre 1947—1952. Geburtsh. u. Frauenheilk. **19**, 201 (1959).

Buttenberg, D., Gutensohn, H.: Die Zunahme der 5-Jahresheilung durch die Antibiotikaprophylaxe bei der Radiumtherapie des Carcinoma colli uteri. Geburtsh. u. Frauenheilk. **24**, 334—338 (1964).

— Kuttig, H.: Zit. nach Buttenberg, D., H. Lau, Kombinierte Behandlung des Ovarialkarzinoms. Geburtsh. u. Frauenheilk. **19**, 308 (1959).

— Lau, H.: Kombinierte Behandlung des Ovarialkarzinoms. Geburtsh. u. Frauenheilk. **19**, 308 (1959).

Carazzone, F. P.: In tempa di isotopoterapia endocaviraria. II. Rilievi scintigrafici in corso di trattamento con 32P endoperitoneale. Minerva ginec. **18**, 795—804 (1966).

Castaño y Almendral, A., Frischkorn, R., Linden, W. A.: Besonderheiten mit 198Au bei der Behandlung des Ovarialkarzinoms. Strahlentherapie, Sonderbd. **55**, 321—329 (1964).

Castro, J. R., Kleith, E. W.: Vorkommen und Erscheinungsformen der röntgenologisch sichtbaren psammomatosen Verkalkungen des papillären Cystadenocarcinom der Ovarien. Amer. J. Roentgenol. **88**, 886—891 (1962).

Cavallero, G., Rossi, R.: Beitrag zum Studium der bösartigen Mischgeschwülste des Eileiters (Carcinosarkome). Ber. ges. Gynäk. Geburtsh. **71**, 233 (1960).

Claus, J.: Tubenkarzinom und Scheidenabstrich. Zbl. Gynäk. **74**, 1672 (1952).

Clausnitzer, W., Albert, H.: Bericht über die Behandlungsergebnisse primärer bösartiger Ovarialtumoren von 1946—1960. Strahlentherapie **129**, 18 (1966).

Cocchi, U.: Betatron und Telekobalttherapie. Berlin-Göttingen-Heidelberg: Springer 1958.

Corscaden, J. A.: Gynecologic cancer. New York: Williams & Wilkins 1951.

Crainz, F.: Die Behandlungserfolge bei den bösartigen Eierstocksgeschwülsten. Strahlentherapie **63**, 434 (1938).

— Schmiemann, R.: Die Bewertung der Behandlungsergebnisse bei den bösartigen Eierstocksgeschwülsten. Zbl. Gynäk. **64**, 794 (1940).

Crisp, W. E.: Choriocarcinoma of the Fallopian tube coincident with viable pregnancy. Amer. J. Obstet. Gynec. **71**, 442 (1956).

CZECH, H., KEPP, R. K., WOLTHAUS, G.: Ergebnisse der Behandlung der bösartigen Genitaltumoren an der Univ.-Frauenklinik Göttingen in den Jahren 1937—1944. Strahlentherapie **82**, 321 (1950).

CZIPRI, M., TOMBOR, J.: Präoperative Diagnose von Primärkarzinom und akuter Drehung des Eileiters. Zbl. Gynäk. **80**, 997 (1958).

DABNEY CERR: Zit. nach BERGMANN, Über die Behandlung der bösartigen Ovarialtumoren und die Behandlungsergebnisse an der Rostocker Univ.-Frauenklinik im Dezennium 1940—1949. Krebsarzt (Wien) **13**, 310 (1958).

DAL CANTON: Beitrag zur Erkennung des primären Tubenkarzinoms. Ber. ges. Gynäk. Geburtsh. **62**, 314 (1957).

DALLEY, V. M.: Is preservation of the uterus worthwhile? Amer. J. Roentgenol. **88**, 867—876 (1962).

DA RUGNA, D., STÄUBLE, K., GÖMÖRI, Z.: Die Therapie des Ovarialkarzinoms. Gynaecologia (Basel) **163**, 247 (1967).

DELFT, H.: Erfolge der Operation und Strahlentherapie bösartiger Ovarialtumoren. Zbl. Gynäk. **65**, 1507 (1941).

DIBBELT, L.: Persönl. Mitteilung.

DIETRICH, H. A.: Die Neubildungen der Eileiter. HALBAN-SEITZ, Biologie und Pathologie des Weibes, Bd. 5, Teil 1. Berlin-Wien: Urban & Schwarzenberg 1953.

DIETZ, W.: Röntgenologische Veränderungen der Harnwege beim Genitalkarzinom der Frau. Tagg der Südwestdtsch. Röntgenges. Baden-Baden 1955.

— Über den röntgenologischen Nachweis von Lungenmetastasen bei Genitalkarzinomen der Frau. Z. Krebsforsch. **62**, 316—322 (1958).

— Strahlentherapie und Heilungsergebnisse beim Kollumkarzinom an der Universitäts-Frauenklinik Freiburg i. Br. 1950—1954. Strahlentherapie **115**, 65—71 (1961).

— Über die Möglichkeit der Erfassung der Strahlenwirkung auf den Organismus aus dem peripheren Blut mit dem Leukozytenresistenzwert. Strahlenschutz in Forschung u. Praxis **4**, 159 (1963).

— BEINERT, W.: Über die Bedeutung des intravenösen Pyelogramms beim Carcinoma colli uteri. Röntgen-Bl. **6**, 339 (1966).

— ENSE, H.: Vergleichende Tierversuche mit dem Leukozytenresistenzwert (LRW) bei Siebbestrahlung. Krebsbehandlung, Strahlenbehandlung und Strahlenforschung. Sonderbde zur Strahlentherapie **43**, 408—416 (1959).

— FISCHER, M.: Über den Wert der Strahlenbehandlung bei Rezidiven und weiterwachsenden Primärtumoren des Kollumkarzinoms unter besonderer Berücksichtigung der Palliativeffekte, S. 117. Dtsch. Röntgenkongr. 1967. 48. Tag der Dtsch. Röntgenges., Teil B, Strahlenbehandlung und Strahlenbiologie, S. 107—113. München-Berlin: Urban & Schwarzenberg 1967.

— POESCHEL, A.: Biologische Untersuchungen über die Siebwirkung. Strahlenforschung und Strahlenbehandlung, Bd. 2. Sonderbde z. Strahlentherapie **46**, 101—107 (1960).

— STARCKJOHANN, J.: Über die Bedeutung der Lochgröße bei der Siebbestrahlung für die Allgemeinreaktion. Strahlentherapie **119**, 620—637 (1962).

D'INCERTI, BONINI: Zit. nach MAURER, H. J., THOMAS, U.: Die Behandlungsergebnisse beim Ovarialkarzinom an der Univ.-Frauenklinik Erlangen während der Jahre 1949—1954. Zbl. Gynäk. **81**, 43 (1959).

DÖRFFEL, E. W., HAI, N. V.: Ergebnisse bei den mit Radiogold (Au^{198}) intraperitoneal behandelten Ovarialkarzinomen an der Geschwulstklinik der Charité, Berlin. Radiobiol. Radiother. (Berl.) **8**, 35—41 (1967).

DUBRAUSZKY, V.: Die Erkrankungen des Eierstocks mit innersekretorischer Funktion. In: TASSILO ANTOINE, Klinische Fortschritte der Gynäkologie. München-Berlin: Urban & Schwarzenberg 1954.

DVORÁK, O.: Primäres Eileiterkarzinom im Material der 1. Gynäk. Klinik der Karlsuniversität Prag in den Jahren 1929—1953. Ber. ges. Gynäk. Geburtsh. **65**, 215 (1958).

DYROFF, R., SIEGERT, A.: Biologie und Pathologie des Weibes, Bd. III, 2. Aufl. Berlin-Innsbruck-München-Wien: Urban & Schwarzenberg 1955.

ELSNER, P., TISCHER, H.: Veränderungen am Ovar bei hormonbehandelten Mammacarcinomen. Arch. Gynäk. **181**, 462 (1952).

ENGSTRÖM, L.: Primäres Tubenkarzinom. [Schwedisch.] Ber. ges. Gynäk. Geburtsh. **64**, 96 (1958).

ENNKER, J.: Zur präoperativen Diagnose des Tubenkarzinoms. Geburtsh. u. Frauenheilk. **15**, 898 (1955).

— Diagnoseförderung der Genitalkarzinome durch die Zytologie. In: v. MIKULICZ-RADECKI, Früherkennung und Behandlung des weiblichen Genitalkarzinoms. Stuttgart: Ferdinand Enke 1957.

ESCHER, F., ROTH, F., COTTIER, H.: Die paranasale transethmoido-sphenoidale Hypophysektomie beim metastasierenden Mammakarzinom. Schweiz. med. Wschr. **88**, 49 (1958).

FALGE, E.: Zur Frage des primären Tubensarkoms. Geburtsh. u. Frauenheilk. **13**, 243—248 (1953).

FARSCHIDPUR, D., BRABAND, H.: Intrakavitäre Curietherapie mit kolloidalem Gold (Au 198). Radiobiol. Radiother. (Berl.) **4**, 323—331 (1963).

FERNÀNDEZ-SUAREZ, J. M.: Primäres papilläres Adenokarzinom der Tube. Ber. ges. Gynäk. Geburtsh. **64**, 307 (1958).

FIDLER, H. K., LOCK, D. R.: Carcinoma of the fallopian tube detected by cervical smear. Amer. J. Obstet. Gynec. **67**, 1103 (1954).

FISCHER, M.: Ergebnisse der Strahlenbehandlung von rezidivierenden, metastasierenden und weiterwachsenden Kollumkarzinomen a. d. UFK Freiburg 1949—1954. Diss. Freiburg 1962.

FOCHEM, K.: Einführung in die geburtshilfliche und gynäkologische Röntgendiagnostik. Stuttgart: Georg Thieme 1967.

— Der Wert der Röntgenroutineuntersuchung für die Diagnostik der weiblichen Genitaltumoren. Fortschr. Röntgenstr., Beih. 40—44 (1966).

— KOFLER, E.: Die Behandlungsergebnisse der primären Ovarialcarcinome in den Jahren 1943—1948 an der I. Univ.-Frauenklinik in Wien. Krebsarzt (Wien) **9**, 215 (1954).

— — Die Behandlungsergebnisse der primären malignen Ovarialtumoren 1948—1955. Krebsarzt (Wien) **17**, 490 (1962).

Fochem, K., Weghaupt, K.: Zur gynäkologischen Strahlenbehandlung mit der Siebmethode. Wien. med. Wschr. 107, 96 (1957).

Forlani: Zit. nach Ries, J., Zum Stand des Ovarialkarzinoms. Krebsarzt (Wien) 13, 121 (1958).

Frankel, A. N.: Primary carcinoma of the Fallopian tube. Amer. J. Obstet. Gynec. 72, 131 (1956).

Frankl, O.: Beiträge zur Pathologie und Klinik des Ovarialkarzinoms. Arch. Gynäk. 113, 29 (1920).

— In: Henke-Lubarsch, Handbuch der speziellen pathologischen Anatomie und Histologie, Bd.VII/1. Berlin: Springer 1933.

Freese, U.: Ein Beitrag zur Zytologie des primären Tubenkarzinoms. Geburtsh. u. Frauenheilk. 17, 179 (1957).

Freund: Zit. nach Schmidt, L., Über primäre solide Tumoren des Beckenbindegewebes. Münch. med. Wschr. 49, 1320 (1953).

Frischkorn, R.: Unsere Erfahrungen mit der Siebbestrahlung gynäkologischer Karzinome. Univ.-Frauenklinik Göttingen. 41. Tagg Dtsch. Röntgenges., Freudenstadt, 11.—14. 5. 1960. Strahlenforsch. und Strahlenbehandlung. Strahlentherapie, Sonderbd. 46, 128—133 (1960).

Froewis, J., Brosch, H.: Die Schwierigkeiten in der Diagnostik maligner Ovarialtumoren. Arch. Geschwulstforsch. 8, 95 (1955).

— Kremer, H.: Frühdiagnose eines Tubenkarzinoms. Krebsarzt (Wien) 13, 141—145 (1958).

Fromme, Heynemann: Zit. nach Wieninger, E., Über das primäre Tubenkarzinom. Zbl. Gynäk. 75, 54 (1953).

Fuchs, W. A.: Lymphographie und Tumordiagnostik. Berlin-Heidelberg-New York: Springer 1965.

Gaebel, E.: Über maligne Ovarialtumoren. Strahlentherapie 114, 225 (1961).

Gauwerky, F.: Persönl. Mitteilung.

Gerteis, W.: Die lymphografische Kontrolle der Supervolttherapie des Genitalcarcinoms. Arch. Gynäk. 202, 320—325 (1965).

Glauner, R.: Die Indikationen zur Röntgen- und Radiumbestrahlung. Stuttgart: GeorgThieme 1948.

Glück, O.: Diagnose und Behandlung bösartiger Ovarialtumoren. Krebsarzt (Wien) 5, 68 (1950).

Goette, U.: Der Einfluß der Gestaltung des Radiumträgers auf den Isodosenverlauf. Diss. Freiburg 1953.

Götz, R.: Drei weitere Fälle von primärem Tubenkarzinom. Zbl. Gynäk. 77, 74—81 (1955).

Goodall, J. R.: In: Curtis, Obst. and Gynec., Saint Louis, Mosley 2, 980 (1933).

Graham, J. B., Graham, R. M.: Method of enhancing effectiveness of radiotherapie in cancer of uterine cervix. Cancer (Philad.) 6, 69 (1953).

Gray, L. A., Barnes, M. L.: Das Carzinom des Ovars. Bericht über 106 Fälle. II. Pathologie, klinischer Verlauf, Behandlung. Ann. Surg. 159, 279—290 (1964).

Grčić, R., Živković, J.: Primäre bösartige Eileitergeschwülste. Med. Pregl. 16, 557—559 mit franz., engl. u. deutsch. Zus.fass. (1963) [Serbo-kroatisch]. (Ber. Gynäk. 86, 282 (1964).

Grünberger, V.: Über den Wert der Palliativoperation des Ovarialkarzinoms. Wien. klin. Wschr. 62, 327 (1950).

Grubisic, S.: Primäres Chorionepitheliom der Tube im Anschluß an Tubargravidität. Ber. ges. Gynäk. Geburtsh. 60, 32 (1956).

Guixa, H. L., Cebollero, L. M. E.: A propositos de dos nuevas observaciones de carcinoma de la trompa. Ber. ges. Gynäk. Geburtsh. 66, 32 (1958—1959).

Guthmann, H., Dörr, H.: Die Behandlungsergebnisse unserer Karzinomfälle vom 1. 1. 1927 bis 31. 12. 1931. Strahlentherapie 66, 440 (1939).

Gutmann, H.: Bericht über die bösartigen Geschwülste der Ovarien an der Univ.-Frauenklinik Freiburg i.Br. in den Jahren 1948—1958. Diss. Freiburg i.Br. 1960.

Guyomar, J.: Tuben-Carcinom. Gynéc. prat. 12, 53—59 (1961).

Hartl, H.: Über Nebenerscheinungen bei gynäkologischer Radiogoldtherapie. Fortschr. Röntgenstr. 85, 610 (1956).

Haselhorst, G.: Ein primäres schleimbildendes Adenokarzinom der Tube. Arch. Gynäk. 134, 489 (1928).

Heiss, H.: Primäres Chorionepitheliom der Tube. Zbl. Gynäk. 76, 870 (1954).

Hess, F.: Erfolge und Mißerfolge bei der Strahlentherapie von Rezidiven des Kollumkarzinoms, S. 114. Dtsch. Röntgenkongr. 1967. 48. Tagg der Dtsch. Röntgenges., Teil B, Strahlenbehandlung und Strahlenbiologie. München-Berlin: Urban & Schwarzenberg 1967.

Hesseltine, H.C., Smith, R.L.: Ovarian malignancy. Amer. J. Obstet. Gynec. 72, 1326 (1956).

Hillemanns, H. G.: Zur Chemotherapie des weiblichen Genitalkarzinoms, Erfahrungen mit der N-Oxyd-Lost-Therapie. Zbl. Gynäk. 80, 181 (1958).

Hofmann-Credner, D.: Tagungsber. 10. Österr. Ärztetagg, Wien 1957.

Hofmeister, F. J., Grothey, R. L.: Problems of ovarian tumors. Postgrad. Med. 20, 393 (1956).

Hohlweg, W.: Schattenseiten der Hormontherapie. Dtsch. med. Wschr. 79, 928 (1954).

Holbrook, M. A., Welch, J. S., Childs, D. S., Jr.: Adjuvants use of radioactive colloids in the treatment of carcinoma of the ovary. Radiology 83, 888—891 (1964).

Holthusen, H.: Zit. nach Kepp, Gynäkologische Strahlentherapie. Grundlagen der Strahlentherapie. Stuttgart: Georg Thieme 1952.

Holzner, J. H., Golob, E., Fischer, P.: Zum Problem der Diagnose von Doppelkarzinomen. Ergänzung der histologischen Methoden durch histochemische und zytogenetische Untersuchungen an einem Doppelkarzinom des weiblichen Genitaltraktes. Krebsarzt 20, 257—265 (1965). Ref. Zbl. ges. Radiol. 90, 219 (1966).

Horálek,F.,Kloc,S. Carcinoma tubae. [Tschechisch.] Ber. ges. Gynäk. 63, 321 (1957—1958).

Hosemann, H.: Persönl. Mitteilung.

Huber, H.: Die multizentrische Karzinomentstehung am weiblichen Genitale und ihre klinische Bedeutung. Geburtsh. u. Frauenheilk. 8, 830 (1948).

— Systemkarzinom am weiblichen Genitale. Ein weiterer Beitrag zur Frage der primären Tumormultiplizität. Dtsch. med. Wschr. 1559 (1952).

HUBER, H.: Ergebnisse der Behandlung des Genitalkarzinoms an Hand des Materials der Univ.-Frauenklinik seit dem Jahre 1922. Karzinom und Karzinombehandlung. Kieler Karzinomtagg 1952. München-Berlin: Urban & Schwarzenberg 1953.

— BESSERER, G.: Über den zytologischen Nachweis östrogener Funktion bei alten Frauen mit gut- u. bösartigen Proliferutionen am Genitalsystem. Geburtsh. u. Frauenheilk. 12, 708 (1952).

— HÖRMANN, G.: Über das Chorionepithelioma malignum. Z. Krebsforsch. 58, 285 (1952).

ISLITZER, E.: Primäres Tubenkarzinom, klinisch diagnostiziert. Zbl. Gynäk. 74, 736 (1952).

ISRAEL, S. L., CRISP, W. E., ADRIAN, D. C.: Preoperativ diagnosis of primary carcinoma of the fallopian tube. Amer. J. Obstet. Gynec. 68, 1589—1593 (1954).

JACKSON, R. L.: Disgerminom des Ovariums. Bericht über 8 Fälle. Div. of Obstetrics and Gynecol., Univ. of Tennessee Coll. of Med., Memphis. Amer. J. Obstet. Gynec. 80, 442—448 (1960).

JAKOBOVITS, A.: Hormone production by miscellaneous ovarian tumors. Amer. J. Obstet. Gynec. 85, 90 (1963). Ref. Ber. Gynäk. 83, 240 (1963).

JÁNOSSY, T., LENGYEL, S.: Experiences with the radiogold therapy of the malignant tumours of the ovary. Magy. Onkol. 9, 83—86 mit engl. Zus.fass. (1965) [Ungarisch]. Zbl. ges. Radiol. 89, 590 (1966).

JOHANNSEN, H.: Spätkomplikationen nach intraperitonealer Radiogoldinfusion. Strahlentherapie 127, 198—205 (1965).

JOHNSON, M. E. K., AMOS, T. G.: Primary carcinoma of the Fallopian tube. Amer. J. Surg. 83, 35—40 (1952).

JOHNSON, W. O.: Primary carcinoma of the Fallopian tube: twenty-five year survey (1930—1955) in six Louisville hospitals. Amer. Surg. 24, 489—491 (1958).

JUNKMANN, K., UFER, J.: Die extragenitalen Wirkungen der Sexualhormone. Med. Klin. 50, 1666 (1955).

KAHR, E., WEISER, G.: Zusätzliche Krebsbehandlung mit dem Faktor AF 2 Guarnieri. Krebsarzt (Wien) 11, 204—210 (1956).

KAISER, H.: E. Mercks Jber. 69, 6 (1955/56).

KAYSER, H. W.: Besondere Verlaufsformen des weibl. Genitalkarzinoms, zugleich ein Beitrag zum Systemkarzinomproblem. Z. Geburtsh. Gynäk. 152, 52 (1959).

KAPP-SCHWOERER, H.: Die Radiogoldseeds-Implantation (Au 198) bei der Behandlung gynäkologischer Malignome. Radiobiol. Radiother. (Berl.) 4, 313—321 (1963).

— Aktuelle Probleme der Strahlentherapie weiblicher Genitalkarzinome. Med. Welt, N. F. 17, 1105—1112 (1966).

KEETEL, W. C., ELKINS, H. B.: Experience with radioactive colloidal gold in treatment of ovarian carcinoma. Amer. J. Obstet. Gynec. 71, 553 (1956).

KEPP, R. K.: Die Therapie mit Radiogold in der Gynäkologie. Geburtsh. u. Frauenheilk. 18, 10 (1958).

— Bisherige Erfahrungen mit der Radiogoldbehandlung im Rahmen der gynäkologischen Strahlentherapie. Zbl. Gynäk. 84, 8—17 (1962).

KEPP, R. K.: Gynäkologische Strahlentherapie. Stuttgart: Georg Thieme 1952.

— Grundlagen der Strahlentherapie. Stuttgart: Georg Thieme 1952.

— CLEMENS, H.: Ergebnisse der postoperativen. Radiogoldtherapie bei bösartigen Ovarialtumoren. Strahlentherapie 126, 65—69 (1965).

KERMAUNER, F.: In: VEIT-STÖCKEL, Handbuch der Gynäkologie, Bd. VII. München: J. F. Bergmann 1932.

KIESLING, F. X.: Zur Chemotherapie des Ovarialcarzinoms. Geburtshilflich Gynäkol. Abtl., Städt. Krankenh. Wien-Lainz. Krebsarzt (Wien) 16, 101—115 (1961).

KIRCHHOFF, H.: Die Bedeutung des Uterus als Radiumträger bei der Therapie des Ovarialkarzinoms, S. 96. Deutscher Röntgenkongr. 1967. 48. Tagg der Dtsch. Röntgenges., Teil B, Strahlenbehandlung und Strahlenbiologie. München-Berlin-Wien: Urban & Schwarzenberg 1967.

KLOC, S.: Das Sarkokarzinom der Tube und des Gebärmutterkörpers. [Tschechisch.] Ber. ges. Gynäk. 62, 314 (1957).

KNOPP, K.: Über die klinische Anwendung des Zytostatikums E 39. Zbl. Gynäk. 79, 1905—1908 (1957).

KÖNIG, P. A.: Zur Differentialdiagnose des primären Tubensarkoms in Klinik und Pathomorphologie. Geburth. u. Frauenheilk. 17, 137—147 (1957).

KOLLER, O., GJØUNAESS, H.: Dysgerminoma of the ovary. A clinical report of 20 cases. Ber. Gynäk. 91, 261 (1965); Acta obstet. gynec. scand. 43, 268 (1964).

KOLLER, TH.: Zur Klinik und Therapie der malignen Ovarialtumoren. Schweiz. med. Wschr. 18, 215 (1937).

KOTTMEIER, H. L.: The classification and treatment of ovarian tumors. Acta obstet. gynec. scand. 31, 313 (1952).

— Aussprache auf der Österr. Krebstagg. Krebsarzt (Wien) 7, 275 (1952).

— In: TASSILO ANTOINE, Klinische Fortschritte der Gynäkologie. München-Berlin: Urban & Schwarzenberg 1954.

— MOBERGER, G.: Experience with radioactive colloidal gold as additional treatment in radiotherapy of uterine cancer. Acta obstet. gynec. scand. 34, 1 (1955).

KREMER, H., ULM, R.: Zur Problematik des primären Tubenkarzinoms. Arch. Gynäk. 185, 609 (1955).

KRUGMANN, PH. I., FISCHER, I. E.: Primary carcinoma of the Fallopian tube. Amer. J. Obstet. Gynec. 80, 722 (1960). Ref. Ber. Gynäk. 74, 44 (1961).

KRUSCHWITZ, S.: Beitrag zur Diagnostik des primären Tubencarzinoms, Univ.-Frauenklinik, Greifswald. Zbl. Gynäk. 96, 615—622 (1964).

LAMBRETHSUN, E., SELL, A.: Palliative treatment of carcinomatons effusions in the pleural and peritoneal cavities with radioactive gold. Acta radiol. (Stockh.) 56, 33 (1961).

LATZKO, W.: Ref. Linksseitiges Tubenkarzinom, rechts karzinomatöse Tuboovarialcyste. Zbl. Gynäk. 30, 599 (1916).

Laughlin, Sharpe: Zit. nach Schmidt, L.: Über primäre solide Tumoren des Beckenbindegewebes. Münch. med. Wschr. 49, 1320 (1953).

Lebherz, Th., Huston, B. J. W., Austin, J. A., Boyce, Ch. R.: Sustained palliation in ovarian carcinoma. Obstet. and Gynec. 25, 475 (1965). Ref. Ber. Gynäk. 91, 261 (1965).

Leonhard, A.: Einseitiges und doppelseitiges Tubenkarzinom. Zbl. Gynäk. 78, 1645 (1956).

Linke, A.: Die Behandlung der Hämoblastosen und malignen Tumoren mit Triäthyleniminobenzochinon. Dtsch. med. Wschr. 44, 1928 (1960).

Lohmeyer, H.: Kasuistischer Beitrag zum primären Tubencarzinom, Klin. Essen, Univ. Münster. Zbl. Gynäk. 86, 622—624 (1964).

Lohse, E.: Die primären malignen Geschwülste der Tuben, Parametrien und Ligamenta rotunda an der Freiburger Univ.-Frauenklinik in der Zeit v. 1. 1. 1937 bis 31. 12. 1959. Diss. Freiburg i. Br. 1961.

Long, R. T. L., Sala, J. M.: Radikales chirurgisches Vorgehen kombiniert mit Strahlentherapie bei der Behandlung von örtlich fortgeschrittenen Ovarialcarzinom. Surg. Gynec. Obstet. 117, 201—204 (1963).

Ludin, H.: Methode zum Einführen von Radiogold in die Bauchhöhle bei Peritonealkarzinose bei fehlendem Ascites. Fortschr. Röntgenstr. 79, 770 (1953).

Luft, R., Olivecrona, H.: Hypophysektomie in the treatment of malignant tumors. Cancer (Philad.) 10, 789 (1957).

Lundgren, N.: Ovarian arrhenoblastoma. Case report and discussion of the steroid metabolism. Acta obstet. gynec. scand. 41, 281 (1962).

Macarini, N., Besio, G. L., Gandolfo, E.: Recenti orientamenti nel trattamento radioterapico delle neoplasie maligne dell' ovaio con particolare riguardo all' impiego della telecobaltoterapia. Riassunto. Minerva med. 53, 1351 (1962).

Malkasian, G. D., Jr., Symmond, R. E.: Die Behandlung des einseitigen, abgekapselten Eierstockdisgerminoms. Sect. of Obstetrics and Gynecol. and Surg., Mayo Clin. and Mayo Found., Rochester. Amer. J. Obstet. Gynec. 90, 379—382 (1964).

Marley, A.: Lymphographie-cavographie exploration conjuguée dans les tumeurs pelviennes. Ann. Radiol. (Paris) 8, 785—795 (1965).

Marquardt, S.: Indikationserweiterung zur Strahlentherapie der Genitalkarzinome durch Siebbestrahlung. Zbl. Gynäk. 76, 91 (1954).

Martius, H.: Fortschritte und Ausblicke in der Strahlentherapie. Arch. Gynäk. 178, 236 (1950).

— Lehrbuch der Gynäkologie, 5. Aufl. Stuttgart: Georg Thieme 1958.

Maurer, H.-J., Thomas, U.: Die Behandlungsergebnisse beim Ovarialkarzinom an der Univ.-Frauenklinik Erlangen während der Jahre 1949—1954. Zbl. Gynäk. 81, 43 (1959).

Meigs, J. V.: Cancer oft the ovary. Surg. Gynec. Obstet. 71, 44 (1940).

— Le traitement du cancer génital chez la femme. Gynéc. prat. 13, 587—600 (1962).

— Zit. nach Pschyrembel, Praktische Gynäkologie. Berlin: W. de Gruyter & Co. 1964.

Merril, J. A.: Carcinoma of the broad ligament. Obstet. and Gynec. 13, 472 (1959).

Meyer, R.: Über verschiedene Erscheinungsformen des als Typus Brenner bekannten Eierstocksgeschwulst, ihre Absonderung von den Granulosazelltumoren und Zuordnung unter andere Ovarialgeschwülste. Arch. Gynäk. 148, 541 (1932).

— In: Henke-Lubarsch, Handbuch der speziellen pathologischen Anatomie und Histologie, Bd. VII/1. Berlin-Heidelberg-New York: Springer 1967.

Möbius, W.: Klinik und Therapie der Ovarialtumoren unter besonderer Berücksichtigung der Ovarialcarcinome. Krebsarzt (Wien) 9, 280 (1954).

Mohr: Zit. nach Heiss, Primäres Chorionepitheliom der Tube. Zb. Gynäk. 76, 870 (1954).

Moraes, A. de: Gegenwärtiger Stand der Behandlung des fortgeschrittenen Genitalkarzinoms der Frau. Ber. ges. Gynäk. Geburtsh. 66, 296 (1958—1959).

Müller, H. J.: Complications vésicales éventuelles après radiothérapie des cancers génitaux de la femme. Urol. int. (Basel) 21, 437 (1966).

— Vermeidung von Früh- und Spätkomplikationen bei der intraperitonealen Applikation von kolloidalem Radiogold Au^{198}. Radioaktive Isotope in Klinik und Forschung 7, 231 (1967).

— Intraaeritoneal Colloidal Radiogold ^{198}Au Therapy in Ovarian Cancer. Privater Vordruck des Autors aus Ovarian Cancer Symposium. Hrsg.: Unio Internationalis Contra Cancrum. Berlin-Heidelberg-New York: Springer 1967.

— Pathologisch-anatomische Gruppierung der malignen epithelialen Ovarial-Tumoren im Lichte der Behandlungsprognose. Mschr. Geburtsh. u. Gynäk. 120, 17 (1945).

— Bisherige Erfahrungen mit der intraperitonealen und intrapleuralen Applikation von künstlich radioaktiven Isotopen (Zn^{63}, Au^{198}) für die Behandlung der vom Ovar ausgehenden Karzinosen seit 1945. Schweiz. med. Wschr. 84, 409 (1954).

— Möglichkeiten und Erfolge der Krebstherapie mit radioaktivem Gold. Geburtsh. u. Frauenheilk. 15, 973 (1955).

Müller-Hummel, P. J.: Über den Wert der Dosismessung an Blase und Rektum bei der Radiumbestrahlung des weiblichen Genitalcarcinoms. Diss. Freiburg 1958.

Navrátil, J.: Geschwülste des Ligamentum rotundum. Ber. ges. Gynäk. Geburtsh. 66, 32 (1958—1959).

Naujoks, H.: Vaginalzytologischer Befund bei primärem Tubenkarzinom. Zbl. Gynäk. 82, 95—99 (1960).

Neeff, Th. C.: Zit. nach Müller-Hummel, P. J.: Über den Wert der Dosismessung an Blase und Rektum bei der Radiumbestrahlung des weiblichen Genitalcarcinoms. Diss. Freiburg 1958.

Neumann, H. O.: In: Henke-Lubarsch, Handbuch der speziellen pathologischen Anatomie und Histologie, Bd. VII/2. Berlin-Heidelberg-New York: Springer 1933.

Neuweiler, W.: Lehrbuch der gynäkologischen Diagnostik, 2. Aufl. Bern: H. Huber 1946.

Nevinny-Stickel, J.: Die hormonanlaktiven Ov.-Tumoren. Dtsch. med. J. 13, 750 (1962).

NOVIKOVA, L. A.: Chemotherapy of malignant Neoplasms of the ovaries. Akush. i Ginek. **3**, 88 (1962). Ref. Ber. Gynäk. **80**, 160 (1962/63).

NÜRNBERGER, L.: In: VEIT-STÖCKEL, Handbuch der Gynäkologie, Bd. VII. München: J. F. Bergmann 1932.

OBERHEUSER, F.: Nebenwirkungen der gynäkologischen Supervolttherapie. Geburtsh. u. Frauenheilk. **26**, 803—806 (1966).

OESER, H.: Strahlenbehandlung der Geschwülste. München-Berlin: Urban & Schwarzenberg 1954.

— SCHLUNGBAUM, W., MEHL, H. G.: Kontrollierte intratumorale und intrakavitäre Radiogoldtherapie. Fortschr. Röntgenstr. **83**, 792 (1955).

ØKLAND, G.: Radioactive gold in ovarian cancer. Nord. Med. **71**, 719—721 mit engl. Zus.fass. (1964) [Norwegisch].

ORTHMANN: Zit. nach WIENINGER, Über das primäre Tubenkarzinom. Zbl. Gynäk. **75**, 54 (1953).

OTTO, G.: Tumor des Ligamentum rotundum und der Mamma. Zbl. Gynäk. **83**, 923 (1961).

OUTERBRIDGE: Zit. nach FRANKL, Beiträge zur Pathologie und Klinik des Ovarialkarzinoms. Arch. Gynäk. **113**, 29 (1920).

PAPAVASILIOU, C., KOSTOUROS, D.: Kombinierte Behandlung des fortgeschrittenen Ovarialkarzinoms mit Telekobalttherapie und Cytostatica (Chlorambucil). Amer. J. Obstet. Gynec. **89**, 691—693 (1964).

PEMBERTON, F. A.: Carcinoma of ovary. Amer. J. Obstet. Gynec. **40**, 751 (1940).

PESCETTO, G., PIPINO, G.: Considerazioni e proposte in tema di terapia dei tumori ovarici maligni. Clin. ostet. ginec. **63**, 379—413 (1961).

PFANNENSTIEL, J.: Über die papillären Geschwülste des Eierstockes. Arch. Gynäk. **48**, 507 (1895).

PFLEIDERER, A., KIYAN, S.: Die Behandlung des Ovarialkarzinoms in der Univ.-Frauenklinik Tübingen seit 1957 und ihre Ergebnisse. Med. Welt **51**, 3097 (1967).

PICARD, J. D., BABINET, J., SZIGETI, B., FORTIER-BEAULIEU, M., SCHWEISGUTH, O., ARVAY, N.: La Lymphographie dans les cancers de l'ovaire Etude diagnostique et thérapeutique à propos de trois cas. Ref. Ber. Gynäk. **91**, 133 (1965). Gynéc. et Obstét. **63**, 585 (1964).

PIERROT, W.: Dauerheilung eines primären Tubenkarzinoms nach Adnexentfernung und supravaginaler Uterusexstirpation. Zbl. Gynäk. **76**, 1051 (1954).

PISANI: Zit. nach GAEBEL, EVA, Über maligne Ovarialtumoren. Strahlentherapie **114**, 225 (1961).

PLASSE, G., BONNEAU, H., SPITALIER, J., AMALRIC, R., AYME, Y.: 3 Beobachtungen gleichzeitig auftretender Genitalcarcinome. Schwierigkeiten der Interpretation. Marseille, 19. 3. 1963. Bull. Féd. Soc. Gynéc. Obstét. franç. **15**, 423—426 (1963).

PORETTI, G. G., GUTEN, H. R. VON, ZIMMERLIUND, B., ZUPPINGER, A.: Die therapeutische Anwendung von ⁹⁰Y. Sonderdruck aus Strahlentherapie **117**, 72 (1962).

POMEROY, TH. C.: Studies of the mechanism of cortisoneinduced metastases of transplantable mouse tumors. Cancer Res. **14**, 201 (1954).

PREDIGER, F.: Über Ergebnisse der Behandlung inoperabler weiblicher Genitalkarzinome mit Plenosol in einem Zeitraum von 5 Jahren. Medizinische **1956**, 1513.

PROTZ, CHRISTA: Ergebnisse in der Behandlung der Ovarialkarzinome an der Städtischen Frauenklinik Charlottenburg (1925—1949). Verl. Med. **8**, 36 (1957).

RANDALL, C. L., GERHARDT, P.: The prohability of the occurence of the more common types of Gynecologic malignancy. Amer. J. Obstet. Gynec. **68**, 1378 (1954).

REED, W. G., WATSON, E. R., CHESTERS, M. S.: A note on the distribution of radioactive colloidal gold following intraperitoneal injection. Brit. J. Radiol. **34**, 323—326 (1961).

REIBER, H.: Primäres Sarkom der Tube. Zbl. Gynäk. **25**, 1428 (1939).

REICHENMILLER, H.: Behandlungsaussichten maligner Ovarialtumoren. Arch. Gynäk. **178**, 263 (1950).

RHU, H.: Primary carcinoma of the Fallopian tube. Report of two cases. Obstet. and Gynec. **9**, 355—357 (1957).

RICHTER, K., MACH, S., LESEWSKI, G.: Die Bedeutung der Pneumopelvigraphie für die Diagnostik gynäkologischer Tumoren. Fortschr. Röntgenstr., Beih. 52—53 (1966).

RIECK: Zit. nach SCHMIDT, L., Über primäre solide Tumoren des Beckenbindegewebes. Münch. med. Wschr. **49**, 1320 (1953).

RIES, J.: Gynäkologie in Praktische Strahlentherapie. Stuttgart: Medica-Verlag 1957.

— Zum Stand des Ovarialkarzinoms. Krebsarzt (Wien) **13**, 121 (1958).

— BLASIU, A. P.: Zur internen Behandlung der Krebskranken durch den praktischen Arzt. Med. Mschr. **9**, 1 (1955).

— BREITNER, J.: Strahlenbehandlung in der Gynäkologie. Sonderbd. zur Strahlentherapie 40. München-Berlin: Urban & Schwarzenberg 1959.

RÖSENER, A.: Vergleichende Tiefendosismessungen am Wasser-Phantom mit der Sieb- und Ohne-Siebbestrahlung. Inaug.-Diss. Freiburg 1956.

RODÉ, I., HAJDU, I.: Massive Siebbestrahlung der gynäkologischen Tumoren. Radiobiol. Radiother. (Berl.) Ref. Zbl. ges. Radiol. **92**, H. 3, 32 (1967).

ROSE, R. G.: Intracavitary radioactive colloidal gold in the management of ovarian carcinoma. Report on 114 cases treated with Au¹⁹⁸. Obstet. and Gynec. **18**, 557—563 (1961).

ROSS, M. W., WARD, C. V., LINDSAY, C. C.: Primary carcinoma of the Fallopian tube. Amer. J. Obstet. Gynec. **83**, 425 (1962).

RUBIN, PH.: A critical analysis of current therapy of carcinoma of the ovary. Introduction to symposium. Amer. J. Roentgenol. **88**, 833—840 (1962).

— GRISE, J. W., TERRY, R.: Has postoperative irradiation proved itself. Amer. J. Roentgenol. **88**, 849—866 (1962).

RUMMEL, A.: Die Therapie des Ovarialkarzinoms an der Univ.-Frauenklinik Würzburg von 1939—1952. Zbl. Gynäk. **79**, 1865 (1957).

— Die Therapie des Ovarialkarzinoms an der Würzburger Frauenklinik. Krebsarzt (Wien) **9**, 286 (1954).

Runge, H.: In: Schmermund, H. J., Welches sind die Vorteile der gynäkologischen Therapie mit dem Betatron. Geburtsh. u. Frauenheilk. 18, 553 (1958).

— Zeitz, H.: Bericht über 2401 Genitalkarzinome (1935—1950). Geburtsh. u. Frauenheilk. 16, 875 (1956).

Sänger, Barth: Zit. nach Nürnberger.

Sänger, M.: Weitere Beiträge zur Lehre von den primären desmoiden Geschwülsten der Gebärmutterbänder, besonders der Ligamenta rotunda. Arch. Gynäk. 21, 279 (1889).

Sagermann, R. H., Hanks, G., Bagshaw, M. A.: Supervoltage radiation therapy. Use of the linear accelerator for treating ovarian adenocarcinoma. Calif. Med. 102, 118—122 (1965).

Schaefer, W., Witte, E.: Über eine neue Körperhöhlenröntgenröhre zur Bestrahlung von Uterustumoren. Strahlentherapie 44, 283 (1932).

Scheffey, L. C., Lang, W. R., Nugent, F. B.: Clinical and pathologic aspects of primary sarcoma of the Fallopian tube. Amer. J. Obstet. Gynec. 62, 904—916 (1946).

Schiller, W.: Concepts of new classification of ovarian tumors. Surg. Gynec. Obstet. 170, 773 (1940).

Schmauss, A. K.: Zur prophylaktischen prä- und postoperativen Hormonbehandlung des Mammakarzinoms. Münch. med. Wschr. 96, 996 (1954).

Schmermund, J.: Moderne Methoden der Strahlen- und Chemotherapie des Ovarialkarzinoms. Krebsarzt (Wien) 13, 305 (1958).

— Oberhäuser, F.: Betatron und Telekobalttherapie. Berlin-Göttingen-Heidelberg: Springer 1958.

Schmid, H. H.: Palliative Operationen beim Eierstockkrebs. Krebsarzt (Wien) 12, 342 (1957).

— Palliative Operationen beim Eierstockkrebs. Krebsarzt (Wien) 13, 279 (1958).

— Klinik der Eierstocksgeschwülste. In: Seitz und Amreich, Biologie und Pathologie des Weibes, 2. Aufl., Bd. V. Berlin-Innsbruck-München-Wien: Urban & Schwarzenberg 1953.

Schmidt, L.: Über primäre solide Tumoren des Beckenbindegewebes. Münch. med. Wschr. 49, 1320 (1953).

Schneider, E.: Ein Beitrag zum primären Tubenkarzinom. Zbl. Gynäk. 5, 184 (1957).

Schroeder, C., Hartl, H.: Die Behandlungsergebnisse bei primären Ovarialkarzinomen im Barmbeker Krankenhaus. Z. Gynäk. Geburtsh. 136, 36 (1952).

Schröder, R.: Gynäkologie. Berlin: Springer 1947.

Schubert, G., Uhlmann, G.: Ergebnisse der Supervolttherapie in der Gynäkologie. Arch. Gynäk. 202, 263 (1965).

Schwach, E.: Zur Diagnose und Therapie des Tubenkarzinoms. Wien. klin. Wschr. 38, 643 (1961).

Schwartz, E. E., Levick, St. N., Cohen, E. A., Sklaroff, D. M.: Combined irradiation and chemotherapy in ovarian carcinoma. Radiology 78, 272—273 (1962).

Schwarz, P.: Beitrag zur Pathologie u. Klinik der Ovarialtumoren. Geburtsh. u. Frauenheilk. 15, 288 (1955).

Shanks: Zit. nach Gaebel, Über maligne Ovarialtumoren. Strahlentherapie 114, 225 (1961).

Shay, H., Sun, D. C. H.: Clinical studies of Triethylenethiophosphoramide in the treatment of inoperable cancer. Cancer (Philad.) 8, 498 (1955).

Snoo, K. de: Chorionepitheliom der Tube, Hormonbildung am isolierten Trophoblasten. Zbl. Gynäk. 52, 2703 (1928).

Spallino, G., Zambarda, E.: Beitrag zum Studium der Tumoren der Lig. rotundum. Ist. di Pat. Spec. Chire. e Propedeut. Clin., Univ., Modena. Quad. Clin. ostet. ginec. 18, 690—703 (1963).

Spechter, H. J.: Pers. Mitteilung.

— Wandlungen in der Therapie des ausgedehnten Ovarialkarzinoms. Med. Welt 16, 893 (1963).

— Neue Wege in der Therapie des ausgedehnten Ovarialkarzinoms. Gynaecologia (Basel) 163, 303 (1967).

— Klinisch maligner Ovarialtumor — ja oder nein? Med. Welt 51, 3103 (1967).

Sramenko, A. J.: Zit. nach Müller-Hummel: Akush. Ginek. 2, 51 (1953). Ref. Zbl. ges. Radiol. 43, 90 (1954).

Staníček, J., Feit, J., Dvorák, K.: Histopathologische Veränderungen nach der Applikation von Radiogold ^{198}Au bei Patientinnen mit Eierstockkrebs. Čs. Gynek. 26 (40), 481—483 mit engl. Zus.fass. (1961) [Tschechisch]; — Ber. Gynäk. 77, 58 (1962).

Staemmler, H. J.: Über die hormonale Zusatzbehandlung beim Genital-Carzinom der Frau. Med. Klin. 53, 1026 (1958).

Sternberg, E.: Biologie und Pathologie des Weibes. In: Halban-Seitz, Bd. V, Teil 2. Berlin-Wien: Urban & Schwarzenberg 1926.

Stoeckel, W., Lax, H.: Stoeckels Lehrbuch der Gynäkologie. Leipzig: Hirzel 1960.

Taylor, H. J., Jr., Greeley, A. V.: Faktors influencing endresults in carcinoma of series of 138 patients treated from 1910 to 1935. Surg. Gynec. Obstet. 74, 928 (1942).

Thaisz, K.: Primäres Tubenkarzinom. Ref. Zbl. Gynäk. 64 (1), 276 (1940).

Thaler, H.: Primäres Chorionepitheliom des rechten Eileiters. Zbl. Gynäk. 28, 576 (1919).

Teschendorf, W.: Über die Bestrahlung des ganzen menschlichen Körpers bei Blutkrankheiten. Strahlentherapie 26, 720 (1927).

— Die Teleröntgentherapie. Stuttgart: Georg Thieme 1953.

Twomboly, G. H., Caceres, E., Corscaden, J. A.: Zit. nach Müller-Hummel: Amer. J. Roentgenol. 68, 779 (1952). Ref. Zbl. ges. Radiol. 40, 202 (1953).

Usadel: Zit. nach Schmidt, L., Über primäre solide Tumoren des Beckenbindegewebes. Münch. med. Wschr. 49, 1320 (1953).

Vavrik, ref. d. Eberle: Die Tuberkulose und das Adenokarzinom der Tube. Ber. ges. Gynäk. Geburtsh. 62, 314 (1957).

Vecchetti, G., Onnis, A.: Isotopentherapie in der Behandlung bösartiger Tumoren des weiblichen Genitalapparates. Attual. Ostet. Ginec. 9, 595—604 (1963).

Verhagen, A.: Vortrag 5. Wiss. Tagg d. Dtsch. Zentralausschusses f. Krebsbeh. u. Krebsforschung, Bad Pyrmont, 5.—7. 4. 1957.

VLADAR, J.: Ein Fall von primärem Tubenkarzinom mit zystischer Metastase in der Vagina. Ber. ges. Gynäk. Geburtsh. 57, 382 (1955—1956).

VOGT, A.: Diagnostik u. Strahlentherapie der Geschwulstkrankheiten. Stuttgart: Georg Thieme 1955.

VULKOV, G., TZANEV, K.: Complications of ovarian carcinoma treatment with radioaktive gold. Akush. i Ginek. 3, Nr 1, 59—63 mit engl. Zus.fass. (1964) [Bulgarisch]. Ref. Zbl. ges. Radiol. 85, 82 (1965).

WALL, H. VAN DER: Vorläufiges Ergebnis eines Blindversuches zwischen Vollfeld- und Siebbestrahlung bei konventioneller Tiefentherapie des gynäkologischen Karzinoms. Krebsarzt (Wien) 21, 101—104 (1966). Ref. Zbl. ges. Radiol. 91, 74 (1967).

WALDEYER, H. W. G.: Die epithelialen Eierstocksgeschwülste, insbesondere die Kystome. Arch. Gynäk. 1, 252 (1870).

WALSER: Zit. nach BUTTENBERG und LAU.

WALTHER, H. E.: Krebsmetastasen. Basel: Benno Schwabe & Co. 1948.

WEEKES, L. R., ANZ, U. E., WHITING, E. B.: Primary carcinoma of the Fallopian tube. Amer. J. Obstet. Gynec. 64, 62—71 (1952).

WEGHAUPT, K.: Hormone als unterstützende Therapie bei der Behandlung des weiblichen Genitalkarzinoms. Wien. klin. Wschr. 30, 364—565 (1958).

— Zur Radiogoldtherapie in der Gynäkologie. Radiobiol. Radiother. (Berl.) 3, 351—354 (1962).

— Spezielle Strahlentherapie des weiblichen Genitalkarzinoms. Wien. klin. Wschr. 78, 348—351 (1966).

WEHNER, R.: Diss. Univ.-Frauenklinik Würzburg 1953.

WEISSHAAR, J.: Pers. Mitteilung.

— Frühergebnisse bei Anwendung der Telekobalttherapie in der Behandlung von Patientinnen mit Kollumkarzinom. Geburtsh. u. Frauenheilk. 1, 3 (1965).

— RIETZ, GERTRAUD: Nebenerscheinungen bei Anwendung von Telekobalt- und Röntgenbestrahlungen bei Patientinnen mit Kollumkarzinom 1960—1962 (vergleichende Gegenüberstellung). Strahlenbehandlung und Strahlenbiologie (Sonderbände z. Strahlentherapie) 60, 147 (1965).

WIENINGER, E.: Über das primäre Tubenkarzinom. Zbl. Gynäk. 75, 54 (1953).

WILHELM, G. P., LLOYD, F. P.: Struma des Ovars. Bericht über einen Fall im Wochenbett mit starkem Ascites. Method. Hosp. Grad. Med. Ctr., Indianapolis/Ind. Obstet. and Gynec. 22, 387—389 (1963).

WIMHÖFER, H.: Pers. Mitteilung.

WINKEL, K. ZUM: Persönliche Mitteilungen.

WOLFF, J. P., ICONIKOFF, L. K.: Die Chemotherapie der malignen Ovarialtumoren. Versuche und Ergebnisse mit Thiotépa im Institut Gustave Roussy. Bull. Féd. Gynéc. Obstét. franç. 15, 315—319 (1963).

ZANETTI, E., TOSCA, L., BOSSOLA, A.: Bemerkungen zur Telekobalt- und Röntgentherapie bei der Behandlung der malignen Ovarialtumoren. Clin. Ostetr. e Ginecol. „L. Mangiagalli", Univ., Milano. 6. Congr., Soc. di Ostetr. e Ginec del Mediterr. Lat., Milano, 2.—4. 5. 1960. Minerva ginec. 13, 389—392 (1961).

ZANGEMEISTER: Zit. nach WIENINGER.

ZEITZ, H.: Pers. Mitteilung.

ZUPPINGER, A.: Pers. Mitteilungen.

B. Tumours of the male genital tract

By

B. Windeyer and S. Dische

With 6 Figures

I. The testis

1. Introduction

Malignant disease of the testis is an uncommon condition and accounts for about one per cent of all cases in cancer registries. It is however a disease which, in the untreated patient, commonly leads to a rapidly fatal outcome and the importance of this subject is out of all proportion to the low incidence, because a young population is affected, more than 80 % of patients being under the age of 50 years when first diagnosed.

A successful plan of treatment can only follow upon a knowledge of the natural history of the disease. The first steps towards this understanding came with the introduction of histo-pathology in the nineteenth century. A multitude of appellations for testicular tumours—sarcoma, endothelioma, fibro-cystic disease, chordoma, chondrosarcoma, etc. were employed. In the first decade of this century CHEVASSU (1906) and NICHOLSON (1907) carefully studied these tumours and were the first to create some order out of this confusion of tumour types.

CHEVASSU showed that there were two common tumours of the testis—the seminoma or carcinoma of the seminal epithelium, and the teratoma, which showed a great variety in structure. NICHOLSON substantially confirmed these findings. The rare chorionepithelioma has been separately classified and recognised as the most lethal variety of teratoma related to the chorionepithelioma in the female.

In 1911 JAMES EWING noted the presence of seminomatous tissue in teratomas and postulated that seminomas did not arise from seminal epithelium but from teratomatous tissue. He gave these tumours the name embryonal carcinoma. According to this view nearly all testicular tumours were teratomas and embryonal carcinomas were a subdivision. Subsequent to EWING's original description the term embryonal carcinoma has been used for a variety of different subdivisions of testicular tumours by different pathologists, and this has led to a great deal of confusion.

In 1949 DIXON and MOORE published their study of over a thousand cases of testicular tumour examined at the United States Armed Forces Institute of Pathology. In addition to seminoma and chorionepithelioma, they recognised terato-carcinoma, embryonal carcinoma and benign teratoma. This study has greatly influenced pathologists and now most contributions from the United States of America and many from elsewhere recognise these tumour types.

Recently, in Great Britain, there has been a great interest in the pathology of testicular tumours, and the British Testicular Tumour Panel has been set up by the Pathological Society of Great Britain in conjunction with the British Empire Cancer Campaign. The Panel has now published its observation upon over 1 000 cases (COLLINS and PUGH, 1964). Teratomatous tumours have been differently classified and the significance of the subdivisions of the teratomas will be discussed below.

The adoption of a system of classification does not mean that exact comparison can be made between series purporting to employ it. Many testicular tumours present problems in diagnosis and diverging opinions are not infrequently expressed on the same specimen by the most eminent pathologists.

The operation of orchidectomy has long been practised for testicular tumour, but for many years the inadequacy of this operation as the only measure of treatment has been generally recognised. ERICKSEN, in 1895, wrote "The only treatment of any avail is removal. The operation is not performed so much with the view of curing the patient of his disease, which will probably return in the lymphatic glands or in some internal organ, as of affording temporary relief from the suffering and encumbrance of the enlarged testicle. It is, therefore, an operation of expedience" (GORDON-TAYLOR and WYNDHAM, 1947).

It was further recognised that recurrence commonly occurred in the lumbar and pelvic nodes, and in the first decade of the 20th century an operation was devised for the removal of these nodes, and became known as the "radical operation". The operation had many advocates, including CHEVASSU and HINMAN, but enthusiasm for this operation waned in the 1920s, as it did not appear to produce sufficient improvement in survival to justify the morbidity and mortality of the procedure (HINMAN, 1933; GORDON-TAYLOR and WYNDHAM, 1947).

Furthermore, anatomical studies revealed the complexity of the lymphatic system in the retroperitoneal region and it became apparent that a radical dissection was a difficult procedure which perhaps could never be performed completely (HANDFIELD-JONES, 1924). Advocates of radical surgery remained in the United States and they received fresh encouragement in the 1940s when advances in surgical technique, anaesthesia and antibiotics made major surgery less hazardous (LEWIS, 1948; STAUBITZ et al., 1958). During recent years the dramatic demonstration of the retroperitoneal nodes by lymphography have reminded surgeons of the anatomical studies of 40 years ago, and further X-rays subsequent to a lymph node dissection have revealed the persistence of lymph nodes in the dissected area (WALLACE et al., 1961).

Radiation therapy was first employed by BECLÈRE in 1905, and it was soon recognised that seminomas were extremely radiosensitive. Although in the early years radium needles and tubes were inserted interstitially by some surgeons to irradiate the retroperitoneal nodes, it was soon recognised that external beam therapy was the only method likely to be successful in the irradiation of the large areas which required treatment.

Effective tumour doses were difficult to attain in the early days because of the low energy of the X-ray beam which was used and the depth of the nodes below the surface. Technical advances led to the so-called deep X-ray apparatus working up to 200 kV in the 1920s, and with it more effective treatment. In the 1940s high energy radiation, using X-ray apparatus working at over 1 million volts and later kilocurie isotope units, became available to treat these patients, and with harder quality of beam it became possible to give an adequate tumour dose to the whole retroperitoneal region in all cases.

During the past 50 years there has been a very marked improvement in survival of patients treated for testicular tumour. The overall survival rate (at 5 years) has improved from about 15 to about 60%. This may be related to a number of factors, but, although it is not possible to define the exact contribution of each, it is quite certain that the dominant one has been the advance of effective radiotherapy.

The outlook in a previously deadly disease has been revolutionized and probably with no other tumour has a comparable improvement in survival been attained.

2. Pathology

The annual incidence of testicular tumours lies between 2 and 3 per 100000 males (COLLINS and PUGH, 1964). This figure can be compared with that of approximately 100 per 100000 males for carcinoma of the bronchus in England and Wales at this time.

We recognize the following malignant tumour types:

Seminoma	Interstitial cell tumour
Teratoma	Orchioblastoma
(Chorionepithelioma)	Metastatic tumours
Malignant lymphoma	

The common tumours are seminoma (40%), teratoma (46%) and malignant lymphoma (7%).

A feature common to all tumours of the testis is a very definite increased incidence of tumours in the right as compared with the left testis—a ratio of 5:4 has been suggested and holds true for all the common tumour types (Collins and Pugh, 1964).

Bilateral tumours occur in 2–3% of all cases, and may present simultaneously or separated by an interval of time. They are usually of similar histological appearance, malignant lymphoma being more commonly found in these cases than seminoma or teratoma. Occasionally a seminoma is found in one testis and a teratoma in the other. In the cases of similar pathology the question as to whether the second tumour is a new primary or a metastasis from the original tumour can never be completely resolved. Even with differing pathologies the second tumour may nevertheless be a metastasis, for varying patterns may be seen in an individual case on histological examination of the primary and of the metastases and furthermore, seminoma and teratoma may coexist in the same tumour (Willis, 1953).

A history of maldescent is recorded in 5–6% of cases. The tumour is found to be a seminoma more commonly than we would expect from a consideration of the overall incidence of seminoma in testicular tumours. Quite commonly a tumour occurs in a testis which was late in descent, finally reaching the scrotum by natural processes or following surgery. The risk of development of a tumour at a later time in such cases compared with that in cases of persistently undescended testis may not be greatly altered by this late descent (Gordon-Taylor and Wyndham, 1947).

Of interest are those recorded cases where with unilateral undescended testis a tumour develops in the other normally descended testis, for here we may postulate a common cause to both maldescent and neoplasia (Gordon-Taylor and Till, 1938; Collins and Pugh, 1964).

In less than 1% of cases a family history of testicular tumour is obtained. In these families there may also be a history of maldescent. Such families are not only of great interest but close observation may lead to early detection of new neoplasms.

Some 77% of all testicular tumours present in the three decades between 20 and 49 years. Tumours are uncommon before the age of 15 and those which do present are usually teratoma or orchioblastoma. Over the age of 50 teratoma are uncommon, but the incidence of malignant lymphoma rises steeply; the remainder are seminoma.

a) Seminoma

The general consensus of opinion is that this tumour has origin from the seminiferous epithelium (Chevassu, 1907; Nicholson, 1907; Deiterman, 1937; Willis, 1953). Tumours quite indistinguishable from testicular seminoma may be found on the posterior abdominal wall, in the ovary (dysgerminoma), the thymus and rarely the pineal body. Although those on the posterior abdominal wall might well be metastases from an occult primary in the testis, it is believed that at least some of these and also those in the thymus have origin from primordial germ cells which have migrated to these areas and, with neoplastic change, have produced tumours identical to those arising in the testis (Collins and Pugh, 1964).

The affected testis is usually enlarged symmetrically, and although in most the surface may be smooth, in some it shows irregularity. Occasionally the testis is smaller than normal and here the tumour is associated with atrophy of the remaining testicular tissue. In the vast majority, however, there is an obvious enlargement which in some may reach massive proportions—for example 30 cm in diameter and 1500 g in weight. A hydrocoele may be present but spread through to the scrotal skin is extremely rare, even with the largest of tumours. The cut surface is pale grey and homogeneous, but some lobulation may be present due to intersections of fibrous tissue. Areas of necrosis can be seen but haemorrhage or cystic degeneration is rare.

The histological appearance is of uniform rounded cells arranged in sheets or solid columns. In the majority of tumours lymphocytic infiltration may be seen and in a number tumour giant cells are observed. A granulomatous reaction in and around the tumour is present quite often. Metastases show a similar appearance to that of the primary.

An examination of reviews of cases treated before the advent or use of effective radiotherapy suggests that orchidectomy may cure about one third of all patients who clinically appear to have disease confined to the testis (TANNER, 1922; CAIRNS, 1926; KEYES, 1926). If no additional treatment is given, the remainder will show metastases usually within two years, the first site being in most cases within the lymphatic drainage, and all or nearly all will be dead in five years. This natural history of disease has been greatly modified by radiotherapy. Some 85–90 % of patients with disease apparently confined to the testis at the time of orchidectomy will now survive five years, and nearly all these will remain free of recurrence indefinitely. Even in the presence of metastases in the retroperitoneal nodes the five year survival is now of the order of 50 %, and some of those with distant metastases may live for a number of years with control of disease when appropriate radiotherapy is given. Further consideration is given to survival figures in the discussion of results of treatment.

b) Teratoma

The histogenesis of this tumour has received much attention. The two most important theories suggest an origin either from embryonic cells or one from abnormal tissue primordia formed during early embryonic life. The second appears more favoured at this time (WILLIS, 1953; COLLINS and PUGH, 1964).

There is a remarkable range of appearance in the teratoma, both to the naked eye and on histological examination. This is observed not only from case to case but also between a tumour and its metastases and in different parts of an individual deposit of tumour. The testicular swelling is usually irregular in shape and the cut surface reveals an admixture of solid yellow or white tissue with areas of haemorrhage or cystic degeneration. Hair, sebaceous material, cartilage and bone may all be identified in the tumour. Under the microscope all types of tissue may be identified and all grades of malignancy observed. The most malignant tumour or the most malignant portion of a tumour consists of closely packed masses of pleomorphic cells with frequent and bizarre mitoses. In the most differentiated tumours all varieties of normal tissue—bone cartilage, mucous glands etc.—may be seen and there be no area showing true malignant characteristics. In the majority of tumours frankly malignant tissue derived from any or all of the three germ layers will be seen.

It is of importance to consider whether the variety of appearance has significance in prognosis and management. One small group can immediately be distinguished and by reason of the presence of syncytio- and cytotrophoblast arranged in villi, associated with a distinctly poor prognosis. These are the chorionepithelioma. Only on occasion will a patient with this deadly tumour survive over two years—this did occur in two of nine cases in the series reported by the British Testicular Tumour Panel (COLLINS and PUGH, 1964) and in one of six in that from the American Armed Forces Institute of Pathology (DIXON and MOORE, 1953). It has been stressed that strict histological criteria must be applied and that the mere presence of trophoblastic tissue does not justify inclusion. The prognosis in a teratoma showing some trophoblastic tissue is similar to that of teratoma in general, and is rather better than that in true chorionepithelioma

At the other extreme there has been argument as to whether a teratoma of the testis is ever benign. There is no doubt that the prognosis in the differentiated tumour which shows no definitely malignant tissue, and which is about as rare as true chorionepithelioma, is much better than with the rest of the teratoma. However, metastases do develop often enough (2 of 13 cases in the British Panel) to justify the management of all as malignant tumours. So-called "differentiated" or "mature" tumours account for between 1 and 20% of all teratoma according to different published series. This wide range must

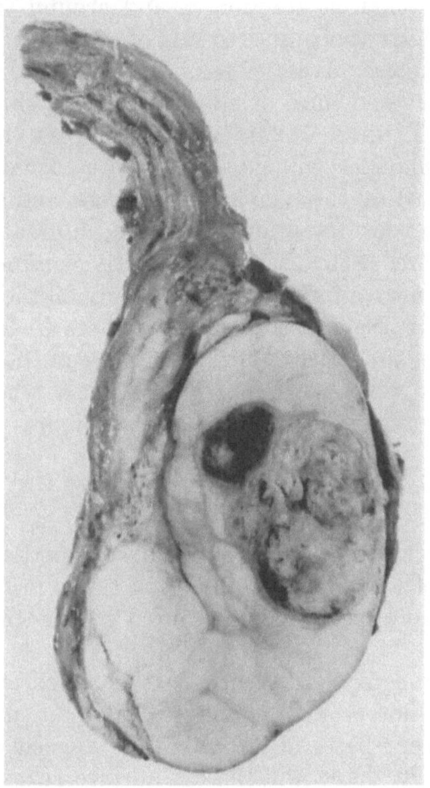

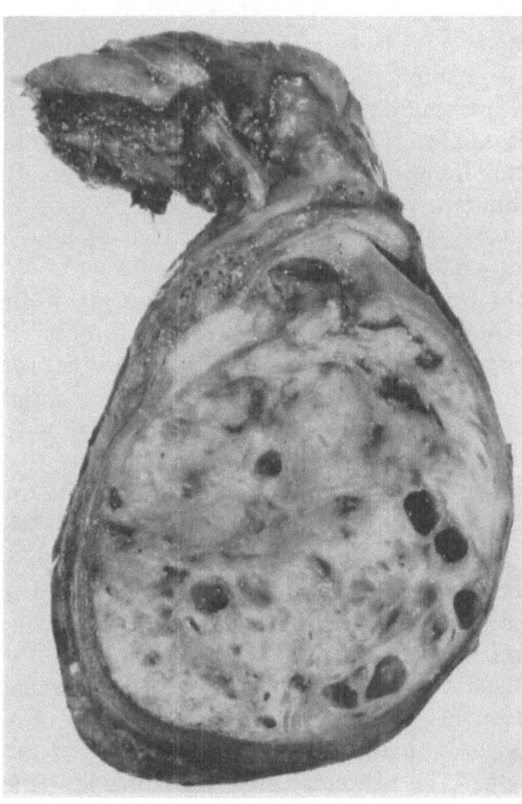

Fig. 1   Fig. 2

Fig. 1. Combined seminoma and teratoma of the testis. The cut surface of the bulk of the tumour shows the typical appearance of seminoma, being pale and homogeneous with some lobulation. In one part of the tumour there is an irregular appearance with areas of haemorrhage and degeneration typical of teratoma

Fig. 2. Teratoma of the testis. The cut surface of the tumour shows a variegated appearance with many areas of cystic degeneration

be accounted to differing histological criteria. It is relevant to this that survival rates for differentiated tumours are lowest for those series where the incidence is highest and conversely highest where very strict criteria are applied and the incidence low. We believe in the strict criteria which limit the number of cases in this category to about 1% of all tumours.

Dixon and Moore (1953) divided the remaining tumours on the basis of differentiation into embryonal carcinoma and teratocarcinoma. They reported that where seminoma and teratoma coexisted the prognosis was that of the teratoma and the presence of seminoma did not modify the natural history. They therefore placed such tumours in their sub-division of teratoma, ignoring the seminomatous element in them. They reported a five year mortality rate of 65% for embryonal carcinoma and of 52.2% for teratocarcinoma.

These figures would give a small difference in prognosis for the two subdivisions, but Buskirk *et al.*, reporting in 1964 upon 698 cases, subdivided using the same system, give survival figures of 44 and 44.7% for these same subdivisions. The identical survival in both groups casts some doubt on the value of the subdivision in clinical practice.

The British Panel subdivide the teratoma in a different way. In addition to the small groups of chorionepithelioma and differentiated teratoma, they separate off those tumours showing seminomatous tissue in addition to teratoma. In the remaining cases they recognise an anaplastic tumour and an intermediate type, which is further subdivided on the basis of differentiation into sub-types A and B. Apart from the chorionepithelioma and the differentiated tumours there is, at the time of their latest review,

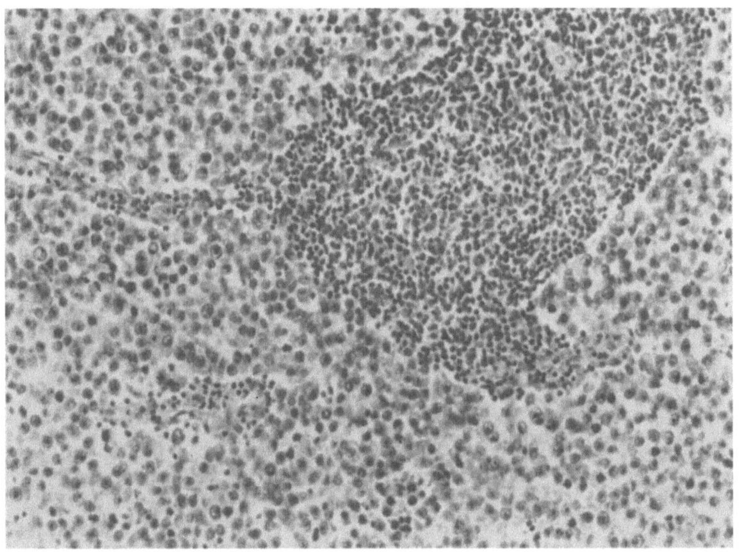

Fig. 3. Histological appearance in seminoma. The tumour is composed of uniform rounded cells. In addition lymphocytic infiltration is seen

no significant difference in survival between the groups of patients with the anaplastic tumour, the intermediate type A and with intermediate type B. Those tumours where seminomatous tissue was seen in addition to teratoma seemed associated with a slightly better survival, but this was nevertheless not statistically significant. The advocates of these subdivisions suggest no other differences in natural history apart from degree of malignancy, which ought to be reflected in the survival rates which have been considered above. We can conclude that, considering the evidence presently available and excluding the small number of chorionepithelioma and differentiated tumours, the subdivisions of teratoma as described by the American Armed Forces Institute and the British Testicular Tumour Panel are of little clinical importance. At this time these subdivisions should not be considered in planning treatment. The teratoma, with the exception of the two small subdivisions noted above, should be considered as a unity.

Although we have rejected rigid subdivisions we do associate a poor outlook with tumours which clinically show a short history, rapid growth rate and a relatively anaplastic histological appearance, while the opposite characteristics—long history, slow growth rate and relatively well differentiated appearances are often associated with a favourable outcome.

The majority of teratoma is certainly less radiosensitive than the seminoma. As we might expect there is a distinct impression that it is inversely related to the degree of differentiation of the tumour. Where masses of metastatic tumour are large it is unusual

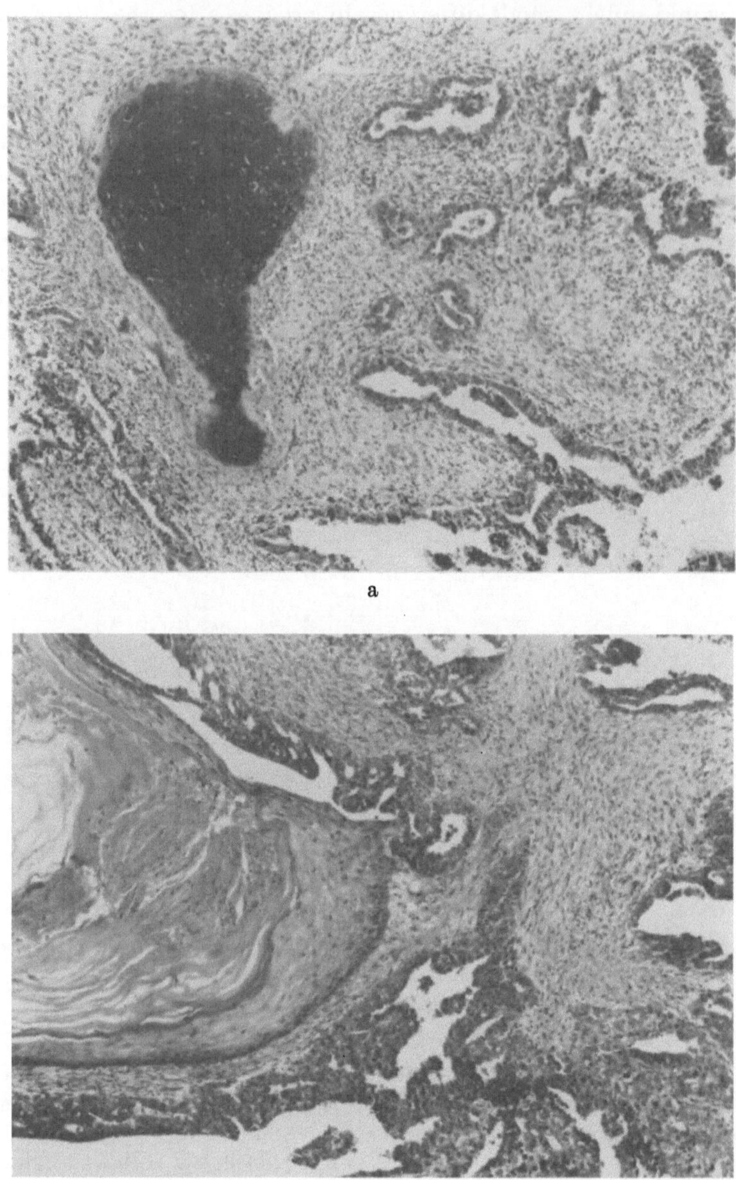

Fig. 4a and b. Histological appearance in teratoma. The photomicrograph (a) shows a well formed stroma and a nodule of cartilage darkly stained, but also areas of poorly differentiated adenocarcinoma. The microphotograph (b) shows a well differentiated keratinised squamous epithelium and regular connective tissue stroma invaded by poorly differentiated adenocarcinoma

to obtain complete regression by radiotherapy. In most, however, there is some reduction in bulk of tumour and palliation of symptoms is gained. Examination of published series of patients treated by orchidectomy alone where tumour was apparently confined to the testis suggests that 75% of such patients will later develop metastases—the first site being most often in the lymphatic drainage (TANNER, 1922; CAIRNS, 1926; KEYES, 1926). In recent years, with the addition of radiotherapy to their management, the survival rate (at 5 years) is in excess of 50%. We may deduce that in a considerable number of cases it is possible for radiotherapy to sterilize lymph nodes containing metastatic teratoma. Comparing these results with those in more advanced cases it seems that a small metastasis

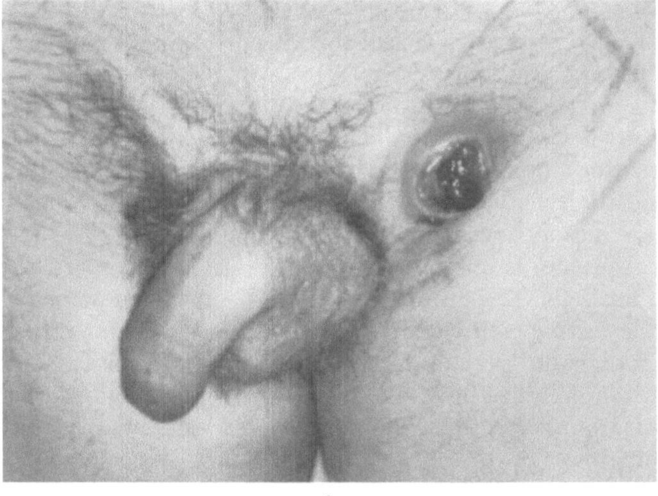

a

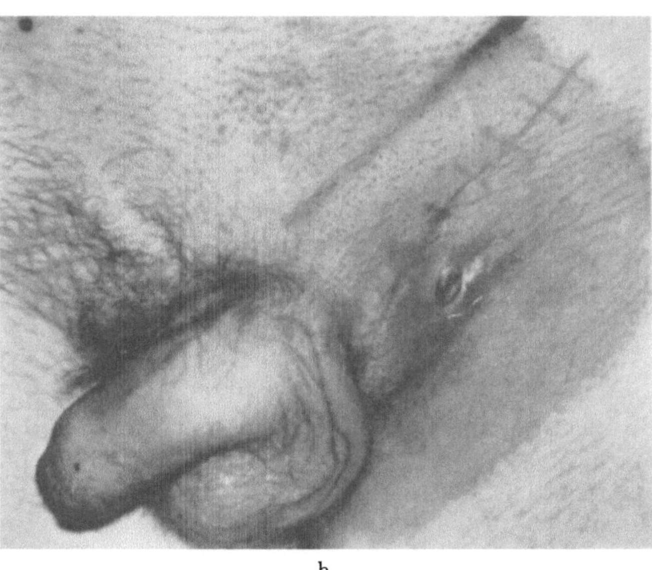

b

Fig. 5a and b. Inguinal node metastasis in teratoma. Metastasis of teratoma of the testis in an inguinal node at the beginning (a) and at the end (b) of radiotherapy. An inguinal node had been removed at orchidectomy, but recurrence occurred within three weeks. There were many invaded retroperitoneal nodes. Patient died at six months with multiple pulmonary metastases

will respond more favourably than a large one. This is probably related to low tissue oxygen tension in areas of a large tumour, showing, as is common in teratoma, necrosis and haemorrhage.

As radiation response seems related to the degree of differentiation, it may be argued that retroperitoneal node dissection should be of value in the occasional case of a well differentiated tumour with known but operable retroperitoneal nodes. The problem here is the selection of such cases. Probably such selection should be made when there is persistance of tumour in the retroperitoneal nodes after radiotherapy of a well differentiated tumour. Operability will be finally assessed only at laparotomy. The majority of tumours in children are considered to be embryonal carcinoma or teratoma. The clinical course seems to be rather similar to that seen in adults and the prognosis seems better than might be expected and no worse than that in adults (ZUPPINGER, 1946; TEFFT et al., 1967).

c) Malignant lymphoma

These tumours have received considerable attention in recent years and it has been shown that they are not as rare as they were formerly thought to be (Ennuyer *et al.*, 1960; Eckert and Smith, 1963; Collins and Pugh, 1964). Some 80% of these tumours are found in men over the age of 50. They are commonly bilateral (22%) and may be associated with past or simultaneous manifestation of a malignant lymphoma elsewhere. A particular association between deposits of malignant lymphoma in the testis and deposits in the nose, nasopharynx and skin is recognised.

The histological picture is one of poorly differentiated cells of the lymphocyte series or of larger reticulum cells. These tumours are best considered as one group of malignant lymphoma and they are not divided into lymphosarcoma and reticulum cell sarcoma. Although these malignant lymphoma are very radiosensitive, generalised disease is commonly seen after orchidectomy and 69% are reported dead within two years of orchidectomy (Collins and Pugh, 1964). A 'plasma cell tumour' may occur as part of generalised myelomatosis.

d) Interstitial cell carcinoma

Interstitial cell tumour arises from the Leydig cells and they usually present because of their endocrine function rather than because of the presence of a tumour in the testis. Gynaecomastia is the common initial symptom. These tumours are rare—about 1% of all testicular tumours, and only one in ten of interstitial cell tumours is considered to be malignant. It is probably wise to treat a malignant interstitial cell tumour as for teratoma.

e) Sertoli cell tumour

The malignant tumours arise from the supporting cells of the seminiferous tubules. The characteristic histological finding is of radially arranged cells which resemble Sertoli cells. These tumours are rare, seem to carry a good prognosis and should be treated as for seminoma.

f) Orchioblastoma

This is a rapidly growing tumour of infants and young children. Histologically it is a tubular or papillary adenocarcinoma, often with mucin production. It is not believed to be of teratomatous origin but appears to have a natural history which is rather similar and they should be treated on the same lines.

g) Metastatic tumours

These may be the cause of a newly presented testicular swelling, but more commonly the primary tumour and other metastases are already known. The common primaries are prostate, kidney, lung and stomach. Orchidectomy alone in most cases is a simple and efficient method of treatment provided that the tumour is not adherent to surrounding structures.

3. Spread of testicular tumours

Testicular tumours in their growth destroy the remaining seminiferous tubules by infiltration or compression. There may be an associated hydrocoele, but penetration of the parietal layers of the tunica vaginalis is uncommon and involvement of the skin of the scrotum rare. This latter complication usually follows a surgical exploration of the testis which in our opinion should never be performed in the management of a testicular tumour (Gordon-Taylor and Wyndham, 1947). Infiltration of the rete testis and epididymis is common. Invasion of the lymphatics in the testis is seen in the majority, and extension along the lymphatics accompanying the spermatic cord is observed in a number of these. It has been reported that tumour can be found at the cut ends of the cord in 7% of orchidectomy specimens of seminoma, and 20% of similar specimens of teratoma.

The lymph drainage of the testis was described by JAMIESON and DOBSON (1910) and HANDFIELD-JONES (1924). These authors showed that the principal drainage of the lymphatics along the spermatic cord is to the para-aortic nodes, particularly in the inter-renal area. There is also some communication with the internal iliac nodes on the affected side. Of further importance is the great intercommunication between lymph nodes lying in front, between and behind the great vessels—the inferior vena cava and the aorta and their principal branches, the common iliac arteries and veins.

From the para-aortic area, spread occurs to the mediastinum and from there to the supraclavicular region. This vast lymphatic plexus from the testis to the left supra-clavicular fossa is considered to be the lymphatic drainage area of the testis. The size of this lymphatic drainage area is quite unparalleled in the field of malignant disease. If metastases within this area can be eradicated then cure is possible and distant metastases may not present. Confirmation of this may be found in the considerable number of patients with many invaded lymph glands through the whole area who have been given treatment with apparent cure.

When unilateral cervical node involvement is observed it is invariably on the left—fourteen patients with unilateral cervical nodes were found to have them on the left side in the series reported by WHITTLE (1957) in the series from St. Bartholomew's Hospital. Two more patients were found to have invaded nodes on the right, but these were associated with similar nodes on the left.

Probably of relevance is the common observation in lymphography that with the formation of the thoracic duct in the upper lumbar region area no more lymphatic glands may be filled with contrast material in the upper abdomen or chest, but commonly left supraclavicular nodes are demonstrated (WALLACE et al., 1961).

Invasion of inguinal nodes is uncommon. It may follow upon invasion of the skin of the scrotum or inguinal area which is sometimes a result of surgery. Retrograde spread from the para-aortic and common iliac nodes through the external iliac nodes certainly accounts for the presence of inguinal node involvement in other cases.

The most common sites for metastases outside the lymphatic drainage area are the lung and liver, where metastases are often present in the later stages of disease. The skeletal system is the third most common site involved by haematogeneous spread.

It is uncommon except in chorionepithelioma to see haematogeneous spread of metastases without past or present evidence of invasion of the lymphatic drainage, and we have a distinct impression that the former nearly always follows upon the latter, and that early direct haematogeneous spread is unusual. These findings encourage early diagnosis and vigorous treatment.

4. Clinical aspects

In the vast majority of patients the initial symptom is due to the primary tumour. Most commonly the patient notices a swelling of the testis, but other complaints include pain, tenderness and heaviness of the testis. Persistent back ache of recent onset should give rise to a strong suspicion that the retroperitoneal nodes are involved.

Although ureteric obstruction, leading to impairment of renal function, often occurs where retroperitoneal nodes are markedly enlarged, urinary tract symptoms are un-common. Very rarely a patient may be found to be in renal failure due to bilateral ureteric obstruction.

Pulmonary and hepatic metastases will more often be suspected because of general deterioration than because of local symptoms. The skeletal system is the third most common site of distant metastases and any persistent bone pain requires X-ray examina-tion (AUERBACH et al., 1946).

Enlargement of the breast, gynaecomastia, may be noted by the patient, who may complain of local tenderness, but more commonly it is first found by the examining physician. Gynaecomastia associated with testicular tumour is often considered of sinister significance, but this has not been our experience. In 15 of 228 patients at the Middlesex Hospital in the years 1929–1956, gynaecomastia was noted at some time in the course of their disease. In nine it was present at the time of initial diagnosis of testicular tumour, but in six it first appeared at a later time. In some it was associated with presence of the primary tumour or metastases, while in others there was no evidence of residual or recurrent neoplasm. Five of the nine patients where the condition was noted at the onset and four of the six patients where it was seen later in their course are alive, free of disease, at the last review. It would seem that, although there appears to be an association of gynaecomastia with presence of tumour in some cases, in a number of others this is not so and further, if disease is present, it is not beyond the stage at which cure is possible.

A careful clinical examination of the patient with a testicular tumour is of great importance. Prior to surgery, all aspects of the primary tumour must be detailed. Spread up the spermatic cord may be shown by continuous induration or irregular nodularity. The unusual spread to the scrotal skin is of much importance, as is also inguinal node involvement.

Palpation of the retroperitoneal nodes is particularly difficult, as most of the patients are young men with well developed muscles in the anterior abdominal wall.

The left lower neck is an important area for glandular metastases and examination should be made with extra special care. An enlarged node may be overlooked because it lies behind the head of the clavicle in a position difficult to palpate.

5. Methods of investigation

A chest X-ray should be performed to determine pulmonary metastases and any inter-current infection. A full blood count must also be performed before treatment is undertaken.

A further study of the retroperitoneal nodes should be performed in all cases. An intravenous pyelogram is the test most commonly employed. Enlarged nodes may be revealed by a lateral displacement of the ureters and by the hydronephrosis and loss of renal function which may follow ureteric obstruction. The study is also of value in treatment planning, for it reveals the exact position of the kidneys which must be known in order that the exposure to radiation be kept down to a minimum.

A simple method of investigating the retroperitoneal region is palpation of the abdomen under general or spinal anaesthesia. Quite often, with good relaxation of the abdominal musculature, enlarged lymph nodes, impalpable under ordinary conditions or only just suspected, may be easily defined.

An inferior venacavagram may demonstrate enlarged nodes in the right para-aortic region, but is likely not to show those on the left unless the enlargement is a considerable one. Lymphangiography has been employed in these patients in recent years (Chiappa et al., 1966; Wallace, 1969). The normal lymphatics and lymph nodes in the retroperitoneal area are clearly shown and evidence of metastatic involvement revealed by replacement or distortion of the pattern of the nodes. Because of the persistence of dye in the nodes check films can be taken and a clear picture of the relationship between lymph nodes and fields of treatment seen (Wallace et al., 1961).

Our feeling at this time is that in the routine case an intravenous pyelogram and an examination under anaesthesia are the methods of choice. The inferior venacavagram does not demonstrate very well nodes in the left para-aortic area, and lymphangiography, a considerable procedure and a cause of much discomfort to the patient, must be shown to have a higher degree of accuracy than we presently credit it before it can be regarded as justified for routine use. In unusual cases, such as where recurrence is suspected in a previously irradiated area, the study is certainly a valuable one.

Some patients with testicular tumours excrete in their urine gonadotrophin in an amount greatly in excess of normal. The percentage of patients presenting this abnormality varies widely from series to series, but in our experience it is limited to a small minority (DEAN, 1935; PATTON *et al.*, 1960; COLLINS and PUGH, 1964). A variety of biological methods has been used in the past and now an immunological technique is employed for detection of abnormally high levels of the hormone in blood or urine. Some of the inconsistencies in published data must be due to the many different methods of assay which have been used. In chorionepithelioma the amount of hormone excreted often reaches high levels and the tumour is considered to be the source. In the case of other tumours, there is the possibility that the hormone is produced by the endocrine system as a response to the presence of the tumour.

In practice a "negative" result has little significance, but where excess hormone is secreted serial observations during and after treatment give another index of response, and also a sign of recurrence. The test should routinely be performed before and, if positive, soon after orchidectomy and at intervals thereafter.

6. Surgery

Orchidectomy must be the standard treatment for the primary tumour. In the past some testicular neoplasms have been irradiated prior to surgery to reduce the bulk of tumour and to determine radiosensitivity (DEAN, 1935). There is no evidence to suggest that these advantages outweigh those of an early, usually easy removal of the primary and the making of an exact histological diagnosis at the earliest possible time, uncomplicated by any radiation change. An inguinal approach should always be used in order to prevent the opening of the scrotum to spread of tumour, also to enable the cord to be tied off at the highest point and, in addition, to obtain a clean, early healing scar which can soon be included in a field of radiation. Most tumours can readily be removed in this way but in some an extension of the incision into the upper scrotum may be required when the very largest tumour masses are to be removed.

The so-called 'radical operation' is directed to the dissection of the lymph nodes of the common iliac and para-aortic groups. The operation may be unilateral or bilateral; the approach may be transperitoneal or retroperitoneal. There is no doubt that the established anatomical studies (JAMIESON and DOBSON, 1910; HANDFIELD-JONES, 1924) and the recent lymphangiographic investigations of these areas have proved the complexity of the lymphatic drainage. The large intercommunicating plexus of lymphatic nodes and channels in this area extends between and behind major vessels into most inaccessible places. A lymph node dissection can never approach the 'en bloc' procedure as practised in the neck and must therefore be inferior as an operation for the invasion of a lymphatic drainage system by a malignant tumour. Lymphangiograms performed prior to surgery and repeat X-rays after radical operation have revealed in some cases residual nodes in the field of surgery (WALLACE *et al.*, 1961).

Despite these defects the operation may still be of value for there are patients shown to have metastases in these nodes at surgery who, without further treatment, have apparently been cured (HINMAN, 1933). These isolated cases can, of course, give little support for routine application, and only statistically sound survival data can be convincing. It is a considerable complication in assessment of series reported in the past twenty years that in all where the operation has been performed and tumour found, radiotherapy has been given in addition. LEWIS operated on 169 of a series of 250 cases (LEWIS, 1948; LEWIS, 1953). Nearly all cases received radiotherapy in addition and there was no controlled trial. Recently, BUSKIRK *et al.* (1964) have brought this series up to date, reporting 698 cases. The plan of management included radiotherapy as a postoperative measure where node dissection revealed invasion with tumour. An examination of LEWIS's survival data for seminoma shows that the figures are similar for patients treated by radiotherapy alone and those by radiotherapy and surgery. As the radiotherapy alone group included a number of patients with such extensive node invasion as to be deemed inoperable, the survival in this group ought to have been worse than in those patients treated by radical surgery and radiotherapy. It is possible that surgical intervention in these patients had an unfavourable influence upon survival. We consider that radical surgery should not be performed in the treatment of seminoma.

Concerning the place of radical surgery in teratoma it is not possible to support any argument with sound statistically significant data. Our feeling is that the radical operation should not form part of the routine management. Where in a teratoma of low grade malignancy deposits in retro-peritoneal nodes persist after adequate radiotherapy the operation may be considered.

7. Radiotherapy

Radiotherapy to the lymphatic drainage of the testis is indicated after simple orchidectomy when the tumour is a seminoma, teratoma (including chorionepithelioma), sertoli cell tumour, malignant interstitial cell tumour, orchioblastoma or lymphoma.

The area to be irradiated should include the surgical scar, the spermatic cord from its cut end upwards, inguinal and external iliac nodes on the affected side, both common iliac nodes and the retroperitoneal nodes up to the level of the body of the 10th dorsal vertebra (xiphoid).

When there is known invasion of the retroperitoneal nodes then the area of treatment must be extended to include the mediastinal nodes and those in the left supraclavicular fossa. These areas are usually irradiated after conclusion of treatment to the retroperitoneal region.

When there is involvement of lymph nodes in the mediastinum or left supraclavicular fossa but no metastases apparent in the areas nearer the testis, it is best to reverse the normal order of treatment. This enables the radiotherapist to exert control on tumour in the region most severely affected and to determine radiosensitivity. Further, when such a large volume is irradiated bone marrow depression commonly slows the rate of treatment and often limits final dosage. It is therefore important first of all to make certain of attaining a satisfactory tumour dose where secondary deposits are known to be present.

The tumour dose which should be set for cases of seminoma, lymphoma and sertoli cell tumour should be 3500 rads using supervoltage given over a period of four weeks. When treating teratoma and the rare interstitial cell carcinoma the dose should be increased to 4500 rads in 5–6 weeks. With orchioblastoma the dose will be reduced, as they occur in infants or young children, and will be of the order of 2000—2500 rads.

Treatment planning

The overall plan which we employ is to use supervoltage for the abdominal and mediastinal treatment and deep X-rays (generated at 250 kV) for inguinal and sometimes the supraclavicular regions. The inguinal field will include the remainder of the extra-abdominal spermatic cord left after surgery and which may in some cases be found in the upper scrotum. Quite often, when the patient arrives in the radiotherapy department, a mass is palpable at the cut end of the cord. This is often extremely hard and well defined and the question of a rapid recurrence of tumour is raised. In nearly all cases it is merely a haematoma, but in order to cover the possibility of tumour it should be included with adequate margin in the treatment area.

The inguinal nodes and scar of the inguinal orchidectomy are included and as the field is in continuity with the lower end of the abdominal field, some of the external iliac nodes may just be within this field. The chief problem in treating this area is the shielding of the remaining testis. The testis must be drawn away from the treatment area, covered by lead rubber and securely kept in its shielded position during treatment. The advantage of using 250 kV X-rays for this region as opposed to supervoltage is the greater ease with which shielding can be arranged with lead. Also, without skin sparing, the scar is

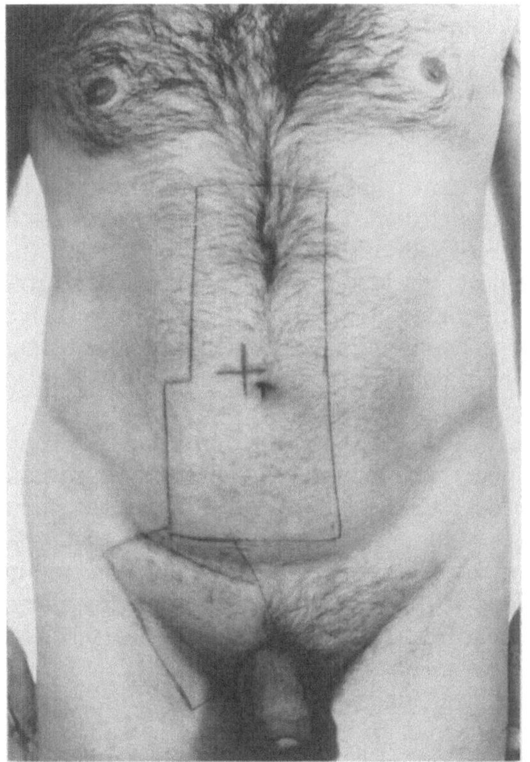

a

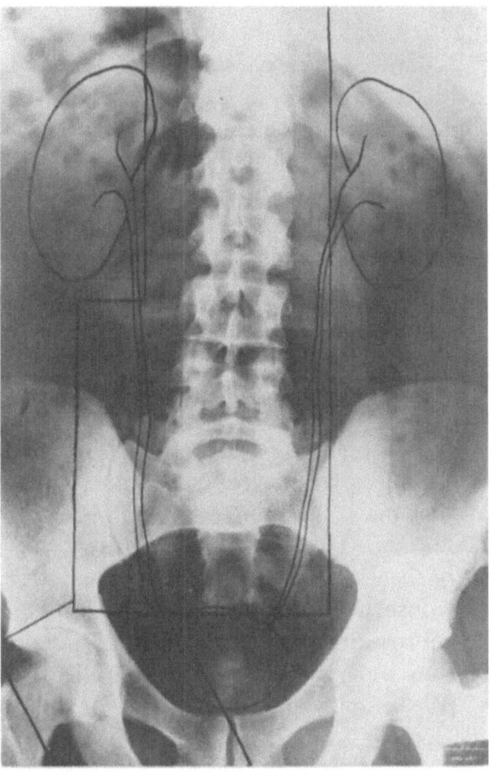

b

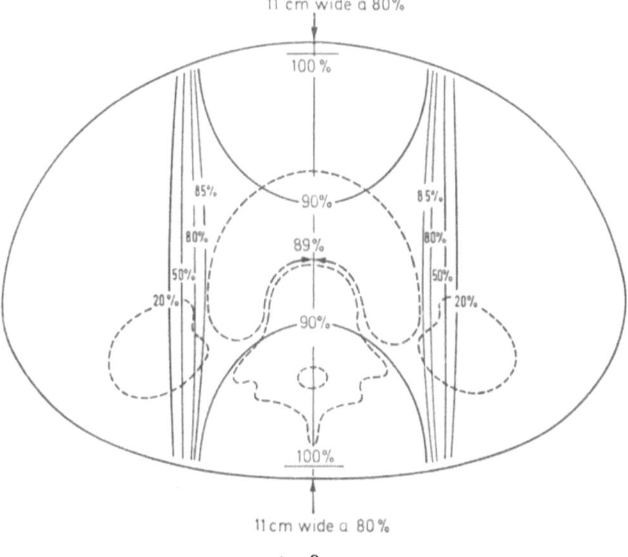

c

Fig. 6a–c. Radiotherapy after orchidectomy for testicular tumour. a Arrangement of fields. The inguinal field is treated with deep X-rays generated at 250 kV. The large anterior field to the retroperitoneal nodes is apposed by a similar posterior field and a cobalt unit operating at 80 cm S.S.D. is employed. A secondary diaphragm with a lead block is used to reduce the width of the upper half of the field. b The areas irradiated superimposed upon an X-ray picture. The position of kidneys, ureters and bladder also shown. c The plan of treatment for the retroperitoneal nodes. The area to be irradiated is shown and the minimum tumour dose is 85% of the maximum dose which occurs in the subcutaneous tissues. The spine and kidneys are also shown. The spinal cord dose is similar to that received by the tumour but the bulk of both kidneys receive less than 20% of the maximum

fully irradiated. Care must be taken that there is no area of under or over dosage at the junction of the fields with the abdominal fields of treatment. A disadvantage is the considerable skin reaction which commonly occurs in the groin. We normally give a total incident skin dose of 3600 rads over a period of four weeks, although with teratoma a slightly greater dose may be given.

The abdominal field of treatment will normally include the retroperitoneal or para-aortic nodes from the level of the body of the tenth dorsal vertebra downwards, the common iliac nodes on both sides and the external iliac nodes on the affected side. In covering this region the spermatic cord and vessels are also irradiated.

The width of the para-aortic region is usually considered to be 8–10 cm. The intravenous pyelogram is of value, as the edges of the field can be brought to the renal pelves on both sides for these and the ureters indicate the lateral edge of the lymphatic plexus. The abdominal field is continuous with the inguinal field and appropriate shielding of the latter allows accurate juncture of the fields.

The problems associated with the treatment of this area are the high radiosensitivity of the kidneys, systemic reaction with leucopenia and bowel reaction. It is important in treatment planning to make sure that the dose to the bulk of both kidneys is below 2000 rads. Occasionally, because of the presence of massive adenopathy, this rule has to be broken, but one kidney must certainly be preserved from radiation damage and this dose not exceeded. Very little can be done to prevent bone marrow depression or bowel reaction except for general supportive measures. These problems will be considered further when we discuss the complications of treatment.

We employ opposing anterior and posterior fields with a cobalt unit or a linear accelerator. It is often necessary, when using a cobalt unit, to increase the source skin distance to obtain a field of required length, commonly 26–30 cm. With lead blocks or a secondary diaphragm the field can be shaped to fit the plan (s. Fig. 6).

When a patient is of an anterior posterior thickness of more than 22 cm and a high tumour dose is required using a cobalt unit or X-ray unit working at 3 MeV or below, it is found that the simple paired anterior and posterior field arrangement leads to irradiation of bowel and spinal cord to doses in excess of the tumour dose and of an order that the chance of morbidity is a real one. Arrangements of 3 and 4 fields can be employed but it is inevitable that with multiple fields the dose to the kidneys is raised. We only employ multiple fields in the treatment of obese patients and where limited volumes are being raised to high tumour doses because of radioresistance or because of recurrence. Where the dose at the spinal cord reaches above 3000 rads we shield the cord, when treating with the posterior field, with a lead block 1.5 cm wide down to the body of the second lumbar vertebra.

The mediastinum can be treated by opposed anterior and posterior fields.

When the para-aortic nodes and mediastinal nodes are to be irradiated during the same course of treatment precautions must be taken to prevent areas of over or under dosage. The borders of adjacent fields are separated in order to allow for divergence of the beam at depth in the tissues and the positions of juncture are placed at different levels anteriorly and posteriorly.

It is usually advisable to include the left supraclavicular region as it is not uncommon for metastases to appear in lymph nodes in this area after successful treatment of the mediastinum. If it does become necessary to treat the supraclavicular area after mediastinal treatment, there is undesirable overlap upon the already irradiated zone in order to obtain a margin round the involved nodes. When anterior and posterior fields are used to treat the mediastinum, it is easy to extend the area to include the left supraclavicular fossa. As the nodes are just below the skin surface the extension can be confined to the anterior field.

When a high tumour dose is required in a patient of unusual thickness, multiple fields, three or four, are employed, and care taken to spare the spinal cord. In these circumstances a left supraclavicular treatment field must then be added with care to avoid overlap or a gap in continuity of the treatment volume. Tumour doses similar to those already discussed for the treatment of the retro-peritoneal nodes are desirable. In all those areas where palpation or special investigation reveals large deposits of tumour extending outside the areas normally treated, modification of plans must be made and larger areas irradiated.

In the treatment of mediastinal and abdominal nodes the greater penetration of supervoltage apparatus as compared with orthovoltage is of tremendous advantage, as also is the reduced systemic disturbance. Orthovoltage can be employed, but in both areas multiple fields, usually four, must be employed. A tumour dose of 3000 rads is achieved in three to four weeks for seminoma, and 4000 rads in five to six weeks for teratoma.

This plan of management is similar to that employed in many radiotherapy centres at this time, but there are a number of variations, some of which are worthy of mention.

In the treatment of the retroperitoneal nodes some radiotherapists offset the treatment fields in the para-aortic area towards the side of the tumour (SMITHERS and WALLACE, 1962). In our experience nodes may be invaded in all parts of the para-aortic region no matter the side of the affected testis, and so our fields in this area are placed centrally. Wide field irradiation of the abdomen as part of the routine post-orchidectomy management must be condemned as serving no advantage and carrying with it a greatly increased chance of morbidity.

In some centres in the treatment of all cases, the entire lymphatic drainage area from spermatic cord to left supracalvicular fossa is irradiated, even if there is no evidence of spread beyond the testis. This is a reasonable plan, knowing how crude is our assessment of lymph node involvement in the retroperitoneal and mediastinal regions. We find, however, that severe leukopenia invariably complicates treatment when so large an area is irradiated and that often the full dosage cannot be achieved. For this reason, when there is no evidence of spread of tumour beyond the testis, we limit radiotherapy to the retroperitoneal and inguinal regions.

The high radiosensitivity of seminoma has influenced some workers to restrict the tumour dose to between 1500 and 2000 rads when treating the para-aortic nodes in the management of this type of tumour (FRIEDMAN, 1950; FRIEDMAN and PURKAYASHTHA, 1960; PATTON et al., 1960). It is our experience when treating easily observed deposits of seminoma that a number of tumours are more resistant to radiation and higher doses must be given in order to obtain complete regression of tumour. In the routine post-orchidectomy treatment radiosensitivity cannot be assessed and the only safe course is to give a tumour dose of 3500 rads in every case. The increase in morbidity due to an elevation of the tumour dose in the para-aortic area to 3500 rads is so small that it does not influence this decision.

8. Complications of radiotherapy

a) Immediate complications

The common immediate complications of radiotherapy to the para-aortic nodes are general radiation reaction, marrow depression and diarrhoea.

Some general malaise, tiredness, anorexia and nausea is inevitable in nearly all patients. In some these symptoms are severe and interruption of treatment or a reduction of the dose rate is necessary. The maintenance of a high fluid intake, administration of drugs to prevent nausea and reassurance will bring nearly all patients through the course without any modification of the plan being necessary apart from, perhaps, some prolongation of the overall duration of treatment.

Depression of the total white cell count is seen in the majority even with the use of supervoltage, where with less scattered radiation, the effect upon the bone marrow

25*

outside the treatment area is reduced. Leucopenia causes us to slow down the rate of treatment in a considerable number of patients. Treatment is given with caution when the total white cell count falls below $4000/mm^3$, and is temporarily suspended at levels below $2000/mm^3$. In some the leucopenia occurs early in treatment and a persistent low count makes it impossible safely to continue the planned course of treatment, a situation which occurs not infrequently in those patients where the mediastinum as well as the para-aortic nodes must be irradiated. Other methods of combating leucopenia in addition to prolongation of the overall period of treatment are the administration of cortico-steroids, which appear to stimulate bone marrow function, or restriction of the volume of tissue treated to the essential minimum.

It is our practice to use cortico-steroids when there is persistent leucopenia, and a dose of 15–20 mg of Prednisone is given daily. If, despite the addition of Prednisone, leucopenia persists, then it becomes necessary to restrict the area of treatment.

Diarrhoea troubles a minority of patients receiving radiotherapy to the para-aortic nodes. It is usually easily controlled with codeine phosphate or kaolin with tinct.opii. Avoidance of foods containing a high residue such as green vegetables, and foods likely to stimulate bowel action, such as fresh fruit, are useful additional measures.

b) Late complications

In the management of patients with testicular tumours, where large deeply placed volumes must be treated, it is inevitable that many normal structures are included and that some changes are induced as a result of the irradiation.

When treatment is given according to the principles which have been described, the incidence of changes severe enough to give rise to symptoms is low. Most of the recorded cases of serious damage leading to considerable morbidity or death, either followed deliberate use of high doses in an attempt to control radio-resistant or recurrent tumour, or could have been avoided if knowledge presently available had been applied.

Serious sequelae may follow radiation changes in the kidneys, gastro-intestinal tract, spinal cord and vertebral column.

The high radio-sensitivity of the kidney was discovered because of the considerable incidence of renal disease in patients with testicular neoplasms who had received treatment at the Holt Radium Institute, Manchester (Kunkler, Farr and Luxton, 1952).

A number of different patterns of radiation nephritis were seen, and ranged from acute renal failure and death shortly after treatment to transient proteinuria with no apparent persistent abnormality. By making certain that both kidneys do not receive more than 2000 rads, this complication can be avoided. Using the techniques described above, the average dose received by the kidneys is kept well below 1000 rads.

It has been reported (Friedman, 1952) that the stomach is the most sensitive part of the gastro-intestinal tract to radiation damage and that the frequency of such damage becomes appreciable above a dose level of 4000 rads. It must be remembered, however, that most of his patients underwent surgery in the form of a retroperitoneal node dissection immediately prior to treatment, and there is no doubt that surgery immediately before or after radiotherapy will considerably increase the chance of morbidity.

Friedman described some cases who developed ulceration and perforation of the stomach wall following radiotherapy to the para-aortic region with tumour doses up to 6000 rads. Other patients had less severe symptoms of dyspepsia and gastritis. The transverse colon was in some cases the site of similar changes and less frequently, perforation of the small intestine occurred.

Surgery may well be indicated for relief of these complications. In our experience, when a lymph node dissection is not performed and a dose level of 4500 rads given over a period of five to six weeks is not exceeded, it is unusual for any significant gastro-intestinal damage to occur.

Marrow depression may persist for some months, and when steroids have been given it is essential that the peripheral blood count should be studied by frequent and regular blood counts, while the dose of steroid is gradually reduced over a prolonged period of time. In most cases the total white cell count in the peripheral blood rises to normal levels within a few weeks or months. Differential counts show that this is due to a rise in the number of neutrophil polymorphonuclear leucocytes to normal levels, but that the absolute lymphocyte count may remain below normal for some years.

As a large volume of bone marrow is irradiated there is an increased risk of the later development of leukaemia. This condition was the cause of death in one of 228 patients treated for testicular tumour at the Middlesex Hospital in the years 1929–1959. Acute myeloid leukaemia was diagnosed seven years after orchidectomy and radiotherapy for seminoma. We can only speculate as to the relationship between radiotherapy and leukaemia in an isolated case of this sort, but it is a reasonable possibility that in this case it was radiation induced.

In addition to the risk of leukaemia, there is the possible risk of radiation induced neoplasms in the areas most heavily irradiated as there is in any heavily irradiated tissue. FRIEDMAN (1952) described four cases of osteogenic sarcoma occurring in patients previously treated for testicular tumour. Two arose in the spinal column, one in a rib and the other appeared to be an extra-skeletal tumour arising in the soft tissues close to the spine. In the Middlesex series there is one case of fibrosarcoma developing in an area of severe radiation fibrosis in the pelvis some nine years after a second course of radiotherapy which was given because of local recurrence.

Spinal cord damage will occur when doses in excess of 5000 rads are applied to the cord (FRIEDMAN, 1952). Care must be taken to avoid overlapping fields when the mediastinal and para-aortic nodes are both being irradiated. We have never seen this complication in our patients.

Sterility is commonly complained of after treatment, and not uncommonly the remaining testis is found to be small and atrophic. There has been some evidence to suggest that atrophy of the other testis is related primarily to the neoplasm of the diseased testis rather than to the treatment, but when the testis was found to be normal in size at the time of treatment but is later found to be atrophic, inadequate shielding of the testis during radiotherapy is the likely cause. Where atrophy is incomplete, hormone therapy may be of value.

When in the follow up period the patient is free of recurrence and there is normal sperm production, there seems no reason to discourage conception. Some increase in the general population burden of genetic change rather than abnormality of the conceived child is to be expected as a result of the inevitable irradiation of the normal testis during radiotherapy, due to scattered radiation. A number of our patients have been successful in begetting children following treatment, including one treated for multiple pulmonary metastases due to seminoma eighteen years ago, who has since become the father of three children.

9. The management of recurrent and advanced disease

In the treatment of malignant tumours of the testis it has been found that in cases with localised recurrence or even generalised metastases, further treatment can frequently be of great benefit. In many of these patients regression of all the deposits of tumour can be attained and in some, control of disease maintained for many years. FRIEDMAN and PURKAYASHTHA (1960) have reported upon the management of 24 cases of "recurrent seminoma". Ten of a possible eighteen patients survived more than five years after treatment for recurrence. In our own series there have been two patients who have survived free of disease for more than twenty years, despite the fact that they had pulmonary metastases when they came for treatment.

Local recurrence of the primary tumour in the scrotum is extremely rare, but recurrence may occur at the cut end of the cord if it was not fully included in the post-orchidectomy course of radiotherapy. Regression can be expected with further radiotherapy.

A tumour of the remaining testis presents in about 3 % of cases. Such a tumour may be a new primary or may be a metastasis from the original tumour. Even if the histological appearance of such a tumour is similar to that of the original in the other testis, it is never possible to conclude that it is a metastasis and not a new primary tumour. Such tumours must be treated as new primaries, by orchidectomy, but routine post-operative radiotherapy is inadvisable because of the great risk of post-radiation sequelae if treatment is given to the para-aortic region on a second occasion in full dosage. With definite involvement of lymph nodes in the lymphatic drainage such treatment, or perhaps lymph node dissection in the case of teratoma, must be performed and the consequent risks must be taken.

The cause for recurrence of tumour within the lymphatic drainage area should be sought with great care. If it can be related to inadequacy of dosage or be due to an unsatisfactory placing of fields, then the outlook is rather better than when recurrence occurs in an area fully irradiated to an adequate tumour dose. In the latter case we can only logically expect that a tumour dose higher than that attained in the original course must be given if there is to be any hope of long term control. This would, however, lead to a high accumulated dose and carry with it a considerable risk of morbidity.

Where there is a localised recurrence in cases of seminoma when the previous dose of radiation has not exceeded 3000 rads, further treatment can be given to a limited volume to the same, or perhaps a slightly greater tumour dose. Multiple fields or a rotational technique may be employed.

Metastases may present in the mediastinal or left supraclavicular nodes months, or even years after an initial treatment which was limited to the para-aortic region. In such cases the prognosis after further radiotherapy is good and "cure" may be obtained. Treatment should be given according to the principles already described.

Even with blood borne metastases in seminoma, thorough treatment can result in local control of disease and a long survival. Such long term survival is possible with bony and also pulmonary metastases, which may be multiple throughout both lung fields; we have in our cases examples of both. The prognosis with hepatic metastases is rather poorer but we have recently obtained apparently complete regression, maintained for eight months, of multiple metastases causing an enlargement of the liver to twice its normal size. The dosage employed in these circumstances must depend on the site, volume to be irradiated and the previous treatment. With multiple pulmonary metastases a dose of 2000 rads may be achieved throughout the chest over a period of four weeks. Isolated metastases in lung, bones and other sites should be given a tumour dose of 3000 rads over a period of three to four weeks.

When local radiotherapy fails to control disease or where the areas involved are too large for radiotherapy reasonably to encompass them, chemotherapy should be considered.

With teratoma the scope for radiotherapy and the chance of local control of disease and long term survival is much reduced. The radiosensitivity of the individual tumour is of great importance, as there is such a wide range in response. If the primary or a single metastasis shows a satisfactory regression, then other metastases are likely to respond in a similar fashion, but such response must not be regarded as an absolute rule. Variations in response may be related to the variations in histological appearance which may be seen between different deposits of the same testicular tumour.

Occasionally a patient with a previously treated teratoma of low grade malignancy presents a solitary pulmonary metastasis after a tumour free period of some years. Surgical exploration and removal of the tumour is then justified to establish the diagnosis and also because such a metastasis is generally radioresistant and may prove to be solitary for a prolonged period of time.

All the cancer chemotherapeutic agents which have been introduced into medicine have been employed upon testicular tumours. Except for a few patients with seminoma, the benefit gained has been rather limited.

The use of Sarcolysin has been advocated by Russian authors who have reported some good responses. However, less satisfactory results have been obtained using an almost identical agent (Melphalan). Lack of success with individual agents has led to the use of two or more in combination. Workers at the Memorial Hospital, New York (Li et al., 1962), have reported on the use of a combination of an alkylating agent (Chlorambucil), an anti-metabolite (Methotrexate) and an anti-tumour antibiotic (Actinomycin D.). The treatment is prolonged and carries with it a high incidence of toxic effects.

About half the patients show some improvement and a number of cases complete or near complete regression of pulmonary metastases has been recorded. These regressions have, however, proved to be short lived; the treatment is palliative and recurrence invariably occurs. The only long term survivor presented a high gonadotropin level in the urine as the only manifestation of recurrent tumour.

10. Results of radiotherapy

Between the years 1929 and 1956, a total of 228 patients were treated for testicular tumour at the Middlesex Hospital. A review of the results obtained gives an indication of the contribution of radiotherapy to the management of malignant disease of the testis.

Of the 228 patients 130 (57%) survived free of disease for at least five years after treatment. When the cases are divided into five groups according to the year of treatment (Table 1) the trend in survival during this period of 28 years can be appreciated.

Table 1. *Results in treatment of all cases of testicular tumour*

	1929–1956	1929–1936	1937–1941	1942–1946	1947–1951	1952–1956
Total	228	30	31	71	44	52
5 year survival	130	9	16	40	30	35
Percentage	57	30	52	55	68	67

It is important to determine whether this gratifying improvement in results is due to advances in treatment or to other factors. If there was an overall reduction in the interval between first symptom and treatment, or if there was an alteration in the incidence of the different types of tumour, or in the stages at which they presented during the period of study, the improvement might be attributable, at least in part, to factors not related to treatment. Examination of our data suggests that during the first eight years from 1929–1936 there was a somewhat higher proportion of unfavourable cases, but that during subsequent years from 1937–1956 no appreciable variation in these factors could be determined.

The improvement in survival is seen both for patients with seminoma and for those with teratoma.

During the whole period 1929–1956, treatment was given to the para-aortic nodes using X-ray apparatus in the 200–250 kV range (with the exception of a few patients in the first few years for whom only 170 kV apparatus was available).

A four field treatment plan (paired antero-lateral and postero-lateral portals) was employed throughout, with very few exceptions.

Two changes in technique did occur during this time. First there was a trend towards an increase in depth dose (especially in the later years in cases of teratoma) and secondly, to an increase in the length of the treatment portals employed when the para-aortic nodes were irradiated. Originally a length of 15 cm was used, but soon this was increased to 20 cm, and later still to 30 cm. We believe that these two changes are to a major extent responsible for the improvement in results of treatment.

Since 1956 supervoltage apparatus has been employed and it is hoped that survival figures will show a further rise.

Table 4 shows the result in patients who received radiotherapy after simple orchidectomy where there was no evidence of metastatic disease.

Table 2. *Results in treatment of seminoma*

	1929–1956	1929–1936	1937–1941	1942–1946	1947–1951	1952–1956
Total	130	10	18	40	31	31
5 year survival	90	6	12	25	23	24
Percentage	69	60	67	62	74	77

Table 3. *Results in treatment of teratoma*

	1929–1956	1929–1936	1937–1941	1942–1946	1947–1951	1952–1956
Total	56	10	7	18	8	13
5 year survival	19	0	0	8	4	7
Percentage	34	0	0	44	50	54

Table 4. *Results in treatment of testicular tumour apparently confined to the testis*

	Seminoma	Teratoma
Total	96	36
5 year survival	74	17
Percentage	77	47

Table 5. *Results in treatment of testicular tumours known to have metastases in the lymphatic drainage*

	Seminoma	Teratoma
Total	27	11
5 year survival	13	1
Percentage	48	(9)

The results of treating patients with metastases within the lymphatic drainage but no distant spread are shown in Table 5. The reduced survival in seminoma where there is definite involvement of lymph nodes in the lymphatic drainage areas can be seen. The chance of survival in teratoma is very poor when there is clinical evidence of spread beyond the confines of the testis.

There have been many reports of the results of treatment for testicular tumour, including those of Dean (1935), Leddy and Desjardins (1938), Cabot and Berkson (1939), Auerbach *et al.* (1946), Gordon-Taylor and Wyndham (1947), Lewis (1948a, 1953), Sauer and Burke (1949), O'Connell and Geschickter (1950), Higgins and Arber (1953), Culp (1953), Cox (1954), Notter (1956), Whittle (1957), Staubitz *et al.*

(1958), Patton *et al.* (1960), Masch (1960), Paul (1961), Thompson *et al.* (1961), Smithers and Wallace (1962), Hope Stone *et al.* (1963), Friedman and Di Rienzo (1963), Prossor (1964), Buskirk *et al.* (1964), Notter and Ranudd (1965), Kurohara *et al.* (1967), Maier *et al.* (1968).

Variations in the composition of the cases in these published series make it difficult to make a useful comparison of the results in one series with another. A review of the literature shows that the survival rate varies inversely as the metastasis rate (percentage known to have disease outside the testis at the time of treatment). Dean (1935) reported a metastasis rate of 72 % and gross five year survival rate of 29 %, and Kelly and Stenstrom (1947), with a metastasis rate of 73 %, also found 29 % as their 5 year figure for survival. At the other extreme Cabot and Berkson (1939) reported a metastasis rate of 26 % and 5 year survival of 51.5 %, and Dixon and Moore a 19 % metastasis rate and 63 % 5 year survival.

When comparison is made with series having a similar metastasis rate and methods of treatment, similar overall survival rates are found.

Table 6

	Metastasis rate	Total	5 years (%)
Cox (1954) Westminster Hospital	30	112	53
Notter (1956) Radiumhemmet	32	214	52
Present (1964) Middlesex Hospital	33	228	56

It is of interest to compare with our series those where different plans of treatment have been employed.

O'Connell and Geschickter (1950) reported a 5 year survival rate of only 32 % in their series of 162 patients from the United States Navy Hospitals. This survival figure is considerably lower than those reported at about this time by other authors from the United States Armed Services, e.g. Dixon and Moore (1953) reported a 63 % 5 year survival in 832 cases recorded at the Armed Forces Institute of Pathology. The patients reported by O'Connell and Geschickter were treated by simple orchidectomy and post-operative radiotherapy. It may however be of significance that the areas irradiated were "inguinal regions, hypogastric and pre-aortic group up to and including the region of the bifurcation of the aorta." This description suggests that the important area in the para-aortic nodes between and below the level of the kidneys was not irradiated, and this might well account for the difference in survival figures.

The largest series of cases where radical surgery has formed an important part of management was originated at the Walter Reed Hospital in Washington, by Lewis, and continued by his successors. Patton and Seitzman reporting this series in 1960 gave 5 year survival figures for 389 patients of 61.5 %. The apparent metastasis rate (prior to surgery) was 13.9 %—considerably lower than our 33 %. Despite this the survival at five years was only 5 % greater than that in our series.

In testicular malignant disease, as in all malignant disease, there is always the great problem of trying to advance knowledge by review of small series of patients, when there are so many factors to complicate and modify the outcome. It is quite impossible to draw any hard and fast conclusion about the big issues of management, such as the place of radical surgery. Only by close co-operation between centres, careful preparation of prospective controlled trials, and by long and detailed observation will knowledge be advanced and further improvements in treatment made.

II. The prostate

Carcinoma of the prostate is one of the more common tumours to present in men. It is responsible for approximately 6% of male deaths due to malignant disease.

A distinction must be drawn in carcinoma of the prostate between latent cancer—not associated with symptoms but found at post mortem or in specimens of benign hyperplasia of the gland—and active or "clinical" cancer that which presents with symptoms and/or signs of its presence. The former is an interesting pathological entity found with great frequency particularly in older men which, though histologically identical with clinical cancer, has little practical significance and will not be considered further (Franks, 1954).

The tumour is usually a fairly well differentiated adenocarcinoma and has origin in the outer portion of the gland, often in the posterior lobe. Local spread occurs through the gland to the urethra, seminal vesicles, bladder and rectum. Metastatic disease is commonly found in the lymphatic drainage in the pelvis and in the bones, particularly the pelvis and spine, where a direct venous pathway is thought to be the method of spread (Batson, 1940; Franks, 1956). The bony metastases are dominantly osteoblastic and may be so widespread as to leave very little normal bone. Production of acid phosphatase by the tumour is reflected in raised levels in the serum in most patients with metastatic disease. Metastases are commonly found in the lung and liver later in the course of the disease (Franks, 1956).

The clinical diagnosis of carcinoma of the prostate is based upon the condition of the prostate found on rectal examination, radiological appearances and serum acid phosphatase estimation. The diagnosis is confirmed by biopsy of the prostate by endoscopic trans-urethral resection or by open or needle aspiration through the perineum or rectum (Mimpriss, 1961). Occasionally biopsy of a metastasis is performed.

It is recognised that in nearly all cases, at the time of first diagnosis of a clinical carcinoma of the prostate, metastasis has already occurred despite the absence of clinical or radiological evidence to give confirmation at the time (Fergusson, 1958). Treatment must therefore be merely palliative. This may be given by surgery, "hormone therapy" or radiotherapy.

1. Surgery

Where the tumour is confined to the prostate the operation of radical prostatectomy by the perineal route is considered. The place for this operation is difficult to establish and there is no convincing evidence that patients treated by radical surgery do better or live longer than those treated conservatively. Often radical surgery for a small tumour is followed by the appearance of extensive metastatic disease, while another similar tumour will follow so benign a course that long term survival occurs without any form of treatment being given. These common occurrences make assessment difficult and there are many urological surgeons who regard the radical operation as unjustified (Fergusson, 1958).

Palliative surgery in the form of per-urethral resection is a satisfactory way of dealing with urethral obstruction, but it may have to be repeated at intervals if there is no response to the administration of oestrogens and other hormonal measures.

2. "Hormone therapy"

The possibilities are administration of oestrogens or corticosteroids, performance of bilateral orchidectomy, bilateral adrenalectomy or hypophysectomy.

The administration of oestrogens and bilateral orchidectomy (using a subcapsular technique) are employed either together or in sequence in nearly every case. The serum acid phosphatase level does not appear to be related to the likelihood of a response to these measures, but a fall in the level is a satisfactory sign of control of disease to support clinical and radiological evidence of response. Treatment with oestrogens is usually initiated with stilboestrol 15 mg daily, but when relapse occurs some believe that further benefit may be obtained by elevation of the dose up to 100 mg daily (FERGUSSON, 1958). Another oestrogen such as diethylstilboestrol diphosphate may also be tried (COLAPINTO and ABERHART, 1961).

Recently the value of oestrogen therapy has been questioned. It has been shown that the high doses given lead to a marked increase in the incidence of death to cardiovascular and cerebrovascular disease. In early cases a controlled trial revealed that survival may be significantly worse in cases of carcinoma of the prostate given 5 mg daily of diethystilboestrol (Veterans Research Group, 1967). It was concluded that oestrogen treatment should be reserved until symptoms warranted its administration and that high doses should be avoided.

Adrenalectomy and hypophysectomy (using a purely surgical technique or by the introduction of a radioactive source) have been employed but their routine use is not established and certainly the impression is gained that these are less likely to aid men with prostatic carcinoma than women with mammary carcinoma.

The administration of corticosteroids (e.g. Prednisone 20–30 mg daily) may achieve symptomatic relief in some patients who have become resistant to other hormone measures.

3. Radiotherapy

With the advent of supervoltage apparatus the position of radiotherapy in the management of a number of tumours previously regarded as completely radio-resistant has been reviewed, and in some an important place for radiotherapy established.

Until recently radiotherapists have found little encouragement to enter this field. In isolated cases where treatment of a primary tumour was undertaken it was associated with severe complications during therapy and a disappointing degree of regression of the tumour. It was inevitable that part or whole of the bladder—in nearly every case previously and often still affected by obstruction to drainage and secondary infection—should be within the treatment volume and that radiation cystitis should be severe. It was also inevitable that a considerable part of the rectum should similarly be included and be the subject of much radiation reaction. Using orthovoltage apparatus skin reactions were added to these complications and it was difficult to reach a satisfactory tumour dose.

The knowledge that in a majority of patients metastasis had occurred by the time of presentation also did not encourage an attempt at cure or long term control of carcinoma of the prostate by the use of radiotherapy.

During the past few years radiotherapists have taken a new look at the treatment of carcinoma of the prostate. Treatment has been given:

1. In early cases where the tumour is confined to the gland radiotherapy may be employed as a radical method with object of cure in place of radical surgery or the palliative use of hormonal measures.

2. With more advanced tumours long term control of the primary tumour and the symptoms caused by it.

3. Radiotherapy has been considered in advanced disease when a patient is suffering severe symptoms, usually pain or bleeding due to the primary tumour, but no response is obtained with all the varieties of hormone treatment. This will be worthwhile if the patient's general condition is good and particularly if there is no evidence of distant metastases.

Urinary obstruction must be relieved before commencing treatment. Supervoltage apparatus should be used, and a 2, 3 or 4 field technique, according to tumour volume and patient size; a tumour dose of 5000–6000 rads in five to six weeks should be the object. Intermittent use of urinary antiseptic is advised during treatment. In a moderate proportion of patients so treated there is relief of symptoms and control of tumour growth for a period of time.

Encouraging results have been reported by Dykhuizen *et al.* (1968). In some centres including our own the hyperbaric oxygen chamber has been employed using a six fractions technique. Early results have been promising.

A technique of infiltrating radioactive colloidal gold into the prostate by direct injection has been described by Flocks and has been employed in several centres in the United States (Flocks *et al.*, 1952; Flocks and Culp, 1960). Some promising results have been reported, but it remains a rather special method with a considerable radiation hazard to the operator, which requires evaluation over a long period before it can be considered for general use.

Metastases, no longer responsive to hormone measures, may also be irradiated, and in some centres this is more frequently performed than is treatment to the primary tumour. Metastases in bone, particularly osteolytic metastases causing or threatening a pathological fracture, may be treated with relief of pain and later sclerosis may be seen on radiological examination of the area. With fracture or impending fracture in a long bone surgical fixation is usually required in addition.

In treating a metastasis from carcinoma of the prostate a fairly high tumour dose must be achieved. A tumour dose of 3000–4000 rads should be given over a period of three to four weeks, using supervoltage apparatus.

Some success in the palliation of multiple metastases in bone no longer influenced by hormones has been reported by Wildermuth using testosterone and radioactive phosphorus (Wildermuth, 1960).

III. The seminal vesicle, spermatic cord and epididymis

Malignant tumours of the seminal vesicle are very rare, and those which do occur are carcinoma clinically indistinguishable, except perhaps by response to hormones, from those arising in the prostate.

A variety of tumours may have origin in the spermatic cord. Approximately one third are malignant and over 90% are sarcoma (Dreyfuss and Goodsitt, 1960). Most appear in children and young adults. The largest group comprises the rhabdomyosarcoma, but leiomyosarcoma, liposarcoma and fibrosarcoma are seen (Prince, 1952). Distant metastases are commonly detected early in the course of the disease and the prognosis is poor, with over 50% of patients dying within a year of diagnosis (Collins and Pugh, 1964). In some there is evidence of retroperitoneal node involvement.

Treatment should be by wide local removal. Surgery should be considered for invasion of the retroperitoneal nodes if there is evidence of invasion without distant metastasis. The value of radiotherapy to the retroperitoneal nodes is difficult to assess. On the whole we would not favour a routine course in all cases, for we recognise the radioresistance of these tumours and the difficulty and dangers in treating the retroperitoneal nodes to a tumour dose likely to be effective in the treatment of a sarcoma. We also take into consideration the dominance of haematogenous as opposed to lymphatic spread with these sarcoma. When metastases are present in the retroperitoneal nodes radiotherapy can be employed as a pre-operative measure or as the sole method of treatment of inoperable nodes. Tumour doses of the order of 5500–7000 rads, given over a period of five to seven weeks are required, except in infants and young children, where some reduction of these levels must be made.

Carcinomas of epididymis, vas deferens and appendix testis are described, but are extremely rare (Collins and Pugh, 1964). They should be treated in the same way as teratoma of the testis.

References

Testicular tumours

AUERBACH, O., BRINES, O. A., YAGUDA, A.: Neoplasms of testis. J. Urol. (Baltimore) **56**, 368–374 (1946).

BUSKIRK, K. VAN, O'SHAUGHNESSY, E., GANGAI, M.: Exhibition—treatment of testicular tumours. Internat. Soc. of Urology, XIIIth Congr., London, 1964.

CABOT, H., BERKSON, J.: Neoplasms of testis; study of results of orchidectomy, with and without irradiation. New Engl. J. Med. **220**, 192–195 (1939).

CAIRNS, H. W. B.: Neoplasms of testicle. Lancet **1926 I**, 845–850.

CHEVASSU, M.: Tumeurs du testicule. Paris 1906.

CHIAPPA, S., USLENGHI, C., GALLI, G., RAVASI, G., BONADONNA, G.: Lymphangiography and endolymphatic radiotherapy in testicular tumours. Brit. J. Radiol. **39**, 498–512 (1966).

COLLINS, D. H., PUGH, R. C. B.: The pathology of testicular tumours. Studies from the testicular tumour panel and registry of the Pathological Society of Great Britain & Ireland in association with the British Empire Cancer Campaign for Research. Brit. J. Urol. **36** (2) Suppl., 1–112 (1964).

COX, R.: Radiotherapy in malignant disease of testicle and penis. Brit. J. Urol. **26**, 350–353 (1954).

CULP, D. A.: Testicular neoplasms: analysis of 113 cases. J. Urol. (Baltimore) **70**, 282–295 (1953).

DEAN, A. L.: Teratoid tumors of testis. J. Amer. med. Ass. **105**, 1965–1971 (1935).

DEITERMANN, J. H.: Zur Kenntnis des Seminoms, seines Wesens und seines Krankheitsverlaufs. Frankf. Z. Path. **50**, 231–251 (1937).

DIXON, F. J., MOORE, R. A.: Testicular tumors; clinicopathological study. Cancer (Philad.) **6**, 427–454 (1953).

ECKERT, H., SMITH, J. P.: Malignant lymphoma of the testis. Brit. med. J. **1963 II**, 891–894.

ENNUYER, A., GRICOUROFF, G., THIVET, M.: The primary and secondary lymphoreticulosarcomas of the testis. Bull. Ass. franç. Cancer **47**, 355–372 (1960).

EWING, J.: Teratoma testis and its derivatives. Surg. Gynec. Obstet. **12**, 230–261 (1911).

FRIEDMAN, M.: Calculated risks of radiation injury of normal tissue in the treatment of cancer of the testis. Proc. 2nd National Cancer Conf. Amer. Cancer Soc., 390–400 (1952).

— PURKAYASHTHA, M. C.: Recurrent seminoma of testis: causes and treatment of late metastasis, recurrence or second primary tumor. J. Urol. (Baltimore) **84**, 360–368 (1960).

— DI RIENZO, A. J.: Treatment of trophocarcinoma (embryonal carcinoma) of the testis. Radiology **80**, 550–565 (1963).

GORDON-TAYLOR, G., TILL, A. S.: On malignant disease of testicle, with special reference to neoplasms of undescended organ. Brit. J. Urol. **10**, 1–45 (1938).

— WYNDHAM, N. R.: On malignant tumours of the testicle. Brit. J. Surg. **35**, 6–17 (1947).

HANDFIELD-JONES, R. M.: Treatment of malignant disease of testicle. Lancet **1924 II**, 850–852.

HIGGINS, C. C., ARBER, F. W.: Malignant tumours of testicle. Canad. med. Ass. J. **69**, 124–131 (1953).

HINMAN, F.: Tumors of testis; 5 year cures following radical operation. Surg. Gynec. Obstet. **56**, 450–461 (1933).

HOPE-STONE, H. F., BLANDY, J. P., DAYAN, A. D.: Treatment of tumours of the testis. Brit. med. J. **1963 I**, 984–989.

JAMIESON, J. K., DOBSON, J. F.: Lancet **1910 I**, 493.

KEYES, E. L.: Malignant tumor of testicle: diagnosis, prognosis and treatment. Amer. J. Roentgenol. **15**, 44–47 (1926).

KUNKLER, P. B., FARR, R. F., LUXTON, R. W.: Limit of renal tolerance to X-rays; investigation into renal damage occurring following treatment of tumours of testis by abdominal baths. Brit. J. Radiol. **25**, 190–201 (1952).

KUROHARA, S. S., GEORGE, F. W., DYKHUISEN, R. F., LEARY, K. L.: Testicular tumours. Cancer (Philad.) 1089–1098 (1967).

LEDDY, E. T., DESJARDINS, A. U.: Radiotherapy for tumors of testis. Radiology **31**, 293–298 (1938).

LEWIS, L. G.: Testis tumours: report on 250 cases. J. Urol. (Baltimore) **59**, 763–772 (1948).

— Radioresistant testis tumors: results in 133 cases; 5 year follow-up. J. Urol. (Baltimore) **69**, 841–844 (1953).

LI, M. C., WHITMORE, W. F., GOLBEY, R., GRABSTALD, H.: Effects of combined drug therapy on metastatic cancer of the testis. J. Amer. med. Ass. **174**, 1291–1299 (1960).

MAIER, J. G., SULAK, M. H., MITTEMEYER, B. T.: Seminoma of testis. Amer. J. Roentgenol. **102**, 596–602 (1968).

MASCH, F.: Klinik, Therapie und Prognose der bösartigen Hodentumoren und ihren Rezidiven. Strahlentherapie **113**, 217–241 (1960).

NICHOLSON, G. W.: New growths of the testicle. Guy's Hosp. Rep. **61**, 249–321 (1907).

NOTTER, G.: Die Behandlung maligner Testistumoren am Radiumhemmet, Stockholm. Acta radiol. (Stockh.) **45**, 483–502 (1956).

— RANUDD, N. E.: Treatment of malignant testicular tumours. (Therapy.) Acta radiol. (Stockh.) **2**, 273–301 (1966).

O'CONNELL, H. V., GESCHICKTER, C. F.: Tumors of testes; 5 year follow-up study. U.S. armed Forces med. J. **1**, 719–732 (1950).

PATTON, J. F., SEITZMAN, D. N., ZONE, R. A.: Diagnosis and treatment of testicular tumors. Amer. J. Surg. **99**, 525–532 (1960).

PAUL, O.: On the radiotherapy of testicular tumors and their metastases. Strahlentherapie **114**, 426–437 (1961).

SAUER, H. R., BURKE, E. M.: Prognosis of testicular tumors. J. Urol. (Baltimore) **62**, 69–74 (1949).

SMITHERS, D. W., WALLACE, E. N. K.: Radiotherapy in the treatment of patients with seminomas and teratomas of the testicle. Brit. J. Urol. **34**, 422–435 (1962).

STAUBITZ, W. J., MAGOSS, I. V., OBERKIRCHER, O. J., LENT, M. H., MITCHELL, F. D., MURPHY, W. T.: Management of testicular tumors. J. Amer. med. Ass. **166**, 751–758 (1958).

TANNER, C. O.: Tumors of testicle. Surg. Gynec. Obstet. **35**, 565–572 (1922).

TEFFT, M., VAWTER, G. F., MITUS, A.: Radiotherapeutic management of testicular neoplasms in children. Radiology 88, 457–458 (1967).

THOMPSON, I. M., WEAR, J., ALMOND, C., SCHEWE, E. J., SALA, J.: An analytical survey of one hundred and seventy-eight testicular tumors. J. Urol. (Baltimore) **85**, 173–179 (1961).

WALLACE, N.: Lymphography in the management of testicular tumours. Clin. Radiol. **20**, 453–458 (1969).

WALLACE, S., JACKSON, L., SCHAFFER, B., GOULD, J., GREENING, R. R., WEISS, A., KRAMER, S.: Lymphangiograms: Their diagnostic and therapeutic potential. Radiology 76, 179–199 (1961).

WHITTLE, R. J. M.: Tumours of the testicle. Brit. J. Radiol. **30**, 7–12 (1957).

WILLIS, R. A.: Pathology of tumours, fourth edition, p. 579—587. London: Butterworths 1953.

ZUPPINGER, A.: Klinik und Therapie der Tumoren im Kindesalter. Rad. clin. (Basel), Suppl. **15**, 5–25 (1946).

Prostate, seminal vesicle, spermatic cord and epididymis

BATSON, O. V.: Function of vertebral veins and their role in the spread of metastases. Ann. Surg. **112**, 138–149 (1940).

COLAPINTO, V., ABERHART, C.: Clinical trial of massive stilboestrol diphosphate therapy in advanced carcinoma of the prostate. Brit. J. Urol. **33**, 171–177 (1961).

COLLINS, D. H., PUGH, R. C. B.: The pathology of testicular tumours. Studies from the testicular tumour panel and registry of the Pathological Society of Great Britain & Ireland in association with the British Empire Cancer Campaign for Research. Brit. J. Urol. **36** (2) Suppl., 1–112 (1964).

DREYFUSS, W., GOODSITT, E.: Tumours of the spermatic cord. J. Urol. (Baltimore) **84**, 658–665 (1960).

DYKHUIZEN, R. F., SARGENT, C. R., GEORGE, F. W., KURAHARA, S. S.: J. Urol. (Baltimore) **100**, 333–338 (1968).

FERGUSSON, J. D.: Cancer, p. 197–209. London: Butterworth & Co. (Publishers) Ltd. 1958.

FLOCKS, R. H.: Combination therapy for localized prostatic cancer. J. Urol. (Baltimore) **89**, 889–894 (1963).

— CULP, D. A.: Radiation therapy of early prostatic cancer. Oxford: Blackwell Sci. Publ., Ltd. 1960.

FRANKS, L. M.: The spread of prostatic cancer. J. Path. Bact. **72**, 603–611 (1956).

MIMPRISS, T. W.: Diagnosis of carcinoma of prostate. Brit. J. Urol. **33**, 167–170 (1961).

PRINCE, C. L.: Malignant tumors of the spermatic cord: brief review, with presentation of case of angioendothelioma. J. Urol. (Baltimore) **47**, 793–799 (1942).

Veterans Administration Co-operative Urological Research Group: Surg. Gynec. Obstet. **124**, 1011–1017 (1967).

C. Tumours of the urinary tract

By

H. J. G. Bloom and D. M. Wallace

I. Tumours of the renal parenchyma

With 52 Figures

1. Introduction

Tumours of the kidney, including the renal paranchyma and the renal pelvis, constitute 1–2% of all malignant tumours in the adult, and approximately 20% of those in children. BADENOCH (1955) found 45 cases among 4700 cases of malignant disease, rather less than 1%, at St. Bartholomew's Hospital, London, during the period 1947–1951.

Renal tumours are classified in Table 1. Those, however, with which we are mainly concerned in clinical practice are:

Table 1. *Classification of renal tumours*

Epithelial

Parenchyma
Adenoma
Adenocarcinoma (Hypernephroma; Grawitz tumour)

Renal pelvis and calyces
Transitional cell papilloma
Transitional cell carcinoma
Squamous cell carcinoma
Adenocarcinoma

Developmental
Nephroblastoma (Wilms' tumour; Embryonal adenomyosarcoma)

Connective tissue
Angioma, fibroma, myoma, lipoma, mixed elements (e.g. angiomyolipoma)
Fibrosarcoma, liposarcoma, mixed elements, reticulosis

Secondary tumours
Direct spread e.g. adrenal carcinoma, retroperitoneal sarcoma
Blood-borne e.g. breast, bronchial and thyroid carcinoma

1. Adenocarcinoma (Hypernephroma),
2. Nephroblastoma (Wilm's Tumour),
3. Transitional cell tumours of the renal pelvis,
4. Squamous cell carcinoma of the renal pelvis.

In the series of some 2300 cases of renal tumour collected by RICHES and his colleagues (1951) adenocarcinoma made up 75% of the series, nephroblastoma 8%, transitional cell carcinoma 7%, and squamous cell carcinoma 2.5%.

The renal pelvis and its calyceal system has a similar histological structure to the ureter and both give rise to transitional cell tumours of identical type and aetiology. We, therefore, regard the renal pelvis and ureter as a single entity from the point of view of neoplasia, and have reviewed this subject in the next chapter, separately from tumours arising from the renal parenchyma which are of a completely different histogenesis and aetiology.

2. Adenocarcinoma

(Synonyms: Hypernephroma, Grawitz tumour)

a) Incidence

This tumour is by far the most frequent type constituting approximately 90% of malignant tumours of the renal parenchyma. It occurs twice as often in men as in women. 80% of cases are found in the fifth, sixth and seventh decades; between 5 and 10% occur under the age of forty. It is a very rare tumour in childhood. Hogan and Simons (1957) who reported such a case in a girl aged five, found only 26 examples of renal adenocarcinoma in children and adolescents in the world literature. The right and left kidneys are affected with equal frequency, and very rarely the tumour is bilateral (Hillenbrand and Hörstebrock, 1957; Hanley, 1945; Bastable, 1960). Seven cases of bilateral adenocarcinoma were encountered by Riches et al. (1951).

b) Aetiology

It has been suggested that at least some renal adenocarcinomas originate in adenomas (Trinkle, 1936; Newcombe, 1937). Cristol et al. (1946), Griffiths and Thackray (1949) and Willis (1948) have pointed out the great difficulty in distinguishing histologically between an adenoma and an adenocarcinoma of low grade malignancy. Both adenomas and adenocarcinomas occur at the same age, are more common in men than women and are often found together in the same kidney. The possibility of a hormonal factor being involved in the development of adenomas and adenocarcinomas of the kidney is suggested by the work of Kirkman and Bacon (1949) and also Horning and Whittick (1954). These authors produced hormone-dependent malignant renal epithelial tumours in male golden hamsters by prolonged treatment with oestrogens.

c) Pathology

α) Macroscopic appearances

The renal adenocarcinoma usually occurs at one or other pole of the kidney. It forms a bulky, well-circumscribed, rounded and lobulated mass, often apparently encapsulated as the result of compression of the surrounding renal tissue. The cut surface has a trabeculated appearance and shows a golden-yellow colour due to the high lipoid content of the cells. There are also areas of cystic change and haemorrhage. As the tumour enlarges it destroys the renal substance and invades the calyces and pelvis.

β) Microscopic appearances

The tumour is composed essentially of either large clear cells with vaculated cytoplasm or smaller cells with a granular cytoplasm. The histological pattern may be papillary or tubular or the cells may be arranged in solid cords. Although the stroma is scanty the vascularity is a prominent feature, many large thin-walled blood vessels being present. Considerable variation in histological structure may exist in different parts of the same tumour, and both clear and granular cells may be present.

d) Mode of spread and natural history

The renal adenocarcinoma involves surrounding structures by direct spread and extends via lymphatics, first to nodes in the renal pedicle and then to the para-aortic chain. Further spread may occur to the mediastinal lymph nodes and occasionally to nodes in the supraclavicular region. There is a special tendency to blood-vessel invasion and to the appearance of distant metastases early in the evolution of the tumour. The renal vein often contains neoplasm which may extend to the inferior vena cava and rarely as far as the right auricle. McDONALD and PRIESTLEY (1943) in some 500 cases of adenocarcinoma found the renal vein involved in 54%.

The behaviour of renal adenocarcinoma is extremely variable. Some tumours may grow slowly to reach a large size without obvious metastases developing, whilst others remain small and symptomless, the first clinical manifestations being due to distant spread. The lungs, skeleton and liver are the most frequent sites for blood-borne metastases, but no organ or tissue is exempt. The heart, for example, was involved in 5 of 17 autopsy cases reported by GRIFFITHS and THACKRAY (1949).

A curious feature of the adenocarcinoma is a tendency to give rise to apparently solitary metastases which, if the presenting feature, may pose a difficult diagnostic problem until a biopsy is performed. For example, an osteolytic deposit, often accompanied by a pathological fracture, at the upper end of the humerus or in the femur, spine or pelvis may masquerade as a primary bone neoplasm. Occasionally such a tumour pulsates and may be mistaken for an aneurysmal bone cyst. Solitary pulmonary or cerebral deposits may also cause errors in diagnosis, and the primary site may be suspected only after their removal and histological examination.

Whilst blood-borne metastase may be the presenting feature in some patients with renal adenocarcinoma, in others they may not become manifest until several years have elapsed following an apparently successful nephrectomy. Such a metastasis, if solitary, is a surgical challenge and its removal by excision from the lung (BARNEY, 1944; ROBB, 1948) or brain (STÖRTEBECKER, 1951) or by amputation of a limb may be followed by a prolonged remission before further deposits occur, and in some cases perhaps even by complete cure. CHUTE *et al.* (1958) have recently reported 5 cases with solitary deposits treated by surgery, 2 of whom are alive and well three and four years post-operatively; the others died with further metastases within eight months to two years of operation.

The renal growth may be present for a number of years before local symptoms arise or before metastases appear. Even when the primary tumour has been found its evolution may be extremely slow. Thus, CARLSON and OCKERBLAD (1941) report a case in whom there was a ten-year history of haematuria and radiological evidence of a renal space-occupying lesion for nine years before the patient would finally consent to nephrectomy, which revealed an adenocarcinoma. A similar case of seven years duration was reported by YOUNG and DEMING (1955). There may be an interval of many years between nephrectomy and local recurrence (fourteen years in the case reported by KUEHN and DAVIS, 1959) or the appearance of distant metastases (twenty-one years in the case reported by STRAUSS and SCARLTON, 1956). Of 8 patients surviving more than fifteen years after nephrectomy reported recently by HUMPHREYS and FOOT (1960) 2 eventually died of metastases.

Metastases from renal adenocarcinoma may show little change over many months. Occasionally, they regress for a time and rarely they disappear for a period of months or even years. This phenomenon has been noted in deposits which have appeared post-operatively (BUMPUS, 1928; BEER, 1937), and soon after nephrectomy in metastases which were present when the patient was first seen (MANN, 1948; ARCOMANO *et al.*, 1958; HOLLAHAN, 1959). MANN'S case was alive and well fifteen years later (personal communication to JENKINS, 1959). The common story with adenocarcinoma, however, is that metastases once they appear slowly advance to bring about a fatal outcome. During a great deal of this time the patient often feels and looks well and is able to continue at work. Unlike transitional cell carcinoma of the renal pelvis, adenocarcinoma does not involve the ureter or the bladder except on extremely rare occasions. Such cases have been reported by MITCHELL (1958) and by SARGENT (1960). Tumours discovered in the ureter in cases of parenchymal carcinoma of the kidney are more likely to be second primaries (GRIFFITHS and THACKRAY, 1949).

e) Clinical features

Unfortunately, symptoms due to adenocarcinoma of the kidney do not generally develop early. The cardinal features are haematuria, pain and tumour occurring singly or in combination. The complete triad, which occurs in 25–30 % of cases, is usually indicative of advanced disease: of 17 patients with all three symptoms 14 were dead within two years (Griffiths and Thackray, 1949). Haematuria, which is commonly regarded as an early symptom, occurred in 62 % of cases in the series studied by Riches and his colleagues (1951) and was the sole symptom in only 21 % of cases. Although haematuria may occur late it is the only symptom likely to bring the patient in time for curative treatment. Constant pain, tumour and especially weight loss and weakness are, of course, symptoms of advanced disease. Pain as a dull ache in the loin or of a colicky nature, due to passage of blood clots, occurs in about 50 % of cases. Tumour is a symptom in approximately one third of patients.

Adenocarcinoma of the kidney may be associated with certain systemic disturbances which have been reviewed by Berger and Sinkoff (1957). A fever of up to 103 or 104° F may occur in the absence of infection and is usually thought to be the result of widespread necrosis or haemorrhage within the tumour (Bleyer, 1944). On the other hand Böttiger (1957), who found pyrexia in 40 % of cases, was not able to correlate this feature with the presence of tumour necrosis or haemorrhage. In a later paper Böttiger and Ivemark (1959) reported that fever was found much more often in association with clear-cell tumours (45 %) than in the granular cell lesions (10 %). These authors held the opinion that certain adenocarcinomas may produce substances responsible for pyrexia and a raised sedimentation rate.

Pyrexia may be accompanied by loss of weight and night sweats and may, therefore, simulate pulmonary tuberculosis, especially if metastatic pulmonary infiltration is present. Occasionally, pyrexia and malaise are the sole manifestations of the disease and give rise to considerable diagnostic difficulties. Following nephrectomy the temperature returns to normal, but may recur with the development of metastases.

Polycythemia vera has been reported in a number of patients with renal adenocarcinoma, and this is of considerable interest in view of the experimental work relating a substance from the kidney to erythropoiesis (Jacobson et al., 1951). Conley and his associates (1957) found 18 cases of renal adenocarcinoma associated with polycythaemia reported in the literature. DeWeerd and Hagedorn (1959) have recently reported 7 new cases from the Mayo Clinic, remission occurring in 5 of the 6 cases who survived nephrectomy. The polycythaemia may recur with the development of metastases.

The presenting symptoms of adenocarcinoma may be related to metastases, there being no hint of the primary renal tumour. This occurred in 20 % of the cases studied by Griffiths and Thackray (1949), 11 cases remaining undiagnosed until autopsy. The commonest sites for metastases are the long bones resulting in pain, swelling and commonly pathological fracture, the spine giving rise to backache, root pain and paraplegia, and the brain, the clinical features of which suggest a primary intracranial neoplasm. A sudden varicocele may occur with left-sided tumours and does not necessarily indicate extension of the growth along the renal vein. Rarely, sudden oedema of the lower limbs and genitalia may signal the development of inferior vena caval obstruction by tumour and superimposed thrombosis.

Non-urological symptoms in patients with renal tumours has recently been the subject of a report by Melicow and Uson (1960). In no less than one-third of 577 cases studied by these authors the classical triad of symptoms, haematuria, flank pain and flank tumour, was absent. In 50 % of this atypical group the presenting symptoms were fever, weakness, anorexia and loss of weight.

The renal tumour may be palpable bimanually as a smooth, rounded mass or the whole kidney may be enlarged. Occasionally, the growth reaches a large size and fills the upper two-thirds of one side of the abdomen. The kidney moves with respiration until it becomes fixed due to perinephric infiltration.

f) Factors influencing prognosis

α) Grade

Prognosis in carcinoma of the kidney, as with carcinoma in general, depends on the inherent malignancy of the tumour and the extent it has reached when the patient is first seen. The degree of malignancy in most tumours is reflected in their microscopic structure, and this has formed the basis of histological grading which is now well-established for such tumours as carcinoma of the breast, mouth, rectum and bladder and for gliomas of the central nervous system. Grading is a measure of the potential malignancy of a tumour and indicates which cases are more likely to have residual tumour or occult distant metastases at the time of treatment. It, moreover, provides a guide to the speed with which local disease and distant metastases become active, produce symptoms and cause death (BLOOM and RICHARDSON, 1957).

McDONALD and PRIESTLEY (1943) and also GRIFFITHS and THACKRAY (1949) related histological grade with prognosis in renal adenocarcinoma, and by combining histological grade and pathological stage (renal vein involvement) these authors obtained a useful guide to possible outcome. GRIFFITHS and THACKRAY (1949) based their grading on three factors, namely, the degree of papillary or adenomatous formation, the irregularity or variability of the cells and the frequency of mitoses and hyperchromatic nuclei. Three grades of malignancy were recognised—low (grade 1), intermediate (grade 2) and high (grade 3). In a later report THACKRAY (1957) gave the following results for a small series of cases (Table 2). Grade 3 tumours tend to have a short history, grow rapidly, invade the

Table 2. *Renal adenocarcinoma, grade and prognosis* (THACKRAY, 1957)

Grade	Survival rate		
	3 years (%)	5 years (%)	10 years (%)
I	92	75	42
II	40	27	20
III	27	9	9

renal vein, infiltrate the surrounding tissues, give rise to lymph node metastases and cause death within one to two years of treatment. Grade I tumours, on the other hand, have a long history and grow much more slowly with less tendency to invade the renal vein. Although metastases are common even with this grade of tumour, they develop slowly (THACKRAY, 1957). HAND and BRODERS (1932) in 193 cases found the average duration of life for their grade I lesions to be 101.4 months and for grade 4 lesions 22.5 months.

β) Structure and cell type

The general structure of renal adenocarcinoma may vary in one and the same tumour, but generally speaking either a papillary, adenomatous or solid pattern predominates. Papillary tumours tend to give rise to early blood-borne metastases whilst those with a tubular pattern appear to involve lymph nodes more frequently. There is, however, no significant difference in the overall survival between the two types of tumour (THACKRAY, 1957). The prognosis also does not appear to be affected by the type of cell. Thus the five-year survival rate was comparable for tumours composed of clear cells and of granular cells (ROYCE and TORMEY, 1955).

γ) Tumour capsule

Tumours of low grade malignancy often appear to be entirely encapsulated. In highly malignant lesions the capsule is absent or found only in isolated areas. Petkovic (1959) in a 110 cases found that a classification based, in part, on the quality of the capsule was important in assessing prognosis.

δ) Perirenal adhesions and local extension

A fixed kidney is not necessarily the result of tumour spread and may be inflammatory in origin. Royce and Tormey (1955) found that fixation in 13 of 35 cases of adenocarcinoma was due to pyelonephritis. Infiltration of tumour through the renal capsule to invade the perinephric fat and muscle occurs more frequently in cases of high grade malignancy and is of serious prognostic significance. Petkovic (1959) reported 19 survivors among 37 cases with absent or moderate perirenal infiltration compared with only 4 of 50 cases with extensive local spread; 30 of these 50 cases were dead within six months of operation.

ε) Size of primary tumour

Generally speaking, the larger the tumour the greater the local extension and the incidence of metastases. Bell (1947) in 149 autopsy cases found that metastases were associated with 2% of tumours less than 3 cm in diameter, 7% of those between 3 and 5 cm and 83% for those greater than 10 cm. Bixler *et al.* (1944) report that patients with tumours less than 5 cm or weighing less than 500 g had a five-year survival rate of 50%, whereas in those with lesions 10 cm or more, or weighing 1000 g or more, the survival was 38%.

ζ) Lymph node involvement

In a series of 80 operable cases Riches (1958) found lymph node metastases in only 6 cases, and these were evenly distributed among the three grades of malignancy. Two of these cases survived for approximately 7 years. Riches (1958) considered that lymph node involvement, although an important fact in prognosis, does not appear to have such an early lethal effect as a high grade of malignancy or venous involvement. On the other hand, in 22 out 84 determinate cases with lymph node metastases reported by Petkovic (1959) there were 5 post-operative deaths and all the remaining cases were dead within two years.

η) Involvement of the renal vein

The incidence of tumour within the renal vein at operation varies in different series. McDonald and Priestley (1943) reported an incidence of 54% at the Mayo Clinic, and Riches and his colleagues (1951) in their series, studied on behalf of the British Association of Urological Surgeons, found the vein involved in 24% of cases. The frequency of renal vein involvement increases with the rise of histological grade (Table 3) and the presence of this complication is of serious significance (Table 4).

Table 3. *Renal adenocarcinoma, grade and renal vein involvement* (Riches et al., 1951)

Grade	Cases	Cases with vein involved
I	26	5 (11%)
II	32	9 (28%)
III	20	9 (45%)
Total	78	23 (29%)

Table 4. *Renal adenocarcinoma, renal vein involvement and prognosis* (RICHES *et al.*, 1951; B.A.U.S. Series)

Renal vein	Survival rate		
	3 years	5 years	10 years
Free	218/434 (50%)	114/308 (37%)	30/138 (22%)
Involved	38/129 (29%)	17/90 (19%)	4/54 (7%)
Total	256/563 (45%)	131/398 (33%)	34/192 (18%)

Table 5. *Renal adenocarcinoma grade, stage and prognosis* (THACKRAY, 1957)

Grade and stage	Survival rate		
	3 years (%)	5 years (%)	10 years (%)
Grade I Vein free	87	75	50
Grade III Vein involved	17	0	0

A useful guide to prognosis is obtained by combining histological grade with the state of the renal vein (Table 5). PETKOVIC (1959) obtained good correlation between stage and prognosis using a system based on the following factors: tumour capsule formation, perinephric invasion, lymph node and renal vein involvement and the presence of distant metastases.

ϑ) Tumour calcification

This is often regarded as indicative of slow growth and a relatively good prognosis. CAHILL and MELICOW (1938), however, found radiological or pathological evidence of calcification in 12 of 82 cases, and only one of the 12 survived 2 years.

ι) Intravenous pyelogram

Absence of secretion on the affected side indicates renal vein involvement, extensive replacement of the renal substance by tumour, or ureteric obstruction by extrinsic pressure due to a large tumour. All these factors influence prognosis adversely, and this is reflected in the reduced 3,5- and 10-year survival rates of cases with absent radiological evidence of secretion (RICHES *et al.*, 1951).

ϰ) Fever

Prolonged pyrexia occurred in 12 of 103 cases reported by GRIFFITHS and THACKRAY (1949) and its presence suggests a poor prognosis. Only 2 of the 12 cases survived five years, 8 dying in less than twelve months.

λ) Duration of symptoms

Patients with symptoms of long duration often have a relatively good prognosis whilst those with a short history often have highly malignant and rapidly advancing growths. Out of 54 cases with a history of less than six months 34 had lymph node or distant metastases, and of 6 cases with a history extending over five to ten years none had such metastases (PETKOVIC, 1959). FLOCKS and KADESKY (1957) in a series of 137 treated cases related duration of symptoms to prognosis. The survival rate is seen to fall with increasing length of history up to two years, after which it steadily rises up to ten years. This merely reflects the natural history of the tumour and relatively good prognosis of the more slowly growing lesions. Similar findings have been obtained in other tumours such as cancer of the breast (Bloom, 1950) and bladder (Payne, 1959).

g) Investigations in cases of suspected renal tumour

Any one of the symptoms of haematuria, pain or tumour should lead to a full investigation of the renal tract. The presence of unexplained pyrexia, of polycythaemia or of a tumour in the lung, bone or elsewhere, suggestive of metastatic origin, should point to the kidney as the possible primary site. In such cases the aim is to establish the site of the lesion, to differentiate between tumour and non-neoplastic conditions, to define the type of renal tumour and to determine the extent of the disease. The following investigations are available:

Cystoscopy during haematuria.
Intravenous pyelography.
Chest radiograph.
Routine cystoscopy.
Retrograde pyelography.
Aortography.
Perirenal gas insufflation.
Exfoliative cytology.
Renal biopsy.

α) Intravenous pyelography

The preliminary roentgen film of the abdomen may reveal enlargement, deformity or displacement of the renal shadow, a calculus and, occasionally, calcification within the tumour itself. Intravenous pyelography will indicate the affected side, suggest the presence of a space-occupying lesion, and show whether the other kidney is functioning normally or not. Absence of secretion on the affected side is of ominous prognostic significance.

β) Retrograde pyelography

This examination is essential if there is no excretion on intravenous pyelography or if the result is doubtful. It will help to distinguish between a parenchymal and a pelvic tumour. The chief changes produced by a parenchymal neoplasm are compression, displacement, elongation and obliteration of the calyces. Secondary dilatation of the pelvis and calyces may result from extrinsic ureteric obstruction. A tumour of the renal pelvis produces a filling defect and seldom gives rise to an enlarged renal outline. An uneven distribution of contrast medium is suggestive of a papillary growth, whilst the presence of stones favours a squamous cell neoplasm. Retrograde pyelography may reveal associated tumours in the ureter, especially if they occur in the upper and middle thirds.

γ) Aortography

This investigation will help to establish the diagnosis when doubt still remains regarding the presence of a tumour following intravenous and retrograde pyelography (see review by Riches, 1955). The chief value of aortography is in differentiating a parenchymal tumour from a solitary cyst. A tumour is vascular and there is pooling of contrast medium in venous spaces. A cyst, on the other hand, is avascular and produces a clear area with displacement of normal vessels.

δ) Perirenal insufflation

Air or oxygen is injected into the retroperitoneal tissues in front of the sacrum and will serve to outline the kidneys and the adrenals. This investigation will help to distinguish between intra and extra-renal lesions and will reveal the presence of perirenal infiltration.

ε) Exfoliative cytology

In cases of unexplained haematuria the sediment of urine obtained by ureteric catheterisation may show clumps of abnormal looking cells suggestive of tumour. Such a finding led BASSOW (1956) to perform a nephrectomy, and on examination of the specimen a small transitional cell carcinoma, a mere 4 mm in diameter, was found in the upper major calyx. The normal transitional cells lining the urinary tract show considerable variation and have been responsible for a large number of false positive examinations of the urinary sediment. It is much more difficult to make a diagnosis of carcinoma of the renal pelvis or parenchyma, especially the latter, based on exfoliative cells, than in the case of bladder tumours (GRAHAM et al., 1950; WEIYRAUCH and PRESTI, 1956). Anaplastic transitional and squamous tumour cells of the renal pelvis can be more readily identified in the urine than the cells shed from well differentiated tumours, which are practically impossible to distinguish from the normal urinary epithelium. Even adenocarcinomas of the kidney frequently give rise to false negative and, occasionally, false positive results (HARRISON et al., 1951).

ζ) Percutaneous renal biopsy

Several authors consider this to be a safe and valuable procedure (BOHNE et al., 1958; MUEHRCKE et al., 1955), but so far it has not been widely used in this country where exploration is preferred for cases where the diagnosis remains in doubt after full radiological investigation. Some authors have condemned needle biopsy as being dangerous owing to the possible risk of dissemination.

h) Differential diagnosis of renal tumours

Carcinoma of the colon, tumours of the adrenal gland, retroperitoneal sarcomas, hepatic enlargement and splenomegaly must be differentiated from renal lesions. Cystic disease of the kidney, hydronephrosis, calculi, tuberculosis and pyelonephritis have to be differentiated from parenchymal or pelvic tumours. Rarely a blood clot, infarct (FRAENKEL, 1956), or dilated calyx in hydrocalycosis may simulate a tumour on the intravenous pyelogram. Leukoplakia, in the absence of a tumour, may give rise to symptoms of ureteric obstruction (POLITANO, 1956). It is most important to remember that although the aortogram may indicate the presence of a solitary cyst this does not exclude tumour, since in some instances adenocarcinomatous tissue will be found in its walls. Such a lesion is more likely to be present in cysts containing blood and has been reported in 25–30% of such cases (WHITMORE, 1936; LOWSLEY, 1955).

Patients with papillary tumours of the bladder should be suspected of having similar lesions elsewhere in the urinary tract, and intravenous pyelography should be carried out in all such cases as a routine. Fortunately, bilateral tumours of the kidney are rare. They have been reported more often in adenocarcinoma and nephroblastoma than in tumours arising from urothelium. Multiple dissimilar tumours have been reported in the same kidney (PENNISI et al., 1957).

i) Treatment

The mortality from renal adenocarcinoma remains high because so many cases are at an advanced stage when they first attend hospital. The inoperability rate in the large series of cases studied by RICHES and his colleagues (1951) was 28%. Although surgery offers the only real hope of cure in these tumours ancillary radiotherapy appears to be of considerable value, especially in cases with tumours of high grade malignancy. Even in the presence of known metastases it is sometimes worthwhile performing nephrectomy to relieve local symptoms. Not infrequently metastases progress very slowly and, on rare occasions, regress following removal of the primary tumour.

Although many deaths take place in the first two years following treatment of the primary tumour local recurrence or the appearance of metastases after five years is quite common. Patients treated for renal adenocarcinoma should be followed up at regular intervals for signs of metastases in order that surgery can be promptly undertaken for a suitable solitary deposit. Extirpation of such a lesion in the brain, lung or skeleton gives a small chance of cure to what is otherwise a hopeless case.

α) Surgery

The principles of treating a case of renal parenchymal carcinoma have evolved over the past two decades so that the operation has now developed into one of minimal operative trauma, combined with control of venous drainage and excision of the lymphatic fields, the so-called radical nephrectomy.

Rough handling through an inadequate incision, unnecessary retraction and compression of the kidney in an attempt to reach the renal pedicle, exposure of the growth by stripping the renal capsule, all lead to dissemination of tumour, particularly when the tumour has already begun to invade the renal vein. Adequate exposure is the first requisite in the operative procedure.

Involvement of the renal vein is a factor of grave prognostic importance. Sometimes the growth is prolapsing along the lumen and sometimes the growth is adherent to the wall of the vein. When there is tumour lying free in the vein it is essential that this be removed with the kidney as a single block. It is, therefore, necessary to expose the renal pedicle and to palpate the renal vein at an early stage in the operation.

The surgical approach may be either purely abdominal, abdomino-thoracic or abdominal with mobilisation of the thoracic cage. Whatever approach is used the early and gentle exposure of the renal pedicle is essential.

The operative mortality for nephrectomy in all adenocarcinoma cases is 4 or 5%. It is considerably greater in patients with growth involving the renal vein than in those without this complication (13% compared with 3% in the series reported by Riches et al., 1951). The major cause of death in these cases is pulmonary embolism.

Lymphatic drainage from the kidney is to the para-aortic nodes around the renal pedicle. When the pedicle is clamped and ligatured with a mass of surrounding tissue it is impossible to get a clear dissection of the para-aortic nodes. The perfect operation aims at the dissection of the vena cava or aorta, both below and above the renal pedicle, the isolation of the components of the pedicle and the separate ligation of vein and artery.

αα) Inoperability

The decision as to whether a tumour is operable or inoperable can frequently be made before operation. Clinical examination may reveal a mass which does not move on respiration. This type of case may be associated with symptoms of back or loin pain. When the tumour has burst through the capsule to become adherent to the back muscles or the lateral aspects of the vertebra there is usually involvement of the renal vein. When this has occurred there may be no evidence of kidney function on intravenous pyelography. The diagnosis will be made on a retrograde pyelogram and then it is essential that pictures be taken both in inspiration and expiration, if possible with the patient supine and erect. A fixed kidney should not be explored without an attempt to improve the chances of operability by a preliminary course of radiotherapy.

ββ) Palliative nephrectomy

Where there is already evidence of metastatic spread this operation will have strictly limited indications. Where the tumour is technically operable and where the course of the disease has not been fulminating, the presence of lung or bone metastases is no contraindication to nephrectomy. There are some recorded cases of apparent disappearance of lung metastases after this operation (Mann, 1948; Arcomano et al., 1958; Hollahan, 1959).

A large adherent renal mass which is producing pain, haemorrhage and perhaps fever is sometimes worth removing even if there has been little change following palliative irradiation, and even in the presence of limited slowly developing metastases. Some authors, however, do not favour nephrectomy for inoperable tumours, nor for patients in whom metastases have been demonstrated (BRAASCH and GRIFFIN, 1936; ROYCE and TORMEY, 1955). Of 28 nephrectomies performed for inoperable cases the last named authors found 72% were dead within 12 months and 93% within 2 years: There were no survivors beyond 3 years. In some circumstances, however, the quality of life may be considerably improved if not actually lengthened by this operation.

β) Radiotherapy

Post-operative irradiation. Nephrectomy should be performed without delay in operable cases and followed by a course of radical external irradiation to the renal bed and regional para-aortic lymph nodes. Although renal adenocarcinoma has generally been regarded as highly radio-resistant, there is now good evidence that such tumours show a limited response to irradiation (BIXLER *et al.*, 1944; RICHES *et al.*, 1951; FLOCKS and KADESKY, 1957).

Post-operative radiotherapy appears to be especially of value in patients with tumours of high grade malignancy, in those showing renal vein or lymph node involvement and where the tumour has infiltrated into the perirenal tissues. It is doubtful whether radiotherapy is of value in cases where the tumour appears clinically to be confined to the kidney. It will not be possible to fully evaluate the role of post-operative irradiation in such cases until a carefully controlled clinical trial has been undertaken. Sufficient cases for such a study could only be collected through the co-operation of a number of large centres. From what information is available at the present time, however, we feel that such cases should not be denied the chance of benefit from supplementary irradiation, in view of the possibility of occult spread or of spill of malignant cells at operation.

RICHES and his associates (1951), in their large series of collected cases, found an increased survival rate at 3,5 and 10 years in those cases given post-operative irradiation (Table 6). Furthermore, this benefit appears to have been greatest in the more unfavour-

Table 6. *Renal adenocarcinoma, prognosis according to stage and treatment* (RICHES et al., 1951; B.A.U.S. Series)

Treatment	Renal vein	Vein involved			Vein free			Total		
		year			year			year		
		3	5	10	3	5	10	3	5	10
Nephrectomy alone	cases	113	79	50	372	266	127	485	345	177
	alive (%)	28	16	6	49	35	21	44	30	17
Nephrectomy and post-operative irradiation	cases	16	11	4	62	42	11	78	53	15
	alive (%)	44	36	25	55	50	27	53	49	27

able group of cases i.e. those with tumours of high grade malignancy and those showing renal vein involvement (RICHES, 1954). FLOCKS and KADESKY (1957) obtained results which also pointed to the value of post-operative irradiation in renal adenocarcinoma (Table 7).

Technique. Adenocarcinoma of the kidney is relatively radio-resistant and a high dose is required to be effective. It is difficult to achieve this satisfactorily, especially in obese people, with conventional roentgen rays in the 200–250 kV range. Supervoltage equipment offers a considerable advantage in the greater depth dose possible, the better definition of the beam, which will enable the dose to the remaining kidney to be reduced even

Table 7. *Renal adenocarcinoma, prognosis according to treatment* (Flocks and Kadesky, 1957)

Treatment	5-year results		10-year results	
	cases	alive	cases	alive
Nephrectomy alone	56	48%	39	23%
Nephrectomy and irradiation	40	53%	27	33%

further, and finally the skin-sparing effect. Using a cobalt-60 unit or roentgen rays in the 2–4 MeV range a maximum tumour dose of between 5500–6000 R is delivered to the renal bed in approximately six weeks. Three to four fields 7.5×15–10×20 cm are used and arranged so as to include the para-aortic nodes, but to avoid the opposite kidney (Figs. 1 and 2). This treatment is generally well-tolerated, even as an out-patient, although some loss of appetite for solid food, nausea and malaise may occur. Such symptoms are seldom severe but, if troublesome, tranquilisor or antihistamine drugs often prove of value. The risk of radiation sickness can be reduced by starting treatment with small doses which are gradually increased until a weekly tumour dose of between 800 and 1000 R is being given. The white blood count should be watched as leukopenia may develop, necessitating a few days rest from treatment.

Pre-operative irradiation. Whereas post-operative irradiation aims at destroying residual malignant cells, the purpose of pre-operative treatment is to prepare the field for surgery by reducing the size and fixity of the tumour, thereby rendering its removal less difficult. The second aim of this treatment is to decrease the viability of tumour cells so that any spilt in the surrounding tissues or dislodged in vessels at the time of operation will fail to take root and perish. Pre-operative irradiation has been advocated for renal adenocarcinoma by Munger (1938), Waters et al. (1934) and Dean (1937). At the present time this is generally not given for operable cases in whom there is no contraindication to immediate surgery. On the other hand, pre-operative irradiation appears to be of considerable value in certain border-line cases, especially those with large tumours and with evidence of perirenal fixation (Riches, 1956). A dose of 3000–4000 R in three to four weeks may be delivered to the greater part of the tumour using either hard quality conventional roentgen rays or supervoltage equipment, after which nephrectomy is performed, if technically possible. When the scar has healed the irradiation is continued to a further tumour dose of 3000 R in three to four weeks. When pre-operative irradiation is indicated we prefer to deliver the entire course of treatment before surgery is undertaken. With 2 MeV roentgen rays a maximum tumour dose of between 5500 and 6000 R is given in 6 weeks.

Irradiation alone. Irradiation as the sole treatment for the primary renal tumour can, at best, be only palliative. Some shrinkage of the mass may occur with reduction in pain and cessation of haemorrhage, and at the same time life may be prolonged. Untreated, inoperable cases have little chance of surviving much beyond a year. Irradiation in such cases appeared to prolong life in the series reported by Riches et al. (1951) (Table 8).

Table 8. *Renal adenocarcinoma, prognosis in advanced cases* (Riches et al., 1951; B.A.U.S. Series)

	Untreated			Radiotherapy		
	year			year		
	1	3	5	1	3	5
Cases	362	330	198	83	70	48
Alive (%)	33	3	0.5	59	13	6

Skeletal metastases should be treated but, although pain is usually reduced or completely relieved following irradiation, the osteolytic deposits rarely show much radiological evidence of tumour regression and recalcification. Pathological fractures of the femoral

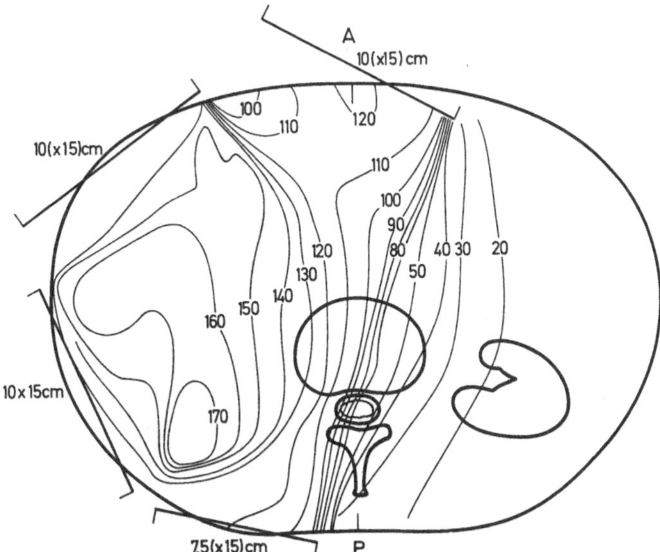

Fig. 1 and 2. Renal adenocarcinoma radical post-operative external irradiation

Fig. 1. Field distribution and summated isodose pattern for four-field conventional roentgen ray technique. Factors: 250 kV; HVL, 3.5 mm Cu; FSD, 50 cm. Dose: renal bed, max. 5000 R/min, 4100 R; para-aortic nodes, 3500 R; contralateral kidney, max. 590 R; skin, incident 3000 R. Time: 6 weeks

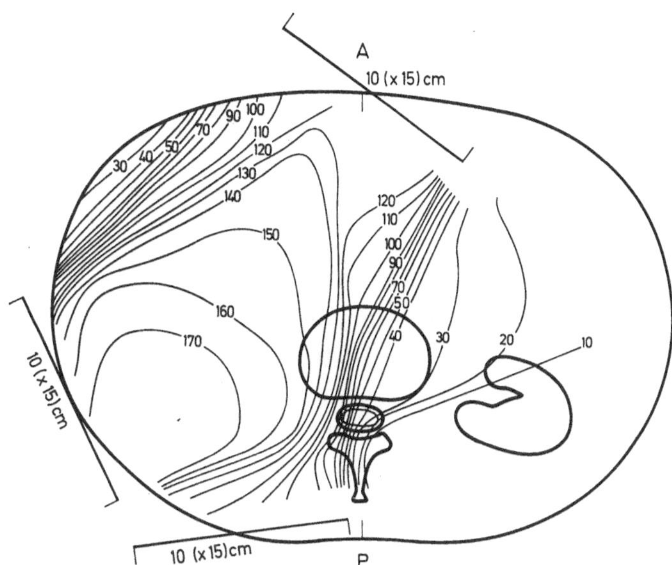

Fig. 2. Field distribution and summated isodose pattern for three-field supervoltage roentgen ray technique. Factors: 2 MeV; HVL, 11.7 mm Cu; FSD, 67 cm. Dose: renal bed, max. 5500 R/min, 5000 R; para-aortic nodes, 4200 R; contralateral kidney, max. 320 R; skin, peak incident 3200 R. Time: 6 weeks

neck can be promptly stabilised by internal fixation using a SMITH-PETERSEN nail or in the case of the shaft of the femur or humerus by a KÜNTSCHER pin. Irradiation is then given to the region of the metastasis in an attempt to arrest further tumour growth and perhaps permit some degree of bone healing. A combination of internal fixation and external irradiation leads to early ambulation (DEVAS et al., 1956). For prolonged relief of pain and disability from skeletal metastases, a dose of 4000–4500 R is required with conventional roentgen rays (HVL. $=3.5$ mm Cu) in approximately four weeks. Doses of less than 3000 R are soon followed by reactivation of the tumour with recurrence of symptoms. If feasible, surgery and not irradiation should be considered for an apparently solitary metastasis, especially if it is the sole manifestation of the disease several years after removal of the primary tumour. Irradiation of peripheral metastatic lymph nodes may be followed by regression, sometimes lasting for several years. There is no doubt that adequate treatment of metastases in cases of slowly progressive renal adenocarcinoma is rewarding, since such cases are often able to return to full employment for a period of one to two years and perhaps even longer.

γ) Chemotherapy

At the present time no useful palliation has been reported following administration of chemotherapeutic agents such as members of the Nitrogen Mustard group of drugs.

j) Results of treatment

The overall survival rate at five years for patients treated for renal adenocarcinoma is between 30 and 45% and for ten years approximately 20–25% (Table 9).

Table 9. *Renal adenocarcinoma, published results of treatment*

Author	5-year results		10-year results	
	cases	alive	cases	alive
PRIESTLEY (1939)	357	38%	253	27%
BIXLER et al. (1944)	64	36%	—	—
FOOT et al. (1949)	37	41%	17	23%
DICK and FLINT (1951)	36	46%	—	—
RICHES et al. (1951)	446	30%	192	18%
GOLDSTEIN (1956)	77	31%	—	—
FLOCKS and KADESKY (1957)	137	41%	101	23%
HUMPHREYS and FOOT (1960)	165	35%	104	18%

3. Nephroblastoma

(Synonyms: Wilms' Tumour; Embryonal Sarcoma)

a) Historical

This tumour was described by GAIRDNER in 1828 under the term "fungus haematoides in the kidney". The first accurate description was given by EBERTH (1872) and in 1899 MAX WILMS wrote a monograph on the subject and suggested the tumour's origin from undifferentiated mesoderm.

b) Incidence

Nephroblastoma constitutes about 10% of all renal tumours and approximately 20% of all malignant tumours in childhood. In approximately 3% of cases the tumour is bilateral. SHEACH (1953) enumerated 19 cases with bilateral tumours reported in the literature and added one of his own. The sexes are affected with equal frequency. The vast majority of tumours occur in the first five years of life, the average age being three. Some 12% of cases are children less than 12 months old, and approximately 5% occur in adults (KLAPPROTH, 1959). Cases of nephroblastoma have been reported in the foetus (NICHOLSON, 1931) and in the new-born infant (WELLS, 1940). ANNAMUNTHODO and HUTCHINGS (1957) report such a tumour in a six-day old male negro infant treated by nephrectomy; the child was alive and well two and a half years later. CAMPBELL (1951) reported a seventeen-year survival following nephrectomy in a child aged six weeks. CULP and HARTMAN (1948) were able to find 89 adult cases in the world literature and added 8 of their own. The tumour has been reported as late as the ninth decade (CLAY, 1930). Adult patients with nephroblastoma are rare, and WILLIS (1948) warns that few such cases reported in the literature withstand critical examination.

FITZGERALD and HARDIN (1955) reviewed five familial cases of nephroblastoma in the literature and reported the tumour appearing in a father and two daughters, being bilateral in one of the children. GAULIN (1951) presented simultaneous nephroblastoma in identical twins aged fifteen months.

c) Histogenesis

The nephroblastoma is of mesenchymal origin and arises from embryonic renal tissue. It is likely that most of these tumours develop during intrauterine life. NICHOLSON (1931) regarded the tumour as being a developmental malformation in which growth is continuous and differentiation aborted. Primitive nephrogenic tissue may be especially susceptible to neoplastic change since nephroblastomas have also been described in white rats (OLCOTT, 1950) swine, and chickens (FELDMAN, 1932).

d) Pathology

α) Macroscopic appearances

A small nephroblastoma is a rarity. Most are large by the time the child is first seen, often occupying a major portion of the abdomen. The tumour replaces the kidney substance forming a smooth, slightly lobulated mass, often with a pseudo-capsule. The cut surface reveals a soft friable growth which is usually greyish-pink in colour and often contains cystic, gelatinous and haemorrhagic areas. The renal pelvis may be compressed, but is usually not directly invaded until late. Rarely, nephroblastoma occurs in association with cystic disease of the kidney (USON et al., 1960).

β) Microscopic appearances

A variety of tissues are present showing varying degress of differentiation. Clumps of undifferentiated epithelial cells are common, in places often showing primitive or abortive glomerular and tubular structures. In some cases well-developed tubules composed of cuboidal of columnar cells are seen. An abundant spindle cell stroma is found with varying degrees of differentiation to connective tissue, muscle fibres, cartilage and bone. A special feature of many of these tumours is the presence of striated muscle fibres. Invasion of blood vessels is common and is of ominous significance. The histological appearance of metastases may differ greatly from that of the primary tumour, but this is to be expected in view of the variety of elements present in the latter.

e) Natural history

Nephroblastoma infiltrates the renal capsule and invades the surrounding structures. Invasion of the renal vein, as in cases of adenocarcinoma, may occur, and rarely the tumour enters the inferior vena cava and may even reach the heart (KRETSCHMER, 1940). Growth had entered the renal vein in 8 % of operated cases reported by RICHES and his colleagues (1951). The most frequent sites for blood-borne metastases are the lungs, liver and skeleton. The para-aortic lymph nodes are involved more frequently than in adenocarcinoma. Recurrences following treatment nearly always appear to develop within a period defined as twice the age at treatment plus nine months (KNOX and PILLERS, 1958).

f) Clinical features

Some 95% of children with nephroblastoma are brought for medical advice within three months of the onset of symptoms (LATTIMER *et al.*, 1958). Abdominal tumour or swelling was a symptom in approximately 70% and the sole complaint in 55% of 189 cases studied by RICHES and his colleagues (1951). Pain was the next most frequent symptom, occurring in 20% of this series. Haematuria is a far less common feature than in adenocarcinoma and was present in only 18% of patients. All three symptoms, tumour, pain and haematuria, were present in 1% of cases. Gastrointestinal symptoms such as nausea and anorexia, vomiting and abdominal distension are often conspicuous and may be accompanied by anaemia, fever and loss of weight. On the other hand, in some cases specific symptoms are much less marked and a doctor is consulted because the child is pale, irritable, listless and fails to thrive.

The abdominal mass may be found accidentally by the mother whilst bathing or dressing the child. Often it is surprising how large the tumour has become before it is noticed by the parents. Occasionally, the mass is a chance finding during a general medical examination. The blood pressure may be raised and in some cases is reversed following nephrectomy. Hypertension was present in 60% of cases reported by LATTIMER *et al.* (1958) and the higher readings were noted in those children with the larger tumours. Pyrexia of a 100° F or more, measured per rectum, was recorded in 44% of the series studied by LATTIMER *et al.* (1958) and in some instances was associated with a leuko-cytosis. Abdominal examination reveals a mass in practically all cases of nephroblastoma. It is usually large and may fill more than half the abdomen. Occasionally, this tumour is associated with congenital malformations such as polycystic kidney, hare-lip, cleft palate and dextrocardia.

g) Factors influencing prognosis

α) Age

Age at the time of treatment has an important bearing on prognosis. Infants less than one year of age have a decidely better prognosis than the older children (GROSS and NEUHAUSER, 1950; HARVEY, 1950; SCOTT, 1956). From the Royal Hospital for Sick Children, Glasgow, SCOTT (1956) reported a survival rate nearly three times greater in patients aged less than one year compared with older children (Table 10). Unfortunately,

Table 10. *Nephroblastoma, age and prognosis* (SCOTT, 1956)

Age	Number of cases		2-year survival rate (%)	
	A	B	A	B
Less than 1 year	17	161	17.6	17.4
Greater than 1 year	46	844	6.5	9.1

A = Cases at Royal Hospital for Sick Children, Glasgow.
B = Collected published cases.

only about 13% of cases fall below the age of twelve months (KLAPPROTH, 1959). The prognosis in adult cases appears to be extremely grave. LIVERMORE (1953) reports that of some 100 adult cases in the literature only 5 cases have survived five years and 9 three years.

β) Duration of symptoms

There is usually little delay in seeking medical advice once the abdominal mass is found. Thus, over 90% of children are brought to the doctor within three months of the onset of symptoms. It is interesting to note that 3 of the 6 survivors reported by Scott (1956) were admitted to hospital within forty-eight hours of the appearance of the first symptom.

γ) Haematuria

This occurs in about 20 % of cases and is a bad omen, indicating involvement of the renal pelvis and, therefore, a late stage in the natural history of the tumour. With few exceptions such cases die within twelve months (Scott, 1956).

δ) Gross pathological factors

The highest survival rate is seen in cases with tumours which appear to be well-encapsulated. Large size, per se, is not necessarily indicative of a bad prognosis, but gross extension, lymph node invasion, penetration of the renal vein and rupture of the capsule at operation are all unfavourable features.

ε) Histology

Attempts to correlate the histological findings with prognosis at the Children's Hospital Boston, have proved fruitless (Gross, 1953).

ζ) Bilateral tumours

Simultaneous or consecutive bilateral tumours occur in 3–4 % of cases (Scott, 1955). The prognosis would appear to be quite hopeless in such cases, but Gross (1953) reports a patient who is alive and well twelve years after a right-sided nephrectomy and radiotherapy to the left kidney.

h) Diagnosis and differential diagnosis

Although nephroblastoma should be suspected in any young child with a unilateral abdominal swelling, a number the other tumours and non-neoplastic conditions will have to be considered in the differential diagnosis. These include neuroblastoma, congenital hydronephrosis, cystic kidney, retroperitoneal tumours and cysts, and splenomegaly or hepatomegaly.

In a series of 653 infants and children with palpable abdominal masses reviewed by Melicow and Uson (1959), 21 % arose in the urinary tract, and of these 40 % were due to hydronephrosis, 30 % to nephroblastoma and 22 % to polycystic disease. Medical conditions causing enlargement of the liver, spleen and lymph glands accounted for 57 % of the entire series.

Neuroblastomas arising in the adrenal medulla occur with approximately the same frequency as nephroblastoma and appear in children of the same age group. This tumour, however, does not usually reach such large proportions as the renal tumour and tends to metastasize at an earlier stage. The liver and skeleton are commonly involved in neuroblastoma, whereas in the case of nephroblastoma the lungs and regional lymph nodes are the site of deposits. Calcification within the primary tumour, which is a common finding in neuroblastoma, is a rare event in the renal tumour. Neuroblastoma tends to produce an irregular mass with a nodular surface and poorly defined borders, and may extend across the mid-line. A nephroblastoma, on the other hand, has a smoother spherical, frequently lobulated, well-defined contour and extends over the mid-line less frequently. Sometimes a neuroblastoma involves the kidney or ureter (Harrison et al., 1950) and may simulate a primary renal tumor.

Excretory pyelography is necessary to assist in establishing the diagnosis of a renal tumour and to assess the presence and normality of the contralateral kidney. In very small infants satisfactory visualisation can be achieved by subcutaneous or intramuscular injection of Diodone with hyaluronidase to increase the rate of absorption. There may be compression of the pelvis and distortion of the calyceal pattern with displacement of the ureter medially. Absence of secretion is rare in nephroblastoma and retrograde pyelographic studies are only necessary in very few cases. Neuroblastoma may invade the kidney and distort the calyces and pelvis, but in so doing usually displaces the kidney downwards and outwards. In some cases the differential diagnosis between renal and adrenal tumour will remain in doubt until exploratory laparotomy is performed.

Adenocarcinoma of the kidney is an exceedingly rare tumour of childhood. Hempstead et al. (1953) reviewed the literature and reported two new cases. In the series of renal tumours collected by Riches and his colleagues (1951) there were 1735 renal adenocarcinomas and only one of these occurred in a child, aged 11. Clinton-Thomas and Robinson (1956) have recently reported a case of a 10-year old Chinese girl with a renal adenocarcinoma, the clinical features of which suggested a diagnosis of neuroblastoma.

i) Treatment

Several treatment regimes have been advocated for nephroblastoma. Surgery alone, irradiation alone, or a combination of surgery and irradiation, which is given either before or after the operation or on both occasions. There is now general agreement that nephrectomy is necessary for cure in these tumours, that irradiation facilitates surgery and reduces the operative risk in patients with large adherent tumours, and that postoperative irradiation is essential if extirpation is suspected of being incomplete. The controversy which exists centres chiefly around the value of pre-operative irradiation in operable cases, and the place of post-operative irradiation in cases in whom the tumour appears to have been completely removed. Abeshouse (1957) carried out a national survey in the United States on the subject of treatment of nephroblastoma, and 81 surgeons replied to his questionnaire covering an experience of 858 cases. Nephrectomy alone was employed in only 5% of cases, nephrectomy and post-operative irradiation in 44%, pre and post-operative irradiation in 22% and pre-operative irradiation in 10%. It is evident that the trend is towards nephrectomy and post-operative irradiation.

Nephroblastoma is remarkably radiosensitive and striking regression usually occurs following treatment. Nevertheless, complete destruction of a large growth is difficult to achieve, probably because of the varying radiosensitivity of the different histological components which are to be found in these tumours. Some twenty years ago the prognosis of nephroblastoma was generally regarded as being hopeless, the mortality being quoted at over 90% (Walker, 1935; Hyman, 1933; Kerr, 1939). Since about 1940 the results of treatment have improved due, no doubt, to the wider use of ancilliary irradiation in adequate doses together with, of course, advances in surgical technique and post-operative care. Scott (1956) reports a two year survival rate of 2.6% prior to 1945 at the Royal Hospital for Sick Children, Glasgow. After this period irradiation was used and the survival rate increased to 20%. The same author reviews the results of treatment in cases collected from the literature according to three different periods (Table 11). Nowadays

Table 11. *Nephroblastoma results in collected cases (treated and untreated)* (Scott, 1956)

Period	Cases	2-year survival rate
Before 1935	458	8.5%
1935—1944	411	18.0%
1945—1954	712	22.2%
Total	1581	17.1%

between 25 and 40% of patients have been reported as surviving two or more years (Riches et al., 1951; Flocks and Kadesky, 1957; Lattimer et al., 1958). The highest rate is given by GROSS and NEUHAUSER (1950) who report 47% for nephrectomy and post-operative irradiation from the Children's Hospital, Boston. Treated cases surviving for periods between 15–30 years are to be found in several reports. Thus RICHES *et al.* (1951) mentions 4 of 11 cases with a prolonged follow-up as surviving 14, 15, 17 and 22 years after nephrectomy. KLAPPROTH (1959) had two survivors, 24 and 29 years after treatment, among 45 cases from the Cleveland Clinic.

α) Irradiation alone

Prolonged survival following treatment by irradiation has been reported in the literature (DEAN, 1945; POHLE and RITCHIE, 1935; KERR, 1939). SAUER (1948) and also NESBIT and ADAMS (1946) each report a ten-year survival in a histologically proven case of nephro-blastoma following irradiation alone. General experience, however, has been that sooner or later recurrence occurs when irradiation has been the sole method of treatment. Most cases treated in this way are advanced and recurrence is, therefore, not surprising. The vast majority of children with nephroblastoma have large masses and to achieve eradi-cation by irradiation is difficult. Examination of the residue following irradiation indi-cates that certain histological elements appear to be more radio-resistant to treatment than others.

Irradiation has not been given the opportunity of demonstrating its effectiveness as the sole method of treatment in operable cases. From what information we have concerning the results of irradiation alone, compared with those for surgery and radiotherapy, and knowing the present day low operative risk of nephrectomy, the concensus of opinion is against irradiation as the chief treatment.

β) Surgery alone

Sole reliance on nephrectomy for the treatment of nephroblastoma is now becoming uncommon, most cases being referred for post-operative irradiation. If a tumour appears to have been completely extirpated and there is no invasion of the renal capsule and no evidence of vascular or lymph node involvement, then ancilliary irradiation appears to be of questionable value. At the present time, however, we do not favour surgery alone as the treatment of choice for operable tumours because of the doubt we feel in being able to achieve complete removal of a large mass of malignant tissue and of being certain that no microscopic, local and lymph node spread has taken place. RICHES and his colleagues (1951) are among the very few authors reporting better results for surgery alone in these tumours. The operative mortality has been reduced from 36% (WALKER, 1897) to no operative deaths in a twenty year period at the Boston Children's Hospital (GROSS, 1953). Generally speaking the overall operative mortality is now between 2 and 3% (ABESHOUSE, 1957). Age is no bar to nephrectomy and the operation has been successfully performed in an infant 72 hours old (BROGAN, 1947).

γ) Pre-operative irradiation

LADD and WHITE (1941) and GROSS and NEUHAUSER (1950) do not favour pre-operative irradiation and claim that it is possible to carry out nephrectomy in all cases of nephro-blastoma without the assistance of preliminary shrinkage. GROSS (1953) is against pre-operative irradiation for two reasons, firstly operation is delayed during which time metastases may develop and secondly, liquifaction of the tumour may increase the risk of dissemination. In his experience pre-operative irradiation is detrimental, the mortality being increased when a dose of 2000—3000 R was delivered in a period of 10–15 days.

The argument that the delay in operation caused by pre-operative irradiation increases the risk of metastases is not tenable, in our opinion, since the three to four weeks required for irradiation is in all probability but a small fraction in the life-time of the tumour, many of which probably arise in utero. There is no doubt that extirpation in some cases is greatly facilitated and the operative risk reduced by preliminary irradiation which reduces the size and vascularity of the tumour and often improves the general condition of the child. Most general surgeons welcome the assistance afforded by irradiation. Furthermore, it is possible that preliminary irradiation reduces the chance of malignant cells which have been disseminated during the operation gaining a footing and developing as local recurrences or distant metastases. During the period of pre-operative irradiation it is important that the child shall not be subjected to frequent abdominal palpation, and that every effort is made to protect it from intercurrent infection.

Operation is usually carried out three to four weeks after completing treatment, but some authors advise an interval of four to six weeks, whilst others, such as Kerr and Flynn (1956) and also Paterson (1948), suggest that at least two to three months should elapse before operation is undertaken. We feel that a tumour which responds rapidly to irradiation is best removed as soon as it is deemed to be more amenable to surgery, and the patient's general condition has improved.

δ) Post-operative irradiation

Published results are generally in agreement that nephrectomy and post-operative irradiation gives better results than surgery alone. Experience at the Boston Children's Hospital supports this view, although the number of cases in each group is small and the follow-up short (Table 12). In "period B" the better results were due to improvements in

Table 12. *Nephroblastoma results of treatment, Boston Children's Hospital* (Gross, 1953)

Period	Cases	2-year cure rate according to age (%)		
		< 12 months	> 12 months	total
A (1914—1930)	27	43	5	15
B (1931—1939)	31	71	21	32
C (1940—1947)	38	80	43	47

surgical technique and operative care, there being no operative deaths after 1931, compared with an operative mortality of 23% for "period A". In "period C" the surgical procedure was essentially the same as in B, but in the former, post-operative irradiation had been given to all but two cases.

Post-operative irradiation should be started as soon as possible. At the Boston Children's Hospital the first treatment is given before the child has recovered from the anaesthetic. Other centres, including ourselves, prefer to wait a few days or at least until the wound is soundly healed.

ε) Pre- and post-operative irradiation

Collected statistics from the literature reviewed by Harvey (1950), Scott (1956) and Abeshouse (1957) suggest that a combination of pre and post-operative irradiation may be the treatment of choice for nephroblastoma. This is supported by the preliminary results of Ng and Low-Beer (1956) who obtained a two-year survival rate of 88% in a small number of cases. These authors advocated nephrectomy three to four weeks after the initial irradiation and they commenced the course of post-operative irradiation one to two weeks after nephrectomy. This method of treatment combines the advantages of pre-operative irradiation (decrease in size, vascularity and viability of tumour) with those of post-operative irradiation (control of residual tumour in the renal bed or local spread to regional lymph nodes).

ζ) Conclusions regarding treatment

From the evidence available at the present time we advise immediate nephrectomy in small to average sized operable tumours, followed by a course of irradiation, starting as soon as the child has recovered from the operation. In the case of larger tumours pre-operative irradiation should be instituted, and nephrectomy performed as soon as the tumour is smaller and more mobile following a maximum tumour dose of 2000–2500 R in three to four weeks. Post-operative irradiation is indicated in such cases, a further dose of 1500 being given in approximately three weeks. When faced with inoperable tumours a radical course of irradiation is given in the first instance to a maximum tumour dose of between 3500 and 4000 R in five to six weeks. If the tumour becomes technically operable following this treatment nephrectomy should be carried out. After such doses no further irradiation should be given in the post-operative period.

η) Technique of treatment

The aim of treatment is to irradiate en bloc the renal tumour or renal bed and the regional para-aortic lymph nodes. A plan is drawn up for each case showing the site and extent of the tumour in relation to a cross-section of the abdomen. The increased depth dose from supervoltage apparatus is not necessary in infants and small children. Treatment can be planned perfectly satisfactorily with roentgen rays generated at 250 kV using a hard quality beam (HVL = 3.5 mm Cu) and two or three fields 8 × 10–10 × 15 cm, depending on the size of the tumour and the dimensions of the child (Fig. 3). It is essential to reduce the dose received by the opposite kidney to a minimum.

Treatment in the first two or three days should be restricted and limited to an anterior field to gain the confidence of the child and to reduce the risk of irradiation sickness. Starting with 50 R the dose is gradually increased until 150 R is being delivered to two fields daily. We aim to give a maximum tumour dose of between 3500 and 4000 R in five to six weeks in post-operative cases. If definite residual tumour is present following nephrectomy it is a good plan to mark its extent with metal clips at the time of operation and to attempt to deliver the maximum dose of irradiation to this restricted region. With pre-operative irradiation a dose of between 2000 and 2500 R is delivered in three to four weeks, and this is followed after nephrectomy by a further 1500 R in three weeks. With very large tumours the greater part of the abdomen may have to be covered, and in such cases it will be necessary to reduce the dose rate and total dose delivered. With two large opposing fields a depth dose of between 1500–2000 R may be given to such cases in five to six weeks. During treatment care is taken to reduce manipulation of the abdomen to a minimum. Blood counts are taken twice weekly and more often if indicated. If the total white cell count falls below 2000 it will be necessary to give a few days rest from treatment to allow the blood to recover. A blood transfusion may be required for anaemia; it is important to maintain the haemoglobin at a high level during the whole course of irradiation. It may be necessary to delay operation until the white cell count returns to normal.

ϑ) Bilateral nephroblastoma

Gross (1953) refers to such a case alive and well twelve years after nephrectomy for one tumour and irradiation for the other. Rickham of Liverpool has performed a nephrectomy on one side and a local excision on the other, the patient being alive three years later (Riches, 1958). It is dangerous to deliver a tumour lethal dose of irradiation to the remaining kidney. A dose of 3000 R, for example, is likely to produce serious renal damage leading to a fatal outcome (Beck, 1958). In the event of nephroblastoma developing in the remaining kidney it would seem best to perform a partial nephrectomy if at all possible, followed by roentgen ray therapy to the regional para-aortic lymph nodes if previous irradiation has not been given.

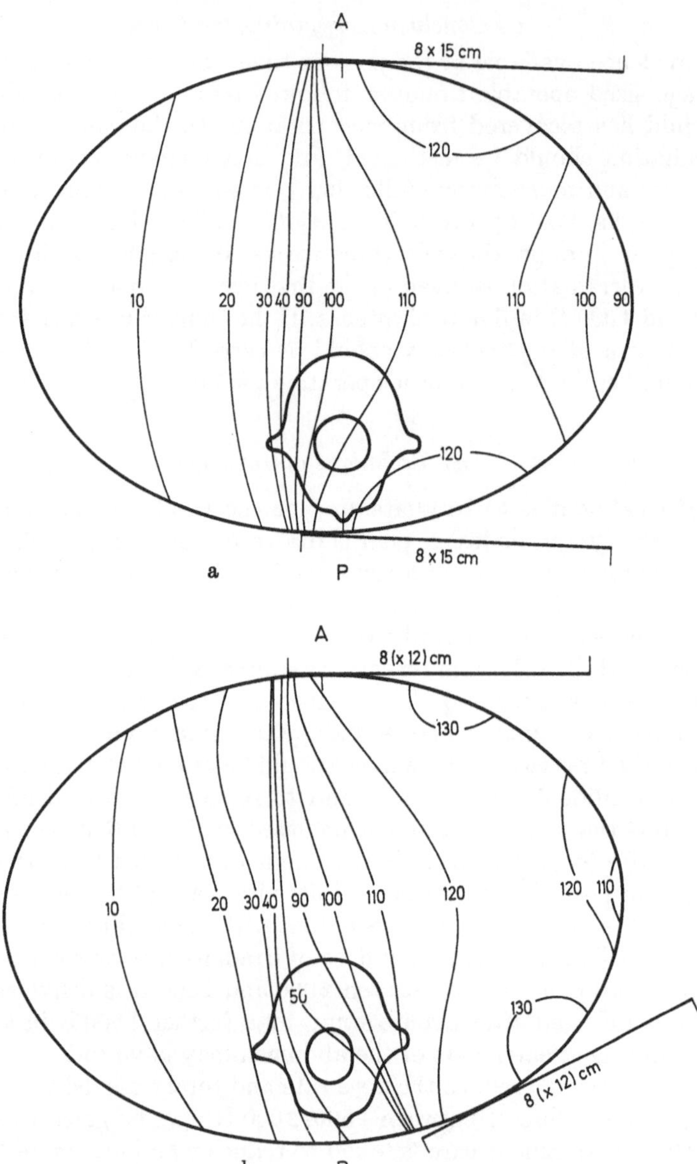

Fig. 3a and b. Nephroblastoma. Pre- and post-operative irradiation. Field distribution and summated isodose pattern for a two opposing conventional roentgen ray technique to give pre- and post-operative irradiation in a child aged 2 years. a Pre-operative irradiation. Opposing parallel anterior and posterior fields to treat large left-sided abdominal mass. Factors: 250 kV; HVL, 3.5 mm Cu; FSD, 50 cm. Dose: tumour, 2000 R; para-aortic nodes, 1800 R; contralateral kidney, max. 360 R; spinal canal, 2000 R; skin, total, 2200 R. Time: 4 weeks. b Post-operative irradiation. Anterior direct and posterior oblique fields. The new position of the posterior field reduces the dose to the contralateral kidney slightly and to the spinal cord substantially. Factors: as above. Dose: renal bed, 1500 R; para-aortic nodes, 1125 R; contralateral kidney, max. 190 R; spinal canal, 560 R; skin, 1500 R. Time: 3 weeks. Total dose: tumour, 3500 R; para-aortic nodes, 3000 R; contralateral kidney, max. 550 R; spinal canal, 2560 R; skin, 3700 R. Total time: 7 weeks

ι) Treatment of local recurrence and metastases

The lungs are the most common site for metastases in nephroblastoma, being present in 34 out of 52 cases reported by Riches and his colleagues (1951). In this series the liver was involved in 17 cases and the lymph nodes in 12. Skeletal metastases were relatively uncommon, being found in only 5 cases. There is no real evidence that pulmonary irradiation for metastases is of anything more than temporary benefit. Prophylactic irradiation of the lungs was advocated at one time in the hope of destroying malignant cells before they were able to gain a firmer footing and produce visible deposits. The amount of irradiation required to destroy such cells throughout both lung fields, however, is likely to ultimately prove lethal to the patient as a result of diffuse pulmonary fibrosis. If widespread pulmonary metastases are present irradiation is probably not worthwhile since such cases soon deteriorate. In cases of metastases localised to *one region* of the lung, however, treatment by means of two opposing fields should be tried. A depth dose of between 2000 and 3000 R may be given in three to five weeks, depending upon the volume being irradiated. NESBIT and ADAMS (1946) reported a ten-year cure following irradiation of pulmonary metastases, and KERR (1939) reported a similar case alive and well four years after such treatment. Although localised deposits in the lung are usually treated by irradiation, BOBBITT and his colleagues (1959) have recently reported the case of a child aged two who, 14 months after pre-operative irradiation and nephrectomy, developed a deposit in the right upper zone of the lung for which a lobectomy was performed; the child was alive and well three years later. No other similar case been reported in the literature.

Although pulmonary metastases usually indicate a hopeless situation the presence of residual tumour or local recurrence in the abdomen following nephrectomy does not necessarily indicate a fatal outcome. Intensive treatment or re-treatment by irradiation may destroy such lesions. FEENEY *et al.* (1955) reported a patient alive and well seven years after nephrectomy in whom excision of several recurrent tumours had been carried out.

j) Post-irradiation sequelae

Gastrointestinal disturbances may occur during treatment, but soon subside when the course of irradiation has been completed. There is often depression of bone marrow with anaemia and leukopenia, and it may be necessary to give the child a rest from treatment for a few days to enable the white cells to recover. The skin of young children is not unduly sensitive to irradiation and wound-healing is not delayed, nor are irradiation sequelae in the skin severe following the doses mentioned. Some irradiation, direct or scattered, will unavoidably be received by the gonads. We have not been able to find any observations reported in the literature on the long-term effects from this in children cured of abdominal malignant disease.

With depth doses of between 2000–3000 R in growing children abnormalities of skeletal development are to be expected. In cases treated for nephroblastoma these are to be seen in the lowest ribs, the vertebrae and ilium but, fortunately, such changes do not lead to serious physical disability (NEUHAUSER *et al.*, 1952; WHITEHOUSE and LAMPE, 1953). To avoid the possibility of scoliosis developing as a late sequelae it is best to include the whole vertebral body in the volume irradiated.

Great care must be taken in treatment planning to avoid the normal kidney. The chief renal changes produced by irradiation are degeneration of the convoluted tubules, atrophy and hyalinization of glomerular tufts and marked increase of interstitial tissue. Thickening of the larger vessels and fibrinoid necrosis of arterioles and glomerular capillaries may also occur. The clinical picture following such changes may be that of acute or chronic nephritis and benign or malignant hypertension (LUXTON, 1953).

k) Chemotherapy

α) Nitrogen mustards

JOHNSON and MARSHALL (1955) have used nitrogen mustard during the post-operative period, prior to radiotherapy, in patients with nephroblastoma. These authors report that of 10 patients surviving two years 4 had received nitrogen mustard. The aim of such chemotherapy is to destroy circulating tumour cells and occult metastases. It is too early to express an opinion as to the value of this group of agents, but on theoretical grounds it would seem justifiable to pursue this study further. Their danger lies in depressing the white cells of the blood and thereby delaying the onset of post-operative irradiation.

β) Vitamin B12

Schneider (1958) has suggested that this vitamin may be of value in cases of nephroblastoma. He bases this view on its use for neuroblastoma (Bodian, 1957) and the fact that the renal tumour is also composed of embryonic cells.

γ) Actinomycin D

This antibiotic, isolated by Wakesman and his associates, has been found to produce a definite therapeutic effect in some cases of nephroblastoma. Pulmonary metastases have shown temporary regression following its administration.

There is also evidence to suggest that actinomycin enhances the effect of ionizing radiations, both with regard to normal as well as neoplastic tissues. The combined treatment has not yet been fully evaluated, but an objective response was noted in 13 of 17 cases of nephroblastoma reported by Tan et al. (1959). Of a further 16 cases treated with actinomycin D alone which were studied by these authors, 6 showed an objective response, in 5 of whom there was substantial clinical benefit. At the present time Tan and his colleagues (1959) feel that this agent should be tried in patients with metastases which are not satisfactorily controlled by roentgen ray therapy. Farber and his associates (1956) have also noted important temporary changes in children with nephroblastoma treated with actinomycin D.

Following the administration of this agent to children with various forms of malignant disease toxic manifestations involving the gastro-intestinal tract may develop in 75% of cases. Skin reactions, loss of hair and depression of bone marrow also occur in up to 40 or 50% of cases (Tan et al., 1959).

l) Results of treatment

Over 50% of treated cases of nephroblastoma die in the first year (Abeshouse, 1957). Because 85% of fatalities occur within 24 months (Klapproth, 1959; Lattimer et al., 1958) the two-year survival rate, without evidence of recurrence, provides a useful gauge of successful treatment. Although metastases may develop after an interval of 5 or more years such an event is uncommon (Flocks and Kadesky, 1957; Falkinberg et al., 1954).

There have been several collective reviews of cases reported in the world literature (Harvey, 1950; Scott, 1956; Abeshouse, 1957). The most recent one by Klapproth (1959) analysed 1351 cases between the years 1940 and 1958. Such a series has the disadvantage of being composed of cases from many centres, small and large, which have been treated by numerous surgeons and radiotherapists with varying degrees of skill and care. Nevertheless, an extensive review such as this probably reflects the overall picture more accurately than does a series from a single centre. It does not, however, reveal the best that can be achieved. In Klapproth's series (Table 13) there was little difference in

Table 13. *Nephroblastoma. Results in collected cases according to treatment.* (After Harvey, 1950)

Treatment	Cases	2-year survival rate (%)
Irradiation alone	63	16
Nephrectomy alone	180	16
Pre-operative irradiation	27	19
Post-operative irradiation	109	30
Pre- and post-operative irradiation	65	32
Total	444	22

results for case treated by irradiation before or after surgery or on both occasions. On the other hand, in the cases collected by HARVEY (1950) (Table 14), SCOTT (1956) and ABESHOUSE (1957) the best results were obtained when pre and post-operative irradiation were administered.

Table 14. *Results in collected cases according to treatment.* (After KLAPPROTH, 1959)

Treatment	Cases	"Cure" rate (%)
Nephrectomy alone	282	21
Pre-operative irradiation	103	27
Post-operative irradiation	423	26
Pre- and post-operative irradiation	145	24
Laparotomy, biopsy and irradiation	38	13
Laparotomy and/or biopsy	21	0
Irradiation alone	93	2
No treatment	117	0
Total	1222	20

4. Miscellaneous renal tumours

a) Adenoma

This is the most common type of benign renal tumour and deserves attention because of its possible relationship to adenocarcinoma. Renal adenomas have been reported as occurring in 0.25–3.87% of routine autopsies (UYS, 1956), but they are probably more common than these figures suggest. They are thought to arise from hyperplastic epithelium of the convoluted tubules in nephrosclerotic kidneys (OLIVER and LUND, 1933; OLIVER and LUEY, 1934).

Adenomas are usually multiple and often bilateral, and are generally a few millimetres in diameter and rarely exceed 2 cm. Microscopically, they show a papillary or alveolar structure and resemble an adenocarcinoma of low grade malignancy. Indeed, a differentiation between the two on purely histological grounds may be extremely difficult. The importance of these adenomas is that at least some adenocarcinomas are considered to arise from them (TRINKLE, 1936). CRISTOL et al. (1946) found adenomas in approximately only 5% of some 500 kidneys containing adenocarcinoma.

Rarely, a solitary adenoma may reach a considerable size and give rise to haematuria and pain and produce a palpable mass. CHILDS and WATERFALL (1953) found 33 cases in the literature requiring surgical removal and reported two of their own. BAUER and his colleagues (1958) reported a further case, the tumour weighing 380 g. Such cases will usually be regarded initially as renal adenocarcinoma, but the smooth outline of the filling defect seen on intravenous pyelography may suggest the presence of a benign growth.

b) Haemangioma

WALLACH and his colleagues (1959) refer to 86 cases of renal haemangioma in the literature and report a further case of their own. In such cases there may be a history of intermittent and painless haematuria extending over several years. More than half the reported cases are under the age of 40. The haemangioma is found in a calyx or at the tip of a papilla, and is usually of a cavernous or capillary type. Nephrectomy has been the usual treatment for such cases, but in about 10% of cases the lesion is multiple and may, occasionally, be bilateral. Thus POLITZ and SEWELL (1951) performed a right nephrectomy for a cavernous haemangioma and, two months after the patient's discharge from hospital, a further episode of haematuria occurred from the remaining kidney. Bleeding stopped following a course of irradiation which was carried out as a last resort, and there has been no recurrence to-date, four years later. Unfortunately, no details of the irradiation treatment were given.

c) Angiomyolipoma

These benign tumours are sometimes referred to as renal hamartomas and may be associated with tuberose sclerosis (Critchley and Earl, 1932). They are usually small symptomless lesions, but may reach a large size and give rise to haematuria (Rusche, 1952). Nephrectomy is curative.

d) Liposarcoma; fibrosarcoma; undifferentiated sarcoma

These are rare tumours which arise from the renal substance or perirenal tissue. They form large smooth or lobulated abdominal masses, often accompanied by backache, pain in the loin and abdominal distension. Where possible treatment is by nephrectomy. The outlook for fibrosarcoma is poor. Weisel et al. (1943) reported 35 cases of renal fibrosarcoma and spindle cell sarcoma treated by nephrectomy at the Mayo Clinic between 1904 and 1940; only 5 living patients could be traced. Radical post-operative supervoltage irradiation to the renal bed and regional paraaortic lymph nodes, on the lines already described for adenocarcinoma, is indicated in such cases to try and reduce the risk of local recurrence. Liposarcoma of the kidney is a very rare tumour, only about 30 cases have been reported in the world literature (see review by Williams and Savage, 1958). These tumours are most frequent in the fourth decade and in about a third of cases are associated with tuberose sclerosis. The prognosis appears to be better than for fibrosarcoma, 11 of the reported cases being alive two to twenty-three years following operation.

e) Malignant reticulosis

Primary malignant lymphoma of the kidney has yet to be proven, all cases apparently having other foci elsewhere. Wentzell and Berkheiser (1955) found renal involvement in 53% of 32 cases of malignant lymphoma among 1047 routine autopsies (Table 15).

Table 15. *Renal involvement in malignant lymphoma* (Wentzell and Berkheiser, 1955)

Type of lymphoma	Number of cases	
	total	with renal involvement
Lymphosarcoma	9	7
Reticulum cell sarcoma	6	1
Hodgkin's disease	6	2
Multiple Myeloma	1	1
Leukaemia	10	6
Total	32 (100%)	17 (53%)

The kidney may show multiple discrete deposits, diffuse infiltration or extension from retroperitoneal lymph nodes. The ureter may also be involved, usually by extrinsic pressure. Any patient with a malignant lymphoma who develops progressive renal failure should be suspected of having renal or ureteric involvement. Contrary to our experience with these tumours when they occur in the bladder, all that can be hoped for in malignant renal lymphomas is a temporary remission induced by external irradiation or chemotherapy (nitrogen mustard, chlorambucil, TEM). In a series of 50 fatal cases of leukaemia in children GOWDEY and NEUHAUSER (1948) found diffuse infiltration of the kidneys in 52%. A dose of 300–400 R from 250 kV roentgen rays was sufficient to reduce the size of the kidney in such cases.

II. Tumours of the renal pelvis and ureter

The modern concept of tumours of the urothelium arising from a field of unstable mucosa, has resulted in such tumours being regarded not as a single entity but as a manifestation of a wide-spread epithelial change. To attempt to divide these tumours into anatomical categories, especially in the case of the renal pelvis and ureter, leads to treatment which is both incomplete or inadequate. Tumours of the renal-pelvis have at the time of operation evidence of tumour formation elsewhere in the urinary tract in 40–50% of cases. Over a period of years following removal of a kidney and ureter on one side, further tumours will develop in the bladder, urethra and in the opposite pelvis and ureter in an appreciable number of patients.

1. Incidence

CABOT and ALLEN (1933) in a series of 527 primary renal tumours at the Mayo Clinic reported 9% as being of pelvic origin. A survey of 2314 renal tumours by RICHES et al. (1951) revealed 315 tumours of the renal pelvis, an incidence of 12.5%, and 21 cases of primary ureteric tumour, an incidence of 0.9%. Transitional cell tumours made up 11% (carcinoma 8%, papilloma 3%) and squamous cell carcinoma 3% of the entire series. The majority of pelvic and ureteric tumours occur in the 5th, 6th and 7th decades. In the case of transitional cell tumours males are affected three to four times more often than females. The sex incidence is approximately equal for squamous cell growths.

2. Aetiology

Since REHN first appreciated the industrial risk in workmen engaged in the manufacture of dye stuffs in 1894, further investigations have implicated a variety of chemical substances, most of which are intermediate compounds in the manufacture of dyes or antioxidants used in the hardening of rubber. Aniline itself is now believed to be non-carcinogenic but β-naphthylamine, the intermediate product, is one of the most powerful carcinogenis at present recognised. Benzidine, auramine, magneta and, more recently, 4-aminodiphenyl xenylamine have also been proved to produce tumours in workmen engaged in their manufacture.

The recognition of these substances has been rendered more difficult by the long latent period between exposure and clinical neoplasia. Thus β-naphthylamine produced tumours in workmen on the average seventeen years after the first exposure.

The institution of cytological examinations of the urine routinely in all workmen who might have been exposed, and cystoscopic examination of any workman whose urine contains malignant cells will result in earlier recognition of the developing lesion.

Although in many countries the manufacture or use of these compounds is prohibited this does not mean that in these countries there is no industrial risk. The substances mentioned are only those substances where there is now positive proof of carcinogenicity; there may be similar substances in use where clinical recognition of carcinogenicity is at present incomplete or where proof is lacking.

Smoking has been suggested as a possible predisposing factor by several authors, but the evidence is not so clear cut as in carcinoma of the lung. When cases are matched not merely for age and sex but also for social group there is little statistical difference between those patients with bladder tumours and the matched controls.

a) Experimental aetiology

β-naphthylamine has been used experimentally to produce bladder tumours in animals. These tumours mimic in every way those tumours that are the result of industrial exposure, but they also resemble those tumours which are believed to be spontaneous, i.e., where no recognised cause has been identified.

The mode of carcinogenesis is by means of metabolic breakdown and subsequent excretion in the urine. Diversion of the urine by uretero-colic anastomosis prevents the development of bladder tumours, but in the presence of a hydroureter or hydronephrosis tumours will form in the renal pelvis or ureter. The presence of stasis produced experimentally predisposes to tumour formation, an observation which has been confirmed clinically.

b) Endogenous carcinogenesis

The similarity between tumours of the urothelium produced experimentally and those which occur apparently spontaneously suggests the possibility of a urogenic factor present in the urine, which is carcinogenic. Such factors, the end products of tryptophane metabolism (3-hydroxykynurenine and 3-hydroxyanthranilic acid) resembling the metabolites of β-naphthylamine, have been identified in the urine of patients with urothelial tumours, and in preliminary work these substances have been demonstrated as being carcinogenic.

3. Pathology

The predominant tumour of the renal pelvis and ureter is a transitional cell papilloma or a papillary carcinoma. Solid infiltrating carcinomas are more commonly found in the lower ureter. Squamous cell carcinoma generally occurs in the renal pelvis, occasionally in association with renal calculus. These calculi may be primary but they can be secondary to a pelvi-ureteric stenosis, the stasis contributing to the development of both the stone and the squamous cell carcinoma.

a) Transitional cell papilloma

The renal or ureteric papilloma is composed of delicate vascular villous processes covered by a uniform layer of transitional epithelium closely resembling that of the normal urinary tract. The tumour may block the ureter and produce hydronephrosis or it may develop silently within a calyx and only give rise to symptoms when it has reached a considerable size. There is no sharp division on histological criteria between papilloma and non-infiltrating papillary carcinoma, and to try and distinguish between the two types of tumour one has to rely on clinical behaviour. It is probably best not to separate these tumours, but to regard the papilloma as potentially malignant. This concept is well-supported by the relatively poor survival rate of patients with what, on histological grounds, is a benign neoplasm. For example, McDonald and Priestley (1944) and also Riches et al. (1951) found only approximately 50 % of patients with renal pelvic papillomas surviving 5 years (see Table 17).

b) Transitional cell carcinoma

These tumours form papillary or solid lesions which in the case of the kidney fill the pelvis and compress and invade the renal substance. Most of these tumours form cauliflower-like masses, the fronds of which are thick and short with irregular epithelium showing obvious mitotic figures. The more solid tumours are composed of anaplastic cells with frequent mitoses. In such tumours areas of squamous metaplasia are common.

c) Squamous cell carcinoma

This type of tumour made up 22 % of the pelvic neoplasms studied by Riches et al. (1951) and 13 % of the series from the Mayo Clinic reported by Utz and McDonald (1957). It is a rare tumour in the ureter. It forms a solid infiltrating and highly malignant growth and is associated with chronic infection. There is ulceration with deposition of calcareous material and often a stone is present, the incidence of which varies from 25–60% in reported series. The kidney is generally immobile due to perirenal inflammatory changes or infiltration by growth. Although the majority of tumours belong to the higher grades of malignancy (Broders' 3 and 4) histological sections often show areas of well-marked keratinization.

d) Adenocarcinoma

This tumour is exceedingly rare and appears to be related to pyelitis glandularis. It is composed of well-differentiated tall mucin-secreting epithelial cells with areas of intra- and extra-cellular mucin. In the small number of cases reported in the literature there was often a long-standing history of renal infection and stone formation, and the glandular metaplasia may have been secondary to prolonged irritation.

e) Associated lesions

The co-existence of hydronephrosis and tumour in the renal pelvis and ureter is frequent. It is difficult, however, to establish which was the primary lesion, although it is generally believed that the tumour is the obstructing factor in the majority of cases.

Pyelitis cystica, pyelitis glandularis and follicularis, and leukoplakia are forms of metaplasia of the epithelium rarely found except in association with tumour. It is believed that such changes are the result of chronic irritation and may predispose to neoplasia.

4. Tumour spread and natural history

a) Transitional cell tumours

Transitional cell tumours of the renal pelvis are often associated with similar tumours in the ureter or bladder which may precede, accompany or follow the discovery of the pelvic lesion. The frequent site of these "secondary" lesions is in the bladder, in the region of the ureteric orifice on the affected side. Multiple urinary tract tumours are more often found with benign or non-infiltrating papillary tumours, less often with the invasive papillary carcinoma, and rarely with the solid infiltrating variety of growth (KAPLAN et al., 1951). Tumours of greater malignancy invade the wall of the pelvis or ureter and soon give rise to lymphatic and distant metastases. Involvement of hilar lymphatics or the renal vein occurred in 45% of 75 cases of renal pelvic carcinoma reported by MCDONALD and PRIESTLEY (1944) from the Mayo Clinic, an incidence which is comparable to the 54% found in cases of hypernephroma from the same centre. The lungs, liver, bone and para-aortic lymph nodes are the most frequent sites for metastases. As a group these tumours have a high recurrence rate unless treated by the most radical surgery, that is total nephro-ureterectomy. It is important to stress that this applies equally well to tumours which appear to be histologically benign or of low grade malignancy and to those which show definite evidence of infiltration.

b) Squamous cell carcinoma

These tumours, unlike transitional cell growths, are invariably solitary, and the majority occur in the renal pelvis. They are highly malignant tumours which soon invade the kidney and perirenal tissue and give rise to distant metastases mainly in the lungs, liver and the para-aortic nodes. The true squamous cell carcinoma of the renal pelvis carries a hopeless prognosis, a survey of the world literature revealing only one five-year survival (CARLSON, 1960).

5. Symptomatology

Bleeding is the commonest presenting symptom of transitional cell tumours of the renal pelvis and ureter and this usually results in a full investigation and the correct diagnosis. Pain or swelling may also be the presenting symptom and may lead to an erroneous diagnosis of idiopathic hydronephrosis. Renal colic may be produced by the passage of clots down the ureter. On the other hand, the cardinal clinical features of squamous cell carcinoma are those of urinary infection and stone, 60–70% of patients complaining of backache or colic. Low grade fever and leucocytosis are common findings, and pyuria is invariably present.

6. Diagnosis

In any cases of haematuria or urinary neoplasia it is not sufficient to identify the source of bleeding, but it is also necessary to demonstrate that the remainder of the urinary tract is normal.

The full clinical investigation, which will include a retrograde pyelogram and ureterogram performed under direct fluoroscopic control, is sufficient to establish the diagnosis. If the investigation is incomplete an error in diagnosis may occur. The common mistake is to remove a hydronephrotic kidney without proof that the lower ureter is normal. The delayed recognition of tumour in the residual stump of the ureter occurs in 20–30% of cases of pelvic or ureteric tumour where a sub-total nephro-ureterectomy is carried out. The second common error is to remove a kidney in the belief that a filling defect is due to an adenocarcinoma of the cortex. In all cases where there has been a deformity of the calyceal system, or where there has been a filling defect in the ureter or pelvis, the ureter and pelvis should be incised at the time of operation to exclude the presence of papillary lesions of the pelvis and ureter.

The five points of diagnosis are:
1. Culture of urine and examination for exfoliated cells.
2. Intravenous pyelography.
3. Cystoscopy under anaesthesia and ureterogram or retrograde pyelogram if there is any abnormality of the intra-venous pyelogram.
4. Biopsy of any suspicious lesion around the ureteric orifice.
5. Bimanual examination under full anaesthesia with complete relaxation.

When these investigations are carried out routinely an error of diagnosis rarely occurs. There is, however, one tumour which is frequently overlooked, the lesion in the lower 2–3 cm of the ureter or its intramural portion. This will present as an obstructed kidney; ureteric catheterisation is difficult or impossible, cystoscopy reveals an abnormal ureteric opening which may be displaced forwards and there may be the suggestion of tumour within a dilated orifice. When a bimanual examination is performed a mass is detected above the prostate, separate from the vesicles and in continuity with a soft dilated ureter. When tumour fronds present through the ureteric orifice, the lesion is frequently mistaken for a bladder growth. If the presenting symptoms are those of a hydronephrosis the kidney may be removed without excision of the lower ureter. Abeshouse (1956) has summarised the position by saying that any obstruction of the ureter in middle age is malignant until proved otherwise.

7. Treatment of pelvic and ureteric tumours

a) Surgery

Where renal function is adequate in the contralateral kidney, lesions of the pelvis and ureter should be treated by complete nephro-ureterectomy, including the intra-mural portion of the ureter and a cuff of bladder wall if the intra- mural portion is involved. The sub-total nephro-ureterectomy, where the intramural portion is left in situ, has a considerably greater recurrence rate in the intramural portion. Not infrequently this operation is very incompletely performed, 5–8 cm of ureter being left as a blind pocket (Table 16). In order to perform a complete nephro-ureterectomy without risking rupture of the ureter due to traction, the vas or uterine artery and the inferior vesical pedicle must be sectioned.

Table 16. *Renal pelvic tumours recurrence rate according to treatment*

Treatment	Recurrence rate	
	TAYLOR (1959)	WALLACE and KINDER (1961)
Nephroureterectomy	bladder 15.4%	bladder 14%
Incomplete removal of ureter	ureter or bladder 33.0%	ureter or bladder 28%

b) Radiotherapy

Little has been recorded on the influence of modern radiotherapy in tumours of the renal pelvis and ureter. It may well be that at least some transitional cell carcinomas at these sites respond to irradiation, in keeping with general experience of similar tumours in the bladder. Post-operative irradiation to the renal or ureteric bed and regional para-aortic lymph nodes would therefore appear to be of possible benefit in cases with lymphatic involvement, or where spill or incomplete excision is suspected.

Squamous cell carcinoma of the renal pelvis is always of high grade malignancy, and at an early stage infiltrates into the surrounding tissues and soon gives rise to lymph node metastases. Microscopic involvement of the hilar vessels is common, and blood-borne metastases are found in a high proportion of cases. We consider that post-operative irradiation should be given to all cases of squamous cell carcinoma of the renal pelvis in the hope of improving the results in this highly lethal tumour.

The technique of treating pelvic tumours is essentially that already described for adenocarcinoma of the renal parenchyma. A course of post-operative irradiation is given by means of three to four fields directed to the renal bed and para-aortic lymph nodes using where possible supervoltage equipment; a maximum tumour dose of 6000 R is given in six to seven weeks.

Radiotherapy appears to have little place in the routine treatment of operable ureteric tumours. In cases where excision is thought to have been incomplete markers may be inserted at operation in the site of suspected residual growth, and post-operative external irradiation given in the hope of delaying or preventing local recurrence. Interstitial therapy using gold 198 grains at the time of operation is an alternative technique in such cases.

External beam irradiation may be of considerable palliative value such as in cases with a large fixed carcinomatous mass of ureteric origin at the pelvic brim. Patients with malignant lymphoma and very rarely Hodgkin's disease may develop unilateral or bilateral ureteric obstruction due to extrinsic pressure from enlarged retroperitoneal lymph nodes (COWEN, 1949; WATSON et al., 1949; GLAY, 1960). The ureter was involved in 14 of 80 cases reported by WATSON et al. (1949) in whom the genito-urinary tract was affected by lymphosarcoma, Hodgkin's disease or leukaemia. As these authors point out, it is important to bear in mind that in patients known to have malignant lymphoma and who develop urological symptoms the urologist should be reluctant to diagnose an apparently unrelated disease of the urinary tract and to undertake surgical treatment. Ureteric obstruction by lymphomatous masses can be readily relieved by external irradiation.

c) Technique

α) Radical treatment

For localized residual or recurrent ureteric tumour following surgery, a multiple beam-directed field technique is employed. Supervoltage apparatus in the 1–4 MeV range is desirable and a maximum tumour dose of 6000 R is delivered in about six weeks.

β) Palliative treatment

Large opposing anterior and posterior fields, preferably with supervoltage apparatus, is used for large fixed abdominal masses causing pain or ureteric obstruction. A midline depth dose of 4000–5000 R is given in 4–5 weeks to patients with ureteric carcinoma, whilst a dose of between 3000–4000 R in 4–5 weeks is adequate for cases with malignant lymphoma or metastases from seminoma testis.

d) Treatment of bilateral lesions

Although rare, more cases of bilateral transitional cell pelvic and ureteric tumours, either occurring simultaneously or at an interval, are being reported every year. When the lesion involves both ureters bilateral ureterectomy with ileal replacement and anastomosis to the bladder maintains function. When one lesion involves the renal pelvis with possible involvement of the calyces, nephro-ureterectomy is carried out with ileal replacement of the contra-lateral ureter.

When the lesions occur at an interval after the primary nephro-ureterectomy, local excision of the tumour in the remaining pelvis or ureter can be carried out successfully, if necessary on several occasions.

In cases with renal insufficiency, where it is necessary to conserve renal function, local excision of a pelvic tumour is preferable to primary radiotherapy because of the risk of irradiation nephritis.

8. Results and after care

The results obtained by surgical treatment of renal pelvic tumours in the series reported by Riches and his colleagues (1951) is shown in Table 17.

Table 17. *Tumours of the renal pelvis. Results of treatment.* (Riches *et al.*, 1951; B.A.U.S. Series)

Tumour type	3-year results		5-year results		10-year results	
	cases	survivals	cases	survivals	cases	survivals
Transitional cell papilloma	35	87%	31	50%	9	44%
Transitional cell carcinoma	81	46%	55	35%	29	25%
Squamous cell carcinoma	32	19%	23	0%	—	—

Patients treated for renal pelvic or ureteric tumours should be carefully followed up and cystoscoped at regular intervals for the rest of their lives for evidence of new or recurrent tumours of urothelial origin.

III. Tumours of the bladder

1. Aetiology

a) Incidence

The incidence of bladder tumours may vary in different countries because of racial characteristics or because of environment. It is extremely low in Japan, Norway and Sweden, and much greater in England and Denmark (Case, 1959). In association with bilharizia it is the second most common form of cancer in Egypt.

The age-specific death rate per thousand living per year in England for all ages is 0.088, but there is a steady increasing rate with advancing age from 0.070 at the age of 50–54 to 0.59 at the age of 70–74.

The sex rate is approximately the same for all countries, a male preponderance of between two and three men to every woman.

b) Industrial factors

Although aniline dye manufacture has been implicated in the aetiology of bladder tumours, there is, in fact, little if any evidence that aniline itself has ever been responsible. The intermediate compounds in the production of the various dye stuffs, especially beta-naphthylamine, have now been shown to be the causal factors. α-naphthylamine (which usually has a small percentage of β-naphthylamine as a contaminent) and benzidine are also believed to be carcinogenic.

Recently a new compound, xenylamine, which had already been forecast as being probably carcinogenic, was responsible for what was virtually an epidemic of bladder tumours amongst the workmen in one factory (MELICK et al., 1955).

It is in industry that the aetiological control of bladder cancer is of greatest value. When a workman has been exposed to an industrial risk it is not feasible or wise to cystoscope him at frequent intervals. It is, however, possible to examine fresh urine for exfoliated cells, and when malignant cells are identified or suspected cystoscopy is indicated. Exfoliated cells can be identified in the urine long before the development of haematuria; in fact they can be identified before there is a recognisable lesion cystoscopically. In nearly every case, however, when cells are positively identified, a lesion can be seen cystoscopically within a few months.

The cytological control of patients with bladder tumours, once treatment has been initiated, is of considerably less value. False position and false negatives are more common than in the untreated case, and although a useful guide, cytological control cannot replace routine follow-up cystoscopy.

α) The industrial risk

In England naphthylamine has not been used commercially since 1949 when its manufacture was voluntarily abandoned by the chemical firms. However, it was used for the period 1928–1949 and therefore considerable numbers of workmen who were exposed to the risk will be expected to develop bladder tumours over the next decade.

Xenylamine (4 amino-di-phenyl) has never been manufactured in England and has only been imported in relatively small quantities. Benzidine has been superceded in the rubber industry but it is still commercially available.

The total industrial risk, where the tumour has been accepted as being of industrial origin, is of the order of 3 %. However, this recognised risk may only be a part of the environmental hazard. Other industries handling similar compounds may still be exposing workmen to a carcinogenic risk. The addition of certain chemicals to food stuffs or cosmetics, as yet only suspected as carcinogenic, may also be responsible for the increasing incidence. Owing to the relatively long latent period between exposure to a carcinogenic hazard and the development of a tumour, the clinicians will inevitably be working a generation behind the organic commercial chemists.

c) Experimental aspects

Since the recognition by REHN in 1895 that certain bladder tumours in men employed in the dye industry were due to a chemical, an immense field of experimental work has been developed. Unlike many other tumours produced experimentally, bladder growths resulting from chemical carcinogenesis, either in man or animals, are similar to those that occur naturally. Single and multiple papillary tumours as well as infiltrating lesions have all been produced in the bladder of animals, but metastases from these experimental lesions are as yet unknown. It is possible that this is due to a shortening of the time factor as once a tumour has been recognised the tendency is to sacrifice the animal rather than to let the disease progress in its natural course.

Experimental bladder tumours are produced by carcinogens in the urine. When the urine is diverted by uretero-colic anastomosis before administering such compounds, tumours fail to develop in the bladder. If, however, there is any stasis in the ureter above the site of anastomosis tumours will appear in the renal pelvis or in the dilated ureter. Confirmation of this observation was obtained by MacDonald and Lund (1954) who constructed a Pavlov pouch of the bladder, a blind sac which was not in contact with the urine but was normal in all other respects. A suitable carcinogenic diet produced tumours only in that portion of the bladder in contact with the urine. In one animal, however, tumours appeared in both portions of the bladder but in this case it was possible to demonstrate the presence of a communicating fistula.

Bonser et al. (1956) have been able to identify carcinogenic substances by an implantation technique in the bladders of mice, a pellet of the test substance being inserted into the bladder cavity. With this technique it was shown that it is not β-naphthylamine itself but probably the metabolic product, 2-amino-1-naphthol, which is the true carcinogenic agent.

The possibility that products of metabolism could also be responsible for the development of the so-called spontaneous tumours was considered when it was shown that animals, fed on a diet of acetoaminofluorene, rarely developed bladder tumours unless the diet was enriched with tryptophane. Tryptophane is metabolised through a number of chemical pathways, several of which result in the production of ortho-amino-phenols, biochemically similar to 2-amino-1-naphthol. These are chiefly 3-hydroxy-kynurenine and 3-hydroxy-anthranilic acid which are structually similar and regarded as being carcinogenic. Using Boyland and Watson's (1956) modification of the Bonser et al. (1956) implant technique, tumours were produced by pellets of both these chemicals as well as by pellets containing substances of similar composition. Unfortunately, the control pellets, consisting of inert base, also produced similar tumours in a few instances.

Both hydroxy-kynurenine and hydroxy-anthranilic acid have been identified in increased amounts in the urine of patients with bladder tumours compared with controls, and this difference can be accentuated by the administration of a test dose of tryptophane.

d) Bilharzia

The association between bilharzia and bladder tumours is recognised but the direct relationship is not generally accepted. Although in Egypt it is believed that the bilharzial ova or miracidia are the direct carcinogenic stimulus, in other centres it is believed that the bilharzia produces a chronic cystitis, and it is the effect of prolonged irritation that eventually produces neoplastic degeneration.

During the acute phase bilharzial disease forms polypoidal masses which will, with treatment, subside and leave a normal unscarred bladder. As the untreated disease progresses the lesions become frankly neoplastic and infiltrative. Unlike other countries, the type of tumour which occurs most commonly in Egypt is a pure squamous cell carcinoma, but there is also a high incidence of glandular metaplasia and adenocarcinoma.

2. Classification

The chief types of tumour occurring in the bladder are shown in Table 18. Tumours arising from transitional epithelium account for over 90% of the lesions seen.

The arbitary division of transitional cell tumours into papilloma and carcinoma has created confusion between various centres. Some pathologists insist that a carcinoma cannot be diagnosed on cytological appearances alone, but must exhibit evidence of infiltration. Others insist that a papilloma is a villous tumour covered with a layer of epithelium, indistinguishable from the normal lining of the bladder. These pathologists are prepared to call a villous tumour a carcinoma if it exhibits nuclear irregularity and hyperchromatin, mitoses in excess and a thickened cell layer. Others will refer to such a lesion as an atypical papilloma while some will call it a "malignant papilloma". Because of this divergence of opinion between pathologists, difficulty is experienced in comparing

Table 18. *Tumours of the bladder*

Primary

Epithelial
    Transitional cell papilloma
    Transitional cell carcinoma
    Squamous cell carcinoma
    Adenocarcinoma

Connective Tissue
    Angioma, fibroma, lipoma
    Fibrosarcoma
    Leiomyosarcoma, rhabdomyosarcoma
    Malignant lymphoma

Miscellaneous
    Phaeochromocytoma

Secondary

Direct Spread
    Prostate, cervix, colon etc.

Metastatic Spread
    Lung, breast, kidney, melanoma etc.

methods of treatment. Even greater confusion is caused by clinicians using the term "papilloma" for a lesions seen cystoscopically, with long papillary processes, but where no histological proof of its nature is obtained.

Transitional cell carcinoma may arise as a papillary lesion or may be a nodular solid ulcerative type of growth. The papillary processes of a transitional cell carcinoma, which are usually thicker and more compact than a papilloma, may be matted together. There may be increased vascularity, sufficient to produce the type of tumour known as a "raspberry lesion". The natural history of these tumours is variable: they may remain as a single non-invasive lesion for many years or they may begin to infiltrate early or late. Blood-borne metastases to lung or bone may occur, or multiple tumours may develop on the bladder mucosa either as an example of multifocal origin or resulting from sub-mucosal lymphatic permeation, or possibly implantation of exfoliated cells. The solid tumours are usually single though they may occur with other papillary lesions or tumours of different histological type. The appearance of a solid nodular tumour is soon followed by invasion and the rate of extension is usually such that, within four months, the tumour has infiltrated bladder muscle, within eight months it has involved the perivesical fat, and by the end of a year the tumour is fixed to the side wall of the pelvis.

Improvement in the results of treatment will occur when these lesions can be recognised early, and prompt and effective treatment instituted. The mucosa of the bladder, surrounding and at a distance from the tumour, frequently shows evidence of abnormal change, either red mossy velvety patches which, if a biopsy is taken, will show carcinoma-in-situ or areas of small cysts. These "cysts" may be examples of VON BRUNNS nests, cystitis cystica, cystitis glandularis, cystitis follicularis or small submucous lymphoid follicles. Cystitis cystica on the base of the bladder is a very common finding but when it occurs elsewhere in the bladder it must be regarded as a manifestation of chronic irritation and therefore a pre-malignant condition.

The squamous cell carcinoma, which is relatively uncommon, its incidence varying between 2–5 % of all tumours, can frequently be recognised clinically. There is usually a history of chronic irritation or stone. The lesion is ulcerated with sharp, solid rolled edges. Occasionally this type of tumour presents with ill-defined margins due to direct and lymphatic spread in the submucosa. The less common and the rarer types of bladder tumour are described later (p. 487).

3. Symptomatology

The classical symptom of bladder tumour is painless haematuria which is the presenting feature in 80% of cases. Haematuria with pain or frequency accounts for a further 12% of cases. It is, therefore, the minority that present with frequency, pain or obstruction without haematuria.

The factor of delay is important in prognosis. Cases of haematuria, irrespective of type of tumour or extent of spread, if treated within a month of the onset of symptoms have a 70% five-year survival rate. With longer periods the prognosis deteriorates. Cases with, for example, a delay of six months between the onset of haematuria and definitive treatment have a five-year survival rate of only 35%. The delay in women is greater than in men, on the average just over a month longer. The main factors in delay before instituting proper treatment are due to errors in diagnosis, treatment for "cystitis", waiting for a hospital bed and protracted investigations.

4. Investigation and diagnosis

Any case of haematuria should be cystoscoped as an emergency if still bleeding at the time of consultation. By so doing, blood may be seen coming from one or other ureteric orifice. If, however, the bleeding has stopped a definite assessment should be made based on the six points of investigation (Fig. 4).

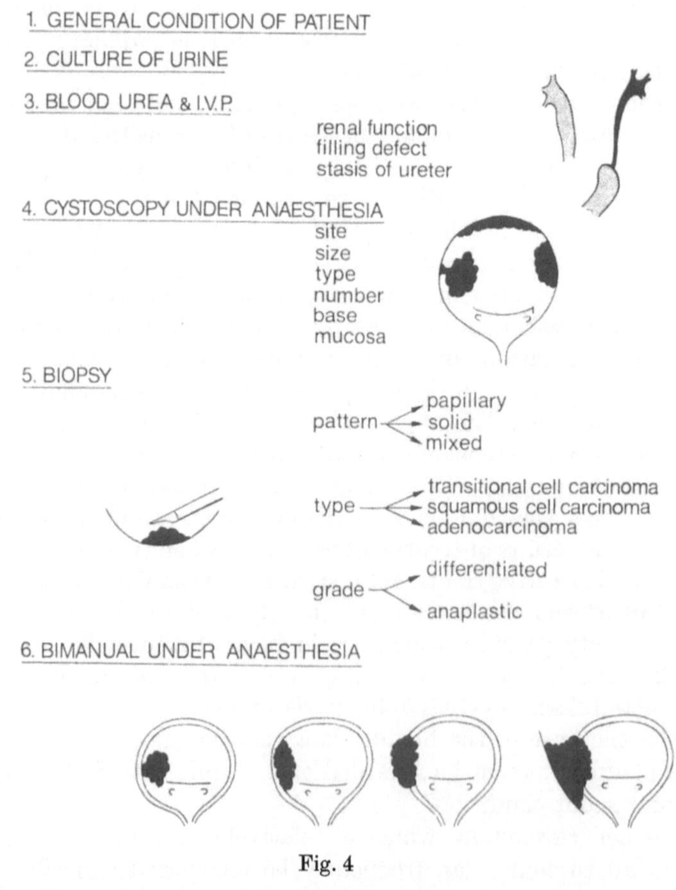

Fig. 4

a) Culture of urine and examination for exfoliated cells

This examination is particularly important in cases where the presenting symptom is frequency or pain, and where there appears to be a sterile pyuria. Frequently these cases are investigated at length on the suspicion of a tuberculous cystitis, when the cytological examination for malignant cells could have given a definite answer without delay.

b) Pyelography

Intravenous pyelography should be performed prior to cystoscopy since, if a filling defect in the renal pelvis or deformity of the calyceal system is demonstrated, a retrograde pyelogram can be done at the time of the first cystoscopy. Apart from deformities of the upper urinary tract pyelography may demonstrate filling defects of the bladder, ureteric dilatation due to infiltration around the intramural ureter, or absence of function of one or other kidney. Pyelography may also demonstrate associated conditions such as diverticulae, calculi or pelvic skeletal metastases.

c) Cystoscopy

The initial cystoscopy should always be performed under a general anaesthetic, since with the one anaesthetic a biopsy and bimanual examination can be carried out without discomfort or pain to the patient. A painful cystoscopy attempted under a local anaesthetic with an inadequate view does not engender confidence for future treatment and follow-up.

A biopsy examination is mandatory in all cases of bladder tumour, except those small papillomas where using a diathermy loop would result in complete charring of the specimen. The possible dangers of biopsy have been stressed by some workers. There is little evidence, however, that the survival rate in mucosal tumours, where a biopsy was taken, is significantly less than a similar group where no biopsy was obtained, allowance being made for the fact that lesions not biopsied were probably too small for this to have been of value.

d) Bimanual examination

The bimanual examination is conducted under full surgical anaesthesia and with an empty bladder. Care must be taken to feel for any tumour immediately behind the pubic symphysis and at the vault. Tumours in the latter position are frequently missed, since the examining finger can be readily approximated below the lesion.

A soft mass, freely mobile within the bladder, or a soft bulky mass occupying the bladder cavity can be palpated in cases of non-infiltrating bladder tumours. A localised thickening in one or other portions of the bladder wall, in the absence of previous operations, usually means early infiltration. Where there is a hard plaque or where definite nodularity can be palpated the tumour has spread to the deep muscle layers or to the perivesical fat. Tethering or fixation to the pelvic wall or to the brim of the pelvis along the vesical pedicles, involvement of an abdominal scar or infiltration of the prostate or vagina indicates advanced disease and carries an extremely grave prognosis.

5. Clinical types of tumour

The bladder perhaps more than any other organ develops neoplastic lesions of pleomorphic character. Tumours may be single or multiple, they may be single with areas of unstable mucosa, or they may form part of a more generalised disease, involving one or both pelvi-ureteric tracts. In an appreciable number of cases carcinoma-in-situ may also be found in the urethra.

Bladder tumours may be sessile or pedunculated and the pattern exhibit a papillary or solid structure or combination of both (Fig. 5). A sessile tumour is for practical purposes always a carcinoma, but a pedunculated lesion may be an anaplastic carcinoma or simply a papilloma. The surface of a pedunculated lesion may consist of long delicate fronds which are pale in colour, or the fronds may be more solid and clumped together forming a mass which has been likened to a "raspberry". Sessile tumours may be nodular, ulcerative or partly papillary and partly nodular. The edge may be well defined or may blend

28*

with submucosal plaques of infiltration, in which case the lesion is usually highly malignant. Necrosis on the surface of a tumour is usually associated with infiltration or at least rapid growth. Oedema at the periphery of the growth always means infiltration, at least into muscle.

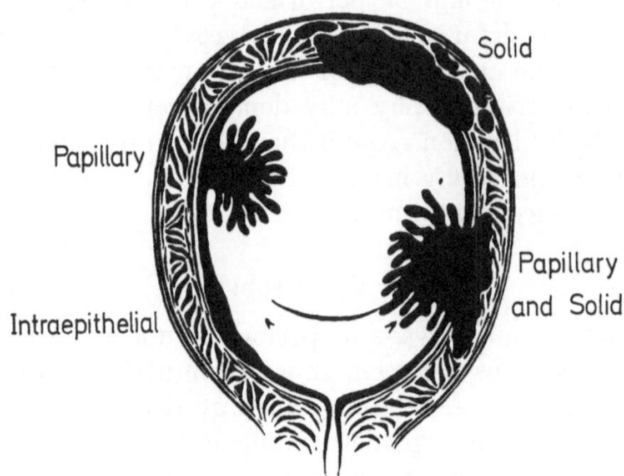

Fig. 5. Patterns of tumour growth

When a tumour in the bladder appears to be surrounded by a sulcus or when its size varies with the degree of vesical distension the lesion may be arising from a diverticulum, especially if the bladder is trabeculated or sacculated. It is important to recognise tumours in a diverticulum at an early stage since the prognosis of such lesions is extremely poor.

Multiple tumours of the bladder are particularly liable to be associated with other urinary tumours, especially in the upper tract, in a stump of the ureter after nephrectomy or in the prostatic urethra. Complete assessment of such cases, which includes urethroscopy at the time of the first examination, intravenous and retrograde pyelography, and radiological screening using an image intensifier, should be repeated if there is any suspicion of a lesion in a ureteric orifice.

Lymphoid tumours form well-defined smooth masses which bulge into the bladder with the overlying mucosa remaining intact. Fibrosarcomas or leiomyosarcomas are occasionally found in the bladder and produce shaggy necrotic lesions with usually more to feel outside than can be seen inside the bladder. Extravesical infiltration from primary tumours of the female genitalia or large bowel can be difficult to recognise, but the appearance of a "bulging in" of the bladder wall, accompanied by minimal polypoidal mucosal change or oedematous fronds, especially when there is a palpable mass in the pelvis, should raise suspicion of secondary bladder involvement.

6. Clinical stage

Clinical staging is defined as the assessment of the extent of tumour spread as judged by clinical and ancillary examinations prior to the initiation of definitive treatment.

Information such as the presence of enlarged lymph nodes, or metastases in the liver which is obtained as a result of laparotomy is not included in clinical staging because laparotomy is not a routine part of clinical assessment, and is not an investigation applicable in every case. If such information were used in staging, all cases submitted to laparotomy would form a selected group and could not be compared with a similar group treated by other methods but not submitted to exploration.

In any series of cases reported on a basis of staging it is essential to define whether the staging is clinical, partly clinical and partly pathological, or entirely pathological. A better method is to show the purely clinical staging separately and to compare this with the subsequent operative and pathological findings. In the majority of cases in large series a correct correlation between clinical and pathological staging can be obtained in 80–90 % of the cases available for study.

At the present time four systems of staging are in common use—that suggested by JEWETT and STRONG (1946) which is similar to the classification used by DUKES (1940) for operative specimens of the rectum; the method of DUKES and MASINA (1949) which made use of clinical or pathological criteria; MARSHALL's (1952) modification of the JEWETT and STRONG (1946) system where the finer points of spread are emphasized; and finally the Tumour, Node, Metastasis (TNM) system based on the principles suggested by the International Committee for Stage-Grouping, which, at the present time, is evolving as a purely clinical method.

The method of staging by JEWETT and STRONG (1946) was originally used for operation specimens but has since been adopted by some centres for clinical use. Tumours of the mucosa or submucosa were classified as A, infiltrating tumours involving muscle were B, and tumours that had spread through the full thickness of the bladder wall were C.

DUKES and MASINA (1949) proposed a classification based on clinical or pathological findings and used the terms 1a for mucosal tumours, 1b for tumours infiltrating muscle, 2 for lesions into the perivesical fat, 3 for the presence of metastatic lymph nodes, and 4 for growth fixation.

As a result of more detailed study of prognosis and spread of bladder tumours, MARSHALL (1952) proposed that purely mucosal tumours, whether papilloma or carcinoma that had not broken through the basement membrane, were classified as 0. When the tumour invaded the submucosa it was called A, superficial muscle B1, deep muscle (i.e. the outer half of the muscular layer) B2, and perivesical tissue C. The stages D1 and D2 indicated local and distant node involvement respectively. This system, although ideal for operative specimens, is difficult to apply clinically for two reasons, firstly because the half way point of the muscle is only capable of definition if the whole thickness is known, and secondly the presence of lymph nodes cannot be accurately determined on clinical examination alone.

a) The T.N.M. Classification (1950—1959)[1]

The principles of T.N.M. staging, suggested by the International Committee for Stage-Grouping for carcinoma of the breast and larynx, have been employed by us to designate the extent of the primary growth in patients with bladder tumours (Fig. 6). Neither the N factor, evidence of local lymph node involvement, nor the M factor, presence of distant clinical metastases, have been used at the time of the clinical assessment.

T1 (Mucosal): This stage comprises all tumours of epithelial origin where there is no evidence of infiltration. The presence of a mild degree of stasis, due to simple mechanical pressure by the tumour on the ureter, is accepted in this group. Biopsy may show invasion of submucosa but not involvement of muscle. Bimanual examination may reveal a soft spongy mass within the bladder.

T2 (Muscular): In this stage there is evidence of infiltration into muscle as a result of biopsy findings, obstruction of the ureter in the intravenous pyelogram, or a rubbery localised thickening on bimanual examination.

T3 (Perivesical): Here the tumour mass is discrete, hard, and nodular and readily palpable on bimanual examination.

T4 (Fixation): The tumour infiltrates an abdominal scar, the prostate or vagina or is adherent to the pelvic wall, either by direct spread or by permeation along the vesical pedicle.

In all cases allowances must be made in staging for previous surgical scarring, radiation fibrosis or inflammatory changes which might result from taking too deep a biopsy on a previous occasion.

---

1 See p. 529 for revised stage classification.

The preliminary trials with the T.N.M. method of staging as a purely clinical system has shown that it can be used as a useful basis of comparison, but that in two respects it can be improved. The so-called mucosal T1 tumours where there is no infiltration into muscle can be divided into those where there is no break-through of the basement membrane, and those where the submucosa is involved. In the first group many pathologists would refuse to consider these tumours as true carcinomas. In stage T1 cases, therefore, there could be a variable proportion of purely benign lesions mixed with those of definite malignant character.

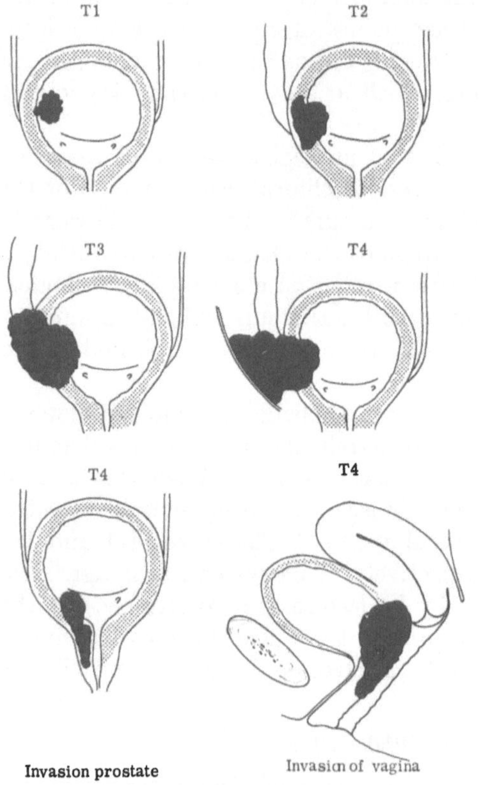

The second point of weakness in this system is the differentiation of deep muscle involvement from perivesical spread. It is a common mistake to classify a case on clinical examination as muscular (T2) but to find at operation that the outer surface of the bladder wall is involved or that there is frank spread into perivesical fat (T3). For practical purposes it is easier to distinguish between purely superficial infiltration of the bladder, accompanied by dilatation of the ureter or muscle involvement in the biopsy specimen, and deep infiltration where there is a palpable mass of firm to hard consistency.

It is hoped that international agreement will soon be reached regarding the classification of cases of bladder tumour, and that clinical and pathological staging will be clearly recognised and their limitations appreciated. It is also to be hoped that the degrees of tumour spread will be clearly defined—the purely mucosal lesion with no infiltration, submucosal infiltration, early muscular involvement, deep muscle involvement or spread into perivesical fat, and finally tumour which has involved the scar, vagina or prostate or become firmly fixed to the pelvic wall. The adoption of an international system of classification would help to clarify the results reported by many centres from various countries. Clinical staging, with practice, can achieve an accuracy of approximately 80%. Pathological staging is more accurate, but is only applicable to cases treated by extirpative surgery.

Fig. 6

7. Histological types of tumour

Tumours of the bladder arise principally from transitional epithelium and, in the main, the cell type remains unchanged. Pure squamous cell carcinoma and pure adenocarcinoma also develop either from an area of transitional epithelium by metaplasia or from an area of leukoplakia or cystitis glandularis. It is necessary to distinguish between those lesions which are primarily transitional, but where areas of squamous change or glandular metaplasia are found, and the true squamous cell carcinoma or the true adenocarcinoma.

The papillary transitional cell lesions form a scale of malignancy ranging from a simple papilloma to a highly anaplastic carcinoma. The borderline between the benign and malignant lesions is difficult to define, some pathologists insisting that until the basement membrane has been transgressed the lesions should be considered as benign. The more generally accepted view is that a benign papilloma is a villous lesion with fronds covered by an epithelial layer of similar appearance to the normal bladder. A tumour exhibiting a grossly thickened cell layer, nuclear irregularity, excessive mitotic activity and polychromasia, which are not typical of a benign lesion, warrants inclusion as a well-differentiated carcinoma. On the other hand, a tumour can be described as a poorly-differentiated carcinoma when papillary processes are short and solid, cell pattern is grossly distorted, marked nuclear irregularity present and the transitional element barely recognised.

8. Natural history

The characteristic behaviour of transitional cell tumours is interesting. There is as yet no evidence that a histologically benign papilloma ever undergoes malignant change or progression. There is, however, ample evidence to show that, although a papilloma may exist unchanged for many years, second, third or even numerous more malignant tumours may develop over a period of time at different sites in the bladder. The modern concept of a papilloma is not that it is a pre-malignant lesion *per se* but that it is an indication of a neoplastic process affecting the entire urothelium.

The well-differentiated papillary carcinoma tends to remain confined to the mucosa for variable but frequently long periods before invasion of the muscle begins. It is, therefore, difficult to define their natural course. These tumours have a tendency to metastasise at any time via the blood stream and give rise to skeletal deposits, rather than by lymphatic spread to the regional nodes. In the case of the solid anaplastic type of tumour, infiltration into the muscle wall develops rapidly. After an average time interval of four months from the onset of symptoms such a tumour is usually into muscle, by eight months into perivesical fat and at the end of a year nearly all have become fixed to the pelvic wall or have developed distant metastases.

Metaplasia may develop in a pure transitional epithelial tumour and may be squamous, glandular or a mixture of both types. This change is especially seen in the more anaplastic types of tumour and its recognition in a biopsy specimen is indicative of a poor prognosis.

9. Factors influencing prognosis

The chief factors influencing the outcome of patients with transitional cell tumours of the bladder are the extent or clinical stage (Table 19a) and the histological pattern and grade of the tumour (Table 19b).

Table 19a. *Transitional cell bladder tumours. Grade, extent and survival*

Histological grade	928 cases		139 autopsy cases		5-year results (all methods)	
	Incidence	infiltra-tion rate (clinical)	vessels invaded	metastases	cases	survival
	(%)	(%)	(%)	(%)		(%)
Papilloma	5	0	—	—	36	72
Papillary differentiated	50	18	21	14	169	52
Papillary anaplastic	9	61	43	14	24	21
Solid differentiated	7	81	70	60	28	18
Solid anaplastic	29	89	84	64	98	16

10. Surgery

The limitations of surgery in the treatment of bladder tumours are well recognised and the types of tumour that can be controlled have been established. What has not been

Table 19 b. *Bladder cancer. Stage, pattern, extent and survival*

Stage	1331 cases incidence	Solid pattern	150 Autopsy cases		5-year results (all methods)	
			vessels invaded	meta-stases	cases	survival
	(%)	(%)	(%)	(%)		(%)
Mucosal	56	8 (67% Ana-plastic)	4	9	262	63
Muscular	17	48 (74% Ana-plastic)	55	27	81	21
Perivesical	14	75 (80% Ana-platic)	86	68	68	10
Pelvic fixation	13	63 (84% Ana-plastic)			42	0 (all dead at 3 years)

established is the correct relationship between surgery and radiotherapy, when they should be used together and when surgery or radiotherapy should be employed as the first stage of the planned treatment.

Table 20. *Methods of treatment for bladder tumours*

I. *Surgery*
  1. Endoscopic diathermy
  2. Open diathermy
  3. Partial cystectomy
  4. Simple total cystectomy
  5. Cysto-prostatectomy
  6. Radical cystectomy
  7. Evisceration
  8. Simple urinary diversion

II. *Radiotherapy*
  1. Intracavitary
     a) Central solid source: Ra, ^{60}Co
     b) Liquid: i) within a balloon: ^{24}Na, ^{60}Co, ^{82}Br
                 ii) direct mucosal contact: ^{198}Au, ^{90}Y
     c) Contact roentgen rays
  2. Interstitial
     Radium, radon, gold grains, tantalum wire, cobalt pellets
  3. External
     Deep roentgen rays (200–500 kV)
     Supervoltage rays: roentgen rays (1–20 MeV); telecurie units: ^{60}Co

III. *Combined*

e. g. 1. Suprapubic cystotomy, diathermy and interstitial therapy
     2. Partial cystectomy and post-operative external irradiation
     3. Interstitial therapy and external irradiation

a) Endoscopic diathermy

Mucosal tumours, whether single or multiple, have been treated by endoscopic diathermy for many years. These tumours, on the whole, tend to be well differentiated papillary carcinomata rather than multiple papillomata. Sooner or later they metastasise or infiltrate the bladder wall. Alternatively, some other part of the bladder mucosa will undergo a more malignant change leading to infiltration.

With endoscopic diathermy, whether coagulation or resection, even quite large tumours can be completely destroyed in one or several treatments. Multiple tumours are equally amenable to repeated endoscopic treatments but these treatments must be prolonged and meticulous in execution. There is no place for a "quick" diathermy coagulation. Complete treatment by endoscopic resection leaves an area of bladder muscle clearly exposed and provides tissue from the base of the lesion for histological study. Coagulation with a large electrode, such as the original Kidd's diathermy cystoscope or the Riches' modification, can be used to destroy not merely a large surface arear, as in the case of multiple tumours with abnormal mucosa, but also to produce thermal necrosis to a considerable depth in the case of localised lesions. The results achieved with cystoscopic diathermy must be considered in relation to the equipment used, the experience of the operator, and the thoroughness of the follow-up. The disasters of endoscopic treatment are due to incorrect assessment, inadequate equipment, inexperienced operators or irregular follow-up. The results of treatment of superficial tumours from the combined records of St. Peter's, St. Paul's and the Royal Marsden Hospitals are presented in Table 21. The influence of histological grade of malignancy on the results of cystodiathermy is shown by RICHES (1958), (Table 22).

Table 21. *Bladder tumours. Mucosal lesions treated by cysto-diathermy. Tumour Registry, Institute of Urology, London*

Tumour	Cases	5-year survival rate
Papilloma	36	72%
Papillary carcinoma	134	60%
Papillary lesion without biopsy[a]	52	78%

[a] This group includes all lesions too small to permit adequate biopsy assessment.

Table 22. *Bladder tumours. Cystodiathermy. Results according to histological grade* (RICHES, 1958)

Histological grade	Cases	5-year survival rate (%)
Localised papillary differentiated tumours	60	72
Localised papillary anaplastic carcinoma	25	32
Total	85	60

Operative mortality, 0.6%.

b) Open diathermy

The role of open diathermy excision is less clear, partly because it is a form of treatment that can be used in centres ill-equipped or inexperienced in cystoscopic treatment, and partly because these cases are selected either because of size or inaccessibility for endoscopic treatment. The major risk in this type of treatment is the implanting of exfoliated cells in the wound. Where adequate care is taken the risk is low (2%). The indications for this method are reasonably well-circumscribed tumours, without extensive areas of abnormal mucosal change, situated far back on the posterior wall or high up on the lateral or anterior walls of the bladder. Bulky tumours with small pedicles are ideally suited for this method of treatment. Where, however, there is suspicion of muscle infiltration or where the entire mucosa is diseased this method is contra-indicated.

Enlargement of the prostate is not a contra-indication to open cysto-diathermy since, if complete removal of all tumours is affected with destruction of abnormal mucosa, the subsequent removal of an adenomatous prostate which interferes with urinary drainage is believed by some to reduce the risk of development of new tumours. There is, however, the danger of implanting tumour cells in the raw prostatic bed if the bladder is not completely treated in the first instance. It is necessary to stress that a prostatectomy performed through a bladder which still contains active viable tumour cells will almost inevitably be followed by an implant in the prostatic bed.

c) Partial cystectomy

Partial cystectomy or segmental resection for bladder tumours is an operation that has been adversely criticised. When cases are correctly chosen and the operation adequately performed the results are surprisingly good. In the wrong type of case or where an inadequate operation has been carried out the results are, as would be expected, poor.

Tumours in the dome of the bladder or high up on the lateral wall, with clearly defined margins and devoid of areas of submucosal infiltration, are suitable for this operation, provided that a two centimetre clearance can be achieved. In tumours of the bladder base or near the trigone this margin of clearance would necessitate excision of both ureteric orifices and often the external meatus. For this reason basal tumours are best treated by diathermy excision supplemented by interstitial irradiation.

Multiple areas of tumour, or of abnormal mucosa, or even a history of multiple tumours arising at different sites of the bladder, are indicative of an unstable mucosa or total mucosal disease. Partial cystectomy in these cases is frequently followed by recurrence or new tumour formation around the line of excision or at the site of the sutures.

The results of partial cystectomy reported by Magri (1961) from the Bladder Tumour Registry of the Institute of Urology on cases treated at St. Peter's and the Royal Marsden Hospitals are shown in Table 23. The importance of an adequate margin of clearance greater than 2.5 cm is illustrated by the survival rates in Table 24.

The apparent benefit of supplementary post-operative external irradiation in cases treated by partial cystectomy is shown in Table 25. It is possible that this difference in survival rates could be explained by several factors of selection. Thus, post-operative

Table 23. *Bladder carcinoma. Partial cystectomy, results according to clinical and pathological stage (St. Peter's and the Royal Marsden Hospitals, 1950–1959).* (Magri, 1961)

	Cases	5-year crude survival rate
Clinical Stage:		
Mucosal	17	3/5 (60%)
Muscular	42	13/29 (45%)
Perivesical	27	4/11 (36%)
Total	86	20/45 (44%)
Pathological Stage:		
Mucosal	28	8/10 (80%)
Muscular	40	10/26 (38%)
Perivesical	34	5/19 (26%)
Total	102	23/55 (42%)

Table 24. *Bladder carcinoma. Partial cystectomy, prognosis according to tumour clearance margin. St. Peter's and the Royal Marsden Hospitals (1950–1959). (MAGRI, 1961)*

Margin	Cases	5-year survival rate
Clearance by 2.5 cm or more	27	10/14 (71%)
Clearance by less than 2.5 cm	70	13/39 (33%)
Line of excision through tumour	5	0/2 (0%)

Table 25. *Bladder carcinoma. Partial cystectomy, results of surgery alone and with radiotherapy. (St. Peter's and the Royal Marsden Hospitals, 1950–1959)*

Treatment	Cases	Survival rate	
		3 years	5 years
Surgery alone	40	11/32 (34%)	7/25 (28%)
Surgery plus post-operative radiotherapy	31[a]	10/22 (45%)	6/13 (46%)
Total	71	21/54 (39%)	13/38 (34%)

[a] External irradition (250–400 kV: 28 cases; 2 MeV: 3 cases).

radiotherapy may have been withheld from the more elderly patients, cases with a suprapubic fistula which failed to heal within a month, and finally because of the opinions of a particular surgeon regarding the value of irradiation in such cases. It is for these reasons that the most favourable cases may have received ancillary radiotherapy. On the other hand, it is the practice of many surgeons to send only those cases in a particular group with the more unfavourable prognostic features for post-operative irradiation.

d) Total cystectomy

Removal of the bladder with deviation of the urinary stream has been in common practice for only the last two decades. Before this, the operation was sporadic, frequently incomplete and the biochemical alterations ill-understood. The work of FERRIS and ODEL (1950) led to a better understanding of the complications of ureteric deviation and to their control.

α) Simple cystectomy

Removal of the bladder without excision of the paravesical tissues, seminal vesicles or prostate is an operation which we largely reserve for cases with irradiation complications such as necrosis and persistent bleeding from telangiectases. Even as an operation for multiple papillary non-infiltrating lesions it is often incomplete, since the prostatic urethra is frequently involved in this type of lesion and local recurrences develop if the prostatic stump is left. Where there is infiltration of the bladder wall by tumour the risk of lymphatic metastases is high, and for these cases simple cystectomy would appear to be inadequate and radical operation indicated.

Total cysto-prostatectomy as advocated by MILLIN and MASINA (1949) is an improvement on simple cystectomy. The former operation removes the entire prostatic urethra, the paravesical nodes and the seminal vesicles, and the peritoneum is reconstructed to form a new pelvic floor. This, however, carries a two-fold hazard since there is a tendency to conserve as much peritoneum as possible to ensure a good closure, which may result in inadequate clearance of paravesical lymphatics, and also there is the danger of intestinal strangulation through peritoneal gaps. The results of this operation are shown in Tables 26 and 27.

Table 26. *Bladder tumours. Cysto-prostatectomy, results according to stage.* (RICHES, 1961)

Stage (pathological)	Cases	5-year survival rate
Mucosal	36	15 (42%)
Muscular	33	3 (9%)
Perivesical	28	1 (4%)
Total	97	19 (20%)

Operative mortality, 12.5%.

Table 27. *Bladder tumours. Cysto-prostatectomy results according to stage and grade* (BRICE, MARSHALL, GREEN and WHITMORE, 1956)

	Cases	5-year survival rate
Stage (pathological):		
Mucosal, sub-mucosal and superficial muscle (O, A, B1)	68	25 (37%)
Deep muscle or beyond (B2, C, D1, D2)	88	8 (9%)
Histological grade:		
Low grade	45	18 (40%)
High grade	111	15 (14%)
Total	156	33 (21%)

β) Radical cystectomy

The place of radical cystectomy as contrasted with simple total cystectomy would appear to be in infiltrating lesions where the risk of lymphatic metastases is high. There is little justification for performing a lymph node dissection in those cases where the risk of metastases is low. Where, however, infiltration has occurred, and especially if radiotherapy has failed to control the disease, a radical clearance of the fore-pelvis is indicated, and is, in fact, technically easier than the more limited total cystectomy.

The extent of the radical operation is considerably greater than total cystectomy. It comprises clearance of the pelvic lymph nodes at the bifurcation of the aorta, and along the iliac vessels. The node in the femoral canal and the obturator node lying on the surface of the obturator internus muscle adjacent to the obturator vessels and nerve must also be removed en bloc with the contents of the fore-pelvis.

Although in the previously irradiated case, dissection of the paravesical planes may be difficult, stripping the lateral walls of the pelvis and dissection of the tissues around the great vessels is relatively simple. When the lateral walls have been cleaned and the great vessels stripped, the internal iliac artery can be ligatured and resected. A ligature is then placed around the internal iliac vein, great care being taken in this procedure, since the vein is extremely fragile and rough handling at this point may precipitate severe haemorrhage.

Once the lymphatic and venous drainage has been controlled the posterior dissection behind the seminal vesicles leads to the retro-prostatic space and the apex of the prostate. In women the posterior dissection opens the posterior vaginal fornix and the excision extends down the vagina on either side so that the tissues removed will include bladder, urethra and external urethral meatus, uterus, broad ligaments with ovaries, and the anterior and lateral vaginal walls. Local recurrence in the stump of the female urethra is by no means uncommon after simple cystectomy.

In the male it has generally been accepted that the line of section should be at the apex of the prostate. However, in view of the recent work by GOWING (1961) and the increasing incidence of urethral tumours in long term survivors after cystectomy, it is probably better to remove the entire urethra with the corpus spongiosum in continuity with the bladder.

The justification for the radical operation, including ligature of the internal iliac vein, is based on the subsequent history of cases who have survived simple cystectomy. In a series of 89 survivors from this operation, 48 died subsequently and in 32 of these the cause of death was lymphatic and/or haematogenous spread (WALLACE, 1960). The early appearance of pulmonary and skeletal metastases, often following cystectomy, suggests that dissemination originated at the time of operation. Pre-operative irradiation, early control of the venous channels during operation and extended lymph node dissection may help to reduce the incidence of lymphatic and blood-borne metastases. At the present time, however, the results of radical cystectomy appear to be comparable to those of supervoltage irradiation (Tables 28 and 38).

Table 28. *Bladder tumours: results of simple and radical cysto-prostatectomy (cases with invasion of deep muscle or beyond)*

Treatment	Cases	Survival rate			
		1 year (%)	2 years (%)	3 years (%)	4 years (%)
Simple (BRICE et al., 1956)	64	41	23	13	11
Radical (WHITMORE and MARSHALL, 1956)	40	50	32	17	15

γ) Disposal of the ureters

There are four major methods of disposal of the ureters, each method having certain advantages and disadvantages.

Uretero-colic anastomosis. Transplantation of the ureters into the sigmoid colon carries the risk of ascending infection if the stoma should become stenosed or if the intra-colonic pressure is high. The second disadvantage is electrolyte imbalance resulting from faulty re-absorption of urinary constituents from the bowel. The advantage of this method is that it is a relatively simple procedure at the end of a prolonged cystectomy operation, and that it leaves the patient without external openings or appliances. Where the ureterocolic anastomosis is performed, ureteric mucosa being sutured to rectal mucosa with a valve to prevent reflux, the risk of immediate complications is slight.

Uretero-cutaneous anastomosis. Bringing the ureters to the skin obviates the risk of intestinal infection, but, as there is a tendency to stricture formation which requires dilatation, the risk of secondary infection and obstruction is high. Furthermore, ureterocutaneous anastomosis requires the patient to wear an appliance for the collection of urine.

Uretero-ileal conduit. This method of using a short ileal loop and implanting the ureters into the blind end minimises the risk of intestinal infection, and as the loop is open at its cutaneous stoma no back pressure changes develop. It is, however, a major surgical undertaking to perform an ileal conduit at the end of an extensive operation, and this is reflected in the operative mortality, which is high. It also leaves the patient with an abnormal fistula which necessitates a skin adhesive rubber collecting appliance.

Rectal bladder. Transplantation of the ureters into the intact bowel is complicated by the risks of reflux if the stoma is incompetent, or stasis and infection if the stoma is too tight. These complications can be partly minimised by transplanting the ureters into a defunctioned rectum which acts as a bladder, devoid of faecal contents and not subjected to waves of colonic pressure. This method of disposal of the ureters, however, leaves the patient with a colostomy.

e) Preservation of renal function

α) Obstruction by tumour

Where there is no evidence of obstruction to the ureters by tumour the risk of early upper renal tract damage is slight, provided cross-infection is minimised and the urine kept sterile if possible. When, however, such obstruction exists, renal failure may develop rapidly with minimal clinical signs. Terminal uraemia is relatively comfortable and before denying a patient with bladder cancer such a death one must try and assess whether therapy will effectively control the tumour. Where the growth has spread to involve pelvic nerves or given rise to multiple skeletal metastases, palliative transplantation of the ureters to the sigmoid colon will merely substitute a much more painful death. In cases where the lesion, as a result of previous injudicious surgery, has begun to fungate through the abdominal wall but where the ureters are not involved by growth, transplantation will improve the patient's comfort since in these cases uraemia develops late.

In less advanced cases where there is impending renal failure prior to treatment by external irradiation or surgery, kidney function can be improved by diversion of the urine, either by uretero-colic anastomosis supplemented by a terminal colostomy or by cutaneous ureterostomy or uretero-ileal conduit with an ileostomy. Failure to ensure free drainage of urine often results in increased obstruction developing in a considerable number of cases treated by irradiation, and death from infective pyelonephritis. Although there are cases where, owing to the response of the growth the drainage improves (Figs. 34 and 35), the incidence of pyelonephritis in the two months following external therapy is sufficiently high to justify ureteric diversion in suitable cases. The ileal conduit, where all the anastomoses are away from the field of treatment, is now the most popular means of diverting urine in cases planned for subsequent radiotherapy.

β) Non-tumour obstruction

The relief of obstruction of the lower urinary tract in patients with bladder tumour by an enlarged prostate, bladder neck stenosis or stricture is a therapeutic problem due to the liability of exfoliated malignant cells to implant onto a raw surface resulting from, for example, the enucleation of a prostatic adenoma. When the bladder tumour is initially treated by cystotomy, diathermy excision and interstitial irradiation, viable exfoliated cells do not appear to form such a risk and therefore enucleation of an enlarged prostate can be carried out at the completion of the bladder operation. More frequently the prostate is not significantly enlarged but there is a tight bladder neck. Once the primary tumour has been controlled in such cases it is safe to excise a wedge from the posterior lip of the stenosis. This manoeuvre facilitates the subsequent removal of tantalum wires, allows better drainage and minimises the risk of suprapubic fistula.

When the irradiation is external it may be impossible to sterilise the bladder from bacteria in the presence of residual urine or necrotic growth. An infected tumour with stagnant residual urine, predisposes to ascending infection. To open the bladder and enucleate the prostate in the presence of active growth invites wound implantation. In such cases prostatectomy can be performed in the middle of a course of radiotherapy, or the bladder can be kept empty by means of an indwelling Foley catheter during the whole irradiation treatment. In this latter method an endoscopic resection of the prostate can be performed immediately the treatment is completed. This allows any further surgery, which may be indicated if the tumour has failed to respond to irradiation, to be conducted in a virgin field.

11. Radiotherapy

a) Intracavitary irradiation

α) Introduction

Intracavitary techniques for radiotherapy of bladder tumours have the advantage that they spare the extra-vesical pelvic tissues and organs from unnecessary irradiation. The use of a central solid source or a liquid isotope within the bladder means that the source-tumour distance will be limited, and consequently this method of treatment is primarily intended for superficial lesions. The whole mucosa is irradiated and the technique is generally employed for multiple wide-spread papillary tumours confined to the mucosa, so called "papillomatosis'" of the bladder.

Three principle methods of intracavitary vesical irradiation have been developed over the past fifteen years: 1. a centrally placed solid source within an inflatible balloon, 2. a liquid isotope within a balloon, 3. a colloidal isotope suspension in direct contact with the mucosa (Table 29).

Table 29. *Radio-isotopes for intracavitary vesical irradiation.* (After DYCHE and MACKAY, 1959b)

Isotope	Physical form	Half-life	Radiation and mean		Depth in tissue for 50% surface dose $(\gamma + \beta)$, mm
			energy	mev	
^{60}Co	a) Solid	5.3 years	γ	1.25	a) 12.0
	b) Solution as $CoCl_2$		β	0.10	b) 7.0
^{24}Na	Solution as NaCl	15 hours	γ	2.10	1.2
			β	0.56	
^{82}Br	Solution as $CaBr_2$	36 hours	γ	0.80	4.5
			β	0.19	
^{198}Au	Colloid	65 hours	γ	0.40	0.4
			β	0.35 (max. 0.96)	
^{90}Y	Colloid	61 hours	γ	nil	1.2
			β	0.9 (max. 2.2)	
^{76}As	Colloid	27 hours	γ	0.7	1.4
			β	1.2	

Central solid source. This technique was first used by FRIEDMAN and LEWIS (1949, 1958) at the Walter Reed Hospital in 1945, for tumours situated in the lower two-thirds of the bladder. A source of 25 mg of radium or 20 mCi of cobalt-60 was placed within a double channel Foley catheter and inserted transurethrally into the bladder. The authors consider it desirable to open the bladder at the time of the first insertion of the catheter to assist in the correct positioning of the source in relation to the tumour, and for providing additional urinary drainage through a suprapubic catheter. At the same time bulky papillary tumours can be resected by diathermy, but FRIEDMAN and LEWIS consider this is best carried out transurethrally, several weeks prior to irradiation, in order to reduce the vesical reaction.

The most frequently employed catheter is of F 26 gauge with a 30 cm³ capacity balloon. The radio-active source is fitted within the main drainage channel of the catheter, urine draining through two holes in the tip and one below the balloon. The position of the radium or cobalt within the balloon is adjusted at cystotomy to suit the demand of the tumour. The balloon is over-distended with 40 or 50 cm³ of diluted radio-opaque material coloured with indigocarmine or methylene blue. This permits radiographic localisation of the balloon, and the dye will serve as a warning in the event of rupture. Antero-posterior and lateral radiographs are taken immediately after the operation and at intervals throughout the treatment to check the position of the bag and source. Further information concerning the accuracy of the "set up" can be obtained by intravenous pyelography or cystography with a small amount of diodone or sodium iodide introduced into the bladder.

The first insertion lasts for four days during which time approximately 4000 γ-roentgens are delivered at the surface of the balloon. After an interval of five to ten days the source is re-inserted for two to six days to give an overall dose of 6000–10000 γ-roentgens. The total dose prescribed is largely determined by the response of the tumour to the first insertion. This is evaluated cystoscopically and by histological changes in biopsy specimens. A shrinkage of 25% or more in tumour volume is regarded by Friedman and Lewis as being indicative of a favourable response. The most common dose was 8000 R in 10–17 days. Severe reactions occurred in 10 of 42 cases in whom reactions were recorded. Severe changes did not occur with doses of less than 7500 R.

Although intracavitary methods of irradiation were generally designed for wide-spread superficial papillary tumours Friedman and Lewis (1958) have treated more advanced growths as well as superficial lesions with their technique. In the series of 50 patients reported by these authors there were 14 cases in whom muscle invasion had taken place and 17 cases with perivesical extension. In 6 cases there was *clinical* evidence of metastases in pelvic lymph nodes. The three-year survival rate in 46 cases was 54% and the five-year survival rate in 34 cases 56%. Primary tumours yielded better results than did recurrent lesions (65% compared with 48% were arrested at three years). It is of considerable interest that among the successful cases at three years were 6 patients with tumours in the perivesical stage and one with *clinical* evidence of pelvic lymph node metastases. Friedman and Lewis (1958) discovered two weaknesses with their treatment. Firstly, there was a proneness to recurrence in the dome of the bladder (6 of 50 cases) and secondly, abdominal wound implants occurred in 3 out of 35 cases.

Duff and Hyman (1951) modified the intracavitary method described by Fried-man and Lewis, and gave 9000 R to the surface of the balloon in 8 days from a central radium source. This was preceded by a dose of 3000 R from external deep roentgen rays administered three to four weeks before the intracavitary treatment. The total dose to the entire bladder mucosa, therefore, was 12000 R. These authors treated 9 cases and, as might have been expected from such high doses, severe reactions were suffered by most patients.

Hinman and his associates (1955) devised their own catheter to hold a cobalt-60 source and treated 35 patients by intracavitary irradiation alone or combined with external deep roentgen rays. A dose of 2500–3000 R was given to the mucosa and repeated after an interval of 7–10 days. Supplementary roentgen rays from four pelvic fields added a further 3500 R in 5–6 weeks, making the total dose 8500–9500 R. The tumour was arrested without recurrence in about 30% of cases, but a contracted bladder developed in 8 of 23 cases receiving what was considered to be adequate irradiation. The authors concluded that infiltrating lesions cannot be properly controlled by intra-cavitary methods because the dose necessary to destroy the deeper parts of the tumour results in too high a mucosal dose.

In England Cones and Gregory (1952) devised an evenly distendable latex balloon catheter for intracavitary irradiation using a central cobalt-60 source. The collapsed balloon was too bulky for introduction through the male urethra and so, in these cases, a perineal urethrostomy was necessary for its insertion into the bladder. A dose of

3 000–3 500 R was delivered to the surface of the balloon in 24 hours and this was repeated after an interval of one week. The depth dose at 0.5 and 1 cm below the surface of the mucosa was approximately 70 % and 50 % respectively. BRATHERTON (1955) also used a latex bag, but this was attached to a metal catheter which could be inserted per urethra. He administered a dose similar to that given by CONES and GREGORY and reported 5 of 16 patients with carcinoma of the bladder as being free from recurrence at two years. The tumours in 9 of 12 cases with wide-spread papillomatosis were sufficiently reduced in size and number to be controlled with diathermy.

A tumour which has extended deeply into the muscularis or through the full thickness of bladder cannot be adequately treated by a technique in which the depth dose in the bladder wall from a central source falls to between 70 and 60 % at 0.5 cm, and approximately 50 % at 1 cm. The method is clearly suitable only for very superficial tumours, that is those confined to the mucosa or infiltrating no more deeply than the submucosa or the most superficial muscle layers. Furthermore, as BRATHERTON (1955) has reminded us, a small displacement of the source may lead to markedly uneven irradiation over the bladder wall. Thus, a mere displacement of 0.25 cm increases the dose to one wall by 40 %, whilst a displacement of 0.5 cm may increase the discrepancy by a factor of 2. These limitations and difficulties, plus the high incidence of bladder complications experienced by some authors, has lead to this method of treatment being abandoned in most centres.

b) Liquid isotopes

Several radio-active isotopes in solution have been used for intracavitary vesical irradiation. MÜLLER (1955) of Zürich was the first to employ this technique with cobalt-60 in 1948. At about the same time WALLACE, WALTON and SINCLAIR (1949) at the Royal Marsden Hospital, London, reported on the use of sodium-24 and later WALTON and SINCLAIR (1952) at the same hospital described their experiences with bromine-82. These isotopes were instilled into a rubber balloon inserted into the bladder. (Fig. 7). ELLIS and OLIVER (1955), on the other hand, used a solution of colloidal gold-198 instilled directly into the bladder.

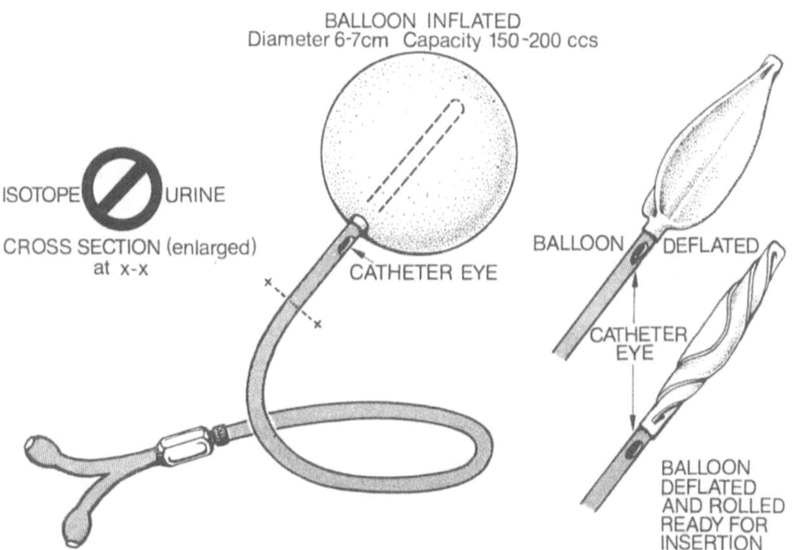

Fig. 7. Diagramatic representation of latex balloon catheter for intra-cavitary sodium-24 and bromine-82 vesical irradiation. Balloon distended, and collapsed ready for insertion

α) *Isotopes within a balloon*

Cobalt-60 solution. Cobalt-60 emits practically monochromatic γ-rays of energy
1.2 MeV. The soft β-rays are largely absorbed by the rubber balloon. Müller (1955)
used a catheter and bag which could be introduced per urethra in both male and female
patients. If the test-filling, lasting 24 hours, with the bag distended with diluted contrast
medium and indigocarmine, proved satisfactory, 70 cm³ of the cobalt solution were
run in. The dose at the surface of the balloon was approximately 10000 R plus or minus
20% over a continuous period of about seven days. Between 1948 and 1955 Müller
treated 96 patients, including 31 cases of infiltrative carcinoma, and of the total, 41%
were free from tumour after an interval of 6 months to $3^{1}/_{2}$ years (Table 30). There were
13 technical accidents in this series and "radio-lesions" were seen in 11 cases and a
seriously contracted bladder occurred in 6.

Table 30. *Intracavitary irradiation using Cobalt-60 solution for tumours of the bladder* (Müller, 1955)

Type of tumour	Cases	Tumour-free $^{6}/_{12}$–$3^{1}/_{2}$ years
Diffuse papillomatosis	25	15 (60%)
Papillary carcinoma	39	16 (41%)
Infiltrative carcinoma (transitional, squamous, adenomatous and undifferentiated types)	31	8 (26%)
Sarcoma	1	0 (0%)
Total	96	39 (41%)

Wildbolz and Poretti (1955) of Bern used a similar technique to Müller, but
gave a much higher dose to the mucosa. The surface of the balloon received 30000 R
continuously over 10 days, the depth dose at 2.5 cm being 7500 R. Exophytic portions
of the tumour were initially removed either transurethrally or at open operation. There
was no treatment mortality and a low morbidity in the 42 cases treated in this way.
The bladder was cleared in 21% of cases, the follow-up being six months to three years.
At the end of this time 19 of 42 cases were dead. By the sixth day of treatment symptoms developed due to irritation within the urethra and bladder, and by the tenth day
a troublesome proctitis had set in. These symptoms usually subsided within one to
six weeks. In 3 of 42 cases severe and incapacitating symptoms developed. In one case
the balloon burst and the circulation became radio-active for two days; elimination
occurred by way of the bowels and urine. No marrow changes were noted in this case
and there were no sequalae two years later.

Sodium-24 and Bromine-82 solutions. The investigators at the Royal Marsden
Hospital, London, tried out different techniques using sodium-24 and bromine-82
solutions (Wallace et al., 1949; Walton, 1950; Walton and Sinclair, 1952; Mackay
et al., 1959). In the early days treatment was given using large amounts of isotope,
up to 300 mCi, the mucosa receiving 2000 R from γ-rays in the course of three to four
hours. Treatment was repeated twice at one to two week intervals. With this programme
the incidence of late complications (haemorrhage and contracted bladder) was high,
occurring in about 25% of cases. Finally, in an attempt to avoid these sequelae, the
dose was reduced and the treatment time extended. A total γ-ray dose of 4500 R and
a β-dose of 1100 R was delivered continuously over a period of 96 hours to the mucosal
surface. The techniques of treatment employed at the Royal Marsden Hospital, together
with a method of dose calculation and the clinical results, have recently been reviewed

by DYCHE and MACKAY (1959a). One third of 71 cases treated with sodium-24 or bromine-82 have survived three to eight years following treatment. In approximately 30% of cases total cystectomy or a uretero-colic transplant alone was carried out for late irradiation changes or persistent or recurrent tumours. The result were more satisfactory in a series of 20 cases treated with bromine-82 in whom the dose was reduced and the treatment time extended. Thus, 8 cases treated in this way were still alive three to four years later and only 3 of the 20 required total cystectomy. In none of the cases in this group were high dose effects noted, but in only 20% of the cases did the bladder remain completely free from tumour over a period of 3 years' observation. It is of interest that there were 13 patients with verified distant blood-borne metastases among the 48 deaths in the entire series.

β) Radio-active liquids without a balloon

ELLIS and OLIVER (1955) were the first to employ a radio-active solution directly in the bladder. They used colloidal gold-198 and showed that the colloid was neither precipitated on the mucosa nor absorbed into the circulation. These workers recommended 300 mCi in 100 ml to be retained for $2^1/_2$–3 hours in order to give a dose of 3000 R (2700 R from β-rays plus 300 R from γ-rays) to the bladder epithelium. Treatment was repeated after an interval of two months. Since the irradiation from gold-198 is chiefly due to β-rays this technique is only suitable for treating the most superficial lesions and would appear to be an ideal method for dealing with diffuse papillary lesions confined to the mucosa. The absence of a bag in this technique has the advantage that it permits the villous processes of the tumours to be bathed directly and from all sides by the radio-active liquid.

Gold-198 emits predominately β-radiation (95%) of 0.96 MeV maximum energy and 5% γ-irradiation of 0.4 MeV. The maximum penetration of the β-particles in soft tissue is approximately 3.8 mm, 50% of the total surface dose being reached at a depth of 0.4 mm.

TUOVINEN and KETTUNEN (1957) of Helsinki also employed gold-198 colloid for superficial papillary tumours of the bladder, and recommended installation of 300 mCi for four to six hours in order to deliver a dose of between 4000–5000 R to the bladder epithelium. DICKSON and LANG (1960) obtained encouraging results in 14 of 17 cases with non-infiltrating lesions of the bladder who remained free from recurrence for six months to $3^1/_2$ years after treatment. There was little benefit from this treatment in the more infiltrating tumours. The dose varied from 3000–12000 R delivered in two applications, separated by an interval of approximately eight weeks. The incidence of complications in this series was low.

In an attempt to deliver a high surface dose with less damage to the bladder wall, gold-198 colloid was used in place of sodium-24 and bromine-82 by the Royal Marsden Hospital group of workers. The technique they employed has recently been reported by DYCHE and MACKAY (1959b) (Fig. 8) who also give details of the method of assessing the dose delivered to the bladder mucosa, and discuss the results of treatment. The total dose delivered in most cases was between 7000 and 8000 R in two to three sessions, each of three hours, using 300 mCi of colloidal gold in an overall time of 4–12 weeks. Between 1954 and 1957, 40 patients were treated in this way and within $2^1/_2$ years serious complications had developed in 10%. In only 20% of cases was the bladder completely cleared of tumour for the period of observation which extended only over 1–$2^1/_2$ years. Total cystectomy for persistent haematuria or tumour was performed in 4 cases. In one case a uretero-colic transplant was carried out for intractable frequency and in one other the internal iliac arteries were ligated for persistent haematuria. In those cases not completely cleared of tumour considerable regression was noted. Small areas of residual or recurrent growth could often be controlled by subsequent careful per urethral diathermy.

Gold-198 has not turned out to be a very satisfactory isotope for treating even the most superficial tumours, presumably because at a depth of only 0.4 mm below the mucosal surface the dose has already fallen to 50%. The more energetic isotope,

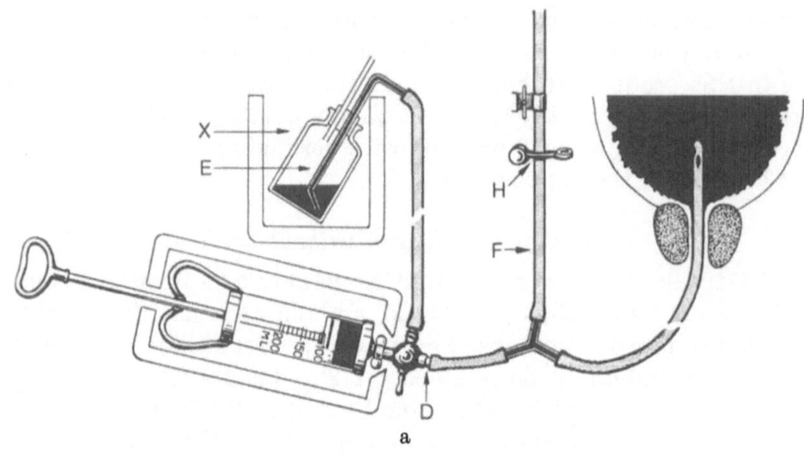

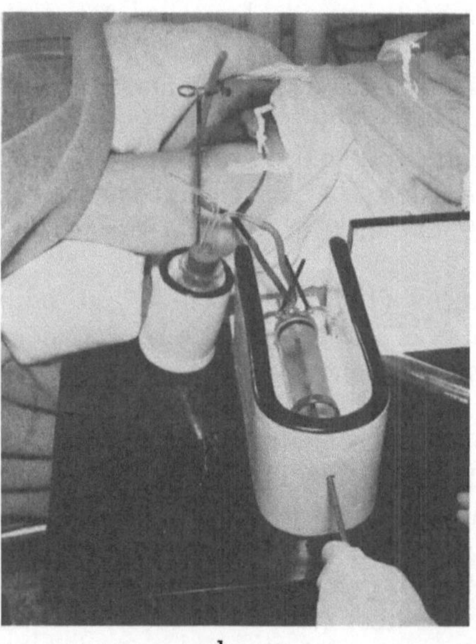

Fig. 8a and b. Apparatus for introducing radioactive colloidal gold directly into bladder (Royal Marsden Hospital). The colloid is aspirated from bottle E into lead protected syringe. The two-way tap D is reversed and clip H opened. By exerting pressure on the extended syringe handle the colloid is displaced into the tubular system. When colloid has risen to height of approximately 15 cm in tube F, clip H is closed and the remaining colloid injected into the bladder. Any air from syringe reaching Y-connection ascends tube F and is excluded from entering bladder

yttrium-90, a pure β-emitter of maximum energy 2.2 MeV, and whose 50% depth dose occurs at 1.2 mm, would appear to hold out greater promise (Einhorn *et al.*, 1955), but at the present time this isotope is not generally available in a suitable stable colloid form. Colloidal radio-active arsenic ($76As_2S_3$) was suggested by Walinder (1955) for the treatment of superficial bladder tumours, but although the energy of the β-rays is similar to those from yttrium-90 the arsenical isotope, in addition, emits γ-rays of 0.7 MeV energy.

c) Other methods of intracavitary irradiation

BECKER and SCHEER (1952) used multiple small sources of radio-active cobalt-60 in the form of gold-plated beads which were packed directly into bladder, on the same principle as the Stockholm technique for intracavitary treatment of carcinoma of the corpus uteri (HEYMAN, 1936). HIGHAM (1952. 1955), with the aim of providing an accurate localised field of uniform irradiation, has used radium needles mounted between adhesive rubber plaques as an intracavitary vesical applicator. The plaque is sutured against the bladder wall after the greater part of the tumour has been removed by diathermy resection. The bladder is distended throughout the treatment by the inflated balloon of a Foley catheter. The minimum dose to an area 8×8 cm and 3 cm thick is 5000 R in six days. HIGHAM (1955) reports no local recurrence in 46 cases treated in this way one to four years later, although the total mortality in the series during this time was 39%.

FLOOD and ABEL treated two cases of bladder cancer with contact roentgen rays at open operation in 1938 at the Royal Marsden Hospital (SMITHERS, 1946). This technique was described in the United States by LEVINE et al. (1939) and developed there by GOIN and HOFFMAN (1941, 1945). The latter authors used a Phillips Metalix apparatus, the technical factors being 50 kV constant potential; 2 ma; target-surface distance, 2.2 cm; H.V.L., 1 mm Al; dose rate, 1143 R per minute. The diameter of the applicator was 3 cm and tumours of the trigone not exceeding this size were selected for treatment. Most cases were treated with 5000 R given on each of two occasions, the interval between each being 7–10 days. The depth dose at 1 cm was 32% and at 3 cm 6%. The early promising results of GOIN and HOFFMAN (1941) were not maintained in a later report by these authors (GOIN and HOFFMAN, 1945). Of 31 cases treated in this way 29% were alive without cancer, but tumour remained in 65%. With a field size restricted to 3 cm diameter and a poor depth dose, this method of treatment was of limited value and has since been abandoned in most centres. LUTTERBECK (1959), however, continues to use this technique, but employs multiple fields for tumours greater than 2.5 cm in diameter. He delivers a single dose of 6000 R to the tumour base after fulgurating the exophytic portion. Supplementary external irradiation to deliver a further dose of 4000–5000 R to the bladder is given for more extensive tumours. Local recurrence was noted only once in 25 cases treated over the past 8 years by this combined procedure.

α) Conclusions

Intracavitary irradiation appears to be an attractive approach to the treatment of bladder cancer of limited extent, since it spares the peri-vesical tissues and other pelvic organs. A solid central source has certain advantages over radio-active liquids in that it is simpler and safer to handle and there is no risk of contamination or absorption following upon leakage or rupture of the bag. Although the depth dose is greater with a central source than with a liquid isotope it is not great enough to deal adequately with lesions infiltrating muscle without inflicting serious damage to the more superficial layers of the bladder (Fig. 9). Intracavitary irradiation would, therefore, appear to be suitable only for very superficial tumours, although certain authors (MÜLLER, 1955, Table 30; FRIEDMAN and LEWIS, 1958) report satisfactory results in some patients with infiltrating growths.

At first it seemed that liquid isotopes such as bromine-82 and sodium-24 or gold-198 could meet the physical requirements necessary for treating superficial tumours. Experience with these isotopes, however, has shown that with doses which can be relied upon to clear the bladder completely of diffuse mucosal papillary tumours there is, unfortunately, a considerable risk of inducing serious bladder injury, whilst with safer doses a high proportion of cases fail to be cured. Preliminary results, with low intensity prolonged irradiation using bromine-82, have been more promising. It may be worth-while exploring colloidal yttrium-90 when it becomes generally available, since it may prove of greater value than gold-198 in the treatment of diffuse mucosal tumours. At the present time we have abandoned intracavitary methods of irradiation and are using external beam techniques with supervoltage equipment for dealing with wide-spread mucosal tumours, and this will be discussed in a later section.

d) Interstitial therapy

The implantation of a bladder tumour with radio-active material was first carried out using radon seeds in the early nineteen twenties by Dr. B. S. BARRINGER at the Memorial Hospital, New York. In 1947 BARRINGER reported the results of twenty-

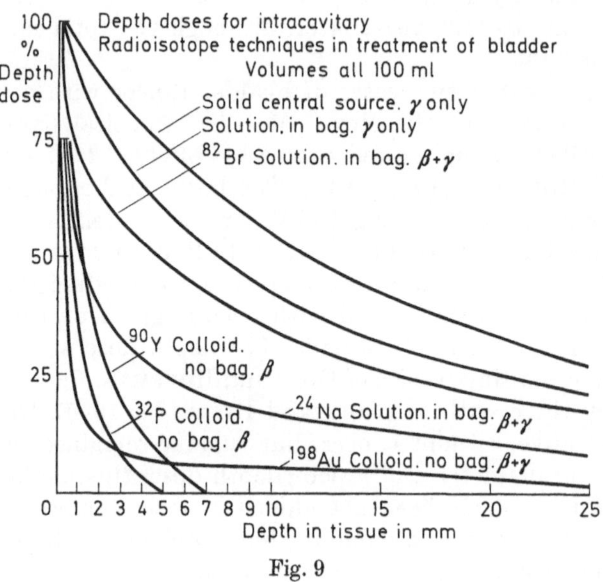

Fig. 9

four years' experience with this treatment for bladder tumours. He obtained a five-year cure rate of 36 % in 221 cases. In 94 cases of non-infiltrating papillary carcinoma the cure rate was 52 % and for 127 cases of infiltrating carcinoma 24 %.

α) Radio-active materials

Radium needles have been used for implanting bladder tumours intra-or extra-vesically with good results (LENZ et al., 1947; JACOBS, 1949). With these sources, however, reactions tended to be severe and a second operation was necessary for their removal.

In spite of a number of difficulties associated with their manufacture and use, radon seeds became popular for treating bladder tumours, and in many centres they completely replaced radium needles. Radon seeds were associated with less reaction in the bladder and less risk of sepsis, and there was no necessity for a second operation to remove them.

The chief disadvantage, however, of using radon seeds lies in the difficulty of performing an accurate implant even by an experienced operator. If the distribution is found to deliver excessive irradiation nothing can be done about it although under-dosage can be supplemented by subsequent external irradiation. It was difficult to make a suitable automatic precision instrument for introducing radon seeds into the tissues owing to their lack of uniformity in size and shape.

About eight years ago radio-active gold-198 grains were introduced as an alternative to radon seeds. Each grain consists of a small gold cylinder ensheathed in platinum, the overall size being 2.5 × 0.8 mm. The grains can be accurately machined, the individual diameter and length being constant within plus or minus 1–1.5 %. The platinum case has an activity due to gold-199 which emits low energy β- and γ-rays, the case activity being approximately one eighth of that of the grains. The uniformity of the individual grains permits the use of a precision instrument to facilitate their introduction into the tissues. The repeating gold grain gun developed at the Royal Marsden Hospital by HODT, SINCLAIR and SMITHERS (1952) carries a magazine holding fifteen grains and enables implants to be carried out with greater accuracy, speed and ease (Fig. 10). Furthermore, the factor of waste is reduced because the grains, if not used, can be returned to the pile for reactivation.

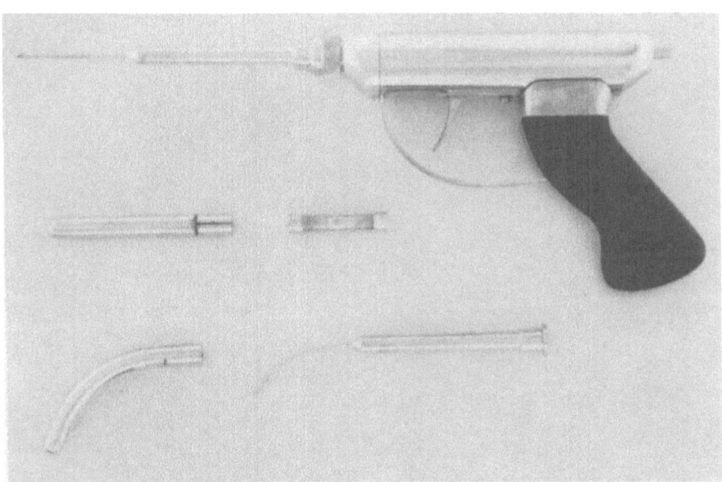

Fig. 10. Repeating gold grain gun (Royal Marsden Hospital pattern), straight and curved introducing needles, needle sheaths and magazine holding fifteen gold-198 grains

Following the suggestion by Professor W. V. MAYNEORD at the Royal Marsden Hospital in 1946 that tantalum-182 with a half life of 111 days would provide a useful alternative to radium, WALLACE, WALTON and TURNER of the same Hospital introduced a technique for implanting bladder tumours with tantalum wire (WALLACE, STAPLETON and TURNER, 1952).

The wire in its platinum sheath is made up into the shape of a hairpin, the limb of each pin being parallel and 1 cm apart (Fig. 15). The pins, which are 0.4 mm in diameter and 6 cm in length, are irradiated in the pile to an activity equivalent to about 0.45 mg of radium per centimetre. The wire is malleable, but sufficiently rigid to retain its shape. It causes little immediate trauma and is well-tolerated by the tissues. Investigations at the Royal Marsden Hospital have shown that unlike cobalt it is not absorbed by the tissues in the event of breakage. Prior to use, the tantalum pins are sterilised in an autoclave at 170° C for one hour.

The chief advantages of tantalum wire over gold grains and radon seeds for implant therapy are as follows:

    a) There is greater accuracy in introducing the radio-active material into the bladder wall.

    b) If for any reason at operation the insertion is unsatisfactory the wires can be removed and reinserted without difficulty.

    c) A considerably more uniform distribution of irradiation is achieved.

    d) There is greater control over dose in that the sources can be removed at any desired time.

    e) Because of the relatively long half-life 111 days tantalum wire can be held in stock for approximately three weeks and made available at short notice. If not used there is no waste.

In general we use tantalum-182 wire for bladder implants. Gold-198 grains are employed for bladders with two or three tumours which cannot be included in one implant, for certain irregular shaped growths and for those patients having a small pelvis with poor access to the bladder. Gold grains are an alternative to tantalum wire for tumours surrounding the internal urethral meatus.

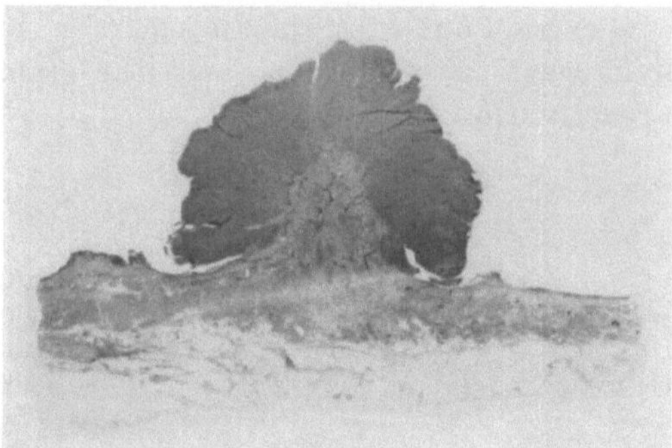

Fig. 11. Solid pedunculated type of carcinoma with early invasion of muscularis (muscle stage), suitable for interstitial therapy. (×2.5)

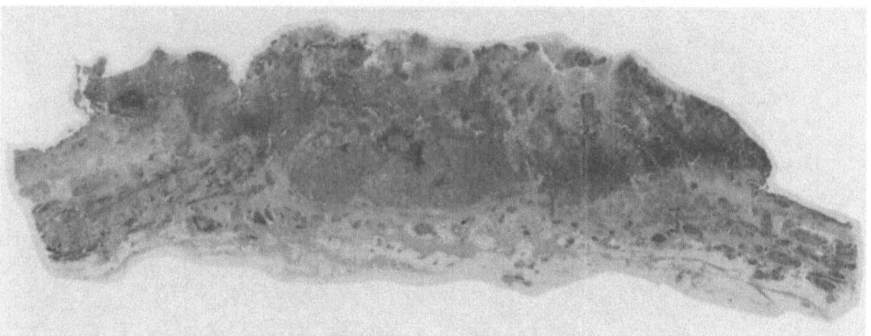

Fig. 12. Rather large solid growth showing deep muscle invasion (muscle stage), but still suitable for diathermy resection followed by interstitial therapy. (×2.5)

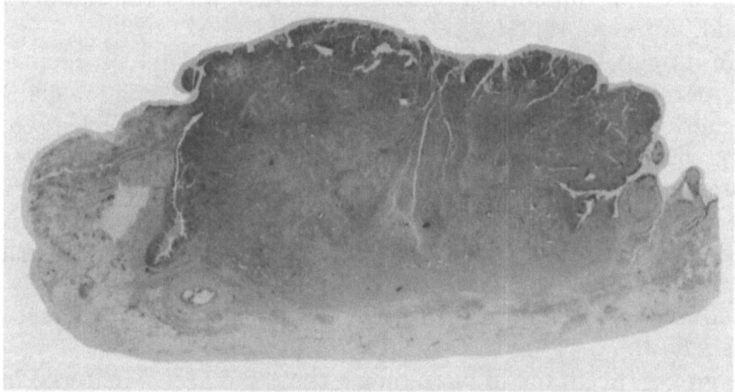

Fig. 13. Solid tumour infiltrating through full thickness of bladder wall (perivesical stage), unsuitable for interstitial therapy. (×2.5)

The ideal case for a radio-active implant is one in which there is a solitary tumour with a base not exceeding 4 or 5 cm in diameter, with early infiltration of muscle and without obvious potential malignant changes elsewhere in the mucosa. Two or three tumours close together may be included in a single tantalum implant. Tantalum pins are unsuitable for multiple implants since the wires may become entangled. More extensive or more numerous tumours, cases with wide-spread pre-malignant mucosal changes, and tumours which have reached the perivesical tissue are not suitable for interstitial radiotherapy (Figs. 11–13). Although limited tumours situated at the vault of the bladder may satisfy the requirements for implantation, they are generally treated by partial cystectomy owing to the good clearance possible at this site.

β) Implant procedure

In cases with infiltrating tumours the first stage of the operation consists of an exploratory laparotomy. A search is made of the peritoneal cavity for metastases, and the bladder and pelvic tissues are examined to re-assess the local extent of the primary

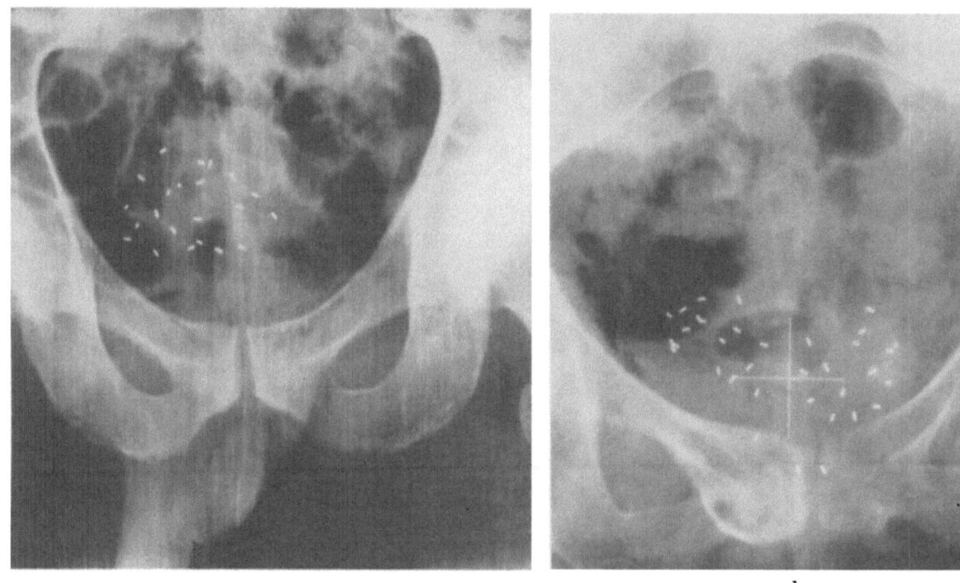

a   b

Fig. 14. a Gold-198 grain implant 4×5 cm for solid tumour infiltrating muscle. Mean dose 7000 R. b Simultaneous double gold-198 implant for two large superficial tumours

tumour. If the disease is found to be too advanced for interstitial therapy it is better not to open the bladder, to abandon the implant and later to refer the patient for external irradiation. In such cases enlarged lymph nodes may be taken for biopsy and a few gold grains can be inserted extravesically into the tumour to act as markers.

If the tumour is suitable for an implant the bladder is opened, care being taken to avoid the incision passing close to the tumour. Pedunculated growths are grasped with Fergusson's forceps and the base cut using diathermy. The projecting portion of more sessile tumours is removed by the diathermy loop, muscle being exposed in the process. Where possible divided mucosa is sutured together to control bleeding and to reduce the risk of calcareous material forming on the bare area. The base, with a surrounding margin of 1–1.5 cm of healthy-looking tissue is treated by means of a single plane implant using either radio-active gold grains or tantalum wire. The implant is planned according to the Paterson and Parker rules (MEREDITH, 1949) to deliver a minimum tumour dose of 6000–7000 R to a slab of tissue 1 cm thick. In the case of tantalum this dose is given in five to seven days. The maximum area in the bladder which can be treated satisfactorily by means of an implant is approximately 7 cm.

To achieve a geometrically satisfying implant using gold grains is not easy, even for an experienced operator. There is the difficulty of inserting them in a regular manner and into the correct plane of the bladder, and in addition, some may fall out. The dose, planned to be 6000 R, may be as low as 4000 R, and occasionally as high as 8000–9000 R. In spite of these difficulties experience has shown us that tumours may disappear and not recur following doses of the order of 4500 R (Fig. 14a and b), and serious sequelae are rare even with doses of 8000 R. In Poole-Wilson's (1954) experience with radon seeds,

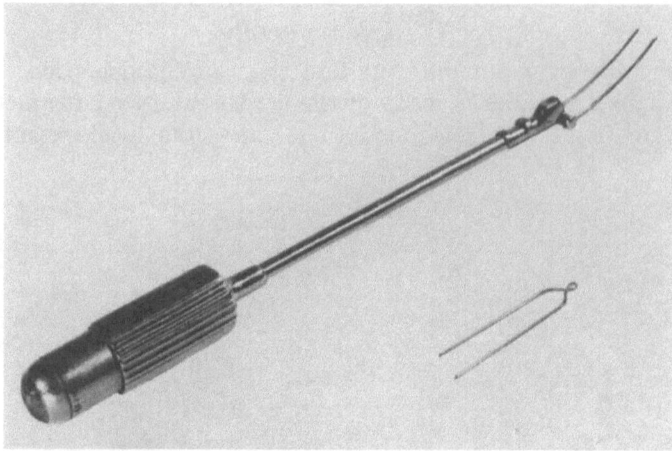

Fig. 15. Tantalum-182 pin and introducer. (Royal Marsden Hospital)

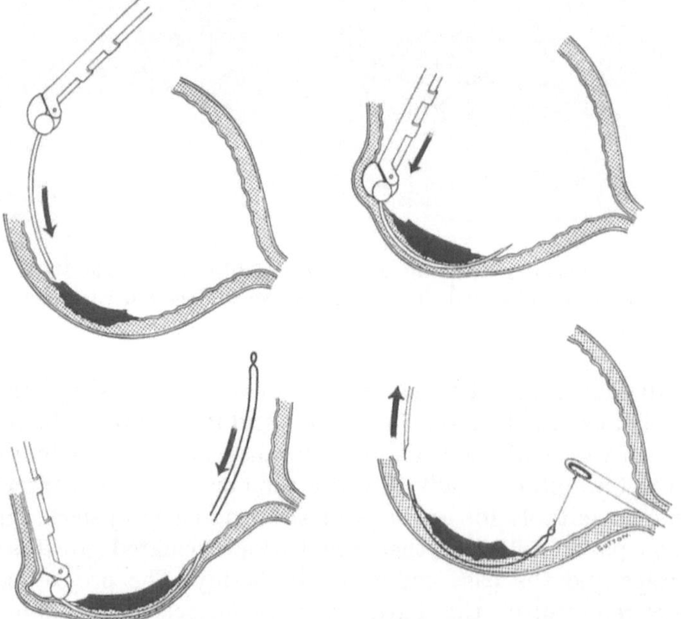

Fig. 16. Diagramatic summary of technique of tantalum-182 pin implantation

tumours treated with less than 4000 R tend to recur and doses in excess of 9000 R often produce local tissue necrosis.

The introducer for the tantalum pin is a modified Harris's boomerang needle holder and consists of a pair of hollow curved needles 5 cm long and 1 cm apart welded to a cross-bar (Fig. 15). The needles are inserted into the bladder wall beneath the site of the tumour, the points emerging towards the internal urinary meatus clear of the tumour region. The position of the needles is checked and an assistant using forceps introduces, as quickly as possible, the ends of the tantalum pin into the lumen of the needles, care being taken to avoid kinking of the wire. On removing the introducer the tantalum wire is drawn into the position previously occupied by the needles (Fig. 16). Depending upon the size of the area to be implanted, a second and perhaps a third pin may be similarly

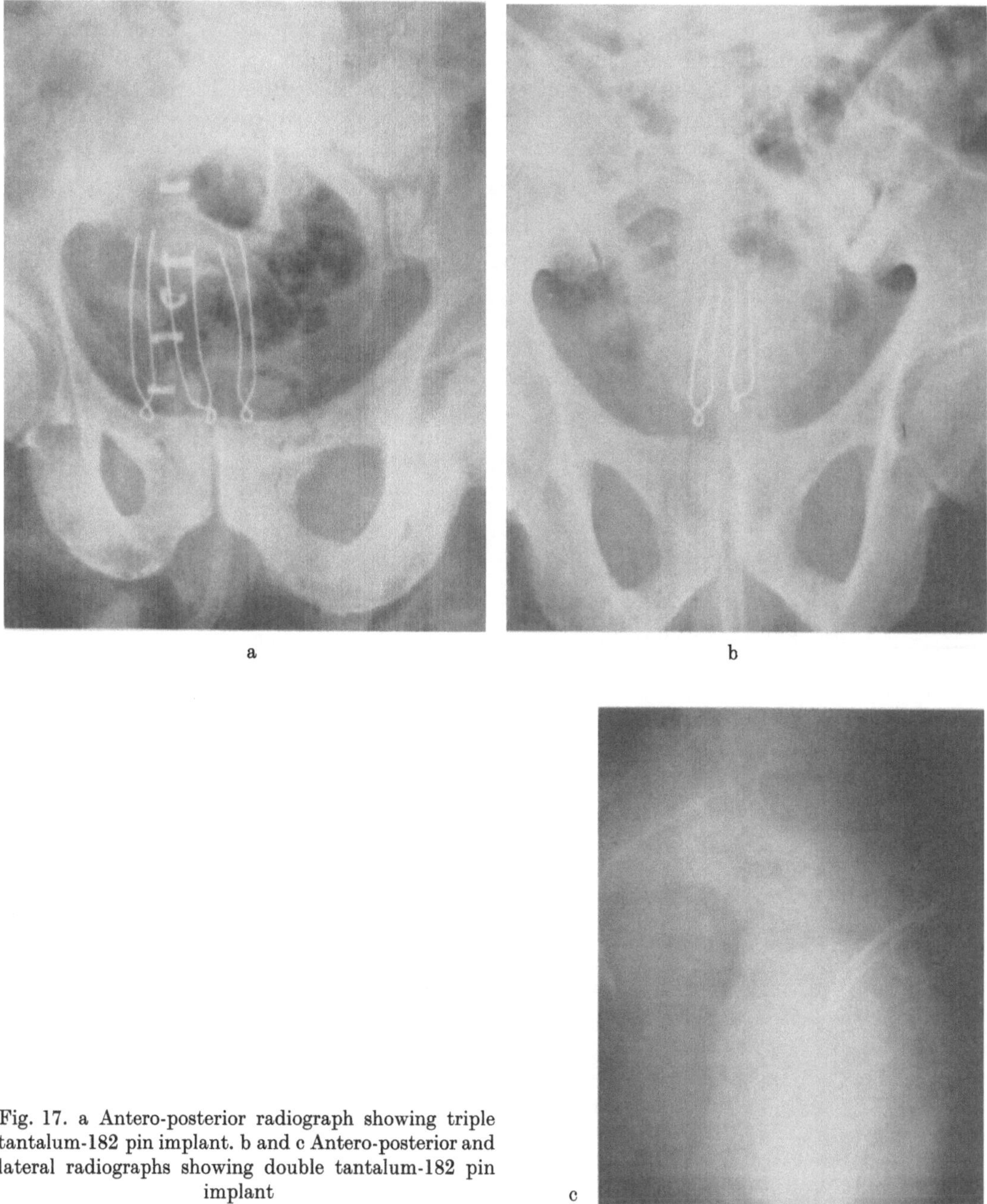

Fig. 17. a Antero-posterior radiograph showing triple tantalum-182 pin implant. b and c Antero-posterior and lateral radiographs showing double tantalum-182 pin implant

introduced. One aims to make the limbs of all wires parallel and 1 cm apart. The strong silk which is attached to the loop of each wire is then knotted to the end of an indwelling urethral catheter which is secured to the bladder by Harris's stitch. The bladder is then closed (WALLACE, STAPLETON and TURNER, 1952). Although the amount of irradiation received by the operating team during a tantalum implant is small, the dose received can be reduced even further by using two teams. The first team exposes the tumour and completes the implant and the second closes the bladder, completes the operation and supervises the removal of the patient from the theatre.

Anterior and lateral plain and double shift radiographs are taken of the pelvis to show the position of the sources (Fig. 17), and from these a three-dimensional model of the implant is reconstructed from which the dose rate is calculated (Fig. 18). The time to deliver 6000–6500 R at 0.5 cm from the plane of the implant is then determined, and at the appropriate time the pins are removed per urethrum by carefully withdrawing the catheter after cutting the Harris's stitch. This can be carried out in the ward and the discomfort of the procedure controlled with morphia, 15 mg. Another urethral catheter is

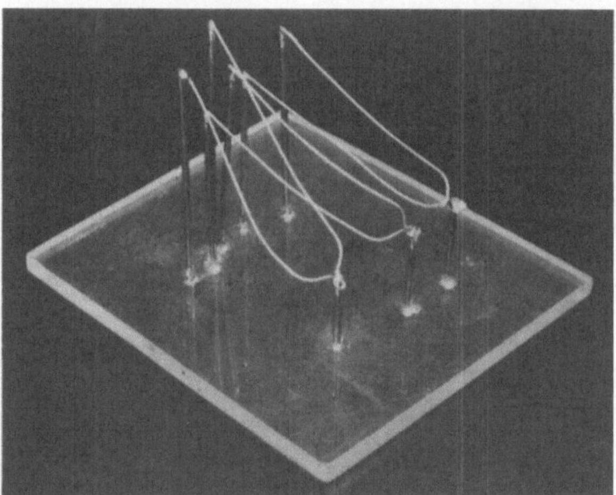

Fig. 18. Three-dimensional model reconstruction of triple tantalum pin implant

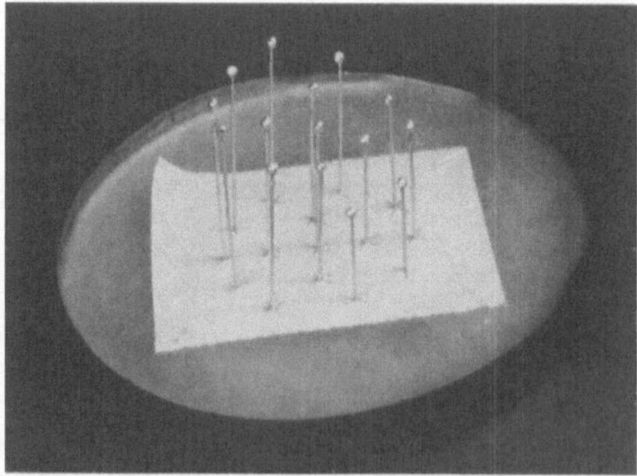

Fig. 19. Three-dimensional model reconstruction of gold grain implant

inserted to remain in position until the fourteenth post-operative day. Rarely, difficulty in removal of the pins may be experienced, and on 4 occasions in some 300 cases it has been necessary to remove them at open operation.

An example of a permanent gold-198 grain implant is shown in Fig. 14 and a three-dimensional reconstruction of such an implant in Fig. 19.

γ) Other methods of interstitial therapy

Some urologists attempt to implant tumours of limited size cystoscopically, using gold grains. It is extremely difficult to achieve a satisfactory implant by the transurethral route, and we have used it only when the patient is unfit for a general anaesthetic. Suprapubic cystotomy permits a more accurate assessment of the extent of the tumour and a more accurate distribution of the grains. It also provides the opportunity to examine the abdomen as well as the pelvic cavity for lymph node and visceral metastases.

YATES-BELL and HENRIQUES (1957) employ suprapubic cystotomy for implanting gold grains in the larger tumours, but smaller ones are dealt with by a closed technique, using suprapubic puncture in the male and the transurethral and transvaginal route in the female. With the closed technique, which is used as a curative treatment in early cases and as a palliative measure in late cases, the patient need be in hospital for only a few days.

A number of jigs have been designed to assist in obtaining geometrically more satisfactory implants with radon seeds (DOUGLAS, 1953) and gold grains (YATES-BELL and HENRIQUES, 1957). None of these, however, have proved very helpful because the position of the tumour often makes it impossible to use them. Furthermore, although a more symmetrical arrangement may be achieved initially, crowding of the grains tends to

ISOTOPE	SOURCE	½ LIFE	RADIATION - ENERGY		METHOD OF INTRODUC-TION	AVAILABILITY	ABSORBED BY TISSUES
			γ	β			
TANTALUM[182]	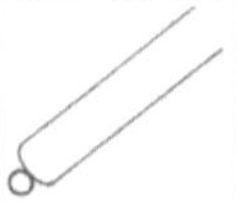	111 days	1,13 Mev	0,5 Mev (max)	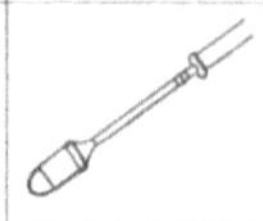	In stock (3 weeks)	No
GOLD[198]	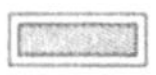	2,7 days	0,41 Mev	0,97 Mev	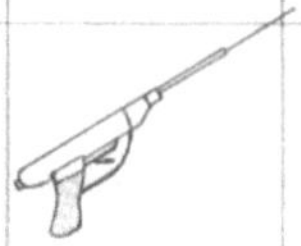	Order from Harwell as required	No
COBALT[60]	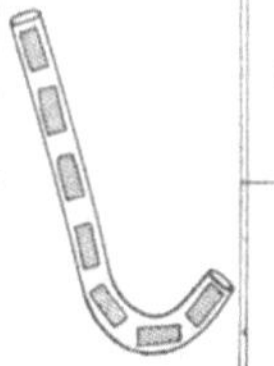	5,3 years	1,25 Mev	0,30 Mev	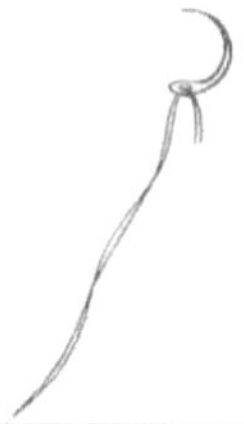	In stock	Yes
IRIDIUM[192]		74 days	0,4 Mev (mean)	0,59 Mev		In stock	No

Fig. 20. Materials for interstitial radiotherapy of bladder cancer

occur when the bladder wall contracts following removal of the jig. So far, it does not appear possible to improve on the combination of a practised eye and the repeating gold grain gun for achieving a good implant.

VERMOOTEN and MAXFIELD (1955) and VERMOOTEN (1955) reported on the use of narrow nylon tubing containing small spaced cobalt-60 pellets for interstitial radiotherapy of bladder cancer (Fig. 20). The tubing is very flexible and is threaded into the bladder wall beneath the tumour, like a suture. RUSCHE and JAFFE (1958), having observed the limitation of total cystectomy in a series of 80 patients with carcinoma of the bladder, are investigating the value of interstitial irradiation using radio-active chromic phosphate in particulate solution. This is injected at open operation and, in some cases, later followed by external supervoltage irradiation using a large cobalt unit. Other workers, such as DOUGLAS (1953) and also HERGER and SAUER (1942a) have combined limited interstitial therapy with supplementary external irradiation.

Radium needles in the past (WARD, 1948; WAYMAN, 1950) and more recently tantalum wire (VAN MIERT and FOWLER, 1956) have been used to carry out extravesical implants for more extensive, but nevertheless localised tumours of the bladder. This technique avoids opening the bladder and so hastens post-operative recovery, reduces the risk of fistula formation and eliminates the danger of implantation of malignant cells in the scar and elsewhere. Jönsson *et al.* (1958) advocate a combination of partial cystectomy and tantalum wire implantation of the bladder scar for mucosal and muscular lesions. In their series of 63 cases there were no deaths attributable to surgery. The time which had elapsed since treatment, however, was too short to evaluate this procedure, but so far there have been no local recurrences.

δ) Radiation reactions and complications

The implant produces a radiation cystitis which gives rise to some frequency of micturition and dysuria. This tends to be more marked when the lesion is situated in the region of the trigone. Symptoms usually subside in the course of three to four weeks, but may last in some degree for two to three months. In due course a slough often develops which persists for three to four months, but is usually not accompanied by troublesome symptoms unless complicated by secondary infection. Healing is sometimes delayed for six to nine months and occasionally for even longer periods. Calcareous material is frequently deposited on the ulcerated area and pultaceous stones may be found lying free in the bladder. When the ulcer has healed the treated area is represented by a flat white scar surrounded by a zone of telangiectasia which is sometimes the cause of repeated bouts of troublesome haematuria.

The duration and fate of irradiation ulcers depends chiefly on the size of the area implanted, the dose of irradiation given, the time in which it has been delivered and the type of radio-active source employed. Other less important factors are the site within the bladder and the type of tumour (Herger and Sauer, 1942).

Herger and Sauer (1942a, 1942b) in a series of 267 cases treated by radon seed implants with or without external irradiation noted vesical ulceration in 74% of cases. At the time of their report just over half had healed, 75% in less than 12 months and 94% within two years. Healing time depended upon the area irradiated, the larger the area the greater the delay in healing. Persistent ulceration occurred in only 11% of cases with implanted areas less than 2 cm in diameter. With increasing area the incidence rose, reaching 63% for an area 4–5 cm and 71% for an area exceding 5 cm in diameter. Ulceration was less likely to heal quickly when situated on the trigone and in the region of the internal urethral meatus. Herger and Sauer (1942b) found a correlation between the type of tumour, the incidence of irradiation ulceration and the delay in its healing. Thus persistent ulceration was found in only 12% of grade 1 papillary carcinomas compared with 63% for cases with grade 3 papillary or solid infiltrating growths.

In our experience a more marked irradiation reaction tends to be associated with tantalum-182 wire than with gold-198 grains. This is, no doubt, due to the presence of continuous linear sources and more uniform irradiation in the case of the tantalum wire, as compared with the multiple small discrete sources of gold which result in intervening areas receiving considerably less irradiation.

The presence of an irradiation ulcer with overlying slough may be interpreted as persistent tumour. This may lead to further treatment, irradiation which would be disastrous, or total cystectomy which may be quite unnecessary. A purely necrotic lesion differs from a neoplastic ulcer in that it shows no surrounding proliferation, oedema or plaques. It forms a discrete ulcer with well-defined flat edges, and although palpable on bimanual examination is rarely felt as a definite mass. If, after a period of observation, doubt still remains regarding the nature of such a lesion, a careful biopsy should be taken.

We have not met cases where there has been irradiation injury to the ureteric orifices leading to fibrosis and stenosis. On the contrary, late irradiation changes involving this region tend to produce a widening or gaping of the ureteric orifice similar in appearance to the "golf-hole" ureter of tuberculous cystitis. Hydro-ureter and hydro-nephrosis caused by tumour may be relieved following interstitial radiotherapy.

ε) *Experience with tantalum-182 wire implants*

Since 1951 approximately 300 cases of carcinoma of the bladder have been treated by interstitial irradiation with tantalum wire at the Royal Marsden Hospital, London, or at St. Peter's and St. Paul's Hospitals with which the Royal Marsden co-operates for radiotherapy. This constitutes about 10 % of all cases of bladder tumour seen at these hospitals. The three-year results for 145 cases treated between 1951 and 1956 are available, one of these cases being lost to follow-up. Five-year results can be presented for 74 patients treated between 1951 and 1954, two cases in this group remaining untraced.

Of the 145 cases, 86 (59 %) were staged as having mucosal lesions and 59 (41 %) muscular lesions. Histology was known in all but three patients and in 90 % of cases the tumour was a transitional cell carcinoma, the remainder being made up of one squamous cell, one glandular and one mixed carcinoma.

Results. The treatment of every case in this series has been in the united hands of surgeon and radiotherapist. The three and five-year results are given in Table 31. All cases treated are shown and no allowance has been made for post-operative deaths and deaths due to other causes. Such cases, including the 2 cases lost to follow-up, are all counted as "tumour deaths".

Table 31. *Bladder cancer:* [182] *Ta interstitial therapy*

Stage	3-year results (1951–1956)		5-year results (1951–1954)	
	cases	survivals	cases	survivals
Mucosal	86	62 (72 %)	44	31 (70 %)
Muscular	59	29 (49 %)	30	12 (40 %)
Total	145	91 (63 %)	74	43 (58 %)

The Royal Marsden Hospital, St. Peter's and St. Paul's Hospitals.

68 % of the cases were considered as having either purely papillary differentiated or solid anaplastic tumours, and the results in these two groups, taken from either end of the histological scale of malignancy, are shown in Table 32a. These cases were further

Table 32a. *Bladder cancer:* [182]*Ta interstitial therapy grade and prognosis*

Transitional cell carc. pattern and grade	3-year results		5-year results	
	cases	survival	cases	survival
Papillary differentiated	67	70 %	39	56 %
Solid anaplastic	31	52 %	11	55 %
Total	98	64 %	50	56 %

Table 32b. *Grade, stage and prognosis*

Transitional cell carc. pattern and grade	3-year results			
	Mucosal		Muscular	
	cases	survival	cases	survival
Papillary differentiated	53	75 %	14	50 %
Solid anaplastic	8	63 %	23	48 %
Total	61	74 %	37	49 %

classified according to their histological grade and clinical stage (Table 32b). It was surprising to find such a small difference between the papillary differentiated and the solid anaplastic groups, since a study of bladder cancer in general has revealed that solid anaplastic tumours are highly malignant growths which rapidly infiltrate the wall and soon give rise to metastases. It is particularly in this group that early diagnosis, with prompt institution of adequate treatment, is essential. After excluding deaths due to other causes and the two cases lost to follow-up, the results bring out perhaps more clearly the possible influence of histology on outcome (Table 33a and b). The number

Table 33a. *Transitional cell carcinoma bladder net results for ^{182}Ta interstitial therapy*

Stage	3-year survivals	5-year survivals
Mucosal	62/79 (78%)	31/39 (79%)
Muscular	29/47 (62%)	12/24 (50%)
Total	91/126 (72%)	43/63 (68%)

Table 33b

Stage	Grade	3-year survivals
Mucosal	pap. diff.	40/49 (82%)
	sol. anap.	5/7 (71%)
Muscular	pap. diff.	7/11 (64%)
	sol. Anap.	11/22 (50%)

Excluding deaths due to unrelated cause and 2 cases lost to F.U.

of cases, however, in each group is small and we shall have to wait for a larger series before drawing conclusions concerning the prognostic significance of histology in these selected cases.

Complications. The operative mortality in our series of cases treated by interstitial tantalum wire was 3.4% (Table 34) which agrees closely with the experience of others who have employed implant therapy at open operation. Thus Riches (1958) and recently also Carver (1959) report an operative mortality of 4% for all cases treated with radio-active gold grains. Ascending infection was the chief cause of post-operative death.

Table 34. *Bladder cancer: ^{182}Ta interstitial therapy complications of treatment. 145 cases (1951—1956)*

Complication		Cases
Post-operative death		5 (3.4%)
Pyelonephritis	3	
Pulmonary embolism	1	
Coronary thrombosis	1	
Scar implant		3 (2.0%)
Total cystectomy		12 (8.3%)
Radionecrosis	3	
Recurrence or new tumour	9	
Total		20 (13.7%)

The Royal Marsden Hospital, St. Peter's and Paul's Hospitals.

Scar recurrence following interstitial therapy is uncommon and occurred in 2% of our cases. MELICOW (1955) reported its occurrence in 6% of 210 cases treated by radium, compared with 20% for partial and 15% for total cystectomy. In 12 patients, which represents 8% of our series, total cystectomy was performed for residual growth, a new tumour or for radionecrosis mistaken for tumour.

Cause of failure in the tantalum series. Most recurrences and deaths from metastases following treatment of bladder cancer occur in the first two years, the majority in the first 12 months. In the 110 cases of JACOBS (1949) treated by interstitial radium, 37 survived five years, after which time 7 died of intercurrent disease and only 1 of bladder cancer in the sixth year, the remaining 29 patients being alive and well six to eleven years after treatment. In our series of 145 cases there were, up to December, 1959, 47 deaths attributable to tumour. Approximately half of these occurred in the first year and almost 80% in the first two years.

In a number of cases treatment by interstitial irradiation will fail because of lymphatic spread, but this is less common than we anticipated. In 32 cases in our series who died with tumour present, and in whom the site of recurrence or metastases was known, lymphatic involvement was present in 11, or 34%. More important than lymphatic spread, however, is the development of blood-borne metastases which were found in 22 of the 32 cases, practically 70%. It is of interest that in no less than 16 of these cases the vascular system appeared to be the sole route of spread (BLOOM, 1960).

ζ) Conclusions

Localised irradiation by interstitial techniques seems to be capable of eradicating the majority of limited mucosal and muscular stage carcinomas in the bladder of both the solid anaplastic as well as the papillary differentiated types. Failure to cure such cases is frequently due to the development of distant metastases which implant therapy and more radical methods of treatment are equally powerless to control. These results, moreover, have been achieved with a low mortality and morbidity rate and by a method of irradiation which spares the extravesical pelvic tissues and the greater part of the bladder itself.

It is not possible at the present time to say whether interstitial irradiation in addition to diathermy resection is necessary for tumours which appear not to have infiltrated muscle. We prefer to treat all such solid tumours and the average-sized broad-based papillary lesions by means of an implant, especially if there is any doubt concerning the depth of invasion, or if the biopsy specimen in such cases shows a high grade of malignancy or invasion of the submucosa. The recurrence rate of tumours of high grade malig-

Table 35. *Localised papillary tumours of the bladder. Results of treatment.* (RICHES, 1958)

Grade of malignancy	5-year survival rate	
	Cysto-diathermy	Radon seeds
Low	43/60 (72%)	26/37 (70%)
High	8/25 (32%)	17/36 (47%)
Recurrence rate	75%	42%

nancy treated solely by cysto-diathermy is greater than that following interstitial therapy (RICHES, 1958), Table 35). Recently, THOMPSON (1960) in a series of 75 non-infiltrating papillary tumours reports a recurrence-free rate of only 33% for patients treated by surgical methods alone, compared with 82% for those receiving ancillary irradiation, chiefly by means of radon seeds. A possible explanation, however, for this striking difference could be that diathermy was used for cases with multiple tumours, whereas radon seeds were employed for single tumours or where the disease was strictly localised.

Radio-active tantalum wire gives a far more satisfactory geometrical implant and a more uniform dose distribution than can be achieved with gold grains. At the present time, however, we have no evidence that the results obtained by tantalum wire are superior to those of gold grains in the best centres. On the other hand, some clinicians may find tantalum wire a more satisfactory material to use, since good gold grain implants are difficult to achieve.

η) *Reported results of interstitial therapy*

The results of this method of treatment will depend upon the proportion of patients with non-infiltrating and infiltrating tumours in a particular series. Millen (1950) and Barringer (1952) report a five-year survival rate of between 50–60% for patients with non-infiltrating lesions and of 20–25% for infiltrating cases. More recently, an overall five-year survival rate in the region of 60% has been achieved for patients with tumours suitable for this method of treatment, with 40–50% for muscle stage cases and approximately 70% for mucosal lesions (Table 36). No attempt has been made in our series of

Table 36. *Interstitial radiotherapy for bladder cancer. Reported results*

Author	Method	Cases	5-year survival rate (crude)		
			mucosal (%)	muscular (%)	total (%)
Herger and Sauer (1942a)	Radon with/without roentgen rays	119	—	—	29
Marshall (1947)	Radon with/without roentgen rays	300	—	—	17
Lenz et al. (1947)	Radium	46	—	—	20
Jacobs (1949)	Radium	110	—	—	34
Emmett and Winterringer (1955)	Radon with/without roentgen rays	118	—	—	29
Poole-Wilson (1957)	Radon	104	—	—	49
		45	71	50	60
Riches (1958)	Radon	73	—	—	59
Carver (1959)	Gold 198 grains	53	61	57	58
Royal Marsden Hospital Bloom (1960)	Tantalum 182 wire	74	70	40	58

cases treated with tantalum-182 wire to differentiate between superficial and deep muscle invasion, and the corrected five-year survival rate for this group as a whole is 50%. We think it highly likely that the poor results reported by some authors for interstitial therapy are due to selecting unsuitable cases, mainly from the peri-vesical group, for this treatment.

e) **External irradiation**

α) *Introduction*

(Principles of treatment. External irradiation v. radical surgery)

Generally speaking, external irradiation for bladder cancer has given poor results, largely because so many of the cases selected for this treatment have advanced and inoperable disease. Furthermore, a high proportion of cases are referred only after other methods of treatment have failed. There is often a large necrotic growth with extensive destruction of the bladder wall and long-standing cystitis. Not infrequently, ureteric stasis or complete unilateral obstruction may be present. Patients are often elderly and in poor general condition. Their haemoglobin is usually low and the blood urea often raised. Such cases are, of course, in the final stages of the disease and will soon die of pyelonephritis and uraemia. Many cases referred for external irradiation are not fit to undergo a course of treatment. In others, radiotherapy can at best be palliative and should often only be given to control bleeding or to relieve pain due to pelvic nerve involvement or skeletal metastases.

It has been argued that as carcinoma of the bladder is only moderately radio-sensitive high doses of irradiation are necessary to try and irradicate this disease, and this can only be tolerated by a limited volume of normal tissue. It is for this reason that some radiotherapists may prefer to confine radical treatment to the bladder, no attempt being made to irradiate the regional pelvic lymph nodes. An alternative view is that if the disease has already spread to these glands there can be no hope of cure, and in such cases, even though the patient's general condition is good, treatment should be regarded as palliative. The Manchester school considers that radical treatment should be given to patients in good general condition with tumours which have not extended outside the bladder proper. Patients in whom the tumour has entered the perivesical tissue are considered incurable and only suitable for palliative treatment.

Such views are contrary to the principles of cancer therapy whereby the regional lymph nodes as well as the primary tumour are taken into account during treatment. In, for example, carcinoma of the cervix it is generally accepted that external irradiation in addition to intra-cavitary radium should be given to all but the earliest cases, in an attempt to control pelvic lymph node deposits. Moreover, there is some evidence to suggest that heavy supervoltage irradiation can destroy or at least reduce the activity of such metastases (GRAY et al., 1958; RUTLEDGE and FLETCHER, 1958). The results of radiotherapy for carcinoma of the cervix from the best centres are highly satisfactory (HEYMAN, 1954; KOTTMEIER, 1955) and the incidence of complications from intracavitary radium and supplementary roentgen rays is low.

The improvement in dose distribution, achieved by supervoltage irradiation compared with conventional roentgen rays has, so far, not been accompanied by an appreciable increase in cure rate when treatment is confined to the bladder (POINTON, 1960).

Irradiation confined to the bladder is comparable in scope to total cystectomy, the results of which, in cases too extensive for diathermy resection or interstitial irradiation, are unsatisfactory. Thus, RICHES (1957) reported a five-year survival rate of only 10% for patients with muscular stage tumours treated by total cystectomy and 4% for cases with perivesical tumours. For patients with mucosal tumours he obtained a survival rate of 39%. BRICE et al. (1956) in a series of 156 cases obtained a five-year survival rate of 37% for superficial tumours (Stage O, A and B1) and 9% for deeply infiltrating lesions (Stage B2, C and D). JEWETT (1958) reported that total cystectomy gave a five-year survival rate of 50% for patients with superficial tumours (Stages O, A and B1) and 9% for those with deep tumours (Stages B2 and C).

According to MARSHALL (1956) approximately 40% of cases with tumours infiltrating deeply into the muscularis or through the full thickness of bladder wall have pelvic lymph node metastases. In a small series of cases BAKER (1955) found that 8 out of 10 cases with deep muscle invasion had at least one regional lymph node involved, compared with only one of 8 cases with infiltration of less than 50% of the muscle layer.

The extent of bladder carcinoma is related to the histological type of tumour and the grade of malignancy (FRANKSSON, 1950; RICHES, 1957; JEWETT, 1958; COOLING, 1959), the higher the grade of malignancy the greater the incidence of lymphatic and blood-borne metastases. JEWETT and BLACKMAN (1946) consider that in the deeply infiltrating tumours the incidence of metastases may be as high as 50% for poorly differentiated papillary tumours, 75% for poorly differentiated squamous cell tumours and practically 100% for undifferentiated growths.

Full pelvic irradiation to treat the bladder and the regional lymph node areas would, therefore, appear to be a rational procedure in cases with undifferentiated tumours infiltrating deeply into the bladder wall, provided that the morbidity rate for such large volume irradiation is not too great. Supervoltage irradiation to the whole pelvis, sparing the rectum as much as possible, is generally well-tolerated and a uniform dose of 6000 R in six to seven weeks with two to four million volt roentgen rays or a large Cobalt-60 unit appears, at present, to be safe. Alternatively, a somewhat higher dose may be given to the bladder and a lower dose to the pelvic wall, on the lines of treatment which have been well-established in the management of carcinoma of the cervix.

If the primary lesion is confined to the lateral wall of the bladder and does not cross the midline, it may be sufficient to raise the bladder and only the hemi-pelvis on the affected side to a high dose. Thus, WHITMORE and MARSHALL (1956) in radical surgical specimens found that unilateral bladder tumours have lymph node metastases confined to the ipsilateral side of the pelvis.

The alternative to full pelvic irradiation for cases with lymph node metastases is radical cystectomy with dissection of the pelvic nodes, but so far this operation has not proved successful. Thus, WHITMORE and MARSHALL (1956) in a series of 100 radical operations (radical cystectomy or pelvic evisceration) found 32 cases with regional lymph node involvement and only one of these cases survived for more than four years. Twenty-five cases failed to survive twelve months and only 3 survived two years. Even the 11 cases with limited lymph node involvement (obturator group only) fared badly, the only survivor being from this group. At least 50% of the cases are known to have died with a local recurrence. Moreover, the operative mortality reported by WHITMORE and MARSHALL (1956) for radical surgery was 17% and the incidence of non-fatal major complications was 13%. The 4-year survival rate for cases with superficial tumours extending no deeper than half way through the muscularis (Stages O, A, B1) was 39%, and for those with deeply infiltrating lesions extending more than half way through the muscularis or infiltrating through the full thickness of bladder wall (Stages B2 and C), but without lymph node metastases, only 15%. For the deeply infiltrating tumours with or without lymph node metastases (Stages B2, C and D) 11% survived four years. For the entire series of 100 cases (47 radical cystectomies and 53 pelvic exenterations) the 4-year survival rate was 18%.

When more than minimal lymph node metastases are present the prognosis following the most radical surgery appears to be practically hopeless as judged even by the two-year survival rate (WHITMORE and MARSHALL, 1956). Even with limited metastases close to the bladder only a small percentage of patients appear to be saved by radical surgery.

There would appear little to lose in employing external supervoltage irradiation to treat the hemi-pelvis or the entire pelvis on the lines suggested here. It remains to be seen whether such a treatment policy will ultimately lead to improved three and five-year survival rates and what price may have to be paid in the way of delayed radiation complications. Unfortunately, many recent reports in the literature on the use of supervoltage roentgen ray of telecurie units are difficult to evaluate because they do not give adequate information concerning such treatment factors as dose, time, depth-dose distribution and the precise volume treated. It would appear, however, from general experience with supervoltage equipment in the 1–4 MeV range that in the treatment of carcinoma of the bladder, rectum and cervix (WILLIAMS and MORGAN, 1955; MELLOR, 1960) a dose of between 6000 and 6500 R in six to seven weeks may be given to the major part of the pelvic cavity without serious complications developing, at least within two to five years. A more prolonged follow-up of patients is, however, necessary before we are able to fully assess the long-term risk.

β) Selection of cases for external irradiation

The best results with external irradiation in bladder cancer have been achieved in cases of multiple or solitary papillary carcinoma, not obviously infiltrating the muscularis. On the other hand, provided that a single tumour is not too large, such cases can be effectively treated by the more limited technique of interstitial therapy, which has the advantage of being able to raise a localised area of the bladder to a high dose whilst completely sparing the extra-vesical pelvic tissues.

External irradiation is best tolerated by patients in good general condition and in whom the growth is neither extensive, necrotic, nor deeply infiltrating and in whom there is a reasonable bladder capacity and good drainage. The cases selected for external irradiation fall into the following groups:

a) Multiple papillomatosis, as the alternative to intra-cavitary irradiation or total cystectomy.

b) Large tumours infiltrating the muscularis and unsuitable for interstitial techniques, as the alternative to total or radical cystectomy.

c) Tumours spreading through the full thickness of the bladder wall, as the alternative to radical cystectomy.

d) As definitive post-operative irradiation following partial cystectomy when the tumour is infiltrating deeply into muscle or when the presence of intramural or extra- vesical lymphatic spread is suspected.

e) Supplementary irradiation in cases treated by interstitial techniques in whom the dose is too low.

f) Palliative treatment for tumours which are fixed to the pelvic wall and in general for those invading adjacent organs. On rare occasions the alternative in the latter is pelvic evisceration.

g) Cases with severe haematuria as a preliminary to other methods of treatment.

h) Where operation is refused or contra-indicated for general medical reasons.

i) In the control of skeletal metastases.

γ) Apparatus and techniques

200–250 kV	Conventional deep roentgen rays.
400–500 kV	Conventional deep roentgen rays.
1– 8 MeV	Supervoltage roentgen rays.
20–30 MeV	Supervoltage roentgen rays.
Caesium-137	Telecurie units.
Cobalt-60	Telecurie units.

Conventional roentgen rays. With 200–250 kV roentgen rays radical treatment of bladder cancer is difficult to carry out. An adequate tumour dose is only possible in thin people with multiple fields utilising practically the whole circumference of the pelvis for ports of entry. Local reactions are often severe, especially in the more obese patients in whom only a poor depth dose is possible at the price of painful skin reactions.

With 400–500 kV roentgen rays (HVL = 5–6 mm Cu) the position is somewhat better. At this voltage it is possible to deliver a tumour dose of between 5500–6000 R in six weeks to the bladder using multiple small fields 6 × 10 to 8 × 12 cm without undue distress to the patient. Two anterior and four posterior oblique fields are usually employed, an alternative arrangement being an anterior direct and two anterior and two posterior oblique fields.

The use of these multiple fields around the circumference of the patient in order to raise the bladder to a high tumour dose results in a considerable dose of irradiation being delivered to the surrounding pelvic tissues. To try and overcome this WINTERNITZ and SMITHERS (1949) used a method of intermittent short axis rotatation with 400 kV roentgen rays. This involves a cluster of eight stationary cirular fields, each 8 cm in diameter,

arranged on the anterior abdominal wall on the circumference of a circle of radius 7 to
9 cm and angled at 55–65 degrees. A cone of irradiation is thus produced with the tumour
at the apex. Four of the eight fields are treated daily and by this technique it is possible

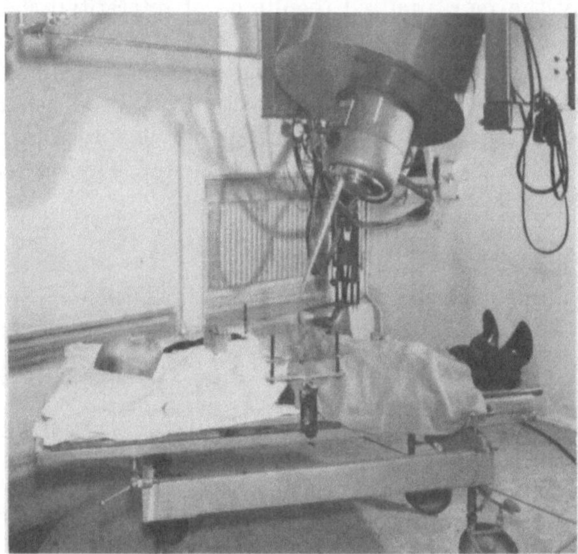

Fig. 21. Supervoltage Roentgen Ray Unit. Van de Graff electrostatic generator (2 MeV) and rotating floor.
Set-up for treatment of bladder cancer using continuous anterior short-axis rotation

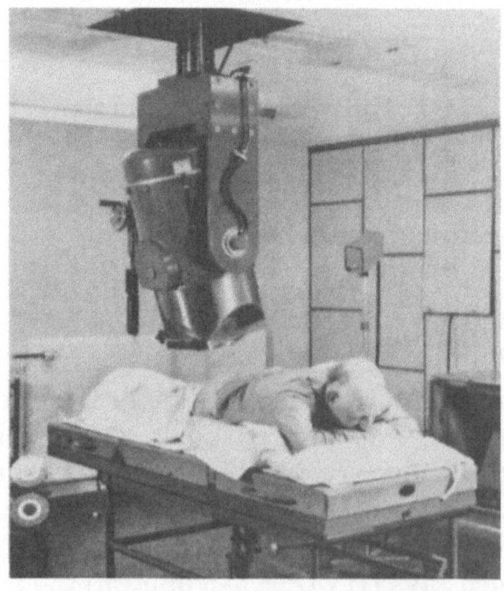

Fig. 22. Telecaesium Unit (1500 Ci)

to deliver a dose of 6000 R in six weeks to a volume 8 cm in diameter at a depth of
8–10 cm below the surface. If the dose falls off too abruptly posteriorly the anterior
cluster of fields may be opposed by a similar cluster from the posterior pelvic wall, or
more simply by two oblique fields avoiding the rectum.

Supervoltage roentgen ray and telecurie units. In the treatment of bladder cancer all
are agreed that supervoltage irradiation is preferable to the use of conventional roentgen
rays because of the improved depth dose, the better beam definition, the skin-sparing

effect, the decreased absorption in bone, the more accurate dosimetry and the improved tolerance.

Higher doses should be given with supervoltage treatment than with conventional roentgen ray therapy, not because the tissues tolerate the irradiation any better, but simply because more irradiation is required at the higher energies to produce the same degree of biological effect at the conventional level. The relative biological efficiency of beams of energy in the 2–8 MeV range compared with 200–250 kV roentgen rays appears to be of the order of 0.8–0.9. In theory this means that for a dose of 6000 R in six weeks to the bladder using conventional roentgen rays, a dose of 6500–7500 R must be given with megavoltage apparatus to produce the same biological effect. Clinical experience is in keeping with this concept, but in practice we do not, at the present time, exceed a maximum tumour dose of 7000 R to a strictly limited volume.

With roentgen rays generated at 1–8 million volts or γ-rays from Cobalt-60 and, to a somewhat lesser extent, from Caesium-137 it is possible to carry out radical treatment for bladder cancer more effectively, more simply, and with less disturbance to the patient than with conventional roentgen rays.

The optimum voltage for general clinical purposes appears to be in the range of 2–4 million. Most experience in the treatment of bladder cancer has been obtained with 2 MeV van de Graaf electro-static generators (Fig. 21) and 4 MeV linear accelerators. Machines for generating roentgen rays at 20–30 million volts have been used for bladder cancer chiefly in the United States, but such therapy is still in the experimental stage.

Massive telecurie units holding between 2000 and 3000 curies of Cobalt-60, which has a half-life of 5.3 years, are now being used for the treatment of bladder cancer in many centres throughout the world. Cobalt units, many of which are capable of rotation, emit beams of energy comparable to that from a roentgen-ray machine working at 3 million peak voltage.

More recently, Caesium-137 has been introduced for telecurie therapy and we have used such equipment for treating cases of carcinoma of the bladder (Fig. 22). This isotope, which has a half-life of 33 years, emits gamma rays which are comparable in quality to roentgen rays generated at 800000 peak voltage. The depth dose and the skin-sparing effect are not so great as with Cobalt-60, but telecaesium units are cheaper and require less protection. The long half-life, the absence of electrical maintainance and the better quality irradiation indicate that caesium units are likely to replace conventional roentgen-ray equipment for palliative therapy in cases with advanced pelvic cancer.

Rotation therapy. This method of treatment was originally introduced to deliver a high dose of conventional roentgen rays to a deep-seated tumour without excessive irradiation of the surrounding tissues, especially the overlying skin. With conventional equipment, however, the dose distribution in rotation techniques was unsatisfactory. The high dose volume was restricted and the depth-dose poor. In recent years this technique has been extended with advantage to the large cobalt units and to 2–4 MeV supervoltage roentgen ray apparatus. Rotation techniques applied to supervoltage radiotherapy not only further improve the depth dose, but also simplify the treatment of deep-seated tumours. Bladder cancer can be treated by long-axis rotation, which implies moving the beam around a fixed patient lying supine, or the patient can be made to move, standing erect with support on a rotating platform, whilst the beam remains fixed in the horizontal position. Short-axis rotation has also been used and here the patient rotates in the supine position with the beam remaining fixed at an angle (Fig. 21).

Short axis continuous rotation therapy with 2 MeV roentgen rays. We have used this method of treatment for irradiating wide-spread multiple papillary tumours of the bladder confined to the mucosa and also limited papillary on solid growths which are too large for interstitial therapy. The advantage of this technique over long-axis rotation for treatment aimed solely at the bladder is that the pelvic tissues are spared unnecessary irradiation. The appropriate radius of rotation and the angle of the roentgen ray beam to the vertical plane is determined for a particular case, depending on the depth and size of the volume to be treated. Generally speaking, we employ a 9 cm diameter field at an angle of approximately 40° moving through full 360° rotation (Fig. 24). For a maximum tumour dose of 7000 R the skin dose is approximately 2500 R.

Technique of radical radiotherapy

Localisation. Accurate localisation is necessary for radical treatment limited to the bladder. The whole bladder is treated, because of the difficulty of localising a tumour within the bladder and because a limited bladder growth may be associated with wide-

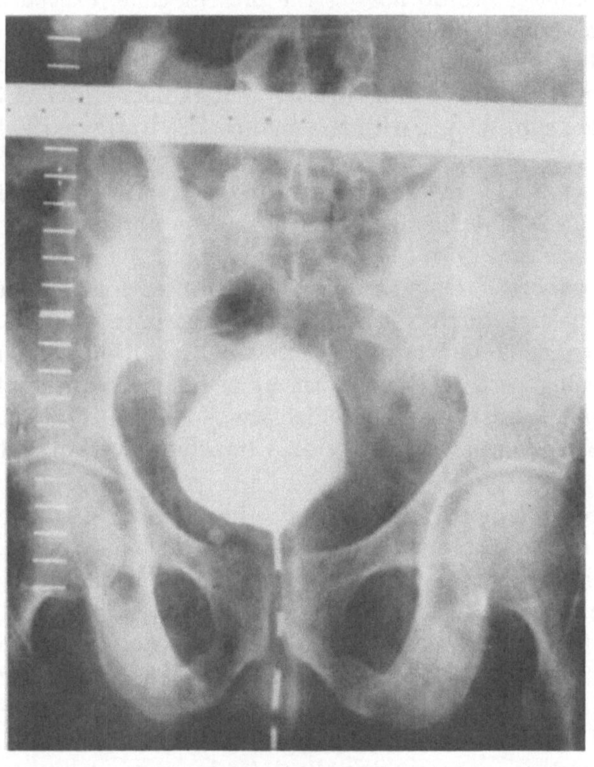
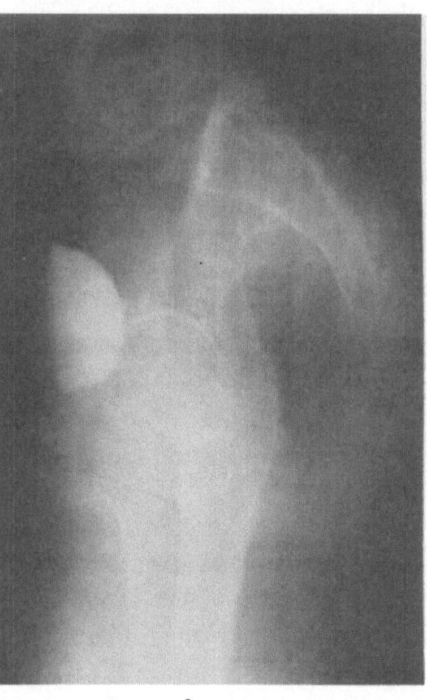

a   b

Fig. 23a and b. Localising cystogram. Antero-posterior and lateral radiographs showing bladder containing radio-opaque medium, and anterior and posterior skin centimetre scales

spread pre-malignant or malignant mucosal change and with a considerable degree of intramural circumferential lymphatic spread, especially in cases with deep muscle invasion (BAKER, 1955). The posterior urethra is included in the volume to be irradiated because of the risk of tumour extension at this site, especially in bladder neck lesions. The position of the bladder within the pelvis is found radiographically, using a suitable contrast medium and relating its position to anterior and posterior skin markers. Some 15–20 cm³ of sodium iodide, Diadone, or Stereopaque are injected into the bladder. Films in the saggital and coronal planes are taken with the patient in the supine and prone position, a radio-opaque button being present over tatoo marks on the skin, one just above the symphysis pubis and the other over the coccyx. A centimetre scale is also placed on the anterior and posterior skin surfaces (Fig. 23). It is necessary to place bolus bags on the skin over the markers if they are to be clearly seen in the lateral views. From the resulting films it is possible to localise the bladder in relation to the skin tatoo marks.

Treatment plan. A transverse outline of the patient is taken at the level of the pubic symphysis and then, using the information obtained from the localisation films together with knowledge of the clinical stage and likely sub-clinical spread of the tumour, a

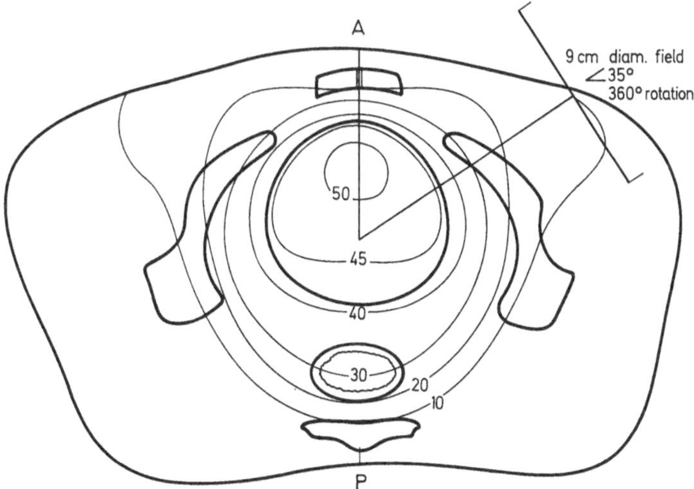

Fig. 24. Radical supervoltage irradiation. Anterior short axis 360° rotation technique for wide-spread papillary mucosal tumours. Factors: 2 MeV; HVL 11.7 mm Cu; FSD 100 cm. Dose: bladder max. 7000 R/min 6000 R; pelvic wall 2800 R; rectum 4200 R (average); skin 2100 R. Time: 6 weeks

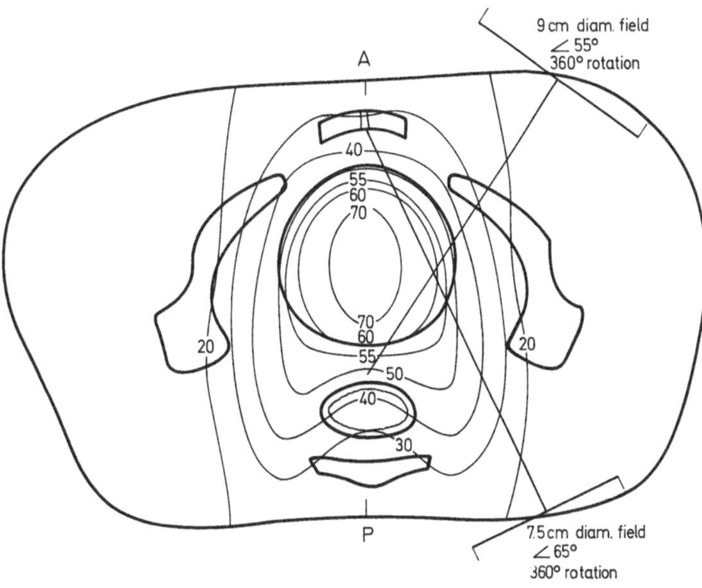

Fig. 25. Radical supervoltage irradiation. Anterior and posterior opposing short-axis 360° rotation technique for wide-spread papillary mucosal tumours. Posterior field is added to raise dose posteriorly in obese patients and in those with elongated bladders in the antero-posterior plane. Factors: 2 MeV; HVL 11.7 mm Cu; FSD 100 cm. Dose: bladder max. 7500 R/min 5900 R; pelvic wall 2150 R; rectum 3750 R (average); skin 2100 R. Time: 7 weeks

treatment plan is drawn up (Figs. 24–31). Three to six fixed fields or a rotation field are employed depending upon the aim of treatment, the size of the patient and the type of equipment available. From the plan the position, size and angles of the fields are noted and suitable marks are made on the patient to enable daily set-ups to be easily reproduced. A maximum bladder dose of between 900 and 1000 R per week is usually well-tolerated. Doses in excess of this are more likely to evoke severe bladder reactions. If distressing symptoms develop during irradiation the patient should be allowed a few days' rest from treatment which, in due course, may be recommenced at a lower dose-rate. Too rapid treatment may aggravate ureteric obstruction due to vesical oedema and precipitate pyelonephritis which is so frequently a fatal complication in this disease.

Treatment confined to the bladder. For example:

i) Wide-spread papillary mucosal tumours.

ii) Tumours with muscle invasion too large for interstitial therapy.

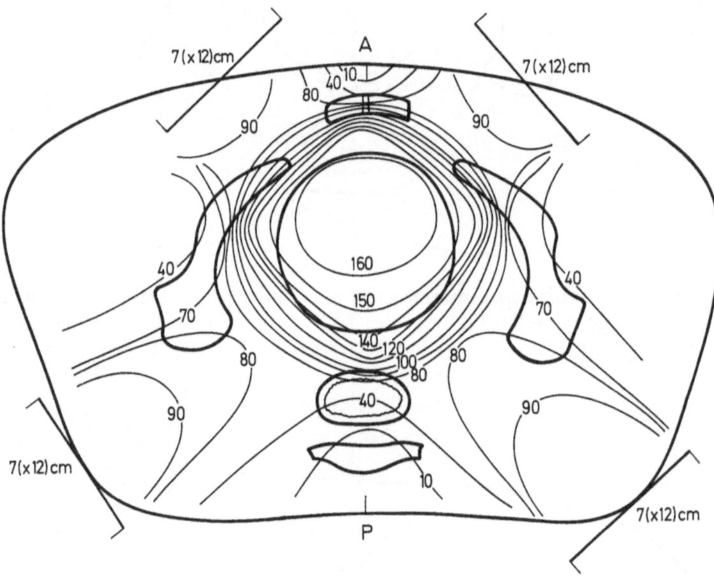

Fig. 26. Radical supervoltage irradiation. Four-field technique for wide-spread papillary mucosal tumours, or a single tumour infiltrating muscle, too large for interstitial therapy. Factors: 2 MeV; HVL 11.7 mm Cu; FSD 67 cm. Dose: bladder, max. 7000 R/min 6125 R; pelvic wall 3000 R; rectum 1750 R (average); skin 4400 R. Time: 7 weeks

The aim of this treatment is to raise a sphere of 8–9 cm to a high dose with minimal irradiation of the surrounding tissues. This can be achieved to some extent using multiple small beam-directed fields or long-axis rotation, but with these techniques the extravesical tissues still receive a considerable amount of irradiation. This can be greatly reduced with a short-axis rotation method. We have treated cases by this technique using a fixed 2 MeV roentgen ray machine or telecaesium unit and a rotating floor or table. To avoid the steep fall-off in dose posteriorly in obese patients and in those with elongated bladders in the antero-posterior diameter two angles may be employed for anterior rotation or, alternatively, posterior rotation (Fig. 25) or two posterior oblique fields may be added. With 2 MeV roentgen rays (HVL = 11.7 mm Cu) we aim to deliver a maximum tumour dose of 7000 R in six to seven weeks. This is usually well-tolerated by the patient. There is no malaise and nausea, no or little rectal reaction and negligible skin changes. Towards the end of treatment frequency and dysuria may prove troublesome, but these usually subside within two to four weeks of completing the course of irradiation.

Rotation techniques have the advantage of simplicity and are time-saving in set-up compared with the use of multiple fixed-field methods. With 2–4 MeV roentgen ray and cobalt-60 units 6500–7000 R in six to seven weeks is usually prescribed and is generally well-tolerated. With 22 MeV apparatus similar doses have been given. FRIEDMAN (1959) using 2 MeV long-axis rotation has delivered doses of up to 8000 to 10000 rads in forty to sixty days to the bladder. These doses, however, refer to the 100% isodose area which is very small. A substantial part of the bladder in these cases is encompassed by the 80% isodose line which represents a dose of 6400–8000 rads. Bladder doses of 5000–5500 R in the shorter period of three to four weeks with supervoltage equipment is more likely to produce troublesome frequency and dysuria.

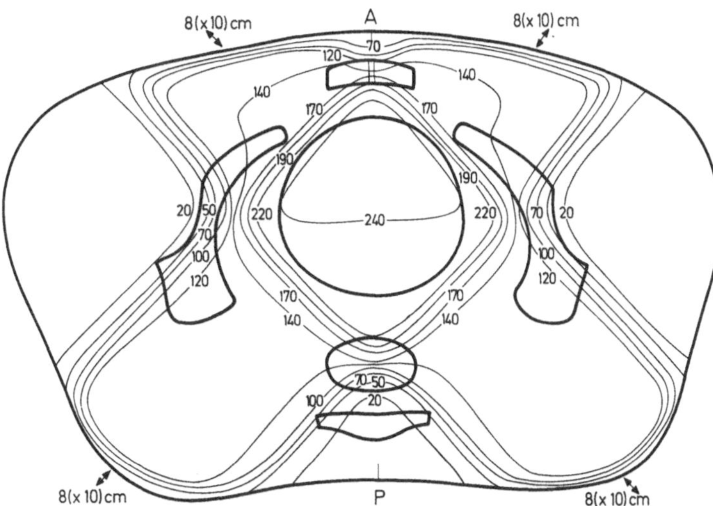

Fig. 27. Radical supervoltage irradiation. Four-field technique for large solitary tumour infiltrating superficial muscle. Factors: 8 MeV; HVL 1.33 cm Pb; FSD 100 cm. Dose: bladder, 7000 R; pelvic wall 3800 R; rectum 3500 R (average); skin 2900 R. Time: 7 weeks

Where multiple small fields with conventional deep roentgen rays have to be employed special care is necessary to obtain accurate beam-direction in the day-to-day treatment. This is greatly facilitated by means of the "protractor" or "pin and arc" methods described by PATERSON (1948). A dose of between 5500–6000 R in six weeks is possible with conventional deep roentgen rays (HVL at least 3.5 mm Cu) using 8 × 10 cm fields.

Irradiation of the hemi-pelvis or full pelvis. For example:

i) Tumours infiltrating through the full thickness of bladder wall.
ii) Solid anaplastic tumours deeply infiltrating the muscularis.

A high proportion of perivesical lesions have lymphatic spread and in such cases it is desirable to consider treatment to not only the bladder, but also the regional lymph node areas. In cases where the growth is clearly situated on the lateral wall of the bladder, treatment may be restricted to the corresponding hemi-pelvis (Fig. 30). The whole bladder and a suitable perivesical margin must be included, but the contra-lateral pelvic wall and its major blood vessels may be spared. For extensive intra-vesical tumours and those crossing over the midline the whole pelvis should be treated. With such a large volume care must be taken to avoid serious irradiation sequelae, especially delayed massive pelvic fibrosis. On the other hand, the prognosis in these cases is so serious that some risk with treatment is justifiable. Certain complications are not necessarily disasterous and may be rectified by judicious surgery. Thus, intractable bladder haemorrhage from telangiectases can be treated by cystectomy and a ureterocolic anastomosis performed or an ileal bladder fashioned for vesical contracture. Once the decision has been made to undertake a radical course of treatment the primary consideration must be to try and eradicate the malignant tumour.

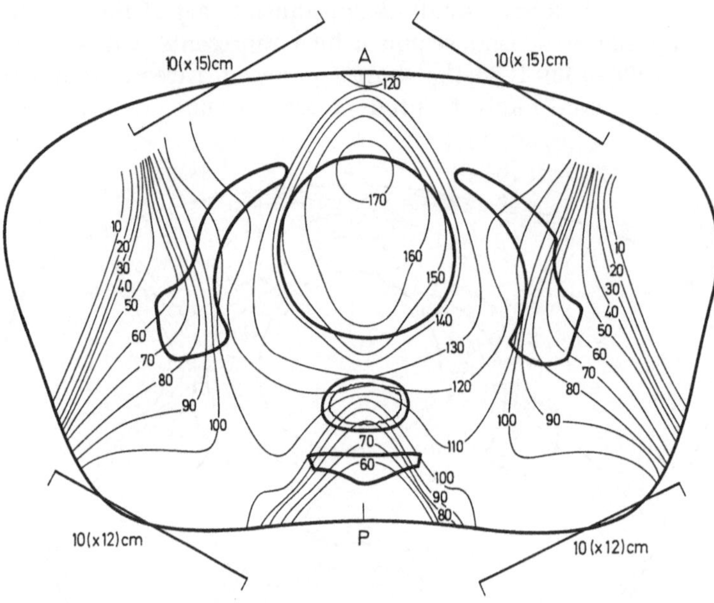

Fig. 28. Radical post-operative supervoltage irradiation. Four-field technique to treat whole pelvis in case of solid anaplastic tumour of bladder fundus removed by partial cystectomy. Surgical specimen revealed deep muscle invasion and involvement of lymphatics. Factors: 2 MeV; HVL 11.7 mm Cu; FSD 67 cm; bladder, max. 7000 R/min 5900 R; pelvic wall 4500 R; rectum 4100 R (average); skin 4100 R. Time: 7 weeks

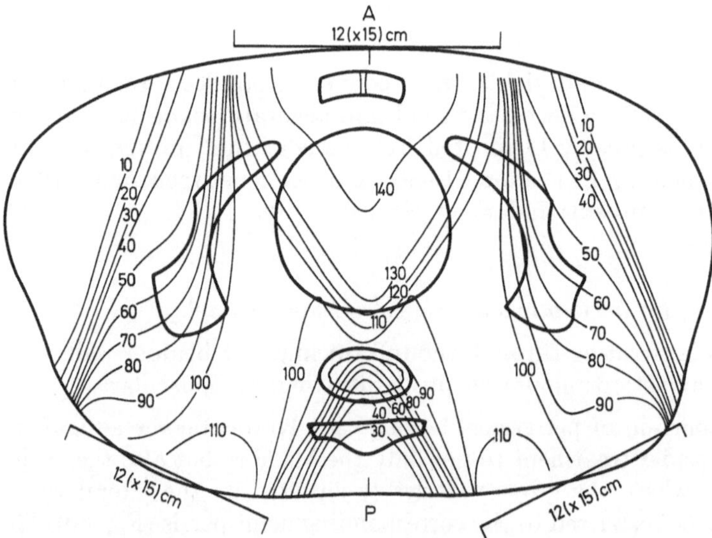

Fig. 29. Radical supervoltage irradiation for recurrent bladder cancer. Three-field technique to treat scar and whole pelvis in patient with recurrent tumour involving anterior wall of bladder and partial cystectomy scar. Factors: 2 MeV; HVL 11.7 mm Cu; FSD 67 cm. Dose: bladder, max. 7000 R/min 5500 R; pelvic wall 4500 R; rectum 3500 R (average); skin (operation scar) 7000 R. Time: 8 weeks

Using rotation cobalt-60 therapy for carcinoma of the cervix Mellor (1960) has delivered a tumour-dose of between 6000 and 7000 R to a volume 6–7 cm in the antero-posterior diameter and 14 cm in the transverses diameter in an overall time of six weeks.

Such treatment was well-tolerated, but it is too early to assess the possible late effects in terms of pelvic fibrosis. Using a 4 MeV linear accelerator and four fixed fields it is the practice of the Manchester school to deliver a dose of 5000 R in three weeks throughout

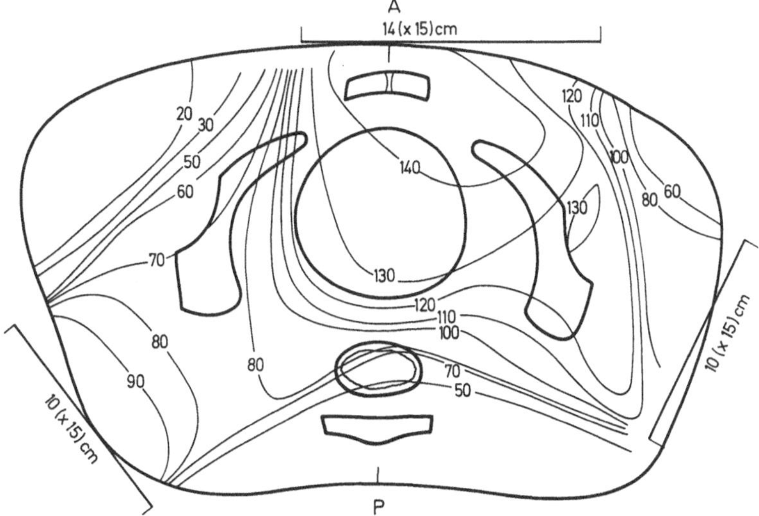

Fig. 30. Radical supervoltage irradiation. Three-field technique to treat hemi-pelvis in patient with solid anaplastic tumour on left lateral bladder wall, infiltrating muscle deeply. Factors: 2 MeV; HVL 11.7 mm Cu; FSD 67 cm. Dose: bladder, max. 6500 R/min 5600 R; pelvic wall, left, 6000 R; right 3700 R; rectum 3000 R (average); skin (max.) 6500 R. Time: 7 weeks

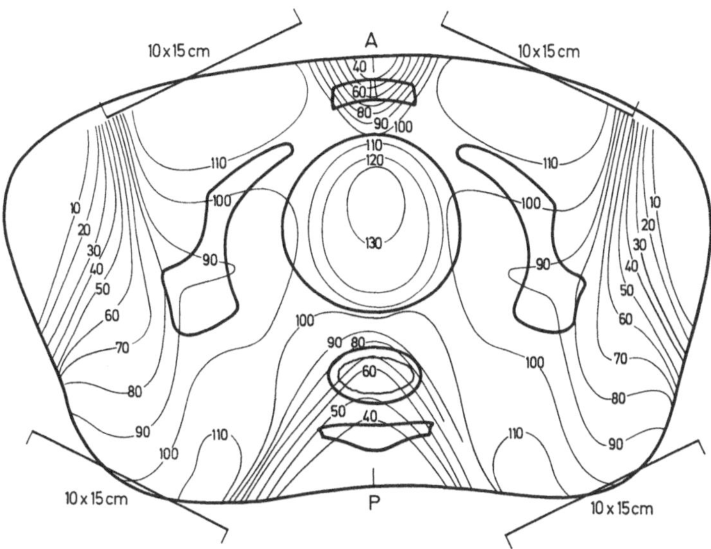

Fig. 31. Palliative external irradiation. Four-field technique to treat whole pelvis. Tumour extends to pelvic wall. General condition of patient good. Factors: 1500 curie caesium unit; HVL 11.0 mm Cu; SSD 40 cm. Dose: bladder, max. 5500 R/min 4250 R; pelvic wall 4000 R; rectum 2900 R (average); skin 4250 R. Time: 4–5 weeks

the whole pelvis for advanced cases of carcinoma of the cervix. The dose to be delivered in advanced cases of carcinoma of the bladder will depend upon the volume to be treated, the general condition and reaction of the patient and the equipment available. Some examples of radical treatment in this disease are presented in Figs. 28–30. With 2–4 MeV roentgen rays or a cobalt-60 unit full pelvic irradiation may be taken to a fairly uniform depth dose of 6000 R in six to seven weeks. Our policy at present in those cases with advanced primary tumours and no gross evidence of lymph node or distant metastases, is to treat the bladder to a maximum tumour dose of 6500–7000 R in six to seven weeks with the dose falling off to between 4500–5000 R at the pelvic wall (Fig. 28). This is based on the assumption that a larger dose of irradiation is required to control the main bulk of tumour at the primary site than occult metastases in the regional lymph nodes.

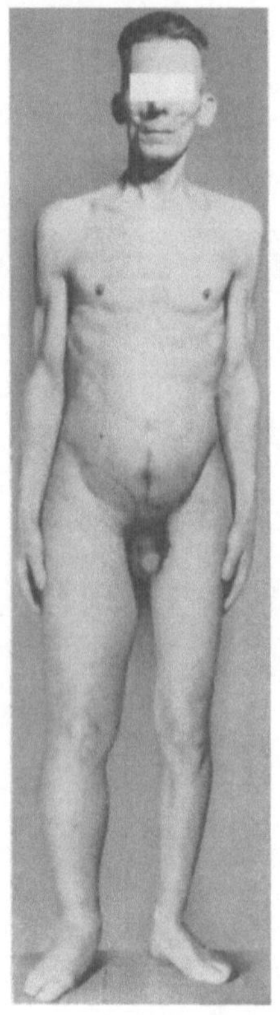
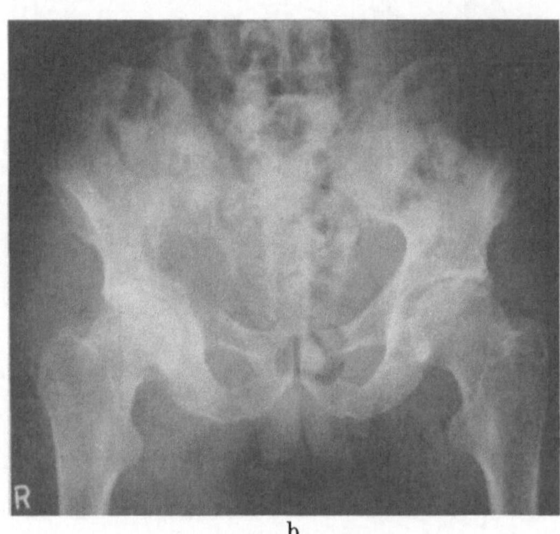
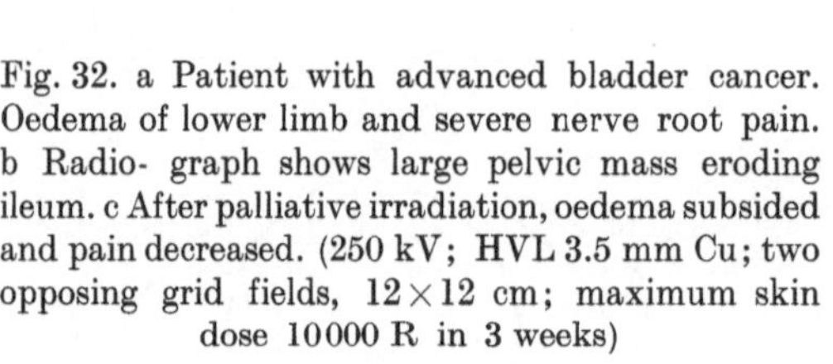
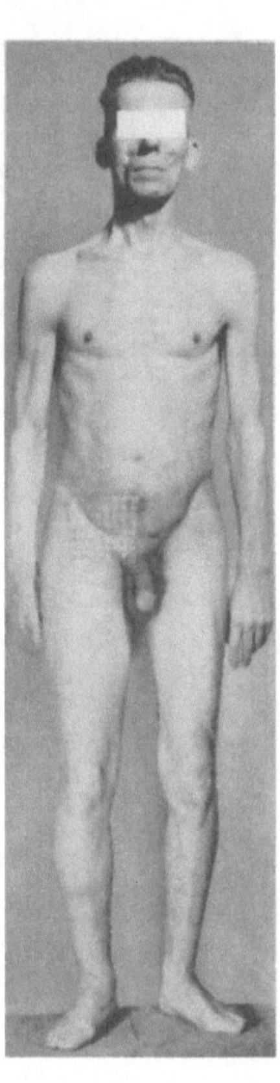

Fig. 32. a Patient with advanced bladder cancer. Oedema of lower limb and severe nerve root pain. b Radio- graph shows large pelvic mass eroding ileum. c After palliative irradiation, oedema subsided and pain decreased. (250 kV; HVL 3.5 mm Cu; two opposing grid fields, 12×12 cm; maximum skin dose 10000 R in 3 weeks)

Palliative radiotherapy. For example:

i) Patients with tumours fixed to the pelvic wall or invading adjacent organs.

ii) Patients in good general condition with extra-pelvic spread or distant metastases.

iii) Patients with limited tumour, but in poor general health.

iv) Painful skeletal metastases.

v) Pain and leg oedema due to nerve and lymphatic involvement by tumour in the pelvis.

The aim of palliative irradiation is to alleviate distressing symptoms or to try and prevent them from developing later by means of a short, but substantial course of irradiation with minimal general and local reactions (Fig. 32). Although palliative irradiation may prolong life it is carried out with the purpose of making what life remains to the patient more tolerable both from the mental as well as the physical aspect. Radiotherapy, however, has no place in the management of the moribund patient nor in the late case where distressing symptoms can be more readily controlled with narcotics and analgesics.

Unfortunately, many cases of bladder cancer when first seen in a urological clinic are hopelessly advanced. Some of these cases are so ill that only analgesics and sedatives are indicated. For many of the others a course of palliative irradiation to the bladder or pelvis may prove of value in reducing pain, in decreasing frequency and dysuria and in stopping haematuria. Pain due to involvement of bone by metastases or direct erosion by a pelvic mass (Fig. 32b) may be reduced or relieved by a short course of treatment. Not infrequently, following palliative irradiation the patients' general condition improves, and when the end does come it appears to be more rapid than in the untreated case. Occasionally, the degree of palliation achieved by irradiation is quite striking, the patient being able to return to full-time employment with minimal symptoms for a period of a year or more.

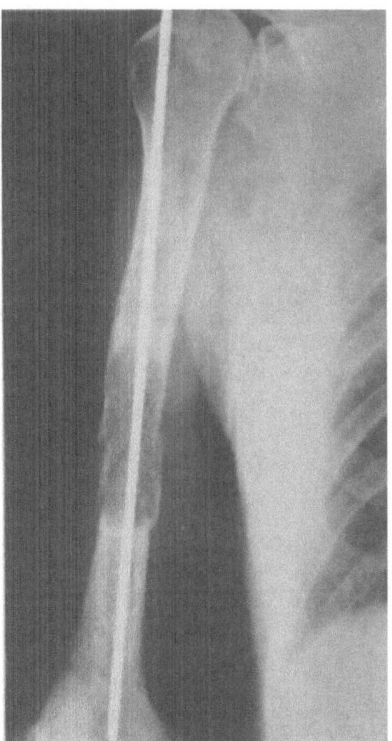

Fig. 33. Pathological fracture of humerus due to bladder cancer metastasis. Treated by internal fixation and external irradiation

Palliative irradiation should be given carefully and with frequent observation of the patient as to clinical progress. Deterioration of the general condition often associated with an ascending urinary infection and rising blood urea is an indication to abandon irradiation. It is important to remember that the treatment of unsuitable cases by irradiation often increases the patient's distress and brings disrepute to radiotherapy for bladder cancer in general.

Palliative external irradiation may be given to the bladder alone or to the entire pelvis by a variety of simple techniques, using ordinary or grid fields. The type of palliative irradiation chosen for a particular patient will depend largely upon his general condition, symptoms and the aim of treatment. Thus, for an elderly debilitated patient with advanced disease who is being looked after at home or in a neighbouring hospital and is distressed by persistent haematuria, a series of four or five consecutive daily treatments will usually suffice to control haemorrhage (e.g. 250 kV, HVL, 3.5 mm Cu, 2 anterior oblique pelvic fields with compression, 10×15 cm; skin dose, 400 R to both fields daily $\times 5$; maximum tumour-dose approximately 1 800 R). On the other hand, a younger man, in reasonably good condition, with a large tumour fixed to the pelvic wall should have the possible benefit of a more substantial course of treatment, afforded by a multiple field technique, extended over three to four weeks (e.g. 250 kV; HVL, 3.5 mm Cu; 2 anterior and 2 posterior oblique pelvic fields, 10×15 cm; skin dose, 350 R to two fields daily $\times 10$; maximum bladder dose approximately 4250 R, pelvic wall dose 3150 R; overall time, 26 days). Although conventional roentgen rays are generally used for palliative treatment there is a definite advantage in using supervoltage equipment for this purpose.

Skeletal metastases in the spine are treated with conventional roentgen rays using a single direct field 12×6 to 15×7.5 cm. A dose of 500 R may be given on five consecutive days. Deposits in the long bones or in the pelvis are treated by two opposing fields 10×12 to 12×15 cm, 300 R being delivered to two fields daily to a tumour dose of 3000 R in

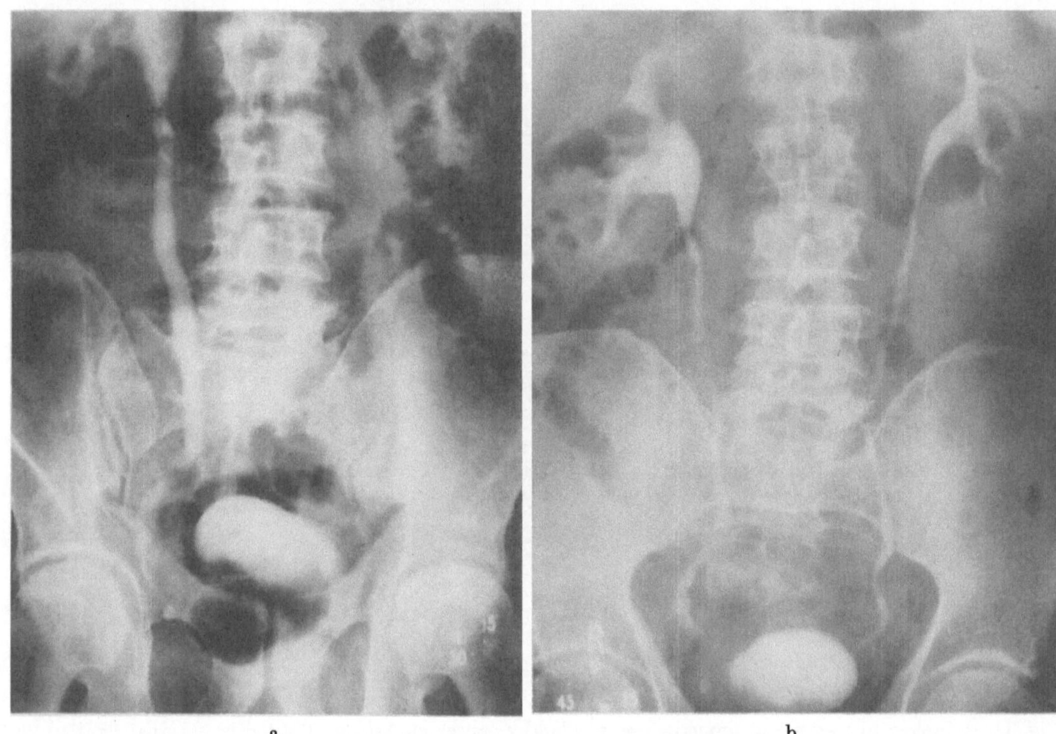

a   b

Fig. 34. a Pyelogram showing right-sided hydro-nephrosis in patient with fixed pelvic mass due to bladder cancer. b Pyelogram showing relief of ureteric obstruction following pelvic irradiation

two weeks. Greater tumour doses such as 3500–4000 R should be given to skeletal deposits when they are solitary or limited in number and the patient's general condition is good. With lower doses in such cases early recurrence of pain is common and further treatment may be required.

A fracture or threatened fracture at the site of a metastasis in the humerus or femur can be treated effectively by internal fixation followed by a course of conventional roentgen rays. This brings relief of pain and leads to early ambulation (Fig. 33).

f) General care of the patient

Prior to commencing radical external irradiation urinary infection is treated with the appropriate antibiotic. Bladder-neck or urethral obstruction by tumour or an enlarged prostate should be relieved endoscopically. In patients with bilateral hydronephrosis ureteric transplantation into the colon or into an ileal loop should be considered before starting treatment, since in such cases there is a great risk of pyelonephritis and renal failure developing during the course of irradiation. In many hopelessly advanced cases, however, the surgical relief of ureteric obstruction is of questionable value, since uraemic death is not associated with undue suffering. Sometimes the degree of ureteric obstruction is reduced following irradiation alone and occasionally even completely relieved with return of the pyelogram to normal (Fig. 34a and b). Anaemia is treated by transfusion; it is best to avoid oral iron during radiotherapy as this may aggravate gut reaction. Plenty of liquids should be taken and every effort should be made to provide an attractive as well as an adequate diet. If there is little desire for solid food extra milk and other liquids containing glucose and "Complan" mixture will help to keep up a satisfactory calorie intake.

Sleep will often be interrupted by frequency of micturition. If this becomes severe and the patient's general condition suffers as a result, a self-retaining urethral catheter may have to be employed, at least during the night. Male cases will often get a good night's rest by sleeping with the penis inserted into a bed urinal.

Patients with troublesome frequency, dysuria and strangury due to irradiation reaction should be rested from treatment for several days. Antispasmodics such as Probanthine (Searle) given in doses of 30 mg every six hours may help to reduce bladder symptoms. For persistent pain a freshly prepared mixture containing acetylsalicylic acid, and nepenthe is of considerable value. For more severe pain Pethidine 100 mg by mouth or by injection will be required.

Irradiation-induced diarrhoea and rectal discomfort should be treated by a low residue diet and by a mixture containing kaolin 2 g, sodium bicarbonate 0.6 g, tincture of chloroform and morphine 0.6 ml every four to six hours. If necessary radiotherapy should be suspended for a few days until symptoms abate. Prednisone in doses of 5 mg thrice daily appears to be of value in reducing the intensity of early vesical and rectal reactions.

With supervoltage irradiation above 2 MeV there is little or no skin reaction and generally speaking no special care of the treated areas is required. However, in obese patients quite severe reactions tend to develop in abdominal folds, especially in the groins, and these areas must be kept clean and dry and free from friction as much as possible. Treatment with conventional roentgen rays is often associated with troublesome reactions and the skin should be dabbed twice daily from the beginning of treatment with a solution of acriflavine 1 in 1000 or a solution containing calomine and tannic acid. With the appearance of an intense dusky erythema with dry desquamation the regular application of a 1% watery solution of gentian violet, which is allowed to dry and form a coagulem, will help to keep the skin intact and comfortable until tolerance is reached. Once moist desquamation appears treatment should be stopped in that area.

Moderately severe bladder reactions cannot be avoided in the radical treatment of bladder cancer. Even in patients that develop a severe irradiation reaction during the treatment of an advanced tumour the subsequent benefit often outbalances the discomfort of the treatment.

g) Results of treatment

A limited number of reports are available in the literature concerning the treatment of bladder tumours with conventional roentgen rays (FERGUSON, 1936; HERGER and SAUER, 1943; MARSHALL, 1947; FRANKSSON, 1950; LOCKWOOD and CHAPMAN, 1956; POOLE-WILSON, 1957). In recent years, with the advent of supervoltage apparatus, more interest has been shown in this subject and many authors have described their experience in the treatment of bladder tumours with roentgen rays in the 1–22 MeV range and with cobalt units (COLBY and SCHULZ, 1943; COLBY and SNIFFEN, 1947; BUSCHKE et al., 1950; HARE et al., 1954; BLOMFIELD, 1954; CORDONNIER and SEAMAN, 1956; SWINNEY, 1957; PLANK et al., 1957; CUCCIA et al., 1958; SMITH and LOTT, 1958; RUBIN and BURAN, 1959; WATSON and BURKELL, 1959; FRIEDMAN, 1959; COX, 1960; MORRISON, 1960; BROWNE and OGDEN, 1960; POINTON, 1960).

Unfortunately, insufficient time has elapsed for an adequate number of three and five year results to be available. Many reports concerning this subject are unsatisfactory in other ways. For example, the authors so often fail to analyse their cases in sufficient detail to permit careful comparison with comparable cases in other series. In addition, dose-time treatment factors are often inadequately reported, and very rarely is the volume given a certain dose adequately defined. The whole issue is further complicated by such variables as the extent of disease, the histological grade of malignancy, the general condition of the patient, the state of the urinary tract and finally the method of treatment used and the skill with which it is applied.

After reviewing the literature the position with regard to external supervoltage irradiation in the treatment of bladder cancer would appear to be roughly as follows. Some 60–75 % of all cases treated derive appreciable subjective benefit. In about 40–50 % of cases there is objective evidence of marked tumour regression. So far, it appears that 30–40 % of cases survive two years, 20–25 % three years and about 15 % five years, no correction being made in these figures for deaths due to other causes.

The results of external irradiation for bladder cancer at the Royal Marsden Hospital are shown in Tables 37 and 38. These survival rates are uncorrected; cases lost to follow-

Table 37. *Carcinoma of the bladder. Results of conventional roentgen beam therapy (250–400 kV). Royal Marsden Hospital, 1949–1956*

Stage	Cases treated	Survival rates			
		1 year	2 years	3 years	5 years
Mucosal	35	23/35 (66%)	15/35 (43%)	10/35 (29%)	5/22 (23%)
Muscular	57	20/56 (36%)	16/56 (29%)	12/56 (21%)	3/39 (8%)
Perivesical	85	32/76 (42%)	10/76 (13%)	6/76 (8%)	5/52 (10%)
Pelvic fixation	80	17/80 (21%)	6/80 (8%)	2/80 (3%)	0/42 (0%)
Unstaged	22	3/22 (14%)	0/22 (0%)	0/22 (0%)	0/12 (0%)
Total	279	95/269 (35%)	47/269 (18%)	30/269 (11%)	13/167 (8%)

Table 38. *Carcinoma of the bladder. Results of supervoltage roentgen beam therapy (2 MeV). Royal Marsden Hospital, 1950–1956*

Stage	Cases treated	Survival rates			
		1 year	2 years	3 years	5 years
Mucosal	21	14/21 (67%)	12/21 (57%)	10/21 (48%)	5/14 (36%)
Muscular	31	17/31 (55%)	14/31 (45%)	10/31 (32%)	3/20 (15%)
Perivesical	41	18/41 (44%)	8/41 (20%)	4/41 (10%)	4/25 (16%)
Pelvic fixation	12	4/12 (33%)	2/12 (17%)	2/12 (17%)	0/6 (0%)
Unstaged	1	1/1 —	1/1 —	1/1 —	1/1 —
Total	106	54/106 (51%)	37/106 (35%)	27/106 (25%)	13/66 (20%)

up and those dying from other causes are counted as "tumour deaths". The improved results with supervoltage irradiation compared with conventional roentgen rays are evident, and the two-year survival rate of 35 % for all treated cases is very similar to that reported by Brice *et al.* (1956) and by Wallace (1959) for simple total cystectomy and by Whitmore and Marshall (1956) for radical cystectomy in highly selected groups of patients.

Treatment by supervoltage roentgen rays in the majority of cases in this series between 1949 and 1956 has been on the principle of delivering a high dose to a limited volume represented by the bladder and immediate perivesical tissue. It remains to be seen whether our present policy of hemi-pelvic or full pelvic irradiation in the more advanced cases will give better results.

Some authors prefer to treat cases of bladder cancer, which we would consider suitable for interstitial therapy, by external supervoltage irradiation. We employ implant techniques for all suitable cases and, as already stated, reserve external irradiation for the larger, the more numerous and the more advanced tumours. To obtain a more accurate picture of the overall radiotherapy results at the Royal Marsden Hospital it is, therefore, necessary to combine the results of tantalum-182 wire implant therapy with those of external irradiation. A sufficient number of mucosal and muscular stage cases treated by tantalum implant or 2 MeV roentgen rays are now available to consider the 3- and 5-year results (Table 39). It is important to note that in this series cases with tumours

Table 39. *Carcinoma of the bladder. Radiotherapy results for tumours limited to bladder wall. Roentgen beam (2 MeV) or interstitial (^{182}Ta) irradiation. Royal Marsden Hospital, 1950–1956*

Stage	Period 1950–1956		Period 1950–1954	
	Cases	3-year survival	Cases	5-year survival
Mucosal	107	72 (67%)	58	36 (62%)
Muscular	90	39 (43%)	50	15 (30%)
Total	197	111 (56%)	108	51 (47%)

infiltrating muscle include those with deep as well as superficial involvement (the B 1 and B 2 stages of JEWETT and STRONG, 1946 and of MARSHALL, 1956).

h) Response of bladder tumours to irradiation

If irradiation fails to eradicate a limited tumour of the bladder and the patient is fit for major surgery, a partial or total cystectomy may save his life. Unfortunately, it is not possible to predict the radiosensitivity and radiocurability of a particular tumour beforehand. These probably depend not only upon intrinsic properties of the tumour itself, but also upon certain local factors in the connective tissue stroma and its vascularity as well as general factors in the host. A tumour may be regarded as showing a favourable response to irradiation if it undergoes a marked or complete regression with doses of irradiation which do not cause excessive damage to normal tissue.

Attempts have been made to correlate pattern, histological type and grade of bladder tumour with response to irradiation. HERGER and SAUER (1942, 1943) studied some 450 cases of bladder cancer which were treated by external irradiation alone combined

Table 40. *Bladder tumours. Response to irradiation.* (HERGER and SAUER, 1943)

Tumour type	Treatment ineffective			
	Cases	2500 R or less	2501–5000 R	5100–5800 R
Papillary	5/25 (20%) ⎫			
Papillary infiltrating	54/91 (59%) ⎭	16/44 (36%)	18/67 (27%)	1/5 (20%)
Solid infiltrating	43/44 (98%)	10/12 (83%)	17/27 (70%)	1/5 (20%)

with a radon seed implant. Papillary tumours were found to respond more favourably than solid infiltrating growths (Table 40). It was concluded that the amount of irradiation required to destroy solid tumours is so large that it cannot be delivered by external means without inflicting irreparable damage to normal tissues. Only by interstitial techniques is it possible to deliver the dose required to destroy some of these tumours with safety.

In 160 cases treated by conventional deep roentgen rays (142 cases) or 1000 kV roentgen rays (18 cases) with or without a subsequent radon seed implant or diathermy, Herger and Sauer (1943) were able to correlate type of tumour with response to irradiation according to dose (Table 40). Of the total series 9% showed complete regression, 52% marked regression and 39% no apparent change. If regression did occur in cases of solid infiltrating cancer it was of short duration. In 15 out of 44 patients with this type of tumour, in whom regression was obtained, recurrence was evident after three to six months in 10 cases and after six to twelve months in the remaining 5 cases. The authors concluded that a satisfactory response to irradiation can be obtained in more than 50% of patients with papillary or papillary infiltrating tumours. In 13 of 57 cases with this type of tumour the lesion completely disappeared (2–5 years follow-up) after external irradiation. In the remaining 44 cases marked regression enabled further limited treatment to be undertaken such as diathermy coagulation with or without radon seed implantation. Unfortunately, in 24 of these 44 cases the response was only of a temporary nature. Of the 44 patients with solid infiltrating tumours a favourable result was obtained in only one case. Herger and Sauer (1943) also noted that smaller papillary tumours responded more satisfactorily to irradiation than did the larger ones. In the case of solid infiltrating growths there was no difference according to size; the response was poor in both small and large lesions. This has not been our experience with solid tumours treated by interstitial irradiation. In most of these cases the bladder has been cleared of tumour, the chief cause of death being distant metastases.

Colby and Schulz (1943) studied 101 cases treated with 1000 kV roentgen rays and correlated histology with response to treatment. These authors concluded that papillary and non-papillary tumours responded almost equally well, and that tumours of high grade malignancy showed the most spectacular initial response although they usually recurred rapidly and responded less well to further measures. The large papillary tumours of low grade malignancy showed the least response.

Swinney (1957) found little difference in the response of well-differentiated transitional cell carcinomas and anaplastic tumours of the bladder treated with the 4 MeV linear accelerator at Newcastle (Table 41). Forty per cent of tumours showing a good initial response to irradiation recurred.

Table 41. *Bladder tumours. Response to 4 MeV roentgen ray therapy* (Swinney, 1957)

Tumour grade	Good response	Unaffected	Recurred after good initial response
Well differentiated	31/51 (60%)	20/51 (40%)	12/31 (39%)
Anaplastic	19/35 (54%)	16/35 (46%)	8/19 (42%)
Total	50/86 (58%)	36/86 (42%)	20/50 (40%)

Friedman (1959) considered that repeated fulguration in the early stages of aggressive types of bladder cancer reduces the effectiveness of subsequent radiotherapy. Thus, in his series of cases treated by 2 MeV roentgen ray rotation therapy the three-year survival rate for 12 previously untreated cases was 42%, whilst that for 33 recurrent cases was only 18%.

In most cases of bladder cancer high doses of irradiation of the order of 6000–7000 R are required to cause marked tumour regression, although occasionally there may be striking shrinkage with doses of the order of 4000 R. On the other hand, many tumours fail to show a satisfactory response to doses as high as 7 000–8 000 R (PLANK *et al.*, 1957; FRIEDMAN, 1959).

Recently, MORRISON (1960) has reported his experience in the treatment of bladder cancer with 8 MeV roentgen rays at the Hammersmith Hospital, London. The tumour response to a dose of 4 500–5 500 R delivered in four weeks is shown in Table 42. Complete tumour regression occurred in 43 % of his stage 1 cases and in 30 % of those in stage 2. It was particularly interesting to find complete regression in 21 % of stage 3 cases and in 24 % of those in stage 4.

Table 42. *Bladder tumours. Response to 8 MeV roentgen ray therapy. 4500–5500 R in 4 weeks.* (MORRISON, 1960)

	Number of cases
At cystoscopy:	
No tumour seen	64 (31%)
Tumour smaller	35 (17%)
No change	19 (9%)
Tumour larger	7 (3%)
No cystoscopy performed	85 (40%)
Total	210 (100%)

i) Complications of radiotherapy

Reactions and complications following radiotherapy for cancer of the bladder, or for other tumours situated in the abdomen or pelvis, have been discussed by WALLACE (1954), FRIEDMAN (1956), BRICK (1955), MACKAY (1956), POOLE (1958), BLOOM (1959) and GOWING (1960). The most common late irradiation sequelae following intracavitary and external methods of radiotherapy for vesical tumours are haemorrhage from telangiectases, and frequency of micturition and incontinence due to a contracted bladder. Delayed healing of necrotic ulcers is the major complication of patients treated by interstitial techniques.

α) Bladder

Haematuria. The telangiectases following irradiation are prone to damage when the bladder is stretched and may give rise to periodic bouts of haematuria which are sometimes severe and occasionally intractable, necessitating total cystetomy to save life.

Necrosis. A well-defined ulcer with overlying slough and calcareous material surrounded by congested and oedematous mucosa is a common sequel to a radio-active implant, and this has already been discussed in the section dealing with interstitial radiotherapy.

Encrustations and calculi. These frequently accompany irradiation reactions, especially following interstitial therapy. The presence of calcareous deposits delays the healing of underlying necrotic areas (HERGER and SAUER, 1942b) and where possible they should be removed by the transurethral route. Because of their pultaceous nature stones are difficult to eradicate.

Contracted bladder. A reduced vesical capacity is a common sequel to irradiation, especially in the presence of chronic infection. A small fibrotic bladder producing intractable frequency of micturition is most often encountered following treatment with intracavitary isotopes. In such cases bilateral hydroureter and hydronephrosis may develop and intercurrent infection is likely to supervene. Ureteric transplantation to the colon or to an ileal loop may be required to bring relief from distressing frequency and incontinence.

Vesico-vaginal and vesico-rectal fistulae. A fistula is a rare complication of properly managed radiotherapy. It was noted in only 4 instances in a series of 229 cases treated

by external irradiation and interstitial radon seeds reported nearly twenty years ago by
Herger and Sauer (1942b). In most cases of fistula tumour is also present. In these
circumstances an evisceration may occasionally save the patient's life.

Irradiation-induced tumours? An undoubted case of an irradiation-induced tumour
of the bladder or the other pelvic organs following radiotherapy for vesical cancer has
yet to be reported. This may be, at least in part, due to the poor survival rate of patients
with bladder cancer who have undergone irradiation in the past, few cases living long
enough to develop such a tumour. It has been suggested that pelvic irradiation to bring
about an artificial menopause may subsequently induce endometrial adenocarcinoma
(Corscaden and Gusberg, 1947; Speert and Peightal, 1949). In such cases, however,
it is more likely that the basic uterine pathology, for which the irradiation was initially
given, is the chief factor responsible for the neoplastic change. The development of a
second or even a third bladder tumour several years after radiotherapy is in keeping
with the natural history of the disease and also occurs in patients treated entirely by
surgical methods.

β) Extra-vesical pelvic tissues

Massive pelvic fibrosis is almost invariably the result of gross irradiation overdosage
and is rarely seen where proper care is taken with regard to dose rate and the total dose
given in the light of the volume treated. It is not uncommon, however, to find pelvic
induration in patients who have been treated for extensive bladder cancer, but in most
of these cases the thickening of the pelvic tissues is the result of malignant infiltration.
With supervoltage equipment and the dose-time factors already referred to in the section
dealing with that subject a serious degree of pelvic fibrosis should be a rare event. Furthermore, those cases coming to total cystectomy or radical cystectomy following pelvic
irradiation do not, in our experience, show a marked degree of pelvic fibrosis, and in the
majority of cases the operation has not been unduly difficult.

γ) Bone necrosis

Irradiation changes in bone may lead to fracture of the pelvis or femoral neck following
treatment with conventional deep roentgen rays. In practice, however, these complications
are rarely seen in patients with bladder cancer, since cases warranting this type of treatment are usually advanced and often fail to survive the two years which usually elapse
before such fractures become evident. With modern supervoltage equipment the risk of
bone necrosis is greatly reduced.

δ) Intestines

Ulceration and stricture of the small or large bowel, which has been described following
abdominal and pelvic supervoltage irradiation, is rare in our experience. Although these
complications may occur with doses as low as 4000 R they are much more likely to follow
doses greater than 6000 R. The risk of inflicting bowel damage is probably greater when
fixed fields are employed and when intra-abdominal adhesions are present which render
the gut immobile. Cases with stricture will require a colostomy or resection operation.
Great care must be taken to assess the viability of the gut before attempting segmental
resection and re-anastomosis.

Although the type of irradiation, the dose and time in which it is delivered and the
volume of tissue treated are the major factors concerned with irradiation reactions and
complications, other factors, about which we know very little, also play a part. For
example, individual sensitivity is important, some cases developing an early and severe
bladder and skin reaction to moderate doses of irradiation. Thus, Poole (1958) in 50 cases
at the Mayo Clinic was unable to find any strict correlation between dose and intensity
of vesical reaction. It is, therefore, important to observe all patients during treatment
at regular intervals and to be prepared to reduce the dose rate, permit periods of rest and,

if necessary, to stop treatment altogether before the prescribed total dose has been delivered in patients showing unduly severe reactions.

12. Non-transitional cell tumours of the bladder and their treatment

a) Squamous cell carcinoma

Only about 2 % of malignant epithelial bladder tumours are of squamous cell origin. This applies to the pure squamous cell tumour as opposed to growths showing areas of squamous cell metaplasia which are quite common in the solid type of transitional cell carcinoma, and were present in 40 % of 513 cases reported by DEAN et al. (1954).

Squamous cell carcinoma is the most unfavourable type of bladder cancer to treat by irradiation. It usually forms a large, ulcerating, deeply infiltrating growth and is accompanied by severe cystitis. It is often associated with leukoplakia and a long-standing urinary infection. Suitable tumours of this type are probably best treated by partial or total cystectomy rather than by interstitial radiotherapy. A course of post-operative supervoltage irradiation is advisable for patients treated by partial cystectomy in order to reduce the risk of local or scar recurrence. More extensive tumours, if operable, should be treated by radical cystectomy or, alternatively, by external supervoltage irradiation in the first instance and, if the response proves to be unsatisfactory, radical surgery can then be undertaken. CUCCIA and his colleagues (1958) had 14 cases of squamous cell carcinoma in their series of bladder tumours treated by supervoltage irradiation, using either a cobalt unit or betatron; 8 patients were alive at the time of their report, 6 for more than a year and 2 for more than two years. SWINNEY (1957) had 3 cases of squamous cell carcinoma in his series of 89 patients treated with 4 MeV roentgen rays, and reports that tumours in two of the three cases were destroyed with no recurrence to date. In a series of 225 cases from the American Bladder Tumour Registry treated by total cystectomy there were 29 cases of squamous cell carcinoma of grade II or grade III malignancy and only one of these patients survived five years (SCHWARTZ et al., 1957).

b) Adenocarcinoma

This tumour which constitutes 1–2 % of bladder cancers arises in exstrophied bladders or from any part of the normal bladder. In the latter the most common sites are the region of the trigone in relation to cystitis glandularis and the apex in connection with the urachus. Direct involvement of the bladder by secondary adenocarcinoma may occur from the body of the uterus, the rectum or the colon. Microscopic differentiation between adenocarcinoma arising from the bladder or from the intestine may be extremely difficult: tumours from either site of origin may show a well-marked glandular structure with mucous secretion.

In a series of 5 324 cases of bladder tumour in the American Bladder Tumour Registry 69 were recorded as being adenocarcinomas (DEAN and ASH, 1950). MOSTOFI et al. (1955) reviewed 44 of these cases which were accepted as being undoubted primary adenocarcinomas of the bladder. The five-year survival rate was 27 %. In general, the prognosis for these tumours is regarded as being more unfavourable than for transitional cell growths. This is probably largely due to the high proportion of urachal lesions which tend to spread widely along remnants of the urachal tract, and also to the fact that symptoms tend to be late when tumours are situated in the "silent area" of the dome.

It is a wide belief that adenocarcinoma of the bladder is radioresistant and that the treatment of choice is total cystectomy. These tumours may in fact respond quite dramatically to irradiation as illustrated by the following case:

Case 035954: Female aged 52 with large bulky tumour invading the whole trigone and most of the right lateral wall of the bladder with extension to the bony pelvis. The tumour was invading the vagina to form a proliferative mass some 4 cm in diameter on the anterior vaginal wall. The bladder contained much mucinous material. Biopsy: well-differentiated, papillary, mucous secreting, columnar-celled adenocarcinoma.

Intravenous pyelogram: bilateral hydroureter and hydronephrosis (Fig. 35a).

The whole pelvis was treated with 2 MeV roentgen rays using one anterior direct 15×15 cm and two posterior oblique 10×15 cm fields. Bladder tolerance was reached when the maximum and minimum depth doses were 5500 and 4800 R respectively, delivered in 6 weeks.

The patient is alive, well and symptom-free 2 years later. There are no signs of tumour in the bladder and the pelvic tissues are soft, apart from some smooth thickening on the right. The vagina is healed and free from tumour[1].

Intravenous pyelogram: previous signs of backpressure have disappeared; poor excretion on right (Fig. 35b).

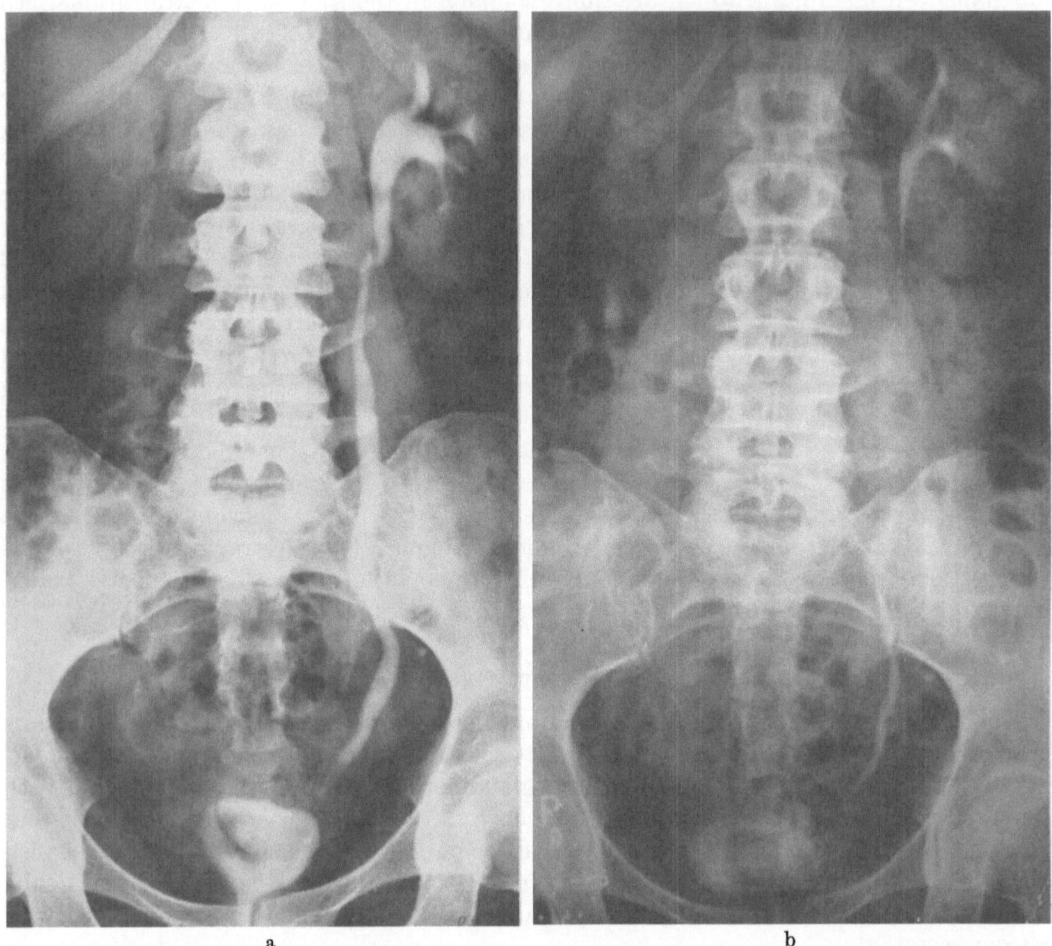

a   b

Fig. 35. a Intravenous pyelogram from a patient with an advanced mucous secreting adenocarcinoma of the bladder causing bilateral ureteric obstruction (Case: 035954). b Same case six months after radical supervoltage roentgen ray therapy to whole pelvis; ureteric obstruction relieved (see text), but poor excretion on right side. Patient alive and well 10 years later

Adenocarcinomas of limited extent, infiltrating no more deeply than the muscularis, should be treated by interstitial radiotherapy. More advanced cases may be treated initially by a radical course of supervoltage irradiation, and if this fails to control the disease a total or radical cystectomy can be undertaken. Seven of the 44 cases reported by MOSTOFI and his colleagues (1955) were treated with radon seeds or roentgen rays; 6 of the 7 survived three years and 4 five years. Two cases survived fourteen years, one being treated with deep roentgen rays alone and the other by local excision and radon seeds. Adenocarcinoma of the bladder associated with the urachus should be treated, in

---

1 This patient is alive and well ten years after treatment.

the first instance, by wide excision of the primary lesion together with the urachus and the umbilicus.

c) Malignant connective tissue tumours

Bladder sarcoma is a rare lesion constituting 0.35–0.50% of all bladder tumours (THOMPSON and COPPRIDGE, 1959; DEAN and ASH, 1950). The world literature of 324 cases of vesical sarcoma was reviewed by POWERS and his associates (1956). The more frequent types were leiomyosarcoma (43 cases), rhabdomyosarcoma (40 cases), and spindle or round cell sarcoma together (52 cases).

Bladder sarcomas, apart from those of lymphoid origin, appear to be radio-resistant lesions, and where feasable treatment should be by surgery. Contrary to general belief these tumours often extend slowly and give rise to blood-born metastases late. Distant metastases were a postmortem finding in only 25% of the cases reported by THOMPSON and COPPRIDGE (1959). Nevertheless the ultimate prognosis in these cases is generally very poor, most patients dying with extensive disease in the pelvis.

Rhabdomyosarcoma (sarcoma botryoides) and myxosarcoma generally occur in infants and young children, and are usually fatal within two years (MOSTOFI and MORSE, 1952). FLOCKS and CULP (1955) report a case of a boy alive and well eight years after total cystectomy at the age of five, and SMITH (1959) refers to a two-year old boy who was alive and well five and a half years after operation.

d) Reticuloses

Bladder involvement is a rare event in Hodgkin's disease, lymphosarcoma and reticulum cell sarcoma, and is then usually part of the general manifestations of a widespread disorder of the reticuloendothelial system. MELICOW (1955) found 17 cases of lymphosarcoma, Hodgkin's disease and leukaemic infiltration of the bladder in a series of 1614 cases of bladder tumour. The majority of cases of urinary tract involvement by such tumours are the result of direct invasion from an adjacent lymph node mass. Occasionally the tumour appears to have originated in the bladder, and is associated with similar foci elsewhere in the body (WATSON et al., 1949; HOFFMAN et al., 1953; GLAY, 1960). The bladder itself rarely appears to be the sole site of origin of a malignant tumour of the reticulo-endothelial system and, in these cases, following adequate radiotherapy, the disease appears to be arrested.

The subject of primary "malignant lymphoma" of the bladder has recently been reviewed by BHANSALI and CAMERON (1960) who collected 23 cases from the literature and reported 8 new ones. These tumours are composed of lymphocytes, lymphoblasts, plasma cells, eosinophils and reticulum cells, all in varying proportion, and these authors found it impossible to sub-divide them into specific categories. Malignant vesical lymphoma generally occurs over the age of forty and is more common in women than in men. The tumour forms a smooth or nodular pink solid mass, usually infiltrating no more deeply than the muscularis and often showing sub-mucosal extension. In most cases the overlying mucosa is intact. These unusual appearances may suggest the diagnosis at the time of cystoscopy. Back-pressure effects, as seen in the intravenous pyelogram, are uncommon with this type of tumour.

Vesical lymphomas are very radio-sensitive and their response to radiotherapy may prove of diagnostic value. The treatment of choice is by irradiation. The entire pelvis should be treated, the fields being made to cover the bladder and the regional lymph nodes up as far as the aortic bifurcation. Supervoltage apparatus is an advantage, but not essential for this type of case as an adequate depth dose can usually be achieved with a conventional roentgen ray or telecaesium unit. A suitable technique is to use two anterior and two posterior oblique pelvic fields each 10×15 cm. We aim to deliver a maximum tumour dose of 4500 R to the bladder in five to six weeks; the dose at the pelvic wall is 3000–3500 R.

The prognosis in this group of cases is surprisingly good. All of the 8 new cases reported by BHANSALI and CAMERON (1960) showed no evidence of dissemination and were alive four months to ten years after treatment. Five of the cases were treated by irradiation, two by surgery and one by surgery and post-operative irradiation.

e) Extra-urinary secondary carcinoma involving the bladder

Direct extension to the bladder may occur from a carcinoma of an adjacent organ such as the uterus, prostate or large intestine. Occasionally, metastases from distant sites involve the bladder, the most frequent primary tumours being carcinoma of the

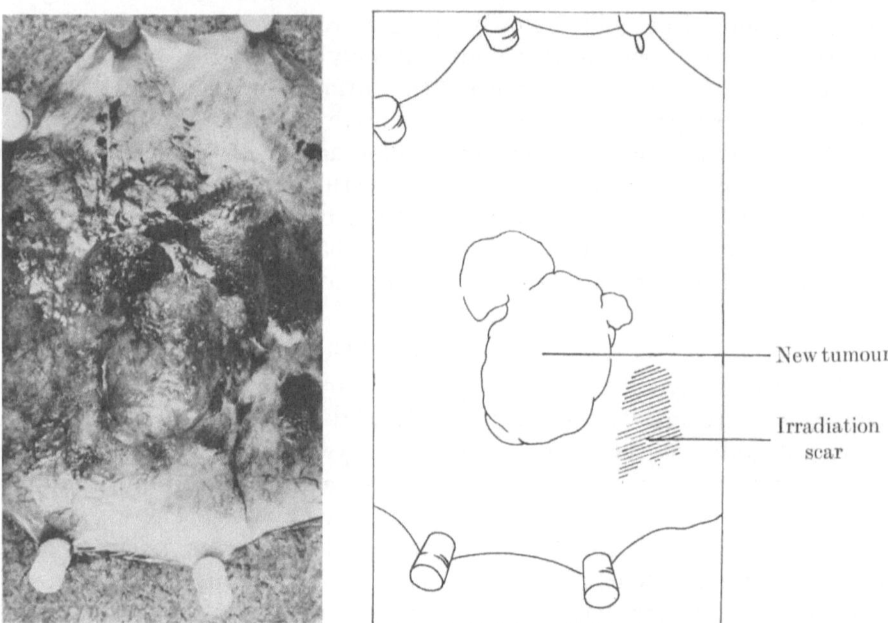

Fig. 36. More than one method of treatment may be required in a patient with bladder cancer. Five years after a tantalum-182 wire implant for a transitional cell carcinoma this tumour, of quite different histological grade to the original lesion, appeared close to the irradiation scar, and was treated by partial cystectomy. The patient is alive and well seven years after the implant

stomach, malignant melanoma, carcinoma of the breast and carcinoma of the lung (KLINGER, 1951; GANEM and BATAL, 1957).

In many cases the secondary involvement of the bladder occurs in the final stages of the disease in a debilitated patient and in whom the only need is for sedatives and analgesics. In some cases, however, such as carcinoma of the rectum, colon and breast the patient's general condition is often good in spite of the advanced malignancy, and the bladder symptoms, especially haematuria, may prove troublesome. A course of palliative irradiation with supervoltage or conventional equipment often stops the bleeding and reduces frequency and dysuria. A maximum depth dose of 3500–3750 R in three to four weeks with four oblique pelvic fields, each 10×15 cm, is usually well-tolerated. Occasionally the bladder is involved by a solitary, slow-growing, local pelvic recurrence from, for example, a carcinoma of the rectum. In such cases a more radical course of treatment is indicated.

13. After care

Except for terminal cases the importance of frequent and regular follow-up examinations under general anaesthesia is stressed to all patients treated for tumours of the bladder before they are finally discharged from hospital, the first appointment being made for two months. Patients are then admitted for a period of thirty-six hours for cystoscopy and bimanual examination by both urologist and radiotherapist. This procedure is repeated at three-monthly intervals during the first year and four-monthly during the second and third years. All being well the interval is finally extended to six months. Any patient who has been treated for a bladder tumour should remain under regular observation for the rest of his life. In this way residual or recurrent growth can be detected and treated at an early stage (Fig. 36).

14. Overall results of treatment of bladder cancer

The results obtained in the treatment of cancer of the bladder at the Royal Marsden Hospital and the main hospitals with which it is associated are shown in Table 43. Our

Table 43. *Bladder cancer. All treated cases. Results according to stage. (Royal Marsden Hospital, St. Peter's, St. Paul's and St. Phillip's Hospitals, London)*

Stage		Term in years				
		1	2	3	4	5
Mucosal	no. cases	743	599	470	369	262
(T1)	crude S. R.	87%	78%	71%	66%	63%
Muscular	no. cases	232	195	148	111	81
(T2)	crude S. R.	57%	41%	35%	26%	21%
Perivesical	no. cases	183	159	128	95	68
(T3)	crude S. R.	38%	19%	13%	11%	10%
Pelvic fixation	no. cases	173	129	95	65	42
(T4)	crude S. R.	15%	5%	1%	0%	0%
Unstaged	no. cases	89	71	50	37	27
	crude S. R.	42%	28%	18%	14%	15%

S. R.: Survival Rate. (PAYNE, 1959).

material includes a large number of cases referred from other hospitals after other methods of treatment have failed to control the disease. Thus there are cases with a long history of multiple diathermy resections, cases with residual or recurrent disease following partial cystectomy, and cases in whom the bladder has been opened and closed without any form of treatment being undertaken because of the extent of the disease. In other words, a high proportion of our cases when first seen are in the later or final stages of the natural history of the disease. In addition, a high proportion of the cases, as in most series, are elderly, in poor general condition, and with evidence of impaired renal function. All this must be remembered when attempting to compare the results of radiotherapy with those obtained in highly selected cases at various surgical centres.

The three and five-year results are suitable yard-sticks with which to assess the value of treatment in the more serious types of bladder tumour since most of these patients, if uncured, die within the first two years following treatment. Untreated cases, chiefly because the disease is hopelessly advanced when the patient is first seen, have a mean duration of life from onset of symptoms of some 18 months (FORBER, 1931; PROUT and MARSHALL, 1956). The 3-year survival rate for 103 untreated cases in our series was approximately 4%. No patients with tumours fixed to the pelvis or invading adjacent organs survived this period. A number of patients, however, in whom the original tumour has been eradicated subsequently develop a recurrence or new tumour several years later, and in such cases a prolonged follow-up is necessary for their full assessment.

15. In conclusion

It is difficult to draw conclusions from reported statistics concerning different methods of treatment for cancer of the bladder since frequently there is no strict comparison between comparable cases. It is only by means of a carefully controlled clinical trial, with cases properly classified, that we shall be in a better position to assess the relative merits of two or more different methods of treatment. Even so there will be other difficulties such as variables in the tumour itself and host resistance which exist in patients with malignant disease, and also such factors as variable medical skill and techniques. All these will cloud such a study unless a large number of cases are collected, and this will require the co-operation of several large medical centres. Until we have statistically significant results arising from such collaborative trials we must formulate a reasonable working policy for treatment based on collected reports in the literature, personal experience and a knowledge of the natural history of the disease. Finally, a balance must be made between the possible gain and the likely morbidity and mortality resulting from a particular line of treatment.

In general, it appears that interstitial and external methods of irradiation can achieve as good or even better results than partial or total cystectomy, with the advantage that the patient retains his bladder. Many patients cured by total cystectomy could have been successfully treated by more conservative procedures. Cystectomy for tumours of low biological potential is generally unnecessary, and for relatively advanced tumours of high grade malignancy of little value[1]. The survival rate for advancing anaplastic tumours of the bladder treated by conventional external irradiation in the past has been low. It remains to be seen whether the results can be appreciably improved by the use of supervoltage apparatus. We have yet to determine more fully the value of a combination of partial or total cystectomy with radiotherapy, and of combining interstitial techniques with supplementary external irradiation. Increasing the oxygen tension of the blood during irradiation and the administration of so-called "radiosensitisors" may ultimately find a place in the treatment of bladder cancer. Meanwhile, every effort must be made to reduce the delay between the onset of symptoms and the institution of definitive treatment.

Surgeon, radiotherapist, radio-biologist and biochemist must all strive together to improve the treatment and management of patients with this disease. In too many centres there is still opposition to one or other method of treatment and no or little collaboration between surgeon and radiotherapist. It cannot be too strongly emphasized that the best results from the treatment of bladder cancer can be expected only where there is close co-operation between the urological surgeon and his radiotherapy colleague in the initial assessment, the planning of treatment and the subsequent follow up of all patients.

16. Summary of treatment for bladder cancer

A single or limited number of well-differentiated papillary mucosal tumours should be controlled for as long as possible by cysto-diathermy. At the present time it would seem that the condition of "papillomatosis" of the bladder is best treated, at least in the first instance, by external supervoltage irradiation, using a technique which reduces the dose to the extra-vesical tissues to a minimum. Following such treatment small residual tumours can be controlled by careful trans-urethral cysto-diathermy. "Papillomatosis" which does not respond to such conservative treatment will require total cystectomy or cystourethrectomy.

A single tumour, not exceeding 4–5 cm in diameter, which is infiltrating muscle is best treated at open operation by interstitial irradiation, using either tantalum-182 wire or gold-198 grains after the bulk of the tumour has been removed by diathermy. This

---

1 This may be no longer true, expecially if pre-operative irradiation is given, chapter VI.

appears to be a satisfactory method of treatment not only for well-differentiated tumours, but also for those of the solid anaplastic variety. We consider that poorly differentiated papillary or solid tumours of moderate size, limited to the mucosa or submucosa, are best treated by interstitial therapy rather than by diathermy alone. Two or three tumours close together may be included in the same implant or, if widely separated, each may be dealt with by gold-198 grains.

Tumours which are unsuitable for interstitial therapy by virtue of their size or multiplicity should be treated in the first instance by external supervoltage irradiation. In the case of well-differentiated tumours infiltrating no more deeply than the muscularis the whole bladder is raised to a high dose, keeping the dose to the extra-vesical pelvic tissues to a minimum. In the solid anaplastic variety of tumour a larger volume should be treated with the aim of controlling possible lymphatic spread.

Tumours which have spread through the full thickness of the bladder wall are also treated by external supervoltage irradiation and in most cases this will mean treating the major part of the pelvic cavity. The prognosis in such cases is extremely poor, but if the patient's general condition is good the treatment should be radical with the aim of saving him from a "pelvic cancer death".

Palliative external irradiation to the whole pelvis is given to patients with tumours adherent to the pelvic wall, to most cases with infiltration of surrounding viscera and to patients with symptoms referable to the growth who are not fit to undergo radical treatment. Palliative irradiation for the patient who is reasonably fit implies a limited but substantial course of irradiation to the whole pelvis, preferably with supervoltage equipment. Palliative irradiation, if judicially administered, is of great value in relieving local symptoms and often enables the final stages of the disease to be endured with considerably less discomfort than in untreated cases.

In our opinion radical surgery for bladder cancer has a strictly limited application. In general, simple total cystectomy is reserved for residual or renewed growth following radiotherapy, for serious radiation sequelae and very occasionally as a palliative procedure. In suitable cases cystectomy is combined with an attempt to remove the pelvic lymph nodes, but when these are found to be invaded there is little chance of curing the patient. Evisceration occasionally saves life, especially when the tumour is invading adjacent organs but is still mobile. This operation carries a high operative mortality and morbidity and should not be undertaken without careful consideration[1].

Partial cystectomy is often performed for tumours of the vesical fundus, and in suitable cases has given satisfactory results. However, in the light of BAKER's (1955) observations concerning circumferential intra-mural lymphatic spread, we consider that post-operative irradiation is indicated in all cases, especially if the growth is of the solid anaplastic variety, or if the margin of clearance is less than 2.5 cm. Post-operative radiotherapy has, in our experience, improved the 5-year survival rate for partial cystectomy by nearly 20%.

Uretero-colic anastomosis as a palliative procedure, may bring welcome relief from distressing urinary symptoms in advanced cancer of the bladder. On the other hand, before performing this operation it is important to consider whether one is going to substitute a relatively comfortable uraemic death for the distress of advancing pelvic cancer in a patient who remains mentally alert.

So far, no chemotherapeutic agent has proved of undoubted value in cancer of the bladder, although quite recently there has been an interesting report by MORROW (1960) on the use of Citral and by DEREN and WILSON (1960) on 5-Fluorouracil in the treatment of advanced carcinoma of the bladder. The possibility that β-glucoronidase activity may be important in the development of bladder cancer in man has encouraged us to initiate

---

1 During the past decade the operative mortality for radical cystectomy has fallen to 5—10%.

a clinical trial of giving 1–4 Saccharolactone and related substances to patients who have been cleared of recurrent papillary tumours, with the object of preventing the formation of new lesions (Boyland et al., 1957; Wallace, 1957; Boyland, 1960).

IV. Tumours of the urethra

1. Carcinoma of the urethra

a) Incidence

Carcinoma of the urethra is generally regarded as a rare disease. It occurs more often in women than in men. McCrea and Furlong (1951) found 223 cases of male urethral cancer reported by various authors and added 7 cases of their own. McCrea (1952) collected 546 verified cases of carcinoma of the female urethra from the literature. To this number, Staubitz and his colleagues (1955) added a further 32 female cases from the Roswell Park Memorial Institute, which represented an incidence of 1 in 1500 female cancer admissions. At the American Oncologic Hospital, Philadelphia, Hahn (1952) found only 3 cases of primary urethral cancer in women among 10851 admissions between the years 1931 and 1952. Sargent (1957) reported an incidence of one in approximately 16000 female admissions over a seven-year period at the Milwaukee County Hospital.

Urethral carcinoma in both men and women generally occurs between the ages of 35 and 75, the average, in most reported series, being between 55 and 60. Riches and Cullen (1951) referred to a male case aged 23 in their series of 34 cases.

b) Aetiology

α) Urethral stricture

A history of chronic urethritis or stricture is present in a high proportion of men with urethral cancer. The incidence of stricture is given as 50% of male cases by Thomson-Walker (1948) and 66% by Lowsley and Kirwin (1956). The highest incidence, 72%, is reported by Kreutzmann and Colloff (1939). The majority of strictures are of gonococcal origin, but a few are traumatic, and occasionally congenital. In contrast to this experience in men, a history of venereal disease or stricture is uncommon among female patients with urethral cancer.

β) Trauma

This may be an important aetiological factor in male patients who have been subjected to repeated dilatations for stricture. The vast majority of women with urethral cancer have had children, and trauma associated with childbirth has been suggested as a factor of aetiological significance.

γ) Caruncle

A caruncle, the commonest urethral "tumour" in the female, is a benign vascular inflammatory lesion usually less than 1 cm in diameter, occurring in the older age groups and arising from the posterior urethral wall, near the meatus. It is sometimes said that malignant change can take place in such a lesion, but it is more likely that some neoplasms, malignant from the onset, simulate caruncles in their presentation at the urethral orifice. Palmer et al. (1948) found no evidence of malignant change in 120 caruncles selected at random from the files of the Mayo Clinic. Occasionally, a woman with urethral cancer gives a previous history of a caruncle. Staubitz et al. (1955) recorded that 5 of their 32 patients with urethral carcinoma gave a history of previous removal of a caruncle. Histological examination of this lesion sometimes reveals epithelial hyperplasia, which may be wrongly interpreted as early malignant change. It is our opinion that caruncles are not pre-malignant, but that every "caruncle" should be subjected to histological examination, since some of these lesions are carcinomas (2.4% in 376 cases reported by MARSHALL and USON, 1960).

δ) Carcinoma of the urinary tract

It is strange that tumours of the urethra are not more frequently reported in patients with transitional-cell neoplasms of the bladder and upper renal tract. Carcinoma of the bladder neck may extend directly into the urethra, and sometimes there is a length of normal urethra between the bladder and the urethral tumour. In these cases, the urethral lesion may be an implant following the trauma of instrumentation, or, alternatively, the urinary tumours may have a multicentric origin, perhaps created by carcinogens in the urine. GOWING (1960) in a careful histological study of the entire urethra of male patients dying of bladder cancer, has found evidence of carcinoma-in-situ in approximately 20% of cases, and in none of his control cases dying of malignant disease other than carcinoma of the bladder. These changes were especially marked in the crypts and folds of the urethral mucosa (Fig. 37), a position where it is unlikely that tumour cells would be implanted or where the mucosa would be abraded. GOWING (1960) suggests that the presence of carcinoma-in-situ in such cases is further evidence for the multicentric origin of urothelial tumours, and indicates that urethral carcinoma associated with bladder cancers are often independant primary growths and not implants.

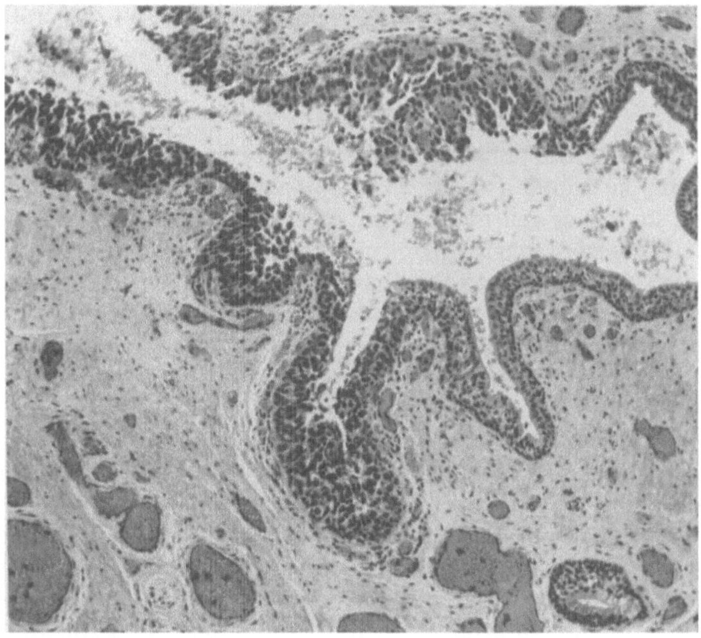

Fig. 37. Urethral carcinoma-in-situ: Section male urethra (×100). Patient died of carcinoma of the bladder with no clinical evidence of urethral involvement. Histology shows abrupt change from normal to irregular hyperplasia of urothelium; the changes are most marked in the crypts

Papillary lesions of the posterior urethra are not infrequent in cases of bladder tumour when the urethra is inspected with a urethroscope. Such lesions are not seen with an ordinary non-irrigating cystoscope and have been noted more frequently since instruments capable of examining the urethra have been used. If patients with cancer of the bladder survived for longer periods, perhaps clinical carcinoma of the urethra in such cases would be seen more often.

c) Clinical classification

A useful clinical classification for carcinoma of the urethra is based on the site of the tumour, and this is related to prognosis and the choice of treatment.

α) Carcinoma of the male urethra

a) Penile urethra.
b) Bulbo-membranous urethra.
c) Prostatic urethra.

β) Carcinoma of the female urethra

a) Anterior urethra and meatus ("vulvo-urethral" carcinoma).
b) Posterior urethra.

The most frequent site for urethral carcinoma in the male is the bulbo-membranous urethra, and in the female, the anterior urethra in the region of the external meatus.

d) Pathology

α) Macroscopic

Carcinoma of the urethra may present as a papillary, nodular or ulcerative lesion. The tumour, especially those occurring at the external meatal region, may be small and localised, and may protrude from the urethral orifice as a dark red indurated mass. More advanced tumours, especially those arising in the deeper parts of the urethra, may extend along the organ, converting it into a thickened, narrowed tube.

β) Microscopic

The mucosal lining of the proximal part of the urethra is composed of transitional-cell epithelium, that of the middle portion of pseudo-stratified columnar epithelium, and the distal portion of squamous-cell epithelium. Malignancy may arise in all three types of epithelium, but the most frequent histological type, in both sexes, is the squamous-cell carcinoma. This is no doubt due to the high incidence of epithelial squamous metaplasia, which occurs in association with chronic urethritis and stricture. Maximow and Bloom (1948) point out that patches of squamous epithelium may be found normally in the penile urethra. 28 of the 32 female cases of urethral cancer reported by Staubitz et al. (1955), 24 of the 30 female cases of Fricke and McMillan (1949), and 101 of the 116 male cases reported by Kreutzmann and Colloff (1939) were of the squamous-cell variety. The majority of squamous-cell tumours are histologically of high grade malignancy, i.e. Broders' grades 3 and 4.

A number of malignant urethral tumours are transitional-cell carcinomas, especially those associated with bladder tumours. Adeno-carcinoma arising from pseudo-stratified columnar epithelium of the urethra or the urethral glands, and occasionally showing mucous secretion, is the most infrequent type of carcinoma. This tumour was seen in 2 of the 23 female cases of Monaco et al. (1958), 1 of the 34 female cases of Ruch et al. (1952) and 4 of the 30 male and female cases reported by Riches and Cullen (1951). In McCrea and Furlong's (1951) review of 230 male cases of urethral cancer, 6 had adeno-carcinomas.

e) Natural history

Urethral carcinoma occurring at the external meatus in both male and female patients presents earlier and appears to be less malignant than carcinoma arising in the deeper portions of the urethra. Deeper placed tumours extend along the length of the urethra and tend to produce a narrowed rigid tube. Growths presenting at the external meatus in the female often extend on to the vulva and involve the clitoris and labia. Carcinoma of the urethra spreads into the peri-urethral tissues, and in the female soon invades the anterior vaginal wall, often to such an extent as to simulate a primary vaginal growth. Urethral carcinomas in the male may extend into the cavernous tissue of the penis with the risk of subsequent widespread dissemination via the blood stream. Secondary infection is common and a peri-urethral abscess in the male, which fails to heal, should arouse suspicion of malignancy.

The lymphatic drainage from the anterior urethra is to the inguinal nodes, and from the posterior urethra direct to the iliac and pre-sacral nodes. Spread from urethral cancer is primarily lymphatic and, generally speaking, between one-third and one half of cases have enlarged inguinal nodes when first seen. In many of these cases, however, this is entirely due to sepsis. For example, of 32 female patients seen at the Roswell Park Memorial Institute, clinical lymph node enlargement was present in 15 cases, but in only 2 of these was there histological proof of metastases (MURPHY, 1959). In 10 cases of carcinoma of the female urethra with enlarged lymph nodes reported by RUCH et al. (1952), in whom the Bassett operation was performed, only 2 were found to have microscopic evidence of metastatic carcinoma. Pelvic and para-aortic node metastases were found in 12 of the 34 male and female patients studied by RICHES and CULLEN (1951).

Blood-borne metastases are uncommon and occur late in urethral cancer. Pulmonary deposits were present in 7 of the 34 cases of RICHES and CULLEN (1951) and occurred in men when there was invasion of the cavernous tissue of the penis. Deposits in liver, bone and brain have also been reported.

Fungating tumour, abscess and fistula formation and ulcerating inguinal nodes make the final stages of urethral cancer particularly distressing. The vast majority of patients who die of their disease do so within one to two years of diagnosis. RUCH and his colleagues (1952) found in their female patients that 94% of the fatal cases died within 2 years, and 77% within 12 months.

f) Prognosis

α) Site

Tumours of the anterior urethra carry a much better prognosis than those occurring in the posterior urethra in both male and female patients. The former give rise to symptoms at an earlier stage, appear to grow and extend at a slower rate, and are more accessible to treatment than the more deeply placed tumours. Furthermore, the lymphatic drainage of the anterior urethra is primarily to the inguinal and not to the pelvic lymph nodes. In the cases of urethral carcinoma studied by RICHES and CULLEN (1951) 7 of the 9 patients with anterior urethral lesions were alive 19 months to 15 years after treatment, compared with only 1 of 19 cases with posterior urethral tumours, who was alive at 2 years. Of these 19 cases, no fewer than 15 developed lymph node metastases, and in 5 the lungs were involved. Only 2 of the 9 patients with anterior lesions had inguinal node deposits. HERGER and SAUER (1942) reviewed 123 cases of male urethral cancer from the literature and reported 55% "cures" for anterior lesions compared with only 15% for posterior tumours.

β) Histological type

The majority of urethral carcinomas are of squamous-cell type. Adeno-carcinomas are rare, and appear to grow and extend at a slower rate than do the squamous-cell tumours.

γ) Histological grade

Most urethral tumours belong to Broders' grades 3 and 4. Twenty-three of the 32 female cases reported by STAUBITZ et al. (1955) were placed in these categories; there were no grade I cases. These authors, however, were unable to find a correlation between grade and survival. We require more information in a larger series of cases concerning histological grade of malignancy and prognosis.

δ) Clinical stage

The stage which the disease has reached when the patient is first seen is the chief factor influencing prognosis. Direct infiltration of the surrounding tissues, and the presence or absence of mobile or fixed inguinal metastases have to be considered in determining the possible outcome. Once the existence of lymphatic metastases has been established, the chance of cure is greatly reduced.

g) Clinical features

Symptoms of carcinoma of the urethra are mainly those of mechanical interference with micturition, tumour formation, ulceration and infection. Staubitz et al. (1955) in their series of female cases, report an average duration of symptoms of 12 months, and Monaco et al. (1958) of 5 months.

A common story in the male is that a stricture which has previously responded well to intermittent dilatation now fails to do so, and instrumentation is followed by an undue amount of bleeding. The patient may complain of difficulty in micturition, a poor stream or retention in the absence of a previous history of stricture. Frequency and painful micturition are common symptoms. The chief complaint, however, in over 80 % of cases is bleeding, and usually consists of intermittent spotting of bright red blood; occasionally frank haematuria occurs. A purulent or sanguinous urethral discharge is present in about 50 % of cases. A few patients complain of priapism or painful intercourse.

A hard tumour may be felt in the shaft of the penis, in the perineum or on the anterior vaginal wall. In a high proportion of cases, especially in the female, the tumour is visible at the external meatus. Occasionally, the chief symptom is an inguinal mass, due to inflammation or secondary deposits in the regional lymph nodes.

h) Diagnosis and differential diagnosis

Unfortunately, in most cases of carcinoma of the urethra the diagnosis is made only when the disease is advanced. Delay in diagnosis occurs especially in those male patients with long-standing strictures which may mask an underlying tumour for a considerable length of time. The possibility of such cases developing cancer should always be borne in mind. The presence of malignant disease should be suspected in these cases when there is increasing difficulty in dilating the stricture, the relief afforded by dilatation becomes increasingly short-lived, an unusual amount of bleeding follows dilatation, a peri-urethral abscess develops and does not heal satisfactorily, or a mass becomes palpable in the penis or perineum.

The diagnosis of urethral cancer is suspected from the history, the clinical examination, and findings on urethroscopy. Occasionally, urethrography, by showing an irregular filling defect, may prove of value. The diagnosis in all cases is confirmed by biopsy.

The differential diagnosis of carcinoma of the urethra includes other malignant urethral tumours and such benign conditions as papilloma, polyp, caruncle, mucosal prolapse, condylomata and urethral varicosities.

i) Treatment of carcinoma of the urethra

Many methods and combinations of treatment have been employed for carcinoma of the urethra, and none have proved entirely satisfactory, the overall results being poor. The most suitable treatment for a particular case depends on whether the tumour occurs in the urethra of a male or female patient, the site within the urethra and the clinical extent. In general, tumours involving the distal portion of the urethra, especially those in the region of the meatus, are more amenable to treatment, and carry a much better prognosis than those which are more deeply placed.

Before the early 1920's treatment for carcinoma of the urethra was mainly surgical. In 1923 Shaw reported 2 cases treated by radium, and ten years later Counseller and

Table 44. *Summary of treatment methods in urethral carcinoma*

A. Primary tumour Female	Male
I. Surgery	
1. Local diathermy excision	1. Local diathermy excision
2. Urethrectomy	2. Segmental resection urethra
3. Cysto-urethrectomy	3. Partial amputation of penis
4. Anterior evisceration	4. Total urethrectomy
	5. Total amputation of penis
	6. Radical amputation of penis and scrotum
	7. Cysto-urethrectomy
	Palliative Surgery
	a) Suprapubic cystostomy
	b) Uretero-colic anastomosis
II. Radiotherapy	
1. Interstitial	1. Interstitial (Gold 198 grains)
a) Gold 198 grains	
b) Radium or cobalt 60 needles	
c) Tantalum 182 wires	
2. Intracavitary	2. Intracavitary (urethral)
a) Urethral	
b) Vaginal	
3. External beam	3. External beam

B. Regional lymph nodes
1. Bilateral inguino-femoral block dissection
    a) Prophylactic
    b) Therapeutic
2. Bilateral ileo-inguino-femoral dissection
3. Pelvic dissection associated with cysto-urethrectomy
4. Palliative external irradiation

PATERSON (1933) decided that the best results in carcinoma of the female urethra were obtained when radium and roentgen rays were used in conjunction with surgery. Since that time, the value of radiotherapy in the management of urethral cancer has become established. TAUSSIG (1935) favoured radium treatment for the primary tumour, combined with bilateral inguino-femoral dissection for the regional lymph nodes. In CADE's (1950) experience, carcinoma of the female urethra is a radio-sensitive tumour, and regression is to be expected following irradiation in those cases which are not too advanced. He reports that even inguinal node metastases may be kept in abeyance for periods of up to 5 or 7 years following teleradium therapy. Male cases of carcinoma of the urethra respond less satisfactorily to irradiation, but this CADE (1950) suggests is probably largely due to the difficulty of achieving a satisfactory implant in the male urethra.

Because of the infrequency of carcinoma of the urethra and the many methods of treatment, both surgical and radiotherapeutic, which have been evolved for this disease, it is extremely difficult at the present time to assess the merits of the various lines of treatment. In general, however, it would seem that irradiation techniques are to be preferred in the female, and surgery in the male. The various methods of treatment for the primary tumour and metastatic lymph nodes in both male and female patients are summarised in Table 44.

α) Treatment of carcinoma of the female urethra

In general, radiotherapy is the initial treatment of choice for infiltrating urethral carcinoma in women. A greater cure rate appears to have been achieved by irradiation than by radical surgery in this sex, and furthermore the latter is attended by a considerable morbidity.

Small localised tumours of the distal urethra are first excised with diathermy, and then the base is implanted with radioactive gold grains. A single plane implant is carried out and the grains are distributed according to the Paterson-Parker rules (Meredith, 1949). Tumours presenting at the urethral meatus resembling caruncles are excised and the urethral orifice surrounded by a plane of gold grains. A less satisfactory alternative to interstitial irradiation at this site is a course of fractionated superficial roentgen rays (100 kV) applied directly to the urethral orifice.

More extensive tumours of the anterior urethra are best treated, where possible, by a curved single plane, or a cylindrical type of radio-active implant using radium or cobalt-60 needles distributed around the urethra according to the Paterson-Parker rules. A cylindrical implant may be combined with fractionated or continuous intracavitary irradiation. Sources such as radium, cobalt-60 or tantalum-182 may be used within the lumen of a self-retaining urethral catheter for this purpose. Alternatively, gold-198 grains or tantalum-182 wire can be mounted on the external surface of the catheter.

Extension of the tumour on to the vulva can be treated separately by interstitial therapy, or by external irradiation using modern telecurie apparatus.

Limited tumours of the posterior female urethra can sometimes be treated satisfactorily by diathermy resection and implantation of the base with gold-198 grains using a suprapubic cystostomy approach. Associated mucosal or muscular stage bladder tumours can be dealt with in the same fashion and at the same time. Because of the curvature of the urethra and the presence of the pubic bone, the posterior part of the urethra cannot be adequately treated by long radio-active needles inserted via the perineum, since this part of the urethra will be at some distance above the ends of the needles. An attempt has been made to treat posterior urethral carcinoma with an intravaginal radium applicator (Cade, 1950). In most patients with operable infiltrating carcinoma of the posterior urethra, however, cysto-urethrectomy will be indicated.

Tumours of the anterior or the posterior urethra which are unsuitable for implantation, or which fail to respond to irradiation, should be treated by radical surgery. This generally implies total urethrectomy, with permanent suprapubic drainage, or cysto-urethrectomy with uretero-colic anastomosis. In a limited number of cases, anterior evisceration may offer the only hope of cure in what appears to be a hopeless situation. In this operation, the urethra, bladder, uterus and vagina are removed, and this is combined with a dissection of the inguino-pelvic lymph nodes.

Patients with advanced inoperable tumours, and those who are unsuitable for radical surgery, are treated by external supervoltage irradiation, using perineal and anterior and posterior pelvic fields. In the vast majority of such cases, although treatment can only be considered palliative, it is of considerable value in reducing distress from fungation, ulceration, haemorrhage and sepsis.

β) Techniques of radiotherapy

Interstitial therapy:

1. Gold-198 grain implant for anterior urethral tumours. This is carried out after diathermy resection of the exophytic portion of the tumour. The repeating gold grain gun is employed, and the lips of the urethral meatus are retracted well apart to permit insertion of the grains. The aim is to give a dose of 6000 R from a single-plane implant. A self-retaining catheter is left *in situ* for 4–5 days.

2. Radium needle cylindrical implant. This type of implant is carried out in the long axis of the urethra, according to the Paterson-Parker distribution rules (Meredith, 1949). A metal urethral sound is kept in position during the implant; this is eventually replaced by a self-retaining catheter. The vagina is packed in order to push the posterior vaginal wall away from the needles. The labia are retracted with mattress sutures, which are fixed to the inner aspect of the thighs. When the implant is completed, radiographs are

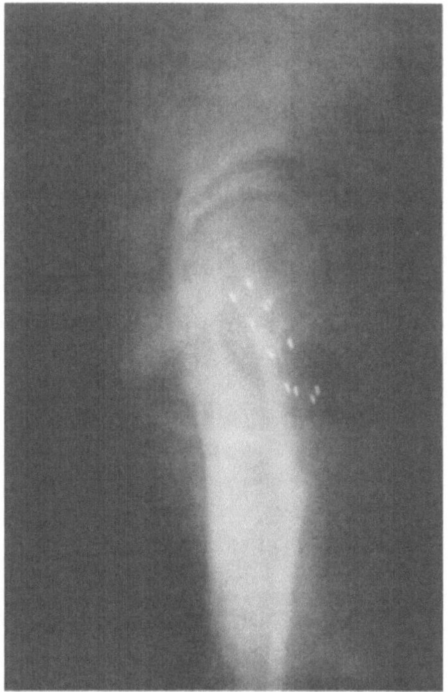 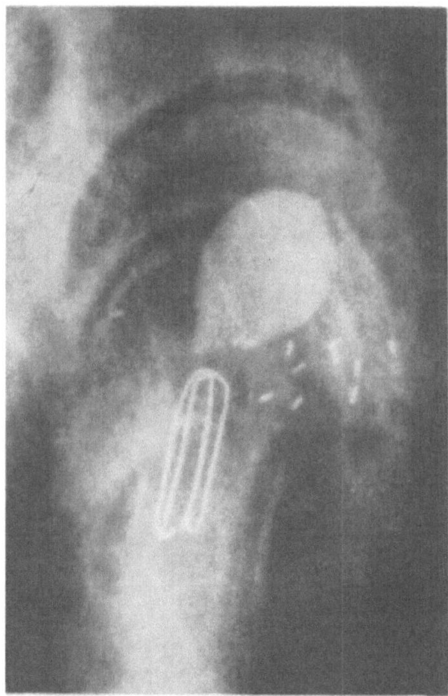

Fig. 38   Fig. 39

Fig. 38. Intracavitary irradiation for carcinoma urethra: Lateral radiograph to show gold-198 grains mounted on external surface of Foley catheter to treat a transitional cell carcinoma of urethra in a woman previously treated for carcinoma of bladder. Each grain 4.0 mCi; dose at 0.5 cm 4500 R in 114 hours

Fig. 39. Intracavitary irradiation for carcinoma urethra: Lateral radiograph to show tantalum-182 wires mounted on external surface of Foley catheter to treat a transitional cell carcinoma of posterior urethra. Male patient previously treated for carcinoma of the bladder with interstitial gold-198 grains. Dose at 0.5 cm 6500 R in 165 hours, following which urethral tumour disappeared. Patient subsequently died with pelvic lymph node metastases

taken in the antero-posterior and lateral planes and include a double-shift film from which the implant can be reconstructed and the dose-rate determined.

A dose of 5500 R is delivered in 5–6 days. Because of the inaccessibility of the inner ends of the implant, differentially loaded needles are a distinct advantage in this situation.

3. Radio-active tantalum-182 wire implant, using modified slotted serum needles. The hollow needles are inserted as for a curved linear or cylindrical radio-active implant, and their position is checked radiographically before a radio-active tantalum wire is passed into each needle. The needles are carefully withdrawn, leaving the wires in position, and these are then secured to the vulva by stitches. The advantage of this method over radium needles is that the inactive hollow needles can be inserted carefully and checked without hurry before the radio-active sources are placed in position.

Intra-cavitary irradiation

Radium tubes, cobalt-60 slugs or tantalum-182 wire, within a polythene tube inserted within the lumen of a self-retaining urethral catheter, can be used for intermittent intra-cavitary irradiation. Alternatively, gold-198 grains or tantalum wire can be mounted on the external surface of the catheter, the former with an adhesive plastic compound and the latter by stitches (Figs. 38 and 39). This will permit the intra-cavitary irradiation to be continuous, since there is free drainage of urine. Unfortunately, because the catheter material, whether plastic or rubber, is profoundly altered by irradiation in the atomic pile, it is necessary to attach the sources to the catheter only after they have been activated, and this results in additional exposure to personnel.

Intracavitary treatment may be employed alone for extensive superficial tumours of the urethra, in which case a dose of 7 000–8 000 R, measured at the surface of the applicator, is given. On the other hand, intracavitary irradiation may be combined with interstitial techniques to take the place of the "core" in a cylindrical implant. The total tumour dose in the treated volume in such cases should be 5 500–6 000 R in 6–7 days.

External irradiation. The initial stages consist of roentgen ray localisation of the tumour-bearing region, using a metal sound in the urethra, and a dye, such as Diodone, in the bladder; a marker may also be placed in the rectum. An outline is taken of the patient's pelvis, and the position of the viscera and the volume to be treated marked. A plan is then drawn up for supervoltage irradiation using either 3 or 4 fixed pelvic fields, or a short or long axis rotation technique, depending largely upon the facilities available. A maximum tumour dose of 6 000–6 500 R is delivered in 6–7 weeks, using roentgen rays

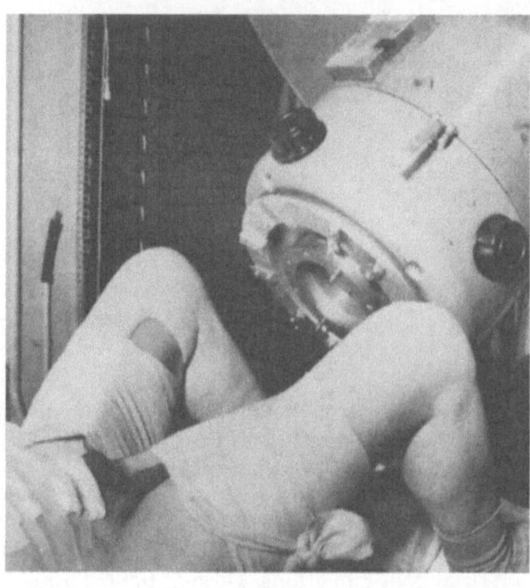
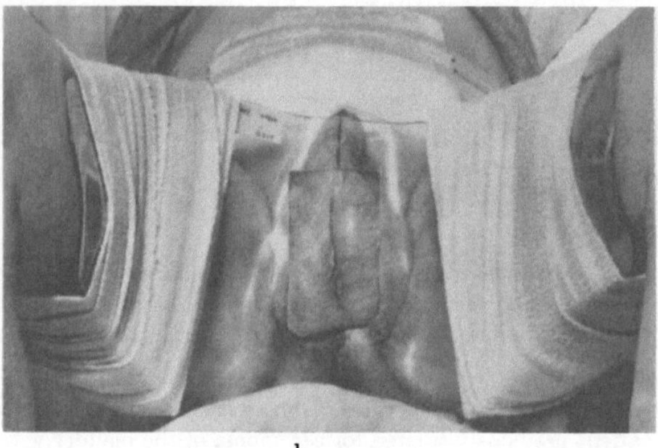

a   b

Fig. 40a and b. External supervoltage irradiation for carcinoma urethra: Male patient with anaplastic squamous cell carcinoma bulbomembranous urethra treated by segmental resection and postoperative irradiation. Direct perineal field 6 × 12 cm (2 MeV; HVL, 11.7 mm Cu; FSD 67 cm). Perspex perineal thigh applicator to displace penis and as much scrotal skin as possible out of beam. Peak skin dose 5 500 R in 6 weeks. Moderate local reaction which healed well. No recurrence at 2 years

generated at 2–8 million volts, or a cobalt-60 beam unit. Tumours of the anterior urethra, too advanced for interstitial therapy, or involving the vulva, can be treated by means of a single direct or a pair of angled supervoltage perineal fields, a maximum tumour dose of 6 000 R being given in 6–7 weeks. With conventional roentgen rays a hard quality beam (HVL = 3.5 mm Cu) should be used; the dose in such circumstances will be limited to approximately 5 000 R in a similar overall time.

γ) Treatment of carcinoma of the male urethra

Small localised tumours of the fossa navicularis can be cured by diathermy excision, followed by a gold grain implant to the base. Superficial tumours of the anterior urethra have been treated by intracavitary techniques. Larger tumours of this part of the urethra should be treated by partial or total amputation of the penis, depending upon the extent of the growth. If amputation is refused, external irradiation is a less satisfactory alternative. A technique similar to that for carcinoma of the penis is employed—two opposing lateral fields or four fields, using a wax or wooden block for field seatings.

It may be possible to treat tumours of strictly limited extent in the bulbo-membranous urethra by resection and re-anastomosis of the affected segment of the urethra. To establish the re-anastomosis it may be necessary to telescope the penis backwards after the manner described originally by YOUNG (1939) and more recently by SPENCE and DENMAN (1957), who report a seven-year cure of carcinoma of the bulbous urethra following this procedure. If the lesion is more extensive, or there is doubt concerning residual local tumour, immediate reconstruction is not done, and a course of post-operative irradiation should be given to the operation field. A direct perineal telecobalt, telecaesium or supervoltage roentgen ray field is employed, and a perspex jig is made to hold the testes and penis out of the irradiation beam. A window is cut in the jig in order to avoid build-up of the beam, and so lose the skin-sparing effect (Fig. 40). In these cases urine is passed via the perineum through the opening into the prostatic urethra. After a period of at least 12 months, provided there has been no tumour recurrence, a urethral reconstruction may be undertaken.

More extensive tumours of the bulbo-membranous and prostatic urethra will require radical surgery, which implies cysto-urethrectomy (emasculation in some cases), prostat-

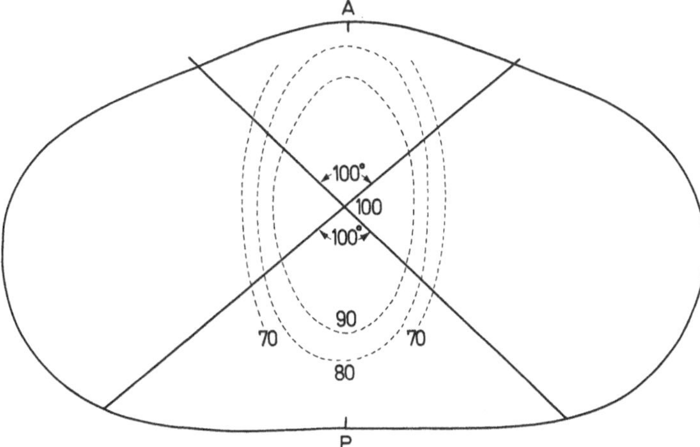

Fig. 41. External supervoltage irradiation: Plan for palliative treatment carcinoma urethra (rotating ⁶⁰Co unit): Summated isodose pattern for two opposing long axis arc therapy fields for male patient with recurrent carcinoma urethra extending widely and deeply over perineum (^{60}Co; HVL, 14.7 mm Cu; SSD, 60 cm; two opposing oscillations each of 100 degrees). Tumour dose at 90%, 5000 R in 6 weeks

ectomy, vesiculectomy, dissection of the pelvic lymph nodes and uretero-colic anastomosis. Three to four weeks later this extensive operation may be followed by a bilateral dissection of the inguino-femoral lymph nodes. Prolonged survival may follow the radical operation, even in the presence of positive external iliac or inguinal lymph nodes (MARSHALL, 1957). If the tumour is inoperable, or the patient is not suitable for such radical surgery, then the alternative is external supervoltage irradiation to the primary tumour, pelvic lymph nodes and inguinal regions, using either anterior and posterior pelvic and perineal fields, or a rotation technique (Fig. 41). Such patients, however, will probably first need a suprapubic cystotomy or uretero-colic anastomosis for the immediate relief of urinary obstruction. In some cases it is possible to perform a resection of the posterior urethra and leave the bladder with a permanent suprapubic cystotomy.

δ) Urethral tumours in cases of bladder cancer

These lesions are usually multiple, well-differentiated, non-infiltrating papillary carcinomas in the posterior urethra, and are amenable to wide endoscopic resection as the first stage of treatment. As the lesions rarely extend beyond the external sphincter, a clean resection of the bladder neck and the posterior urethra, leaving bare the prostate muscle, is adequate to clear these lesions even in the presence of superficial infiltration.

This, however, should not be undertaken unless the bladder has been rendered tumour-free, since the risk of implantation of malignant cells from higher up in the urinary tract, although small, is still a real one, and a raw granulating prostatic cavity filled with urinary deposits is the ideal bed for such an implant.

Tumours of the anterior urethra cannot be treated by endoscopic resection, but can be controlled by urethro-diathermy through a pan-endoscope or a direct vision urethroscope. When the urethral tumours are superficial and of low grade malignancy, diathermy alone is adequate, but in the presence of infiltration ancillary, interstitial or intracavitary radiotherapy is indicated. If urethral tumours co-exist with bladder lesions, which are to be treated by total cystectomy, the urethra should also be removed in a monobloc excision in continuity with the bladder. When the urethral lesions develop after a cystectomy the most effective therapy is excision of the non-functioning urethra, including the stump behind the compressor urethra; local recurrence in the perineum after cystectomy results from incomplete excision at the time of cystectomy or spill of tumour cells as the urethra is cut. There is no curative surgery for this complication once it develops and external radiation is at best purely palliative.

ε) Management of inguinal lymph nodes

Riches and Cullen (1951) considered that metastases to the inguinal lymph nodes are sufficiently common in carcinoma of the urethra to warrant consideration of their treatment in all cases. At the present time, however, it would seem reasonable to adopt a policy of "wait and see", as in cases of carcinoma of the penis, provided that the patient agrees to remain under regular observation at frequent intervals, and that there is no delay once it becomes evident that nodes are likely to be involved by metastases. In such cases a bilateral block dissection of the inguino-femoral lymph nodes is carried out. A number of surgeons in the United States favour extending the block dissection to include the external iliac nodes. The value of this operation, however, has yet to be determined. So far, it has not been practised widely in Great Britain and the majority of surgeons here are content to restrict their operation to the groins. Marshall (1957) reports one case of prolonged survival in urethral cancer with limited external iliac node involvement following radical pelvic surgery. When the lymph nodes are fixed, and therefore inoperable, or when the patient is not fit for radical surgery, then external irradiation may provide worthwhile palliation, and hold lymph node metastases in abeyance for a considerable time. Where possible, supervoltage roentgen ray or telecurie apparatus should be employed, primarily because of the skin sparing effect. With 2–4 MeV roentgen or telecobalt γ-rays a maximum skin dose of between 5000 and 5500 R may be given through a direct inguinal field 10×15 cm in 5–6 weeks. With conventional roentgen ray apparatus in the 200–250 kV range a hard quality beam of HVL. 3.5 mm of copper should be employed; the skin dose will be limited to approximately 4500 R in 5 weeks.

2. Miscellaneous urethral tumours

The female urethra is the most frequent site of primary malignant melanoma of the urinary tract. Up to 1955, however, only 15 cases had been reported in the world literature (Abrams, 1955). It is a tumour of elderly women, and in most cases is situated at the urethral orifice, and may simulate a caruncle. The clinical diagnosis may be difficult when there is no evidence of pigmentation. Malignant melanomas should be treated by surgery. Urethrectomy may be performed for small localised tumours in the anterior urethra, combined with bilateral block dissection of the inguino-femoral lymph nodes. In patients with more deeply placed or more extensive tumours anterior evisceration, including pelvic lymph node dissection, offers the only real hope of cure, and this major procedure will only be possible in selected cases. The prognosis is extremely grave in all cases of urethral melanoma: a 5-year survival has yet to be reported.

The principles of treatment for malignant melanoma are also applicable to those rare cases of spindle-cell sarcoma, fibrosarcoma and leiomyosarcoma of the urethra. Since, however, these tumours usually metastasize via the blood-stream a block dissection of the inguino-femoral lymph nodes may be delayed until there is evidence suggesting their involvement. The primary site and the regional lymph nodes in lymphosarcoma of the urethra should be treated by external irradiation.

Involvement of the urethra by direct tumour spread is seen in patients with carcinoma of the penis, vagina and anal canal. Such cases of penile cancer should be treated by partial or total amputation of the organ. The only hope of saving life in the cases of vaginal or anal canal cancer is by anterior or total pelvic evisceration. For inoperable cases, palliative irradiation may be of considerable value. In most instances this will be by external methods, but in some female patients a gold grain implant via the anterior vaginal wall is a simple procedure and will control the tumour for a time.

3. Reactions and complications of radiotherapy for urethral tumours

Severe skin and mucosal irradiation reactions tend to occur at this site, especially from external irradiation. During treatment the vulva is kept as clean and as dry as possible, and friction from clothing is reduced to a minimum. In the early stages, 1:1000 acriflavine lotion should be dabbed on to the vulva twice daily. When the irradiation reaction develops, a 1% watery solution of gentian violet, applied as a paint or from a spray, twice daily, will help to delay the onset of moist desquamation. In the later stages, bed rest, with no clothing, and a heated cradle, will be found comforting. An acute urethral irradiation reaction will give rise to frequency and painful micturition. In such cases a mixture containing aspirin and nepenthe will be found of value, but in more severe cases Pethidine or Physeptone, will be required.

Late irradiation reactions include urethral stricture, which will require repeated dilatation, incontinence of urine resulting from damage to the external sphincter, and which may require uretero-colic anastomosis, or the formation of an ileal bladder, and finally vulval oedema or necrosis. Occasionally, urethro-vaginal or vesico-vaginal fistulas may develop, but these are usually the result of tumour and not of treatment.

Table 45. *Carcinoma of the urethra, published results of treatment*

	Author	Methods	Cases	5-year cure or survival rate (%)
Female urethra	Fricke and McMillan (1949)	Local excision. Radium with or without roentgen rays	35	43
	Cade (1950)	Interstitial radium	11	55
	Murphy (1959)	a) Radiotherapy	32	28
		b) Interstitial technique with or without roentgen rays	20	40
	Ruch et al. (1952)	Local surgery. Radiotherapy	25	37
	Flocks (1956) (Collected cases from the literature)	Various	218	25
	Monaco et al. (1958)	Local surgery alone or with radiotherapy	23	30
Male urethra	Kreutzmann and Colloff (1939) (Collected cases from the literature)	Mostly surgery:		
		a) Penile urethra	65	54
		b) Bulbo-membranous and prostatic urethra	77	12
	Herger and Sauer (1942) (Collected cases from the literature)	Various:		
		a) Anterior urethra	123	55
		b) Posterior urethra		15

4. Results of treatment

See Table 45.

V. Tumours of the penis

The vast majority of malignant tumours of the penis are squamous-cell carcinomas. Other primary malignant tumours of this organ are extremely rare (Table 46). Occasionally the penis is the site of metastases from distant organs, usually the prostate, bladder and rectum.

Table 46. *Malignant tumours of the penis*

Primary	1. Squamous cell carcinoma.
	2. Basal cell carcinoma.
	3. Adenocarcinoma.
	4. Angiosarcoma, fibrosarcoma, myosarcoma, Kaposi's sarcoma.
	5. Melanoma.
Secondary	1. Direct spread from urethral carcinoma.
	2. Metastases from such sites as prostate, bladder, rectum and kidney.
	3. Leukaemic infiltration.

1. Carcinoma of the penis

a) Incidence

In great Britain and the United States cancer of the penis is a rare disease constituting 0.5–2% of all malignant tumours in men. In England and Wales there are some 150 deaths each year from this disease. Harnett (1952) in his survey of cancer in London reported an incidence of 1% compared with the Registrar General's figure of 0.5% for England and Wales as a whole. In Continental Europe the incidence may reach 5%. The disease in America is said to be five times more common among negroes than in white men (Lenowitz and Graham, 1946). Penile cancer is much more common in Asia, especially among the Chinese and Javanese (Ngai, 1933). This tumour accounts for 10% of all male cancers in India (Lowsley and Kirwin, 1956) and nearly 20% in China, Siam and Java. Noble (1933) found 52 cases of carcinoma of the penis among the 231 male cancer cases during a four-year period at Bangkok, Siam, an incidence of 23%. Bercovitz (1919) reports a similar incidence from Hainan, China. The highest incidence is found in North Vietnam, where Lavedan et al. (1954) report an incidence of 40%. There is, therefore, a progressive increase in the incidence of cancer of the penis as one travels eastwards.

The peak incidence of carcinoma of the penis appears between the ages of sixty and seventy. In the West, a few cases appear under the age of forty. The number of cases in the lower age groups is greater in the Far East, where the peak incidence occurs a decade earlier than in the West. Kini (1944) has described penile cancer occurring in a two-year old child.

b) Aetiology

α) Phimosis

A tight foreskin has long been regarded as of major importance for the development of cancer of the penis, and has been reported as occurring in 50–80% of cases. In a personal series of 795 cases of cancer of the penis treated by Chu and Tam (1954) in Vietnam, pre-existing phimosis was present in 90% of cases. Retained stagnant smegma and chronic balanitis appear to be the underlying factors responsible for initiating the malignant change. There is evidence that smegma is a carcinogen. PLAUT and KOHN-SPEYER (1947) found that horse smegma was capable of inducing local tumours and also a high incidence of tumours at distant sites in the Paris R. 3 strain of mice.

Circumcision in early infancy (8th day) as practised by the Jewish race confers absolute immunity against this disease, except when the growth appears on the shaft, which is seldom the primary site. This operation does not merely remove the cancer-bearing area, since carcinoma of the penis occurs most often on the glans. On the other hand, circumcision performed in later childhood, as practised by Moslems and certain African tribes in Kenya, between the ages of 3 and 14, does not confer immunity, although it does reduce the incidence of this disease. Thus, the train of events leading to the development of cancer of the penis appears to be initiated early on in life, and later removal of the cause does not prevent the development of malignant disease (KENNAWAY, 1947). In 16 cases of cancer of the penis occurring among non-Jews collected from the literature that were circumcised between the ages of 14 and 45, the tumour developed after an interval of 8–41 years (average 23 years) following the operation (KENNAWAY, 1947). The incidence of penis cancer in Moslems is approximately 3% of all cases of malignant disease in males, and in Hindus, who do not practice circumcision at all, it is 10–20%. At the Tata Memorial Hospital, Bombay, KHANOLKAR (personal communication to KENNAWAY, 1947) saw 86 cases of carcinoma of the penis in 2511 male Hindus with cancer, compared with only two cases among 835 male Moslems. WOLBARST (1932) reports that of 7692 cases of male cancer seen at Indian hospitals there were 1200 cases of cancer of the penis; the incidence among Hindus was 19.2%, and among Moslems only 1.5%.

In 1936 DEAN reported the first case of cancer of the penis arising in a Jew who had been circumcised in infancy. The lesion arose in the region of the external urethral meatus. BLEICH (1950) reviewed the world literature and could find only two cases of carcinoma of the penis in Jews, one being Dean's case, and the other occurring in an uncircumcised patient. As KENNAWAY (1947) points out, it is possible for an Orthodox Jew to be uncircumcised. The Talmud states that if two sons of the same father, or a son of each of three sisters have died as a result of circumcision, the next son, or the son of the fourth sister shall not be circumcised. These exemptions may have resulted perhaps from observations in haemophiliac families. In 1953, MARSHALL reported a second case of carcinoma of the penis in a circumcised Jew. LEDLIE and SMITHERS (1956) have reported carcinoma of the penis occurring in a fifty-one year old Gentile who had been circumcised at three weeks; the tumour developed at the site of trauma.

SMITHERS (1960) points to the doubtful value of recommending routine circumcision of the entire male population to prevent carcinoma of the penis in this country, where the disease is rare. On the other hand, this prophylactic measure would appear to be of real value in certain Far Eastern countries, such as Vietnam, where cancer of the penis may constitute as much as 40% of all malignant tumours in males.

Circumcision may not be the whole story behind the immunity of the Jewish race to this disease. The possibility of a hereditary racial immunity cannot be excluded.

β) Venereal disease

Traditionally, venereal disease is blamed for a share in the development of cancer of the penis, and there is certainly a higher incidence among patients with this disease compared with the general population. Thus, among 204 cases of cancer of the penis reported by STAUBITZ et al. (1955) 20% had a history of venereal disease or a positive Wassermann reaction. Among 139 cases reported by LENOWITZ and GRAHAM (1946) venereal disease occurred in 92% of 39 negroe patients and 52% of 100 white patients. Several authors, such as BARNEY (1907), CUNNINGHAM (1914), NGAI (1933) and HANSSON (1938) have reported carcinoma of the penis arising at the site of a syphilitic chancre. Nevertheless, it is now generally agreed that syphilis and gonorrhoea are of no or little significance in this disease. It is probable that lack of cleanliness and the likelihood of veneral disease are to be found in the same patient.

γ) Trauma

A history of trauma is given by about 5% of patients (Ngai, 1933; Hansson, 1938) and is of doubtful significance.

δ) Occupation

In all countries carcinoma of the penis mainly affects members of the poorer classes. In the Far East, the disease is most frequently found among farm workers and coolies where neglect of personal hygiene may be the underlying factor (Ngai, 1933).

ε) Pre-malignant dermatoses

Such conditions of the skin as Bowen's disease, Paget's disease and Erythroplasia of Queyrat are probably all examples of carcinoma-in-situ and will be dealt with later.

c) Pathology
α) Macroscopic

In most text-books the division is made between proliferative and infiltrating cancer of the penis, but the distinction between these is often not clear-cut. A single tumour may, in fact, show both proliferative and infiltrating features. Superimposed sepsis often complicates the picture further, the inflammatory induration simulating neoplastic infiltration. In spite of these difficulties, most lesions can usually be classified as being either proliferative or ulcerative. The former type grows slowly and may reach a huge size. It rarely invades the corpora cavernosa, and metastases to the inguinal lymph nodes when the patient is first seen are uncommon. The ulcerative form, on the other hand, is much more malignant, invades deeply, and is not infrequently associated with metastases in the inguinal nodes. A superficial infiltrating type of lesion is sometimes seen, and in these cases invasive changes have usually supervened on a pre-malignant skin condition, such as Erythroplasia of Queyrat.

β) Microscopic

Cancer of the penis is generally a squamous-cell growth. The majority are well-differentiated tumours showing marked keratinization, over 70% belonging to Broders' grades I and II. Marked lymphocytic and plasma cell infiltration is often present, and evidence of secondary infection is usual.

d) Natural history

Squamous-cell carcinoma of the penis commences as a small wart, nodule, plaque, ulcer or scaly patch on the glans or the inner surface of the prepuce, and generally remains localised for a considerable time. The disease would carry a much better prognosis if it were not for prolonged delay, though fear or ignorance, before patients seek medical advice. The untreated tumour extends slowly over the surface of the penis and invades the tunica of the corpora cavernosa. Eventually, infiltration of the corpora cavernosa occurs, and this was present in approximately 50% of the cases reported by Ngai (1933). In the late stages urethral involvement may occur with fistula formation. Finally, practically the whole penis may be destroyed, the tumour extend on to the pubic and scrotal skin and invade the perineum.

Once the cavernous spaces are invaded, the tumour often extends rapidly and the whole shaft soon contains growth. It is strange that blood-borne visceral metastases are rare in this disease, even at death. These were found in only 10% of the series reported by Staubitz et al. (1955).

The chief mode of spread in cancer of the penis is via lymphatics to the inguinal lymph nodes. Because cancer of this organ is so often associated with infection, it is often very difficult to assess clinically the significance of enlarged nodes. It has been estimated that approximately 75% of patients with penis cancer have easily palpable inguinal nodes when first seen, but that only half of these (37% of the total) actually contain metastatic deposits (JORSTAD, 1941). The incidence of inguinal metastases in various reports ranges between 30–50% (BARNEY, 1907; NGAI, 1933; DEAN, 1935; LENOWITZ and GRAHAM, 1946; BASSETT, 1952; STAUBITZ et al., 1955; EKSTRÖM and EDSMYR, 1958). In general, it may be said that approximately one-third of cases have definite lymph node metastases when first seen. Of 48 cases with inguinal metastases in a series of 139 patients reported by LENOWITZ and GRAHAM (1946) bilateral involvement was present in 37 or 77%.

The incidence of inguinal metastases is greater in the larger, the more extensive tumours, those which are of the ulcerative or infiltrative types and in those classified in Broders' grades III and IV. Involvement of iliac or retroperitoneal lymph nodes is uncommon, being found in only some 5% of cases (STAUBITZ et al., 1955). Spread to pelvic nodes usually occurs from the inguinal nodes, occasionally directly from the deep lymphatics of the penis or those accompanying the dorsal vein of this organ.

The final stages of the neglected case are particularly distressing. The greater part of the penis may be destroyed, and the neoplastic inguinal glands become matted together and ulcerate the overlying skin. Pain, sepsis and haemorrhage produce much misery. The absence of distant metastases permits patients with advanced disease to linger for many months before finally being released by death.

Cancer of the penis may have a long natural history. The disease occasionally takes more than 5 years from clinical onset to kill the host (BASSETT, 1952). An interval varying from several months to five or more years may intervene between the treatment of the primary tumour and the appearance of the inguinal node deposits.

e) Site of tumour

Carcinoma of the penis almost invariably arises from the prepucial sac i.e. the glans, coronal sulcus or the inner surface of the prepuce. The shaft is the primary site in only 1% of cases, but is involved much more frequently due to direct extension. In 204 cases reported by STAUBITZ et al. (1955) the tumour involved the glans in 39%, the prepuce in 7%, the glans and prepuce in 17%, the coronal sulcus in 12%, and the shaft in 1%. In a further 24% three-quarters or more of the organ was occupied by tumour. Rarely, the tumour arises at the external urethral meatus.

f) Clinical classification

Cancer of the penis has been divided into 3 stages by HANSSON (1938) depending upon the clinical state of the inguinal lymph nodes—Stage 1, no significant lymphadenopathy; Stage 2, enlarged lymph nodes which are operable; Stage 3, inoperable lymph nodes.

The disadvantage of this type of classification is that there may be histological metastases without palpable lymph nodes, and enlargement of the lymph nodes may be purely inflammatory. Nevertheless, this method of grouping cases serves to provide a useful guide to prognosis and treatment and permits comparison of different methods of treatment between one centre and another.

g) Clinical features and diagnosis

The usual clinical picture in cancer of the penis is that of a painless, firm swelling beneath an unretracted, tight, oedematous prepuce. Secondary infection is common, producing an offensive discharge, which on occasion may be blood-stained. Very occasionally priapism occurs as the result of occlusion of the cavernous spaces, due either to neoplasm or superimposed thrombosis.

Patients with penis cancer so often appear to be of poor intellect, and allow minor symptoms, such as irritation, discharge, difficulty in retracting the foreskin, swelling of the penis and swollen inguinal glands to continue unheeded for many months before seeking medical advice. By this time the tumour is often advanced. Sometimes the responsibility for delay rests with the physician, such cases often being treated over a considerable period for "chronic balanitis".

Any patient with disease beneath a tight foreskin should have a dorsal slit or circumcision performed, to enable a proper examination of the lesion to be carried out. The presence of malignant disease is established on clinical grounds, and confirmed by biopsy.

The clinical differential diagnosis includes carcinoma of the urethral meatus and the following benign conditions of the penis: syphilitic chancre, condylomata acuminata, soft chancre, papilloma, the pre-malignant dermatoses, herpes simplex and tuberculosis. To avoid any possible error in diagnosis a biopsy should be taken of all penile lesions.

h) Prognosis

Duration of symptoms, actual site on the penis and also size of tumour *per se* all have no significant relationship to the incidence of inguinal metastases (Staubitz *et al.*, 1955; Ekström and Edsmyr, 1958). Ekström and Edsmyr (1958) in their series of 229 cases found that the incidence of inguinal metastases was greatest in the younger age groups, 59% for ages 20–39, 30% for 40–69, and 24% for 70–89. On the other hand, Staubitz *et al.* (1955) found that the average age for patients with and without metastases was comparable.

Tables 47 and 48. *Cancer of the penis: Stage and prognosis*

Table 47				Table 48		
(Hansson, 1938)				(Ekström and Edsmyr, 1958)		
Clinical stage	Number of cases	5-year cures (%)		Pathological stage	Number of cases	5-year cures (%)
1	27	85		1	127	80
2	12	58		2	57	42
3	7	0		3	10	10
Total	46	65		Total	194	65

The chief factors influencing prognosis are: 1. extent of involvement of the penis, 2. histological grade of malignancy and 3. clinical stage with regard to the state of the inguinal lymph nodes. The larger lesions tend to be associated with a higher incidence of inguinal deposits, and a less favourable outcome. Some authors, in fact, consider that a carcinoma of the penis more than 2 cm in diameter, irrespective of other local factors, should be treated by surgery and not by irradiation (Bowing *et al.*, 1934; Dean, 1935; Engelstad, 1948; Zausner, 1948). On the other hand, Bassett (1952) could find no evidence to support this view. The incidence of inguinal metastases rises with increasing involvement of the penis, both with regard to area and also depth of invasion. Undifferentiated tumours belonging to Broders' grades 3 and 4 have a greater incidence of metastases than the more differentiated lesions belonging to grades 1 and 2. The most important single factor in prognosis is whether the inguinal nodes are involved or not, and if they are, whether they are mobile or fixed (Tables 47–48).

i) Treatment

Opinions differ greatly regarding the role of surgery and radiotherapy in the management of cancer of the penis. In the American literature, surgery, partial or total amputation, is generally advocated for the management of the primary tumour. In this country, radiotherapy is more widely used for this disease than in the United States and the results, in suitable cases, carefully treated and followed up, are satisfactory, with the advantage over surgery that the patient retains a useful organ. Some authors prefer surgery, some radiotherapy and others a combination of both.

An extreme view concerning treatment of carcinoma of the penis is expressed by SAUER and LEIGHTON (1944) who consider that squamous cell cancer at this site is "inherently unresponsive to irradiation", and favour total amputation as the treatment of choice, even in patients with limited lesions. These authors mention only 10 cases treated by radium or roentgen rays, in 2 of whom there was no follow-up; 6 cases died with recurrence. No details of radiotherapy are given. Even more recently, LOWSLEY and KIRWIN (1956) advocate amputation as the treatment of choice and consider that irradiation is of little value as penile carcinoma is radioresistant. There is, however, ample evidence that squamous-cell carcinoma of the penis does, in fact, respond to irradiation. Thus, five-year survival rates, ranging from 41—68 % (Table 49), have been reported for cases where the primary tumour was treated by irradiation, with amputation held in reserve for radiotherapy failures (up to 30–40 % of cases largely because of recurrence, and in a few necrosis). ENGELSTAD (1948) reports a five-year survival rate of no less than 89 % for patients without lymph node enlargement in whom the primary tumour was treated by radiotherapy at the Norwegian Radium Hospital.

α) Treatment of the primary tumour

Partial amputation for a limited tumour of the penis is the simplest and quickest method of treatment, and the one least likely to be followed by local recurrence. BASSETT (1952) reviewed the results of this operation reported in four papers, covering more than

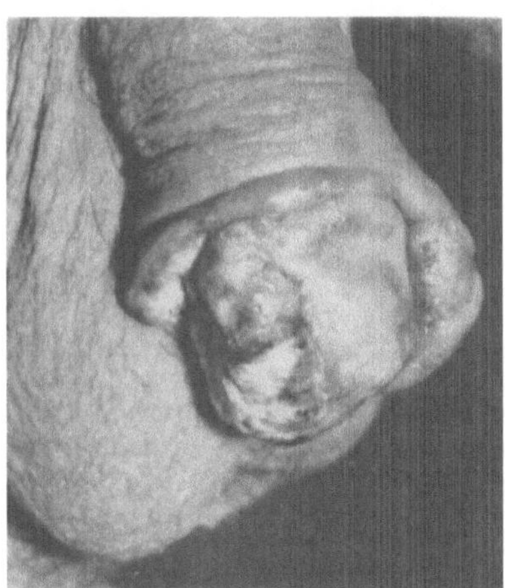

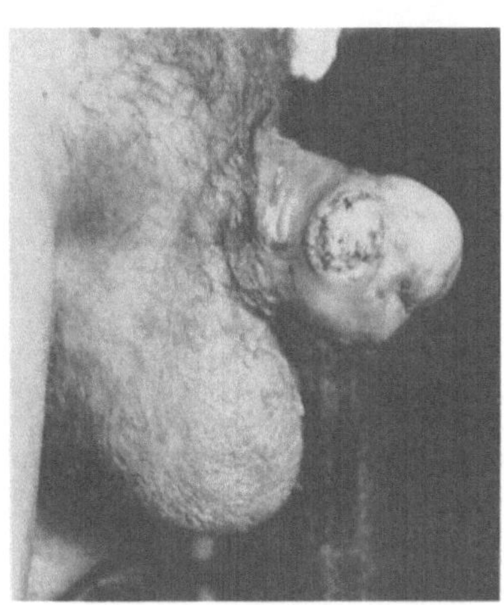

Fig. 42   Fig. 43

Fig. 42. Ulcerating penile carcinoma with extensive infiltration of the glans, prepuce and terminal portion of shaft; suitable for partial amputation

Fig. 43. Advanced ulcerating carcinoma of penis involving glans and lateral aspect of shaft. Deep infiltration of entire organ producing enlargement, rigidity and shortening of shaft. Urethral fistulae present and suprapubic skin involved. One enlarged firm node in groin. Case suitable for radical amputation. Excision penis, scrotum and suprapubic skin performed. Patient alive and well 6 years later

250 cases, and only 2 developed local recurrence. A case suitable for partial amputation (Fig. 42) must have at least 2 cm clearance of the tumour and sufficient of the shaft, at least 1.5–2.0 cm, should be left for directing the urinary stream. If this is not possible

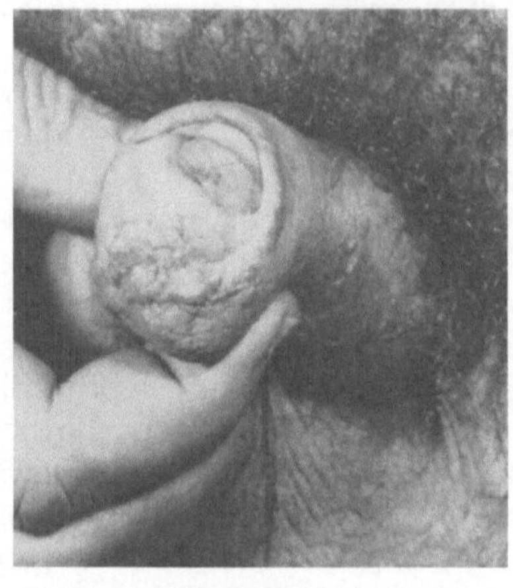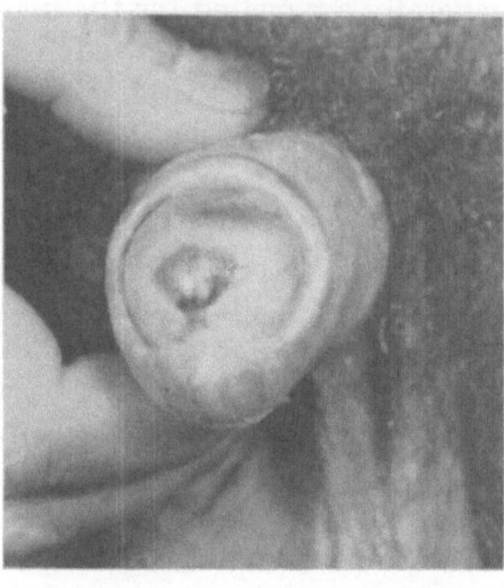

a   b

Fig. 44a and b. Papillary carcinoma of penis involving glans with area of superficial ulceration. Treated by external irradiation using two opposing lateral fields 10 × 6 cm (220 kV; HVL, 1.5 mm Cu); maximum tumour dose 4800 R in five weeks. Subsequent dilatation of urethral stricture. Patient alive and well 6 years later. a Before treatment; b two months after treatment

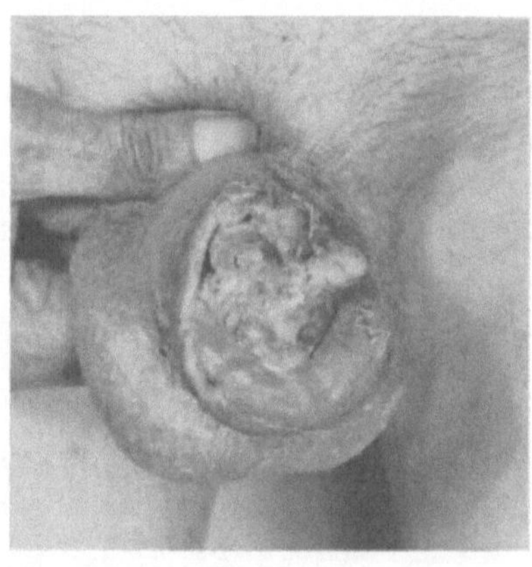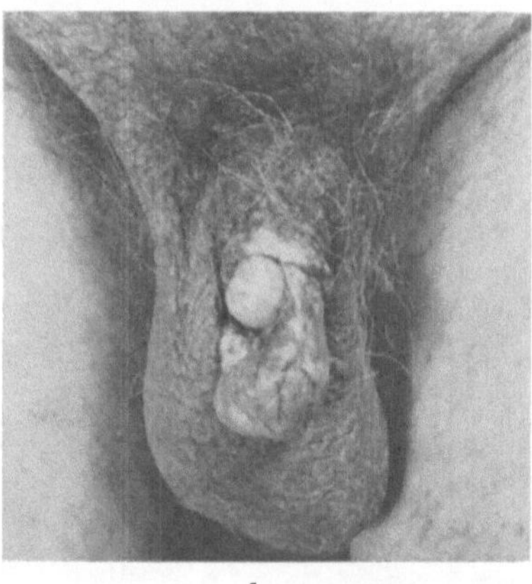

a   b

Fig. 45a and b. Papillary carcinoma of penis replacing glans and involving the anterior distal half of shaft. Prepuce infiltrated and oedematous. Treated with roentgen rays using two pairs of opposing fields (100 kV; HVL, 2 mm Al). Maximum tumour dose 5500 R in 6 weeks. Patient alive and well 6 years after treatment. Post-irradiation thickening and scarring of prepuce; glans atrophied. Micturition satisfactory. a Before treatment; b 6 years after treatment

(Fig. 43), it is better to perform a total amputation and a perineal urethrostomy. Attempts to carry out a simple removal of a small tumour by local excision or diathermy coagulation is likely to be followed by local recurrence, and should not be undertaken. Having decided to treat a case solely by surgery, nothing less than a partial amputation should be performed.

It is a wide belief amongst surgeons that radiotherapy gives poor results in cancer of the penis. It is believed that this is largely the result of the alleged radio-resistance of cancer at this site, the liability to necrosis because of the low tolerance of the normal penile tissues to irradiation, and the presence of sepsis, which reduces radiosensitivity and may complicate treatment. The fact is that carcinoma of the penis, as in squamous-cell tumours at other sites, is a radiosensitive growth, and in many cases potentially curable (Figs. 44–45). With care and attention to details of technique, serious over-dosage effects can be avoided. Sepsis can be reduced with antibiotics and local dressings and, where indicated, a preliminary circumcision or a dorsal slit operation. Whilst it must be admitted that irradiation is a less certain method of curative treatment for this disease than amputation, the former gives the patient a chance to retain his organ, and its normal function, thus avoiding mutilation and often profound psychological disturbance. No less than 43 patients out of a series of 138 reported by SAUER and LEIGHTON (1944) who advocated total amputation, refused to have treatment. If radiotherapy fails, the patient's life is not jeopardised, since surgery can always be undertaken, provided, of course, that the patient is kept under careful and regular observation, and that there is no prolonged delay once it is evident that the disease has not responded satisfactorily or is recurring (Fig. 46).

Generally speaking, radiotherapy is the treatment of choice, for relatively small superficial primary carcinomas, especially those not greater than 2 cm in diameter.

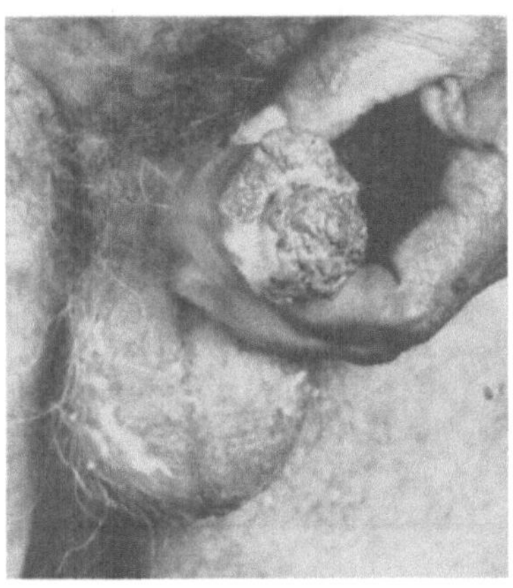 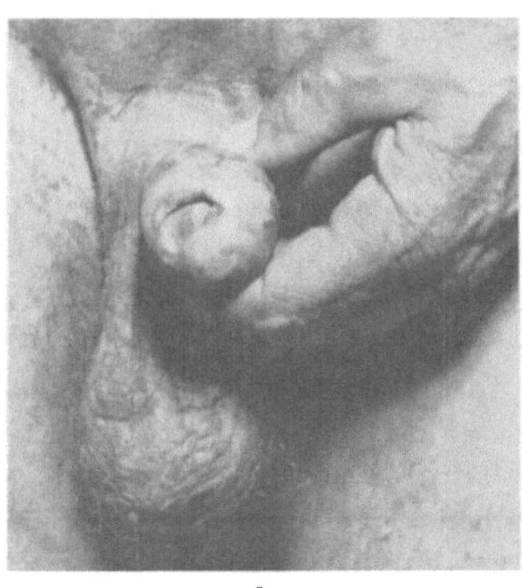

a   b

Fig. 46a and b. Papillary carcinoma of penis involving entire circumference of glans and distal part of shaft. Treated with teleradium unit using two pairs of opposing fields. Maximum tumour dose 5500 R in 5 weeks. Apparent complete resolution of tumour nine months after treatment. Recurrence developed three months later for which partial amputation performed. Patient died 11 years later, aged 81, from myocardial degeneration: no evidence of recurrence. a Before treatment; b 9 months after treatment

Surgery is indicated for those tumours which are larger, deeply infiltrating, involve the corpora cavernosa or the urethra, and for those cases with recurrence or necrosis following irradiation. In borderline cases, irradiation can be tried in the first instance. In elderly patients, in whom the loss of the penis is of less significance than in younger men, lesions suitable for radiotherapy may be more satisfactorily dealt with by surgery, this being a quicker method and producing less physical discomfort than radiotherapeutic techniques.

In some cases with advanced disease, a palliative amputation of the penis may be the quickest and simplest method of saving the patient from the distress of a fungating and advancing primary tumour.

β) Treatment of the inguinal lymph nodes

Clinical assessment of whether the inguinal lymph nodes contain metastases or not is unreliable, especially in the presence of sepsis. About 75 % of all patients have enlarged lymph nodes when first seen, but only about half of these (i.e. 30–40 % of the total) contain metastases. Some 20 % of patients with impalpable nodes have occult metastases. Aspiration biopsy may be helpful in determining involvement (BARRINGER and DEAN, 1924), but a negative result does not exclude this complication. Biopsy of a suspicious lymph node is also of limited value, because here again a negative result does not exclude the possibility of small deposits in other nodes.

The absence or presence of inguinal node metastases means all the difference between hope and despair, since very few cases with this complication are cured, in spite of the most radical treatment. In the past, irradiation with conventional deep roentgen rays has not proved effective in controlling inguinal metastases. This has been partly due to the limitation imposed on treatment by the poor skin tolerance at this site. With super-voltage equipment, the skin effect is greatly reduced, and perhaps better results may be achieved. At the present time, however, it is generally accepted in most centres that the management of inguinal lymph node metastases should, where possible, be entirely surgical, and that radiotherapy should be reserved for patients who are unfit for operation, and for those with inoperable nodes. Engelstad (1948) of the Norwegian Radium Hospital, and also Hansson (1938) of the Radiumhemmet are among the very few authors who report routine irradiation to the inguinal nodes whether or not metastases are suspected. Only in the presence of persistent or recurrent tumour is dissection undertaken.

The surgical management of inguinal node metastases involves a bilateral inguino-femoral block dissection performed in either one or two stages. Ekström and Edsmyr (1958) report that of 30 patients with unilateral metastases undergoing bilateral dissection, 18 had spread to both sides, and of a further 17 cases undergoing unilateral dissection, at least 4 patients subsequently developed contralateral deposits. Some surgeons extend the operation to include removal of the external iliac nodes. Kuehn and Roberts (1953) advocate removal of the entire chain of iliac nodes up as far as the aortic bifurcation. Hudson and his colleagues (1953) employ an extended radical operation in which the inguinal, iliac and the lowermost peri-aortic nodes are all removed *en bloc*, and this is combined with partial amputation of the penis. No results, however, for this procedure were available. The value of these extended lymph node dissections, which carry a considerable morbidity, has yet to be determined, and at the present time most surgeons restrict their operation to the inguino-femoral region. Dissection confined even to the groins should not be undertaken without good reason, since healing at this site is often delayed and incomplete, and oedema of the legs a frequent complication.

Because of the low incidence of histological metastases in clinically free nodes, the morbidity of the operation (protracted wound infection, necrosis of skin flaps and oedema of the lower limbs) and, above all, because the results appear to be no better than when we wait for clinical evidence of metastases before operating, bilateral prophylactic block dissection of the groins is not advised by many writers in this country, including the present authors. A number of surgeons, especially in America, such as Jorstad (1941), Sauer and Leighton (1944), Barnofsky (1948), Hovnanian (1952) and Staubitz et al. (1955) all advocate routine bilateral block dissection, together with amputation of the penis, where possible, in all cases. Colby and Smith (1931) reported that prophylactic block dissection was carried out in 11 patients, and 4 of these had histological metastases. Only 1 of the 4 patients lived more than 5 years. Bassett (1952) found that in 26 patients in whom a "wait-and-see" policy for inguinal metastases was adopted, tumours became manifest in only 5 cases, and all these died in spite of treatment. Prophylactic dissection was carried out in 15 other patients in Bassett's series, and only 3 of these were found to have occult metastases. These 3 cases also died. Dean (1935) reports 43 of 112 cases as having histologically positive nodes with only 2 survivors.

Prophylactic lymph node dissection may be considered for young patients, in those with large tumours, especially if they are anaplastic, and in those who are not able to undergo regular frequent follow-up examinations. Routine prophylactic irradiation to the inguinal regions is contraindicated, since, if the nodes enlarge subsequently, surgery may be difficult and healing greatly delayed.

When palpable nodes are present, the primary tumour is dealt with first, and the nodes watched. With reduction in sepsis of the penis, the nodal enlargement, if inflammatory, will subside. If the nodes remain enlarged, then operative treatment is undertaken, but not until control of the primary tumour has been established. If the nodes, from their number, size and consistency, are considered to be malignant and advancing, but operable, and the treatment of the primary tumour is likely to take some time, then a limited course of pre-operative irradiation to the groins may be undertaken with the aim of a "holding action". If the nodal prominence is of doubtful significance the patient should be seen at regular intervals, not exceeding 3–4 weeks during the first few months. At the first sign of further enlargement, or if there is failure to subside, bilateral inguino-femoral dissection should be undertaken without delay, provided the nodes are mobile and the patient's general condition satisfactory for major surgery.

γ) Radiotherapy techniques

Interstitial.
Applicator or mould.
External beams:
Superficial roentgen rays; 60–100 kV.
Medium voltage roentgen rays: 140 kV.
Deep roentgen rays; 200–250 kV.
Telecurie Units; Radium, Cobalt-60, Caesium-137.

In general, small superficial tumours can be successfully treated either by a course of superficial roentgen rays or by means of a radioactive implant. Larger tumours, suitable for irradiation, are treated either by a radium mould, or more simply by conventional roentgen rays or by γ-rays from a telecurie apparatus.

Interstitial

Radium needle implants have been widely used for carcinoma of the penis by CADE (1950) and by COX (1954) at the Westminster Hospital, London. In suitable cases these authors consider this to be the method of choice. The advantages are that it delivers a high dose localised to the area where it is required, reduces the dose to the surrounding normal tissues to a minimum, and is a quick method usually well-tolerated by the patient. Great care is required to bring about a reasonably uniform dose distribution, which is achieved by arranging the needles in accordance with the Paterson and Parker rules for single plane implants (MEREDITH, 1949). There are technical difficulties in carrying out a satisfactory implant in the penis owing to the contour of the organ and the toughness of the normal tissues through which the needles are inserted. A dose of between 5500 to 6500 R is given in 6–7 days depending upon the size of the area implanted; the smaller dose being given in the case of the more extensive implants. The risk of localised radionecrosis is greater with radioactive implants than with other methods, but CADE (1950) considers this justifiable since he regards the chance of cure as being greatest with interstitial techniques.

Applicator or mould

The treatment of penile cancer using a radium mould to encircle the entire organ was first described by HUTCHISON (1935). This is the chief technique employed by the Manchester School (PATERSON, 1948) where very satisfactory results have been obtained. WINDEYER (1939) and also LEDERMAN (1953) report cases treated in this manner. The method is particularly suited for cases in whom the tumour encircles a greater part of the circumference of the organ, but does not extend nearer to the base than the radium skin distance (THURGAR, 1955).

A simple cylinder of the correct diameter is made from sponge rubber, cork, beeswax or columbia paste, and is split into two interlocking parts. Alternatively, a plaster cast of the penis can be made with the organ maintained in the vertical position. The cylinder can then be made more accurately from the cast, and this is an advantage when the organ is deformed by tumour.

33*

The radium needles are mounted on the outer surface of the mould, which is 1.5 to 2.5 cm thick in "belt-form", either as circular rings or a series of parallel lines. The number, strength and distribution of the needles are chosen in accordance with the Paterson and Parker rules for cylinder mould treatments (MEREDITH, 1949). The aim is to deliver a skin dose of between 5500–6000 R and a central axis dose of between 4500–5000 R in 10–14 days. To achieve this the applicator has to be worn for 6–8 hours per day. The Manchester School advocates a similar dose, but chooses to deliver the treatment in the shorter time of 8–10 days (PATERSON, 1948).

To ensure accuracy in this treatment, the whole penile shaft should be irradiated, the active length of the moulded cylinder extending several centimetres beyond the end of the organ. During treatment a lead plate, with a hole through which the penis is passed, can be rested on the abdomen and thighs to reduce the dose to these parts and to the scrotum. Disadvantages of the mould technique are:

1. Time-consuming in preparation and treatment.
2. Technicians, medical and nursing personnel are exposed to stray irradiation.
3. Treatment is uncomfortable for the patient.
4. Scattered irradiation is received by the scrotum and thighs.

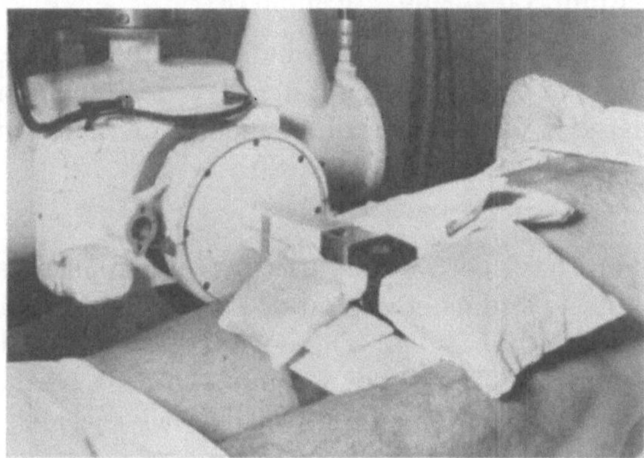

Fig. 47. To show technique for external irradiation of entire penis using conventional roentgen rays (250 kV; HVL, 3.5 mm Cu) and prior to adding final bolus bags. A lead shield protects the scrotum

The dose delivered to the scrotum, abdomen and thighs of the patient and the quantity of irradiation received by the medical and nursing staff, can be reduced considerably by mounting the radium on a special carrier bearing a handle, which is placed over a positioning cylinder fitted to a base plate (McKIE, 1959).

Because of the irradiation of the entire organ, the reaction with this method is severe. The cure rate, however, is most satisfactory, and the cosmetic result excellent.

Roentgen and gamma beam therapy

Primary tumour. Small superficial tumours of the penis, as in the case of squamous and basal cell cancer of the skin elsewhere, can be treated with roentgen rays generated at 60–100 kV. In these cases a dose of 4000–4500 R in two to three weeks is adequate. The use of a lead "cut-out" will help to flatten the tumour site and ensure greater accuracy of the set-up.

In more advanced tumours, those which are still superficial but extend round the glans, and those which are localised but associated with patches of carcinoma-in-situ (e.g. Bowen's disease), treatment must be directed to the whole or greater part of the shaft. This requires the use of a suitable box-jig made of wax, cork or wood. Perspex is a good material for this purpose, since it enables the penis to be visualised when treatment is to be directed to less than the entire organ. The penis is supported within the cavity of the box at right-angles to the supine patient. The box rests on a lead plate which protects the scrotum from scattered irradiation. The lateral sides of the box serve as seatings for the roentgen ray unit applicator (Fig. 47). With such a cross-fire arrangement, a fairly uniform through-and-through dose is obtained. A similar two-field technique can be used for a telecurie unit containing caesium-137 or cobalt-60, the physical factor of the unit being such as to bring about an isodose distribution similar to that from 200 to 250 kV roentgen rays. With teleradium units containing 5–10 g of element, it is necessary to use 4 fields to obtain a satisfactory dose distribution throughout the organ. With conventional roentgen rays (200–250 kV; Thoraeus III filter; HVL = 3.5 mm Cu) a dose of between 5000 and 5500 R is given in an overall time of five to six weeks. With γ-ray beams the equivalent dose is in the region of 6000–6500 R in a similar period of time.

Treatment of inguinal regions. Irradiation is chosen to treat metastatic inguinal lymph nodes only when they are inoperable or when the patient is unfit for radical surgery. Because of the poor skin tolerance of the groins the use of supervoltage roentgen ray or telecurie therapy is desirable at this site. The treatment field may be increased to include the iliac lymph nodes, since with supervoltage equipment in the 2–8 MeV range, a reasonable depth dose can be achieved. Patients with advanced penile cancer often linger for many months, and it is important to deliver an adequate dose of irradiation, even when the aim is palliation, if the activity of the disease is to be reduced for an appreciable time.

If only 200–250 kV apparatus is available, then a hard quality beam should be employed (HVL = 3.5 mm of Cu) and a dose of approximately 4500 R may be given to the inguinal region through a 10×15 cm field in five weeks. A useful way of employing conventional roentgen rays to the best advantage in this region is by means of grid therapy, when a skin dose of between 6000 and 8000 R may be given to the open areas in approximately 3 weeks. With supervoltage equipment in the 2–4 MeV range between 5000 and 5500 R may be given in five to six weeks.

δ) Local recurrence after partial amputation

External irradiation to the entire remaining shaft may be tried, failing which total amputation or emasculation will be necessary.

ε) Preparation and care of patient during radiotherapy

An essential preliminary to the treatment of carcinoma of the penis is to expose the lesion completely by performing a circumcision if the prepuce is free of tumour, or a dorsal slit if it is involved. This enables the full extent of the tumour to be determined and, by allowing free drainage, sepsis can be controlled. The radiotherapist should be present in the theatre when this is done to assess the case jointly with his surgical colleague. If the decision is in favour of surgery, then it is convenient to proceed at once with amputation. If the case is suitable for radiotherapy, laying bare the growth will permit cleanliness and reduce the risk of subsequent phimosis.

During a course of external irradiation, either by means of a mould, roentgen rays or a telecurie beam, the penis should be bathed two to three times daily with a 1:1000 aqueous solution of proflavine. In the later stages of treatment, friction from clothing and movement should be avoided as much as possible. When the penis becomes sore, proflavine cream, hydrocortisone ointment or an anaesthetic ointment may be substituted for the solution. If there is much discharge, a wet dressing of 1 % eusol is employed. The appropriate antibiotic is given for infection. A scrotal and penile cotton or linen support may reduce discomfort and serve to keep dressings in place.

If the groins are to be given palliative irradiation, then the skin should be kept clean and dabbed two to three times daily with a 1:1000 solution of proflavine or with surgical spirit, and then powdered with talc. When a deep erythema is developing the skin should be treated with a 1% aqueous solution of gentian violet to delay the onset of moist desquamation for as long as possible. When treatment has been completed, applications of cream of proflavine, zinc peroxide or calamine may be found comforting. Dysuria can be reduced by regular medication with disprin, codis or a mixture containing disprin and nepenthe.

j) Complications of radiotherapy

Phimosis and adhesive balanitis can be prevented by circumcision which should be performed, where possible, in all cases prior to radiotherapy. When the tumour involves the prepuce a dorsal slit is performed. Atrophy or chronic oedema of the penis are occasional sequelae to radical radiotherapy. Sterility may occur and this of greater importance in the East, where cancer of the penis is a more common disease, than in the West, and tends to occur in younger age groups. The use of a lead shield will help to reduce the dose to the gonads, but even if sterility is avoided, there is the possible hazard of defective embryonic development which may follow the fertilisation of an ovum by an irradiated spermatozoon. Embryonic abnormalities have, in fact, been reported in the frog following a dose as low as 15 R to the sperm prior to fertilisation (Henshaw, 1943). Urethral stricture and meatal stenosis resulting from radiotherapy are treated by dilation at intervals. Necrosis of the penis is the most frequent and troublesome complication and is a sequel to over-dosage, generally following interstitial techniques. In such cases partial amputation is indicated. In a series of 21 cases treated by irradiation and reported by Windeyer (1939) amputation for necrosis was performed in three.

k) Results of treatment

The survival rate and recurrence-free rate at five years are suitable yardsticks with which to measure the results of treatment in carcinoma of the penis. In view of the advanced age of so many men with this disease allowance for the natural death rate in such figures is justifiable. In all reports, however, the overall picture must be given in addition to any corrected results.

Although some patients with carcinoma of the penis may survive more than five years before succumbing to the disease, the vast majority of untreated cases die within two years of first attending hospital. Furlong and Uhle (1953) reported that of 40 patients who received either no treatment or palliative surgical or irradiation therapy, all but two died within eighteen months. These authors also reported that 60% of recurrences in treated cases occurred within twelve months, and 15% after three years. Barney (1907) found that of 26 cases with recurrences all but four developed within five years.

It is difficult to compare the results of radiotherapy with those of surgery reported in the literature because many surgical series contain few cases followed for an adequate period. At least two centres have employed a combination of irradiation and surgery to treat the inguinal regions. In some centres, dissection is carried out as a routine procedure whilst in others a "wait-and-see" policy is adopted, and dissection undertaken only when there is good clinical evidence of metastases. Finally, the indications for treating the primary tumour by a particular method are often not clearly stated.

Authors reporting series containing a reasonable number of cases followed for at least five years are shown in Table 49. The results obtained at the Royal Marsden Hospital are shown in Table 50. It appears that radiotherapy for suitable cases, with surgery held in reserve for failures, can achieve comparable results to those of primary amputation with the added advantage that a considerable proportion of the survivors in irradiation cases retain the penis (54% in the Royal Marsden series).

Table 49. *Cancer of penis: Published results*

Author	Treatment	5-year results	
		no. cases	survivals
HANSSON (1938)	Majority amputation and teleradium for nodes. Dissection for persistent nodes	46	30 (65%)
a) No nodes		27	23 (85%)
b) Operable nodes		12	7 (58%)
c) Inoperable nodes		7	0 (0%)
HUDSON et al. (1948)	Radical surgery	46	21 (46%)
a) No nodes		27	15 (55%)
b) Nodes		19	6 (31%)
TAILHEFER and COURTIAL (1943)	Radium for primary tumour. Surgery for nodes	49	23 (41%)
ENGELSTAD (1948)	Radium mould or telecurie therapy	57	38 (67%)
a) No nodes		27	24 (89%)
b) Operable nodes		22	14 (64%)
c) Inoperable nodes		8	0 (0%)
PATERSON et al. (1950)	Mould or roentgen rays. Surgery for nodes	41 corrected	22 (54%) (67%)
CADE (1950)	Radium implant	56	25 (45%)
LEDERMAN (1953)	Radiotherapy or surgery depending upon general and local factors. Surgery for 19 irradiation failures	55	28 (52%)
BASSETT (1952)	Amputation. Dissection nodes in 41 cases	61 corrected 43	24 (39%) 24 (53%)
STAUBITZ et al. (1955)	Radiotherapy or amputation with or without inguinal irradiation or dissection	204	84 (41%)
a) No nodes		105	63 (60%)
b) Nodes		99	21 (21%)
SANJUNIO and FLORES (1960)	Partial amputation with or without inguinal or inguino-ileo-femoral dissection	24	7 (29%)
EKSTRÖM and EDSMYR (1958)	Chiefly amputation. Dissection for definite nodes. Irradiation for doubtful nodes	194	127 (65%)
a) No nodes		127	102 (80%)
b) Nodes		57	24 (42%)
c) Inoperable nodes		10	1 (10%)
THURGAR (1955)	Radiotherapy. Amputation for recurrence or radionecrosis in 17	57	39 (68%)

Table 50. *Cancer of the penis: Results of treatment Royal Marsden Hospital* (LEDERMAN, 1953)

Survival period	Amputation and irradiation groins	Irradiation initial treatment	Irradiation with surgery for failures	Total cases
3 years (1929—49)	7/13 (54%)	16/46 (35%)	30/46 (65%)	37/59 (62%)
5 years (1929—47)	4/11 (36%)	13/44 (30%)	24/44 (54%)	28/55 (52%)
10 years (1929—42)	1/8 (12%)	4/33 (12%)	11/33 (33%)	12/41 (30%)

2. Miscellaneous malignant tumours of the penis

a) Sarcomas

Malignant connective tissue tumours of the penis are rare. ASHLEY and EDWARDS (1957), after reviewing the literature, found 54 proven cases of sarcoma, re-classified them, and added a personal case of leiomyosarcoma (Table 51).

Table 51. *Malignant connective tissue tumours of the penis* (ASHLEY and EDWARDS, 1957)

	Number of cases
Angioendothelioma	20
Fibrosarcoma	19
Kaposi's sarcoma	7
Myosarcoma	6
Undifferentiated sarcoma	3
Total	55

α) Haemangioendothelioma or angiosarcoma

WAUGH (1953) reviewed the subject of haemangioendothelioma of the corpus cavernosum penis and suggested the existence of benign as well as malignant forms of the tumour. He was able to collect 12 reported cases and added 2 of his own; 5 of these cases were regarded as having benign tumours.

Malignant haemangioendothelioma or angiosarcoma of the penis is a highly lethal tumour, the prognosis following either local excision or amputation being very poor. Most cases reported in the literature have died with distant metastases within a few months of treatment. Of 11 recorded cases only 2 were without evidence of recurrence after a few months (BARNETT and LOW, 1960). The tumour, which is of endothelial origin, produces one or more nodules or involves the corpora cavernosa diffusely. These tumours are radiosensitive and may show marked regression following moderate doses of irradiation. A course of pre-operative radiotherapy to the whole organ would seem to be worth trying before proceeding to total amputation, the aim of such treatment being to reduce the risk of local recurrence and of dissemination at the time of operation. A suitable dose with 250 kV roentgen rays (HVL, 3.5 mm Cu) would be 5000–5500 R in five weeks.

β) Fibrosarcoma of the penis

This tumour appears as a localised swelling of the glans, shaft or root of the organ. The degree of undifferentiation varies but most tumours appear to be of relatively low malignancy. The chief danger of this tumour appears to be from local recurrence rather than from early blood-borne metastases. There is a high incidence of recurrence in cases reported in the literature following local excision, and the treatment of choice would appear to be partial or total amputation, depending upon the site and extent of the tumour. In cases of partial amputation, there may be a place for pre-operative irradiation to reduce the risk of recurrence in the stump, a dose of between 5000 and 5500 R in five weeks being given with conventional roentgen rays.

γ) Kaposi's sarcoma

This lesion, which has histological features suggestive of a vascular origin, is now usually grouped with the malignant reticuloses and may be found in association with chronic myeloid or chronic lymphatic leukaemia, Hodgkin's disease and lymphosarcoma. It is a multicentric disorder, arising primarily in the skin and generally first appearing in the lower limbs. It is often chronic, lasting up to 15 or 20 years, but when viscera become involved the prognosis is much more serious. Kaposi tumours occur on the penis as part of the generalised disease, but occasionally this organ is the site of the initial lesion. In such cases, removal of the penile lesion may be followed by freedom from other manifestations of the disease for five or more years (MCCARTHY and PACK, 1950). These authors give examples of cases treated by local excision or partial amputation of the penis. The Kaposi lesion, however, is very radiosensitive, and, certainly if it is part of a more widespread disorder, should be treated by irradiation and not by surgery, a dose of 2500 R from 140–250 kV roentgen rays in two weeks being adequate.

δ) *Muscle sarcoma*

Four of the six examples of malignant muscle tumours in the literature were leiomyosarcomas, the remaining two being rhabdomyosarcomas. The treatment of choice would appear to be partial or total amputation. There is no reported experience with radiotherapy in such cases.

b) Malignant melanoma

This is a rare tumour of the penis, only some 14 cases having been reported in the world literature (MACDERMOTT and KENNEDY, 1955). A recent case has been described by REID (1957). The tumour presents as a black or red nodule, mass or ulcer of the glans, and in most cases grows quickly and soon gives rise to metastases. Occasionally the natural history extends over many years (REID, 1957). The penile malignant melanoma is probably best treated by partial or total amputation, with bilateral block dissection of the inguinal lymph nodes. Deposits in the iliac nodes, however, were not a feature in the cases reviewed by MACDERMOTT and KENNEDY (1955).

c) Metastases

In view of the rich blood supply to the penis it is perhaps surprising that secondary deposits are not more frequently seen in this organ. MCCREA and TOBIAS (1958) found only 69 cases reported in the literature and described one of their own. The most frequent

Table 52. *Metastases to the penis: Primary site and survival* (MCCREA and TOBIAS, 1958)

Primary site	Number of cases	Average survival
Prostate	22	5.6 months
Bladder	15	2.8 months
Rectum	13	22.3 months
Kidney	7	1.0 months
Testis	6	6.6 months
Others	6	2.8 months
Total	69	6.9 months

primary sites are in the pelvis i.e. prostate, bladder and rectum (Table 52). No doubt this is due in most cases to direct extension or to retrograde blood flow from the pelvic venous plexus (PAQUIN and ROLAND, 1956). The prognosis in metastatic disease of the penis is very poor, the average survival being approximately 7 months; it was longest in carcinoma of the rectum and shortest in carcinoma of the kidney (Table 52). Priapism is a presenting or subsequent symptom in approximately 50% of cases. Frequency, dysuria and retention may occur. Patients may develop nodules, plaques and ulcerative lesions on the penis, chiefly in the corpora cavernosa, or the entire organ may be enlarged and indurated.

In many cases the penile manifestations will be overshadowed by the generalised nature of the disease and will not call for any special treatment. In cases of prostatic cancer, which is the most frequent primary site for metastases to the penis, treatment by orchiectomy and oestrogen therapy may be rewarding. In those cases with local discomfort palliative external irradiation may help to reduce symptoms. Occasionally, the penile deposit appears to be the sole manifestation of metastatic spread, such as in the cases of carcinoma of the rectum reported by Cattell and Mace (1951) and by Boyd (1954). In such cases a partial amputation of the penis appears to be worthwhile. The case reported by Cattell and Mace (1951) was alive and well nine years following local excision of the penile deposit, which occurred two-and-a-half years after abdominoperineal resection. Boyd's case developed the penile metastasis five years after the primary operation. A local excision was performed, but ten months later amputation of the penis had to be carried out for recurrence: the patient was alive and well seven-and-a-half years after removal of the rectum.

Priapism is usually the result of superimposed thrombosis in the corpora cavernosa which generally requires incision with evacuation of the clot to bring relief.

d) Leukaemia

It is often stated that priapism is a symptom of leukaemia, but it occurs rarely in this disease. Craver (1933), for example, found only one case among 100 male patients with leukaemia and Lower and Christoferson (1945) found only two cases in a fifteen-year period in 309 cases of leukaemia.

The cause of priapism in these cases may be leukaemic infiltration of the corpora cavernosa with or without superimposed thrombosis. Irradiation and perhaps chemotherapy may be of value in relieving this distressing symptom. Haar et al. (1960) have recently reported a case of chronic myeloid leukaemia with priapism in whom there was no improvement with myleran, but a response was obtained with an ethyleneiminoquinone compound.

3. Pre-malignant skin conditions of the penis

A number of local chronic skin diseases of the penis have been described which may remain quiescent for a number of years, but which are prone, sooner or later, to progress to invasive carcinoma. These diseases have been collectively called the "pre-malignant dermatoses" and according to Willis (1948) are probably all variants of intradermal carcinoma-in-situ. They include the following conditions:

1. Bowen's disease.
2. Erythroplasia of Queyrat.
3. Paget's disease.
4. Leukoplakia.

Atypical proliferation of the epidermal cells is the essential feature of all these disorders. Generally speaking, the clinical picture is that of a slowly-extending brownish-red patch or plaque (white in the case of leukoplakia), some with crusted surface, others with a moist, velvety appearance. Warty projections may be present in some cases. The patches are frequently multiple, and finally coalesce to form extensive irregular areas of skin change over the glans and inner surface of the prepuce. The duration of the disease varies greatly and may be present for several years before the patient receives adequate treatment.

Histologically the epidermis is thickened and the intercapillary processes are deep and broad. Nuclear hyperchromatism and mitotic figures are a feature. Large vacuolated cells are sometimes seen. Chronic inflammatory cells are abundant in the dermis. These lesions may remain without evidence of infiltration for many years. Invasive properties, however, supervene during the lifetime of the host in a considerable proportion of cases.

Some 40% of patients with penile Bowen's disease develop invasive carcinoma (MULLIGAN, 1951), and MERRICKS and COTTRELL (1953) consider that between 20–40% of patients with Erythroplasia of Queyrat develop epitheliomas.

a) Treatment

Circumcision is the first step to be taken in any of these conditions and, if the disease is confined to the foreskin, the operation is curative. If the lesions are situated on the glans a biopsy is taken, from one or more areas. Partial amputation of the penis has been advocated by some authors such as PAUL (1952) and MERRICKS and COTTRELL (1953). On the other hand, EDSMYR and EKSTRÖM (1959) consider that amputation is curative only at the cost of mutilation, and that conservative measures are justifiable in the first instance. If these fail amputation can be carried out, nothing having been lost. Although recurrence of the pre-malignant skin condition is not uncommon following conservative measures, change to frank malignancy as a result of such treatment was not noted in any of the 25 cases studied by EDSMYR and EKSTRÖM (1959). The cases reported by these authors were treated by local excision, electrocoagulation or radiotherapy. Fifteen cases were followed for more than 5 years, of which 11 were alive nine to fourteen years after treatment: there were no recurrences and none developed invasive carcinoma. The remaining 4 cases died of intercurrent disease at intervals of up to twelve years. Of the 10 cases with shorter periods of observation one died of lung cancer and the others were asymptomatic for eighteen months to over four years after treatment. The authors concluded that radiotherapy was the most effective conservative treatment available.

A trial of radiotherapy would appear to be worthwhile as the first measure in most cases with partial amputation held in reserve for irradiation failures. Small lesions may be treated with superficial roentgen rays generated at 60 kV, a dose of 500 R being given on eight consecutive days to a total of 4000 R. More extensive lesions should be treated by means of a radium mould or by external irradiation using deep roentgen rays or telecurie apparatus. With roentgen rays generated at 200–250 kV a through-and-through dose of 4500 R in three weeks, or 5000 R in four weeks, may be given to the glans using two opposing lateral fields with a wax or perspex block to assist in the 'set-up'.

4. Peyronie's disease or plastic induration of the penis

This curious non-neoplastic condition was first described in 1743 by FRANCISCURA DE LA PEYRONIE, court physician to Louis XIV of France. It is characterised by the formation of indurated areas in the sheath of the corpora cavernosa which lead to painful deformity of the erect organ. It is an uncommon disorder, generally occurring between the ages of 40–70 (90% of cases), but may occur in the twenties. Reference to this disease is made here because, of the many different methods of treatment advocated, irradiation is the only one which has given consistently good results in the relief of pain. The treatment of Peyronie's disease is especially important in younger men: although the condition sometimes appears to be self-limiting or capable of spontaneous regression, in many untreated cases it seems to herald the end of effective sexual life (ASHWORTH, 1960).

a) Aetiology

The disease is a chronic, sclerosing condition, perhaps allied to Dupuytren's contracture of the hand. HEITE and SIEBRECHT (1950) found Dupuytren's contracture in 10% of patients with Peyronie's disease, BURFORD et al. (1951) in 3 of 124 cases, and ASHWORTH (1960) in 5 of 32 cases. It has been suggested that both Peyronie's disease and Dupuytren's contracture may be due to poor general nourishment and vitamin deficiency, especially vitamin E. HEITE and SIEBRECHT (1950) found 455 cases of Dupuytren's contracture, 14 of Peyronie's disease and 10 cases with both conditions among 6038 male inmates of a German prison camp. Trauma has been blamed as an aetiological factor in Peyronie's disease and such a history was present in a third of 186 cases reported by BURFORD and BURFORD (1957).

b) Pathology

The indurated areas consist of grey, glistening, scar-like tissue resembling keloid, which may contain calcium, cartilage and bone. Histologically, compact bundles of relatively avascular connective tissue are present containing sparse nuclei.

c) Clinical features

In contrast to more serious conditions approximately 90% of patients with Peyronie's disease seek medical advice within the first year of onset, the average delay being eight months (BURFORD and BURFORD, 1957). The chief symptoms are deformity or lump, painful erection and painful and difficult coitus. Over 35% of the patients seen by LOWSLEY and KIRWIN (1956) were impotent.

The indurated area consists of a well-defined hard plaque, cord or nodule of average size 2×3 cm, situated most often in the midline on the dorsal aspect of the penis, in the region of the mid-shaft or near the glans. Occasionally, multiple plaques are present and are then often connected by some degree of intervening thickening. The differential diagnosis of Peyronie's disease includes traumatic fibrosis, os penis and benign and malignant neoplasms.

d) Treatment

The wide variety of treatments advocated for Peyronie's disease serves only to emphasize that no entirely satisfactory method has been established. A high proportion of successful results has been claimed following the administration of vitamin E or tocopherols (SCOTT and SCARDINO, 1948; SCARDINO and SCOTT, 1949; THOMSON, 1949; WIJN-BLADH, 1949; DAHL, 1954), potassium para-aminobenzoate (ZARAFONETIS and HORRAX, 1959), oral cortisone (ASHWORTH, 1960), the local injection of hydrocortisone (TEASLEY, 1954; FUREY, 1957; BOLADO and LAVIN, 1957) or hydrocortisone and hyaluronidase (BODNER et al., 1954).

LOWSLEY and BOYCE (1950) reported cures in 39 of 50 cases treated by surgical excision of the plaques. No other surgeon, however, has reported such a high cure rate by this method, and surgery, in general, has been abandoned. Operation may lead to further deformity and recurrence is not uncommon.

Radiotherapy, which has been found of value in Dupuytren's contracture, appears to be the most reliable method of treatment in Peyronie's disease, consistently giving a high proportion of cures or improvement. SAILAND et al. (COSTOLOW, 1951) employed a radium mould in 32 cases and obtained 31% cures and 88% cures or improvement. Similar results were obtained by BURFORD and BURFORD (1957) who also used a radium mould in 96 patients and obtained 41% cures and 77% cures or improvement. DAHL (1954) reported pronounced improvement in 20% of cases and a moderate improvement in a further 35% among 96 cases treated by radium or roentgen rays at the Radiumhemmet.

e) Radiotherapy techniques

α) Radium mould

This technique is similar to the one used for treating carcinoma of the penis, but the dose is considerably less, 1500–2000 R being delivered to the surface of the organ in two weeks.

β) Deep roentgen rays

Using a wax or perspex block and two lateral opposing fields, a mid-line dose of between 1500–2000 R is given in two to three weeks from roentgen rays generated at 200–250 kV (HVL = 3.5 mm Cu).

With either of these techniques the whole shaft is treated because the plaques may be multiple and because recurrence at a new site may follow localised treatment.

The use of roentgen rays rather than radium is recommended in this disease, since with the former protection from stray irradiation is much easier to achieve. In younger men this is of especial importance in relation to the gonads; these should be carefully covered during treatment with a suitable lead shield.

A successful result in Peyronie's disease is characterised by reduction of pain or discomfort during erection and intercourse. The degree of induration is often reduced but penile deformity usually shows little change.

Acknowledgements

We are indebted to the many surgeons who have referred cases to us. We wish to thank the Editor of the British Journal of Radiology for permission to reproduce Figs. 4, 11–13, 15–18 and 36; Messrs. E. & S. Livingstone Ltd. for Figs. 7, 8a, 9–10, 21 and 22; and Dr. R. Morrison for Fig. 27.

We wish to thank Dr. M. Lederman for Figs. 43, 44 and 45.

We are grateful to Dr. N. F. C. Gowing and the Editor of the British Journal of Urology for kind permission to reproduce Fig. 37.

VI. Some current views on treatment of urological cancer[1]

1. Renal cell carcinoma

a) Aetiology

Over the past decade much interest has been focused on the production of experimental renal tumours in the hope of finding clues to the causes and control or renal cancer in man (see reviews by Bloom, 1967; and Pavone-Macaluso, 1967).

b) Investigations

With high-dose or infusion pyelography retro-grade studies of the kidney are rarely necessary and are only required when there is complete absence of function of the involved organ. The technique of pedal lymphography for outlining the para-aortic nodes has been of special interest. Good correlation exists between the radiological appearances and the operative findings in renal carcinoma, since the factor of chronic infection which may confuse the picture in other primary sites, such as the bladder, is not present. Routine lymphography is indicated before exploration of the kidney, and may prove helpful in assessing the extent of the disease and in planning treatment (Higgs and MacDonald, 1968). Selective arteriography should be preceded by free-flowing aortography, which will outline the contra-lateral kidney and also demonstrate one or more renal arteries on the affected side. Using a Seldinger catheter the artery to the affected kidney and, on occasions, the artery to the suspected segment of the kidney, can be catheterised. Better definition and greater contrast can be achieved by this technique.

c) Radiotherapy

The value of routine post-operative irradiation for renal carcinoma, widely advocated in the past, is now being questioned. Most published series continue to suggest that post-operative radiotherapy improves prognosis compared with nephrectomy alone (Riches, 1963; Ringleb and Rommel, 1963; Bratherton, 1964). The comparison between case-groups in these retrospective studies has not been on the basis of similar lesions. In a recent report by Peeling *et al.* (1969), in which efforts were made to compare comparable groups of cases, but where 31% of the material was rejected because of

---

1 Submitted July 1970 as appendix to chapters on "Tumours of the urinary tract".

inadequate information, post-operative irradiation appeared to worsen the prognosis. This unusual result finds no support in the latest study on the subject by Rafla (1970). In 244 cases, with only one patient excluded, a substantial and significant increase in survival rate was found for patients receiving irradiation in whom there was involvement of the renal pelvis or capsule. The local recurrence rate in 94 cases treated by nephrectomy and post-operative irradiation was only 7%, compared with 25% in 96 cases treated by surgery alone.

Pre-operative irradiation would appear to be a more rational approach to combined cancer therapy (see reviews by Nickson and Glicksman, 1966; Herbst et al., 1966; Cady, 1968; and the radiobiological considerations presented by Powers and Palmer, 1968). Riches (1970) from personal experience, continues to advocate this therapeutic approach for renal carcinoma. Cooperative clinical trials have now been set up in London, Holland and the United States, in which pre-operative irradiation followed by nephrectomy is being compared with surgery as the initial treatment.

The place of megavoltage radiotherapy in renal cell carcinoma continues to be a subject of controversy, partly because the number of cases referred to individual clinicians, and even to single institutions, is usually limited, and because the results of treating this capricious tumour are often based on incomparable groups of cases. Cooperative clinical trials are required in which the cases, even though randomised, are classified by an agreed system of staging (such as that proposed by the UICC, 1968) and histological grading. Until the results of such trials become available there can be no objection to recommending irradiation post-operatively in cases with gross or suspected residual disease following nephrectomy, and pre-operatively for particularly large or tethered tumours.

Attempts to achieve a greater response to treatment through additive or synergistic effects has led to the concept of combining irradiation with the administration of cytotoxic or radiosensitising agents. This approach for renal carcinoma would hardly seem worthwhile, however, until more effective chemical compounds have been discovered. The value of irradiation under hyperbaric oxygen for this tumour is not known.

d) Radical nephrectomy

Para-aortic node involvement is found in about 25% of cases of renal carcinoma. The incidence is related to primary tumour size (Hultén et al., 1969). A high ten-year survival rate (49%) has been obtained by Robson et al. (1969) for nephrectomy combined with lymphadenectomy; his latest five-year result (52%), however, is comparable to that reported by other authors for simple nephrectomy. It should be noted that an unusually high proportion (62%) of Robson's cases had tumours of low grade malignancy. In Rafla's (1970) recent study simple nephrectomy gave better results than nephrectomy combined with lymphadenectomy. Because of significant variables, such as tumour size, extent and histological grade, it will require a prospective randomised trial, in which cases are classified by stage and grade, to assess the value of the more extensive operation.

e) Chemotherapy and hormone therapy

Though occasional limited responses have been reported for a variety of cytotoxic agents, no useful compound against this disease has so far been discovered. Woodruff et al. (1967) reviewed some 60 reports concerning 33 different cytotoxic agents, in which the overall objective response rate was only 9%. Talley et al. (1969) obtained objective improvement in 3% of 57 cases treated with various compounds including alkylating agents, antimetabolites, and vinblastine. Research must continue for more effective, more selective and less toxic drugs.

In recent years, attention has been drawn to the value of sex hormones, particularly progestogens, in the treatment of far advanced renal carcinoma (Bloom, 1964; Bloom and WALLACE, 1964; BLOOM, 1967). Reports from elsewhere have confirmed these observations (MELANDER *et al.*, 1967; SAMUELS *et al.*, 1968; TALLEY *et al.*, 1969). In our experience with Provera (Upjohn Ltd.) or testosterone propionate objective improvement may occur in seriously ill patients within four weeks, and last for up to two or three years. In a total of some 100 collected hormone-treated cases from the literature, the overall objective response rate was 18%. More frequent and more effective responses are seen in male patients. In the present state of our knowledge, hormones should be reserved for cases with advancing metastatic disease for which neither surgery nor radiotherapy are feasible.

2. Nephroblastoma

There has been a decrease in the incidence of inoperable cases and a substantial improvement in treatment results for nephroblastoma in specialised centres. At the Children's Hospitals in Boston, Toronto and London, the two-year cure rate has increased from approximately 15–50% (GROSS, 1953; WILLIAMS, 1964; DARTE, 1965). This has been achieved by advances in operative techniques and the wider use of radiotherapy. At present most authorities advocate post-operative irradiation for all cases with the possible exception of the youngest children with limited tumours showing no evidence of local spread.

The optimum time for radiotherapy in relation to surgery for operable cases is still debated. Though appealing radiobiological arguements can be advanced for pre-operative irradiation, experience with this approach in a small number of cases at the Children's Hospital in Boston and also in London has been disappointing. Remarkably good results for a combination of pre- and post-operative irradiation has been reported by VAETH and LEVITT (1963). The distribution of prognostic variables such as age, tumour stage (GARCIA *et al.*, 1963) and histological type and grade (BODIAN and RIGBY, 1964) may account for different results obtained in retrospective studies. Randomised trials will be required to determine the optimum time for irradiation and its value in children with no evidence of tumour spread. Until these results are available it would seem reasonable to recommend pre-operative irradiation for large and tethered tumours, and post-operative irradiation as a routine procedure for all cases, except infants in whom there is no evidence of tumour spread and total removal of the disease appears to have been accomplished.

a) Chemotherapy

Actinomycin D remains the principal cytotoxic drug against nephroblastoma. It has been suggested that this agent potentiates the effect of irradiation, but this concept is by no means established. The benefit observed from this combined treatment in many desperate cases may be due merely to an additive rather than a synergistic effect.

α) Primary treatment

Following a combination of surgery, irradiation and Actinomycin D, a number of authors have reported results so good that some investigators may now feel quite unable to participate in clinical trials in which randomised children would be denied prophylactic chemotherapy (Table 53a). Experience with Actinomycin D, however, has not always been encouraging. This agent administered to operable cases was without value in the series reported by SUKAROCHANA and KIESWETTER (1966) and possibly even harmful to the children treated by MAIER and HARSHAW (1967) and by STONE and WILLIAMS (1969) (Table 53b). The last authors reported a high incidence of pulmonary metastases following adjuvant treatment with Actinomycin D, compared with surgery and post-operative irradiation without chemotherapy.

Conflicting treatment results in non-randomised retrospective studies are not surprising. Cases of nephroblastoma can be classified by patient's age and tumour extent, both of

Table 53a. *Nephroblastoma. Survival rate after nephrectomy and radiotherapy*

Author	With Actinomycin D		Without Actinomycin D	
	Cases	%	Cases	%
Fernbach and Martyn (1966)	13	92	14	43
Burgert and Glidewell (1967)	49	63	136	44
Johnson et al. (1967)	34	62	30	47
Cases over age 1	32	67	17	18
Howard (1965)	18	62	26	11
Schneider et al. (1970)	9	89	14	50

Table 53b

Author	With Actinomycin D		Without Actinomycin D	
	Cases	%	Cases	%
Sukarochana and Kiesewatter (1966)	16	62	21	62
Maier and Harshaw (1967)	17	29	24	54
Stone and Williams (1969)	13	38	15	67

All survival rates at 2 years except those of Burgert and Glidwell which are at 4 years.

which influence prognosis. For example, the encouraging results reported by Fernbach and Martyn (1966) have to be considered in the light of extrarenal spread in only four of their 30 cases. The timing and frequency of courses of Actinomycin D also appear to be of some importance. Repeat courses at intervals of eight to twelve weeks seem to be more effective than single courses (Wolff et al., 1968).

Even in cases with no evidence of extra-renal spread or in whom total tumour removal appears to have been accomplished, remarkably high cure rates have been reported for prophylactic chemotherapy (Fernbach and Martyn, 1966; Johnson et al., 1967; Schneider et al., 1970). The work of Johnson and his colleagues (1967) is particularly interesting since these authors showed Actinomycin D to be of value as an adjunct in all case-groups classified by age and tumour stage.

The clinical trials already set up in England and the United States will, no doubt, lead to the correct evaluation of Actinomycin D. In the meantime, the present authors recommend the administration of intermittent courses of Actinomycin D post-operatively for one to two years in all cases not committed to clinical trials, except those less than 18 months of age, in whom complete tumour removal appears to have been accomplished.

β) Metastases

Distant metastases from nephroblastoma, especially in the lung, respond well to either Actinomycin D or to irradiation. Better results appear to be achieved when both modalities are employed. In recent years some of the gloom surrounding advanced cases has been lifted. Following bilateral whole lung irradiation for pulmonary metastases. Pearson et al. (1964) report a three-year survival rate of 14% among 35 patients. Farber (1966) obtained a two-year survival rate of 58% for 31 cases in whom metastases were present at or after diagnosis and who were treated by a combination of irradiation and Actinomycin D. This combined treatment achieved a two-year survival rate of 30% in the series reported by Koop (1970) and a three-year survival rate of 35% in 18 cases studied by Burgert and Mills (1967).

In cases with pulmonary metastases we irradiate the whole chest shielding the humeral heads and the larynx, to a dose of 1500 R over three to four weeks. Additional local treatment may be given for residual disease to bring the maximum dose to 2 500–3 000 R, depending upon the treated volume. We prefer to delay the administration of Actinomycin D until irradiation has been completed and the blood count has returned to normal. Intermittent courses of this agent (15 µg per kilo per day for five days) are given every two months for one to two years.

Vincristine Sulphate is another highly active agent against nephroblastoma which may prove to be equally or even more effective than Actinomycin D. Complete regression of metastases was observed in 16 of 22 children treated with vincristine combined with irradiation: ten of the 22 (45%) were alive and well at two years (VIETTI *et al.*, 1970).

Though many authors report cure rates of 60–80% for nephroblastoma, the results in some centres are far less satisfactory, falling between 30 and 50%. Encouraging survival rates often relate to special case-groups, whereas the overall picture for a particular centre or geographical region may be gloomy. Thus, BAERT *et al.* (1966) report a three-year survival rate of 67% for 23 cases treated by nephrectomy and postoperative irradiation, compared with only 20% for their entire series of 54 cases. Most hospitals see but few cases, and the experience of any one surgeon must be even more limited. The organisation for the treatment of nephroblastoma (as well as for other solid tumours in children) on a regional basis supported by Federal funds is long overdue. Such an arrangement would lead to the more efficient management of this uncommon tumour and bring together sufficient cases with which to explore more effective lines of treatment, particularly through randomised trials.

The value of hyperbaric oxygen should be explored for cases of nephroblastoma undergoing whole lung irradiation for pulmonary metastases. The increased tissue oxygen tension may render such metastases more susceptible to the limited dose of irradiation without additional risk to the normal pulmonary tissue.

3. Bladder

a) Aetiology

An association between smoking and bladder cancer has been reported from many countries. The mortality from this disease appears to be linked with the number of cigarettes smoked (FRAUMENI, 1968). The absence of a strict control group makes the epidemiological interpretation difficult, but non-smokers form a very small percentage of patients with bladder tumours. KERR (1970) believes that smoking may increase the concentration of ortho-aminophenols in the urine. SCHLEGEL *et al.* (1970) has suggested that a deficiency of ascorbic acid, more common in smokers, may influence the biochemical change at the mucosal-urine interface. Prognosis and recurrence in patients with bladder tumours may be both affected by smoking (ANTHONY and THOMAS, 1970).

b) The TNM staging of the International Union against Cancer (1963)

Although this is a system of clinical staging, information concerning depth of tumour invasion in the biopsy report may be used to modify the clinical assessment. Neither histological grade nor lymphatic involvement, however, influences stage.

The TNM system may be used for pathological staging of operative specimens, the depth of tumour invasion being indicated by the same numerals, but preceded by the letter 'P' rather than by 'T'. It is not possible to assess the condition of the regional nodes in the pelvis by clinical examination but, when the patient has been subjected to laparotomy, nodes can be removed for histological examination. Such information can be recorded in the 'P' classification.

I.S. In-situ, non-invasive stage: Any tumour that has not broken through the basement membrane into the suburothelial layers is included in this stage. The difference between a histological papilloma (X) or a non-invasive carcinoma (IS) depends largely on the pathological interpretation.

T1 Sub-urothelial stage: There is definite evidence in the biopsy specimen of invasion into connective tissue. Cases in this stage can be sub-divided into those where the invasion is into the tumour stroma only, and those where the sub-urothelial connective tissue of the bladder wall is invaded. These tumours may be palpable, but they are soft and freely mobile within the bladder cavity.

T2 Superficial muscle stage: There is invasion of superficial muscle in the biopsy specimen. These tumours are more rubbery to palpation; there may be a localised thickening of the bladder wall, but there should be no nodularity or hardness.

T3 Deep muscle and perivesical stage: The biopsy shows invasion deep into the muscle layer. Because deep biopsies are exceptional and because the thickness of the bladder wall varies between patients, and at different degrees of distention, the biopsy here is less reliable than the bimanual examination. This examination reveals a hard nodular but freely mobile mass. (In pathological staging some workers are drawing a distinction between deep muscle and perivesical spread.)

T4 Fixation stage: The tumour is fixed to the pelvic wall or to scar or it involves the rectum, vagina, or prostate. (A distinction is now being made by some pathologists between tumour invading the prostate where the prognosis is bad, and in-situ changes in the prostatic ducts where the prognosis is good.)

It is still necessary to make a general plea for treatment results to be presented in a manner which permits comparison between different centres. There has been increasing use of the UICC staging system, and it is hoped that this trend will continue.

c) Investigations

The role of lymphography in bladder cancer is being studied by Higgs and Mac-Donald (1968) who consider this examination to be of value in determining treatment policy, in radiotherapy planning, and in judging radio-responsiveness from serial x-ray films.

Interest has been shown in the possible relationship between tumour cytogenetic factors and histological grade, invasive properties and prognosis in urothelial tumours (Tavares et al., 1966; Lamb, 1967). So far, no correlation between ploidy and radio-sensitivity of bladder tumours has been demonstrated. By means of hamster cheek pouch studies (Kaufman et al., 1969) and perhaps organ tissue culture techniques (Tchao et al., 1968), it may be possible to assess the likely sensitivity of bladder tumours from individual patients to irradiation, cytotoxic drugs, or to a combination of agents.

Therapeutic failure in carcinoma of the bladder is usually due to inability to control the local disease, but as survival rates are increasing so it has become evident that failure may also be due to the development of new primary urothelial tumours in the bladder, lower ureter or urethra. Premature death may also occur from urinary sepsis resulting from ureteric diversion or from reflux and not from cancer itself.

d) Treatment
α) Intracavitary

Interest in the intracavitary treatment of multiple small superficial tumours has been transferred from liquid radio-isotopes to cytotoxic chemicals such as thiotepa (Gibson, 1969; Veenema et al., 1969) and epodyl (Abassian and Wallace, 1966). The latter agent, due to its heavy molecular weight, is less readily absorbed into the circulation and is, therefore, safer to use than thiotepa, following which a number of deaths from marrow failure have been reported. Evidence of ureteric, urethral or prostatic duct involvement is a contra-indication to intracavitary techniques.

Attempts to prevent the development of new superficial tumours with 1–4 gluco-saccharolactone on the basis of a randomised trial have not proved successful (Boyland et al., 1964).

β) Interstitial

The use of low energy caesium 131 seeds (HENSCHKE and LAWRENCE, 1965) and the modifications to the Royal Marsden Hospital gold grain gun to permit more rapid and safer loading (JONES *et al.*, 1965) will lead to greater radiation protection during interstitial techniques.

In the case of superficial bladder tumours, it is difficult to compare results of transurethral diathermy with those of open interstitial irradiation because of the undoubted selection of the more favourable lesions for the transurethral approach. In our experience both methods give comparable results for well-differentiated tumours confined to mucosa or to the superficial muscle layers (Stages TIS, T1 and T2), whereas superficial tumours of high grade malignancy, especially with early muscle invasion, are best treated by interstitial irradiation. The inadequacy of transurethral diathermy alone for undifferentiated lesions is evident in the recent report by MILLER *et al.* (1969): 37% of such cases died with tumour extension within five years, compared with only 2% of patients with differentiated tumours treated by the same technique.

γ) External beam therapy

Though some radiotherapy centres have reported three year survival rates for deeply infiltrating tumours of between 30 and 40% (CRIGLER *et al.*, 1966; EDSMYR *et al.*, 1967; CALDWELL *et al.*, 1967; POINTON and EVANS, 1969), and these undoubtedly constitute more than a challenge for radical cystectomy, results for this tumour are more often in the range of 10–20% and have been equally poor for surgery (WERF-MESSING, 1965; KUROHARA *et al.*, 1965; MACKENZIE *et al.*, 1965; RAVASINI, 1966). Our three-year survival rate for 140 unselected cases with deeply infiltrating tumours (Stage T3) treated by orthovoltage or 1 MeV X-rays (prior to the opening of our new megavoltage department) was 20%.

Bearing in mind the extent to which cases are selected for radical operation and the unfavourable condition of many patients referred for radiotherapy, the results of megavoltage irradiation may, in fact, be superior to those of surgery.

In a recently reported controlled trial from the Christie Hospital (POINTON and EVANS, 1969) cases of bladder cancer were carefully selected for radical radiotherapy so that they also appeared suitable for major surgery. The crude five-year survival rate for 81 patients with tumours clinically invading the peri-vesical tissue and treated with 4 MeV X-rays was 27%, whereas only 11% of cases with similar stage tumours treated by radical surgery at the Memorial Hospital (WHITMORE and MARSHALL, 1962) survived this time. When only new cases were considered, including some with less advanced tumours invading deep muscle but not the perivesical tissue, the survival rate following primary radical cystectomy was still limited to 20% (WHITMORE *et al.*, 1968).

The wide range in results reported for deeply infiltrating tumours following external beam therapy is probably due more to case-selection, or to differences or errors in clinical staging, than to specific techniques and skills. Inconsistencies in treatment results by clinical stage are evident in several reported series (EDSMYR *et al.*, 1967; DONKER, 1967; POINTON and EVANS, 1969).

The maximum tumour dose used most frequently for bladder cancer is 6000–6500 R over five to seven weeks. Though this is close to normal tissue tolerance, not more than 50% of cases will show complete tumour regression within three months following treatment. LAING and DICKINSON (1965) and JOMAIN (1966) have shown that tumour doses exceeding 6500 R in six weeks do not appear to improve results and are associated with substantially more severe acute reactions and late complications.

e) Complications

The potential hazards associated with pelvic megavoltage irradiation for bladder cancer have now been more accurately defined. The incidence of major complications ranges between 5 and 20%, and is generally between 5% and 8%, consisting chiefly of contracted bladder, vesical haemorrhage and bowel stenosis or perforation. Such complications occur more frequently with high-dose, short-time schedules, especially when there is a history of pelvic surgery, repeated diathermy or infection.

Vesico-ureteric reflux has been described by Edsmyr and Nilson (1965) as a possible sequel to beam therapy, and it has been observed in our clinic following interstitial techniques. The chief cause of the valvular dysfunction appears to be tumour itself in the region of a ureteric orifice. Reflux of sterile urine is probably harmless, but recurrent infection in patients with this complication may lead to chronic pyelonephritis and renal failure. This is undoubtedly responsible for death in some patients otherwise cured of bladder cancer. Special care, including a micturating cystogram and excretory pyelogram, is therefore necessary in the follow-up of patients treated for periureteric tumours if lives are not to be needlessly lost. Meatotomy and re-implantation of the ureter may be required.

f) Pre-operative irradiation

From many animal experiments supported by preliminary clinical observations, it appears that the concept of pre-operative irradiation represents the most promising contribution made in recent years to the treatment of cancer (Herbst et al., 1966; Nickson and Glicksman, 1966; Cady, 1968; Powers and Palmer, 1968).

Because of the generally poor results for deeply infiltrating bladder cancer following radical radiotherapy or surgery, the idea arose of employing both modalities as a planned combined treatment. Wizenberg and his colleagues (1966) introduced a scheme of total cystectomy one to three months after 6000 R in five to six weeks, but at this dose level the operative mortality was 22%.

Limited pre-operative irradiation (i.e. 4000 R in 4–6 weeks) with radical cystectomy one to three months later has been practised at the Memorial Hospital since 1959. Post-operative complications and deaths were no greater than following surgery alone. Early reports gave hope of improvement in the three-year results for deeply infiltrating tumours compared with radical surgery or radical radiotherapy alone (MacKenzie et al., 1965). In a more recent analysis of this material (Whitmore et al., 1968), however, any advantage of the combined approach was seen only when cases were classified by subsequent pathological stage. These results are, nevertheless, encouraging, especially as they concern cases with no "down-staging" following the pre-operative irradiation.

During the last few years controlled clinical trials have been set up to evaluate the merits of various treatments. Special interest is being focused on pre-operative irradiation followed by cystectomy, compared with surgery alone, or radical radiotherapy alone. The clinical material in these trials is good, because the patients have not been subjected to previous surgery, renal function is preserved and the patients are fit for radical treatment whether by surgery or irradiation. Results from such studies will, therefore, be expected to reflect the best that can be achieved by the various methods of treatment.

Though it is too early to consider results, certain facts are emerging. The operative mortality for radical cystectomy following planned pre-operative irradiation is extremely low, and there is certainly no appreciable increase in major complications, providing that the irradiation does not exceed 4000 R in 4 weeks, and the operation is performed within 4–8 weeks of completing radiotherapy. With this programme some 20% of patients show no tumour, or only *in-situ* changes in the subsequent surgical specimen. In a study at the Royal Marsden Hospital, the incidence of positive nodes following whole pelvic pre-operative irradiation to 4000 R in 4 weeks has been only 14%, compared with at least 40% reported for purely surgical cases (Bloom, 1970).

In some cancer studies the dose of pre-operative irradiation has been limited to about 2000 R delivered over a few days, and followed immediately by radical operation. Schlienger and Dutreix (1968) have been using two fractions, each of 870 R, separated by 48 hours, with operation three to four days later. If this type of brief pre-operative treatment proves to be as effective as more prolonged courses, then the lengthy incapacity associated with some current combined treatment programmes could be easily reduced (e.g. from 12–5 weeks).

Recent results reported by WERF-MESSING (1969) support the value of pre-operative, low dose, external beam irradiation in patients with infiltrating bladder tumours treated primarily by radium implant: a total dose of 1050 R to the pelvis over three consecutive days immediately prior to operation resulted in total eradication of scar recurrences, fewer distant metastases and superior survival rates.

g) Post-operative irradiation

Planned post-operation radical radiotherapy following partial cystectomy appears to be of particular value in cases of deeply infiltrating, poorly differentiated tumours. In a retrospective study at the Royal Marsden Hospital the five-year survival rate for this type of lesion was substantially improved by the combined treatment (26% of 41 cases), compared with operation alone (8% of 35 cases).

h) Apparatus

The general introduction of megavoltage equipment is usually considered responsible for the improved results in bladder cancer reported from a number of centres during the past decade. An equally and perhaps more important factor is the care with which cases have been selected for treatment by better trained radiotherapists working in closer collaboration with urologists. Comparable results were obtained for bladder cancer treated by orthovoltage (400 kV) and megavoltage (4 MeV) X-irradiation in a controlled trial reported by POINTON and EVANS (1969). Megavoltage treatment, however, being simpler and less wearing for the patient, has displaced conventional X-ray therapy for this disease.

In a few centres, betatrons, producing X-rays in the 20–30 MeV range, have been used for bladder cancer. Only a prospective randomised trial will indicate whether this type of equipment can produce significantly better results, especially in more advanced lesions requiring large volume irradiation, than telecobalt and 4–6 MeV X-ray machines.

i) Oxygen

The results of treating patients with cancer of the bladder by irradiation in oxygen have proved disappointing, and do not reflect the promise of the convincing experimental data. CADE and McEWAN (1967), in a controlled trial, compared orthodox fractionated cobalt irradiation in hyperbaric oxygen and in air, and found that survival was shorter and distant metastases more frequent in the oxygen series. RIDER et al. (1970), also in a randomised trial, found no difference in the crude survival rate of 75 patients treated in orthobaric oxygen and 75 treated in air.

j) 5-Flurouracil

So far, no cytotoxic agent is of proven value in the treatment of infiltrating tumours of the bladder. Citral, reported by MORROW (1960), did not improve prognosis nor palliate symptoms in advanced cases. STEIN and KAUFMAN (1968) have claimed that pre-operative irradiation to 3500 R combined with 5-Flurouracil produced a greater incidence of bladder cancer regression than was anticipated from either agent alone. Practically 50% of 32 cases with muscle infiltrating lesions were rendered tumour-free, which is considerably greater than that expected from sub-radical doses of irradiation alone. 5-Flurouracil combined with irradiation appears to enhance the regression rate of various tumours, either by synergistic or by additive action, but a greater permanent local control rate and a substantial increase in patient-survival have yet to be demonstrated.

k) Palliation

Palliative treatment, generally by external beam irradiation, is indicated for tumours fixed to the pelvic walls. In such circumstances, the aim is to achieve maximum relief in the shortest possible time. Optimum dose-time-volume factors are still being explored (Schlienger and Dutreix, 1968; Vargha et al., 1969).

Uretero-colic anastomosis as a palliative measure is now rarely employed because of the risk of double incontinence of urine and faeces in terminal patients. Tractotomy or phenol nerve block for root pain may also render a patient with a uretero-colic diversion completely incontinent. When a urinary diversion is indicated an ileal conduit or a skin-ureterostomy with a nipple have considerable advantage over the intestinal diversion.

The co-operative approach to treatment by urologist, radiotherapist, and chemotherapist, often working together in joint clinics, and the increasing acceptance of randomised trials, represent two of the most significant advances in recent years towards the more effective control of urological cancer.

4. Current supervoltage treatment plans

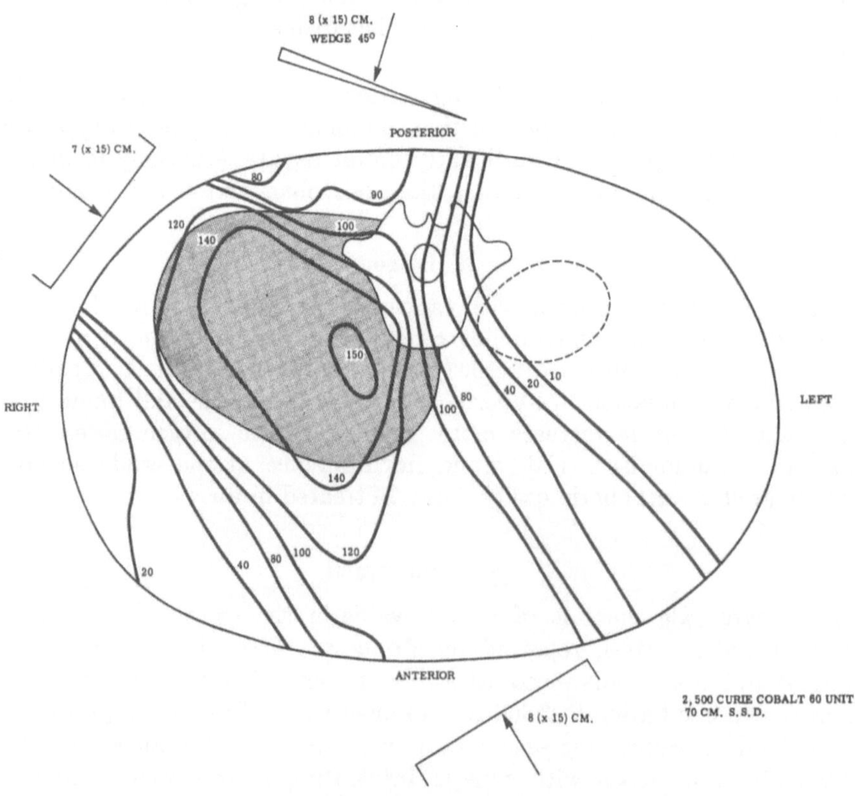

Fig. 48. Plan I. 3000 Curie Cobalt-60 Unit: post-operative irradiation for carcinoma of the kidney; 5000 R at 140% isodose line in 6 weeks

The following figures are complete print-out plans by Digital Equipment PDP 8/1 Computor System developed at the Royal Marsden Hospital and Institute of Cancer Research by Dr. R. E. BENTLEY *and* Mr. J. MILAN.

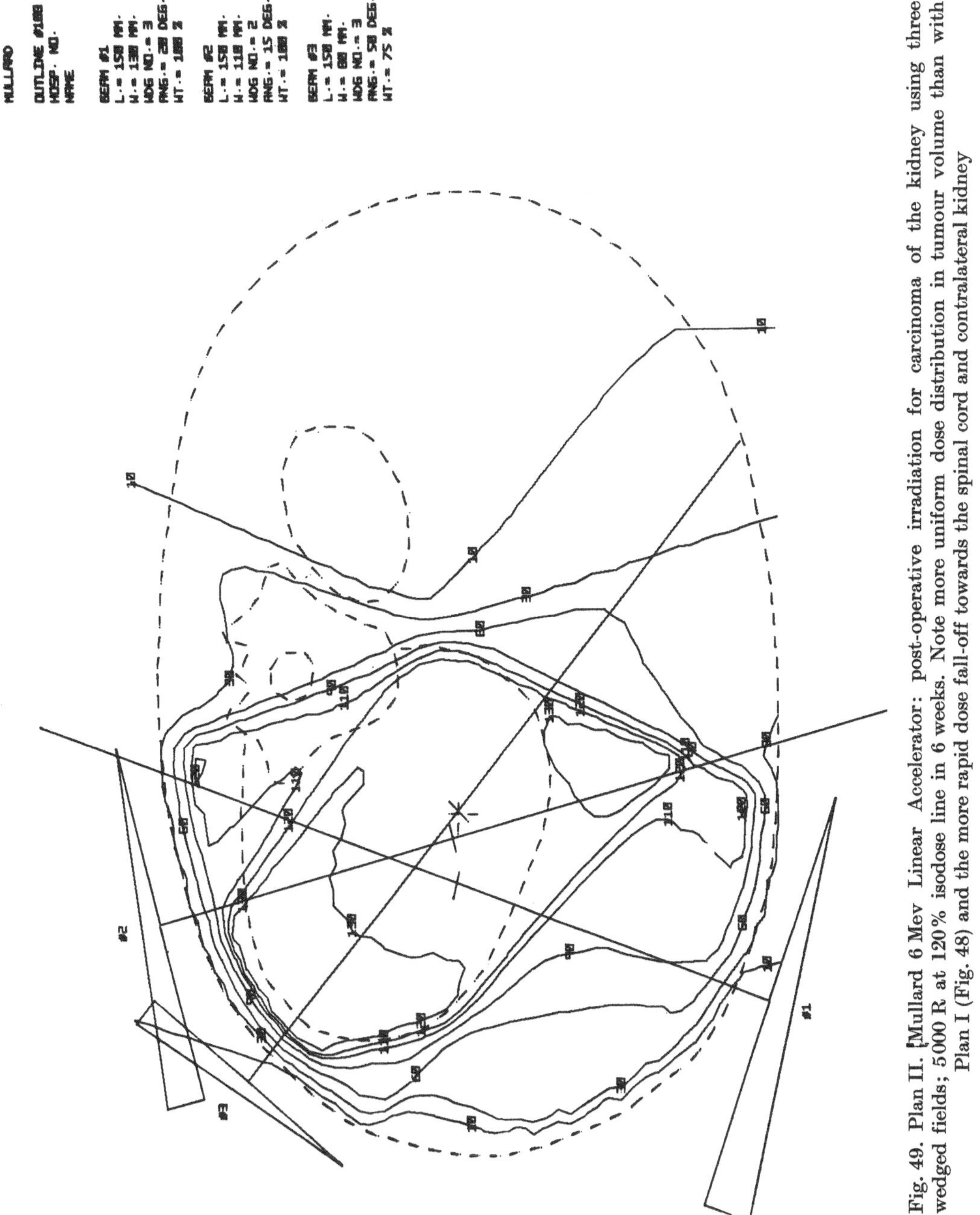

Fig. 49. Plan II. [Mullard 6 Mev Linear Accelerator: post-operative irradiation for carcinoma of the kidney using three wedged fields; 5000 R at 120% isodose line in 6 weeks. Note more uniform dose distribution in tumour volume than with Plan I (Fig. 48) and the more rapid dose fall-off towards the spinal cord and contralateral kidney

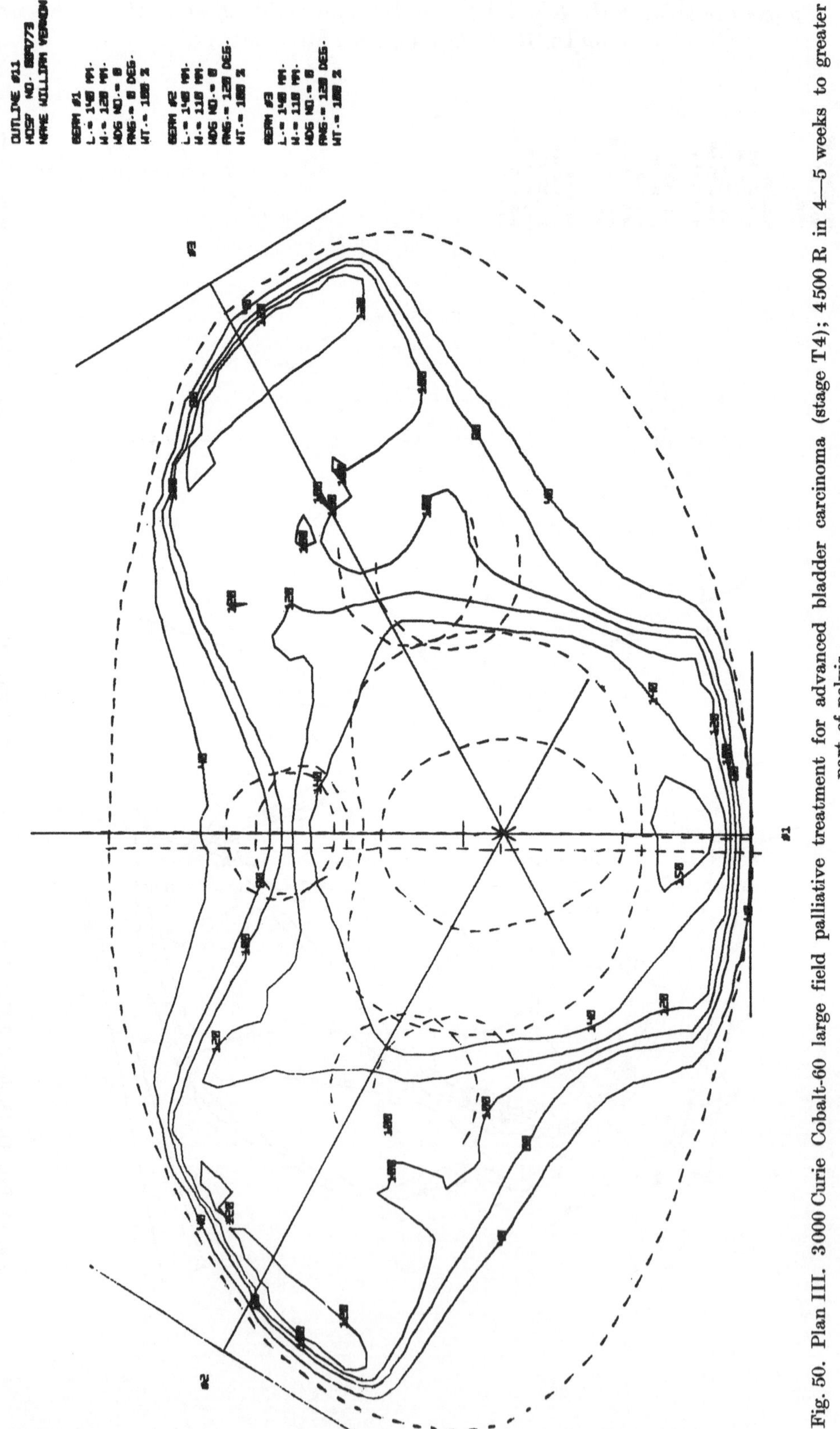

Fig. 50. Plan III. 3000 Curie Cobalt-60 large field palliative treatment for advanced bladder carcinoma (stage T4); 4500 R in 4—5 weeks to greater part of pelvis

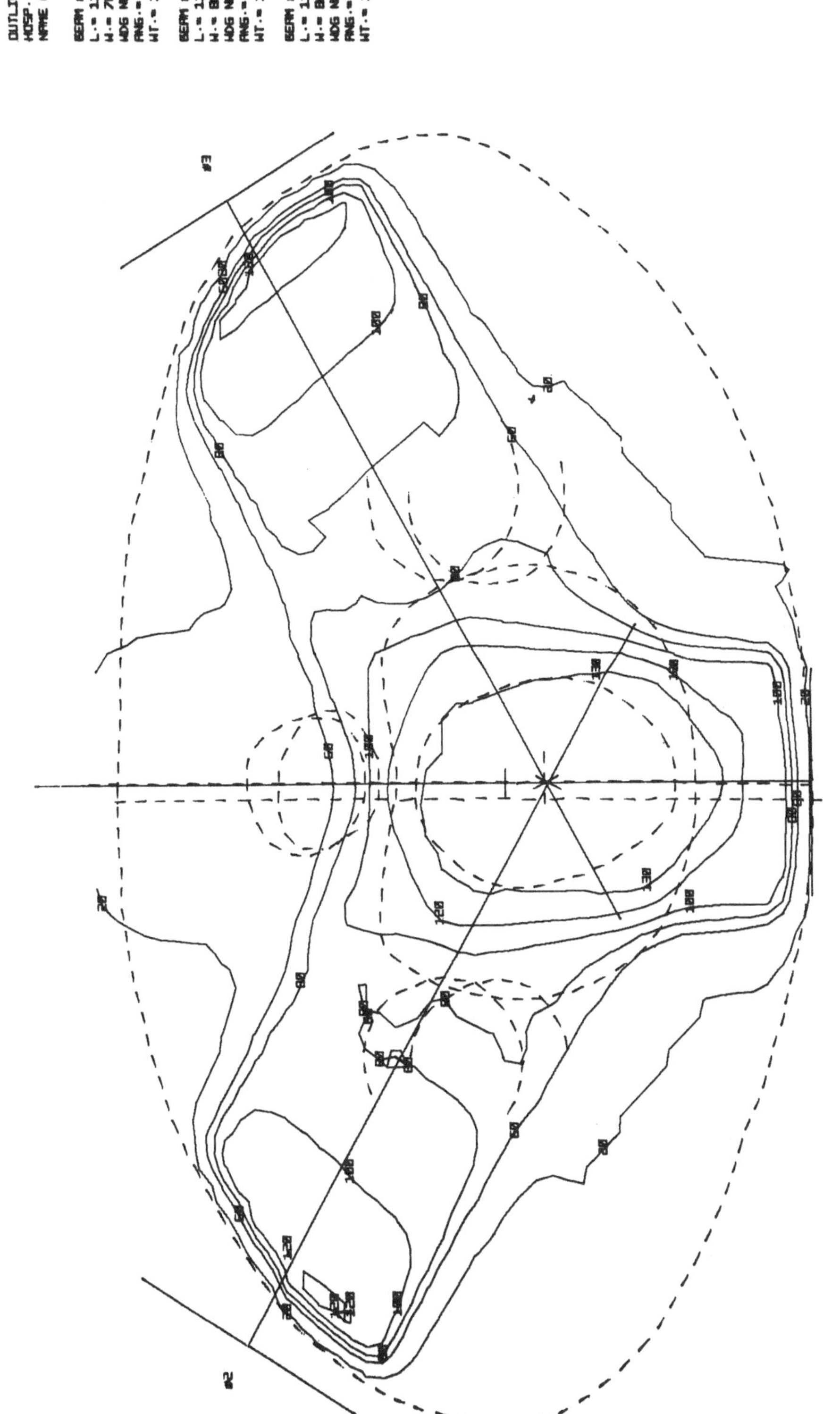

Fig. 51. Plan IV. 3000 Curie Cobalt-60 small field radical treatment for limited infiltrating bladder carcinoma (stage T2, too large for interstitial therapy); 6000 R in 6 weeks to whole bladder: dose to pelvic side walls limited to 3700 R

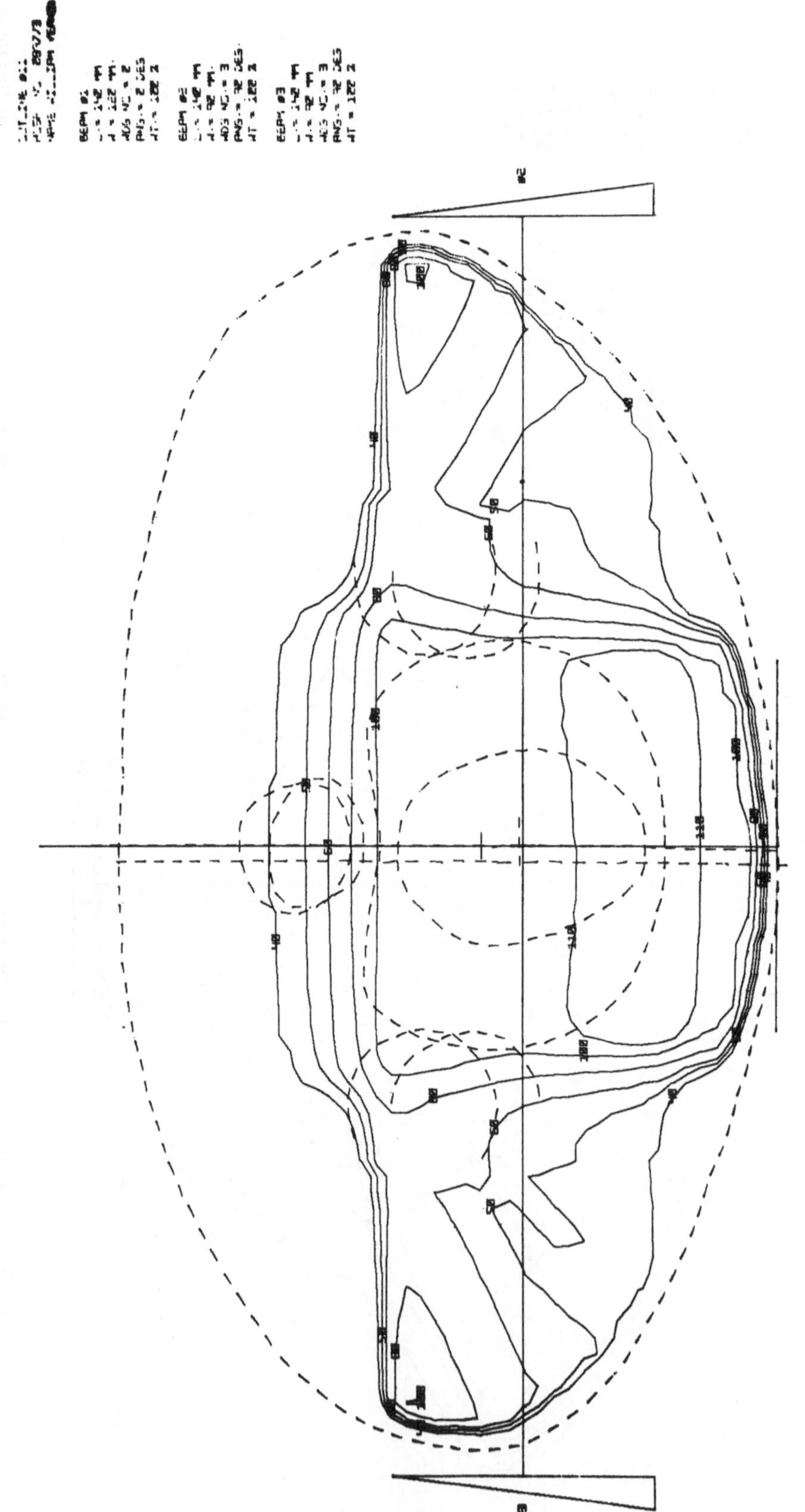

Fig. 52. Plan V. 3000 Curie Cobalt-60 "box" treatment given pre-operatively for deeply infiltrating mobile bladder carcinoma (stage T3): 4000 R in 4 weeks to greater part of pelvis. Radical cystectomy after interval of 4 weeks. This plan may also be use as the first phase of radical radiotherapy when treatment is entirely by irradiation: the second phase consists of administering an additional 2000 R in 2 weeks to the bladder with Plan IV (Fig. 51)

References

Tumours of the renal parenchyma

ABESHOUSE, B. S.: The management of Wilms' tumour as determined by national survey and review of the literature. J. Urol. (Baltimore) 77, 792–813 (1957).

ANNAMUNTHODO, H., HUTCHINGS, R. F.: Nephroblastoma (Wilms' tumour): Case report. J. Urol. (Baltimore) 78, 197–204 (1957).

ARCOMANO, J. P., BARNETT, J. C., BOTTONE, J. J.: Spontaneous disappearance of pulmonary metastases following nephrectomy for hypernephroma. Amer. J. Surg. 96, 703–704 (1958).

BADENOCH, A. W.: Tumours of the kidney. Ann. roy. Coll. Surg. Engl. 16, 163–174 (1955).

BARNEY, J. D.: A twelve year cure following nephrectomy for adenocarcinoma and lobectomy for solitary metastasis. J. Urol. (Baltimore) 52, 406–407 (1944).

BASSOW, S. H.: Exfoliative cytology as an aid in the diagnosis of early renal carcinoma. J. Urol. (Baltimore) 76, 47–52 (1956).

BASTABLE, J. R. G.: Bilateral carcinoma of the kidneys. Brit. J. Urol. 32, 60–68 (1960).

BAUER, F. C., MURRAY, D. E., HIRSCH, E. F.: Solitary adenoma of the kidney. J. Urol. (Baltimore) 79, 377–382 (1958).

BECK, J. S.: Acute radiation nephritis in childhood. Brit. med. J. 1958 II, 489–490.

BEER, E.: Some aspects of malignant tumours of the kidney. Surg. Gynec. Obstet. 65, 433–446 (1937).

BELL, E. T.: Diseases of the kidney. London: Kimpton 1947.

BERGER, L., SINKOFF, M.: Systemic manifestations of hypernephroma: review of 273 cases. Amer. J. Med. 22, 791–796 (1957).

BIXLER, L. C., STENSTROM, K. W., CREEVY, C. D.: Malignant tumours of the kidney: Review of 117 cases. Radiology 42, 329–345 (1944).

BLEYER, L. F.: Clinical-pathological review of tumours of urinary tract with relationship to age and sex incidence and functional disturbance. Urol. cutan. Rev. 48, 516–522 (1944).

BLOOM, H. J. G.: Prognosis in carcinoma of the breast. Brit. J. Cancer 4, 259–288 (1950).

— RICHARDSON, W. W.: Histological grading and prognosis in breast cancer: A study of 1409 cases of which 359 have been followed for 15 years. Brit. J. Cancer 11, 359–377 (1957).

BOBBITT, R. M., HARWOOD, I. R., PECK, F. M.: Behaviour of certain metastatic malignant diseases arising in the urinary tract. J. Urol. (Baltimore) 81, 629–632 (1959).

BODIAN, M.: The management of neuroblastoma with vitamin B12. Seminar, University of Texas Medical Branch, Galveston, September 23rd, 1957.

BÖTTIGER, L. E.: Fever of unknown origin. IV. Fever in carcinoma of the kidney. Acta med. scand. 156, 477–485 (1957).

— IVEMARK, B. I.: The structure of renal carcinoma correlated to its clinical behaviour. J. Urol. (Baltimore) 81, 512–514 (1959).

BOHNE, A. W., ACKLES, R. C., DREW, D. R., URWILLER, K. L.: Needle biopsy of the kidney. J. Urol. (Baltimore) 79, 393–396 (1958).

BRAASCH, W. F., GRIFFIN, M.: Prognosis in renal carcinoma and clinical and pathological data affecting it. J. Amer. med. Ass. 106, 1343–1346 (1936).

BROGAN, R. E.: Successful nephrectomy in 3 day old infant. Lancet 67, 274–277 (1947).

BUMPUS, H. C.: Apparent disappearance of pulmonary metastases in case of hypernephroma following nephrectomy. J. Urol. (Baltimore) 20, 185–191 (1928).

CAHILL, G. F., MELICOW, M. M.: Calcification of renal tumours and its relation to prognosis. J. Urol. (Baltimore) 39, 276–286 (1938).

CAMPBELL, M. F.: Clinical pediatric urology. Philadelphia: Saunders & Co. 1951.

CARLSON, H. E., OCKERBLAD, N. F.: A case of unoperated hypernephroma of ten years duration. Amer. J. Roentgenol. 45, 221–222 (1941).

CHILDS, P., WATERFALL, W. B.: Renal adenoma: A review with a report of two further cases. Brit. J. Urol. 25, 187–194 (1953).

CHUTE, R., IRELAND, E. F., HOUGHTON, J. D.: Solitary distant metastases from unsuspected renal carcinomas. J. Urol. 80, 420–424 (1958).

CLAY, J.: Developmental mixed tumour of kidney in a patient aged 80. Brit. med. J. 1930 II, 1083.

CLINTON-THOMAS, C. L., ROBINSON, T. M.: Adenocarcinoma kidney in childhood. Report of a case and review of literature. Brit. J. Urol. 28, 132–136 (1956).

CONLEY, C. L., KOWAL, J., D'ANTONIO, J.: Polycythaemia associated with renal tumours. Bull. Johns Hopk. Hosp. 101, 63–73 (1957).

CRISTOL, D. S., McDONALD, J. R., EMMETT, J. L.: Renal adenoma in hypernephromatous kidneys: Study of their incidence, nature and relationship. J. Urol. (Baltimore) 55, 18–27 (1946).

CRITCHLEY, M., EARL, C. J. C.: Tuberose sclerosis and allied conditions. Brain 55, 311–346 (1932).

CULP, O. S., HARTMAN, F. W.: Mesoblastic nephroma in adults: clinico-pathologic study of Wilms' tumours and related renal neoplasm. J. Urol. (Baltimore) 60, 552–576 (1948).

DEAN, A. L.: Radiation treatment of more common kidney tumours. Amer. J. Surg. 38, 80–84 (1937).

— Wilms' tumours. N.Y. St. J. Med. 45, 1213–1217 (1945).

DeWEERD, J. H., HAGEDORN, A. B.: Hypernephroma associated with polycythaemia. J. Urol. (Baltimore) 82, 29–36 (1959).

DEVAS, M. B., DICKSON, J. W., JELLIFFE, A. M.: Pathological fractures. Treatment by internal fixation and irradiation. Lancet 484–487, 1956 II.

DICK, U. S., FLINT, L. D.: The prognosis of renal tumours. Surg. Clin. N. Amer. 31, 633–643 (1951).

EBERTH, C. J.: Myoma sarcomatodes renum. Virchows Arch. path. Anat. 55, 518–520 (1872).

FALKINBERG, L. R. W., KAY, M. N., SAYER, E. A.: Recurrence of nephroblastoma (Wilms' tumour) 8 years after nephrectomy. J. Amer. med. Ass. 155, 1228–1229 (1954).

FARBER, S., TOCH, R., SEARS, E. M., PINKEL, D.: Advances in chemotherapy of cancer in man. in Advances in cancer research, vol. 4, ed. GREENSTEIN, J. P. and HADDOW, A., N. YORK: Academic Press 1956.

FEENEY, M. J., MULLENIX, R. B., PRENTISS, R. J., WHISENAND, J. M.: Clinical experience with Wilms' tumour. J. Urol. (Baltimore) 74, 301–311 (1955).

FELDMAN, W. H.: Neoplasms of domesticated animals Philadelphia: Saunders & Co. 1932.

FITZGERALD, W. L., HARDIN, H. C.: Bilateral Wilms' tumour in Wilms' tumour family: case report. J. Urol. (Baltimore) 73, 468–474 (1955).

FLOCKS, R. H., KADESKY, M. C.: Malignant neoplasms of the kidney: An analysis of 353 patients followed five years or more. Trans. Amer. Ass. gen.-urin. Surg. 49, 105–110 (1957).

FOOT, N. C., HUMPHREYS, G. A., WHITMORE, W. F.: Importance of accurate pathological classification in prognosis of renal tumours: second report. J. Urol. (Baltimore) 61, 477–487 (1949).

FRAENKEL, G. J.: Renal infarct as space-occupying lesion. Brit. J. Urol. (Baltimore) 28, 145–146 (1956).

GAIRDNER, E.: Case of fungus haematodes in kidneys. Edinb. med. Surg. J. 29, 312–315 (1828).

GAULIN, E.: Simultaneous Wilms' tumours in identical twins. J. Urol. (Baltimore) 66, 547–550 (1951).

GOLDSTEIN, A. E.: Longevity following nephrectomy. J. Urol. (Baltimore) 76, 31–41 (1956).

GRAHAM, R. M.: The cytologic diagnosis of cancer. Philadelphia: Saunders & Co. 1950.

GRIFFITHS, I. H., THACKRAY, A. C.: Parenchymal carcinoma of the kidney. Brit. J. Urol. 21, 128–151 (1949).

GROSS, R. E.: Surgery of infancy and childhood: its principles and techniques. Philadelphia: Saunders & Co. 1953.

— NEUHAUSER, E. B. D.: Treatment of mixed tumours of kidney in children. Pediatrics 6, 843–852 (1950).

HAND, J. R., BRODERS, A. C.: Carcinoma of the kidney: the degree of malignancy in relation to factors bearing on prognosis. J. Urol. (Baltimore) 38, 199–216 (1932).

HANLEY, H. G.: Bilateral renal carcinoma. Brit. J. Surg. 32, 399–402 (1945).

HARRISON, F. G., WARRES, H. L., FUST, J. A.: Neuroblastoma involving the urinary tract. J. Urol. (Baltimore) 63, 598–612 (1950).

HARRISON, J. H., BOTSFORD, T. W., TUCKER, M. R.: Use of the smear of the urinary sediment in the diagnosis and management of neoplasms of the kidney and bladder. Surg. Gynec. Obstet. 92, 129–139 (1951).

HARVEY, R. M.: Wilms' tumour: Evaluation of treatment methods. Radiology 54, 689–696 (1950).

HEMPSTEAD, R. H., DOCKERTY, M. B., PRIESTLEY, J. T., LOGAN, G. B.: Hypernephroma in children: report of two cases. J. Urol. (Baltimore) 70, 152–158 (1953).

HILLENBRAND, H. J., HÖRSTEBROCK, R.: Doppelseitige Nierenkurginome. Z. Urol. 50, 396–401 (1957).

HOGAN, J. F., SIMONS, C. E.: Renal cell adenocarcinoma in a five year old girl with a reduplicated collecting system and ectopic ureter opening into urethra. J. Urol. (Baltimore) 78, 212–215 (1957).

HOLLAHAN, J. D.: Spontaneous remission of metastatic renal cell adenocarcinome. Case report. J. Urol. (Baltimore) 81, 522–525 (1959).

HORNING, E. S., WHITTICK, J. W.: The histogenesis of stilboestrol-induced renal tumours in the male golden hamster. Brit. J. Cancer 8, 451–457 (1954).

HUMPHREYS, G. A., FOOT, N. C.: Survival of patients following nephrectomy for renal cell and transitional cell tumours of the kidney. J. Urol. (Baltimore) 83, 815–819 (1960).

HYMAN, A.: Clinical study of malignant tumours of the kidney. Surg. Clin. N. Amer. 13, 347–364 (1933).

JACOBSON, L. O., GOLDWASSER, E., FRIED, W., PLZAK, L.: Role of the kidney in erythropoiesis. Nature (Lond.) 179, 633–634 (1951).

JENKINS, G. D.: Regression of pulmonary metastasis following nephrectomy for hypernephroma: eight year follow-up. J. Urol. (Baltimore) 82, 37–40 (1959).

JOHNSON, S. H., MARSHALL, M.: Kidney tumours in childhood. J. Urol. (Baltimore) 74, 707–720 (1955).

KERR, H. D.: Treatment of malignant tumours of kidney in children. J. Amer. med. Ass. 112, 408–411 (1939).

— FLYNN, R. E.: The role of irradiation in the treatment of Wilms' tumour in children. Amer. J. Roentgenol. 75, 971–976 (1956).

KIRKMAN, H., BACON, R. L.: Renal adenomas and carcinomas in diethyl-stilboestrol treated male golden hamsters. Anat. Rev. 103, 59–60 (1949).

KLAPPROTH, H. J.: Wilms' tumour: A report of 45 cases and an analysis of 1,351 cases reported in the world literature from 1940 to 1958. J. Urol. (Baltimore) 81, 633–648 (1959).

KNOX, W. E., PILLERS, E. M. K.: Time of recurrence or cure of tumours in childhood. Lancet 1958 I, 188–191.

KRETSCHMER, H. L.: Adenomyosacroma of kidney (Wilms' tumour); report of three cases. Arch. Surg. 41, 370–384 (1940).

KUEHN, C. A., DAVIS, P.: Carcinoma of renal parenchyma: long term survival: report of a case and 5 year review of literature. J. Urol. (Baltimore) 81, 519–521 (1959).

LADD, W. E., WHITE, R. R.: Embryoma of kidney (Wilms' tumour). J. Amer. med. Ass. 117, 1858–1863 (1941).

LATTIMER, J. K., MELICOW, M. M., USON, A. C.: Wilms' tumour: a report of 71 cases. J. Urol. (Baltimore) 80, 401–416 (1958).

LIVERMORE, G. R.: Wilms' tumour in adult: report of 10-year cure. J. Urol. (Baltimore) 70, 141–145 (1953).

LOWSLEY, O. S.: Malignant cyst of the kidney. J. Urol. (Baltimore) 74, 586–590 (1955).

LUXTON, R. W.: Radiation nephritis. Quart. J. Med. 22, 215–242 (1953).

MANN, L. T.: Spontaneous disapearance of pulmonary metastases after nephrectomy for hypernephroma. Four-year follow-up. J. Urol. (Baltimore) 59, 564–566 (1948).

McDonald, J. R., Priestley, J. T.: Malignant tumours of the kidney. Surg. Gynec. Obstet. **77**, 295–306 (1943).

Melicow, M. M., Uson, A. C.: Palpable abdominal masses in infants and children: Report based on review of 653 cases. J. Urol. (Baltimore) **81**, 705–710 (1959).

— — Nonurologic symptoms in patients with renal cancer. J. Amer. med. Ass. **172**, 146–151 (1960).

Mitchell, J. E.: Ureteric secondaries from a hypernephroma. Brit. J. Surg. **45**, 392–394 (1958).

Muehrcke, R. C., Kark, R. M., Pirani, C. L.: Technique of percutaneous renal biopsy in the prone position. J. Urol. (Baltimore) **74**, 267–277 (1955).

Munger, A. D.: Experiences in treatment of certain urinary tract malignancies with supervoltage roentgen therapy. Amer. J. Surg. **41**, 220–227 (1938).

Nesbit, R. M., Adams, F. M.: Wilms' tumour; review of 16 cases. J. Pediat. **29**, 295–303 (1946).

Neuhauser, E. B. D., Wittenborg, M. H., Berman, C. Z., Cohen, J.: Irradiation effects of roentgen therapy on the growing spine. Radiology **59**, 637–650 (1952).

Newcombe, W. D.: The search for truth with special reference to the frequency of gastric ulcer-cancer and the origin of Grawitz tumours of the kidney. Proc. roy. Soc. Med. **30**, 113–136 (1937).

Nicholson, G. W.: Embryonic tumour of kidney in foetus. J. Path. Bact. **34**, 711–730 (1931).

Ng, E., Low-Beer, B. V. A.: The treatment of Wilms' tumour. J. Pediat. **48**, 763–769 (1956).

Olcott, C. T.: Transplantable nephroblastoma (Wilms' tumour) and other spontaneous tumours in a colony of rats. Cancer Res. **10**, 625–628 (1950).

Oliver, J., Luey, A. S.: Plastic studies in abnormal renal architecture II. Arch. Path. **18**, 777–816 (1934).

— Lund, E.: Plastic studies in abnormal renal architecture I. Arch. Path. **15**, 755–774 (1933).

Paterson, R.: The treatment of malignant disease by radium and X-rays. London: Arnold & Co. 1948.

Payne, P.: In tumours of the bladder, ed. Wallace, D. M., Edinburgh: Livingstone 1959.

Pennisi, S. A., Russi, S., Bunts, R. C.: Multiple dissimilar tumours in one kidney. J. Urol. (Baltimore) **78**, 205–211 (1957).

Petkovic, S. D.: An anatomical classification of renal tumours in the adult as a basis for prognosis. J. Urol. (Baltimore) **81**, 618–623 (1959).

Pohle, E. A., Ritchie, G.: Malignant tumours of the kidney in children. Radiology **24**, 193–203 (1935).

Politano, V. A.: Leukoplakia of renal pelvis and ureter. J. Urol. (Baltimore) **75**, 633–642 (1956).

Politz, B. E., Sewell, G.: Renal angioma: suspected bilateral involvement. J. Urol. (Baltimore) **65**, 9–14 (1951).

Priestley, J. T.: Survival following the removal of malignant renal neoplasms. J. Amer. med. Ass. **113**, 902–906 (1939).

Riches, E. W.: Irradiation therapy in urology: The kidney. Brit. J. Urol. (Baltimore) **26**, 319–323 (1954).

Riches, E. W.: The present status of renal angiography. Brit. J. Surg. **42**, 462–470 (1955).

— Radiotherapy in renal new growths. J. Fac. Radiol. (Lond.) **8**, 19–27 (1956).

— Factors in the prognosis of carcinoma of the kidney. J. Urol. (Baltimore) **79**, 190–195 (1958a).

— Malignant disease of the urinary tract—Kidney and ureter. Trans. med. Soc. Lond., **74**, March 3rd (1958b).

— Griffiths, I. H., Thackray, A. C.: New growths of the kidney and ureter. Brit. J. Urol. **23**, 297–356 (1951).

Robb, D.: Pulmonary resection for metastatic malignancy. Three cases secondary to hypernephroma. Brit. J. Surg. **36**, 200–202 (1948).

Royce, R. K., Tormey, A. R.: Malignant tumours of the renal parenchyma in adults. J. Urol. (Baltimore) **74**, 23–35 (1955).

Rusche, C.: Renal hamartoma (angiomyolipoma): Report of three cases. J. Urol. (Baltimore) **67**, 823–831 (1952).

Sargent, J. W.: Ureteral metastasis from renal adenocarcinoma. J. Urol. (Baltimore) **83**, 97–99 (1960).

Sauer, H. R.: Wilms' tumours. N.Y. St. J. Med. **48**, 497–501 (1948).

Schneider, M.: Renal embryoma in Progress in radiation therapy, ed. Buschke, F. New York: Grune and Stratton 1958.

Scott, L. S.: Bilateral Wilms' tumour. Brit. J. Surg. **42**, 513–516 (1955).

— Wilms' tumour: Its treatment and prognosis. Brit. med. J. **1956 I**, 200–203

Sheach, J. M.: Bilateral Wilms' tumour: case report with review of literature. Brit. J. Urol. **25**, 109–113 (1953).

Störtebecker, T. P.: Metastatic hypernephroma of the brain from neurosurgical point of view. J. Neurosurg. **8**, 185–197 (1951).

Strauss, F. H., Scarlton, E. F.: Five year survival after hepatic lobectomy for metastatic hypernephroma. Arch. Surg. **77**, 328–331 (1956).

Tan, C. T. C., Dargeon, H. W., Burchenal, J. H.: The effect of actinomycin D on cancer in childhood. Pediatrics **24**, 544–561 (1959).

Thackray, A. C.: Ten year follow-up of cases of adenocarcinoma of the kidney. Proc. roy. Soc. Med. **50**, 362–366 (1957).

Trinkle, A. J.: The origin and development of renal adenomas and their relation to carcinoma of the renal cortex. Amer. J. Cancer **27**, 676–689 (1936).

Uson, A. C., Del Rosario, C., Melicow, M. M.: Wilms' tumour in association with cystic disease: Report of two cases. J. Urol. (Baltimore) **83**, 262–266 (1960).

Uys, C. J.: Tumours of the kidney in the Ba tu races of South Africa. Brit. J. Urol. **28**, 75–78 (1956).

Walker, G.: Sarcoma of the kidney in children. Ann. Surg. **26**, 529–602 (1897).

Walker, K.: Prognosis of renal growths. Lancet **1935 I**, 565–566.

Wallach, J. B., Sutton, A. P., Claman, M.: Haemangioma of the kidney. J. Urol. (Baltimore) **81**, 515–518 (1959).

Waters, C. A., Lewis, L. G., Frontz, W. A.: Radiation therapy of renal cortical neoplasm with special reference to preoperative irradiation. Sth. med. J. (Bgham, Ala.) 27, 290–299 (1934).

Weisel, W., Dockerty, M. B., Priestley, J. T.: Sarcoma of the kidney. J. Urol. (Baltimore) 50, 564–573 (1943).

Weiyrauch, H. M., Presti, J. C.: Papanicolaou examinations of urine in diagnosis of urinary cancer: 2 false positives in diagnosis of renal neoplasms. J. Urol. (Baltimore) 75, 551–575 (1956).

Wells, H. G.: Occurrence and significance of congenital malignant neoplasms. Arch. Path. 30, 535–601 (1940).

Wentzell, R. A., Berkheiser, S. W.: Malignant lymphomatosis of the kidneys. J. Urol. (Baltimore) 74, 177–185 (1955).

Whitehouse, W. M., Lampe, I.: Osseous damage in irradiation of renal tumours in infancy and childhood. Amer. J. Roentgenol. 70, 721–729 (1953).

Whitmore, E. R.: Hypernephroid tumours of the kidney. Sth. med. J. (Bgham, Ala.) 29, 1051–1062 (1936).

Williams, J. P., Savage, P. T.: Liposarcoma of kidney. Brit. J. Surg. 46, 225–231 (1958).

Willis, R. A.: Pathology of tumours. London: Butterworth & Co. 1948.

Wilms, M.: Die Mischgeschwülste der Niere. Leipzig: A. Georgi, 1899.

Young, M. O., Deming, C. L.: Nephrectomy for carcinoma seven years after demonstration of the tumour. J. Urol. (Baltimore) 74, 36–41 (1955).

Tumours of the renal pelvis and ureter

Abeshouse, B. S.: Primary benign and malignant tumours of the ureter: a review of the literature and report of one benign and twelve malignant tumours. Amer. J. Surg. 91, 237–271 (1956).

Cabot, H., Allen, R. B.: Epithelioma primary in the renal pelvis: report of 45 cases. Lancet 1933 II, 1301–1309.

Carlson, H. E.: Squamous cell carcinoma renal pelvis: a 5 year cure. J. Urol. (Baltimore) 83, 813–814 (1960).

Cowen, R. L.: Lymphadenomatous ureteral obstruction. Report of first case. Urol. cutan. Rev. 53, 521–522 (1949).

Glay, A.: Roentgen manifestations of Hodgkin's disease involving the urinary tract. Amer. J. Roentgenol. 84, 227–231 (1960).

Kaplan, J. H., McDonald, J. R., Thompson, G. J.: Multicentric origins of papillary tumours of the urinary tract. J. Urol. (Baltimore) 66, 792–804 (1951).

McDonald, J. R., Priestley, J. T.: Carcinoma renal pelvis: Histopathologic study of 75 cases with special reference to prognosis. J. Urol. (Baltimore) 51, 245–258 (1944).

Riches, E. W., Griffiths, I. H., Thackray, A. C.: New growths of the kidney and ureter. Brit. J. Urol. 23, 297–356 (1951).

Taylor, W. N.: Tumours of the kidney pelvis. J. Urol. (Baltimore) 82, 452–458 (1959).

Utz, D. C., McDonald, J. R.: Squamous cell carcinoma kidney. J. Urol. (Baltimore) 78, 540–552 (1957).

Wallace, D. M., Kinder, H.: Recurrent carcinoma in the ureteric stump. Brit. J. Surg., 50, 202–205 (1962).

Watson, E. M., Sauer, H. R., Sadugor, M. G.: Manifestations of the lymphoblastomas in the genito-urinary tract. J. Urol. (Baltimore) 61, 626–642 (1949).

Tumours of the bladder

Baker, R.: Correlation of circumferential lymphatic spread of vesical cancer with depth of infiltration: relation to present methods of treatment. J. Urol. (Baltimore) 73, 681–690 (1955).

Barringer, B. S.: Twenty-five years of radon treatment of cancer of the bladder. J. Amer. med. Ass. 135, 616–618 (1947).

— Radium therapy of bladder cancer, retrospect and prospect. J. Urol. (Baltimore) 68, 280–282 (1952).

Becker, J., Scheer, K. E.: Strahlentherapeutische Anwendung von radioaktivem Kobalt in Form von Perlen. Strahlentherapie 86, 540–547 (1952).

Bhansali, S. K., Cameron, K. M.: Primary malignant lymphoma of the bladder. Brit. J. Urol. 32, 440–454 (1960).

Blomfield, G. W.: Irradiation therapy in urology. Brit. J. Urol. 26, 301–316 (1954).

Bloom, H. J. G.: Complications following radiotherapy of the thorax and abdomen. Proc. roy. Soc. Med. 52, 495–500 (1959).

— Treatment by interstitial irradiation using tantalum 182 wire. Carcinoma of the bladder: Brit. J. Radiol. 33, 471–479 (1960).

Bonser, G. M., Clayson, D. B., Jull, J. W., Pyrah, L. N.: Carcinogenic activity of 2-naphthylamine. Brit. J. Cancer 10, 533–538 (1956).

Boyland, E.: Aetiology of cancer of the bladder. Extrait de Acta Un. int. Cancr. 16, 273–276 (1960).

— Wallace, D. M., Williams, D. C.: Enzyme activity in relation to cancer. Inhibition of urinary β-glucoronidase of patients with cancer of the bladder by oral administration of 1:4 saccharolactone and related compounds. Brit. J. Cancer 11, 578–589 (1957).

— Watson, G.: 3-Hydroxyanthranilic acid, carcinogen produced by endogenous metabolism. Nature (Lond.) 177, 837–838 (1956).

Bratherton, D. G.: The treatment of bladder growths by a solid intravesical cobalt source. Brit. J. Radiol. 28, 508–513 (1955).

Brice, M., Marshall, V. F., Green, J. L., Whitmore, W. F.: Simple total cystectomy for carcinoma of the urinary bladder. Cancer (Philad.) 9, 576–584 (1956).

Brick, I. B.: Effects of million volt irradiation on the gastro-intestinal tract. Arch. intern. Med. 96, 26–31 (1955).

Browne, H. H., Ogden, R. T.: Rotational cobalt 60 teletherapy of vesical cancer. Amer. J. Roentgenol. 83, 107–115 (1960).

BUSCHKE, F., CANTRIL, S. T., PARKER, H. M.: Supervoltage roentgentherapy. Springfield: Thomas 1950.

CARVER, J. H.: Interstitial radiation in the treatment of selected cases of cancer of the bladder. Brit. J. Urol. 31, 313–316 (1959).

CASE, R. A. M.: In Tumours of the bladder, ed. WALLACE, D. M. Edinburgh and London: E. & S. Livingstone Ltd. 1959.

COLBY, F. H., SCHULZ, M. D.: A review of carcinoma of the bladder treated by supervoltage X-rays over a five-year period. Radiology. 41, 371–376 (1943).

— SNIFFEN, R. C.: Carcinoma bladder: a classification of epithelial tumours and a study of the effects of external radiation. J. Urol. (Baltimore) 57, 133–139 (1947).

CONES, D. M. T., GREGORY, C.: A technique for intracavitary radiation of the bladder. Brit. J. Radiol. 25, 597–600 (1952).

COOLING, C. I.: Review of 150 Post-mortems of carcinoma of the urinary bladder. In: Tumours of the bladder, ed. WALLACE, D. M. Edinburgh and London: E. &. S. Livingstone Ltd. 1959.

CORDONNIER, J. J., SEAMAN, W. B.: Betatron therapy in advanced carcinoma of the urinary bladder. J. Urol. (Baltimore) 76, 256–262 (1956).

CORSCADEN, J. A., GUSBERG, S. B.: Background of cancer of corpus. Amer. J. Obstet. Gynec. 53, 419–431 (1947).

COX, R.: Treatment of carcinoma of the bladder by 2 MeV X-rays. Brit. J. Radiol. 33, 480–483 (1960).

CUCCIA, C. C., JONES, S., CRIGLER, C. M.: Clinical impressions in 100 consecutive cases of carcinoma of the urinary bladder treated by supervoltage. J. Urol. (Baltimore) 79, 99–109 (1958).

DEAN, A. L., ASH, J. E.: Study of the bladder tumours in the registry of the Amer. Urol. Assoc. J. Urol. (Baltimore) 63, 618–621 (1950).

— MOSTOFI, F. K., THOMSON, R. V., CLARK, M. L.: A restudy of the first fourteen hundred tumours in the bladder tumour registry, Armed Forces Institute of Pathology. J. Urol. (Baltimore) 71, 571–590 (1954).

DEREN, T. L., WILSON, W. I.: Use of 5-fluorouracil in treatment of bladder carcinomas. J. Urol. (Baltimore) 83, 390–393 (1960).

DICKSON, R. J., LANG, E. K.: Treatment of papillomata of the bladder with radioactive colloidal gold. Amer. J. Roentgenol. 83, 116–122 (1960).

DOUGLAS, M.: Uniformity of dosage in bladder carcinoma. Proc. roy. Soc. Med. 46, 465–466 (1953).

DUFF, J., HYMAN, R. M.: The intravesical radium bomb. A therapeutic failure in bladder tumours. Urol. cutan. Rev. 55, 683–688 (1951).

DUKES, C. E.: Cancer of the rectum. An analysis of 1000 cases. J. Path. Bact. 50, 527–539 (1940).

— MASINA, F.: Classification of epithelial tumours of the bladder. Brit. J. Urol. 21, 273–295 (1949).

DYCHE, G. M., MACKAY, N. R.: Techniques for the intracavitary treatment of bladder neoplasms with radioactive solutions contained in a rubber balloon. Brit. J. Radiol. 32, 752–756 (1959a).

— — The intracavitary treatment of the bladder with radioactive colloidal gold. Brit. J. Radiol. 32, 757–763 (1959b).

EINHORN, J., LARSSON, L. G., RAGNULT, I.: Radioactive yttrium (Y 90) as possible adjunct in treatment of papillomatosis of urinary bladder. Acta radiol. (Stockh.) 43, 298–304 (1955).

ELLIS, F., OLIVER, R.: Treatment of papilloma of bladder with radioactive colloidal gold Au[198]. Brit. med. J. 1955 I, 136–139.

EMMETT, J. L., WINTERRINGER, J. R.: Experience with implantation of radon seeds for bladder tumours compared with results with other forms of treatment. J. Urol. (Baltimore) 73, 502–515 (1955).

FERGUSON, R. S.: Treatment of cancer of the bladder by divided doses of roentgen rays at long distances. Amer. J. Roentgenol. 36, 73–78 (1936).

FERRIS, D. O., ODEL, H. M.: Electrolyte pattern of the blood after bilateral ureterosigmoidostomy. J. Amer. med. Ass. 142, 634–640 (1950).

FLOCKS, R. H., CULP, D. A.: Polypoid fibromyxosarcoma of the urinary bladder in a child. J. Urol. (Baltimore) 73, 299–306 (1955).

FORBER, J. E.: Rep. Publ. Hlth Med. Subj., No 66. London: H. M. Stationery Office 1931.

FRANKSSON, C.: Tumours of the urinary bladder. Acta chir. scand., Suppl. 151 (1950).

FRIEDMAN, M.: The superior value of supervoltage irradiation in special situations: carcinoma of the mouth and testis. Radiology 67, 484–497 (1956).

— Supervoltage (2-MVP) rotation irradiation of cancer of the bladder. Radiology 73, 191–208 (1959).

— LEWIS, L. G.: A new technique for the radium treatment of carcinoma of the bladder. Radiology 53, 342–361 (1949).

— — Irradiation of carcinoma of the bladder by a central intracavitary radium or cobalt 60 source. (Walter Reed Technique.) Amer. J. Roentgenol. 79, 6–31 (1958).

GANEM, E. J., BATAL, J. I.: Secondary malignant tumours of the bladder. J. Urol. (Baltimore) 75, 965–970 (1957).

GLAY, A.: Roentgen manifestations of Hodgkin's disease involving the urinary tract. Report on a case with Ureteral and Bladder Localizations. Amer. J. Roentgenol. 84, 227–231 (1960).

GOIN, L. S., HOFFMAN, E. F.: The use of intravesical low voltage contact roentgen irradiation in cancer of the bladder. Radiology 37, 545–548 (1941).

— — Contact roentgen therapy in cancer of the bladder. Amer. J. Roentgenol. 54, 392–394 (1945).

GOWING, N. F. C.: Pathological changes in the bladder following irradiation. Brit. J. Radiol. 33, 484–487 (1960a).

— Urethral carcinoma associated with cancer of the bladder. Brit. J. Urol. 32, 428–438 (1960b).

GRAY, M. J., GUSBERG, S. B., GUTTMAN, R.: Pelvic lymph node dissection following radiotherapy. Amer. J. Obstet. Gynec. 76, 629–633 (1958).

HARE, H. F., SMEDAL, M. I., JOHNSTON, D., COTE, M., TRUMP, J. G., WRIGHT, K. A., GRANKE, R. C., BEIQUE, R. A.: Observations on rotational therapy with two million volt roentgen .... J. Amer. med. Ass. 154, 890–894 (1954).

HERGER, C. C., SAUER, H. R.: Radon treatment of cancer of the bladder. Report of 267 cases. Amer. J. Roentgenol. **47**, 909–915 (1942a).

— — Occurrence and clinical course of reactions following use of radon implants in carcinoma bladder. J. Urol. (Baltimore) **47**, 141–147 (1942b).

— — Consideration of the response of bladder tumours to external irradiation. J. Urol. (Baltimore) **50**, 310–321 (1943).

HEYMAN, J.: The Radiumhemmet method of treatment and results in cancer of the corpus of the uterus. J. Obstet. Gynaec. Brit. Emp. **43**, 655–666 (1936).

— Annual report of results of radiotherapy, vol. 9. Stockholm: Norstedt and Söner 1954.

HIGHAM, A. R. C.: Treatment of vesical neoplasms by closed radium applications. Proc. roy. Soc. Med. **45**, 484–485 (1952).

— Treatment of growths of the bladder. Diathermy followed by intravesical radium. Brit. J. Urol. **27**, 211–220 (1955).

HINMAN, F., SCHULTE, J. W., LOW-BEER, B. V. A.: Further experience with intracavitary radiocobalt for bladder tumours. J. Urol. (Baltimore) **73**, 285–291 (1955).

HODT, H. J., SINCLAIR, W. K., SMITHERS, D. W.: A gun for interstitial implantation of radioactive gold grains. Brit. J. Radiol. **25**, 419–421 (1952).

HOFFMAN, G. T., ROTTINO, A., SUMMERILL, F.: Genito-urinary tract lesions in Hodgkin's disease. Bull. N.Y. Acad. Med. **29**, 655–657 (1953).

JACOBS, A.: The treatment of cancer of the bladder by radium. Brit. J. Radiol. **22**, 393–398 (1949).

JEWETT, H. J.: Surgical treatment of carcinoma of the bladder. J. Urol. (Baltimore) **79**, 87–93 (1958).

JEWETT, H. J., BLACKMAN, S. S.: Infiltrating carcinoma of the bladder: histologic pattern and degree of cellular differentiation in 97 autopsy cases. J. Urol. (Baltimore) **56**, 200–210 (1946).

— STRONG, G. H.: Infiltrating carcinoma of the bladder: relation of depth of penetration of the bladder wall to incidence of local extension and metastases. J. Urol. (Baltimore) **55**, 366–372 (1946).

JÖNSSON, G., MANSSON, B., RÖHL, L.: Tantalum 182 in the treatment of bladder tumours. Acta chir. scand. **115**, 111–119 (1958).

KLINGER, M. E.: Secondary tumours of the genito-urinary tract. J. Urol. (Baltimore) **65**, 144–153 (1951).

KOTTMEIER, H. L.: The places of radiation therapy and of surgery in the treatment of uterine cancer. J. Obstet. Gynaec. Brit. Emp. **62**, 737–751 (1955).

LENZ, M., CAHILL, G. F., MELICOW, M. M., DONLAN, C. P.: The treatment of cancer of the bladder by radium needles. Amer. J. Roentgenol. **58**, 486–491 (1947).

LEVINE, S., PACK, G. T., GALLO, J. S.: Intravesical roentgen therapy of cancer urinary bladder. J. Amer. med. Ass. **112**, 1314–1317 (1939).

LOCKWOOD, I. H., CHAPMAN, S. B.: Therapy of carcinoma of the urinary bladder. Amer. J. Roentgenol. **75**, 519–524 (1956).

LUTTERBECK, E. F.: Contact roentgen radiation of bladder tumours. J. Urol. (Baltimore) **82**, 90–91 (1959).

MACKAY, N. R.: Tolerance of the bladder to intracavitary irradiation. J. Urol. (Baltimore) **76**, 396–400 (1956).

— SMITHERS, D. W., WALLACE, D. M.: In: Tumours of the bladder, ed. WALLACE, D. M. Edinburgh and London: E. & S. Livingstone Ltd. 1959.

MAGRI, J.: Partial cystectomy: A review of 104 cases. Brit. J. Urol., **34**, 74–78 (1962).

MARSHALL, V. F.: A comparison of radiation and surgery for cancer of the bladder. J. Amer. med. Ass. **134**, 501–507 (1947).

— The relation of the preoperative estimate to the pathological demonstration of the extent of vesical neoplasms. J. Urol. (Baltimore) **68**, 714–723 (1952).

— Current clinical problems regarding bladder tumours. Cancer (Philad.) **9**, 543–550 (1956).

McDONALD, D. F., LUND, R. R.: Role of the urine in vesical neoplasm. I. Experimental confirmation of the urogenous theory of pathogenesis. J. Urol. (Baltimore) **71**, 560–570 (1954).

MELICK, W. F., ESCUE, H. M., NARYKA, J. J., MEZERA, R. A., WHEELER, E. P.: The first reported cases of human bladder tumours due to a new carcinogen xenylamine. J. Urol. (Baltimore) **74**, 760–766 (1955).

MELICOW, M. M.: Tumours of urinary bladder: clinico-pathological analysis of over 2500 specimens and biopsies. J. Urol. (Baltimore) **74**, 498–521 (1955).

MELLOR, H. M.: Carcinoma of Cervix uteri: Treatment by supervoltage irradiation only. Brit. J. Radiol. **33**, 20–27 (1960).

MEREDITH, W. J.: Radium dosage: The Manchester system, Edinburgh: Livingstone 1949.

MIERT, P. J. VAN, FOWLER, J. F.: The use of tantalum 182 in the treatment of early bladder carcinoma. Brit. J. Radiol. **29**, 508–512 (1956).

MILLEN, J. L. E.: Results of treatment of bladder cancer by radiotherapy. Brit. J. Urol. **22**, 430–433 (1950).

MILLIN, T., MASINA, F.: Total cystectomy, consideration of technique. Brit. J. Urol. (Baltimore) **21**, 108–127 (1949).

MORRISON, R.: Carcinoma of the bladder: Its treatment by supervoltage x-ray therapy. J. Fac. Radiol. (Lond.) **11**, 125–129 (1960).

MORROW, J. W.: Chemotherapy of carcinoma of the bladder: Preliminary report of 44 cases treated with citral. Brit. J. Urol. **32**, 69–78 (1960).

MOSTOFI, F. K., MORSE, W. H.: Polypoid rhabdomyosarcoma (sarcoma botryoides) of bladder in children. J. Urol. (Baltimore) **67**, 681–687 (1952).

— THOMSON, R. V., DEAN, A. L.: Mucous adenocarcinoma of the urinary bladder. Cancer (Philad.) **8**, 741–758 (1955).

MÜLLER, J. H.: Radiotherapy of bladder cancer by means of rubber balloons filled in situ with solutions of radioactive isotope (Co^{60}). Cancer (Philad.) **8**, 1035–1042 (1955).

PATERSON, R.: The treatment of malignant disease by radium and X-rays. London: Arnold 1948.

PAYNE, P.: In: Tumours of the bladder, ed. WALLACE, D. M. Edinburgh and London: E. & S. Livingstone Ltd. 1959.

PLANK, L. E., GROSSMAN, J. W. CAMPANELLA, S. D.: Cobalt 60 teletherapy for urinary bladder carcinoma: two and one half years experience. J. Urol. (Baltimore) 78, 402–409 (1957).

POINTON, R. C. S.: Bladder carcinoma. In: Symposium on some clinical aspects of megavoltage. Proc. roy. Soc. Med. 53, 244–246 (1960).

POOLE, T. L.: Irradiation cystitis. J. Amer. med. Ass. 168, 854–856 (1958).

POOLE-WILSON, D. S.: The treatment of malignant tumours of the bladder by irradiation therapy. Brit. J. Urol. 26, 326–342 (1954).

POOLE-WILSON, D. S.: Surgery and irradiation in the treatment of bladder cancer. Brit. J. Urol. 29, 244–250 (1957).

POWERS, J. H., HAWN, C. V. Z., CARTER, R. D.: Osteogenic sarcoma and transitional cell carcinoma arising simultaneously in the urinary bladder. J. Urol. (Baltimore) 76, 363–369 (1956).

PROUT, G. R., MARSHALL, V. F.: The prognosis with untreated bladder tumours. Cancer (Philad.) 9, 557–558 (1956).

REHN, L.: Blasengeschwülste bei Juskin-Arbeiten. Langenbecks Arch. Klin. Chir. 50, 588–600 (1895).

RICHES, E. W.: Carcinoma of the bladder: the place of total cystectomy. Brit. J. Urol. 29, 232–235 (1957).

— Malignant disease of the urinary tract (Lettsomian lectures). Trans. med. Soc. Lond. 74, 77–140 (1958).

— WINDEYER, B. W.: In: Modern trends in urology (second series), ed. RICHES, E. W. London: Butterworth & Co. 1960.

RUBIN, P., BURAN, R.: Supervoltage irradiation in bladder carcinoma 1952–1958. Radiology 73, 209–255 (1959).

RUSCHE, C. F., JAFFE, H. L.: Treatment of bladder and prostatic cancer by combined interstitial isotope radiation and the cobalt bomb. J. Urol. (Baltimore) 79, 474–489 (1958).

RUTLEDGE, F. N., FLETCHER, G. H.: Transperitoneal pelvic lymphadenectomy following supervoltage irradiation for squamous cell carcinoma of the cervix. Amer. J. Obstet. Gynec. 76, 321–334 (1958).

SCHWARTZ, J. W., MOSTOFI, F. K., REED, J. F., DEAN, A. L.: Total cystectomy: Analysis of 225 cases from the bladder tumour registry. J. Urol. (Baltimore) 78, 41–53 (1957).

SMITH, B. A.: Sarcoma botryoides: rhabdomyosarcoma of the bladder. J. Urol. (Baltimore) 82, 101–104 (1959).

SMITH, I. H., LOTT, J. S.: Some observations on the effect of cobalt 60 beam therapy on epidermoid carcinoma during the first 5-year study period. Amer. J. Roentgenol. 79, 406–414 (1958).

SMITHERS, D. W.: The X-ray treatment of accessible cancer. London: Edward Arnold 1946.

SPEERT, H., PEIGHTAL, T. C.: Malignant tumours of uterine fundus subsequent to irradiation for benign pelvic conditions. Amer. J. Obstet. Gynec. 57, 261–273 (1949).

SWINNEY, J.: Treatment of bladder cancer by megavoltage irradiation. Brit. J. Urol. 29, 241–243 (1957).

THOMPSON, I. M., COPPRIDGE, A. J.: Bladder sarcoma. J. Urol. (Baltimore) 82, 329–332 (1959).

THOMPSON, N.: Bladder papilloma: An analysis of 74 cases. Brit. J. Surg. 47, 419–424 (1960).

TUOVINEN, P. I., KETTUNEN, K.: Superficial malignant lesions in bladder treated by radioactive colloidal gold (198 Au). Brit. med. J. 1957 I, 1090–1092.

VERMOOTEN, V.: Use of radioactive cobalt (Co 60) in treatment of bladder tumours. J. Urol. (Baltimore) 74, 85–92 (1955).

— MAXFIELD, J. G. S.: The use of radioactive cobalt in nylon sutures in the treatment of bladder tumours: Technique and case reports. J. Urol. (Baltimore) 74, 767–776 (1955).

WALINDER, G.: Colloidal $As_2 76 S_3$. Its production and possible use in treatment of papillomatosis of urinary bladder. Acta radiol. (Stockh.) 44, 521–526 (1955).

WALLACE, D. M.: The ill-effects of radiotherapy. Brit. J. Urol. 26, 364–368 (1954).

— Aetiological factors in bladder tumours. Postgrad. med. J. 33, 494-498 (1957).

— Aetiological factors in bladder tumours (1957) Postgrad. med. med. J., 33, 494-498.

— Tumours of the bladder. Edinburgh and London: E. & S. Livingstone Ltd. 1959.

— Surgery in the treatment of bladder tumours. Brit. J. Radiol 33, 487–490 (1960).

— STAPLETON, J. E., TURNER, R. C.: Radioactive tantalum wire implantation as a method of treatment for early carcinoma of the bladder. Brit. J. Radiol. 25, 421–424 (1952).

— WALTON, R. J., SINCLAIR, W. K.: Intracavitary irradiation of the bladder mucosa by radioactive isotope solution. Brit. J. Urol. 21, 357–364 (1949).

WALTON, R. J.: Therapeutic uses of radioactive isotopes in the Royal Cancer Hospital. Brit. J. Radiol. 23, 559–566 (1950).

— SINCLAIR, W. K.: Radioactive solutions (24 Na and 82 Br) in the treatment of carcinoma of the bladder. Brit. med. Bull. 8, 158–165 (1952).

WARD, R. O.: Extravesical radium therapy in cancer of the bladder. Brit. J. Urol. 20, 191–202 (1948).

WATSON, E. M., SAUER, H. R., SADUGOR, M. G.: Manifestations of lymphoblastomas in the genito-urinary tract. J. Urol. (Baltimore) 61, 626–645 (1949).

WATSON, T. A., BURKELL, C. C.: Five-year results of betatron X-ray therapy. Brit. J. Radiol. 32, 143–151 (1959).

WAYMAN, T. B.: Treatment of infiltrating carcinoma of bladder by retrograde method of interstitial radiation. J. Urol. (Baltimore) 64, 469–483 (1950).

WHITMORE, W. F., MARSHALL, V. F.: Radical surgery for carcinoma urinary bladder. Cancer (Philad.) 9, 596–608 (1956).

WILDBOLZ, E., PORETTI, G. G.: The treatment of cancer of the bladder by radioactive cobalt. J. Urol. (Baltimore) 74, 93–103 (1955).

WILLIAMS, I. G., MORGAN, C. N.: Carcinoma of the rectum and anal canal. In: British practice in radiotherapy, ed. CARLING, E. R., WINDEYER, B. W., and SMITHERS, D. W. London: Butterworth & Co. 1955.

Winternitz, J. G., Smithers, D. W.: A multiple small field technique, in Symposium on small field X-ray therapy for deep-seated tumours with special reference to rotation techniques. Brit. J. Radiol. **22**, 197–204 (1949).

Yates-Bell, J. G., Henriques, C. Q.: The use of radioactive gold grains in the treatment of bladder growths. Brit. J. Urol. **29**, 97–111 (1957).

Tumours of urethra

Abrams, M.: Primary melanoma of the female urethra. J. Urol. (Baltimore) **74**, 371–374 (1955).

Cade, S.: Malignant disease and its treatment by radium. 2nd ed., vol. 111. Bristol: John Wright & Sons 1950.

Counseller, V. S., Paterson, S. J.: Carcinoma of the female urethra. J. Urol. (Baltimore) **29**, 587–595 (1933).

Flocks, R. H.: The treatment of urethral tumours. J. Urol. (Baltimore) **75**, 514–526 (1956).

Fricke, R. E., McMillan, J. T.: Radium therapy in carcinoma of the female urethra. Radiology **52**, 533–537 (1949).

Gowing, N. F. C.: Urethral carcinoma associated with cancer of the bladder. Brit. J. Urol. **32**, 428–438 (1960).

Hahn, G. A.: Primary carcinoma of the female urethra. J. Urol. (Baltimore) **67**, 319–325 (1952).

Herger, C. C., Sauer, H. R.: Primary carcinoma of the male urethra: Report of one case. Urol. cutan. Rev. **46**, 346–348 (1942).

Kreutzmann, H. A. R., Colloff, B.: Primary carcinoma of the male urethra. Arch. Surg. **39**, 513–529 (1939).

Lowsley, O. S., Kirwin, T. J.: Clinical urology, vol. 1. Baltimore: Williams & Wilkins 1956.

Marshall, F. C., Uson, A. C.: Neoplasms and caruncles of the female urethra. Surg. Gynec. Obstet. **110**, 723–733 (1960).

Marshall, V. F.: Radical excision of locally extensive carcinoma of the deep male urethra. J. Urol. (Baltimore) **78**, 252–264 (1957).

Maximow, A. A., Bloom, W.: Textbook of histology. Philadelphia: W. B. Saunders 1948.

McCrea, L. E.: Malignancy of the female urethra. Urol. Surv. **2**, 85–149 (1952).

— Furlong, J. H.: Primary carcinoma of the male urethra. Urol. Surv. **1**, 1–30 (1951).

Meredith, W. J.: Radium dosage—The Manchester system. Edinburgh, E. & S. Livingstone Ltd. 1949.

Monaco, A. P., Murphy, G. B., Dowling, W.: Cancer of the female urethra. Cancer (N.Y.) **11**, 1215–1221 (1958).

Murphy, W. T.: Radiation therapy. Philad.: W. & B. Saunders 1959.

Palmer, J. K., Emmett, J. L., McDonald, J. R.: Urethral caruncle. Surg. Gynec. Obstet. **87**, 611–620 (1948).

Riches, E. W., Cullen, T. H.: Carcinoma of the urethra. Brit. J. Urol. **23**, 209–221 (1951).

Ruch, R. M., Frericks, J. B., Arneson, A. N.: Cancer of the female urethra. Cancer (N.Y.) **5**, 748–753 (1952).

Sargent, J. S.: Total urethrectomy for carcinoma of female urethra. J. Urol. (Baltimore) **77**, 843–849 (1957).

Shaw, W. F.: Carcinoma of female urethra with notes of 2 cases treated with radium. J. Obstet. Gynaec., Brit. Emp. **30**, 215–219 (1923).

Spence, H. M., Denman, J.: Primary carcinoma of the male urethra. Seven-year cure by radical surgery. J. Urol. (Baltimore) **78**, 414–420 (1957).

Staubitz, W. J., Carden, L. M., Oberkircher, O. J., Lent, M. H., Murphy, W. T.: Management of urethral carcinoma in the female. J. Urol. (Baltimore) **73**, 1045–1053 (1955).

Taussig, F. J.: Primary cancer of the vulva, vagina and female urethra. Five-year results. Surg. Gynec. Obstet. **60**, 477–478 (1935).

Thomson-Walker, J. W.: Genito-urinary surgery. London: Cassell & Co. 1948.

Young, H. H.: A new radical operation for carcinoma bulbous urethra: a new use for the penis. Surg. Gynec. Obstet. **68**, 77–86 (1939).

Tumours of the penis

Ashley, D. J. B., Edwards, E. C.: Sarcoma of the penis: leiomyosarcoma of the penis. Report of a case with review of the literature on sarcoma of the penis. Brit. J. Surg. **45**, 170–179 (1957).

Ashworth, A.: Peyronie's disease. Proc. roy. Soc. Med. **53**, 692–694 (1960).

Barnett, C. P., Low, J. R.: Haemangio-endothelioma of the corpus cavernosum penis. Case report. J. Urol. (Baltimore) **83**, 160–162 (1960).

Barney, C. D.: Epithelioma of the penis. Ann. Surg. **46**, 890–914 (1907).

Barnofsky, I. D.: Technique of inguinal node dissection. Surgery **24**, 555–567 (1948).

Barringer, B. S., Dean, A. L.: Epithelioma of the penis. J. Urol. (Baltimore) **11**, 497–514 (1924).

Bassett, J. W.: Carcinoma of the penis. Cancer (N.Y.) **5**, 530–538 (1952).

Bercovitz, N.: Cancer in Hainan, China. A preliminary statistical study of 131 operations with special reference to age, incidence, anatomical distribution and aetiology. J. Cancer Res. **4**, 229–234 (1919).

Bleich, A. R.: Prophylaxis of penile carcinoma. J. Amer. med. Ass. **143**, 1054–1057 (1950).

Bodner, H., Howard, A. H., Kaplan, J. H.: Peyronie's disease: cortisone-hyaluronidase-hydrocortisone therapy. J. Urol. (Baltimore) **72**, 400–403 (1954).

Bolado, J. L. I., Lavin, P. D.: Sobre circo casos de enfermedad de Peyronie. Arch. esp. Urol. **13**, 260–265 (1957).

Bowing, H. H., Fricke, R. E., Counseller, V. S.: Results of treatment of carcinoma of the penis. Radiology **23**, 574–579 (1934).

Boyd, H. L.: Metastatic carcinoma of the penis secondary to carcinoma of the rectum: a review of the literature and report of a case. J. Urol. (Baltimore) **71**, 82–90 (1954).

Burford, E. H., Burford, C. E.: Combined therapy for Peyronie's disease. J. Urol. (Baltimore) **78**, 265–268 (1957).

BURFORD, E. H., GLENN, J. E., BURFORD, C. E.: Therapy of Peyronie's disease. Urol. cutan. Rev. 55, 337–338 (1951).

CADE, S.: Malignant disease and its treatment by radium, 2nd edit., vol. 3. Bristol: Wright 1950.

CATTELL, R. B., MACE, A. J.: Metastases to the penis from carcinoma rectum. J. Amer. med. Ass. 146, 1230–1231 (1951).

CHU, N. X., TAM, P. B.: Le cancer de la verge chez les vietnamiens. Presse méd. 62, 125–126 (1954).

COLBY, F. H., SMITH, G. G.: Carcinoma of the penis. J. Urol. (Baltimore) 25, 461–467 (1931).

COSTOLOW, W. E.: Radiation therapy in diseases of the genito-urinary tract. Urol. cutan. Rev. 55, 324–327 (1951).

COX, R.: Radiotherapy in malignant disease of the testicle and penis. Brit. J. Urol. 26, 350–361 (1954).

CRAVER, L. F.: Priapism in leukaemia. Surg. clin. N. Amer. 13, 472–477 (1933).

CUNNINGHAM, J. H.: The operative treatment of carcinoma of the penis. Surg. Gynec. Obstet. 19, 693–699 (1914).

DAHL, O.: Treatment of plastic induration of the penis. Acta radiol. (Stockh.) 41, 290–301 (1954).

DEAN, A. L.: Epithelioma of the penis. J. Urol. (Baltimore) 33, 252–276 (1935).

— Epithelioma of the penis in a Jew who was circumcised in early infancy. Trans. Amer. Ass. gen.-urin. Surg. 29, 493–499 (1936).

EDSMYR, F., EKSTRÖM, T.: Precancerosis of the penis. A clinical study of 25 cases. Acta chir. scand. 116, 296–305 (1959).

EKSTRÖM, T., EDSMYR, F.: Cancer of the penis; a clinical study of 229 cases. Acta chir. scand. 115, 25–45 (1958).

ENGELSTAD, R. B.: Treatment of cancer of the penis at the Norwegian Radium Hospital. Amer. J. Roentgenol. 60, 801–806 (1948).

FUREY, C. A.: Peyronie's disease: treatment by local injection of prednisolone and hydrocortisone. J. Urol. (Baltimore) 77, 251–266 (1957).

FURLONG, J. H., UHLE, C. A. W.: Cancer of the penis: a report of 88 cases. J. Urol. 69, 550–555 (1953).

HAAR, H., SHANBROM, E., MILLER, S.: Treatment of leukaemic priapism with A-139. J. Urol. (Baltimore) 83, 429–432 (1960).

HANSSON, C. J.: Cancer of the penis and its treatment. Acta radiol. (Stockh.) 19, 443–457 (1938).

HARNETT, W. L.: Survey of cancer in London. London: British Empire Cancer Campaign 1952.

HEITE, H. J., SIEBRECHT, V. H. H.: Beitrag zur Pathogenese der induratio penis plastica. Derm. Wschr. 121, 1–10, 25–34 (1950).

HENSHAW, P. S.: Peculiar growth lesions in frogs induced by irradiation of sperm cells with x-rays. J. nat. Cancer Inst. 3, 409–417 (1943).

HOVNANIAN, A. P.: Radical ilio-inguinal lymphatic excision. Ann. Surg. 135, 520–527 (1952).

HUDSON, P. B., CASON, J. F., SCOTT, W. W.: The value of radical operation for carcinoma of the penis. South. med. J. 41, 761–765 (1948).

— HOPKINS, J. A., FISH, G. W.: Carcinoma of the penis: evaluation of recurrence following limited surgery. Presentation of an extended surgical attack. Amer. J. Surg. 85, 519–522 (1953).

HUTCHISON, R. G.: Radium treatment of epithelioma of the penis. Brit. J. Radiol. 8, 306–314 (1935).

JORSTAD, L. H.: Carcinoma of the penis. Amer. J. Roentgenol. 46, 232–236 (1941).

KENNAWAY, E. L.: Cancer of the penis and circumcision in relation to the incubation period of cancer. Brit. J. Cancer 1, 335–344 (1947).

KINI, M. G.: Cancer of the penis in a child aged two years. Indian med. Gaz. 79, 66–68 (1944).

KUEHN, C. A., ROBERTS, R. R.: Amputation and radical lymph gland dissection in carcinoma of the penis: an operative technique. J. Urol. (Baltimore) 69, 171–180 (1953).

LAVEDAN, J., ENNUYER, A., BAUDOUIN, M.: Les cancers de la verge; étude pathologique et therapeutique basée sur 74 observations, Fondation Curie 1922–1947. Bull. Ass. franc. Cancer 41, 149–200 (1954).

LEDERMAN, M.: Radiotherapy of cancer of the penis. Brit. J. Urol. 25, 224–232 (1953).

LEDLIE, R. C. B., SMITHERS, D. W.: Carcinoma of the penis in a man circumcised in infancy. J. Urol. (Baltimore) 76, 756–757 (1956).

LENOWITZ, H., GRAHAM, A. P.: Carcinoma of the penis. J. Urol. (Baltimore) 56, 458–484 (1946).

LOWER, W. E., CHRISTOFERSON, L. A.: Priapism in leukaemia; report of 2 cases. Cleveland Clin. Quart. 12, 133–137 (1945).

LOWSLEY, O. S., BOYCE, W. H.: Further experiences with an operation for the cure of Peyronie's disease. J. Urol. (Baltimore) 63, 888–899 (1950).

— KIRWIN, T. J.: Clinical urology. Baltimore: Williams & Wilkins 1956.

MACDERMOTT, E. N., KENNEDY, J. D.: A case of melanoblastoma of the penis. Brit. J. Surg. 43, 213–214 (1955).

MARSHALL, V. F.: Typical carcinoma of the penis in a male circumcised in infancy. Cancer (N.Y.) 6, 1044–1045 (1953).

McCARTHY, W. D., PACK, G. T.: Malignant blood vessel tumours: a report of 56 cases of angiosarcoma and Kaposi's sarcoma. Surg. Gynec. Obstet. 91, 465–482 (1950).

McCREA, L. E., TOBIAS, G. L.: Metastatic disease of the penis. J. Urol. (Baltimore) 80, 489–500 (1958).

McKIE, J.: A radium applicator for treatment of the penis. Brit. J. Radiol. 32, 210–213 (1959).

MEREDITH, W. J.: Radium dosage. The Manchester system. Edinburgh: E. & S. Livingstone Ltd. 1949.

MERRICKS, J. W., COTTRELL, T. L. C.: Erythroplasia of Queyrat. J. Urol. (Baltimore) 69, 807–812 (1953).

MULLIGAN, R. N.: Syllabus of human neoplasms. London: Kimpton 1951.

NGAI, S. K.: The aetiological and pathological aspects of squamous cell carcinoma of the penis among Chinese. Amer. J. Cancer 19, 259–284 (1933).

NOBLE, T. P.: Carcinoma of the penis in Siam. Brit. J. Urol. 5, 242–248 (1933).

PAQUIN, A. J., ROLAND, S. I.: Secondary carcinoma of the penis. Cancer (N.Y.) 9, 626–632 (1956).

PAUL, M.: Carcinoma of the penis. Post. Grad. med. J. 28, 615–618 (1952).

PATERSON, R.: The treatment of malignant disease by radium and X-rays. London: Edward Arnold 1948.

Paterson, R., Tod, M., Russell, M.: The results of radium and X-ray therapy in malignant disease. Third Statistical Report from the Christie Hospital and Holt Radium Institute, Manchester Edinburgh: Livingstone 1950.

Plaut, A., Kohn-Speyer, A. C.: The carcinogenic action of smegma. Science 105, 391–392 (1947).

Reid, J. D.: Melanosarcoma of the penis; report of a case. Cancer (N.Y.) 10, 359–362 (1957).

Sanjunio, L. A., Flores, B. G.: Carcinoma of the penis. J. Urol. (Baltimore) 83, 433–437 (1960).

Sauer, D., Leighton, W. E.: Clinic on carcinoma of the penis based on clinical study of 138 cases. Surg. Clin. N. Amer. 24, 1211–1219 (1944).

Scardino, P. L., Scott, W. W.: Use of tocopherols in treatment of Peyronie's disease. Ann. N.Y. Acad. Sci. 52, 390–396 (1949).

Scott, W. W., Scardino, P. L.: New concept in treatment of Peyronie's disease. South. med. J. 41, 173–177 (1948).

Smithers, D. W.: A clinical prospect of the cancer problem. Edinburgh: Livingstone 1960.

Staubitz, W. J., Lent, M. H., Oberkircher, O. J.: Carcinoma of the penis. Cancer (N.Y.) 8, 371–378 (1955).

Tailhefer, A., Courtial, J.: Le traitement des cancers primitifs de la peau et des orifices cutanéo-muqueux à la Fondation Curie. Bull. Ass. franc. Cancer 31, 85–115 (1943).

Teasley, G. H.: Peyronie's disease: a new approach. J. Urol. (Baltimore) 71, 611–614 (1954).

Thomson, G. R.: Treatment of Dupuytren's contracture with vitamin E. Brit. med. J. 1949 II, 1382–1383.

Thurgar, C. J. L.: Carcinoma of the penis. In: British practice in radiotherapy, ed. Carling, E. R., Windeyer, B. W., and Smithers, D. W. London: Butterworth 1955.

Waugh, T. R.: Endothelioma of corpora cavernosa of penis. Arch. Path. 55, 98–117 (1953).

Wijnbladh, H.: Behandling av Dupuytren's Kontraktur ach induratio plastica penis med alfato-coferolacetat. Nord. Med. 42, 1644 (1949).

Willis, R. A.: Pathology of tumours. London: Butterworth 1948.

Windeyer, B. W.: Discussion on radiotherapy in urology. Proc. roy. Soc. Med. 32, 1504–1509 (1939).

Wolbarst, A. L.: Circumcision and penile cancer. Lancet 1932 I, 150–153.

Zarafonetis, C. J. D., Horrax, T. M.: Treatment of Peyronie's disease with potassium para-amino-benzoate. J. Urol. (Baltimore) 81, 770–772 (1959).

Zausner, J.: Penile carcinoma: a review of 43 cases treated at Bellvue Hospital during the past 25 years. Radiology 50, 786–790 (1948).

Current views on urological cancer

Abassian, A., Wallace, D. M.: J. Urol. (Baltimore) 96, 461 (1966).

Anthony, H. M., Thomas, G. M.: Int. J. Cancer 5, 266 (1970).

Baert, L., Verduyn, H., Vereecken, R.: J. Urol. (Baltimore) 96, 871 (1966).

Bloom, H. J. G.: In: Tumours of the kidney and ureter, ed. Sir E. Riches, p. 311. London: E. & S. Livingstone, Ltd., 1964.

— In: Renal neoplasia, ed. J. S. King, p. 605. Boston: Little, Brown & Co. 1967.

— In: The prevention of cancer, eds. R. W. Raven and F. J. C. Roe, p. 226. London: Butterworths 1967.

— at 10th Internat. Cancer Congr. Houston 1970.

— Wallace, D. M.: Brit. med. J. 1964 II, 476.

Bodian, M., Rigby, C.: In: Tumours of the kidney and ureter, ed. Sir. E. Riches, p. 219. London: E. & S. Livingstone Ltd. 1964.

Boyland, E., Wallace, D. M., Avis, P. R. D., Kinder, C. H.: Brit. J. Urol. 36, 563 (1964).

Bratherton, D. G.: Brit. J. Radiol. 37, 141 (1964).

Burgert, E. O., Glidewell, O.: J. Amer. med. Ass. 199, 464 (1967).

— Mills, S. D.: CA, N.Y. 17, 15 (1967).

Cade, I. S., McEwen, J. B.: Cancer (Philad.) 20, 817 (1967).

Cady, B.: Surg. Gynec. Obstet. 126, 851 and 1091 (1968).

Caldwell, W. L., Bagshaw, M. A., Kaplan, H. S.: J. Urol. (Baltimore) 97, 294 (1967).

Crigler, C. M., Miller, L. S., Guinn, G. A., Schilaci, H. G.: J. Urol. (Baltimore) 96, 55 (1966).

Darte, J. M.: In: Progress in Radiation Therapy, ed. F. Buschke, vol. 3, p. 141. New York: Grune and Stratton 1965.

Donker, P. J.: Arch. chir. neerl. 19, 179 (1967).

Edsmyr, F., Jacobsson, F., Dahl, O., Walstam, R.: Acta radiol. (Stockh.) 6, 81 (1967).

— Nilson, A. E.: Acta radiol. (Stockh.) 3, 449 (1965).

Farber, S.: J. Amer. med. Ass. 198, 826 (1966).

Fernbach, D. J., Martyn, D. T.: J. Amer. med. Ass. 195, 1005 (1966).

Fraumeni, J. F.: J. nat. Cancer Inst. 41, 1205 (1968).

Garcia, M., Douglass, C., Schlosser, J. V.: Radiology 80, 574 (1963).

Gibson, G. R.: Aust. N.Z. J. Surg. 38, 281 (1969).

Gross, R. E.: Surgery of infancy and childhood: its principles and techniques. Philadelphia: Saunders & Co. 1953.

Henschke, M. K., Lawrence, D. C.: Radiology 85, 1117 (1965).

Herbst, W. E., Cooley, R. N., Ozarda, A. T.: Amer. J. med. Sci. 252, 603 (1966).

Higgs, B., MacDonald, J. S.: Brit. J. Urol. 40, 727 (1968).

Howard, R.: Arch. Dis. Childh. 40, 200 (1965).

Hultén, L., Rosencrantz, M., Seeman, T., Wahlqvist, L., Ahrén, Ch.: Scand. J. Urol. Nephrol. 3, 129 (1969).

Johnson, D. G., Maceira, F., Koop, C. E.: J. pediat. Surg. 2, 13 (1967).

Jomain, J.: J. Urol. Néphrol. 72, 279 (1966).

Jones, C. H., Taylor, K. W., Stedeford, J. B. H.: Brit. J. Radiol. 38, 622 (1965).

Kaufman, J. J., Kaneshiro, W., Roux, F.: J. Urol. (Baltimore) 101, 559 (1969).

Kerr, W. K.: In: Modern trends in urology, ed. Sir E. Riches, vol. 3, p. 163. London: Butterworths 1970.

KOOP, C. E.: at 10th Internat. Cancer Congr. Houston, 1970.

KUROHARA, S. S., RUBIN, P., SILON, N.: Amer. J. Roentgenol. **95**, 458 (1965).

LAING, A. H., DICKINSON, K. M.: Clin. Radiol. **16**, 154 (1965).

LAMB, D.: Brit. med. J. **1967**I, 273.

MACKENZIE, A. R., WHITMORE, W. F., NICKSON, J. J.: Cancer (Philad.) **18**, 1255 (1965).

MAIER, J. G., HARSHAW, W. G.: Cancer (Philad.) **20**, 96 (1967).

MELANDER, O., NOTTER, G., SCHREEB, T. VON: Nord. Med. **78**, 1309 (1967).

MILLER, A., MITCHELL, J. P., BROWN, N. J.: Suppl. to Brit. J. Urol. **41**, 13 and 48 (1969).

MORROW, J. W.: Brit. J. Urol. **32**, 69 (1960).

NICKSON, J. J., GLICKSMAN, A. S.: Amer. med. Ass. **195**, 922 (1966).

PAVONE-MACALUSO, M.: In: Renal neoplasia, ed. J. S. KING, p. 247. Boston: Little, Brown & Co. 1967.

PEARSON, D., DUNCAN, W. B., POINTON, R. C. S.: Brit. J. Radiol. **37**, 154 (1964).

PEELING, W. B., MANTELL, B. S., SHEPHEARD, B. G. F.: Brit. J. Urol. **41**, 23 (1969).

POINTON, R. C. S., EVANS, C. M.: Clin. Radiol. **20**, 95 (1969).

POWERS, W. E., PALMER, L. A.: Amer. J. Roentgenol. **102**, 176 (1968).

RAFLA, S.: Cancer (Philad.) **25**, 26 (1970).

RAVASINI, G.: J. Urol. Néphrol. **72**, 240 (1966).

RICHES, SIR E.: Ann. roy. Coll. Surg. Engl. **32**, 201 (1963).

RICHES, SIR E.: In: Modern trends in urology, vol. 3, p. 216. London: Butterworth 1970.

RIDER, W. D., KERESTECI, A. G., HAWKINS, N. V., BUSH, R. S.: Personal communication prior to publication (1970).

RINGLEB, D., ROMMEL, K.: Strahlentherapie **121**, 323 (1963).

ROBSON, C. J., CHURCHILL, B. M., ANDERSON, W.: J. Urol. (Baltimore) **101**, 297 (1969).

SAMUELS, M. L., SULLIVAN, P., HOWE, C. D.: Cancer (Philad.) **22**, 525 (1968).

SCHNEIDER, B., SAGERMAN, R. H., WOLFF, J. A., SANTULLI, T. V.: Amer. J. Roentgenol. **108**, 92 (1970).

SCHLEGEL, J. M., PIPKIN, G. E., NISHIMURA, R., SCHULTZ, G. N.: J. Urol. (Baltimore) **103**, 155 (1970).

SCHLIENGER, M., DUTREIX, J.: In: Front. Radiation Ther. Onc., vol. 3, p. 220, ed. J. VAETH. Basel: Karger 1968.

STEIN, J. J., KAUFMAN, J. J.: Amer. J. Roentgenol. **102**, 519 (1968).

STONE, J., WILLIAMS, I. G.: Clin. Radiol. **20**, 40 (1969).

SUKAROCHANA, K., KIESWATTER, W. B.: J. Pediat. **69**, 747 (1966).

TALLEY, R. W., MOORHEAD, E. L., TUCKER, W. G., SAN DIEGO, E. L., BRENNAN, M. J.: J. Amer. med. Ass. **207**, 322 (1969).

TAVARES, A. S., COSTA, J., CARVALHO, A. DE, REIS, M.: Brit. J. Cancer **20**, 438 (1966).

TCHAO, R., EASTY, G. C., AMBROSE, E. J., RAVEN, R. W., BLOOM, H. J. G.: Europ. J. Cancer **4**, 39 (1968).

Union Internationale Contre le Cancer: T.N.M. classi-fication of malignant tumours, Geneva, p. 59, 1968.

VAETH, J. M., LEVITT, S. H.: J. Urol. (Baltimore) **90**, 247 (1963).

VARGHA, Z. O., GLICKSMAN, A. S., BOLAND, J.: Radiology **93**, 1181 (1969).

VEENEMA, R. J., DEAN, A. L., USON, A. C., ROBERTS, M., LONGO, F.: J. Urol. (Baltimore) **101**, 711 (1969).

VIETTI, T. J., SULLIVAN, M. P., HAGGARD, M. E., HOLCOMB, T. M., BERRY, D. H.: Cancer (Philad.) **25**, 12 (1970).

WERF-MESSING, B. VAN DER: Clin. Radiol. **16**, 165 (1965).

— Europ. J. Cancer **5**, 277 (1969).

WHITMORE, W. F., GRABSTALD, H., MACKENZIE, A. R., ISWARIAH, J., PHILLIPS, R.: Amer. J. Roentgenol. **102**, 570 (1968).

— MARSHALL, V. F.: J. Urol. (Baltimore) **87**, 853 (1962).

WILLIAMS, D. I.: In: Tumours of the kidney and ureter, p. 267, ed. Sir E. RICHES. London: E. & S. Livingstone, Ltd. 1964.

WIZENBERG, M. J., BLOEDORN, F. G., YOUNG, J. D., GALLEHER, E. P.: Amer. J. Roentgenol. **96**, 113 (1966).

WOLFF, J. A., KRIVIT, W., NEWTON, W. A., D'ANGIO, G. J.: New Engl. J. Med. **279**, 290 (1968).

WOODRUFF, M. W., WAGLE, D., GAILANI, S. D., JONES, R.: J. Urol. (Baltimore) **97**, 611 (1967).

Sachverzeichnis

Bei gleicher Schreibweise in beiden Sprachen sind die Stichwörter nur einmal aufgeführt

Subject Index

Where English and German spelling of a word is identical, the German version is omitted

HANDBUCH DER MEDIZINISCHEN RADIOLOGIE
ENCYCLOPEDIA OF MEDICAL RADIOLOGY

HERAUSGEGEBEN VON

L. DIETHELM   **O. OLSSON**   **F. STRNAD**   **H. VIETEN**   **A. ZUPPINGER**
MAINZ   LUND   FRANKFURT/M.   DÜSSELDORF   BERN

BAND XIX/3

REDIGIERT VON

A. ZUPPINGER, BERN

SPRINGER-VERLAG, BERLIN · HEIDELBERG · NEW YORK 1971
(PRINTED IN GERMANY)

CARCINOMA OF THE VULVA

BY

F. EDSMYR AND H.-L. KOTTMEIER

SONDERDRUCK AUS

HANDBUCH DER MEDIZINISCHEN RADIOLOGIE
ENCYCLOPEDIA OF MEDICAL RADIOLOGY

HERAUSGEGEBEN VON

L. DIETHELM   **O. OLSSON**   **F. STRNAD**   **H. VIETEN**   **A. ZUPPINGER**
MAINZ   LUND   FRANKFURT/M.   DÜSSELDORF   BERN

BAND XIX/3

REDIGIERT VON

A. ZUPPINGER, BERN

SPRINGER-VERLAG, BERLIN · HEIDELBERG · NEW YORK 1971
(PRINTED IN GERMANY)

TUMOREN DER VAGINA

VON

F. GAUWERKY

HANDBUCH DER MEDIZINISCHEN RADIOLOGIE
ENCYCLOPEDIA OF MEDICAL RADIOLOGY

HERAUSGEGEBEN VON

L. DIETHELM **O. OLSSON** **F. STRNAD** **H. VIETEN** **A. ZUPPINGER**
MAINZ LUND FRANKFURT/M. DÜSSELDORF BERN

BAND XIX/3

REDIGIERT VON

A. ZUPPINGER, BERN

SPRINGER-VERLAG, BERLIN · HEIDELBERG · NEW YORK 1971
(PRINTED IN GERMANY)

DIE STRAHLENBEHANDLUNG DES KORPUSCARCINOMS

VON

R. FRISCHKORN

SONDERDRUCK AUS

HANDBUCH DER MEDIZINISCHEN RADIOLOGIE
ENCYCLOPEDIA OF MEDICAL RADIOLOGY

HERAUSGEGEBEN VON

L. DIETHELM   **O. OLSSON**   **F. STRNAD**   **H. VIETEN**   **A. ZUPPINGER**
MAINZ   LUND   FRANKFURT/M. DÜSSELDORF   BERN

BAND XIX/3

REDIGIERT VON

A. ZUPPINGER, BERN

SPRINGER-VERLAG, BERLIN · HEIDELBERG · NEW YORK 1971
(PRINTED IN GERMANY)

NICHT IM HANDEL

DIE STRAHLENBEHANDLUNG DES COLLUMCARCINOMS

VON

H.-J. FRISCHBIER

SONDERDRUCK AUS

HANDBUCH DER MEDIZINISCHEN RADIOLOGIE
ENCYCLOPEDIA OF MEDICAL RADIOLOGY

HERAUSGEGEBEN VON

L. DIETHELM **O. OLSSON** **F. STRNAD** **H. VIETEN** **A. ZUPPINGER**
MAINZ LUND FRANKFURT/M. DÜSSELDORF BERN

BAND XIX/3

REDIGIERT VON

A. ZUPPINGER, BERN

SPRINGER-VERLAG, BERLIN · HEIDELBERG · NEW YORK 1971
(PRINTED IN GERMANY)

NICHT IM HANDEL

MALIGNE TUMOREN DER TUBEN, OVARIEN, PARAMETRIEN UND DER LIGAMENTA ROTUNDA

VON

W. DIETZ

SONDERDRUCK AUS

HANDBUCH DER MEDIZINISCHEN RADIOLOGIE
ENCYCLOPEDIA OF MEDICAL RADIOLOGY

HERAUSGEGEBEN VON

L. DIETHELM   **O. OLSSON**   **F. STRNAD**   **H. VIETEN**   **A. ZUPPINGER**
MAINZ   LUND   FRANKFURT/M.   DÜSSELDORF   BERN

BAND XIX/3

REDIGIERT VON

A. ZUPPINGER, BERN

SPRINGER-VERLAG, BERLIN · HEIDELBERG · NEW YORK 1971
(PRINTED IN GERMANY)

NICHT IM HANDEL

TUMOURS OF THE MALE GENITAL TRACT

BY

B. WINDEYER AND S. DISCHE

TUMOURS OF THE URINARY TRACT

BY

H. J. G. BLOOM AND D. M. WALLACE